AIIMS-MAMC-PGI IMAGING SERIES

DIAGNOSTIC RADIOLOGY

Gastrointestinal and Hepatobiliary Imaging

Pioneers of AIIMS-MAMC-PGI Imaging Series

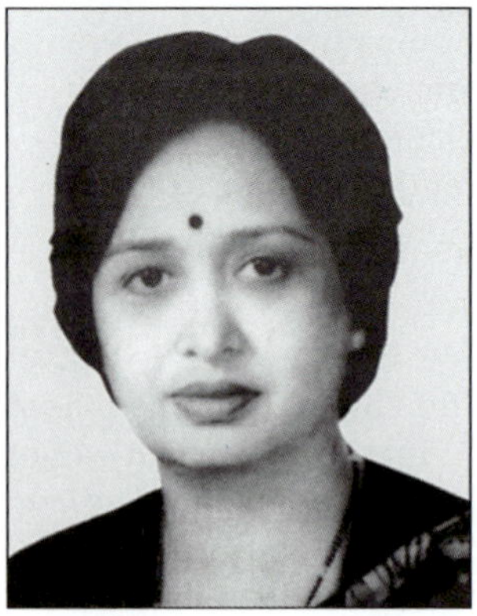

Manorama Berry

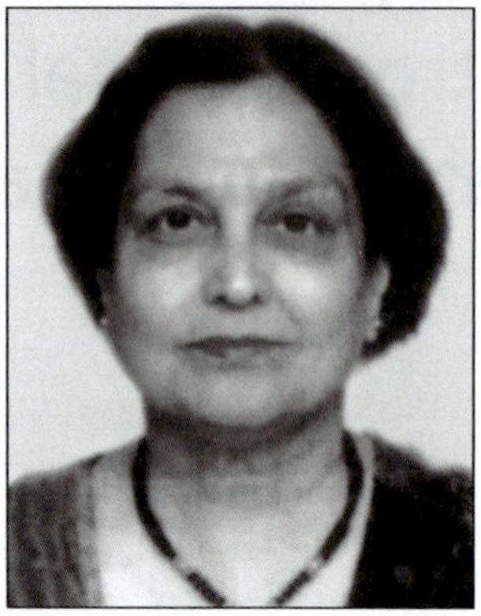

Sudha Suri

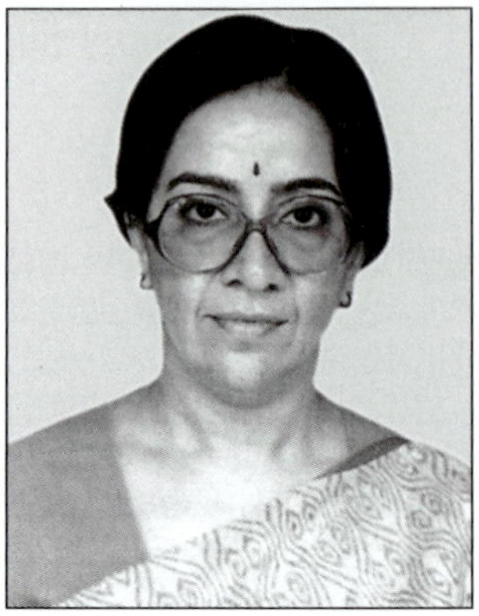

Veena Chowdhury

Past Editors

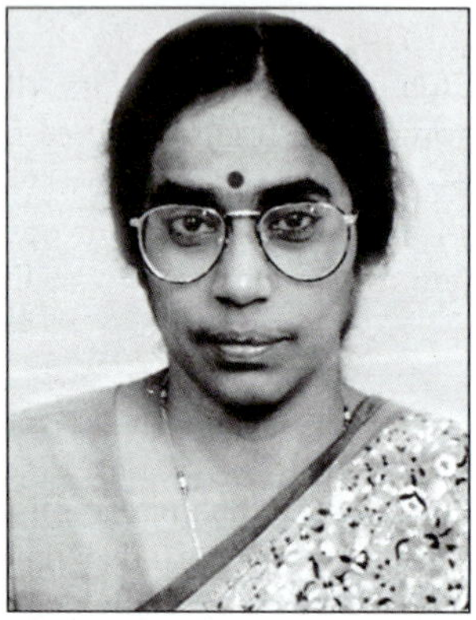

Sima Mukhopadhyay

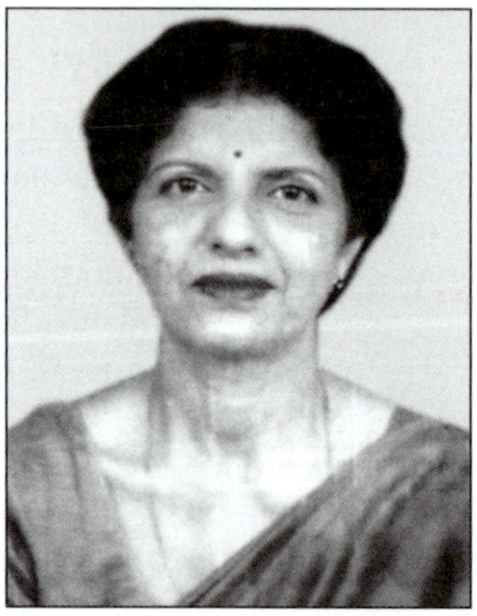

Sushma Vashisht

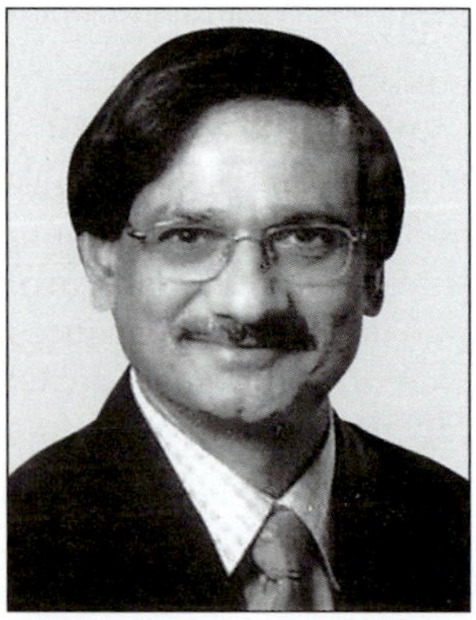

Niranjan Khandelwal

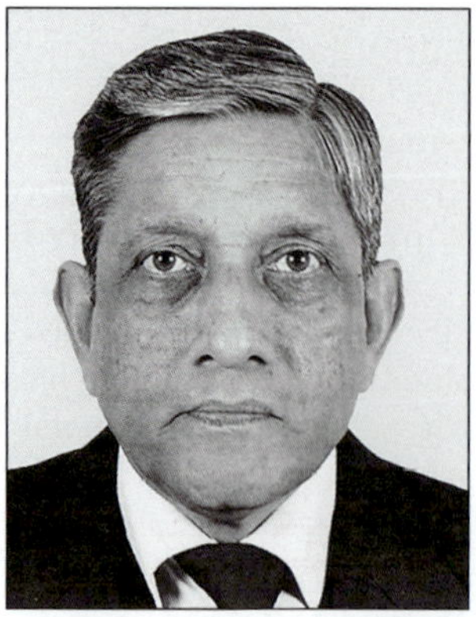

Arun Kumar Gupta

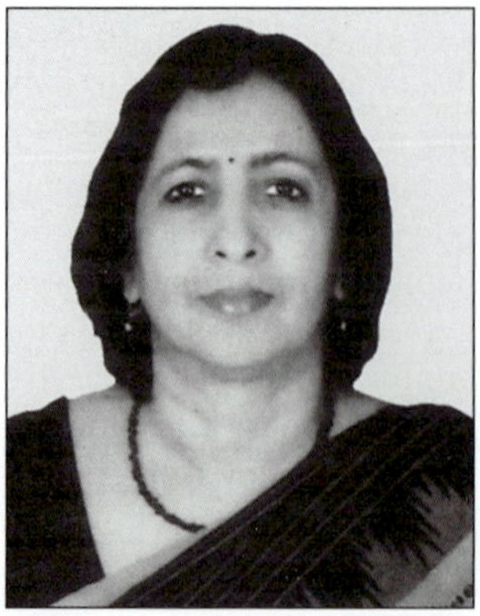

Anju Garg

AIIMS-MAMC-PGI IMAGING SERIES

DIAGNOSTIC RADIOLOGY

Gastrointestinal and Hepatobiliary Imaging

Fifth Edition

Editors

Raju Sharma MD MAMS FICR
Professor and Head
Department of Radiodiagnosis and Interventional Radiology
All India Institute of Medical Sciences (AIIMS)
New Delhi, India

Gaurav Shanker Pradhan DMRD DNB
Director Professor and Head
Department of Radiodiagnosis
Maulana Azad Medical College (MAMC) and Lok Nayak Hospital
New Delhi, India

Manavjit Singh Sandhu MD FICR CCST(UK)
Professor and Head
Department of Radiodiagnosis and Imaging
Postgraduate Institute of Medical Education and Research (PGIMER)
Chandigarh, India

Associate Editors

Shivanand Gamanagatti MD MAMS FICR
Professor
Department of Radiodiagnosis and Interventional Radiology
Jai Prakash Narayan Apex Trauma Center
All India Institute of Medical Sciences (AIIMS)
New Delhi, India

Rashmi Dixit MD
Director Professor
Department of Radiodiagnosis
Maulana Azad Medical College (MAMC)
New Delhi, India

Mandeep Kang MD MAMS FICR
Professor
Department of Radiodiagnosis and Imaging
Postgraduate Institute of Medical Education and Research (PGIMER)
Chandigarh, India

Ankur Goyal MD DNB MNAMS FICR FESUR(Europe)
Additional Professor
Department of Radiodiagnosis and Interventional Radiology
All India Institute of Medical Sciences (AIIMS)
New Delhi, India

Anjali Prakash DMRD DNB MNAMS FICR
Director Professor
Department of Radiodiagnosis
Maulana Azad Medical College (MAMC) and Associated Hospitals
New Delhi, India

Naveen Kalra MD FAMS FICR FINASL
Professor
Department of Radiodiagnosis and Imaging
Postgraduate Institute of Medical Education and Research (PGIMER)
Chandigarh, India

JAYPEE

JAYPEE BROTHERS MEDICAL PUBLISHERS
The Health Sciences Publisher
New Delhi | London

JAYPEE Jaypee Brothers Medical Publishers (P) Ltd

Headquarters
EMCA House
23/23-B, Ansari Road, Daryaganj
New Delhi 110 002, India
Landline: +91-11-23272143, +91-11-23272703
+91-11-23282021, +91-11-23245672
E-mail: jaypee@jaypeebrothers.com

Corporate Office
Jaypee Brothers Medical Publishers (P) Ltd.
4838/24, Ansari Road, Daryaganj
New Delhi 110 002, India
Phone: +91-11-43574357
Fax: +91-11-43574314
E-mail: jaypee@jaypeebrothers.com

Overseas Office
JP Medical Ltd.
83, Victoria Street, London
SW1H 0HW (UK)
Phone: +44-20 3170 8910
Fax: +44(0)20 3008 6180
E-mail: info@jpmedpub.com

Website: www.jaypeebrothers.com

Website: www.jaypeedigital.com

Inquiries for bulk sales may be solicited at: jaypee@jaypeebrothers.com

***Diagnostic Radiology: Gastrointestinal and Hepatobiliary Imaging* / Raju Sharma, Gaurav Shanker Pradhan, Manavjit Singh Sandhu**

First Edition: 1997

Fifth Edition: **2025**

ISBN: 978-93-5696-917-9

Printed at: Samrat Offset Pvt. Ltd.

Contributors

Ajay Gulati MD MAMS FICR Fellowship Abdominal Imaging(Canada)
Professor
Department of Radiodiagnosis and Imaging
Postgraduate Institute of Medical Education and Research (PGIMER)
Chandigarh, India

Alpana Manchanda MD
Director Professor
Department of Radiodiagnosis
Maulana Azad Medical College (MAMC)
New Delhi, India

Amarinder Singh Malhi MD DM(Cardiovascular Radiology and Endovascular Interventions)
Assistant Professor
Department of Radiodiagnosis and Interventional Radiology
All India Institute of Medical Sciences (AIIMS)
New Delhi, India

Anindita Sinha MD MAMS
Professor
Department of Radiodiagnosis and Imaging
Postgraduate Institute of Medical Education and Research (PGIMER)
Chandigarh, India

Anjali Prakash DMRD DNB MNAMS FICR
Director Professor
Department of Radiodiagnosis
Maulana Azad Medical College (MAMC) and Associated Hospitals
New Delhi, India

Anjali Sah MD
Senior Resident
Department of Radiodiagnosis and Interventional Radiology
All India Institute of Medical Sciences (AIIMS)
New Delhi, India

Anju Garg MD
Director Professor
Department of Radiodiagnosis
Maulana Azad Medical College (MAMC)
New Delhi, India

Ankita Aggarwal MD
Assistant Professor
Department of Radiodiagnosis and Interventional Radiology
All India Institute of Medical Sciences (AIIMS)
New Delhi, India

Ankur Goyal MD DNB MNAMS FICR FESUR(Europe)
Additional Professor
Department of Radiodiagnosis and Interventional Radiology
All India Institute of Medical Sciences (AIIMS)
New Delhi, India

Anmol Bhatia MD(Radiodiagnosis) and Fellowship PGI(Pediatric Radiology)
Additional Professor
Department of Radiodiagnosis and Imaging
Postgraduate Institute of Medical Education and Research (PGIMER)
Chandigarh, India

Anupam Lal MD
Professor
Department of Radiodiagnosis and Imaging
Postgraduate Institute of Medical Education and Research (PGIMER)
Chandigarh, India

Anuradha Sharma MD
Fellow in GI Radiology
Department of Radiodiagnosis and Interventional Radiology
All India Institute of Medical Sciences (AIIMS)
New Delhi, India

Arun Sharma DM
Assistant Professor
Department of Radiodiagnosis and Imaging
Postgraduate Institute of Medical Education and Research (PGIMER)
Chandigarh, India

Ashu Seith Bhalla MD FICR MAMS
Professor
Department of Radiodiagnosis and Interventional Radiology
All India Institute of Medical Sciences (AIIMS)
New Delhi, India

Atin Kumar MD DNB MNAMS
Professor
Department of Radiodiagnosis and Interventional Radiology
Jai Prakash Narayan Apex Trauma Center
All India Institute of Medical Sciences (AIIMS)
New Delhi, India

Chandan Jyoti Das MD DNB PhD MAMS FICR FRCP
Professor
Department of Radiodiagnosis and Interventional Radiology
All India Institute of Medical Sciences (AIIMS)
New Delhi, India

Chandrashekhara SH MD DM DNB
Professor
Department of Radiodiagnosis and Interventional Radiology
Dr BR Ambedkar Institute Rotary Cancer Hospital (IRCH)
All India Institute of Medical Sciences (AIIMS)
New Delhi, India

Deeksha Bhalla MD DNB MNAMS
Assistant Professor
Department of Radiodiagnosis
Maulana Azad Medical College
(MAMC)
New Delhi, India

Devasenathipathy Kandasamy MD DNB FRCR
Professor
Department of Radiodiagnosis and Interventional Radiology
All India Institute of Medical Sciences (AIIMS)
New Delhi, India

Dipin Sudhakaran MD
Fellow in GI Radiology
Department of Radiodiagnosis and Interventional Radiology
All India Institute of Medical Sciences (AIIMS)
New Delhi, India

Ekta Dhamija MD
Additional Professor
Department of Radiodiagnosis and Interventional Radiology
Dr BR Ambedkar Institute Rotary Cancer Hospital (IRCH)
All India Institute of Medical Sciences (AIIMS)
New Delhi, India

Gaurav Shanker Pradhan DMRD DNB
Director Professor and Head
Department of Radiodiagnosis
Maulana Azad Medical College (MAMC) and Lok Nayak Hospital
New Delhi, India

Harish Bhujade MD FVIR(PGI)
Assistant Professor
Department of Radiodiagnosis and Imaging
Postgraduate Institute of Medical Education and Research (PGIMER)
Chandigarh, India

Jyoti Kumar MD DNB MNAMS FICR
Director Professor
Department of Radiodiagnosis
Maulana Azad Medical College (MAMC)
New Delhi, India

Krithika Rangarajan MD DNB FRCR
Associate Professor
Department of Radiodiagnosis and Interventional Radiology
Dr BR Ambedkar Institute Rotary Cancer Hospital (IRCH)
All India Institute of Medical Sciences (AIIMS)
New Delhi, India

Madhurima Sharma MD DNB
Assistant Professor
Department of Radiodiagnosis and Imaging
Postgraduate Institute of Medical Education and Research (PGIMER)
Chandigarh, India

Mahesh Prakash MD MAMS FIACM FICR
Professor
Department of Radiodiagnosis and Imaging
Postgraduate Institute of Medical Education and Research (PGIMER)
Chandigarh, India

Mandeep Garg MD FRCR
Professor
Department of Radiodiagnosis and Imaging
Postgraduate Institute of Medical Education and Research (PGIMER)
Chandigarh, India

Mandeep Kang MD MAMS FICR
Professor
Department of Radiodiagnosis and Imaging
Postgraduate Institute of Medical Education and Research (PGIMER)
Chandigarh, India

Manisha Jana MD DNB FRCR
Professor
Department of Radiodiagnosis and Interventional Radiology
All India Institute of Medical Sciences (AIIMS)
New Delhi, India

Manphool Singhal MD DNB MAMS FICR FSCCT FSCMR
Professor
Department of Radiodiagnosis and Imaging
Postgraduate Institute of Medical Education and Research (PGIMER)
Chandigarh, India

Mukesh Kumar Yadav MD
Additional Professor
Department of Radiodiagnosis and Interventional Radiology
Dr BR Ambedkar Institute Rotary Cancer Hospital (IRCH)
All India Institute of Medical Sciences (AIIMS)
New Delhi, India

Naveen Kalra MD FAMS FICR FINASL
Professor
Department of Radiodiagnosis and Imaging
Postgraduate Institute of Medical Education and Research (PGIMER)
Chandigarh, India

Nidhi Prabhakar MD DNB
Assistant Professor
Department of Radiodiagnosis and Imaging
Postgraduate Institute of Medical Education and Research (PGIMER)
Chandigarh, India

Pankaj Gupta MD
Associate Professor
Department of Radiodiagnosis and Imaging,
Postgraduate Institute of Medical Education and Research (PGIMER)
Chandigarh, India

Priyanka Naranje MD DNB MNAMS EBIR
Additional Professor
Department of Radiodiagnosis and Interventional Radiology
All India Institute of Medical Sciences (AIIMS)
New Delhi, India

Radhika Batra MD DNB
Associate Professor
Department of Radiodiagnosis
Maulana Azad Medical College (MAMC)
New Delhi, India

Rajendra Behera MD
Assistant Professor
Department of Radiodiagnosis and Interventional Radiology
All India Institute of Medical Sciences (AIIMS)
New Delhi, India

Raju Sharma MD MAMS FICR
Professor and Head
Department of Radiodiagnosis and Interventional Radiology
All India Institute of Medical Sciences (AIIMS)
New Delhi, India

Rashmi Dixit MD
Director Professor
Department of Radiodiagnosis
Maulana Azad Medical College (MAMC)
New Delhi, India

Sanchita Gupta MD
Fellow in GI Radiology
Department of Radiodiagnosis and Interventional Radiology
All India Institute of Medical Sciences (AIIMS)
New Delhi, India

Sanjay Kumar Meena MD
Assistant Professor
Department of Radiology
National Cancer Institute, Jhajjar Campus
All India Institute of Medical Sciences (AIIMS)
New Delhi, India

Sapna Singh MD DNB MNAMS
Director Professor
Department of Radiodiagnosis
Maulana Azad Medical College (MAMC)
New Delhi, India

Satyam DNB MNAMS
Senior Specialist
Department of Radiodiagnosis
Lok Nayak Hospital and Associated Maulana Azad Medical College (MAMC)
New Delhi, India

Shivanand Gamanagatti MD MAMS FICR
Professor
Department of Radiodiagnosis and Interventional Radiology
Jai Prakash Narayan Apex Trauma Center
All India Institute of Medical Sciences (AIIMS)
New Delhi, India

Shrea Gulati MD
Senior Resident
Department of Radiodiagnosis and Interventional Radiology
All India Institute of Medical Sciences (AIIMS)
New Delhi, India

Smita Manchanda MD DNB FICR
Additional Professor
Department of Radiodiagnosis and Interventional Radiology
All India Institute of Medical Sciences (AIIMS)
New Delhi, India

Smriti Hari MD MAMS
Professor
Department of Radiodiagnosis and Interventional Radiology
All India Institute of Medical Sciences (AIIMS)
New Delhi, India

Sreedhara BC MD FVIR EBIR
Associate Professor
Department of Radiodiagnosis and Imaging
Postgraduate Institute of Medical Education and Research (PGIMER)
Chandigarh, India

Stanzin Spalkit MD DNB EDiR
Assistant Professor
Department of Radiodiagnosis and Interventional Radiology
All India Institute of Medical Sciences (AIIMS)
New Delhi, India

Stuti Chandola MD
Senior Resident
Department of Radiodiagnosis and Interventional Radiology
All India Institute of Medical Sciences (AIIMS)
New Delhi, India

Surabhi Vyas MD DNB MNAMS
Professor
Department of Radiodiagnosis and Interventional Radiology
All India Institute of Medical Sciences (AIIMS)
New Delhi, India

Swati Gupta MD DNB FRCR
Associate Professor
Department of Radiodiagnosis
Maulana Azad Medical College (MAMC)
New Delhi, India

Ujjwal Gorsi MD DM
Additional Professor
Department of Radiodiagnosis and Imaging
Postgraduate Institute of Medical Education and Research (PGIMER)
Chandigarh, India

Uma Debi MD
Additional Professor
Department of Radiodiagnosis and Imaging
Postgraduate Institute of Medical Education and Research (PGIMER)
Chandigarh, India

Preface to the Fifth Edition

This latest edition of *"AIIMS-MAMC-PGI Imaging Series Diagnostic Radiology: Gastrointestinal and Hepatobiliary Imaging"* builds upon the strong foundation established by its predecessors, first published in 1997.

Over the last four editions, this book has been widely acclaimed as an essential and comprehensive reference for radiologists, gastroenterologists, and gastro-surgeons, and this new edition carries forward that tradition. Recognizing the ever-changing landscape of radiology, every chapter has been meticulously updated to incorporate the latest advancements, new guidelines, and evolving concepts. New terminology and concepts in metabolic-associated steatotic liver disease (MASLD), magnetic resonance (MR) elastography, updated Barcelona Clinic Liver Cancer (BCLC) and National Comprehensive Cancer Network (NCCN) guidelines, Liver Imaging Reporting and Data System (LI-RADS) nomenclature, recent advances in "interventional radiology" options for hepatocellular carcinoma, etc., have been suitably highlighted. The content has been trimmed to keep it concise and readable. The book has 27 Chapters covering all the important entities. Readers can expect an enriching and informative experience, ensuring their practice stays current and their knowledge updated.

This book represents a collaborative effort by distinguished faculty from India's premier institutions: AIIMS (New Delhi), MAMC (New Delhi), and PGIMER (Chandigarh). We extend our heartfelt gratitude to each contributor for their dedication and hard work over the past few months, which made this edition possible.

We also express our sincere appreciation to our publishing partner "Jaypee Brothers Medical Publishers (P) Ltd" for their continuous and unwavering support.

Raju Sharma
Gaurav Shanker Pradhan
Manavjit Singh Sandhu

Preface to the First Edition

There has been a tremendous change in the approach to the diagnosis of abdominal diseases in the last decade, making the imaging of gastrointestinal and hepatobiliary system as one of the most interesting and challenging specialties to the radiologists. New imaging and therapeutic techniques that have revolutionized the diagnosis and treatment of many abdominal diseases, have also given us the added responsibility of defining the proper role of these techniques, evaluating their efficacy against earlier and more established methods, and providing guidance to clinicians through the judicious use of newer technology.

It is with this goal in mind, the faculty of Departments of Radiodiagnosis at the All India Institute of Medical Sciences, Maulana Azad Medical College, New Delhi, India, and Postgraduate Institute of Medical Education and Research, Chandigarh, India, present this third book in the series of Diagnostic Radiology, devoted to gastrointestinal and hepatobiliary imaging.

The book comprises twenty-nine chapters covering the radiological and imaging aspects of hepatobiliary and gastrointestinal systems in detail. In spite of advancements in various imaging techniques, conventional radiology still remains the mainstay as the initial imaging modality for many abdominal disorders and its interpretation continues to be a great challenge. The importance of plain radiography and barium studies has been described in depth. Techniques of US, CT and the potential role of MRI in evaluation of these disorders have also been explicitly elaborated upon. There are separate sections dedicated to imaging of the liver, biliary tract and pancreas. Clinicopathological aspects with radiological correlation have been discussed in the section on liver with special reference to focal and diffuse, benign and malignant lesions. Biliopathy and pancreatic disorders have been covered at length, with two separate chapters dealing with interventions. Portal hypertension has been discussed in great detail with authors explaining the role of various radiological modalities, including US, color Doppler, angiography and newer imaging techniques. The status of conventional techniques and advances in imaging have been described in an attempt to provide a comprehensive overview of all regions of the GI tract involved by infective, benign, and malignant lesions with special reference to the evaluation of the patients with GI bleed.

We hope, the reader shall find this book—both instructive and informative—for the improved use of imaging resources, which will help to serve the common goal of good healthcare and management of patients everywhere.

We wish to take this opportunity to thank our faculty colleagues from AIIMS, MAMC and PGIMER for their active support, cooperation and timely submission of the manuscripts. We owe immense gratitude to Prof K Subbarao, Prof A Gajaraj, Prof Ratni B Gujral and Prof B Nagi, who have been very kind to contribute their experience into this book. We specially like to thank Dr Sumedha Pawa, Dr Mona Bhatia, Dr Anju Garg, Dr Sima Mukhopadhyay, and Dr Sushma Vashisht for their help and untiring efforts in bringing out this volume. We also express our sincere thanks to the publishers of the series of these books, M/s Jaypee Brothers, for timely publication of this volume as always, in the present form.

Manorama Berry
Veena Chowdhury
Sudha Suri

Contents

Section 1: Bowel

Section 2: Liver

SECTION

1

Bowel

CHAPTER 1

Alpana Manchanda, Jyoti Kumar, Gaurav Shanker Pradhan

Imaging Approach to Dysphagia

INTRODUCTION

Dysphagia is a common manifestation of many of the disorders affecting the esophagus. It is a nondescriptive term that literally means "difficulty in swallowing". It is defined as the subjective awareness of difficulty in swallowing or perception of obstruction of a solid or liquid bolus as it passes from the mouth to the stomach.[1] Dysphagia is considered to be clinically significant when such symptoms occur a minimum of several times a month. It can result from functional or structural abnormalities of the oral cavity, pharynx, esophagus or gastric cardia. It may be further classified as oropharyngeal or esophageal (substernal), depending on the anatomic site of involvement. It is of utmost importance to differentiate between the two as their etiology, radiologic evaluation, and management may vary greatly.[1]

EPIDEMIOLOGY

Dysphagia has a prevalence of 20%, affecting up to 50% of the population > 60 years of age.[2]

The diagnosis of dysphagia is important because of its associated morbidity and mortality. The elderly are at the highest risk of subsequent complications of dysphagia such as dehydration, weight loss, and airway obstruction; the most dangerous being aspiration, which can be silent in up to 55% of patients.[3]

There are also psychosocial consequences in the form of social isolation, depression, anxiety, resulting in reduced quality of life.

PHYSIOLOGY OF SWALLOWING

Swallowing is a complex activity which occurs in a coordinated manner to transport the ingested material from the mouth to the stomach. Normal swallowing is divided into oral, pharyngeal, and esophageal stages and involves both voluntary and involuntary neuromuscular contractions starting from the mouth to the stomach.[3]

Oropharyngeal Stage

This stage is initiated by the contractions of the tongue and striated muscles of mastication which mix the food bolus with saliva and propel it from the oral cavity into the oropharynx. Once the food has left the oral cavity, swallowing is no longer under voluntary control. The bolus then activates the oropharyngeal sensory receptors initiate the deglutition reflex which is a centrally-mediated wave of inhibition which precedes the peristaltic contraction. It not only propels the food through the pharynx and esophagus, but also prevents its aspiration (i.e., entry into the airway) and nasal regurgitation (retrograde flow into the nose). This is achieved in the following sequence of events—elevation of the soft palate which closes the nasopharynx, closure of the laryngeal vestibule which is critical for airway protection. This occurs as a result of upward and anterior movement of the larynx by the suprahyoid muscles. The epiglottis moves downward to cover the airway. Finally, the upper esophageal sphincter (UES) including the cricopharyngeus muscle relaxes due to which the bolus enters the cervical esophagus. The pharynx is cleared of the bolus by the sequential contraction of the pharyngeal constrictor muscles. The deglutition reflex lasts for approximately one second.[4]

Primary esophageal peristalsis is induced by a swallow at the pharyngoesophageal junction. Caudad progression of a bolus is achieved by deglutitive inhibition.

Secondary peristalsis is induced by esophageal distention and initiates around the level of the aortic arch. It is a propulsive wave that occurs to clear the esophagus of any retained bolus.

Tertiary contractions are nonpropulsive and cause a variable degree of narrowing of the lumen. Between swallows, the esophagus is collapsed and the upper and lower esophageal sphincters (LES) are closed.

Esophageal Stage

The esophageal stage of swallowing begins once the bolus passes through the UES. In this phase, the peristaltic contractions of the smooth muscle of the thoracic esophagus propels the food toward the LES and stomach. The LES relaxes as soon as the swallow is initiated, which persists until the food bolus is propelled into the stomach.[4]

PATHOGENESIS OF DYSPHAGIA

The normal passage of the ingested bolus through the pharynx and esophagus depends on the size of the ingested bolus, size of the lumen, the force of peristalsis, deglutitive inhibition along with normal relaxation of the upper and LES during swallowing. When there is mechanical or structural cause to the dysphagia it is called *mechanical dysphagia*.

In contrast, *motor dysphagia* occurs due to weak peristaltic contractions or impaired deglutitive inhibition, causing nonperistaltic contractions and impaired relaxation of sphincters.[5]

Clinical Presentation

Dysphagia is a very nondescriptive term that can result from any problem from the proximal oral cavity to the proximal stomach.

A carefully taken history helps a physician to identify 80–85% of the causes of dysphagia. Specific questions such as the onset, duration, severity of dysphagia and any associated symptoms may help in narrowing the differential diagnosis to a specific diagnosis or to an anatomic or a pathophysiologic-related diagnosis.[6]

It is important to know if dysphagia is present during swallowing or at all times. Dysphagia which occurs during swallowing at all times without any organic cause is suggestive of globus hystericus. Dysphagia that occurs only for solids is likely due to a mechanical obstruction, while dysphagia for both solids and liquids is more likely to indicate a motility disorder.

Symptoms such as delayed or absence of swallow initiation, postswallow cough, nasopharyngeal regurgitation, and repeated swallows to clear the bolus are indicative of oropharyngeal dysphagia.[7]

Oropharyngeal dysphagia can be predicted with 80% accuracy if any one of the above four symptoms are associated. **Flowchart 1** depicts the clinical approach to dysphagia.[2]

Abnormality of the oral phase of swallowing results in food dribbling from the mouth, difficulty in drinking or chewing, or difficulty in initiating a swallow. Soft-palate insufficiency results in a nasal quality of voice or nasal regurgitation. Coughing or choking during swallowing indicates laryngeal penetration. Patients with pharyngeal dysphagia typically complain of a "lump in the throat" or of food "sticking in the throat" during swallowing. It may be caused by a functional abnormality such as cricopharyngeal dysmotility, amyotrophic lateral sclerosis or by a morphologic abnormality such as Zenker's diverticulum or pharyngeal tumor.[8]

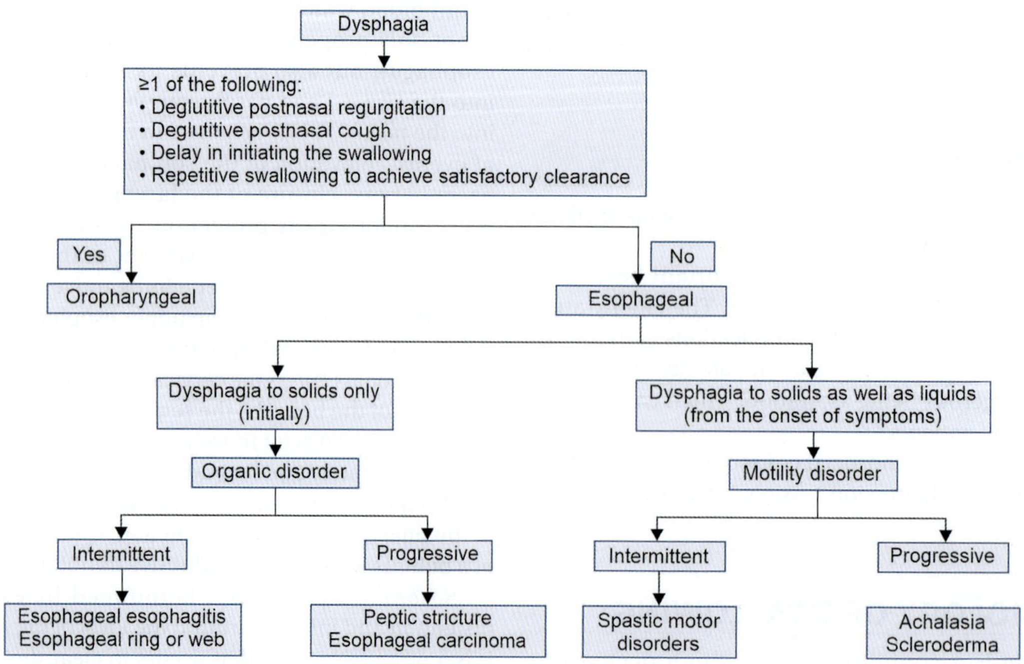

FLOWCHART 1: Flowchart depicting clinical approach to dysphagia.

A sensation of blockage at the level of the suprasternal notch or thoracic inlet raises the possibility of a cervical esophageal web, tumor or of extrinsic compression of the cervical or upper thoracic esophagus by an enlarged thyroid, mediastinal lymphadenopathy, or other mass lesion.[8] Substernal localization of dysphagia is usually due to a structural disorder such as reflux esophagitis, peptic stricture or Schatzki ring or motility disorder of the esophagus such as achalasia. A distal lesion (even carcinoma of the gastric fundus) may refer dysphagia proximally as far as the pharynx. The patient may complain of odynophagia (pain on swallowing) or chest pain. These symptoms may be due to esophageal spasm or other motor disorders, but may also be caused by infectious esophagitis, gastroesophageal reflux disease (GERD) and ulcerated pharyngeal or esophageal tumors.

The duration and progression of symptoms also provide a clue to the etiology. Chronic and stable symptoms are suggestive of benign conditions such as peptic strictures, Schatzki's ring, while rapidly progressive symptoms associated with weight loss are suggestive of a malignant etiology. The timing of regurgitation in relation to swallowing or meals is also indicative of the underlying cause, e.g., regurgitation in-between meals is suggestive of an underlying Zenker's diverticulum, while immediately after swallowing suggests esophageal retention of food.[7] **Table 1** lists the associated symptoms with possible etiologies of dysphagia.[5,6]

Dysphagia is also more common in patients with a history of GERD than in those without GERD.[1]

Patients who develop dysphagia after a long history of reflux symptoms and those with poor control of symptoms may develop complications such as peptic stricture, Barrett's esophagus (BE) and even esophageal adenocarcinoma.[7] In young patients with history of atopy who present with dysphagia or obstruction to food bolus, eosinophilic esophagitis (EoE) must be suspected and ruled out by endoscopic biopsy.

TABLE 1: Symptoms associated with possible etiologies of dysphagia.[5,6]

Symptoms	Possible diagnoses
Progressive dysphagia	Neuromuscular dysphagia
Sudden dysphagia	Obstructive dysphagia
Episodic dysphagia to solids	Lower esophageal ring
Difficulty in initiating swallow	Oropharyngeal dysphagia
Food sticks after swallow	Esophageal dysphagia
• Cough/choking-before, during or after swallow • In early phase of swallowing • In late phase of swallowing	• Indicative of aspiration • Neuromuscular dysphagia • Obstructive dysphagia
Weight loss: • In the elderly • With regurgitation	Carcinoma and achalasia
Progressive symptoms: • Heartburn • Intermittent symptoms of dysphagia • Odynophagia	• Peptic stricture and scleroderma • Rings and webs and diffuse esophageal spasm • *Esophagitis*: - Postradiation - Infectious - Pill induced
Chest pain with dysphagia	DES and related motor disorders
Worsening of pain by: • Solid food only • Solids and liquids	• Obstructive dysphagia • Neuromuscular dysphagia
Regurgitation of old food	Zenker's diverticulum
Weakness and dysphagia	Stroke, muscular dystrophies, and myasthenia gravis
Halitosis and dysphagia	Zenker's diverticulum
Dysphagia relieved with repeated swallows	Achalasia

(DES: diffuse esophageal spasm)

CAUSES OF DYSPHAGIA

These can be divided into two broad groups—mechanical and motor, involving oropharynx and esophagus **(Tables 2A to D)**.[5]

TABLES 2A TO D: Causes of dysphagia.

A: *Mechanical oropharyngeal dysphagia*
• Zenker's diverticulum
• Cricopharyngeal bar or stenosis
• Cervical (mucosal) web-Plummer–Vinson syndrome
• Retropharyngeal abscess
• Oropharyngeal tumor
• Head and neck surgery
• Stricture-caustic and postradiation

Continued

IMAGING TECHNIQUES IN THE EVALUATION OF DYSPHAGIA

As the anatomic structures and causes responsible for oropharyngeal and esophageal dysphagia are different, the approach to their evaluation also differs.[7]

Continued

B: *Motor oropharyngeal dysphagia*[7,9]	
1. Central nervous system	• Stroke • Parkinson's disease • Brainstem tumors • Alzheimer's disease • Drugs (phenothiazines and benzodiazepines)
2. Degenerative diseases	• Amyotrophic lateral sclerosis • Huntington's chorea • Multiple sclerosis
3. Peripheral nervous system	• Spinal muscular atrophy • Guillain–Barré syndrome • Postpolio syndrome
4. Myogenic	• Drugs (Botulinum toxin and cytotoxics) • Myasthenia gravis • Dermatomyositis and polymyositis • Thyrotoxic myopathy • Drugs (amiodarone, alcohol, and cholesterol lowering drug)
C: *Mechanical esophageal dysphagia*	
1. *Intrinsic narrowing*	
i. Inflammatory/ Infective esophagitis	• Viral • Bacterial • Fungal
ii. Webs and rings	• Congenital esophageal stenosis • Lower esophageal mucosal ring (Schatzki's ring)
iii. Benign strictures	• GERD and Barrett's esophagus • Peptic stricture • Caustic injury • Pill-induced • Inflammatory (*Candida*, mucocutaneous lesions) • Postoperative or anastomotic • Postradiation
iv. Malignant stricture	
v. Foreign body	
2. *Extrinsic narrowing*	• Substernal thyroid • Posterior mediastinal mass • Vascular compression (aberrant right subclavian artery, right-sided aorta, and aortic aneurysm) • Enlarged vertebral osteophytes

Continued

Continued

D: *Motor esophageal dysphagia*[5]	
1. *Diseases of smooth muscles*	
i. Weak muscle contraction or LES tone	• Idiopathic • Scleroderma and related collagen vascular disease • Myotonic dystrophy • Metabolic neuromyopathy (amyloid/alcohol/diabetes) • Drugs (anticholinergics and smooth muscle relaxants) • Hypertensive peristalsis (nutcracker esophagus) • Hypercontracting lower esophageal sphincter (LES)
ii. Enhanced muscle contraction	
2. *Disorders of inhibitory innervation*	
i. Diffuse esophageal spasm (DES)	Primary, secondary (Chagas disease, carcinoma, lymphoma leading to pseudoachalasia)
ii. Achalasia	
iii. Contractile (muscular/lower esophageal ring)	

(GERD: gastroesophageal reflux disease)

Oropharyngeal dysphagia is evaluated by:

- Plain film
- Barium swallow
- Modified barium swallow/videofluoroscopic swallowing study (VFSS)
- Nasopharyngeal-endoscopy
- Pharyngomanometry
- Cross-sectional studies (CT/MRI)

Esophageal dysphagia is evaluated by:

- Barium swallow
- Upper gastrointestinal (GI) endoscopy
- Esophageal manometry
- Scintigraphy
- Cross-sectional studies (CT/MRI)
- Endoscopic ultrasound (EUS)
- Intraesophageal pH measurement

Barium studies and endoscopy are complementary investigations, but barium swallow is a useful first-line investigation for dysphagia. Its wide availability, noninvasiveness, and it being a relatively inexpensive investigation are some of its advantages. It allows real-time continuous viewing of the bolus during transit from the oropharynx to the stomach and allows a good qualitative and functional assessment of the esophagus including the upper and LESs and esophageal peristalsis.

A barium swallow can demonstrate structural abnormality such as a stricture or mass lesion and is found to be more sensitive than esophagoscopy in detecting esophageal webs and rings.[7] It can help in identifying major esophageal motility disorders; however, the reported sensitivity for it is low, around 56–69%.[2]

Examination Technique

Preparation: The pharynx, esophagus, and stomach should be as free of fluid and secretions as possible to permit optimal mucosal coating during the barium study. The patient is instructed to fast overnight before the examination. The patient should avoid smoking or chewing gum as these activities may stimulate salivary and/or gastric secretions and impair mucosal coating.[8]

Plain Films

Although scout films are not obtained routinely, frontal and lateral plain films of the neck and chest may be helpful in cases of suspected foreign body, abscess, or fistula formation, and in the postoperative patient. The plain film may show fluid levels in the esophagus in a patient with achalasia. In major esophageal dilatation, the esophagus expands to the right, producing a mediastinal edge that runs from the neck to the diaphragm with a single indentation produced by the azygos vein.

Barium Studies

Examination of the pharynx and esophagus requires a dynamic evaluation of motility as well as double-contrast spot films to detect morphologic abnormalities. Cineradiography or videofluoroscopy should be used to study swallowing dynamics. The recordings may be reviewed later to analyze tongue movement, soft-palate elevation, epiglottic tilt, laryngeal closure, cricopharyngeal opening, and pharyngeal peristalsis.

The routine barium examination of the esophagus should be a biphasic study combining upright double contrast and prone single contrast technique. In the double-contrast phase, the aim is to achieve adequate gaseous distention of the lumen with a thin layer of high-density barium coating the mucosa. Gaseous distention is improved by the patient swallowing effervescent agents. The patient is also instructed to swallow rapidly the high-density barium. Rapid drinking causes air swallowing and thus, esophageal distention. In addition, it interrupts the esophageal peristalsis, thus resulting in esophageal hypotonia.

The effervescent agent may be omitted in patients with suspected esophageal infections or obstructing lesions (because it is painful and may cause artifacts).

Prone views of the upper esophagus best show esophageal webs and indentations by aortic arch anomalies. Barium-filled views of the distal esophagus are important for the detection of hiatal hernias, strictures, webs or rings as these may not be visible in the erect double-contrast phase. Next, the patient is turned to the right and gastroesophageal junction (GEJ) is monitored fluoroscopically to elicit spontaneous gastroesophageal reflux. The cardia is best shown in double contrast with the patient in the recumbent right lateral position.

Provocative testing in an attempt to reproduce symptoms may be useful in a patient with solid food dysphagia who has a normal study with liquid barium. A barium impregnated solid bolus may hold up at a subtle stricture or induce spasm not seen with liquid bolus.

A tube esophagogram may be performed if there is marked aspiration or penetration.

Evaluation of a patient presenting with dysphagia includes detailed evaluation of the pharynx, esophagus, GEJ and the cardia using double-contrast and single-contrast barium examinations.[8]

Evaluation of Pharynx

The patient is positioned erect in the right lateral position with the fluoroscopy table being vertical and asked to swallow approximately 10 mL of 250% w/v of barium sulfate (high density) suspension. A cine recording of the oral and pharyngeal phases of swallowing is done both in full-field lateral views as well as collimated views of the pharynx. In addition to this, two lateral spot films are obtained during phonation (patient is asked to say "*eeeeeee...*") and during suspended respiration respectively.[10]

The patient's position is then changed to a frontal position and the head tilted backward till the mandible is superimposed over the occiput. In this position, cine recording of two additional swallows is done. Two frontal spot films are obtained during Valsalva maneuver and during suspended respiration respectively **(Figs. 1A and B)**.

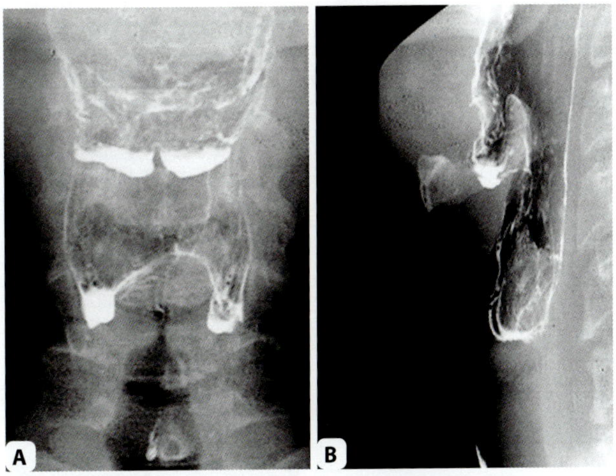

FIGS. 1A AND B: Spot views of the normal pharynx. (A) Frontal view shows normal smooth mucosal outline of the paired valleculae, pyriform sinuses, and lateral walls of the hypopharynx; (B) Lateral view shows normal smooth mucosal outline of superimposed bilateral valleculae and pyriform sinuses.

Evaluation of the Esophagus, Gastroesophageal Junction, and Cardia

The patient is positioned erect in the left posterior oblique position with the fluoroscopy table being vertical and asked to swallow effervescent granules with approximately 10 mL of water. The patient is then asked to rapidly swallow a mouthful of 250% w/v of barium sulfate suspension. Spot films of the proximal and distal esophagus are obtained. In order to get proper double-contrast views, the spot exposures should be timed with periods of optimal distention and coating **(Figs. 2A and B)**.

The fluoroscopy table is then made horizontal and the patient is asked to lie down in the right lateral position and spot films of the double-contrast views of gastric cardia and fundus are obtained.

The patient is then turned prone in a right anterior oblique (RAO) position and asked to swallow 100% w/v suspension of barium sulfate. Fluoroscopic examination of esophageal motility is done, along with spot exposures to obtain single contrast views of proximal and distal esophagus. In case of any abnormal esophageal motility detected, cine recording of additional swallows can also be done.

The patient is then asked to turn to his left side and then on to his back. The GEJ is focused and monitored fluoroscopically as the patient is asked to slowly turn toward his right side in order to look for any spontaneous gastroesophageal reflux. If no spontaneous reflux is seen, then straight leg raising maneuver or Valsalva maneuver can be done to increase intra-abdominal pressure and gastroesophageal reflux is looked for.

Thus, there are several important principles in the evaluation of patients with dysphagia:[11]

- Radiographic evaluation of patients with dysphagia must include all structures involved in swallowing.
- If possible, the examination should be biphasic.
- Every patient should be examined in both the erect and recumbent positions.
- Each patient with dysphagia is different. Although there is a routine or basic examination, studies of patients with swallowing problems lend themselves to tailoring. Each examination is subtly altered on the basis of a short patient history taken by the radiologist. The routine examination is also modified by the clinical condition of the patient. The sicker the patient, less routine and more tailored the examination should be. The examination should be focused on answering a specific question such as "does the patient aspirate". The answer should not be just "yes" or "no" but "yes, for the following reasons". Aspiration may occur during swallowing due to a failure of laryngeal protection or after swallowing, e.g., pharyngeal paresis may result in progressive retention of liquid in the pyriform sinuses and subsequent overflow aspiration, or gastroesophageal reflux may produce aspiration from esophagopharyngeal regurgitation of the refluxed material. Aspiration may also occur before swallowing if there is premature leakage from the mouth when the larynx is open and unprotected. The other important observation is whether the patient coughs during aspiration. With loss of sensory feedback, aspiration may be silent and not suspected clinically.

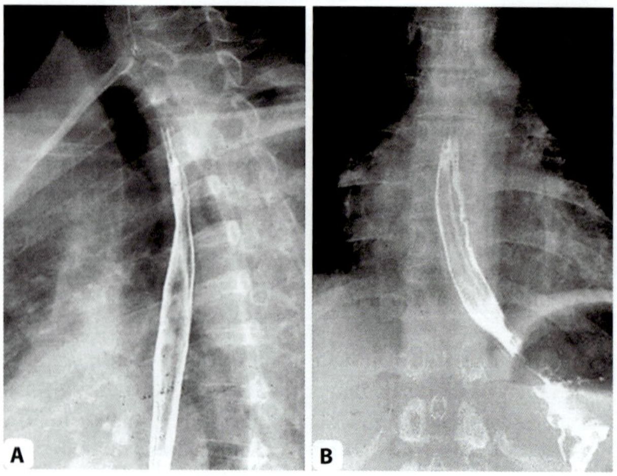

FIGS. 2A AND B: (A) Normal appearance of mid and (B) lower dorsal esophagus and gastroesophageal junction on barium swallow study.

The Tailored Examination[8]

Recommended Approach

Patients with pharyngeal dysphagia or other symptoms localized to the pharynx, neck or suprasternal notch should undergo a careful radiologic examination of the pharynx with videofluoroscopic recordings and double-contrast spot films. If the patient aspirates a substantial amount of barium, the examination should be terminated. If marked swallowing dysfunction occurs, particularly in stroke patients, a detailed study of the esophagus is unwarranted. However, patients with pharyngeal carcinoma have a significantly increased risk of synchronous esophageal carcinoma. Therefore, a double-contrast examination of the esophagus should be performed in these cases. A normal pharyngeal study should always be followed by a careful examination of the esophagus and cardia to rule out more distal abnormalities causing referred dysphagia to the pharynx.

Conversely, patients with substernal dysphagia, odynophagia, reflux symptoms, or nonspecific chest pain should first undergo a detailed radiologic examination of the esophagus and cardia. Some esophageal disorders such as achalasia and GERD may be associated with pharyngeal or cricopharyngeal dysfunction. However, pharyngeal abnormalities virtually never cause referred dysphagia below the level of the thoracic inlet, so a limited pharyngeal study may be performed in patients with substernal symptoms.

Videofluoroscopic Swallowing Study

It is also known as modified barium swallow and is the standard of reference for evaluating the swallowing mechanism. VFSS is a dynamic fluoroscopic study performed with high-frame rate image capture and is useful for evaluating the motility of oropharynx and hypopharynx. The study is often performed in conjunction with a swallowing therapist and provides information about swallowing function in response to therapeutic measures and necessary dietary requirements. The images can be reviewed later with referring physicians, speech language pathologist, patients and their family members to explain the management recommendations.[4] VFSS provides real-time visualization of the oropharyngeal and esophageal structures, movement, and coordination of swallowing. The study best detects aspiration during swallow. Even though VFSS is a gold standard for dysphagia, it can be normal in patients with early or slowly progressive disease. Hence, if patient's discomfort persists in spite of normal VFSS, they should be followed up.

Nasopharyngoscopy

It is also known as fiberoptic endoscopic swallowing study. This technique allows direct visualization of lingual, pharyngeal, and epiglottic movements during swallowing and also assesses the presence of any pharyngeal retention of fluids after swallowing.[7]

Pharyngeal/Esophageal Manometry

Manometry is the most sensitive and accurate technique to assess esophageal motility and diagnose esophageal motility disorders. The study entails positioning a pressure sensing catheter within the esophagus. Test swallows are given to the patient following which esophageal contractility is observed. The upper and LESs appear as zones of high pressure that relax on swallowing while the intersphincteric esophagus shows peristaltic contractions.[12]

With advancements in technology, the conventional manometry has been replaced by high-resolution manometry (HRM) with substantial improvement in its recording power and fidelity. Pressure measurement of 1 cm or less can be measured along the entire esophagus thereby providing detailed mapping of esophageal motor function including upper and LESs.

The traditional line plot in manometry has further largely been replaced by the topographical or contour or color plot which aids in more rapid interpretation of results. The combination of HRM with topography, also called high-resolution esophageal pressure topography allows more precise measurement of esophageal pressures **(Fig. 3)**. It has been shown to have higher sensitivity (72%) for achalasia as compared to conventional manometry (56%).[7]

High-resolution manometry is thus the "gold standard" test for diagnosing esophageal motility disorders with high sensitivity in detecting pressure changes and its good correlation with bolus transit in these conditions.

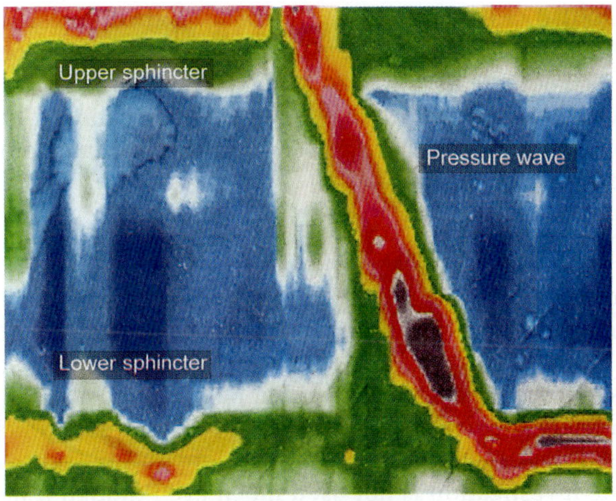

FIG. 3: Color plot depicting pressure waves of a normal swallow by esophageal manometry, also called high-resolution esophageal pressure topography.

Upper Gastrointestinal Endoscopy

It is recommended as the first-line diagnostic investigation which should be performed in the workup with esophageal dysphagia after a detailed history and physical examination.

Upper GI endoscopy not only provides direct visualization of the esophagus but also the oropharynx, stomach and duodenum. It is useful in identifying intraluminal mass lesion, strictures, inflammatory disorders such as reflux disease, EoE, and pill-induced ulceration.[7]

Endoscopes also have an instrumentation channel through which biopsy forceps, sclerotherapy catheters or balloon dilators can be passed and various therapeutic procedures can be performed simultaneously. Some of the advantages of endoscopy over contrast radiographic studies are:[12]

- Increased sensitivity for detection of mucosal lesions.
- Increased sensitivity in the detection of Barrett's metaplasia which is mainly identified by its abnormal color.
- Obtaining biopsy specimen of suspected abnormalities for histopathological evaluation. At least six biopsies from the distal and proximal esophagus should be taken in the absence of structural lesions.
- The ability to effectively dilate strictures, which may be peptic, anastomotic or radiation induced or esophageal web or Schatzki's ring is a therapeutic capability of this technique. Endoscopic-guided pneumatic dilatation and botulinum toxin injection at the LES are some of the therapeutic alternatives which can be performed in patients of achalasia who are not suitable for surgical myotomy.[7]

Though upper GI endoscopy has relatively low sensitivity and specificity in the evaluation of underlying motility disorder, it can suggest underlying achalasia in the presence of a dilated esophagus with features of reduced contractions which occlude its lumen and a tight LES. In the setting of achalasia, endoscopy provides direct visualization of the GEJ and gastric cardia to detect any underlying carcinoma causing pseudoachalasia.

Esophageal Scintigraphy

Scintigraphy is a screening test used to detect an abnormality in the esophageal transit time. It involves the ingestion of a liquid or solid bolus labeled with a radionuclide such as ^{99m}Tc-DTPA (diethylene-triamine-pentaacetate). The radionuclide movement is recorded by a γ-camera which measures the esophageal bolus time and clearance. The investigation is not used much even though it has been reported to have a high sensitivity and specificity in detecting esophageal motor abnormalities.[7] Handling of radioactive material and radiation exposure, poor anatomical definition compared with barium swallow and a lack of well-defined diagnostic criteria are some of the reasons why scintigraphy is rarely used in the investigation of dysphagia.

Intraesophageal pH Monitoring

This investigation is done in the setting of suspected GERD. It can be performed in either of the two ways—a wireless pH—sensitive transmitter is anchored to the esophageal mucosa or a wire electrode is passed transnasally with the tip in the distal esophagus and an ambulatory 24–48 hours esophageal pH recording is done. The outcome is expressed as percentage and a pH value of <4 is indicative of recent acid reflux with values $>5\%$ indicative of GERD. Intraluminal impedance monitoring can be added to pH monitoring to detect reflux irrespective of whether it is acidic or not thereby increasing the sensitivity of the study.[12]

Endoscopic Ultrasound

Endoscopic ultrasound combines an endoscope with an ultrasound transducer to create a transmural image of the tissue surrounding the endoscope tip. Its most important advantage is greater resolution attributable to the proximity of the ultrasound transducer to the tissue being examined. There are two types of endoscopic probes-side viewing for imaging and at the tip for interventional purposes. The main esophageal application of EUS is in the staging of esophageal cancer, in the evaluation of dysplasia in BE, and in the assessment of submucosal tumors.

Cross-sectional Imaging Studies

Imaging of the esophagus is challenging because the esophagus is a long tube, and poorly distensible, with a close relationship to many vital organs.[13]

Pharynx

Although the mucosal detail of the pharynx is studied best with barium contrast, the extraluminal anatomy is demonstrated in detail by CT, MRI, and sonography. Cross-sectional investigations are therefore most useful as an adjunct to barium studies, particularly for tumor staging and the delineation of central and peripheral nervous system lesions producing pharyngeal dysfunction.

Esophagus

Although there is no absolute size of normal wall thickness, some authors define that the thickness should not exceed 3 mm in a well-distended esophagus. Also, an eccentric thickening of the wall is suggestive of an underlying pathology.[7] With increasing age, the esophageal caliber may increase, an anteroposterior (AP) diameter >10 mm and a transverse diameter >24 mm are considered abnormal. Air may be seen in the esophagus in around 65% of normal population. However, an air-fluid level, fluid-filled lumen or a lumen caliber >10 mm usually indicate obstruction or severe dysmotility.

Proper distention of the esophagus and stomach (by oral administration of effervescent granules and water) and optimally timed administration of intravenous contrast material are required to detect and characterize disease. Preoperative staging of esophageal carcinoma appears to be the main indication for multidetector computed tomography (MDCT). CT provides considerable information on the intramural and extramural extent of esophageal malignancy and is also an indispensable part of the planning for radiation therapy. CT and MRI have been used to stage esophageal carcinoma, because these techniques can reveal extraesophageal extension into adjacent mediastinal structures, including the trachea, bronchi, aorta, and pericardium, and can detect lymphadenopathy in the mediastinum. For assessing unresectability, CT and MRI have comparable accuracy when using criteria such as tracheobronchial invasion and aortic invasion. However, CT appears more sensitive for detecting lymphadenopathy, particularly in the mediastinum.[14]

Though MRI is not routinely performed for esophageal pathology, the normal esophagus is well visualized in its entire length except the mid-part which may be difficult to visualize as it is flattened behind the left atrium. On T1-weighted (T1W) images, the normal esophagus appears as a low signal intensity (SI) structure contrasted by high SI of periesophageal fat. On T2-weighted (T2W) images, it appears as low SI in contrast to high SI of internal contents. On postcontrast MRI, the muscle layer of the esophagus shows moderate enhancement. Use of phase array surface coils can provide high-resolution MR images of individual layers of the esophageal wall. On high-resolution T2W images the esophagus is seen as intermediate SI mucosa surrounded by high SI submucosa and low SI muscularis propria.[15]

FUNCTIONAL OROPHARYNGEAL ABNORMALITIES

Functional neuromuscular disorders (enlisted in **Table 2B**) can lead to the following pathophysiologic conditions with oropharyngeal dysphagia.

Laryngeal Penetration

During fluoroscopy, when the contrast material enters the laryngeal vestibule but does not pass below the level of the glottis through the true vocal cords, it is indicative of laryngeal vestibular penetration. In healthy people, spontaneous clearing of the contrast occurs from the laryngeal vestibule which is known as transient penetration or high penetration. It can arise from poor oral control of the bolus or from delayed initiation of the pharyngeal swallow.[4]

Aspiration

The term aspiration is used to describe the passage of foreign material including food and liquid through the true vocal cords into the trachea. Prevention of aspiration requires superior and anterior elevation of the larynx, closure of larynx, and epiglottic tilt. These mechanisms can be evaluated at videofluoroscopy.[4] Aspiration can occur before, during, or after swallowing and is the most threatening symptom of oropharyngeal dysphagia.

Once aspiration has occurred, the immediate expected reflex is a cough due to excitation of recurrent laryngeal nerve receptors. In patients with dysphagia who present with aspiration, the cough response may be immediate, delayed, or absent. The cough may also not be effective in throwing out material back into the hypopharynx. The severity of aspiration is determined subjectively by:

- The amount of material aspirated, i.e., minimal, moderate, or severe
- Quantification of the depth of aspiration
- Response in terms of coughing

The standard measure of severity of aspiration is the "8-point penetration aspiration scale" which includes both the depth of airway invasion (above or below the true vocal cords) and whether the material is ejected back into the hypopharynx or not. Silent aspiration is represented by a score of 8 in which material is aspirated below the true vocal cords without any overt clinical signs.

Post-swallow Residue in the Pharynx

Following a swallow, the bolus may collect and remain in the valleculae and pyriform sinuses. This may be due to weak propulsion of bolus or inadequate opening of the UES. The residue in the pharynx may lead to secondary post-swallow aspiration.

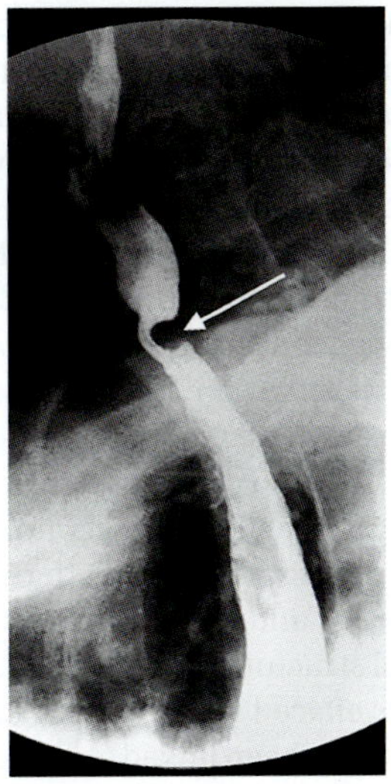

FIG. 4: Prominence of the cricopharyngeus muscle seen as posterior indentation (arrow) on barium swallow study with mild proximal dilatation.

Cricopharyngeal Bar or Prominent Cricopharyngeus Muscle

The posterior indentation at approximately C5–C6 level by cricopharyngeus muscle normally effaces as a bolus passes through. Mild persistent indentation may be normal but more obvious prominence may be seen in patients with gastroesophageal reflux or functional or mechanical esophageal obstruction. It is postulated that acid reflux leads to edema, spasm, and/or hypertrophy of cricopharyngeus. On a contrast study on the lateral view, it is seen as a smooth posterior bar-like or band-like protrusion into the lumen of the barium column at the junction of the hypopharynx and cervical (C5–C6 level) esophagus **(Fig. 4)**. It may mimic a web, but webs are seen along the anterior wall.[16] Cricopharyngeal bar may be seen in 5–10% of patients who are asymptomatic.

Extrinsic pharyngeal indentation caused by a cervical osteophyte may simulate cricopharyngeal prominence. Osteophytic impressions are fixed in position in relation to the spine, whereas cricopharyngeal indentations move with the pharynx and esophagus during swallowing.

STRUCTURAL OROPHARYNGEAL ABNORMALITIES

Postcricoid Webs

Webs are thin mucosal folds that are located in the anterior wall of the lower hypopharynx and proximal few centimeters of the esophagus. They typically present with dysphagia to solids but deglutitive aspiration may occur due to their proximal location. They have been reported to be twice as common in women than men and more easily appreciated on barium swallow than on endoscopy[9] wherein they are seen as eccentric but occasionally circumferential 1–2 mm wide shelf-like filling defect **(Figs. 5A and B)**. Characteristic "jet effect" may be seen on contrast swallow when a large bolus passes through a web. Jet phenomenon is usually seen in case of partial obstruction.[16] They arise on the anterior wall and never on the posterior wall and are best seen on the lateral projection. As rapid peristalsis allows cervical webs to be visualized only for fraction of a second, cineradiography is required to demonstrate them. Differentiation must be made between webs and the submucosal venous plexus which is a normal structure on anterior wall and causes an impression that is effaced as the bolus distends the lumen.

Cervical webs have been linked to underlying conditions such as GERD, epidermolysis bullosa and possibly associated with iron-deficiency anemia (Plummer-Vinson syndrome).

Pharyngeal Diverticula and Pouches

Several types of diverticula may be seen on oropharyngeal and upper GI barium studies such as pharyngeal diverticula and pouches, Zenker's diverticulum and Killian-Jamieson diverticulum. Zenker's diverticulum has been found to be the most common of them and frequently implicated in pharyngeal dysphagia. This develops secondary to fibrosis and loss of compliance of the cricopharyngeus muscle.[9] It occurs as a result of increase in intraluminal pressure associated with distal obstruction in the form of a stenotic cricopharyngeus muscle (UES). Zenker's diverticulum is a false-diverticula which involves herniation of the mucosa and submucosa through the muscular layer of esophagus. It is a pouch that develops as an area of anatomic weakness in the posterior hypopharyngeal wall between the horizontal and oblique fibers of the cricopharyngeus muscle.

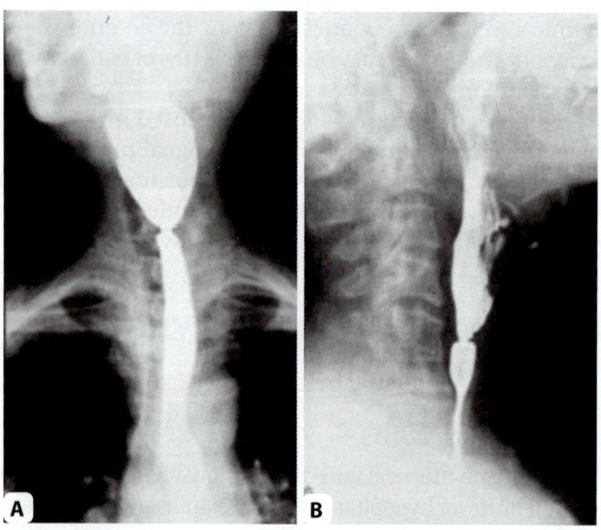

FIGS. 5A AND B: Barium swallow shows well-defined localized circumferential narrowing seen at the level of C5–C6 with minimal proximal dilatation—cricopharyngeal web.

On the lateral view it is seen as a bulge or true sac extending posteriorly from the posterior hypopharyngeal wall just above the cricopharyngeal impression. On the frontal view a Zenker's diverticulum is seen as a barium-filled sac below the arcuate lines of the pyriform sinuses. This area is known as the triangle of Killian or Killian dehiscence. The mouth of the Zenker's diverticulum is present immediately above the cricopharyngeal muscle. Imaging in three projections is required for confirmation and assessment of the severity of a Zenker's diverticulum, i.e., AP, lateral, and oblique. In contrast, the Killian-Jamieson diverticula originate below the cricopharyngeus muscle.

Small Zenker's diverticula are usually asymptomatic. Dysphagia occurs as the diverticulum fills preferentially with food and obstructs the lumen of the esophagus. There is regurgitation of pouch contents and often, aspiration as its overflows. Recurrent chest infections are hence common.

The treatment of choice for Zenker's diverticulum is cricopharyngeal myotomy, either alone or in combination with pouch resection. In the elderly with significant comorbidity, cricopharyngeal dilatation can provide symptomatic relief and can be performed as an alternative treatment.

Oropharyngeal Tumors and Their Surgery

Tumors of the head and neck such as those arising from the tongue, palate, pharynx, tonsil, and glottis may present with dysphagia. The surgical resection of these cancers can cause complications such as anastomotic leak, vascular injury, and cranial nerve damage which can result in dysphagia. The effect of head and neck cancer surgery on swallowing can vary markedly from person to person and depends on many factors such as the extent of surgical resection, whether flap reconstruction is required, the nature of component structures removed, i.e., cartilaginous, muscular, or bony or whether surgery has resulted in damage to neural innervations.

In those undergoing surgery for oral cancer, the extent of tongue resection is the most important factor which determines the severity of dysphagia. This is because tongue-base motion is very important in generating pharyngeal propulsive forces. Also, following laryngeal surgery, the degree of preservation of tongue base motion is an important prediction of recovery of swallow function.[9]

The majority of malignant pharyngeal tumors are squamous cell carcinomas (SCCs). They metastasize to cervical nodes which typically appear necrotic. Small tumors may be seen as a nodular mucosal surface en face or as an irregular contour. Radiographic findings in large, advanced tumors include intraluminal mass, mucosal irregularity and asymmetric distensibility. An intraluminal mass may be seen as an abnormal luminal contour, abnormally located extra-barium-coated lines, a focal area of increased radiodensity, or a filling defect in the barium pool. Mucosal irregularity is recognized by abnormal barium collections due to ulceration or by a nonuniform nodular surface pattern. Asymmetric distensibility may be due to an infiltrating tumor or extrinsic mass **(Figs. 6A and B)**. The value of double-contrast pharyngography in patients with a known carcinoma is to determine the size, extent, and inferior limit of the pharyngeal tumor and the degree of functional impairment. Pharyngoesophagograms are also useful for detecting separate coexisting carcinomas of the pharynx and esophagus. Extraluminal extent of the tumor (e.g., invasion of the preepiglottic space or cartilage destruction) and lymphadenopathy are best assessed by CT and MRI **(Figs. 7A to C)**.

Radiation-induced Esophagitis

Esophageal damage can occur secondary to high-dose external beam radiotherapy used for treatment of malignant tumors of the lung, esophagus or mediastinum. Severe esophagitis with irreversible damage is known to occur following a radiation dose of 45–60 Gy. A milder form of self-limiting esophagitis without permanent sequelae can be caused by small doses of radiation in the range of 20–45 Gy. Acute radiation esophagitis usually occurs 2–4 weeks after completing radiotherapy and is self-limiting, seen as granular appearance of mucosa with ulceration and reduced distensibility. In contrast, chronic esophagitis presents at 4–8 months after completion of radiotherapy as radiation strictures, appearing as long segments of concentric and smooth narrowing of the esophagus.[16]

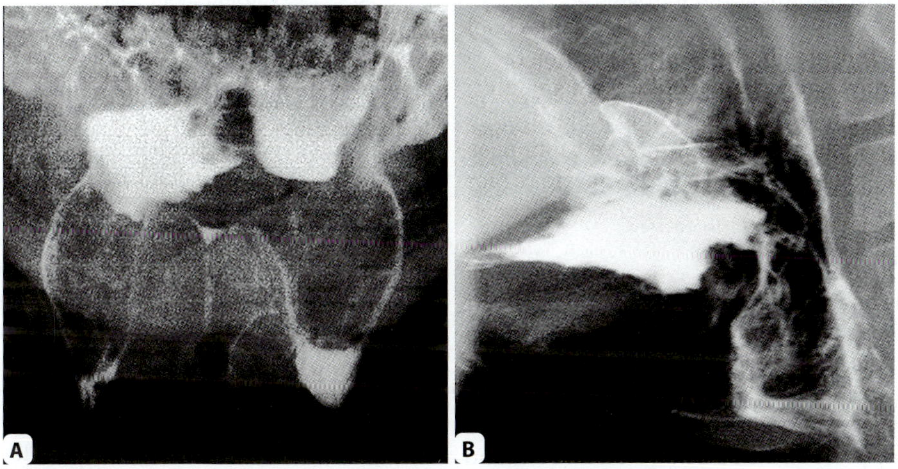

FIGS. 6A AND B: Contrast swallow: (A) Frontal; and (B) Lateral spot views of the hypopharynx showing expansion and mucosal irregularity of the right vallecula by a malignant mass. The left vallecula and pyriform sinuses appear normal—malignant right vallecular mass [squamous cell carcinoma (SCC)].

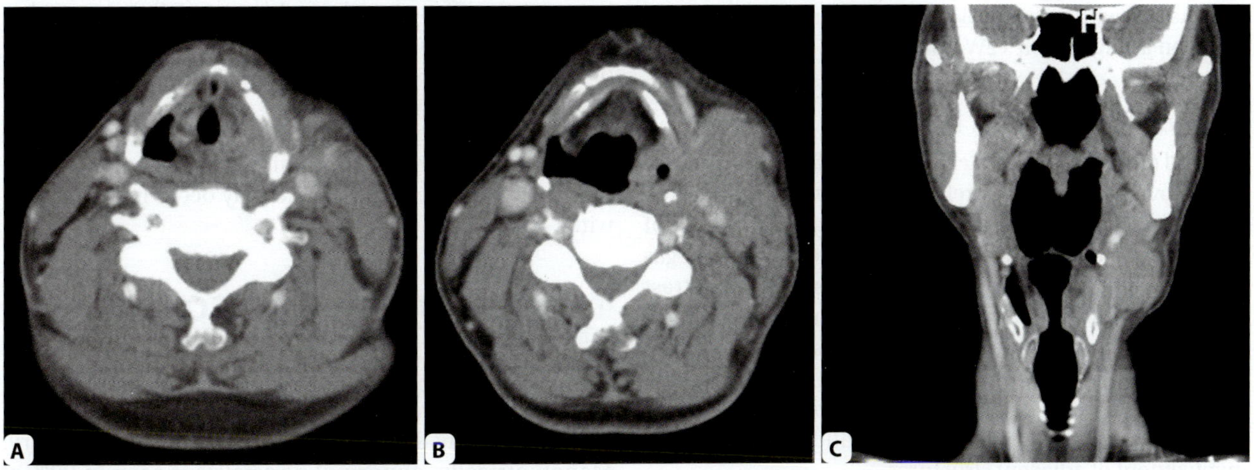

FIGS. 7A TO C: Contrast-enhanced axial (A and B) and coronal (C) CT scan of the neck reveals a heterogeneously enhancing soft-tissue mass in the left pyriform sinus causing thickening of the left aryepiglottic fold with enlarged level II cervical lymph nodes—carcinoma left pyriform sinus.

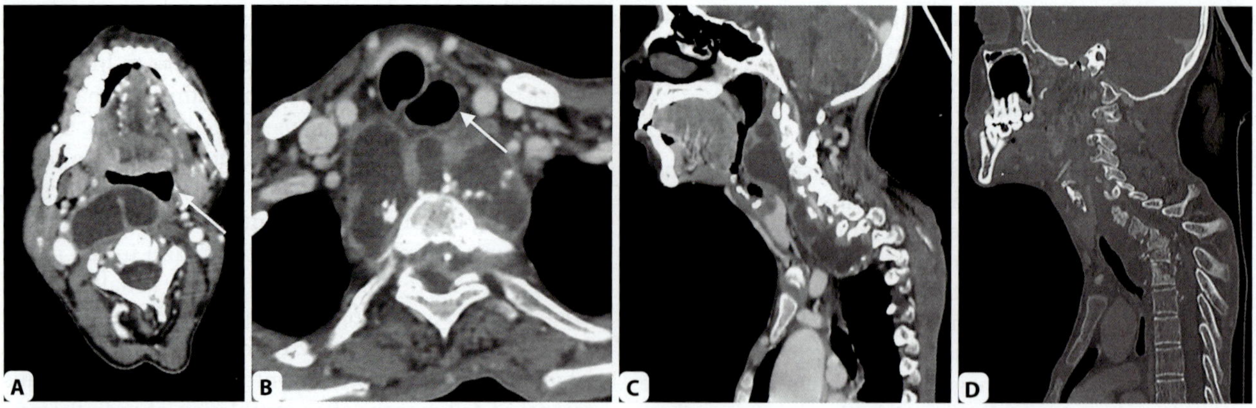

FIGS. 8A TO D: Contrast-enhanced computed tomography (CECT) neck reveals multiloculated peripherally enhancing intercommunicating collection in pre- and paravertebral locations extending from C1 to D4 levels with multiple calcific foci within. The lesion is causing attenuation and mass effect on oropharyngeal airway and esophagus (arrows in A and B). Sagittal sections in soft tissue and bone window (C and D) reveal the complete extent of the abscess with D2 vertebral body collapse and multiple vertebral involvement: Tubercular spondylodiscitis with large pre- and paravertebral abscesses causing dysphagia.

It is important to take a history of radiotherapy for an oral or neck surgery in the past as radiation-induced dysphagia is known to manifest clinically > 10 years post-treatment.[9]

Retropharyngeal Abscess

Retropharyngeal abscess may occur secondary to tonsillar infection, suppurative lymphadenopathy, spread of tubercular infection from the prevertebral space to the retropharyngeal space or from perforating injury of the pharynx or esophagus. It is more often seen in small children who may present with fever, neck stiffness, and dysphagia. On lateral plain radiograph of the neck, findings are an increase in the retropharyngeal space, reversal of cervical lordosis and anterior displacement of the airway. The abscess may contain air and an air-fluid level may be seen. On CT, the abscess appears as an area of low attenuation with peripheral rim enhancement and on MR it is seen as high-SI on T2W images **(Figs. 8A to D)**.

Pharyngeal Foreign Bodies

A lateral radiograph of the neck taken at soft-tissue exposure may show a radiopaque foreign body, but many impacted fish or chicken bones are poorly opaque. Evidence of perforation should be sought, including extraluminal gas and widening of the prevertebral soft tissues. A contrast swallow is performed with a small volume of low-density barium, or water-soluble nonionic contrast if perforation is suspected. CT is an excellent investigation in localizing and identifying a foreign body, detecting complications such as perforation, collection or abscess formation, and depicting involvement of adjacent structures.

ESOPHAGEAL MOTILITY DISORDERS

These disorders are those which are attributable to esophageal neuromuscular function and are commonly associated with dysphagia, chest pain, or heart burn. The dysphagia is slowly progressive and occurs to both liquid and solid foods. The esophageal motility can be easily assessed at fluoroscopy with the patient in the prone RAO position. Two to five individual swallows should be observed at fluoroscopy as the bolus passes. It is important to remember that in patients suspected of having an esophageal motility disorder, individual swallow should be evaluated, as a second or double swallow would interfere with primary peristalsis and limit evaluation of esophageal motility.

Motility disorders can be categorized into primary or secondary types. The esophagus is the main organ involved in primary motility disorder and includes achalasia and its variants, diffuse esophageal spasm (DES), nutcracker esophagus. Secondary esophageal motility disorder occurs due to systemic diseases such as scleroderma or secondary to injury to esophagus.[16]

Specific motility disorders consist of DES, achalasia, and scleroderma. However, the motility disorders may not fall into any of these categories and may occur in association with GERD.

PRIMARY MOTILITY DISORDER

Nonspecific Esophageal Motility Disorder

Motility abnormalities that do not meet the criteria of specific motility disorders fall into this broad category. Manometrically, abnormal peristalsis is seen in 20% of

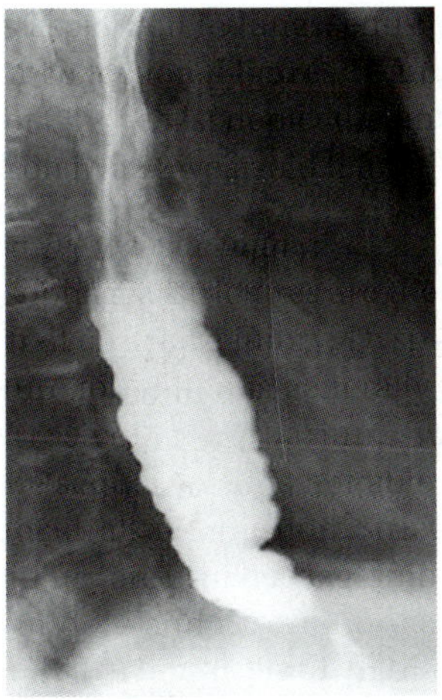

FIG. 9: Nonspecific esophageal motility disorder.

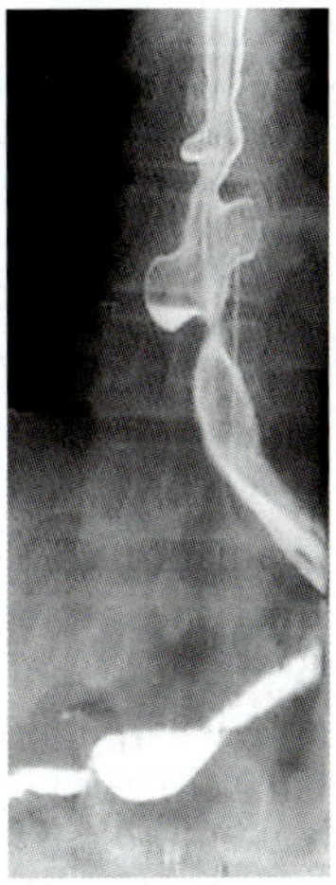

FIG. 10: "Corkscrew" esophagus—nonpropulsive segmental contractions producing multiple areas of pronounced luminal narrowing with areas of sacculation.

such cases. Peristalsis may be intermittently absent or of low amplitude. LES dysfunction (incomplete relaxation) and frequent spontaneous or repetitive contractions are also detected. Radiologically, a nonspecific disturbance of primary peristalsis and tertiary contractions are seen in 40–50% of cases **(Fig. 9)**.

Diffuse Esophageal Spasm

Clinical Presentation

Diffuse esophageal spasm is manifested by episodes of dysphagia and chest pain occurring due to abnormal esophageal contractions with normal LES relaxation on deglutition. Esophageal chest pain may closely mimic pain of angina. Features which suggest a pain of esophageal origin are it being unrelated to exertion, pain of prolonged duration which interrupts sleep, its relation to meals, relief with antacids and being accompanied by heartburn, dysphagia or regurgitation. All these presenting features also show overlap with cardiac pain. Both chest pain and dysphagia are also characteristic of peptic or infectious esophagitis. Hence, only after the most common entities mentioned above are excluded, that a diagnosis of DES should be considered.[12]

Imaging Features

Diffuse esophageal spasm is characterized by the absence of primary peristalsis with simultaneous, spontaneous, repetitive, and nonperistaltic uncoordinated esophageal contractions on manometry. The LES usually functions normally, although high-resting pressures and incomplete relaxation may occur. It occurs in patients over 50 years of age and may be intermittent and noted mostly in the distal two-thirds of esophagus. Radiographically, there is loss of primary peristalsis in the distal esophagus. Nonperistaltic tertiary contractions are usually repetitive and simultaneous and may produce a classic "corkscrew" or "rosary bead" appearance on barium swallows **(Fig. 10)**. The findings are similar to those seen in nonspecific esophageal motility disorder. The clinical picture helps to distinguish the two conditions, because DES is associated with chest pain. The esophagus is not usually dilated and the LES functions normally.

The radiological appearance of DES is also known as pseudodiverticula or curling phenomena which can also be found with spastic achalasia.

Treatment

Various trials/treatment options for DES have been reported such as use of nitrates, calcium-channel blockers, anxiolytics, with varying response. Surgery in the form of long myotomy or esophagectomy is generally not done.

Achalasia

Achalasia is an uncommon motility disorder of the esophagus characterized by a loss of primary esophageal peristalsis, incomplete relaxation of the LES in response to deglutition, increased resting LES pressure, and increased intraesophageal pressure on manometry.

All these lead to esophageal dilatation or megaesophagus. Of all the conditions associated with esophageal dilatation like achalasia, inflammatory narrowing, progressive systemic sclerosis (PSS) and carcinoma; achalasia causes the most severe generalized dilatation.[17]

Clinical Presentation

Achalasia can be present at any age but is most common in the 30–50 years age group. Dysphagia is usually worse with liquids than with solids, may initially be intermittent and eventually is persistent. It is diagnosed manometrically as esophageal aperistalsis and LES dysfunction, primary incomplete relaxation, and elevated resting pressure. Esophageal dilatation is mild in the early stages, which may make radiographic diagnosis difficult.

Although the pathogenesis of achalasia is not known, the most accepted theory is related to the paucity or absence of ganglion cells in the Auerbach's plexus in the distal esophageal wall.

Imaging Features

Plain chest radiographs are frequently sufficient for the diagnosis of achalasia. The esophagus is dilated with large amounts of retained food and fluid which may become markedly tortuous and present as a widened mediastinum mainly on the right side, adjacent to the cardiac shadow, often with an air-fluid level. Aspiration of the retained food from the dilated esophagus frequently leads to episodes of pneumonia. On an erect radiograph, air bubble of the gastric fundus is small or absent **(Figs. 11A and B)**.

Barium swallow with the patient erect demonstrates a variable degree of dilatation of the esophagus above a beak-like narrowing at the LES **(Figs. 12A and B)**. The sphincter opens intermittently under the force of the hydrostatic pressure of the barium column above it to allow bolus passage. A gradual, tapered, smooth, and conical narrowing of the distal esophageal segment extending for 1–3 cm in length is known as "bird's beak appearance" and is the hallmark of achalasia. With the patient in erect position, sequential radiography can show small spurts of barium entering the stomach through the narrowed distal segment. The distal two-thirds of the esophagus, which contains smooth muscle is aperistaltic. Secondary to stasis esophagitis is common. Esophageal carcinoma may develop which may be seen in 2–7% of patients with long-standing achalasia. The carcinoma may develop in the mid-esophagus secondary to stasis and irritation of esophagus. Whenever there is a worsening of symptoms in patients of achalasia, possibility of superimposed esophageal carcinoma is to be ruled out.[14]

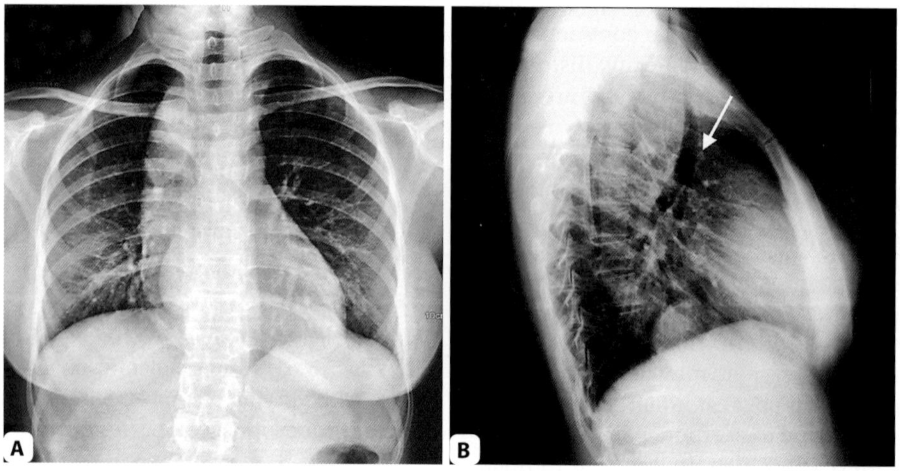

FIGS. 11A AND B: Chest posteroanterior (PA) erect (A) in a 21-year-old female with achalasia reveals a mediastinal shadow extending from the neck to the diaphragm on the right side due to markedly dilated esophagus. There is absence of air in the fundus of the stomach. Chest lateral (B) shows anterior displacement of the trachea (arrow) by the dilated esophagus.

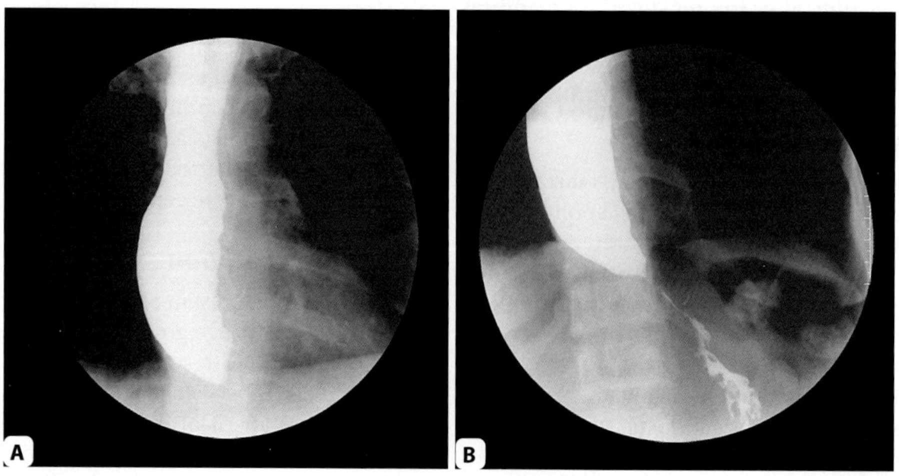

FIGS. 12A AND B: Barium swallow depicts: (A) A moderately dilated esophagus, (B) with a smooth conical narrowing of the distal esophagus: "Bird beak" appearance-achalasia.

It is essential that the patient with achalasia is examined in the recumbent position because in the erect position, gravity can simulate the effect of peristalsis and hide subtle abnormalities. Evaluation in the upright position is also necessary for the barium column to provide adequate hydrostatic pressure to force even small amounts of contrast into the stomach. In patients of achalasia, complete emptying of the esophagus does not occur even in the erect position. This is an important point to remember to differentiate from scleroderma radiologically, where emptying is usually normal in the erect position.[18]

Achalasia is diagnosed on barium swallow studies or esophageal manometry while the role of endoscopy is only in ruling out pseudoachalasia. Manometry is the most sensitive test in diagnosing achalasia as it identifies early disease before esophageal dilatation and food retention **(Fig. 13)**.[12] HRM identifies three subtypes of achalasia on the basis of pattern of pressurization in the aperistaltic esophagus: (1) Classic achalasia, (2) achalasia with compression, and (3) spastic achalasia. All are characterized by impaired relaxation of the LES with absent peristalsis.

CT features of achalasia have been described by Rabuschka and colleagues[19] which consist of a moderate dilatation of the esophagus with a mean diameter of 4.5 cm at the carinal level, but having a normal wall thickness. They found a normal wall thickness to be the most important feature that differentiates patients of achalasia from other esophageal diseases **(Figs. 14A to C)**. CT is routinely not

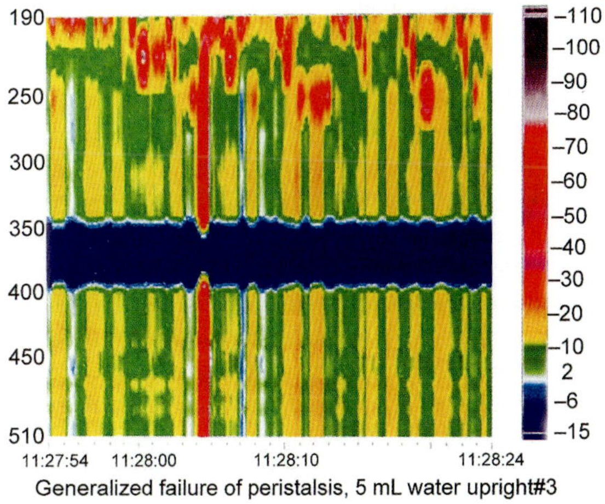

FIG. 13: Esophageal manometry in the patient with achalasia reveals absent esophageal peristalsis with incomplete relaxation of lower esophageal sphincter (LES) with high basal pressure.

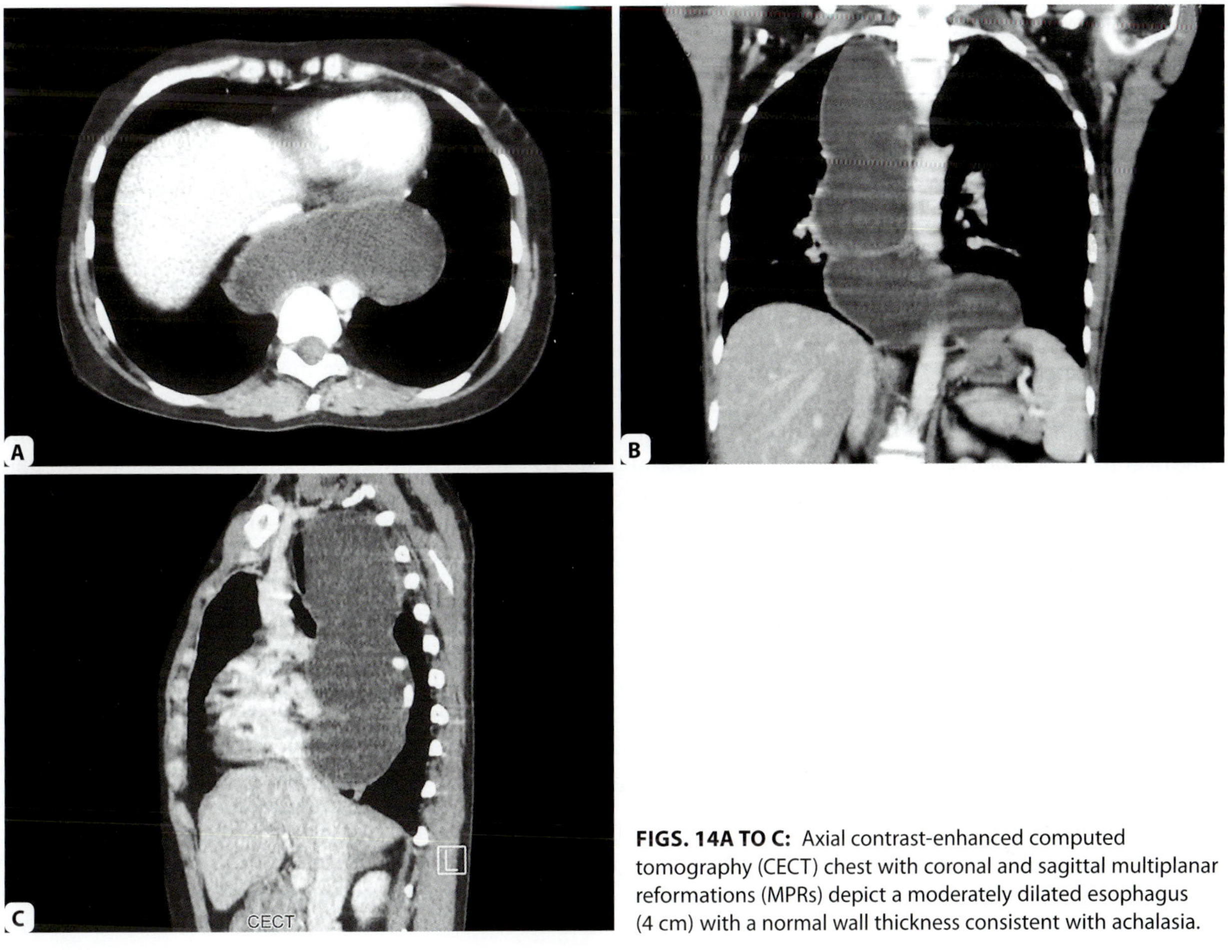

FIGS. 14A TO C: Axial contrast-enhanced computed tomography (CECT) chest with coronal and sagittal multiplanar reformations (MPRs) depict a moderately dilated esophagus (4 cm) with a normal wall thickness consistent with achalasia.

indicated for the diagnosis of achalasia, but may be useful in confirming the diagnosis and detecting its complications. It may also suggest the presence of other diseases or superimposed benign or malignant processes.[17] The other causes of narrowing of the LES that may mimic achalasia are intrinsic or extrinsic neoplasm, peptic stricture, and complications of scleroderma.

Secondary achalasia refers to carcinoma of the gastric cardia or metastases involving the GEJ resulting in a radiographic picture simulating achalasia. It is related to destruction of the intramural myenteric plexus. Secondary achalasia should be considered in older patients if symptoms are acute or if the tapered GEJ shows mucosal nodularity or mass effect. In contrast, primary achalasia is seen in younger patients with long-standing dysphagia showing smooth narrowing of distal esophagus on contrast study. The length of the narrowed segment is >3.5 cm in secondary achalasia compared to a shorter narrow segment in primary achalasia.[16] Repeating the esophagogram after patient inhales amylnitrate may help to distinguish this entity from achalasia. This smooth muscle relaxant relaxes the LES in achalasia while in secondary achalasia the LES remains rigid and unchanged.

Treatment

Achalasia cannot be prevented or reversed. Therapy is directed at reducing LES pressure, so that gravity and esophageal pressurization promote esophageal emptying. Peristalsis is rarely known to return. LES pressure can be reduced by pharmacological therapy, forceful dilatation, or surgical myotomy. Pharmacological therapy in the form of nitrates or calcium-channel blockers are used as temporary therapies and are administered before eating. Botulinum toxin injected under endoscopic guidance into the LES inhibits acetylcholine release from the nerve endings and is known to improve dysphagia in about 66% of cases for at least 6 months.[12]

The most reliable therapies for achalasia are pneumatic dilatation and Heller's myotomy. Pneumatic dilatation is an endoscopic technique which uses a noncompliant, cylindrical balloon dilator positioned across the LES and inflated to a diameter of 3–4 cm. The reported accuracy of this technique ranges from 32 to 98%. Esophageal perforation is the major complication which can occur rarely. Heller's myotomy is the most effective surgical procedure for achalasia. It is performed laparoscopically, usually in conjunction with partial Nissen's fundoplication, with good to excellent results being reported in 62–100% of cases. The surgery involves incising the circular muscle fibers down to the mucosa and allowing the mucosa to protrude through.

In patients with advanced achalasia who fail to respond to the above surgical measures, esophageal resection with gastric pull up or interposition of a segment of transverse colon may be the only option other than a feeding gastrostomy.

SECONDARY MOTILITY DISORDER

Scleroderma

Scleroderma results from atrophy or degeneration of smooth muscle in the lower half to two-thirds of the esophagus with subsequent replacement of esophageal musculature by fibrosis. Neural elements and ganglion cells are normal. The upper third of the esophagus is composed of striated muscles which are usually not affected by scleroderma. Hence, on a barium swallow, a normal peristaltic wave may be seen in this region. In the distal two-thirds esophageal region as the disease progresses, mild uncoordinated tertiary contractions seen early in scleroderma may disappear. As the LES tone is severely decreased in scleroderma, drinking in the erect position allows the bolus to the propelled down the esophagus by the striated muscles, i.e., pharyngeal constrictors and carried by gravity into the stomach. Due to the incompetent LES, there is reflux of acid secretions into the distal esophagus leading to peptic esophagitis and stricture formation, resulting in heartburn and severe dysphagia. Distal esophageal peristalsis is absent or diminished which contributes to the severity of reflux esophagitis **(Figs. 15A and B)**.

STRUCTURAL ESOPHAGEAL DYSPHAGIA

Esophagitis

Numerous etiologic factors may cause esophagitis. The most common cause is gastroesophageal reflux.

Reflux Esophagitis and Barrett's Esophagus

Reflux esophagitis is the most common inflammatory condition of the esophagus, occurring secondary to GERD.[16] Patients with GERD usually complain of a variety of symp-3toms such as heartburn, regurgitation, substernal pain, and also dysphagia in some cases. Double-contrast barium swallow has shown to have high sensitivity, approaching 90% in diagnosing reflux esophagitis.[16] Early changes of reflux esophagitis may be recognized as a fine mucosal nodularity or granular appearance of the mucosa in the distal third or half of the thoracic esophagus, occurring due to the presence of mucosal edema and inflammation during the early stages of reflux esophagitis. As the disease progresses, double-contrast esophagography may demonstrate shallow ulcers and erosions, thickened longitudinal folds, inflammatory polyps, and scarring. Reflux esophagitis may be recognized also on mucosal relief views as lobulation or nodularity of slightly thickened longitudinal folds. Superficial ulceration occurs with increasing severity, seen as tiny, punctate, linear or irregular collection of barium associated with

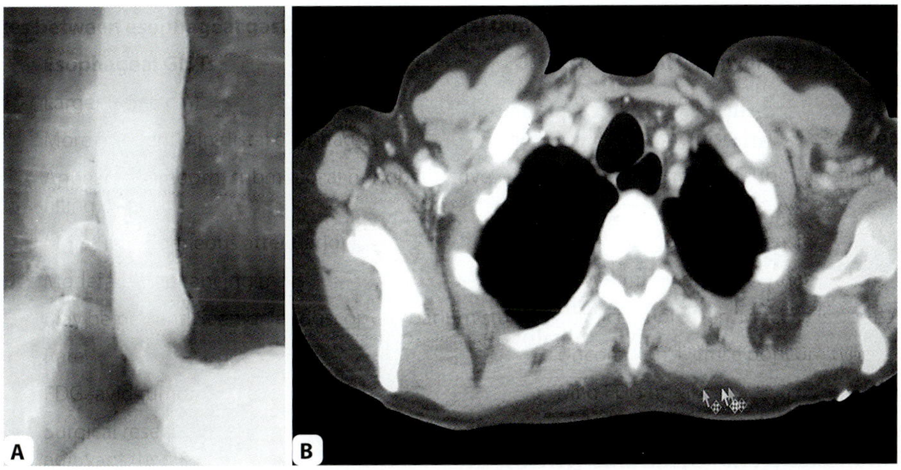

FIGS. 15A AND B: (A) Barium swallow spot film of lower dorsal esophagus showing dilated esophagus with patulous lower esophageal sphincter; (B) CT of chest in the same patient shows dilated esophagus in a patient of scleroderma.

mounds of edema and fold thickening and distortion. The changes of reflux esophagitis involve a continuous area in the distal esophagus extending proximally from the GEJ. Sparing of distal esophagus indicates another cause for the radiographic abnormalities.[19]

A peptic stricture may develop with chronic GERD, which is a smooth, tapered and concentric narrowing in the distal esophagus with associated sliding hiatus hernia. Occasionally, the benign stricture is asymmetric due to scarring. A peptic stricture may mimic a Schatzki's ring in patients with dysphagia wherein it can appear as a ring-like narrowing. Sacculation may form with severe scarring Esophageal dysmotility and dilatation of the esophagus due to atony may also be seen in GERD.

Barrett's esophagus represents acquired progressive columnar metaplasia of the squamous epithelium in the distal esophagus due to reflux esophagitis, i.e., when the normal squamous epithelium within the esophagus changes to columnar epithelium. The length and extent of metaplasia can be short (< 3 cm) or long (> 3 cm) depending on the presence and type of cellular changes in the columnar epithelium, it is referred as BE (no dysplasia present), low-grade dysplasia (LGD), or high-grade dysplasia (HGD). It is a premalignant condition and occurs in about 15% of patients with long-standing GERD.[20,21] Obesity and hiatus hernia are the known risk factors of development of BE, with BE being the single largest risk factor identified for the development of esophageal adenocarcinoma. Most strictures of BE appear as peptic-type distal esophageal stricture. However, a more specific but less common finding is a mid to upper esophageal stricture, often associated with a sliding hiatal hernia or gastroesophageal reflux. Most specific finding in BE is a reticular mucosal pattern which is however seen in only 5–10% of patients. If BE is suspected, patient should be kept under endoscopic surveillance with endoscopic biopsy performed as it carries a 100-fold increased risk of adenocarcinoma.[22]

Schatzki Ring

A lower esophageal ring is common finding on barium swallow in an asymptomatic patient. Schatzki ring is seen in patients presenting with dysphagia. A Schatzki ring is a thin, smooth, and concentric, symmetric mucosal ring-like narrowing of the distal esophagus which marks the junction between the esophageal and gastric mucosa. The ring is constantly present and it does not change its position. However, Schatzki's ring is only seen on contrast swallow studies when the esophagus above and below it is dilated more than the width of the ring. It may be the result of scarring due to GERD. These usually cause dysphagia when < 13 mm in diameter but are usually asymptomatic when > 20 mm in diameter.[18]

The lower esophageal ring has been considered to be a transverse mucosal fold of noninflammatory origin. On barium studies, it needs to be differentiated from a variant of ring-like peptic stricture with which it bears a resemblance. However, the ring-like peptic stricture is more asymmetric with tapered borders and generally longer than (> 4 mm) a Schatzki ring.[23]

Congenital Esophageal Stenosis

It is a rare condition which produces smooth fusiform narrowing of the esophageal lumen with varying degree of obstruction and proximal dilatation. Severe stenosis occurs in newborns and infants and usually requires surgery. However, a milder form of narrowing may go on till adulthood as patients adapt themselves to their eating habits to compensate for the stenosis. Its diagnosis can be made if a long concentric narrowing is seen in a patient with a long history of dysphagia often associated with recurrent food impaction with no other risk factors for developing esophageal stenosis.[18] On barium swallow, the stenotic segment, usually in the mid-esophagus, may show mild narrowing with distinctive ring-like indentations ("ringed esophagus") in the region of the stricture. There are two schools of thought for this appearance. Some believe that the ring-like indentations represent tracheobronchial remnants or cartilaginous rings in the wall of the esophagus. While others believe that it is an acquired condition which occurs secondary to GERD.[23]

INFECTIOUS ESOPHAGITIS

Involvement of the esophagus by infective organisms such as *Candida* species, herpes virus, and cytomegalovirus (CMV) have become relatively common with the increase in use of immunosuppressive drugs for organ transplant as well as chronic inflammatory diseases, chemotherapy, and acquired immunodeficiency syndrome (AIDS). In AIDS patients, infectious esophagitis is common when the CD4 count falls to < 100. CMV esophagitis occurs only in immunocompromised patients, especially transplant patients.

Regardless of the cause of the infectious agents, odynophagia (painful deglutition) is a characteristic symptom of infectious esophagitis with dysphagia, chest pain, and hemorrhage also being common. Odynophagia is uncommon with reflux esophagitis; hence, its presence should always raise the suspicion of an alternative etiology.[12]

On CT scan, esophagitis appears as a long segment, uniform, circumferential esophageal wall thickening, often with a "target sign". The thickening is as a result of edema, infiltration by inflammatory cells, and muscular spasm. The mediastinal fat plane is preserved in esophagitis while esophageal carcinoma usually shows asymmetrical wall thickening with extension into mediastinum.

Candida Esophagitis

Candida albicans is the most common cause of infectious esophagitis. It usually occurs opportunistically in immunocompromised patients. *Candida* is normally present in the throat but can become pathogenic and produce esophagitis in the compromised host and is thought to result from downward spread of the fungus from the oropharynx to the esophagus. *Candida* esophagitis can also result from local esophageal stasis caused by severe esophageal motility disorders such as achalasia and scleroderma. Symptoms range from asymptomatic to severe dysphagia.

Imaging Features

Since it is a mucosal disease, it can be identified on double-contrast barium examination. In the diagnosis of *Candida* esophagitis, double-contrast esophagography shows a sensitivity of about 90%. The findings include discrete, linear, or irregular plaque like filling defects with intervening normal mucosa **(Fig. 16)**. These plaques are oriented longitudinally within the esophagus and may slough off resulting in ulcerations scattered on a background of plaques. In advanced disease, there may be coalescent plaques, which have been likened to a "cobblestone" or "snakeskin" appearance that correspond to the distinctive white plaques seen at endoscopy. Patients with AIDS may get a severe form of this disease, resulting in a grossly irregular or shaggy appearance secondary to extensive plaques and pseudomembranes that trap barium between them.

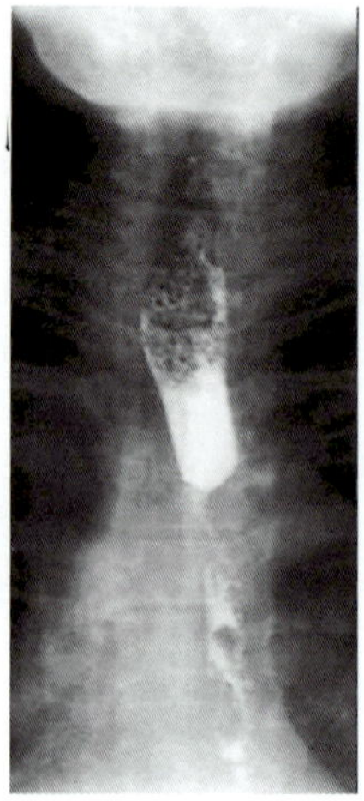

FIG. 16: *Candida esophagitis*: Esophagogram shows a shaggy contour with irregular plaque-like filling defects, seen above a stricture.

"Foamy" esophagus can be seen on double-contrast barium swallow study in the immunocompromised and in 25% of patients of esophageal stasis such as scleroderma and achalasia. It is characterized by the presence of multiple tiny, smooth, round lucencies (bubbles) of around 1–3 mm size that are intermingled with the barium suspension along the top of the barium column on upright views producing a layer of foam. The layer of foam may have a length ranging from 3 to 16 cm in the barium column. The pathophysiologic basis of the "foamy esophagus" is uncertain, but has been postulated to be produced directly by the fungal organisms that colonize the esophagus. These round lucencies in the foamy esophagus are bubbles, hence mobile and are usually distinguished radiographically from retained food or debris in the esophagus or diffuse nodularity of the esophageal mucosa. Undissolved effervescent granules used in a double-contrast swallow may mimic the round lucencies seen in *Candida* esophagitis and hence should not be used in the initial swallows when candidal involvement is suspected.[24]

The CT findings of *Candida* esophagitis, though nonspecific and commonly seen in various kinds of esophagitis, are circumferential esophageal wall thickening of > 5 mm, with relatively long segmental involvement. Enhanced scans may also depict the target sign (circumferential wall thickening and enhancing internal mucosa).[25]

Viral Esophagitis

Herpes esophagitis occurs as opportunistic infection in immunocompromised patients. On double-contrast barium swallow it appears usually as multiple discrete superficial ulcers separated by normal mucosa. The ulcers may be punctate, linear or stellate and are surrounded by radiolucent halos due to edema. In the appropriate clinical setting, the presence of small, discrete ulcers without plaques should be highly suggestive of herpes esophagitis, because ulceration in candidiasis almost always occurs against a background of diffuse plaque formation. When CMV and HIV infect the esophagus, large, and shallow ulcers up to several centimeters in size are seen in the mid- and sometimes the distal esophagus. The ulcer is usually solitary, ovoid in shape and longitudinal in orientation with smooth margins and often surrounded by a thin radiolucent rim of edematous mucosa. Since the treatment of CMV and HIV esophagitis differs widely, endoscopy with biopsies and cultures is required to differentiate the two infections.[20]

Tuberculosis

Tuberculous involvement of the esophagus is rare. When present, it is usually secondary to current or previous tuberculous infection in other sites. The esophagus may become infected as a result of direct extension from adjacent mediastinal or hilar lymph nodes, vertebral bodies, aortic aneurysms, tuberculous pharyngitis or laryngitis, or by inoculation of swallowed sputum, hematogenous, or lymphatic spread.[26]

Tuberculous lesions can occur in any segment of the esophagus. However, they are most common in the middle third, just proximal to the tracheal bifurcation, because of its proximity to the mediastinal lymph nodes around the bifurcation of the trachea.[27] The changes in the esophagus may result from pressure, adhesions, or actual involvement of mucosal surface.[26] The most common feature is extrinsic compression of the esophagus, usually by a mass of lymph nodes **(Fig. 17)**. Although the esophageal mucosa is often intact in such cases, the adventitia is usually implicated and this may produce classical traction diverticulum. A traction diverticulum is a true diverticulum seen in mid-esophagus usually caused by scarring in perihilar lymph nodes. On barium swallow, it has a triangular and tented appearance and shows emptying with collapse of esophagus. In contrast, a pulsion diverticulum is a false diverticulum which lacks a muscular layer. It occurs in lower esophagus and is usually associated with motility disorder. On barium swallow, they appear as broad-based contrast-filled outpouchings with retention of barium after emptying of esophagus.[16] When the disease process involves the esophageal mucosa, a tumorous lesion or an ulcer may result. Sinus or fistula as a result of rupture of caseous lymph nodes may also occur. Tracheoesophageal or bronchoesophageal fistula and subsequent aspiration pneumonia or lung abscess may occur. A constricting lesion or kinking of the esophagus may be seen as a result of fibrosis.[27]

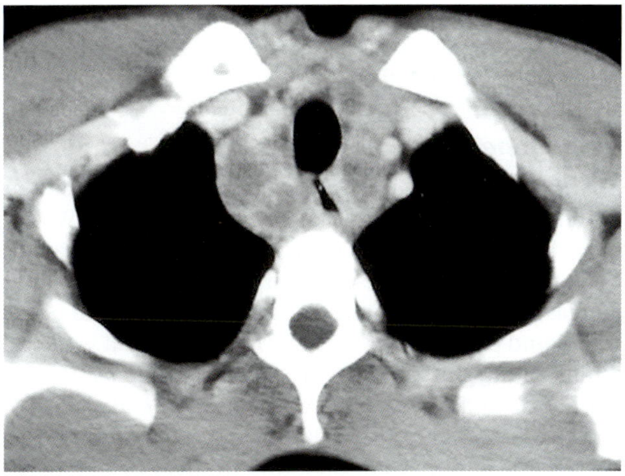

FIG. 17: Contrast-enhanced computed tomography (CECT) of chest mediastinal window showing multiple variable sized rim enhancing necrotic mediastinal lymph nodes in bilateral paratracheal regions causing extrinsic compression of the esophagus—tuberculosis.

Computed tomography of the chest enables complete evaluation of the caseous mediastinal lymph nodes which surround and displace the esophagus and also depicts any fistulous tract extending from the esophagus to the nodal mass. The presence of amorphous gas in enlarged mediastinal lymph nodes in patients with tubercular lymphadenitis is suggestive of an esophageal nodal fistula.[12]

INFLAMMATORY ESOPHAGITIS

Corrosive/Caustic Esophagitis

Corrosive ingestion can cause severe injury to the esophagus and stomach. The severity and extent of damage depends on the type, concentration, volume, physical form (solid or liquid) of the agent, and duration of contact with the mucosa. Ingestion is usually accidental in children < 5 years of age and intentional in adults. The most common cause is ingestion of a strong alkali (sodium or potassium hydroxide) present in drain cleaners, disk batteries, etc. The term "lye" refers to substances which contain sodium or potassium hydroxide. Highly concentrated acids such as hydrochloric and sulfuric acid are contained in toilet cleaners, anti-rust compounds. Button batteries are highly concentrated alkaline solution which when lodged in the esophagus can cause burns within 4 hours and perforation within 6 hours.

The conventional school of thought is that acids preferentially damage the stomach as they are somewhat neutralized by the alkaline pH of the esophagus and alkalis injure the esophagus and spare the stomach. But extensive esophageal damage and perforation have been known to occur after acid ingestion.

Pathogenesis

Alkali ingestion results in a penetrating injury called liquefactive necrosis due to its viscous nature which spreads rapidly within seconds through the mucosa and wall of the esophagus resulting in esophageal perforation, mediastinitis, and even death. This is most likely to occur with liquid preparations that coat larger mucosal surfaces. While solid lye preparation or alkaline batteries induce a more localized injury to the esophagus. The liquefactive necrosis usually lasts for 3–4 days with vascular thrombosis, mucosal inflammation, resulting in focal or extensive sloughing or ulceration. The esophageal wall becomes thinner in the next few weeks because of sloughing and development of granulation tissue and fibrosis. It takes 1–3 months for re-epithelialization to complete. The likelihood of a stricture to develop depends on the depth of damage and the degree of collagen deposition.

Acid-induced injury produces a superficial coagulation necrosis that forms a protective layer over the mucosa, thereby preventing further penetration of acid limiting the depth of injury. Acid ingestion has a tendency to cause pylorospasm with resultant stasis and prolonged contact of the inciting agent in the prepyloric region, leading to a stricture formation in the antropyloric region.[28] Being less viscous than alkaline solutions, they tend to pass quickly into the stomach. Patients of corrosive ingestion may complain of oropharyngeal, retrosternal, or epigastric pain, and odynophagia or dysphagia. Severe and persistent retrosternal or back pain may be indicative of esophageal perforation with mediastinitis.

Management of patients of corrosive ingestion requires a multidisciplinary approach with imaging having a role both in acute and chronic setting.

Diagnosis and Staging

Based on the history of corrosive intake and clinical examination findings, radiological investigations have a role in assessing the severity of injury, thereby guiding in further management. Plain radiographs of the chest and abdomen performed in the emergency may reveal pleural effusion, pneumomediastinum, pneumothorax or nodules, and consolidation secondary to aspiration pneumonitis. An upper GI endoscopy should be performed during the first 24 hours after caustic corrosive ingestion to assess the damage, establish the prognosis and guide further treatment. It should not be performed after 96 hours of corrosive ingestion as the injured esophagus is in the phase of ulceration and granulation tissue formation hence is fragile and prone to perforation. Endoscopy has a limitation of not being able to differentiate between superficial and transmural necrosis. Hence, based on endoscopic findings alone, unnecessary surgery should not be performed. Endoscopy is contraindicated in a hemodynamically unstable patient, if there is severe respiratory distress or there is evidence of perforation.

An endoscopic grading system for corrosive esophageal injury has been developed for predicting clinical outcome is the Zargar classification with grades 1 and 2A having an excellent prognosis while at the other end, grade 3B carrying a risk of early mortality in 65% cases. Patients with grades 2B and 3A are known to develop strictures in 70–100% cases.

Esophageal or gastric perforation can occur anytime during the first 2 weeks of corrosive ingestion. Water soluble contrast swallow should be performed to rule out the same. CT has been regarded more useful than endoscopy in assessing transmural damage and extent of necrosis and detecting perforation. CT being advocated in the emergency, Ryu et al. have proposed a CT grading of acute corrosive injury which has been found to be better than the endoscopic grading in predicting long-term complications.

Table 3 depicts the CT grading of acute corrosive injury of the upper GI tract (GIT).[28]

Another classification of esophageal injury which determines viability, has been proposed by Chirica et al. which is based on the presence and extent of esophageal and gastric wall enhancement on CT scan.

Table 4 gives the CT classification of corrosive injury based on viability of the GIT.

Computed tomography scan should be performed from the neck to the iliac crest after intravenous contrast administration when evaluating for corrosive injury. Apart from detecting the esophagus and stomach, CT allows assessment of the chest and abdomen for associated

TABLE 3: Computed tomography (CT) grading of acute corrosive injury.

CT grade	Extent of involvement on CT
I	Normal wall thickness (<3 mm) and enhancement
II	Wall edema (>3 mm thick) with hypoenhancement
III	Wall edema (>3 mm thick) with surrounding soft-tissue stranding, with maintained sharp interface with serosa
IV	Wall edema (>3 mm thick) with surrounding soft-tissue stranding and ill-defined interface with serosa, with or without collection

TABLE 4: Computed tomography (CT) classification of corrosive injury based on viability of the gastrointestinal tract (GIT).

CT grading	Extent of esophageal and gastric wall enhancement on CT
I	Normal appearing organs
II	Wall edema with surrounding soft-tissue inflammation and postcontrast wall enhancement
III	Absence of postcontrast wall enhancement suggestive of transmural involvement

findings such as aspiration in lungs, effusion, mediastinal inflammation, or collection. **Figures 18A to G** of axial and sagittal images of CT of chest depict the findings following corrosive ingestion in a 22-year-old female.

Sequelae of corrosive/caustic injury:

- *Strictures*: Esophageal strictures are the most common complication of corrosive injury. Dysphagia occurring due to stricture formation is generally seen 2 months after the corrosive injury. Barium swallow helps in evaluating the sequelae but is not able to differentiate if it is due to acid/alkali ingestion. Strictures secondary to corrosive injury are usually long, smooth, and mostly involve the middle and distal esophagus **(Figs. 19A to C)**. But, variable appearances of caustic/corrosive strictures have been described. They can be short, long, or multiple with a smooth outline with nodular defects or scalloping due to focal areas of submucosal fibrosis. Short-segment strictures are often amenable to endoscopic or fluoroscopic balloon dilatation. It is important to perform a contrast study up to the pylorus to rule out concomitant gastric injury which can occur from 20 to 62.5% cases in the form of antral ulceration, pyloric stenosis or frank gastric outlet obstruction.
- *Hemorrhage*: Bleeding from the site where the corrosive agent erodes the viscera is a rare complication, associated with high mortality. It usually presents in the 3rd to 4th week of injury, resulting in active leak or pseudoaneurysm formation requiring surgery or endovascular embolization.

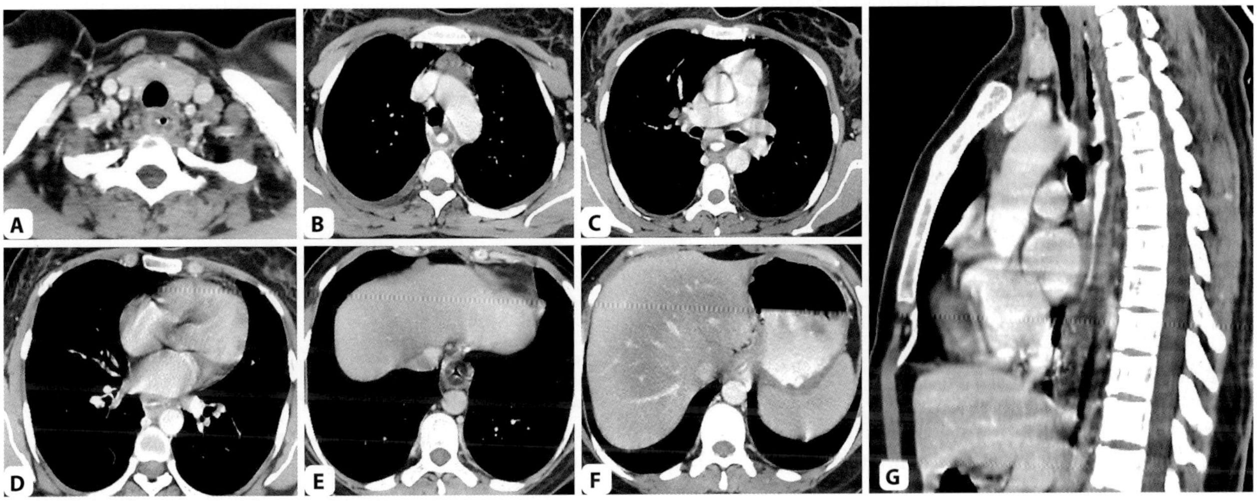

FIGS. 18A TO G: Contrast-enhanced computed tomography (CECT) chest and abdomen (A to G) in a 22-year-old female with alleged history of corrosive poisoning reveals edematous mural thickening of 10 mm of entire esophagus with hypoenhancing wall showing postcontrast enhancement with mild mural thickening of the cardia of stomach with no periesophageal collection or free air or oral positive contrast extravasation: Grade 2 esophageal injury.

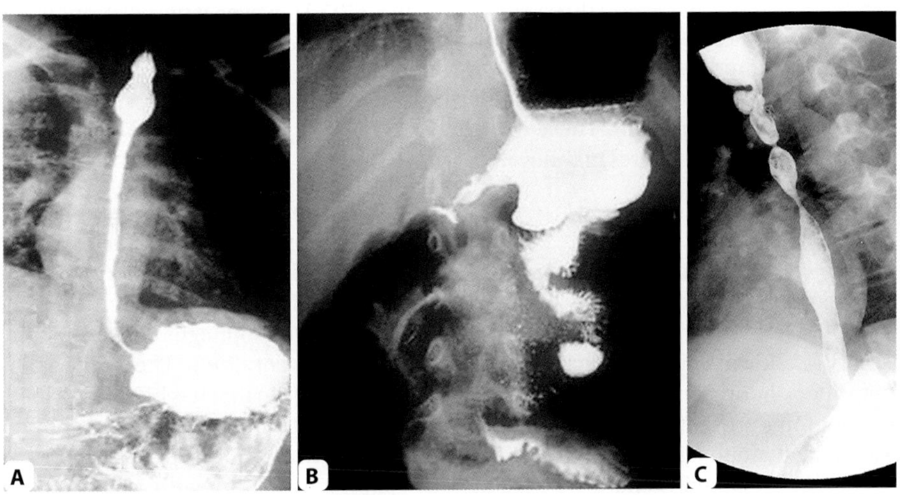

FIGS. 19A TO C: (A) Barium swallow showing a long stricture with nodular defects due to focal areas of submucosal fibrosis in a case of caustic esophagitis; (B) The stomach shows narrowing of distal body and antrum with mucosal irregularity; Corrosive strictures in another patient showing (C) multiple, short, and smooth strictures with proximal dilatation with diverticulum formation.

- Pulmonary complication which occurs are pneumonia secondary to aspiration. Various fistulas, though rare, have been reported such as esophageal-bronchial, esophageal-pulmonary or esophageal-pleural fistula, especially in the acute phase.
- *Perforation and collections*: They typically occur in the acute phase and are associated with full thickness necrosis of the esophagus. A mediastinal abscess can result secondary to pneumomediastinum and mediastinitis following esophageal perforation.

Management

Management depends on when the patient presented following corrosive injury and consists of resuscitation, airway management, and hemodynamic stabilization. A nasogastric tube when required to be inserted, should be placed under endoscopic guidance. Esophageal strictures are treated by esophageal dilatations which should be performed 3–6 weeks after the initial injury because of the associated high incidence of perforation if attempted early. The goal is to dilate the esophageal lumen to 15 mm and to completely relieve dysphagia. Long and eccentric strictures may be managed by endoscopic dilatation under fluoroscopic guidance so as to minimize the risk of perforation.

There is an increased risk for the development of esophageal SCC in patients of caustic/corrosive ingestion. This risk is substantially higher in victims of chronic lye ingestion as compared to the general population.[23] The latent period is generally in decades. Hence, these patients should be followed up periodically to rule out the same with endoscopic surveillance for cancer recommended for 15–20 years after ingestion.

Drug-induced or Pill Esophagitis

Drug-induced esophagitis is caused most commonly by ingesting antibiotics, such as tetracycline and doxycycline which cause only superficial ulceration. Other medications include potassium chloride, quinidine, ferrous sulfate, and anti-inflammatory drugs. They generally get lodged in the esophagus at sites of extrinsic compression. These drugs may result in severe esophagitis and strictures may develop.

Clinical Presentation

When such drugs dissolve in the esophagus, they cause mucosal injury by creating an acid pH or by a direct irritant effect in the epithelium. Hold up of tablets in the esophagus is favored by swallowing pills while lying down, taking them without water, abnormal esophageal motility, and cardiomegaly. Symptoms are usually sudden in onset and consist of chest pain, odynophagia, or dysphagia. The pain of drug-/pill-induced esophagitis characteristically develops over a period of hours or will awaken the patient from sleep. A history of ingesting the pill obviates the need for any diagnostic testing. Endoscopy when performed reveals localized ulceration or inflammation.

Drug-induced esophagitis usually involves the proximal or middle esophagus. A typical location is the aortic arch level, where tablets are delayed because of the aortic indentation on the esophagus and the low contractile force of peristalsis.

Imaging Features

The radiographic findings consist of small and superficial ulceration in upper or mid esophagus. The ulcers are usually ovoid, occasionally linear and clustered circumferentially. A repeat study 7–10 days after withdrawal of the offending agent will show healing of ulcers. CT of the chest may sometimes show esophageal thickening consistent with transmural inflammation. The condition usually resolves within days to weeks, but symptoms may persist for months. In severe cases, stricture may develop, which may require dilatation.[20]

Eosinophilic Esophagitis

Eosinophilic esophagitis is an inflammatory condition characterized pathologically by eosinophilic infiltration of the esophagus that is thought to occur as an inflammatory response to food allergens in susceptible individuals.

Clinical Presentation

The condition should be strongly considered in children and adults with long-standing dysphagia and recurrent food impaction. Majority of the patients present with an atopic history of food allergy, asthmas, eczema, allergic rhinitis or peripheral eosinophilia.

The diagnosis of EoE is based on a combination of typical esophageal symptoms and esophageal mucosal biopsies demonstrating infiltration of the esophageal squamous epithelium with eosinophils. It can also be seen with GERD. However, if the eosinophils are > 20 eosinophils per high power field on endoscopic biopsy, a diagnosis of EoE should be made.[29]

Imaging Features

Eosinophilic esophagitis may cause segmental or diffuse esophageal strictures that can be diagnosed with esophagoscopy. Strictures may occur most often in the upper to mid thoracic esophagus. It may be associated with distinctive ring-like indentation known as "ringed esophagus". An esophagus with a small caliber may instead be seen in this condition. The "small caliber esophagus" is a radiographic sign that has been described in 2010 by White, Levine et al. at barium esophagography and is defined as an esophagus with a caliber of < 20 mm. The involved segment of esophagus is long with variable length of narrowing having a mean length of 15.4 cm with smooth contours and tapered margins.[29]

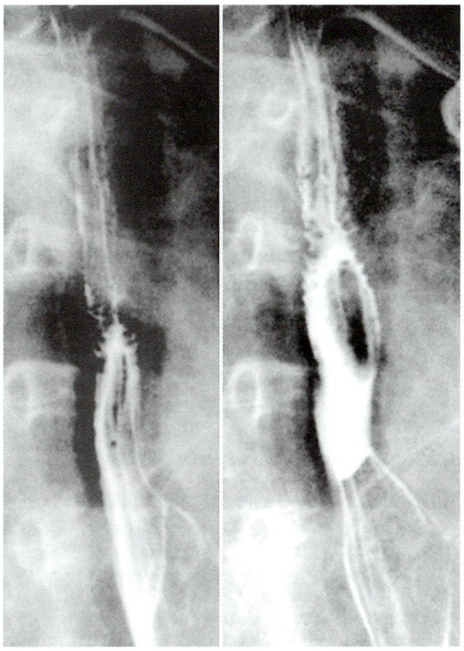

FIG. 20: Intramural pseudodiverticulosis: Tiny, flask-shaped outpouchings arranged in longitudinal rows produced by barium entering dilated esophageal glands, seen in the thoracic esophagus.

Endoscopy needs to be performed for a definitive diagnosis.

Treatment

Treatment includes dietary modification, proton pump inhibitors, steroid therapy, dilatation of strictures. Esophageal dilatation must be cautiously performed in patients with strictures because of increased risk of esophageal mural disruption and perforation.[1,12]

Intramural Pseudodiverticulosis

It is an unusual condition in which inflammation leads to dilatation of the ducts of the deep mucous glands. Intramural pseudodiverticulosis may occur as a consequence of scarring and is associated with strictures in 90% of patients. It can also occur in isolation wherein the patients are asymptomatic.

Imaging Features

Radiologically, they appear as tiny, flask-shaped outpouchings of contrast material, 1–4 mm in size arranged in clusters or longitudinal rows **(Fig. 20)**. Often the necks of the pseudodiverticulae are not opacified and they appear to be separated from the esophageal lumen by 1 or 2 mm and appear to float outside the esophagus. The condition may be segmental or diffuse, and may be seen in association with a peptic stricture in the lower esophagus.

ESOPHAGEAL NEOPLASMS

Benign Esophageal Neoplasms

Benign tumors comprise 20% of esophageal tumors. The most common benign intramural neoplasm of the esophagus is leiomyoma. Others such as hemangioma, schwannoma, neurofibroma, and glomus tumor are very rare.

Mucosal-based benign tumors of the esophagus are squamous papilloma and adenoma.

Leiomyoma

They are neoplasms of mature smooth muscle cells and account for >50% of all benign esophageal neoplasms.[14] Leiomyomas are also the most common mesenchymal tumors of the esophagus in contrast to the rest of the GIT, where gastrointestinal stromal tumors (GISTs) are more common.

Clinical Features

They occur mostly in adults, being twice more common in males than females. However, rarely they may also be seen in children. Most patients are asymptomatic, but dysphagia and pain may develop depending on the size of the lesion and how much the esophageal lumen is getting compromised. Those affected generally have symptoms of more than 2 years duration[30] and dysphagia to solids is the predominant symptom. On immunohistochemistry, esophageal leiomyomas can be distinguished from GISTs as leiomyomas are negative for CD117 and CD34.

Esophageal leiomyomas mostly involve the mid (60%) and lower (30%) third of the esophagus, where smooth muscle is present.[27] They may arise from the muscularis mucosa or muscularis propria layers of the esophageal wall. Majority of the leiomyomas (97%) are intramural with 10% of them showing circumferential growth pattern. These tumors are mostly solitary with a size of <3 cm. Multiple leiomyomas (leiomyomatosis) can be familial and often associated with Alport syndrome in children. Esophageal leiomyomatosis can occur on its own or be associated with leiomyomas of the tracheobronchial tree and genital tract in the pediatric age group.

Imaging Features

On double-contrast barium studies, esophageal leiomyomas appear as smoothly marginated filling defect that forms an obtuse angle with the adjacent esophageal wall. This appearance is characteristic of a submucosal mass.[30] On cross-sectional imaging, it appears as a smoothly marginated exophytic intraluminal mass or as an eccentric esophageal wall thickening **(Figs. 21A and B)**. It shows soft-tissue homogeneous attenuation which may occasionally contain calcification. Leiomyomas are iso to hypodense to muscle on noncontrast CT and slightly hyperintense

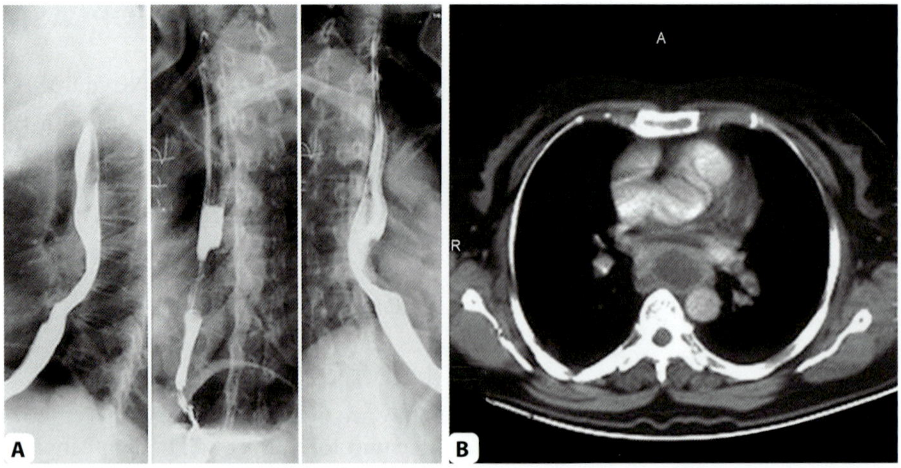

FIGS. 21A AND B: (A) Leiomyoma in the distal thoracic esophagus seen as a semilunar mass with intact mucosa, narrowing the barium column, and widening the esophageal diameter; (B) Contrast-enhanced computed tomography (CECT) shows smooth hypodense mass indenting the esophageal lumen with intact fat planes around esophagus—leiomyoma.

on T2W MRI. They show homogeneous enhancement on contrast imaging without any necrosis.[14]

Endoscopic ultrasound has a diagnostic accuracy of 89% in the diagnosis of esophageal leiomyomas as it is able to depict which layer of the esophageal wall is involved.[7] On EUS, leiomyoma is seen as homogeneous hypoechoic mass in the muscularis mucosa, submucosa, or muscularis propria.

On positron emission tomography (PET)-CT, leiomyomas do not usually show avid uptake as these tumors have a low mitotic rate.[30]

Differential diagnosis of esophageal leiomyomas includes duplication cysts, GISTs, lymphoma, and hematogenous metastases. Duplication cysts usually manifest in childhood and appear as cysts on all imaging modalities. Calcification is a feature of leiomyomas, but may be seen in GISTs. Small GISTs may mimic leiomyomas as they too appear as homogeneous intramural masses. However, small leiomyomas are relatively more common. Large GISTs may be differentiated on the basis of necrosis or cyst formation in them. Esophageal lymphoma and metastatic disease generally occur in a setting of contiguous invasion or widespread disease.[30]

Treatment

Treatment for esophageal leiomyomas consists of removal in the form of endoscopic resection or surgical enucleation or conservative follow-up. These lesions have a benign course and usually do not recur after surgery.

Gastrointestinal Stromal Tumors

Esophageal GISTs are uncommon mesenchymal tumors as compared to leiomyomas of the esophagus. Esophageal GISTs, similar to other GISTs in the GIT, are positive for C-KIT (a cell surface transmembrane tyrosine kinase also known as CD117) and CD34. These tumors have a malignant potential and have overlapping imaging features with esophageal leiomyomas. Hence, it is important for the radiologist to be familiar with the clinicopathologic and imaging features of these tumors for appropriate patient management.

Clinicopathological Features

Esophageal GISTs are more commonly encountered than previously thought. They occur more often in the lower dorsal esophagus, the site for abundant intrinsic distribution of the GIST progenitor cells, the interstitial cells of Cajal. The patients generally present late with symptoms of dysphagia because of their submucosal, exophytic location, and are usually large at presentation. Patients may also have pain and cough due to the mass effect exerted by the tumor on adjacent mediastinal structures.

Imaging Features

On barium studies, GIST appears as a submucosal smoothly marginated mass. Ulceration may be seen in large GISTs on endoscopy or barium swallow study, while it is not a feature of esophageal leiomyomas.

On CT, esophageal GISTs appear as large, heterogeneous intramural soft-tissue masses that are isoattenuating to muscles and show moderate postcontrast enhancement. Cystic areas are common in tumor > 4.5 cm while calcification is rare. GISTs show uniform ^{18}F-fluorodeoxyglucose (FDG) uptake on PET scan.[31]

Treatment

Treatment consists of surgery alone or along with adjuvant imatinib (tyrosine kinase inhibitor) or radiation therapy. The following table **(Table 5)** lists the differentiating features between esophageal GIST and esophageal leiomyomas.[31]

TABLE 5: Differences between esophageal gastrointestinal stromal tumors (GISTs) and leiomyomas.

	Esophageal GISTs	Esophageal leiomyomas
Tumor size	Larger (~5–6 cm)	Smaller (<3 cm)
Location	More frequently in distal esophagus	Mid (40%) and distal (50%) esophagus both locations
Barium swallow	Appears as smooth, submucosal nonobstructive filling defect	Appears as smooth, submucosal nonobstructive filling defect
CT scan	More heterogeneous attenuation	More homogeneous density
CECT	Moderately enhancing mass	Shows minimal to no enhancement
Ulceration	May be present. Seen on endoscopy or barium study	No ulceration seen. Mucosa is normal
Calcification	Rare	Uncommon. Diffuse popcorn type
PET scan	FDG–avid tumor	Mild FDG uptake
Treatment	Surgical resection because of malignant potential/ adjuvant therapy or radiation	Resection/conservative follow-up if asymptomatic

(CECT: contrast-enhanced computed tomography; FDG: ^{18}F-fluorodeoxyglucose; PET: positron emission tomography)

Fibrovascular Polyp

Fibrovascular polyp is a rare, benign, tumor-like lesion of the esophagus composed of loose or dense fibrous tissue, adipose tissue and vascular structure. The polyp is covered by normal squamous epithelium. The components of fibrovascular polyp may vary from lesion to lesion and in different parts of the same lesion.

A fibrovascular polyp usually arises in the cervical esophagus near the level of the cricopharyngeus. It probably originates in the loose submuscular tissue of the cervical esophagus and gradually elongates over many years as it is dragged into the middle or distal third of the esophagus by esophageal peristalsis, until the intraluminal portion of the tumor becomes massive in size. Occasionally, it may even prolapse through the cardia into the gastric fundus.[32]

Clinical Features

Fibrovascular polyps generally occur in elderly with slowly progressive dysphagia over years. Other symptoms include vomiting, weight loss, and respiratory difficulty likely due to compression of the adjacent trachea by the distended esophagus. Very rarely fibrovascular polyp with a long stalk may regurgitate into the pharynx or mouth, resulting in sudden death from laryngeal occlusion.[14]

Imaging Features

On plain chest frontal radiographs, fibrovascular polyps may be detected as a right-sided superior mediastinal mass and on a lateral view may cause compression and anterior bowing of the trachea. It can be differentiated from achalasia due to lack of distention of the distal esophagus.

On barium swallow studies, it typically appears as a smooth, expansile, and sausage-shaped intraluminal mass that arises in the cervical esophagus and extends to the middle or distal third of the esophagus. It can show a lobulated appearance which, if marked, can mimic a malignant neoplasm radiographically. The CT appearance can vary depending on the amount of fat and fibrovascular tissue in the lesion. If fat is the predominant tissue, the presence of an intraluminal esophageal mass with fat attenuation in it is considered a typical sign of a fibrovascular polyp. When oral contrast surrounds the mass on CT, it may help in determining the intraluminal location of the lesion.

Magnetic resonance further aids in characterizing the composition of a fibrovascular polyp. Fat within the mass, mucoid secretion, and nonacute blood depict a high SI on T1W images while soft tissue and muscle within the tumor appear as low SI on T2W images.[14]

Treatment

Fibrovascular polyps do not usually undergo malignant degeneration. But, still these lesions warrant a removal because of the progressive and debilitating nature of the symptoms. Also, because of the known risk of asphyxiation and sudden death due to the gigantic sizes it can grow to in the esophagus, it is imperative to surgically remove these tumors.

MALIGNANT ESOPHAGEAL NEOPLASMS

Majority (~80%) of the esophageal neoplasms are malignant. More than 90% of these are SCCs or adenocarcinomas which are epithelial neoplasms.

Esophageal Cancer: Squamous Cell Carcinoma and Adenocarcinoma

As per GLOBOCAN 2020 data, esophageal cancer is the seventh most common cancer in the world. In India, it ranks fifth in terms of incidence and mortality. Based on tumor location, the American Joint Committee on Cancer (AJCC) has divided esophageal cancer as being located in the cervical, upper thoracic, mid thoracic, and lower thoracic esophagus including the GEJ and up to 2 cm of the gastric cardia. Esophageal-gastric junction tumors with epicenters 2 cm beyond GEJ are staged as gastric cancers. The distance of the tumor epicenter from the incisors on endoscopy defines the tumor location, rather than its upper edge.[33]

Both SCC and adenocarcinoma are very aggressive malignant epithelial neoplasms which disseminate early because of lack of serosa in the esophagus. The nonepithelial malignant neoplasms are rare in comparison and include sarcomas, particularly leiomyosarcoma. Lymphoma, malignant melanoma, and metastasis also involve the esophagus rarely.

Clinical Presentation

Histologically, the most common esophageal cancer is SCC and accounts for around 85% cases.[33] However, there has been a marked increase in the prevalence of esophageal *adenocarcinoma* (EAC) due to increasing weight gain and obesity and it has been recently found to be the most predominant type of esophageal carcinoma in the UK, the USA, and Western Europe, with BE seen in many of these patients.[1,14] BE is the most important risk factor which is implicated in the development of esophageal adenocarcinoma. It is a premalignant condition where the normal stratified squamous epithelium of the esophagus is replaced by columnar epithelium secondary to chronic gastroesophageal reflux and reflux esophagitis. These patients may present with symptoms secondary to underlying GERD. However, most patients have advanced malignancy at the time of presentation with symptoms of dysphagia, odynophagia, rapidly progressive weight loss being similar to that seen in patients with advanced SCC. Esophageal adenocarcinoma is seen predominantly in males in the seventh decade. Most of them involve the distal third of the esophagus with consequent invasion of the stomach by direct extension across the GEJ.

Major risk factors of SCC are tobacco chewing and smoking and alcohol intake with other predisposing factors being achalasia, lye strictures, Plummer–Vinson syndrome, celiac disease, and tylosis. Patients with achalasia have a much higher risk of developing esophageal cancer which is 9–28 times that of a person without achalasia. The secondary cancers developing in achalasia patients usually present late in the disease course and have a poor prognosis. They may appear as large, bulky mass within a markedly dilated esophagus. SCC is more common in males than females with peak age group of involvement being 60–74 years.[14,30] They are most commonly located in the upper and middle third of esophagus.[34] Patients present with progressive dysphagia more to solids than liquids and by the time dysphagia develops, the esophageal lumen is >50% compromised and two-thirds of the circumference of the esophageal wall is invaded by the tumor. Ulceration in the tumor can produce odynophagia and patients may have chest pain unrelated to swallowing if the tumor has invaded the mediastinum.[17]

Independent of staging, the prognosis of both esophageal squamous cell and adenocarcinoma is poor with a reported 5-year survival rate of 12% for SCC and 15% for adenocarcinoma.[34]

Imaging Features

On barium contrast studies, esophageal adenocarcinoma may be indistinguishable from SCC on the basis of morphological findings. The reported sensitivity of double-contrast barium swallow in diagnosing esophageal cancers has been reported to be >95%. Early cancers may appear as plaque like lesions, small lobulated sessile polyp, or focal wall irregularity on double-contrast barium swallow.[16] Advanced esophageal carcinoma present with a variety of morphologic abnormalities. They may appear as annular apple-core lesion with overhanging margins **(Figs. 22A and B)**, irregular narrowed segment, smooth tapering stricture, bulky endophytic mass **(Figs. 23A and B)**, large

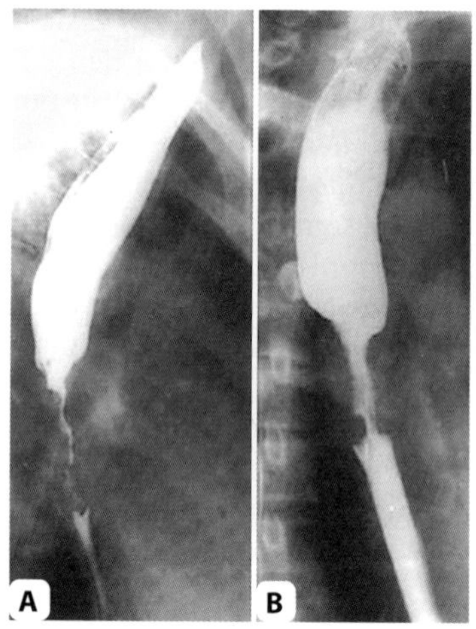

FIGS. 22A AND B: Annular carcinoma in midportion of esophagus with circumferential infiltration and overhanging margins.

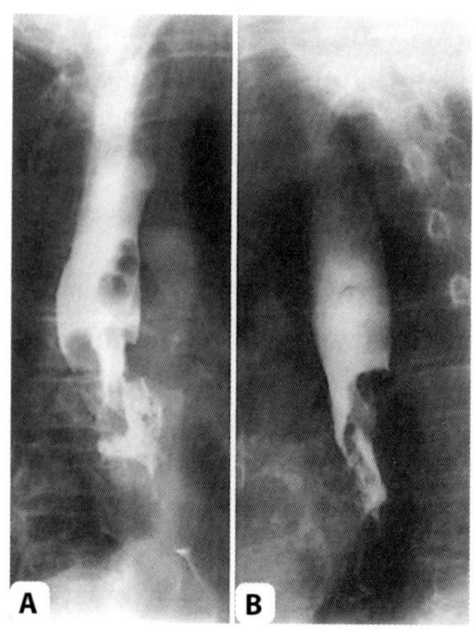

FIGS. 23A AND B: Polypoidal filling defects with shouldering and irregular narrowing of lumen-carcinoma involving the mid and lower esophagus.

ulceration, varicoid infiltrate **(Figs. 24A and B)**, or diffuse nodularity **(Figs. 25A and B)**. Varicoid carcinomas are those in which submucosal spread of tumor produces thickened, tortuous, longitudinal defects that mimic the appearance of varices. Varicoid tumors have a fixed configuration, whereas varices change in size and shape at fluoroscopy. In some cases, esophageal carcinoma spreads submucosally via the lymphatics and reappears at another site in the esophagus **(Figs. 26A and B)**. These satellite metastases may appear as polypoid, plaque-like, or ulcerated lesions separated from the primary tumor by normal mucosa.[20] Tumor also spreads subdiaphragmatically to the proximal stomach via submucosal lymphatics. Fistulization may occur spontaneously, or after radiotherapy.

On CT scans, esophageal carcinoma appears as a mass or wall thickening of soft-tissue attenuation **(Figs. 27A to C)**. A study on dynamic CECT has shown that the optimal phase in depicting esophageal carcinoma is the late arterial phase as it best depicts the tumor enhancement and the attenuation difference between the tumor and the normal esophageal wall compared to early arterial and venous phases.[35]

On MRI, the mass appears isointense to the residual esophageal wall on T1W images and intermediate or high SI on T2W images. CT and MRI are both used for staging esophageal carcinoma and are both considered comparable for assessing resectability in terms of mediastinal invasion, lymph node involvement, and distant metastasis.[27] However, in routine clinical situations, CT is recommended.[14]

LEIOMYOSARCOMA

Leiomyosarcoma of the esophagus are rare, low-grade malignant lesions accounting for < 1% of all esophageal malignant neoplasms. They are characterized by slow growth and late metastasis, hence, have a better prognosis than SCC.

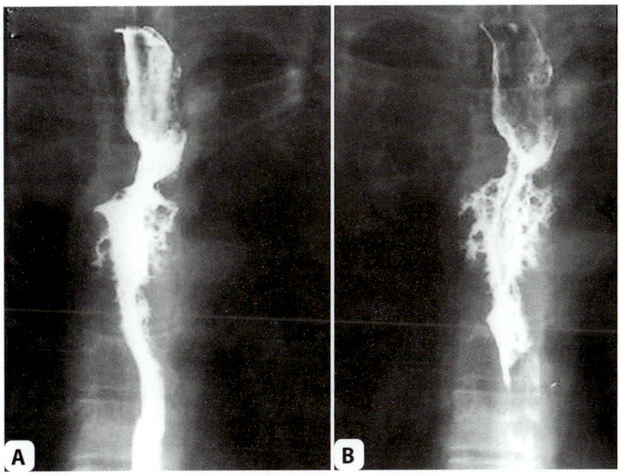

FIGS. 24A AND B: Spot film of the esophagus at the level of aortic arch shows irregularity and nodularity of the mucosa with lymphatic infiltration—varicoid appearance in squamous cell carcinoma.

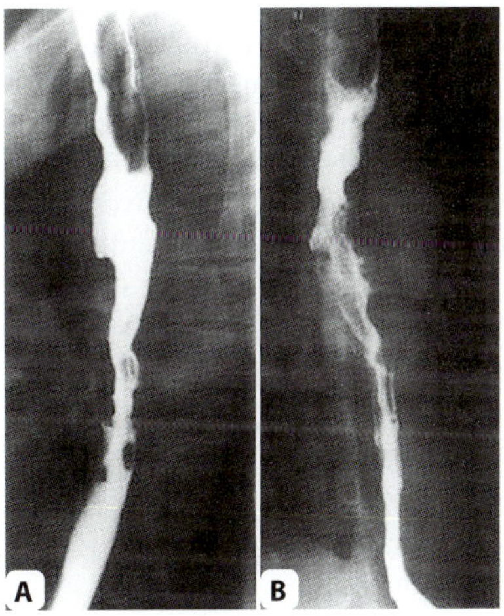

FIGS. 25A AND B: Carcinoma involving mid esophagus with narrowing of lumen and diffuse nodular filling defects.

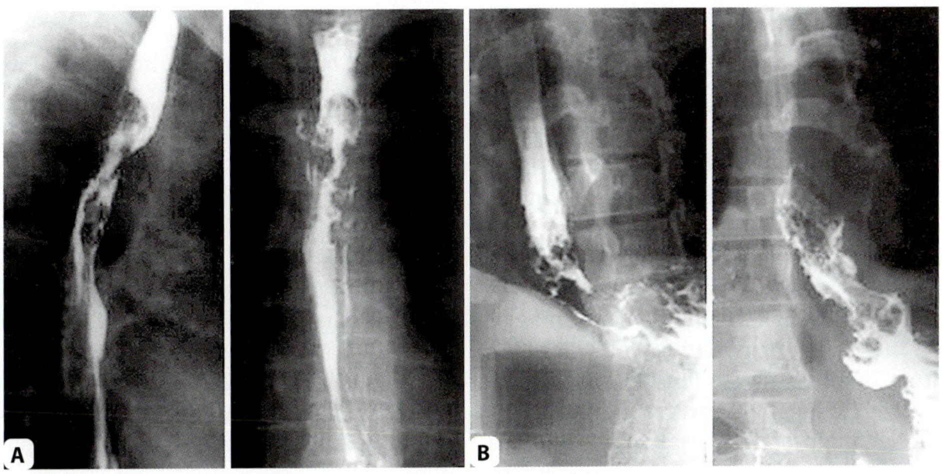

FIGS. 26A AND B: Carcinoma involving upper and mid esophagus in a circumferential manner. Another lesion is seen just above the esophagogastric junction—multicentric carcinoma.

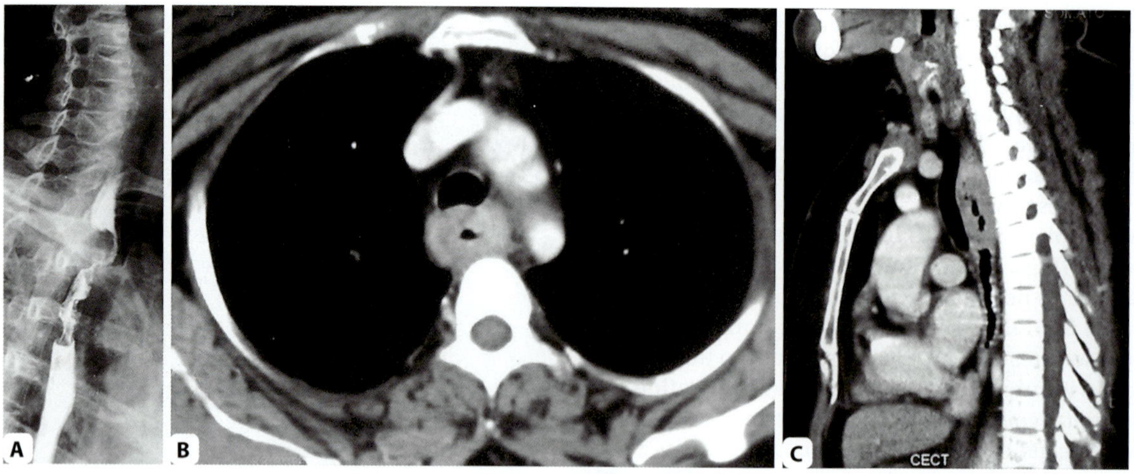

FIGS. 27A TO C: Barium swallow study (A) showing irregular area of luminal narrowing, ulceration with polypoid filling defect and shouldering involving upper dorsal esophagus. (B and C) axial and sagittal contrast-enhanced computed tomography (CECT) reveals homogeneously enhancing circumferential mural thickening of the upper dorsal esophagus (D2–D5 level) with indentation of the trachea anteriorly. The periesophageal triangular fat pad is preserved: Carcinoma esophagus.

Leiomyosarcoma are seen in middle aged or older adults. Most of them are thought to arise de novo rather than from pre-existing leiomyomas.[35] They are usually located in the middle and distal thirds of the esophagus as the esophagus here is lined by smooth muscle. Leiomyosarcoma generally spreads by direct extension into the mediastinum or by hematogenous metastases.

Clinical Presentation

Patients present clinically with slowly progressive dysphagia and weight loss. But, if tumor has a significant exophytic growth pattern without encroachment on the esophagus, dysphagia can be minimal or absent. GI bleeding can occur, if the tumor ulcerates.

Imaging Features

Leiomyosarcoma may sometimes be detected on plain chest radiographs when they show a large exophytic component extending into the mediastinum. Two types of growth patterns have been described—polypoid or infiltrating. The typical appearance on barium studies is a submucosal mass that appears as an intramural polypoidal filling defect that tends to be larger and more lobulated than benign leiomyoma and may sometimes contain areas of ulceration, cavitation, or calcification **(Figs. 28A and B)**.[16]

On CT, leiomyosarcomas of the esophagus are seen as thickening of the esophageal wall with a large soft-tissue exophytic component showing central areas of low attenuation due to necrosis and extraluminal air due to ulceration. An infiltrating type of lesion may be indistinguishable from an infiltrative esophageal cancer.[14] On MRI, the tumor may appear as a mass that is isointense to skeletal muscle on T1W images and hyperintense on T2W images.

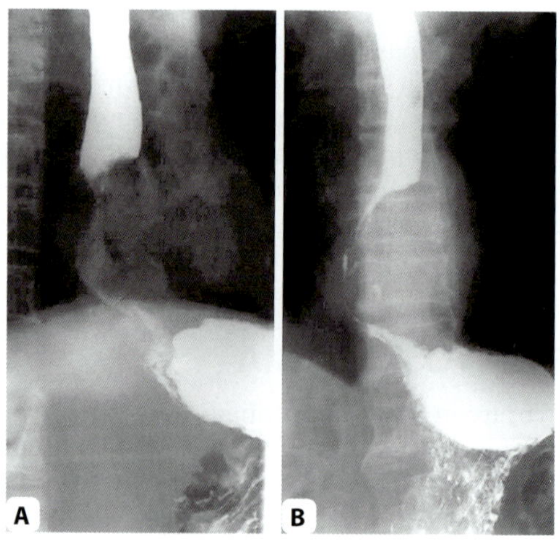

FIGS. 28A AND B: Barium swallow shows a smooth extrinsic impression on the distal esophagus with a large exophytic component suggestive of an intramural mass—leiomyosarcoma.

Early treatment is essential as leiomyosarcomas have a better prognosis than SCC.

LYMPHOMA

Esophageal lymphomas are very rare, are more commonly of non-Hodgkin type accounting for < 1% of all GI lymphomas. Esophageal involvement usually occurs secondary to contiguous spread of lymphoma from the gastric fundus or direct invasion by adjacent lymphomatous lymph nodes. Primary lymphoma has been reported in patients of AIDS.[30]

Clinical Presentation

Patients may present with dysphagia but often these tumors may not produce symptoms and have known to be discovered at autopsy with widespread disease.[14]

Imaging Features

Lymphomas most often occur in the distal esophagus with variable appearance on imaging. On barium studies, they are commonly seen as irregular narrowing of the distal esophagus due to direct spread of the tumor from the proximal stomach. They may also appear as multiple submucosal nodules, polypoid or ulcerated lesions, enlarged folds, strictures or rarely as aneurysmal dilatation of the esophagus.[30]

On cross-sectional imaging, lymphomas can cause concentric or asymmetric thickening of the esophageal wall with or without mediastinal lymphadenopathy. A helpful point to remember is that an intact fat plane between the esophageal tumor and adjacent structures goes in favor of an esophageal lymphoma **(Figs. 29A to C)**.[30]

On EUS, the tumor most commonly appears as homogeneously hypoechoic transmural thickening. On PET scan, it mostly demonstrates avid FDG uptake.

Treatment

Esophageal lymphomas are treated by a combination of chemotherapy and radiotherapy which have been found to be as effective as surgery.

SPINDLE CELL CARCINOMA

These tumors of the esophagus have both carcinomatous and sarcomatous components and are currently considered as a variant of SCC.

Imaging Features

Majority of the spindle cell tumors are located in the middle and distal esophagus and are characterized by intraluminal growth rather than esophageal wall invasion.[30] On esophagography, it is seen as a large irregular polypoid filling defect in the mid and distal esophagus. It mainly expands the esophagus without causing obstruction and may show scalloped margins.[16] The CT appearance is of a large intraluminal mass without proximal dilatation or localized wall thickening. On MRI, these tumors show greater enhancement than the esophageal wall.

The differential diagnosis of spindle cell carcinoma includes leiomyosarcoma, fibrovascular polyp, primary malignant melanoma, and SCC. Fibrovascular polyp also appear as polypoid intraluminal masses. This can be differentiated from spindle cell carcinoma as they have a very smooth contour and arise from the cervical esophagus while spindle cell carcinomas are more lobulated and arise from mid-dorsal esophagus.

PRIMARY MALIGNANT MELANOMA

These are very rare tumors of the esophagus which arise from malignant degeneration of the pre-existing melanocytes in the esophageal mucosa.

Imaging Features

On barium studies, primary malignant melanoma of the esophagus appears as polypoid intraluminal masses which expand the esophagus without causing significant obstruction. It may be indistinguishable from spindle cell carcinoma on double-contrast barium swallow.[16] CT scan appearance is of a large intraluminal mass, surrounded by a rim of intraluminal air or contrast. They are not usually associated with lymphadenopathy.

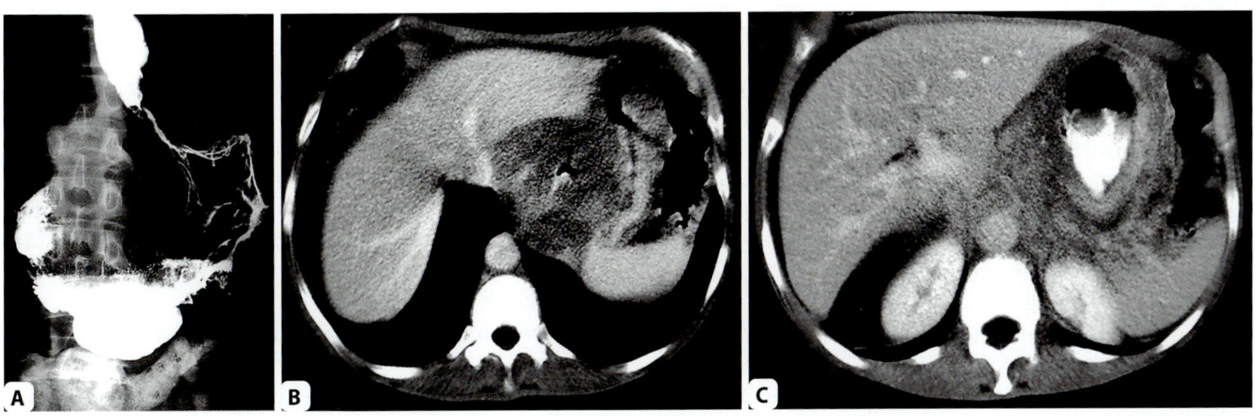

FIGS. 29A TO C: Barium swallow study (A) shows smoothly tapered narrowing of lower end esophagus with contiguous involvement of the proximal stomach. On contrast-enhanced computed tomography (CECT) (B and C), there is bulky circumferential mass in the distal esophagus with diffuse infiltration into the stomach with preservation of fat planes: Primary esophageal lymphoma of lower end esophagus with contiguous involvement of proximal stomach.

SMALL CELL CARCINOMA

Small cell carcinoma is the most common histologic subtype of neuroendocrine carcinoma. It is a rare but aggressive malignant tumor of the esophagus which metastasizes early and resembles its counterpart in the lung.[27] The tumor usually expands the lumen of the esophagus.

Imaging Features

On contrast swallow, it appears as a smoothly marginated, polypoid or fungating mass with ulceration. On CT, it shows irregular eccentric esophageal wall thickening and extensive lymph node metastasis to the mediastinum, supraclavicular region and abdomen. As spindle cell carcinoma is associated with extensive and distant metastasis, CT examination should include both the thorax and the abdomen.

STAGING OF ESOPHAGEAL CANCER

Staging of esophageal cancer is by the TNM classification which has been proposed by the 8th edition of the American Joint Committee on Cancer (AJCC) and Union for International Cancer Control (UICC) in use since 2018 **(Table 6)** where T represents tumor, N represents lymph node, M represents metastasis, and is independent of the histologic cell type. It is an imaging based clinical TNM (cTNM) staging system followed for esophagus and GEJ epithelial cancers.

Accurate preoperative staging of esophageal cancer is difficult due to its proximity to other structures (aorta, trachea, and left bronchus). The malignant nodes may arise some distance away from the tumor and may not be enlarged. Also, at time of diagnosis, unsuspected metastases may be present in 50% of cases. Hence, a number of different imaging modalities may be required for accurate staging such as endoscopy, CT, EUS, and PET-CT. The multidisciplinary approach is crucial for planning appropriate treatment in patients of esophageal cancer.[36]

Initial diagnosis is usually with endoscopy as histological confirmation with biopsy is possible. A good quality double-contrast swallow study can detect even early tumors. On a contrast swallow, if the appearance is of a symmetrical smooth narrowing, with gradual tapering to a normal caliber it is indicative of a benign stricture and malignancy can be ruled out safely. On the other hand, if a stricture shows ulceration, irregular mucosa, shouldering and shelf-like margins at fluoroscopy, it can be considered to be malignant at imaging.

Most of the patients undergo a CECT scan at initial evaluation for staging. Even though CT is less sensitive than EUS and PET-CT, it is relatively specific for detecting locally advanced or metastatic disease. If these findings are picked up on CT, patient need not undergo further investigation for staging.

TABLE 6: Eighth edition (2018) of TNM staging system for esophageal cancer.

TNM category	Description
T category	
Tx	Tumor cannot not be assessed
T0	No evidence of a primary tumor
Tis	High-grade dysplasia with no invasion of the basement membrane
T1	Tumor cells invading the lamina propria, muscularis mucosae or submucosa
T1a	Tumor cells invading the lamina propria, muscularis mucosae
T1b	Tumor cells invading the submucosa
T2	Tumor cells invading the muscularis propria
T3	Tumor cells invading the adventitia
T4	Tumor cells invading the adjacent structures
T4a (resectable)	Tumor cells invading the pleura, pericardium, azygos vein, diaphragm, or peritoneum
T4b (unresectable)	Tumor cells invading the aorta, vertebral body or trachea
N category	
Nx	Regional lymph nodes could not be assessed
N0	No regional lymph nodal metastasis
N1	1–2 regional lymph nodes involved
N2	3–6 regional lymph nodes involved
N3	≥7 regional lymph nodes involved
M category	
M0	No metastasis to distant organs
M1	Distant organ metastases seen

The changes from the 7th edition which have been incorporated in the 8th TNM staging of esophageal cancer are:

- T1a is tumor confined to the mucosa while T1b is involvement of the submucosa.
- As stated earlier, tumors 2–5 cm from GEJ even if they involve the lower end of esophagus in continuity, are reclassified as gastric cancers. **Figures 30A to D** depict the same.
- There is no change in the remaining T stages, N and M stages.
- T4 disease remains as resectable (T4a) and non-resectable (T4b) disease.
- Positive nodal disease is similar to that used in cancer of stomach where N describes the number of cancer

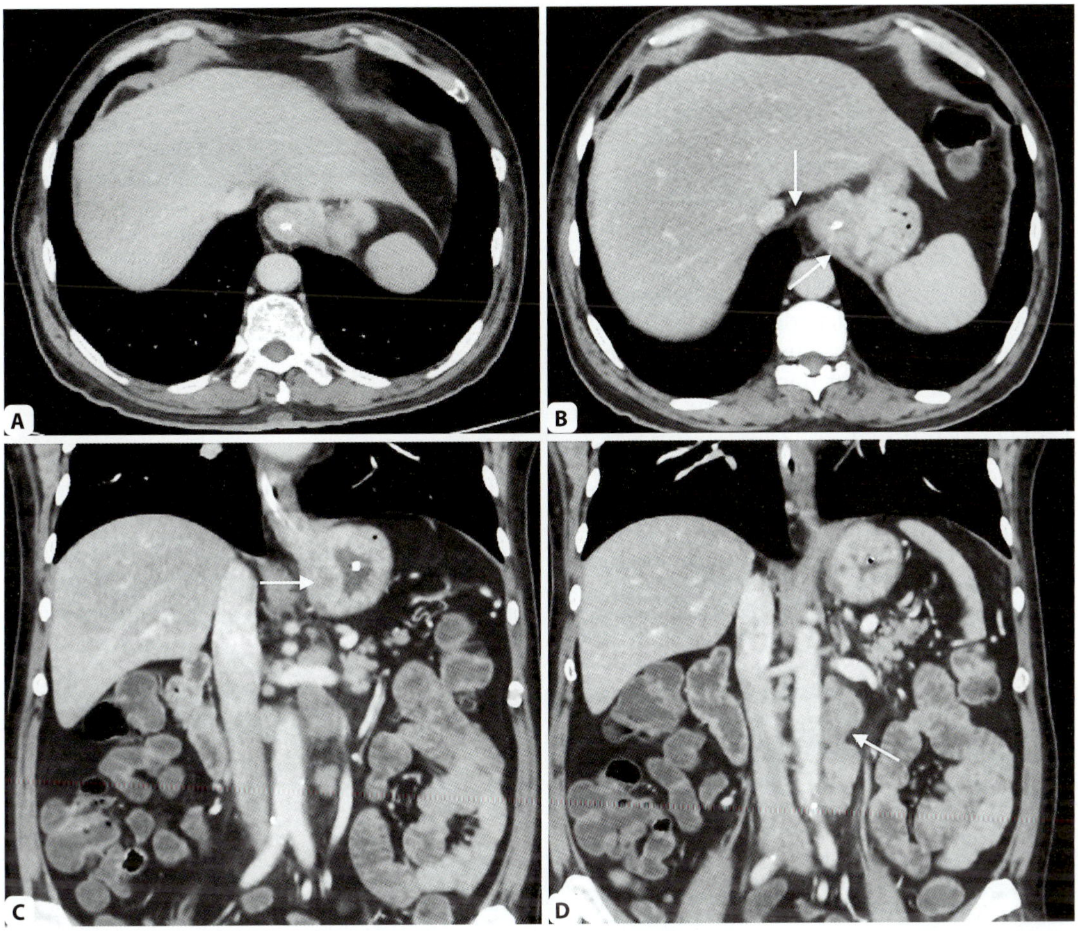

FIGS. 30A TO D: Contrast-enhanced computed tomography (CECT) images through the lower chest (A and B) and abdomen (C and D) in axial and coronal planes reveal circumferential thickening in the distal esophagus, GEJ, extending to the cardia and proximal body along the lesser curvature of stomach (arrow) causing luminal narrowing (A to C) with loss of fat planes with bilateral diaphragmatic crura (arrows in B). Multiple heterogeneously enhancing lymph nodes are seen in the perigastric and para-aortic regions (arrow in D): Ca stomach as per 8th TNM staging as involving >2 cm distal to GEJ with distal esophageal involvement.
(GEJ: gastroesophageal junction)

positive nodes.[37] It is subdivided into N1, N2, and N3 where N1 is 1–2 regional LNs, N2 is 3–6 regional LNs and N3 is ≥7 regional lymph nodes **(Fig. 31)**.

The spread of esophageal cancer to nodes occurs because of the longitudinal nature of lymphatic drainage. Hence, it defines regional lymph nodes which includes any paraesophageal lymph node from the cervical nodes to the celiac nodes.

Computed Tomography for Esophageal Cancer

Contrast-enhanced CT of the chest and abdomen with oral and intravenous contrast is the primary radiological investigation for esophageal cancer staging, usually performed after endoscopy and biopsy. CT helps in identifying patients with metastatic disease to liver or lung which if present precludes definitive treatment, with only

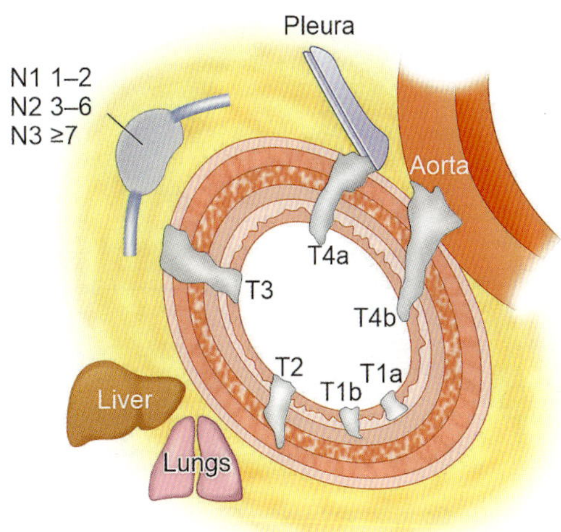

FIG. 31: Drawing illustrating the revised TNM staging system for esophageal cancer (8th edition).

palliative therapy. The layers of the esophageal wall cannot be identified on CT, hence CT is inaccurate for the early T (tumor) staging as differentiation between T1 and T2 stage is not possible.[38] T1–2 tumors depict an esophageal wall thickness of > 5 mm on CT. T3 stage on CECT is recognized by mural thickening > 15 mm with periesophageal fat infiltration without any loss of fat planes or invasion of adjacent structure. Invasion of adjacent structures is categorized as T4 tumors. CT has an important role in assessment of T4 stage of the tumor. Esophageal cancer is staged 4a when there is pleural, pericardial, azygous vein, diaphragm or peritoneal involvement. Stage 4b is one in which aorta, vertebral body or trachea is involved. For tumor involving proximal and middle third of the esophagus staging should include bronchoscopy to rule out invasion of the airway.[39]

The accuracy of CT for T staging varies widely in various studies, ranging from 43 to 92%.

Signs of T4 disease on CT are:

- Tumor having an arc of contact of > 90° with aorta.
- Loss of the triangular fat which is normally seen between the esophagus, aorta and vertebral column and
- Nodular protrusion of the tumor into the airways.

CT and MR both detect macroscopic periesophageal fat invasion by the tumor with accuracy ranging from 88 to 100%. However, microscopic invasion of the same is not discernible on cross-sectional imaging. Periesophageal fat invasion on CT appears as strand-like areas of soft-tissue attenuation in the periesophageal fat plane **(Figs. 32A to D)**. On MRI, it appears as focal loss of bright signal of fat with periesophageal invasion having ill-defined, irregular margins. Though periesophageal fat infiltration adversely effects prognosis, it is not a contraindication to en-bloc resection of the tumor.[14]

While assessing mediastinal involvement on CT or MRI, accurate assessment of the tracheobronchial tree and aorta (T4 disease) is important as their invasion is a contraindication to surgical resection. The features of tracheobronchial invasion are displacement or indentation of the posterior wall of the trachea or the bronchus by the

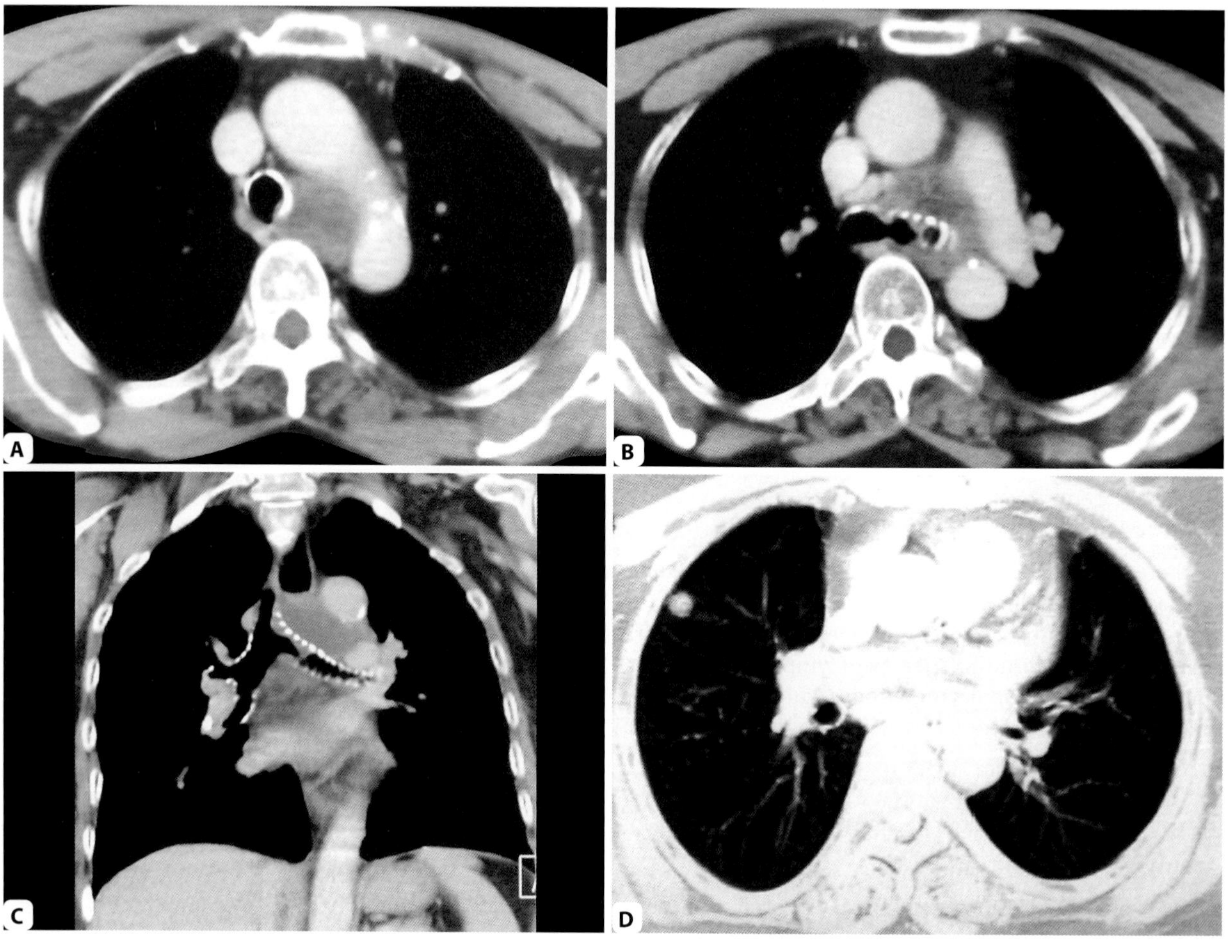

FIGS. 32A TO D: Contrast-enhanced CT of the chest in axial (A and B) and coronal planes reveals circumferential thickening of the esophagus with complete narrowing of its lumen with proximal dilatation at the level of carina (C). It is closely abutting the adjacent carinal wall, left pulmonary artery, and descending aorta. (D) CT of the chest depicts a well-defined nodular opacity in the right upper lobe suggestive of a metastatic nodule. Carcinoma esophagus—Stage IV.

tumor mass as well as evidence of direct extension of the tumor into the lumen of the airway **(Figs. 33A to D)**. The reported overall accuracy of tracheobronchial tree invasion which has been described ranges from 88 to 97%. It is important to remember that an absent intervening fat plane can also be seen in normal persons and does not always suggest tumor invasion.

Picus et al., in 1983, defined the criteria for aortic invasion on CT which has an accuracy of > 90%. Aortic invasion is diagnosed when the area of contact between the esophageal cancer and aorta is an arc of > 90°. When area of contact is < 45°; aortic invasion is considered to be absent while an area of contact of 45–90° is considered indeterminate.[40]

The presence of pleural, pericardial, and diaphragmatic or gastric invasion are not considered contraindications to surgery as the involved area can be removed with the tumor at the time of surgery.

Computed tomography is relatively insensitive in nodal staging of esophageal cancer as majority of the malignant nodes are not enlarged (i.e., appear < 1 cm in short-axis diameter). Also, benign inflammatory nodes may be larger than the cut-off criteria, nodes may not be detectable if inseparable from the primary tumor and it may not be possible to accurately measure the number of lymph node metastasis if they are matted. The periesophageal, subcarinal, left gastric, and celiac regions are the common sites of nodal involvement by an esophageal cancer. The supraclavicular and retroperitoneal abdominal lymph nodes are the most frequently involved nonregional lymph nodes, i.e., metastatic nodes. The liver, lungs, bones, and adrenal glands are the sites for distant metastasis.

Endoscopic Ultrasound for Esophageal Cancer

Endoscopic ultrasound is considered standard in the workup of esophageal cancer and is the only modality which distinguishes various layers of the esophagus. The esophageal wall appears as alternating concentric hypoechoic and hyperechoic layers on EUS with tumor appearing as a hypoechoic lesion involving the wall

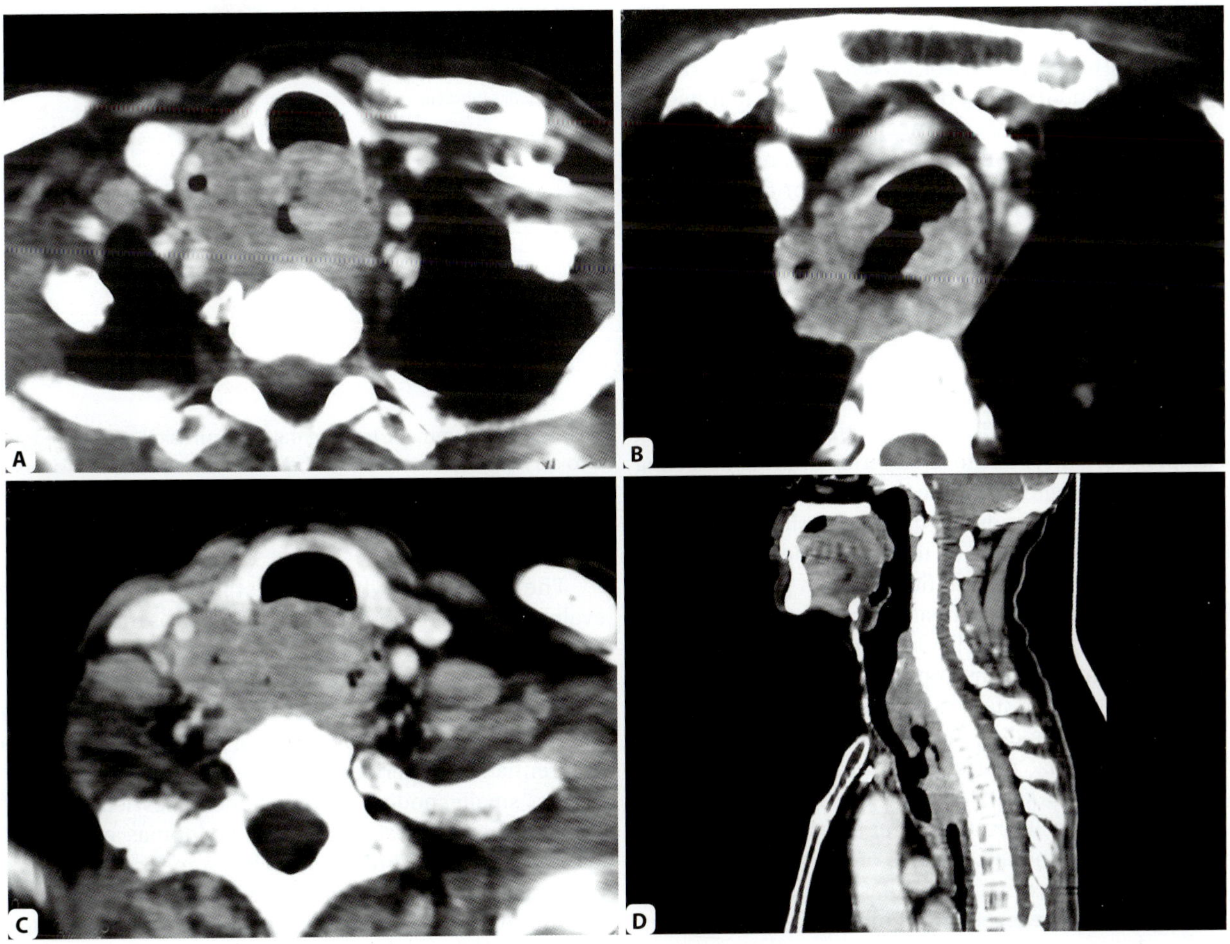

FIGS. 33A TO D: Axial (A to C) and sagittal (D) contrast-enhanced CT (CECT) reveals long-segment asymmetric mass like mural thickening (~2.2 cm) of cervical, upper, and mid-thoracic esophagus (C6 to D5 level) with infiltration and fistulous communication with posterior wall of trachea (B and D). There is partial encasement with loss of fat planes with right subclavian and proximal common carotid arteries (A and C): Squamous cell carcinoma (SCC) with tracheoesophageal fistula.

layers. A very high frequency probe such as 20 MHz radial miniprobe may be needed to differentiate mucosal (T1a) from submucosal (T1b) lesions. It is important to differentiate between T1a and T1b categories because lymph node metastasis is associated with submucosal invasion, requiring esophagectomy. EUS is able to differentiate between T1 and T2 categories on the basis of invasion of the fourth hypoechoic layer, that is muscularis propria. The reported accuracy of EUS in differentiating T1–T2 from T3–T4 esophageal cancer is 81–85%.[28] Fine needle aspiration (FNA) of suspicious nodes can be performed via guidance of EUS. However, lack of wider availability, expertise, and inability to traverse a stenotic lesion are some of the limitations of this modality. EUS provides a general roadmap as to the longitudinal length of the tumor, presence of Barret's disease, the tumor morphology and the anatomic site at which it is affected, i.e., distance from the incisor. Based on the approximate distance from incisors on endoscopy, the esophagus can be divided into various regions as depicted in **Table 7** and **Figure 34**. It is superior to CT/MRI and PET-CT for locoregional or T-staging of the tumor as the individual layer from which the tumor arises is well- visualized. In advanced tumor, if the stricture is too tight the EUS probe may not be negotiable. This indicates that the stage to be almost T3 or T4. Hence, a combination of CT and EUS should usually be performed for initial staging of patients with esophageal cancer.

For nodal disease, EUS has a higher sensitivity than PET-CT or CT, but a lower specificity. *For evaluation of metastatic disease, EUS* does not have whole body coverage, hence it is to be used along with cross-sectional imaging for identifying the same.

TABLE 7: Depicts the various parts of the esophagus based on distance from incisors on endoscopy.

Division of esophagus	Approximate distance from incisors
Cervical esophagus (upper esophageal sphincter to sternal notch)	15–20 cm
Upper thoracic esophagus (sternal notch to azygos vein)	20–25 cm
Middle thoracic esophagus (azygos vein to inferior pulmonary vein)	25–30 cm
Lower thoracic esophagus or GEJ (inferior pulmonary vein to stomach)	30–40 cm

(GEJ: gastroesophageal junction)

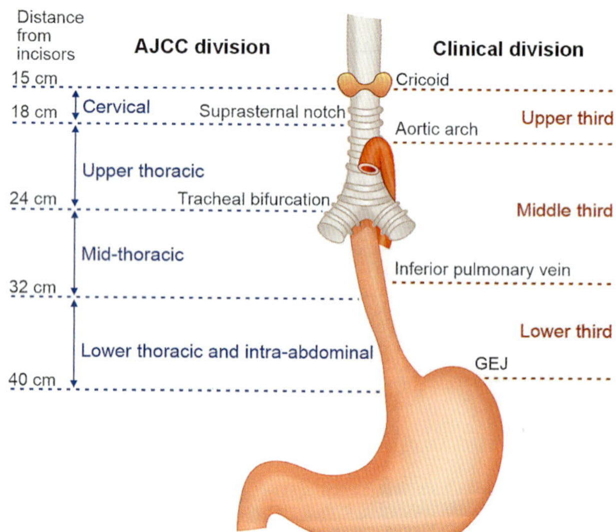

FIG. 34: Diagrammatic representation of divisions of esophagus into cervical and thoracic parts based on distance from incisors on endoscopy as per AJCC and clinical divisions.
(AJCC: American Joint Committee on Cancer; GEJ: gastroesophageal junction)

Positron Emission Tomography–Computed Tomography for Esophageal Cancer

The main role of PET-CT scanning is in the initial staging of esophageal cancer due to its superior ability in detecting metastatic and regional disease even when no metastasis is detected on a CECT study. The metastatic sites can be liver, bones, or distant nodes. In up to 50% of patients at the time of diagnosis, distant metastatic disease is present, which then rules out any surgical treatment.[34]

The esophagus has a rich lymphatic drainage system with development of lymph node metastases anywhere along its length.[34] N staging is based on the number of affected nodes extending from the supraclavicular region to paragastric/celiac nodes. Nodal status can be assessed noninvasively by EUS, CT, and PET-CT, with each modality having their own limitations. Features suggestive of a metastatic lymph node are a size of >1 cm, round shape with hypoechoic texture. However, size criteria cannot be relied upon with enlarged nodes often being reactive and small nodes may contain micro-metastases.[33]

The criteria by which metastatic lymph nodes are evaluated by PET-CT are parameters such as mean standardized uptake value (SUV mean), metabolic tumor volume (MTV), intratumoral metabolic heterogeneity.[33]

The reported sensitivity of PET-CT for periesophageal nodes is poor due to its poor spatial resolution limiting the differentiation of periesophageal nodes from the primary tumor,[34] smaller nodes (2–10 mm), and nodes near the GEJ.[33]

Even though most esophageal carcinomas appear FDG avid at PET-CT, the investigation has some limitations.[37]

- Positron emission tomography-CT has reduced spatial and contrast resolution which limits the entire anatomic extent of the primary mass to be evaluated.

- Not possible to assess the depth of local tumor invasion in most cases.
- May not be possible to detect early-stage cancer on PET-CT.
- It has limited role in assessing spread to locoregional lymph node.

However, for T or local staging, PET is not the investigation of choice. If a tumor is not detected on PET-CT, it is likely to be T2 or less in 70% of cases.[36]

In patients of esophageal cancer, use of PET-CT has been found to improve patient stratification, reduce relapse rate and increase overall survival after esophagectomy. It should be considered in all patients prior to radical treatment as it has the ability to correctly upstage up to 20% of patients.

Treatment

A primary tumor that is T1 or T2, i.e., confined to the esophageal wall is potentially curable by esophagectomy. However, most of the patients present with locally advanced disease and ~50% have distant metastasis at the time of presentation. Those with periesophageal involvement (T3 stage) are treated with combined therapy in the form of neoadjuvant chemotherapy and radiotherapy followed by esophagectomy. T4 tumors are treated with definitive chemoradiotherapy, while patients with distant metastasis undergo palliative therapy.

As per the National Comprehensive Cancer Network (NCCN) guidelines, surgical treatment in the form of esophagectomy is the standard of care for esophageal cancer. Endoscopic treatment in the form of endoscopic mucosal resection (EMR) and submucosal dissection (SMD), for stage T1a and T1b tumors are being performed at specialized centers and found to be effective in achieving curative rates only for preinvasive and superficial esophageal cancer.

Even though surgical resection is the mainstay for management of locoregional esophageal cancer, the reported 5-year survival postsurgery is poor ~20–33%.[41] Definitive chemoradiation is the treatment of choice for locoregionally advanced esophageal SCC, while multimodal therapy including surgery is the preferred treatment for EAC.

Trimodality therapy, i.e.,—combination of neoadjuvant concurrent chemoradiation followed by surgery is the standard of care for locally advanced thoracic esophageal cancer. For SCC of cervical esophagus, definitive chemoradiation is the treatment recommended. As per literature, there is significant difference in the response of tumor and recurrence pattern of esophageal SCC compared to EAC. Adenocarcinoma has been found to be less sensitive to chemoradiation compared to SCC with higher rates of metastases.

Patients presenting with advanced stage disease of esophageal cancer require palliative intervention which involves multidisciplinary approach to improve their quality of life for management of digestive obstruction, tracheoesophageal fistulas, malnutrition and pain. Endoscopic stenting should be considered in all patients with complete dysphagia for infiltrating tumors < 12 cm in length and at least 3 cm below the upper esophageal sphincter (UES).[42]

FOREIGN BODIES

Foreign body ingestion is most commonly seen in children with psychiatric disorders, developmental delay, and those < 6 years of age.[43] In children, coins are the most frequently ingested foreign bodies. Bones from fish and chicken are the second most common foreign body in both children and adults. Most frequently they get lodged in the hypopharynx or cervical esophagus and may be difficult to visualize endoscopically. Patients with history of foreign body ingestion and impaction may present with symptoms such as dysphagia, odynophagia, and foreign body sensation or food refusal.

Majority of the foreign bodies in the GIT are seen to pass spontaneously without intervening, with 10–20% requiring endoscopic removal and only 1% requiring open surgery, secondary to complication. Imaging has an important role to play in the diagnosis in predicting outcome and in detecting complications especially in pediatric patients as often the ingestion is not witnessed and children are not able to give a history.[43] They are initially evaluated with plain radiographs of the neck, chest and abdomen. Barium studies are generally discouraged as they may hinder with attempts at endoscopic examination and retrieval later on. CT may be useful in select cases for definitive diagnosis or localization, prior to endoscopy, when perforation or another complication is suspected or assess for radiolucent objects **(Figs. 35A to E)**.

Coin ingestions are most common around 1–3 years of age and account for around 80% of all foreign body ingestions. They usually do not cause major injury as they are inert and blunt, unless they get lodged in the esophagus and cause obstruction. Most often, once the ingested coin reaches the stomach, it is likely to pass without intervention. Button battery ingestion is known to cause serious harm as they react with saliva to produce an electric current. The caustic injury can occur even when the batteries are dead. Batteries of size > 20 mm are frequently used in household products, toys, etc., and are associated with poorer outcomes, as they can get lodged in UES.

Food impaction is more commonly seen in adults, and it is more challenging to diagnose as food being organic in nature appears radiolucent on plain radiographs.

Sharp objects such as fish bones, needles, pins, and metals or glass fragments can injure or perforate the esophageal mucosa.

Smooth foreign bodies, such as coins, buttons, and dental crowns generally pass through the esophagus but may lodge in areas of normal anatomic narrowing at the thoracic inlet, aortic arch, or diaphragmatic hiatus. Sharp

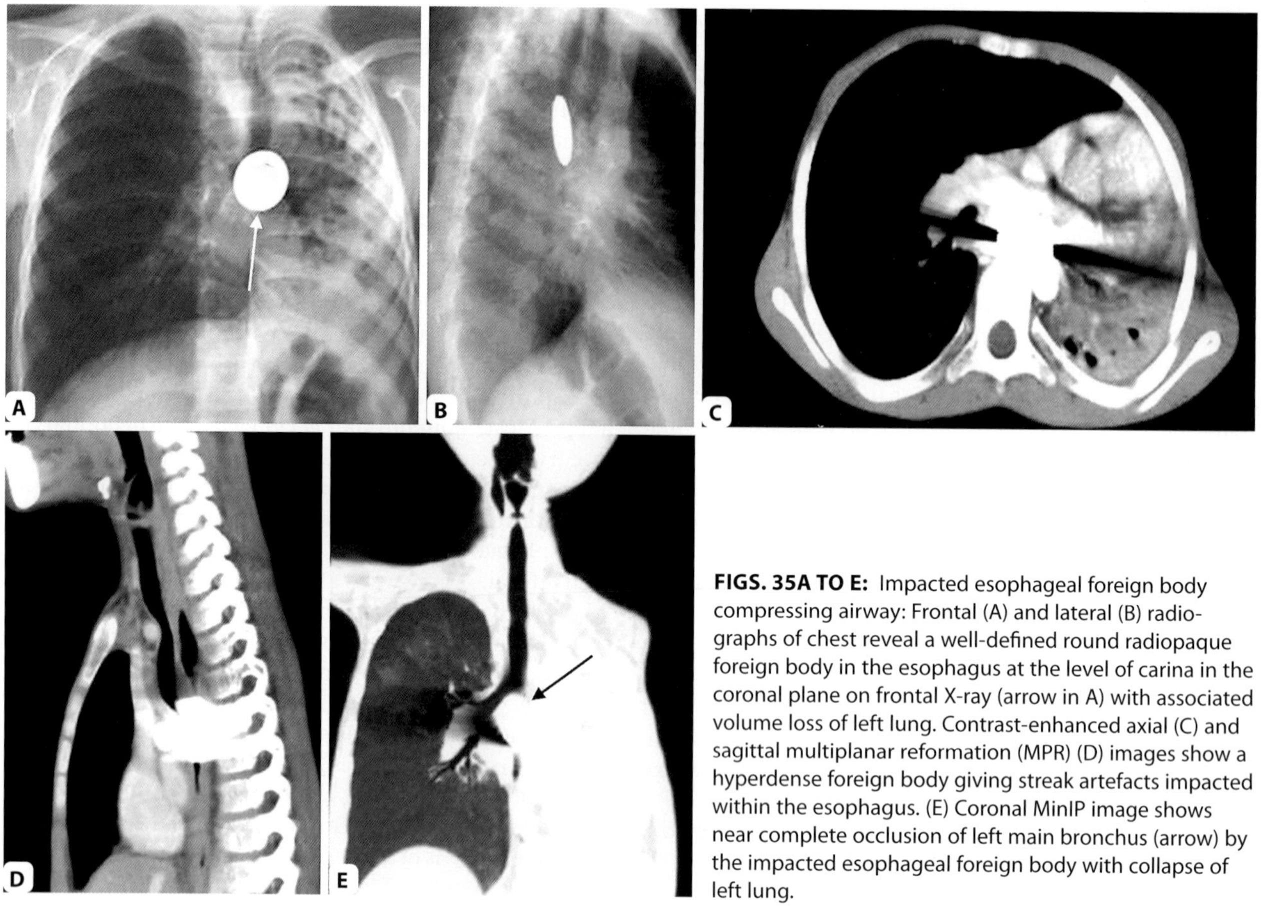

FIGS. 35A TO E: Impacted esophageal foreign body compressing airway: Frontal (A) and lateral (B) radiographs of chest reveal a well-defined round radiopaque foreign body in the esophagus at the level of carina in the coronal plane on frontal X-ray (arrow in A) with associated volume loss of left lung. Contrast-enhanced axial (C) and sagittal multiplanar reformation (MPR) (D) images show a hyperdense foreign body giving streak artefacts impacted within the esophagus. (E) Coronal MinIP image shows near complete occlusion of left main bronchus (arrow) by the impacted esophageal foreign body with collapse of left lung.

objects may arrest at any esophageal level. Metallic or dense foreign bodies are recognized on plain films of the neck or chest with a positive predictive value of 100%. It is much lower for radiolucent objects such as fish, bone, and wood. Flat objects such as coins are oriented in the coronal plane of the esophagus in contrast to the sagittal plane orientation in the trachea. Obstructing foreign bodies may cause a gas-fluid level in the esophagus or tracheal displacement.

Water-soluble contrast is indicated for the initial swallow to exclude perforation. Barium may be used for subsequent swallows. Cotton balls or marshmallows soaked in barium may be useful to demonstrate a small and hard to detect foreign body. 80% of foreign bodies pass through the GIT spontaneously. If the diameter of the foreign body is too large to pass through the areas of esophageal narrowing, it lodges frequently at one of the three abovementioned areas of esophageal narrowing. Endoscopic removal of the obstructing foreign body may be required in such cases.

On plain frontal radiographs, coins can be differentiated from button batteries by their radiographic densities. While coins show homogeneous radiodensity, the ingested battery shows a central area of decreased density with a rim of increased density.[44]

Computed tomography is a sensitive modality for the detection of a foreign body, especially those that are radiolucent on plain radiography, such as wood, plastic, chewed food, fish, and chicken bones. In adults, fish bone ingestion is commonly encountered in the emergency department.[45]

Plastic is mostly not detected on plain radiographs as it lacks contrast with soft tissues. On CT, it is often seen as an object distending the esophagus with trapped air in the form of bubbles due to secretions cranial and caudal to the ingested object. Evaluating in sagittal and coronal planes in both soft tissue and lung window is useful as it may provide a clue to the localization of the foreign body which may be missed when viewed only in the axial plane.[45]

A simple coin can be allowed to pass through the esophagus without worrying for any corrosive esophageal injury. However, button battery ingestion is a medical emergency and needs to be removed immediately by endoscopy, so as to prevent substantial damage to the esophagus. Due to its electrochemical properties, they can cause local cell death and mucosal necrosis. Complications secondary to ingestion of a button battery may range from local erosion to esophageal perforation to tracheoesophageal fistula. Fatal aortoesophageal fistulas have also been reported.

One must remember that proper history and physical examination of the patient is very important as chronic impaction of a foreign body in the esophagus may produce features of erosion, fistula formation, and inflammatory reaction which may be similar to findings produced by a malignant process.[46]

EXTRINSIC NARROWING

Vascular Ring

Vascular ring is an aortic arch anomaly in which the trachea and esophagus are surrounded by vascular structures. The most common aortic arch anomaly is the left aortic arch with an aberrant right subclavian artery which occurs in 1 in 200 individuals.[47] The aberrant right subclavian artery arises from the diverticulum of Kommerell which is a persistence of the embryologic right aortic arch. In most cases, the aberrant right subclavian artery crosses posterior to the esophagus **(Figs. 36A to C)**. Patients are symptomatic at extremes of age with children usually presenting with tracheal obstruction or dysphagia. While in adults, aneurysms of aberrant subclavian artery or a prominent diverticulum of Kommerell can occur resulting in dysphagia, classically known as "dysphagia lusoria".[44]

Enlarged Thyroid Gland

Mass effect due to enlarged thyroid gland is most often seen at the level of cervical esophagus. When the enlarged thyroid extends into the superior mediastinum it can result in a mass effect on the upper thoracic esophagus at esophagography. High-resolution ultrasonography of the neck can confirm thyroid disease and CT neck apart from confirming helps in determining its extent **(Figs. 37A to C)**.

Enlarged Cervical Osteophytes

Cervical osteophytes are seen in around 20–30% of the elderly who may have neck stiffness and localized or radiating pain. However, large osteophytes have been known to cause dysphagia, odynophagia and globus symptoms. Dysphagia has also been found in patients of diffuse skeletal hyperostosis. The large osteophytes may impinge and mechanically compress the pharynx or upper esophagus causing obstruction **(Fig. 38)**. Another factor that can lead to dysphagia is the impaired tilting of the epiglottis over the laryngeal inlet by the mid cervical (C3–C4) osteophytes.

Retention of food and aspiration has been more often seen in patients with increased osteophytic size (> 10 mm) that impinge on the pharynx than those without enlarged osteophytes.[48]

Cervical osteophyte-induced dysphagia is treated depending on the nature and severity of the disease. Sedation, anti-inflammatory drugs, muscle relaxants, and appropriate soft diet are known to provide substantial relief. Surgical excision of large osteophytosis is reserved for patients with severe symptoms or those whose conservative treatment fails.

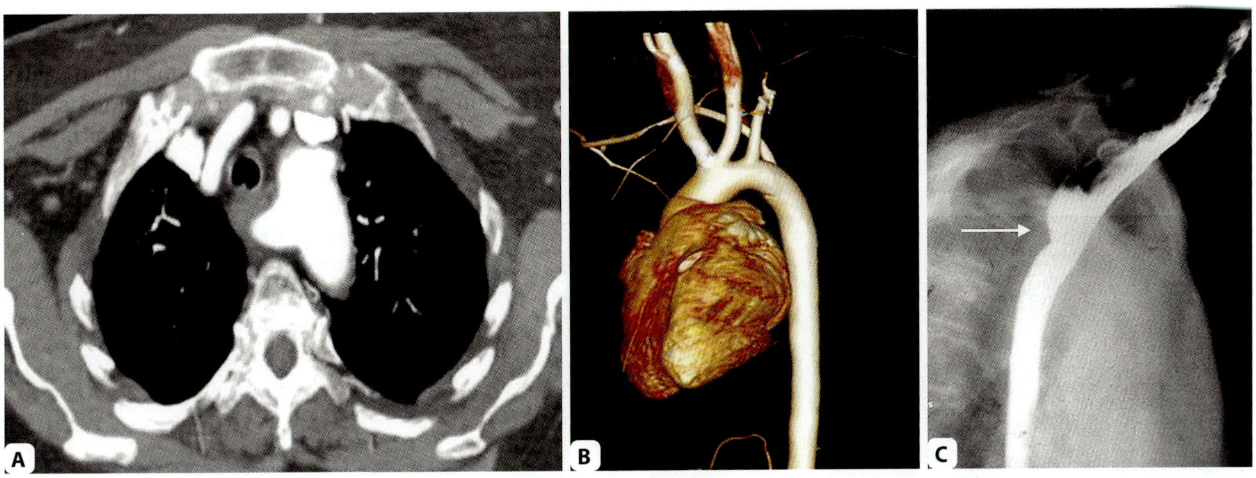

FIGS. 36A TO C: (A) Axial contrast-enhanced computed tomography (CECT) image shows left aortic arch with aberrant origin of the right subclavian artery coursing behind the esophagus; (B) Volume rendering technique (VRT) image depicts the aberrant origin of the right subclavian artery behind the origin of the great vessels; (C) Barium swallow study shows oblique indentation (arrow) on the upper esophagus-dysphagia lusoria.

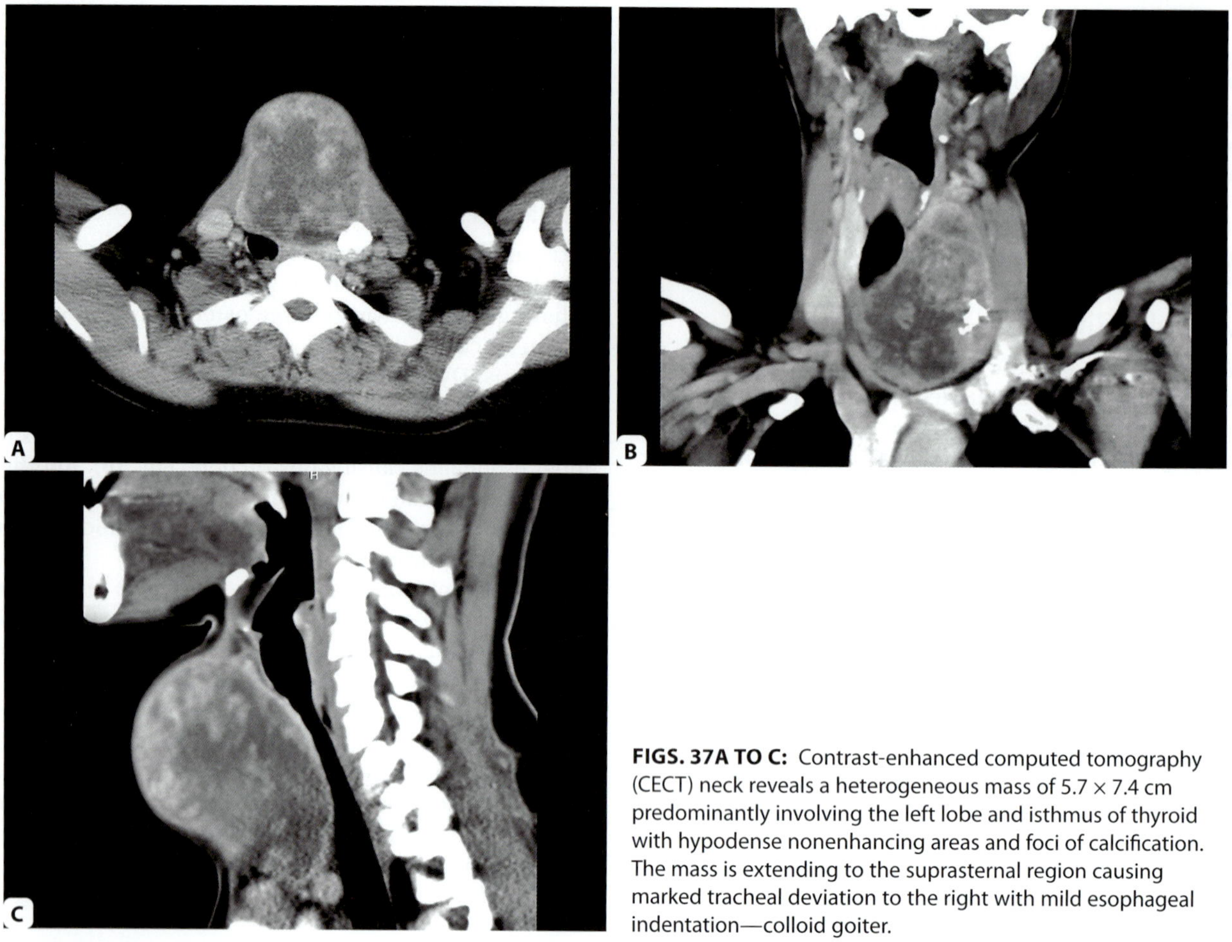

FIGS. 37A TO C: Contrast-enhanced computed tomography (CECT) neck reveals a heterogeneous mass of 5.7 × 7.4 cm predominantly involving the left lobe and isthmus of thyroid with hypodense nonenhancing areas and foci of calcification. The mass is extending to the suprasternal region causing marked tracheal deviation to the right with mild esophageal indentation—colloid goiter.

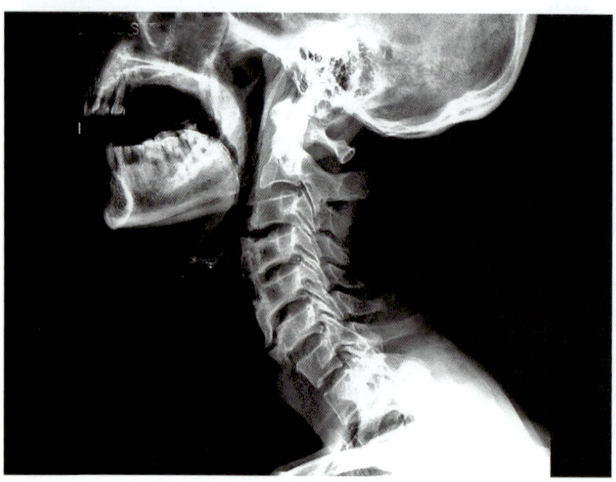

FIG. 38: X-ray lateral view cervical spine reveals enlarged osteophytes of C5, C6 vertebrae impinging on the esophagus.

CONCLUSION

Dysphagia is a common problem and is generally due to an obstruction which may be either mechanical or functional. Patient demographics and symptomatology have an important role in determining the likely cause (i.e., oropharyngeal or esophageal) in around 85% of patients which help in guiding subsequent investigation and management **(Flowchart 2)**.

Knowledge of the radiological evaluation and imaging spectrum of the possible causes of dysphagia is essential for treatment planning.

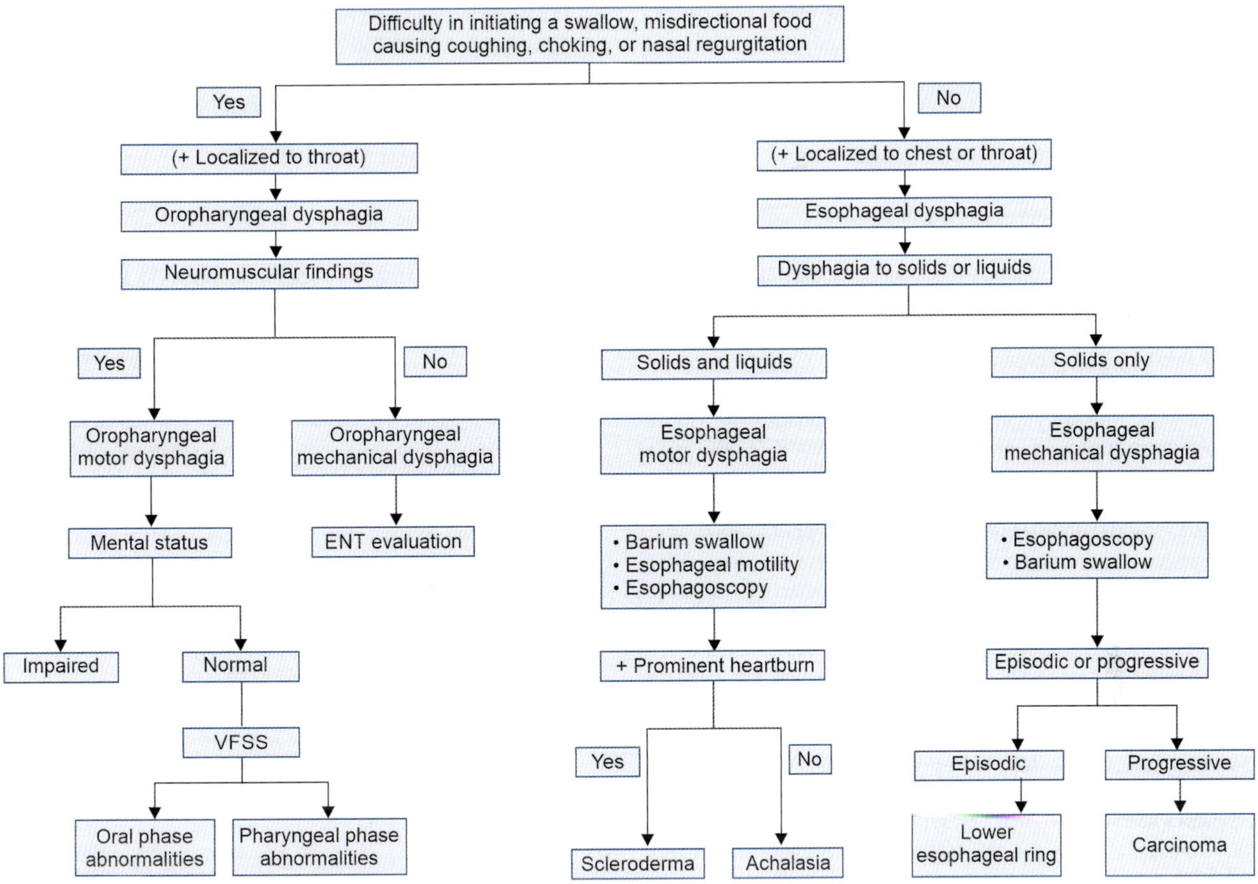

FLOWCHART 2: Algorithmic approach to a patient with dysphagia.
(VFSS: videofluoroscopic swallowing study)

REFERENCES

1. Carucci LR, Turner MA. Dysphagia revisited: Common and Unusual causes. Radiographics. 2015;35:105-22.
2. Mascarenhas A, Mendo R, O'Neill C, Franco AR, Mendes R, Simão I, et al. Current Approach to Dysphagia: A Review Focusing on Esophageal Motility Disorders and Their Treatment. GE-Portuguese J Gastroenterol. 2023;30(6): 403-13.
3. Dodds WJ, Stewart ET, Logemann JA. Physiology and radiology of the normal oral and pharyngeal phases of swallowing. AJR Am J Roentgenol. 1990;154:953-63.
4. Jaffer NM, Ng E, Au FW, Steele CM. Fluoroscopic evaluation of oropharyngeal dysphagia: anatomic, technical, and common etiologic factors. AJR Am J Roentgenol. 2015;204:49-58.
5. Goyal RK. Alteration in gastrointestinal function. Dysphagia. In: Fauci AS, Braunwald E, Kasper DL, Hauser S, Longo DL, Jameson J, Loscalzo J (Eds). Harrison's Principles of Internal Medicine, 17th edition. United States: McGraw Hill (Medical); 2008. pp. 237-42.
6. Spieker MR. Evaluating dysphagia. Am Fam Physician. 2000;61(12):3639-48.
7. Kuo P, Holloway RH, Nguyen NQ. Current and future techniques in the evaluation of dysphagia. J Gastroenterol Hepatol. 2012;27:873-81.
8. Levine MS, Rubesin SE. Radiologic Investigation of Dysphagia. AJR Am J Roentgenol. 1990;154:1157-63.
9. Cook IJ. Oropharyngeal Dysphagia. Gastroenterol Clin N Am. 2009;38:411-31.
10. Tao TY, Menias CO, Herman TE, McAlister WH, Balfe DM. Easier to swallow: Pictorial review of structural findings of the pharynx at barium pharyngography. Radiographics. 2013;33:E189-E208.
11. Jones B, Donner MW. Examination of the patient with Dysphagia. Radiology. 1988;167:319-26.
12. Kahrilas PJ, Hirano I. Disease of the esophagus. In: longo DL, Kasper DL, Jameson JL, Hauser S, Jameson J, Loscalzo J (Eds). Harrison's Principles of Internal Medicine, 18th edition. United States: McGraw Hill Professional; 2012;292:2427-37.
13. Ba-Salamah A, Zacheri J, Noebauer-Huhmann IM, Uffmann M, Matzek WK, Pinker K, et al. Dedicated multi-detector CT of the esophagus: Spectrum of diseases. Abdom Imaging. . 2009;34(1):3-18.
14. Ha HK, Park SH, Lee SS, Kim AY. Gastrointestinal tract–Esophagus In: Hagga JR, Dogra VS, Forsting M, Ha HK, Gilkeson RC, Sundaram M (Eds). CT and MRI of the Whole Body, 5th edition. Philadelphia, PA: Mosby (Elsevier); 2009. pp. 1213-371.

15. Riddell AM, Hillier J, Brown G, King DM, Wotherspoon AC, Thompson JN, et al. Potential of surface-coil MRI for staging of esophageal cancer. AJR Am J Roentgenol. 2006;187:1280-7.
16. Debi U, Sharma M, Singh L, Sinha A. Barium esophagogram in various esophageal diseases: A pictorial essay. Indian J Radiol Imaging. 2019;29(02):141-54.
17. Jang KM, Lee KS, Lee SJ, Kim EA, Kim TS, Han D, et al. The spectrum of benign esophageal lesions: imaging findings. Korean J Radiol. 2002;3:199-210.
18. Eisenberg RL. Esophagus (Section-1). In: Eisenberg RL (Ed). Gastrointestinal Radiology. A Pattern Approach, 4th edition. United States: Lippincot Williams & Wilkins; 2003. pp. 3-150.
19. Rabushka LS, Fishman EK, Kuhlman JE. CT evaluation of achalasia. J Comput Assist Tomogr. 1991;15(3):434-9.
20. Pawa S, Prakash A. Imaging of the esophagus. In: Gupta AK, Chowdhury V, Khandelwal (Eds). AIIMS–MAMC–PGI's Comprehensive Textbook of Diagnostic Radiology, 1st edition. New Delhi: Jaypee Brothers Medical Publishers (P) Ltd. (The Health Sciences Publisher); 2016. pp. 1139-57.
21. Fabian T, Leung A. Epidemiology of Barrett's esophagus and esophageal carcinoma. Surg Clin North Am. 2021;101(3):381-9.
22. Leslie P, Carding PN, Wilson JA. Investigation and management of chronic dysphagia. BMJ. 2003;326:453-6.
23. Luedtke P, Levine MS, Rubesin SE, Weinstein DS, Larfer I. Radiologic diagnosis of benign esophageal strictures: A pattern approach. RadioGraphics. 2003;23(4):897-909.
24. Sam JW, Levine MS, Rubesin SE, Laufer I. The "foamy" esophagus: A radiographic sign of Candida esophagitis. AJR Am J Roentgenol. 2000;174:999-1002.
25. Berkovich GY, Levine MS, Miller WT. CT findings in patients with esophagitis. Am J Roentgenol. 2000;175(5):1431-4.
26. Rosario MT, Raso CL, Comer GM. Esophageal tuberculosis. Dig Dis Sci. 1989;34:1281-4.
27. Nagi B, Lal A, Kochhar R, Bhasin DK, Gulati M, Suri S, et al. Imaging of esophageal tuberculosis. Acta Radiol. 2003;44: 329-33.
28. Agarwal A, Srivastava DN, Madhusudhan KS. Corrosive injury of the upper gastrointestinal tract: the evolving role of a radiologist. Br J Radiol. 2020;93(1114):20200528.
29. White SB, Levine MS, Rubesin SE, Spencer GS, Katzka DA, Laufer I. The small-caliber esophagus: radiographic sign of idiopathic eosinophilic esophagitis. Radiology. 2010;256: 127-34.
30. Lewis RB, Mehrotra AK, Rodriguez P, Levine MS. From the radiologic pathology archives: Esophageal neoplasms: radiologic-pathologic correlation. Radiographics. 2013;33: 1083-108.
31. Winant AJ, Gollub MJ, Shia J, Antonescu C, Bains MS, Levine MS. Imaging and clinicopathologic features of esophageal gastrointestinal stromal tumors. AJR Am J Roentgenol. 2014; 203:306-14.
32. Levine MS, Buck JL, Pantongrag-Brown L, Buetow PC, Hallman JR, Sobin LH. Fibrovascular polyps of the esophagus: clinical, radiographic, and pathologic findings in 16 patients. AJR Am J Roentgenol. 1996;166:781-7.
33. Jayaprakasam VS, Yeh R, Ku GY, Petkovska I, Fuqua III JL, Gollub M, et al. Role of imaging in esophageal cancer management in 2020: update for radiologists. Am J Roentgenol. 2020;215(5):1072-84.
34. Withey SJ, Goh V, Foley KG. State-of-the-art imaging in oesophago-gastric cancer. Br J Radiol. 2022;95(1137): 20220410.
35. Umeoka S, Koyama T, Togashi K, Saga T, Watanabe G, Shimada Y, et al. Esophageal Cancer: Evaluation with triple-phase dynamic CT-initial experience. Radiology. 2006;239(3): 777-83.
36. Godfrey EM, Freeman AH. The esophagus. In: Adam A, Dixon AK, Gillard JH, Schaefer-Prokop CM (Eds.). Grainger and Allison's Diagnostic Radiology (A textbook of Medical Imaging), 6th edition. 2015;26(1):610-26.
37. Hong SJ, Kim TJ, Nam KB, Lee IS, Yang HC, Cho S, et al. New TNM staging system for esophageal cancer: What chest radiologists need to know. radiographics. 2014;34:1722-40.
38. Chakrabarty N, Mahajan A, Patil P, Chowhan M, Munmmudi N, Niyogi D, et al. Imaging recommendations for diagnosis, Staging, and management of esophageal cancer. Indian J Med Paediatr Oncol. 2023;44(02):229-40.
39. Shemmeri E, Fabian T. Staging of esophageal malignancy. Surg Clin. 2021;101(3):405-14.
40. Picus D, Balfe DM, Koehler RE, Roper CL, Owen JW. Computed tomography in the staging of esophageal carcinoma. Radiology. 1983;146:433-8.
41. Watkins AA, Zerillo JA, Kent MS. Trimodality approach for esophageal malignancies. Surg Clin. 2021;101(3):453-65.
42. Federico JA, Martin JT. Surgeons' Role in Local Palliation of Esophageal Cancer. Surg Clin North Am. 2021;101(3):489-97.
43. Powers K, Baldassari C, Lucas J. Pediatric Esophageal Foreign Bodies and Caustic Ingestions. Otolaryngologic Clin North Am. 2024:S0030-6665.
44. Hryhorczuk AL, Lee EY, Eisenberg RL. Esophageal abnormalities in pediatric patients. AJR Am J Roentgenol. 2013;201:W519-32.
45. Seghers VJ, Herman Kan J, Somcio R, Sher AC, Paul Guillerman R, Sammer MB. CT imaging of esophageal foreign bodies in children: a pictorial essay. Japanese J Radiol. 2021:1-9.
46. Young CA, Menias CO, Bhalla S, Prasad SR. CT features of esophageal emergencies. Radiographics. 2008;28(6): 1541-53.
47. Gilkeson RC, Kolodny S. Thoracic Aorta. in: Hagga JR, Dogra VS, Forsting M, Ha HK, Gilkeson RC, Sundaram M. (Eds). CT and MRI of the Whole Body, 5th edition. Philadelphia, PA: Mosby (Elsevier). 2009;1:1091-132.
48. Strasser G, Schima W, Schober E, Pokieser P, Kaider A, Denk DM. Cervical osteophytes impinging on the pharynx: importance of size and concurrent disorders for development of aspiration. AJR Am J Roentgenol. 2000;174(2):449-53.

CHAPTER 2

Gaurav Shanker Pradhan, Rashmi Dixit, Radhika Batra

Imaging Approach to Gastric and Duodenal Pathologies

INTRODUCTION

A wide spectrum of pathological conditions affecting the stomach and duodenum can be detected and evaluated at imaging. These conditions vary from benign etiologies such as inflammation to malignant etiologies like carcinoma or lymphoma. Radiologists should be familiar with the imaging features of various gastric and duodenal lesions. Cross-sectional imaging modalities, especially multidetector computed tomography (MDCT) and magnetic resonance imaging (MRI), enable comprehensive evaluation of the stomach, duodenum, and adjacent abdominal organs with MDCT being the first-line imaging for such patients. Contrast-enhanced computed tomography (CECT) is the preferred modality for the staging of malignant gastric lesions. Neutral or negative oral contrast material can aid in the detection of mucosal and submucosal enhancing masses. Dual or triple phase scans after intravenous contrast administration can be used to diagnose active bleeding, delineate hypovascular and hypervascular masses and look for metastases. Other imaging modalities such as single photon emission computed tomography (SPECT)/CT and positron emission tomography (PET)/CT can also provide useful information in specific scenarios. Endoscopy is the standard modality for the definitive diagnosis of most gastric and duodenal pathologic conditions with the ability to perform tissue sampling. It helps to diagnose small gastric ulcers and areas of induration and differentiate between mucosal, submucosal, and intramural masses.

STOMACH

The stomach, deriving from the foregut, is anchored in place by five ligaments: the gastrohepatic ligament, hepatoduodenal ligament, gastrosplenic ligament, splenorenal ligament, and gastrocolic ligament. The gastrohepatic and hepatoduodenal ligaments collectively form the lesser omentum, extending between the liver hilum and the lesser curvature of the stomach and proximal duodenum. Meanwhile, the gastrocolic ligament connects the greater curvature of the stomach to the transverse colon, constituting the greater omentum. The gastrosplenic ligament links the hilum of the spleen to the gastric fundus along the greater curvature of the stomach. The splenorenal ligament, a misnomer, spans between the spleen hilum and the anterior pararenal space, housing the pancreatic tail and splenic vessels.[1,2]

Peritoneal lining covers the gastric ligaments, encompassing adipose tissue, nerves, lymphatics, and blood vessels. On CT scans, blood vessels coursing through these ligaments serve as reference points. The left and right gastric arteries form an arcade within the gastrohepatic ligament. The portal triad (hepatic artery, portal vein, and common bile duct) traverses the hepatoduodenal ligament. Similarly, the right and left gastroepiploic arteries create an arcade within the gastrocolic ligament. The gastrosplenic ligament, located near the splenic hilum, contains the short gastric and left gastroepiploic arteries. Within the splenorenal ligament reside the distal splenic artery and vein.[2]

Lymphatics within the gastric ligaments facilitate the spread of gastric cancer, draining into the para-aortic lymph nodes. Alternatively, tumors penetrating the subserosal connective tissue of the stomach can disseminate directly through the adipose tissue of gastric ligaments, termed "subperitoneal dissemination". **Table 1** lists the various conditions that can affect the stomach and the duodenum.

GASTRIC NEOPLASMS

Gastric Polyps

Gastric polyps can arise from the mucosa or submucosa or even be extrinsic. Gastric polyps can be epithelial, mesenchymal, and hamartomatous; the epithelial polyps

TABLE 1: Gastric pathological conditions.

Neoplastic	Inflammatory and infectious	Emergencies
Adenocarcinoma	Gastritis	Emphysematous gastritis
Lymphoma	Anisakiasis	Gastric hemorrhage
Neuroendocrine tumor	Ménétrier disease	Bouveret syndrome
Mesenchymal tumors • Gastrointestinal stromal tumor (GIST) • Non-GIST sarcoma • Lipoma • Lipomatosis • Leiomyoma • Schwannoma • Glomus tumor	Gastric pneumatosis	Gastric rotations and volvulus
Metastasis		Bezoars

includes hyperplastic, fundic gland, and adenomatous subtypes. The prevalence and the type of the polyps also depend on the risk factors in the population under consideration. Hyperplastic and adenomatous polyps are encountered more often in a *Helicobacter pylori (H. pylori)*-infected territory while fundic gland polyps (FGPs) are seen with increased proton pump inhibitor (PPI) usage.[3] In most cases, they are asymptomatic but may present with bleeding, anemia, obstruction, or abdominal pain when large. The clinical importance of these polyps is because of the variable malignant potential and their cooccurrence with other risk factors for gastric malignancy. For these reasons, polyps need to be biopsied or resected wherever possible, along with multiple biopsies from surrounding flat gastric mucosa.[4]

Fundic Gland Polyps

Fundic gland polyps are one of the most common polyps found in the stomach on upper GI (UGI) endoscopy.[5] Sporadic FGPs are sessile polyps and are distributed exclusively in the body and fundus of the stomach with the lesions varying from 1 to 8 mm in size, most commonly noted in middle-aged women.[6] Hypergastrinemia associated with a gastrinoma, Zollinger–Ellison syndrome, or long-term therapy with PPIs has been shown to be associated with FGPs. Few studies also conclude that sporadic FGPs are not associated with atrophic gastritis and have low prevalence of *H. pylori* infection.[7] About 30–100% of patients with familial adenomatous polyposis (FAP) have been reported to have gastric polyps.[8] Majority (95%) are FGPs while only remaining 5% are actually adenomatous polyps and arise from a mutation in the *APC* gene.[9]

Dysplasia is not common and usually of low grade. The risk factors for dysplasia include large polyp size, and presence of antral gastritis.[10] Polyps associated with PPI use have virtually no malignant potential.[3] As per current guidelines, polypectomy is not required for sporadic FGPs because of their low malignant potential.[8] Biopsy is usually indicated at the initial endoscopy to rule out dysplasia or adenocarcinoma. FGPs > 1 cm in size are resected assuming sampling error from forceps biopsy alone.[6]

On double-contrast barium studies, polyps on the dependent gastric surface appear as smooth, round filling defects in the pool of barium while polyps on the nondependent surface are seen as ring shadows etched in white. In cases of pedunculated polyps, the stalk is seen en face as an inner ring shadow overlying the head of the polyp giving rise to the "Mexican hat" sign.

Hyperplastic Polyps

These are the second most common gastric polyps after FGPs and typically occur in the sixth and seventh decades. These polyps are usually sessile or pedunculated, smooth, dome-shaped, usually < 2 cm.[8] These are usually multiple and are randomly distributed anywhere in the stomach, although antrum is commonly involved.

These polyps have a strong tendency to occur in the setting of inflammatory disorders such as chronic gastritis, *H. pylori* gastritis, pernicious anemia, gastric surgical site, bile reflux disease, and chemical gastritis.[11,12] They appear as radiolucent filling defects if present on dependent posterior wall or as ring shadows with white rim of barium, if present on nondependent anterior wall. Large hyperplastic polyps often become pedunculated and can present with gastric outlet obstruction because the polyp may obstruct or prolapse through the pylorus.

Like FGPs, hyperplastic polyps also seem to have low neoplastic potential but they have a tendency to have synchronous cancers in the adjacent gastric mucosa especially if associated with chronic gastritis.[13] Because of low risk of dysplasia and synchronous cancers there is confusion regarding the management of hyperplastic polyps. Recommendations of size criteria for polypectomy range from > 2 cm as per few authors and > 0.5 cm as per others.[14] Because of more risk of adenocarcinoma in the surrounding nonpolypoid flat tissue as compared to polyps per se, multiple biopsies from the flat uninvolved mucosa are recommended.[8]

Adenomatous Polyps

Adenomatous polyps are premalignant and are histologically divided into tubular, villous, and tubulo-villous subtypes. These polyps are usually solitary and seen in the antrum; however, these can be seen anywhere in the stomach. They vary in size from millimeters to centimeters and larger size > 2 cm and villous histology increases the risk of neoplasia (28–40%).[15]

They are commonly seen as sessile or flat lesions but the pedunculated form may be seen uncommonly. They are also seen in various polyposis syndromes like FAP, Gardner's syndrome, and Turcot syndrome. These lesions are usually seen in relation to atrophic gastritis and in the background of intestinal metaplasia. *H. pylori* infection is not associated with these polyps. They are premalignant with high-grade dysplastic changes and are currently redefined as noninvasive intraepithelial neoplasia (NiN).[16] It is hence recommended to remove the adenoma with further examination of entire gastric mucosa and biopsy, if necessary.

Hamartomatous Polyps

These are mucosal polyps but can arise from any of the embryonic layers and are composed of disorganized tissue in situ. These polyps are seen sporadically, though occasionally they occur as part of a syndrome such as Peutz–Jeghers syndrome, juvenile polyposis, etc. Although hamartomatous means non-neoplastic, they can coexist with adenomatous polyps.[17]

Peutz–Jeghers syndrome is an autosomal dominant hereditary disorder which characteristically has multiple hamartomatous polyps along the entire gastrointestinal (GI) system and mucocutaneous hyperpigmentation at the lips.[18] Gastric polyps are seen in 15–30% of the cases. Gastric syndromic polyps are however often indistinguishable from nonspecific gastric hyperplastic polyps and hence endoscopic, pathologic, and clinical correlation is required for proper diagnosis.

Juvenile polyps and juvenile polyposis syndrome: These are mucosal tumors that consist of excess lamina propria and dilated cystic glands and hence are occasionally called inflammatory polyps or retention cysts due to these distended glands, inflammatory cells, and edema. These lesions are typically solitary pedunculated polyps and range from 3 to 20 mm in size. However, when multiple, a syndrome of juvenile polyposis should be considered.

The different subtypes are difficult to differentiate radiologically. These polyps, if small, are well circumscribed with smooth, nodular surface if seen en face and are seen to form acute angle with the gastric wall when viewed in profile on barium studies. Larger polyps have a lobulated surface and areas of erosion or ulceration mimicking malignant growth.[19]

Gastric Cancer

Gastric cancer is presently the fifth most common cancer in the world accounting for nearly 8.2% of all cancer related deaths globally.[20] Incidence of gastric cancer varies with a significant geographic heterogeneity between high-risk and low-risk countries. The reason behind this is a difference in *H. pylori* infection rates, cigarette smoking, and use of salt and salt preserved foods which are established carcinogens for gastric cancer. Other risk factors include a low intake of fruit and vegetables, a high consumption of processed meat, alcohol or tobacco, metabolic syndrome or a previous partial gastrectomy. Anisakiasis is also considered a hazard in areas such as Japan, Italy, and Spain where consumption of raw fish is high. It is a parasitic infection caused by Anisakis which causes persistent local inflammation. The principal risk factors for gastric cardia adenocarcinomas are obesity and gastroesophageal reflux. The average age at diagnosis is 68 years and it is more common in men than in women (2:1 ratio). The highest age standardized incidence rates have been reported in Mongolia and Afghanistan as 37.6 and 33.6 per 100,000 population, respectively. High-age standardized incidence rates are also seen in Asia-Pacific region (Japan and South Korea) with incidence of 29.5 per 100,000 population followed by Eastern Europe and Andean Latin America. India has relatively low-age standardized incidence rate of 7.5 per 100,000 population.[21]

The signs and symptoms of gastric cancer are non-specific and the diagnosis is often delayed. Weight loss and persistent abdominal pain are the most common symptoms at initial diagnosis. Nausea or early satiety may result from tumor involving the gastric lumen. Some patients may present with occult GI bleeding which may result in iron-deficiency anemia. Advanced cancer of the proximal stomach is a cause of pseudoachalasia, which can cause dysphagia. Patients with metastatic disease can present with palpable left supraclavicular node (Virchow's node), periumbilical nodule (sister Mary Joseph node), ascites or rarely with jaundice resulting from metastatic disease. Gastric adenocarcinoma is also associated with deep venous thrombosis, which may cause UGI bleed from the gastric mass when treated with anticoagulants.

There are many classification systems proposed to describe gastric carcinoma. Differentiation between cancers involving the gastric cardia (gastroesophageal junction, GEJ) and cancers involving the noncardia (more distal) portions of the stomach is important clinically. The incidence of noncardia gastric cancer has been steadily declining over the last several decades in most populations and is likely influenced by extrinsic factors such as *H. pylori* infection and food preservatives. Cancers of the gastric cardia, on the other hand, have epidemiological characteristics similar to esophageal adenocarcinoma like obesity and gastroesophageal reflux disease.

The Lauren classification is an important classification system which differentiates gastric carcinoma into intestinal and diffuse types based on microscopic growth pattern.[22] Diffuse cancers exhibit deep infiltration of the gastric wall and show little or no gland formation, and they are associated with inflammation and desmoplasia with relative sparing of the mucosa. They are seen mainly in younger individuals probably due to genetic predisposition. The intestinal type shows glandular proliferation, similar to that seen in the large intestine. These can be well- to poorly differentiated and tend to show an expansile growth pattern rather than an infiltrative pattern. They are related to environmental factors and are more common in high-risk regions.

Gastric cancers can be classified as epithelial, mesenchymal, neuroendocrine tumors and lymphoma, based on histopathology and cell origin. Malignant epithelial tumors are the most common, about 90% of which are adenocarcinomas. Gastric carcinomas are pathologically further subclassified, based on histological appearance into tubular, papillary, mucinous, and signet-ring cell carcinomas.

According to Borrmann's classification, they can be classified into four types based on gross macroscopic appearance.

- *Type I*: Polypoid and fungating variety
- *Type II*: Polypoid tumor with central ulceration
- *Type III*: Ulcerated tumor with infiltrative margins
- *Type IV*: Diffuse infiltrative type or linitis plastica

Staging of Gastric Cancer

The prognosis of gastric cancer correlates with the stage of the cancer determined at diagnosis according to the depth of tumor invasion (T), lymph node involvement (N), and metastasis (M). Gastric cancer is classified into two groups: early gastric cancer (EGC) and advanced gastric cancer (AGC). EGC involves the mucosa and submucosa (T1), irrespective of tumor size and lymph node involvement with a 5-year survival rate of >90%. AGC affects deeper layers (T2–T4) and has a 5-year survival rate of 7–27%.[23] The TNM staging classification is the most widely accepted system for staging gastric cancers and the 8th edition of the American Joint Committee on Cancer (AJCC) and Union for International Cancer Control TNM staging system, published in 2017, applicable to adenocarcinomas, poorly differentiated neuroendocrine carcinomas and mixed adenoneuroendocrine carcinomas is presently used.[23]

The Japanese Research Society for Gastric Carcinoma has categorized regional lymph nodes into four compartments, numbered 1 through 4.[24] Compartment 1 comprises perigastric lymph nodes situated immediately adjacent to the stomach along unnamed arteries. Compartment 2 includes nodes along the left gastric artery, the common hepatic artery, the celiac axis, and the splenic artery. Compartment 3 encompasses nodes along the hepatoduodenal ligament, nodes posterior to the head of the pancreas, and nodes at the root of the small bowel mesentery. Compartment 4 consists of para-aortic lymph nodes. Surgeons determine the extent of lymph node dissection based on the dissections of these compartments. D1 dissection involves compartment 1, D2 dissection involves compartments 1 and 2, D3 dissection involves compartments 1, 2, and 3, while D4 dissection entails the dissection of all four compartments. Surgical practices vary widely and are mainly based on the extent of lymph node dissection. Understanding nodal anatomy in gastric carcinoma is crucial for accurately staging patients and guiding appropriate treatment decisions. The International Committee on Gastric Carcinoma recommends including a minimum of 16 lymph nodes in the surgical specimen for accurate staging and prognostic prediction.[25] The N stage serves as an independent variable for survival. N0 disease is associated with a 10-year survival rate of 70%, N1 has a survival rate of 41%, and N2/N3 exhibit a 10-year survival rate of < 30%.[26]

The three main changes in the 8th TNM staging manual compared to the 7th edition are that it features three separate staging systems for gastric cancer: pretreatment clinical staging (cTNM), pathological staging assigned after surgery (pTNM), and pathological staging assigned after resection following neoadjuvant therapy (ypTNM). A change is made to the classification of tumors of the GEJ: in the current staging manual, tumors that involve the GEJ with epicenters located > 2 cm away from the GEJ or, those which having epicenters within 2 cm of it and not involving the GEJ are classified and staged as gastric cancers.[23] **Box 1** lists the essential findings to be reported for staging of gastric cancer.

Imaging Evaluation of Gastric Carcinoma

Various imaging techniques can be used in the diagnosis and staging of gastric cancer, these include double-contrast UGI barium examinations, MDCT, MRI, PET-CT, and endoscopic ultrasound (EUS). Optimal gastric distention is vital for imaging of gastric cancer and this can be achieved through administration of effervescent granules or 800 mL of water which acts as a negative contrast agent. Dynamic multiphasic CT scanning is performed after injection of approximately 85 mL of intravenous contrast at a rate of 2.5–3.0 mL/s. Arterial phase images are acquired 25–40 seconds after starting the injection of IV contrast, the venous phase images are acquired at 60–80 seconds, and

BOX 1 Essential findings to report for staging of gastric cancer.

- *Primary tumor (T)*:
  - Morphology of lesion: Polypoid, ulcerated or diffuse
  - Location: Cardia, fundus, body, antrum, pylorus, greater curvature, and lesser curvature
  - Tumor size (not a feature of staging system but is an important prognostic factor)
  - Depth of tumor invasion
  - Distance to gastroesophageal junction
  - Local extent: Presence of any extraluminal extension into the adjacent ligaments, direct invasion of nearby organs
- *Lymph Node (N)*: Presence, size, location, and number of lymph nodes in the expected nodal basins that drain the site of the primary tumor
- *Metastases (M)*:
  - Liver metastases
  - Peritoneal deposits (presence of ascites is suggestive for peritoneal involvement)
  - Nodes posterior to the head of pancreas, in the para-aortic region and in the supraclavicular region are considered distant metastases

delayed phase at 3–4 minutes.[27] MRI is not recommended for local staging of gastric cancer; however, it is useful for characterization of indeterminate liver lesions that are suspicious for metastasis. Double-contrast UGI examination can be used as a screening tool for gastric cancer. The prerequisite is 6 hours of fasting and it involves distending the gastric lumen using effervescent granules and coating its mucosal lining with high-density (210–250% wt/vol) barium suspension. Barium UGI examination can provide functional and anatomic information of the esophagus, stomach, and duodenum.

Tumor Detection and Staging

High-income East-Asian countries with a high incidence of gastric cancer have implemented screening programs for gastric cancer. Both endoscopy and double-contrast UGI barium studies were found to be effective for gastric cancer screening, and Japanese guidelines recommend these modalities for screening adults > 50 years of age. Malignant gastric ulcer is the most common presentation of gastric cancer on UGI barium studies **(Fig. 1)**. Malignant ulcers are usually nonprojecting, with ulcer brim being wide and thick with central ulceration (Carman–Kirklin meniscus sign), distorted irregular radiating folds stopping well short of ulcer brim **(Figs. 2A to C)**.[9] As opposed to malignant ulcers, a typical benign ulcer shows a projecting ulcer **(Fig. 3A)** with an ulcer collar or mound with symmetrical radiating folds reaching up to brim of the ulcer **(Fig. 3B)**. Correlative axial CECT image shows mild wall thickening in the region of the gastric antrum **(Fig. 3C)**. There is also undermining of gastric mucosa noted in benign ulcers which is seen as a filling defect/lucent line rimming the ulcer crater on double-contrast barium meal known as Hampton's line. However, the use of double-contrast UGI barium studies has been declining.

Polypoid carcinomas are lobulated masses that protrude into the lumen. They may contain one or more areas of ulceration. With ulcerated carcinomas, an irregular crater is located in a rind of malignant tissue. On profile view, these lesions are seen to be intraluminal as opposed to benign projecting ulcers, and on enface view, nodular distorted mucosal folds are seen converging to the edge of the ulcer **(Figs. 4A and B)**.

Infiltrative cancers, on the other hand, can have nonscirrhous or scirrhous (desmoplastic) histology. Nonscirrhous lesions have stomach wall thickening as well as rugal-fold thickening in the form of nodularity or spiculation of the mucosa. On the contrary, aggressive scirrhous lesions exhibit wall thickening with loss of mucosal folds. If diffuse, scirrhous lesions are called

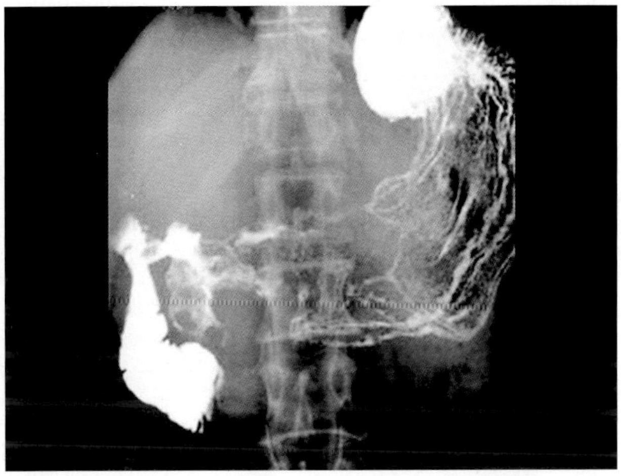

FIG. 1: Mass like intraluminal filling defect with ulcerations in antropyloric region on DCBM with extension into first part of duodenum in a patient with adenocarcinoma of stomach.
(DCBM: double-contrast barium meal study)

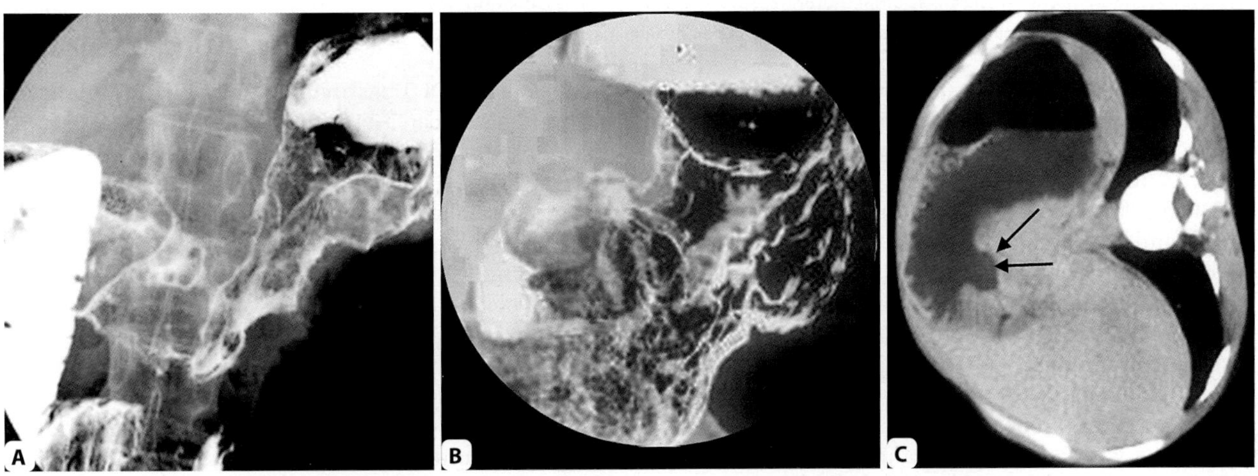

FIGS. 2A TO C: (A) DCBM shows polypoidal filling defects in body and antrum of stomach with fold destruction and ulcerations; (B) DCBM in profile view shows irregular filling defect with ulceration along the lesser curvature with asymmetric radiating folds stopping short of the ulcer crater; and (C) CECT axial image in decubitus view of the same patient reveals soft-tissue mass along lesser curvature with ulceration (arrows).
(CECT: contrast-enhanced computed tomography; DCBM: double-contrast barium meal study)

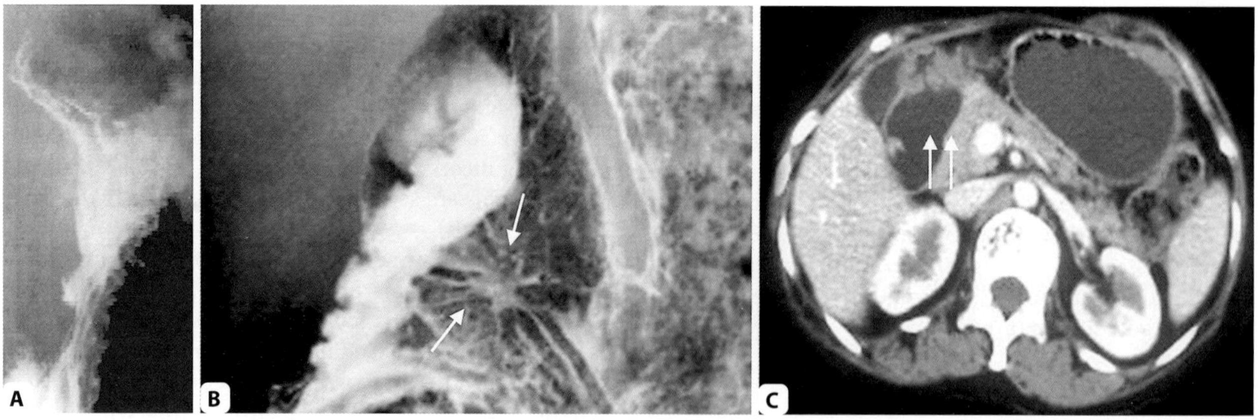

FIGS. 3A TO C: (A) Barium-filled crater seen projecting beyond the line of gastric contour on profile view; (B) Double-contrast barium meal study en-face view showing a contrast-filled benign gastric ulcer along the anterior wall of stomach with the gastric folds seen reaching up to the ulcer margin; and (C) CECT of the same patient reveals mild gastric wall thickening in the antrum with ulceration.
(CECT: contrast-enhanced computed tomography)

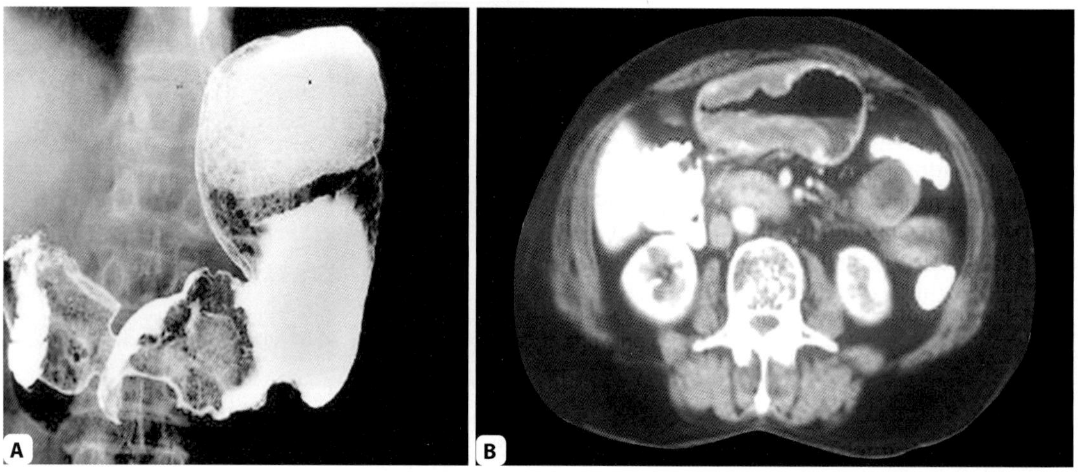

FIGS. 4A AND B: (A) Irregular polypoidal filling defect noted along greater and lesser curvature of the stomach distally on DCBM study with narrow string like pyloric canal and shouldering proximally. Visualized duodenum shows normal mucosal outline; (B) Heterogeneously enhancing polypoidal mural thickening noted in the gastric antrum on CECT. No epigastric extension is noted.
(CECT: contrast-enhanced computed tomography; DCBM: double-contrast barium meal study)

linitis plastica. They cause narrowing of the stomach with a rigid structure (leather bottle stomach) and are better appreciated on fluoroscopic imaging than endoscopy **(Figs. 5A and B)**.[19]

Presently, endoscopy is the modality of choice to detect and diagnose gastric carcinoma due to its high specificity, ability to diagnose the disease at an early stage, and the added advantage of obtaining tissue samples. It also provides access to perform EUS, which is reliable to T-stage the tumor at the time of diagnosis. EUS provides exquisite delineation of the layers of gastric walls and is the most accurate preoperative staging modality for gastric carcinoma with an accuracy ranging between 78 and 94%. The layers of the gastric wall are seen as alternating hyperechoic and hypoechoic bands—superficial mucosa, deep mucosa, submucosa, muscularis propria, and serosa. This layered appearance is disrupted in the presence of a tumor which may appear hypoechoic or hyperechoic.

The use of MDCT has improved the ability of CT scan for staging of gastric carcinoma, although, it remains inferior to EUS. A two- to three-layered structure of the normal gastric wall is seen on MDCT: a markedly enhancing mucosa layer, a submucosal layer with lower attenuation, and an outer muscular layer invested with serosa, showing moderate enhancement in the arterial and early portal venous phase of contrast enhanced CT. Macroscopically, gastric adenocarcinoma can be classified as superficial, mass forming, ulcerative, and diffuse infiltrative or unclassifiable. Superficial tumors, if flat, may be undetectable on cross-sectional imaging, but they can be visualized when they have a polypoid configuration. T1 and T2 lesions are confined to the gastric wall. T3 lesions may show slight blurring of the outer contour with perigastric fat stranding **(Figs. 6A to D)**. T4 lesions can spread via ligamentous attachments and peritoneal reflections or directly invade adjacent structures **(Figs. 7A to D)**.[27] MDCT performs better

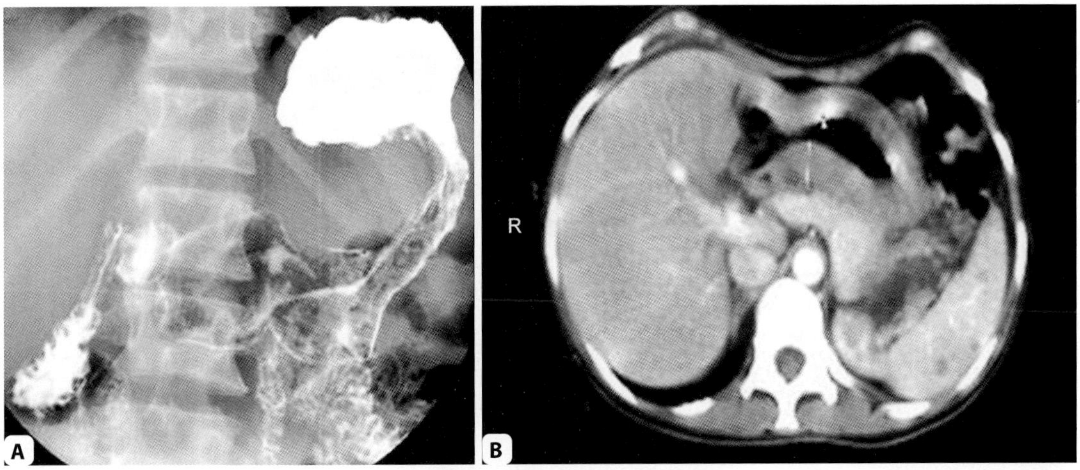

FIGS. 5A AND B: (A) DCBM reveals markedly reduced distensibility of body and antrum of stomach in a case of adenocarcinoma (Scirrhous type); (B) CECT of the same patient reveals diffuse circumferential mural thickening (~2 cm) in the region of body and antrum of stomach, note made of few hypodense lesions in the spleen suggestive of metastases.

(CECT: contrast-enhanced computed tomography; DCBM: double-contrast barium meal study)

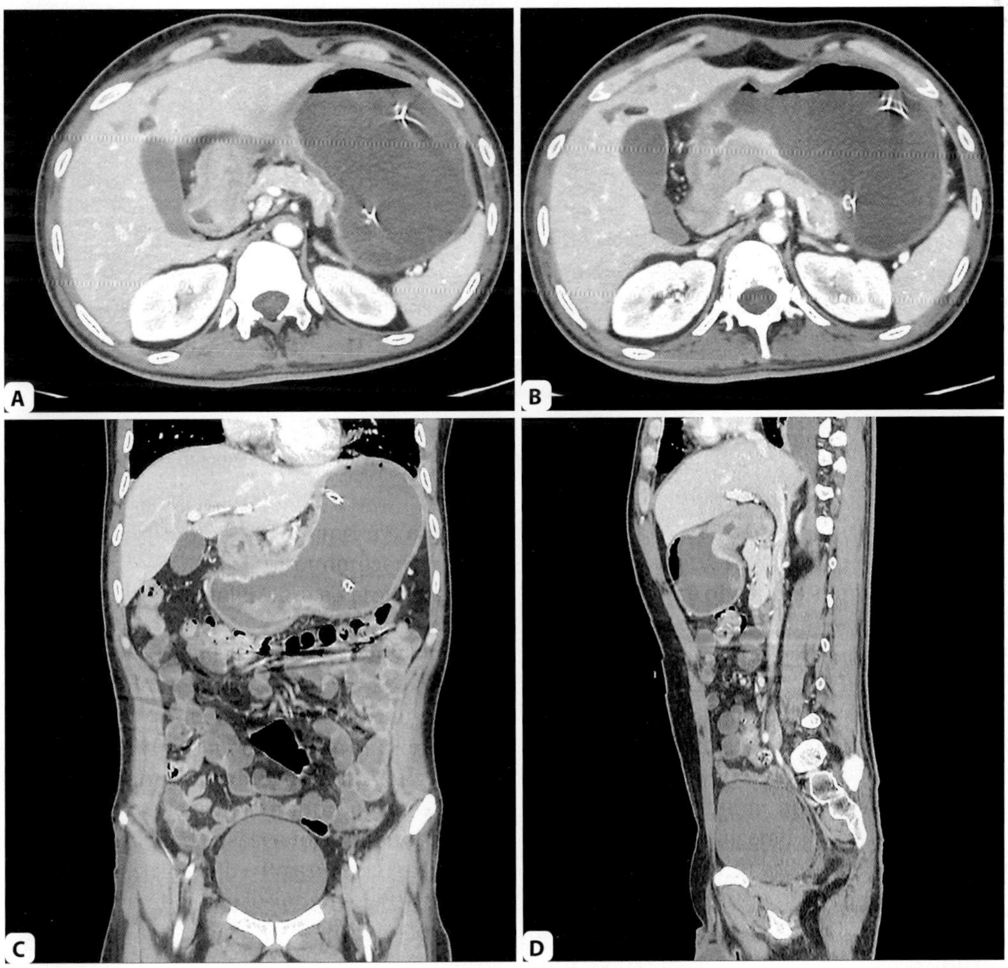

FIGS. 6A TO D: Gastric carcinoma—CECT axial (A and B), coronal (C), and sagittal (D) images show irregular, circumferential, enhancing mural thickening involving the distal gastric body, antrum, pylorus with loss of rugal folds and mural stratification. There is surrounding perigastric fat stranding and heterogeneity (T3 tumor).

(CECT: contrast-enhanced computed tomography)

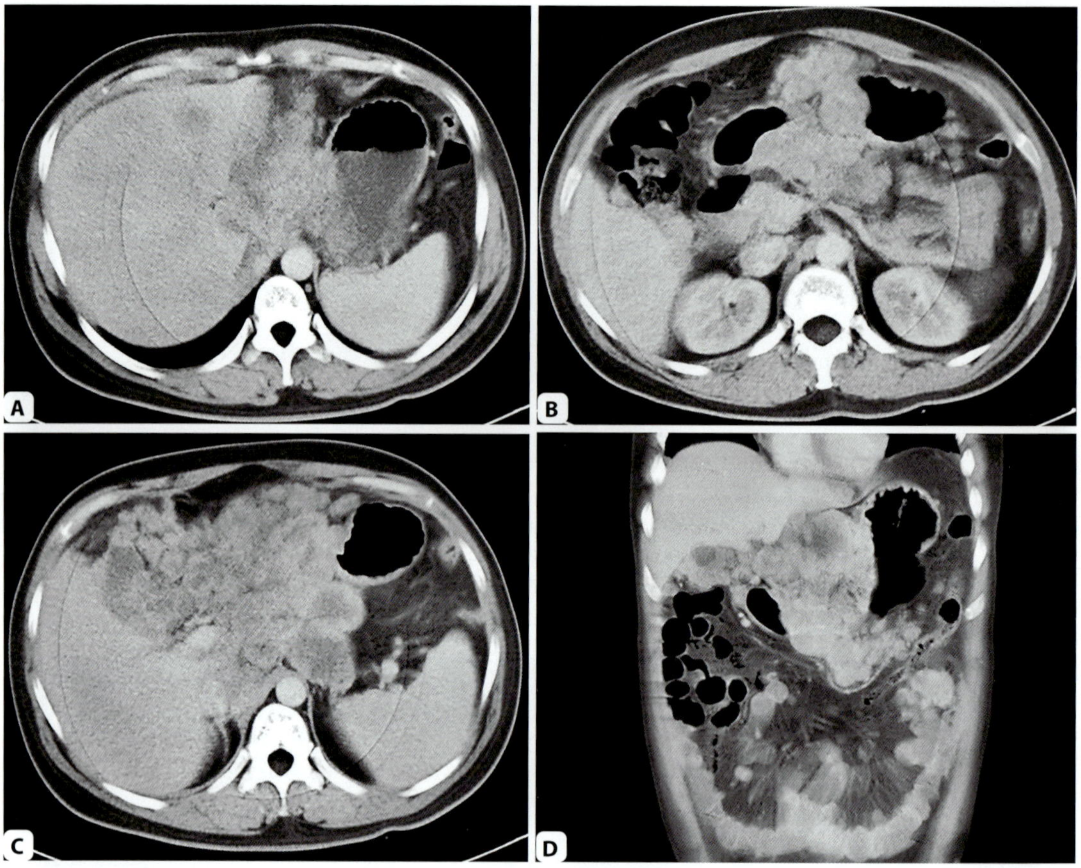

FIGS. 7A TO D: Gastric carcinoma—CECT axial (A to C) and coronal (D) images show a large, ill-defined, heterogeneously enhancing mass lesion replacing the distal gastric body, antrum, pylorus, and duodenum with extensive perigastric nodular deposits and perigastric and retroperitoneal lymphadenopathy. Note is also made of a hypodense lesion in the liver parenchyma (A) suggestive of hepatic metastases.

(CECT: contrast-enhanced computed tomography)

at T-staging of advanced (T3 and T4) carcinomas (98% and 82%, respectively) versus early (T1 and T2) carcinomas (23% and 15%, respectively). Multiplanar reconstructions in coronal and sagittal planes help to improve the detection and staging. The role of MRI in staging of the primary tumor is limited due to respiratory, cardiac, and peristalsis motion artifacts. Fluorodeoxyglucose (FDG) PET-CT performs inconsistently in the detection of gastric carcinoma, as there is physiologic uptake of FDG in the gastric mucosa. Also, the FDG uptake varies according to the histologic subtype of gastric cancer with signet ring cell carcinoma and poorly differentiated adenocarcinoma showing little or no radiotracer uptake.

Lymph Node Staging

Lymph nodal staging in gastric carcinoma is challenging due to limitations in detecting microscopic metastases by currently available imaging modalities. Nodes which are larger than 8–10 millimeters in short axis are considered as suspicious. However, the size parameter has certain drawbacks, while 80% of the lymph nodes < 5 millimeters in size were noted to be benign, 55% of metastatic nodes were also < 5 millimeter in short axis. CT is slightly better at staging lymph nodes compared to MRI. EUS can detect metastatic nodes in the perigastric region, however, nodal stations such as station 3 or station 4 which are essential for surgical planning cannot be staged using this modality **(Figs. 8A to F)**. Nodes which are avid on FDG PET-CT are likely malignant and therefore PET-CT has a higher specificity than CT or MRI. However, the limitations of PET-CT are that smaller nodes may not be detectable and signet cell carcinomas do not show FDG uptake with probable understaging of such lymph nodes on PET-CT.[27]

Metastatic Gastric Cancer

According to the AJCC staging system, involvement of the hepatoduodenal ligament, retropancreatic, mesenteric or paraaortic lymph nodes are considered distant metastases (i.e., M1 disease). Hepatic metastases are commonly seen due to hematogenous spread of gastric carcinoma with the lesions best seen on portal venous phase images on CT. Lung metastases are less common, and are well visualized

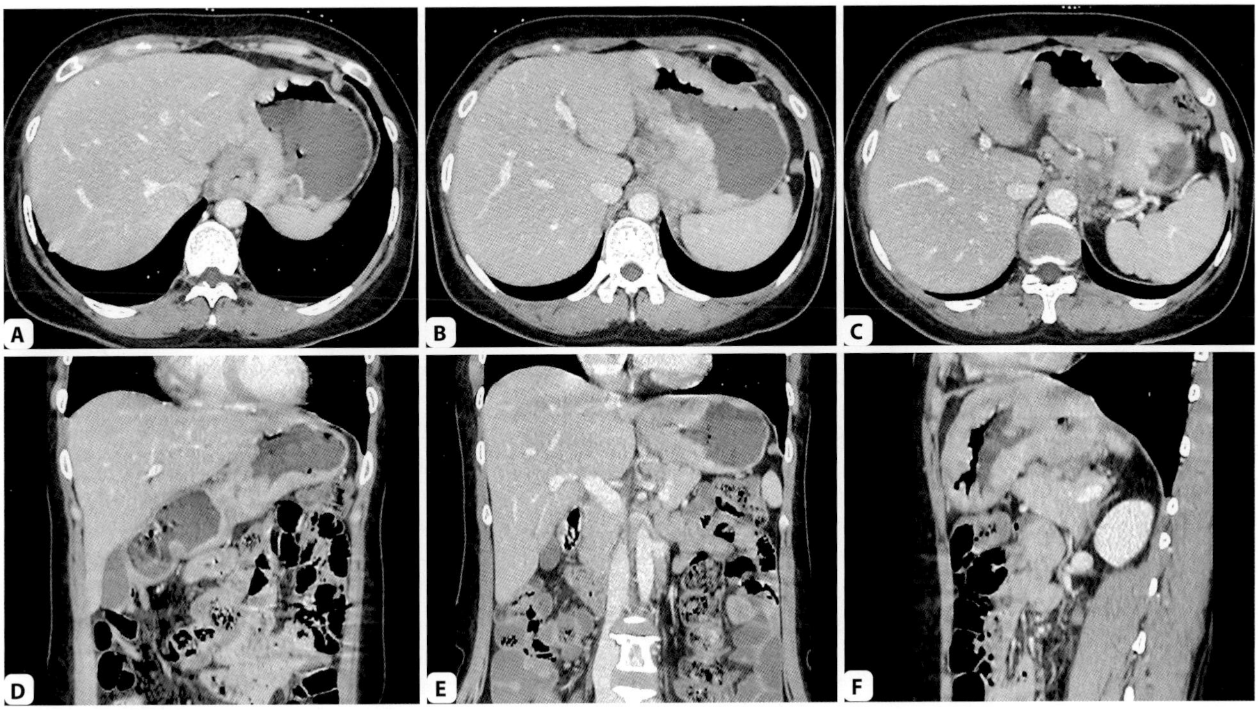

FIGS. 8A TO F: In an elderly male patient with early satiety and weight loss, CECT axial (A to C), coronal (D and E) and sagittal images (F) show ill-defined heterogeneously enhancing circumferential thickening of the gastric wall involving the region of the fundus and body with enlarged perigastric, celiac, peripancreatic and retroperitoneal lymph nodes.

(CECT: contrast-enhanced computed tomography)

on CT appearing as solid lung nodules. Bone metastases are more common in advanced cases. On CT, these lesions may be sclerotic, lytic, or isodense to bone marrow. Involvement of distant lymph nodes such as left supraclavicular node (Virchow's node) can also be seen. Advanced gastric carcinoma frequently metastasizes to the peritoneum, typically involving the omentum, the ovaries (Krukenberg tumor) **(Fig. 9)**, and rectovesical pouch (Blumer's shelf tumor). The presence of ascites in a patient with gastric carcinoma is usually associated with positive free tumor cells, which is suspicious for peritoneal carcinomatosis.

Table 2 shows the 8th edition of the AJCC staging for gastric cancer with corresponding CT imaging features.

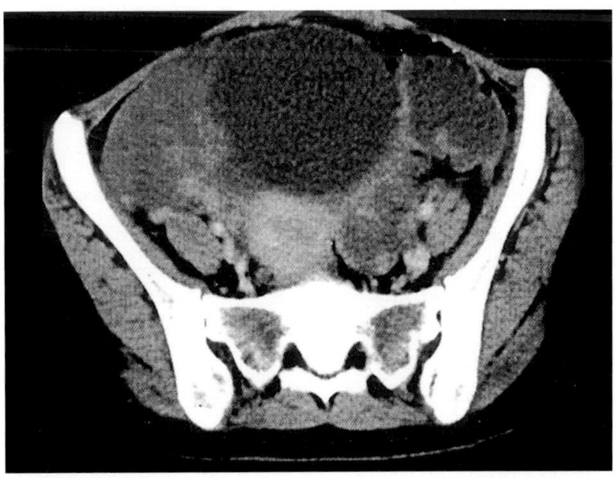

FIG. 9: In a known case of carcinoma stomach, axial contrast-enhanced image reveals multicystic masses in bilateral adnexa suggestive of Krukenberg tumor.

Treatment of Gastric Cancer

Treatment options for patients with gastric cancer have expanded, with therapeutic approaches tailored according to the stage of the tumor. Early, superficial tumors (T1a) often benefit from endoscopic mucosal resection/submucosal dissection. Surgical resection becomes the preferred choice for early-stage cancers unsuitable for endoscopic procedures. Total/distal gastrectomy, paired with neoadjuvant chemotherapy is the standard treatment for locally AGC (≥ T3, any N or ≥ T2, N^+). In cases of advanced, unresectable, or metastatic gastric cancer (35–40% of initial diagnoses), chemotherapy remains the primary approach. Thus, accurate staging is vital for selecting the optimal treatment pathway, with imaging playing a crucial role in this determination.[28]

TABLE 2: Eighth edition of the American Joint Committee on Cancer (AJCC) staging for gastric cancer with corresponding CT appearances.

Staging category	Definition	CT appearance
T0	No evidence of primary tumor	
Tis	High-grade dysplasia, defined as malignant cells confined to the epithelium by the basement membrane	
T1a	Tumor invades lamina propria or muscularis mucosae	Not visible on CT
T1b	Tumor invades submucosa	• Mucosal thickening and enhancement • Hypodense submucosal stripe remains visible
T2	Tumor invades muscularis propria	Loss of submucosal hypoattenuating stripe but smooth outer gastric wall
T3	Tumor penetrates subserosal connective tissue	• Inability to discriminate between gastric mass and the outer enhancing layer of stomach • Mildly blurred but generally smooth outer gastric wall • Few small linear areas of fat stranding • Nodular or sheet-like soft-tissue thickening within perigastric ligaments
T4a	Tumor invades the serosa (visceral peritoneum)	• Nodular or irregular serosal surface infiltration of surrounding peritoneal fat • Hyperattenuating serosa sign
T4b	Tumor invades adjacent structures (spleen, transverse colon, liver, diaphragm, pancreas, abdominal wall, adrenal gland, kidney, small intestine, and retroperitoneum)	Direct invasion into adjacent organs and structures, deformity or irregular contour or loss of fat planes between tumor and adjacent organ
N0	No regional lymph node metastases	
N	N1: Metastases in one or two regional lymph nodes N2: Metastases in three or six regional lymph nodes N3: Metastases in seven or more regional lymph nodes	• >6 mm in perigastric lymph nodes • >8 mm in extraperigastric lymph nodes • Rounded shape • Heterogeneous or intense enhancement • A cluster of three or more nodes
M0	No distant metastases	
M1	Distant metastases involving distant nodes, nondirect extension into other organs or peritoneal carcinomatosis	Distant (nonregional) lymph nodes, nondirect extension into other organs or peritoneal carcinomatosis (ascites, peritoneal nodules, plaques, thickening, fat stranding and/or peritoneal enhancement)

New Frontiers

CT Volumetry

In recent years, CT volume rendering techniques have been increasingly utilized for generating three-dimensional (3D) volume-rendering images, facilitating precise calculations of solid organ or tumor volumes. There are two primary methods of CT volumetry. Two-dimensional volumetry relies on manually segmented regions of interest (ROI), with the final gastric volume determined by multiplying the ROI areas with the slice thickness. Conversely, 3D volumetry involves a semiautomatic segmentation process necessitating specialized postprocessing software. Studies have demonstrated that CT volumetry results are comparable to those of EUS in terms of accuracy for T2–T4 staging (83–95%). Moreover, tumor volume has been proposed as supplementary information for predicting metastatic disease and assessing the risk of peritoneal spread. It has also been reported that the tumor volume of the esophagogastric junction is an independent risk factor for node metastasis. Based on these factors, some authors have demonstrated that the tumor volume, using pathological data as the reference standard, is correlated with survival, and it has been suggested as a significant prognostic factor.

Perfusion CT

Perfusion computed tomography (pCT) is a technique enabling the quantitative and qualitative assessment of tissue perfusion. This is achieved by administering iodinated contrast agents and conducting consecutive acquisitions to estimate time enhancement curves. Several studies have explored the potential utility of pCT in gastric cancer patients, suggesting that computed parameters can furnish crucial insights into tumor angiogenesis. A significant correlation has been reported between the blood volume (BV) in gastric cancer and microvessel density, offering valuable preoperative assessment data. Malignant tumors, including gastric cancer, often exhibit leaky vessels due to neoangiogenesis, and pCT can detect such vascular abnormalities, particularly increased permeability surface (PS), which holds diagnostic significance.[28]

Furthermore, pCT-derived tumor perfusion parameters tend to decrease in AGC cases, indicating their potential role in identifying more aggressive subtypes, as previously noted. In one study, authors compared three gastric cancer groups with varying degrees of differentiation, observing significant disparities in blood flow (BF), BV, and PS among well-, moderately, and poorly differentiated gastric cancer cases.

Radiomics and Artificial Intelligence

Over recent decades, radiomics has emerged as a versatile technique applicable to various pathological conditions, including its potential role in detecting gastric cancer.[28] In a study involving 171 patients, radiomics showed promise in aiding the differential diagnosis of gastric cancer subtypes, with respective automatic classifier (AUC) values of 0.755, 0.710, and 0.712 in training, internal, and external validation cohorts. A systematic review of 25 studies, encompassing over 10,000 patients, highlighted the predominance of CT imaging (96% of studies) in radiomics research. Notably, radiomics was found particularly valuable in assessing treatment response. For instance, in a study of 292 patients, a CT-based radiomics model accurately predicted pathological downstaging postneoadjuvant chemotherapy in AGC.

Similarly, in a study of 955 patients, radiomics showed promise in predicting peritoneal dissemination in gastric cancer, serving as an independent predictor in both test and validation cohorts. Artificial intelligence (AI) also shows promise in evaluating gastric cancer patients, especially in diagnosing gastric cancer using techniques like EUS. Various AI systems contribute to enhancing the accuracy of primary tumor detection, while deep learning methods improve the identification of peritoneal dissemination. In a recent multicenter retrospective study of 1,978 patients, an AI model achieved an impressive AUC of 0.946, with sensitivity and specificity levels surpassing clinicopathological factors. AI's utility extends to predicting treatment outcomes. In a study published in 2021 involving 2,209 patients, a deep-learning model demonstrated high diagnostic accuracy in assessing tumor stroma (AUC = 0.960), an independent predictor of disease-free survival (DFS) and overall survival (OS) in both test and validation cohorts.

Gastric Lymphoma

Lymphoma may involve the gastrointestinal tract (GIT) as primary malignancy or more commonly as a part of systemic illness and is considered the most common extranodal site for lymphoma. GI lymphoma accounts for 5–20% of extranodal lymphoma with the stomach being the most common site of involvement followed by the small intestine and colorectal region. Primary gastric lymphoma constitutes 1–5% of the gastric malignancies and approximately 50–70% cases of primary GI lymphoma. Primary GIT lymphoma does not involve liver or spleen and is confined to stomach and the regional lymph nodes. Majority of lymphomas are non-Hodgkin lymphoma of B-cell type and there are only a few case reports of Hodgkin disease involving GI system in literature.[29]

Primary GI lymphomas usually affect one site. There are five diagnostic criteria, which have been described by Dawson[30] to make the diagnosis of a primary GI lymphoma:

1. No palpable superficial lymph nodes
2. No adenopathy on chest radiograph
3. Normal values of white cells in blood count
4. Involvement of GI tract predominantly with involvement of drainage lymph nodes only if at all on laparotomy
5. No lesions in the liver and spleen

Patients frequently present with abdominal pain associated occasionally with malabsorption, abdominal mass and weight loss. Modified TNM staging by the European Gastrointestinal Lymphoma Study Group and Lugano staging[31] are two most commonly used staging protocols used for primary GI lymphoma.

Most of lymphomas arise from mucosa-associated lymphoid tissue (MALT) and have good prognosis as they remain localized for a long time. It is usually a low-grade MALT lymphoma; however, it can transform into intermediate or higher grade if not treated timely.[32] MALT lymphomas are now referred to as extranodal marginal zone B cell lymphoma (ENMZCL), as they arise from the marginal zone of lymph node. Chronic *H. pylori* infection is associated with MALT lymphomas, and many low-grade MALT lymphomas undergo regression with treatment of *H. pylori* infection. Low-grade lymphomas tend to spread superficially, accompanied occasionally by ulceration and manifest as small nodules with minimal mucosal thickening. Tumors < 5 in size with < 5 mitoses per high power field suggest low-grade lymphoma. On the other hand, high-grade lymphomas are usually large tumors, often > 5 cm in size, polypoidal and associated with marked rugal-fold thickening and have > 5 mitoses per high-power field. There is commonly necrosis within the tumor which may give rise to septated appearance and excavation may lead to communication with rest of the GIT or peritoneal cavity. Occurrence of hemorrhage may produce fluid-fluid level within the tumor. Direct invasion of adjacent organs or distant, omental and peritoneal metastasis may also occur.

T-cell lymphomas associated with enteropathy, Burkitt's lymphoma, etc., are rare. Other risk factors for gastric lymphoma include inflammatory bowel disease, celiac disease, HIV infection, and immunosuppression after solid organ transplant.[33]

Diagnostic Imaging

Lymphoma can be focal or diffuse and involve any portion of the stomach. Though early lymphoma is confined to the mucosa and submucosa, gastric lymphomas are usually advanced at presentation and may mimic the appearances of gastric carcinoma. Double-contrast barium studies may reveal ulcerative, polypoidal or infiltrative patterns, findings that favor a diagnosis of lymphoma include presence of multiple polypoidal tumors showing central ulceration giving rise to bull's eye appearance, giant cavitating lesions or extensive gastric fold thickening **(Figs. 10A to C)**. Gastric distensibility is preserved. EUS can show giant rigid gastric folds which may reveal a polypoid appearance, localized or diffuse hypoechoic infiltration and thickening with superficial stellate-shaped ulcerations. EUS is superior to CT for assessment of T and N parameters; however, it cannot demonstrate the true extraluminal extent of the disease (M) and involvement of distant lymph nodes.

Multidetector computed tomography reveals preservation of the perigastric fat planes even with a massive tumor. This favors the diagnosis of lymphoma over adenocarcinoma. Adenocarcinoma and lymphoma both are associated with lymphadenopathy; however, bulky lymph nodes extending below the renal hila favor the diagnosis of lymphoma **(Figs. 11A and B)**.[34] CT is also a better technique to diagnose complications such as perforation, obstruction, and fistulization. Moreover, despite extensive infiltrative lesions stomach remains pliable and gastric outlet obstruction is uncommon in contrast to gastric adenocarcinoma.

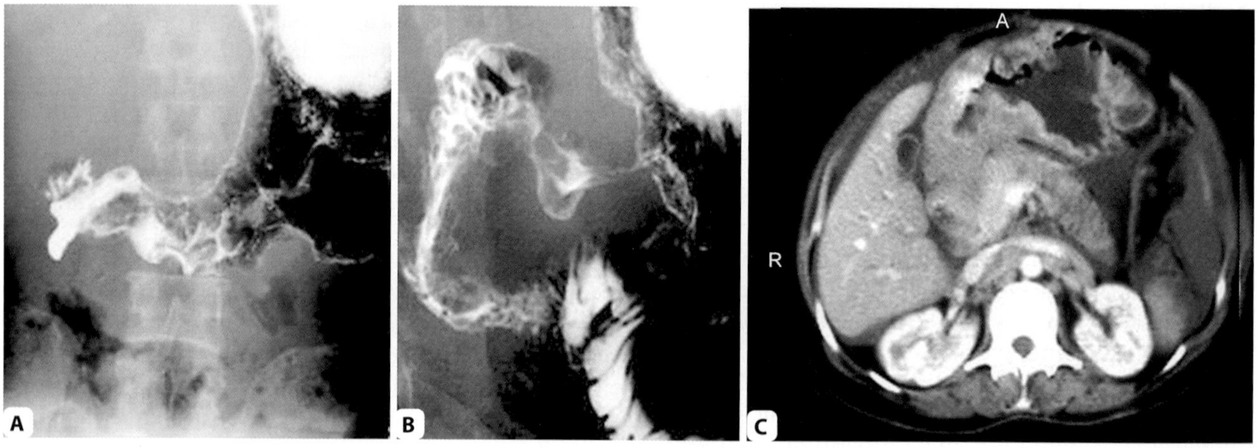

FIGS. 10A TO C: (A and B) Nodular filling defects noted on DCBM study in the distal body and antropyloric region with extension into duodenum in a patient of gastric lymphoma; (C) CECT of the same patient reveals enhancing mural thickening of distal body and antropyloric region. Enlarged aortocaval lymph nodes with ascites are also seen.

(CECT: contrast-enhanced computed tomography; DCBM: double-contrast barium meal study)

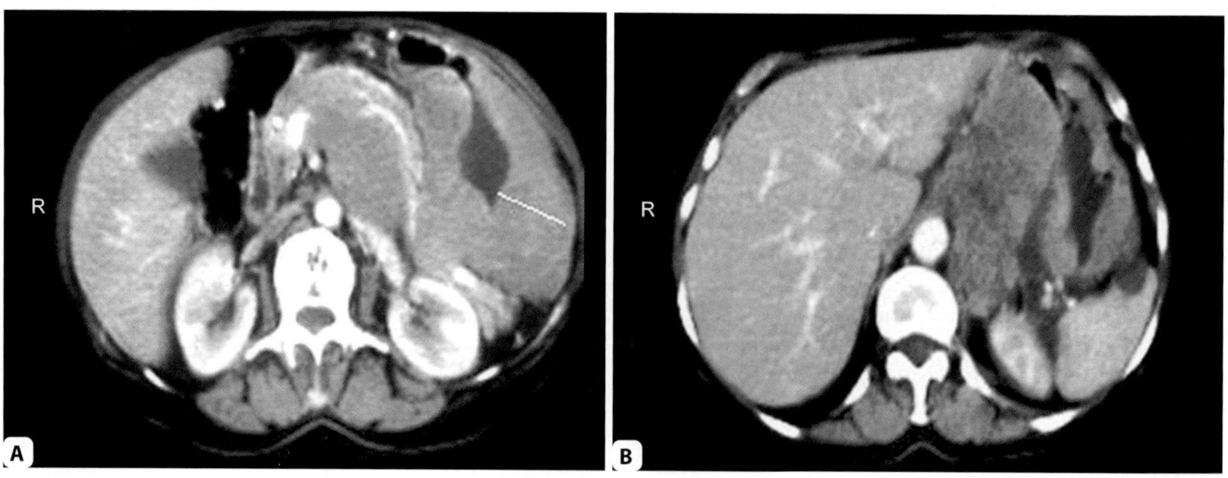

FIGS. 11A AND B: Marked homogeneously enhancing wall thickening (5 cm) noted in a patient with gastric lymphoma on CECT with multiple enlarged retroperitoneal nodes reaching up to the renal hilum (A). In another patient with gastric lymphoma, axial CECT abdomen reveals thick nodular folds in the region of gastric body along with enlarged lymph nodes noted in gastrohepatic ligament and paraaortic region. Note is also made of hypodense lesion in spleen (B).

(CECT: contrast-enhanced computed tomography)

The type of involvement can be infiltrative, ulcerative, polypoidal, nodular or a combination of these types.

- *Infiltrative form*: Infiltration can be local or diffuse. It is associated with thick and nodular folds which are not effaced after hypotonic agent administration. Distensibility of stomach is maintained which helps in differentiation from linitis plastica due to adenocarcinoma. These patients are therefore less prone to develop gastric outlet obstruction.[35] Differential diagnosis includes Ménétrier disease, hypertrophic, lymphocytic, and eosinophilic gastritis.
- *Ulcerative form*: Presence of ulcer accompanied by a polypoidal mass, absence of areae gastricae and associated rugal-fold thickening are pointers of ulcerative form of lymphomatous involvement.
- *Polypoidal form*: There can be an intraluminal mass which may be lobulated or may present as submucosal mass. It may be associated with ulceration.
- *Nodular form*: These present as multiple submucosal masses. These often ulcerate giving "target or bull's eye" appearance.

Extension to involve duodenum may be seen in about 40% cases. Esophageal involvement is less common and seen in about 10% cases.[3]

MRI is useful in evaluating bowel wall-thickening along with organ and lymph node involvement. Lymphomatous masses are hypointense on T1- and hyperintense on T2-weighted images as they have high free water content. MR is helpful in evaluating treatment due to reduction in signal intensity on T2 as a result of reduced cellular and water content. However, longer scan times and susceptibility to artifacts due to respiration and peristalsis limit the use of MRI. Radionuclide imaging using FDG PET-CT is helpful in evaluating lymph nodes as involved nodes show increased uptake, FDG-PET is also found helpful in predicting the treatment response.

Gastric Neuroendocrine Tumors

Gastrointestinal carcinoids are well-differentiated endocrine neoplasms arising from specialized endocrine cells that populate the mucosa and submucosa of the GI system. Hence, theoretically, they can be seen arising from any part of the GI system and produce clinical symptoms depending on the type of the hormone they are secreting. Carcinoids arise most commonly from the distal ileum from enterochromaffin cells which produce serotonin. They usually present as lymph nodal or liver metastasis.

Carcinoids of the stomach, duodenum, or colon are, however, a relatively rare entity. Gastric carcinoids account for 1-2% of all gastric neoplasms. Majority of the gastric carcinoids arise from gastric body and fundus from enterochromaffin-like cells of the oxyntic mucosa.[36]

Gastric carcinoids are primarily divided into three types depending on their clinical, imaging, and pathological differences by Bordi et al.[37]

- *Type I*: Most common (75%), female predominance at an older age, are usually associated with autoimmune chronic gastritis and usually encountered during endoscopy performed for dyspepsia or anemia. Achlorhydria, pernicious anemia, or gastric G-cell hyperplasia may be seen.

  On imaging, they are seen as multiple, small (1–2 cm), circumscribed, smoothly marginated, hypervascular mural masses in the body and fundus of stomach.
- *Type II*: Least common (5–10%) is associated with Zollinger–Ellison syndrome in patients of multiple endocrine neoplasia type 1 (MEN type-I). They are usually present as recurrent nonhealing gastric or duodenal ulcers with marked mucosal fold and rugal thickening, abdominal pain, bleeding, or diarrhea due to hypergastrinemia by gastrin producing neoplasms. Imaging features include diffuse mural thickening with multinodular enhancing mucosal and mural masses **(Fig. 12)**. The gastrinoma triangle must be evaluated carefully to assess for a primary enhancing lesion.
- *Type III*: Type III subtype represents 10–15% of the gastric carcinoids and are mostly malignant. They are not associated with hypergastrinemia or atrophic gastritis and usually present with signs and symptoms of aggressive lesions like anorexia, weight loss, bleeding, or pain abdomen.

Imaging features include a large, invasive, hypervascular mural mass in the body and/or fundus with the stomach which can show ulceration. The perigastric region and liver should be inspected for signs of metastatic disease[36,37] **(Fig. 13)**. ^{68}Ga-DOTATATE PET/CT and ^{111}In-pentetreotide SPECT/CT have high sensitivity in localizing the primary tumor (> 1 cm) and are helpful in staging of the disease.

The differentials for types I and II gastric carcinoids include multifocal polypoidal masses like multiple hyperplastic polyps, adenomatous polyps in FAP syndrome, hamartomatous polyps in Peutz–Jeghers syndrome and juvenile polyposis. Type III carcinoids can mimic adenocarcinoma, lymphoma, and gastrointestinal stromal tumors (GISTs).

Gastric Metastases

Common tumors that metastasize to stomach include breast, malignant melanoma, lung, lymphoma, and Kaposki sarcoma. These may present as multiple small submucosal masses which may show "target or bull's eye" appearance in the presence of central ulceration **(Figs. 14A and B)**. Differential diagnosis includes neurofibromas, pancreatic rest cells, and leiomyomas.

Mesenchymal Tumors

Mesenchymal tumors of the stomach arise from the mesenchymal cells in the gastric wall and include gastrointestinal

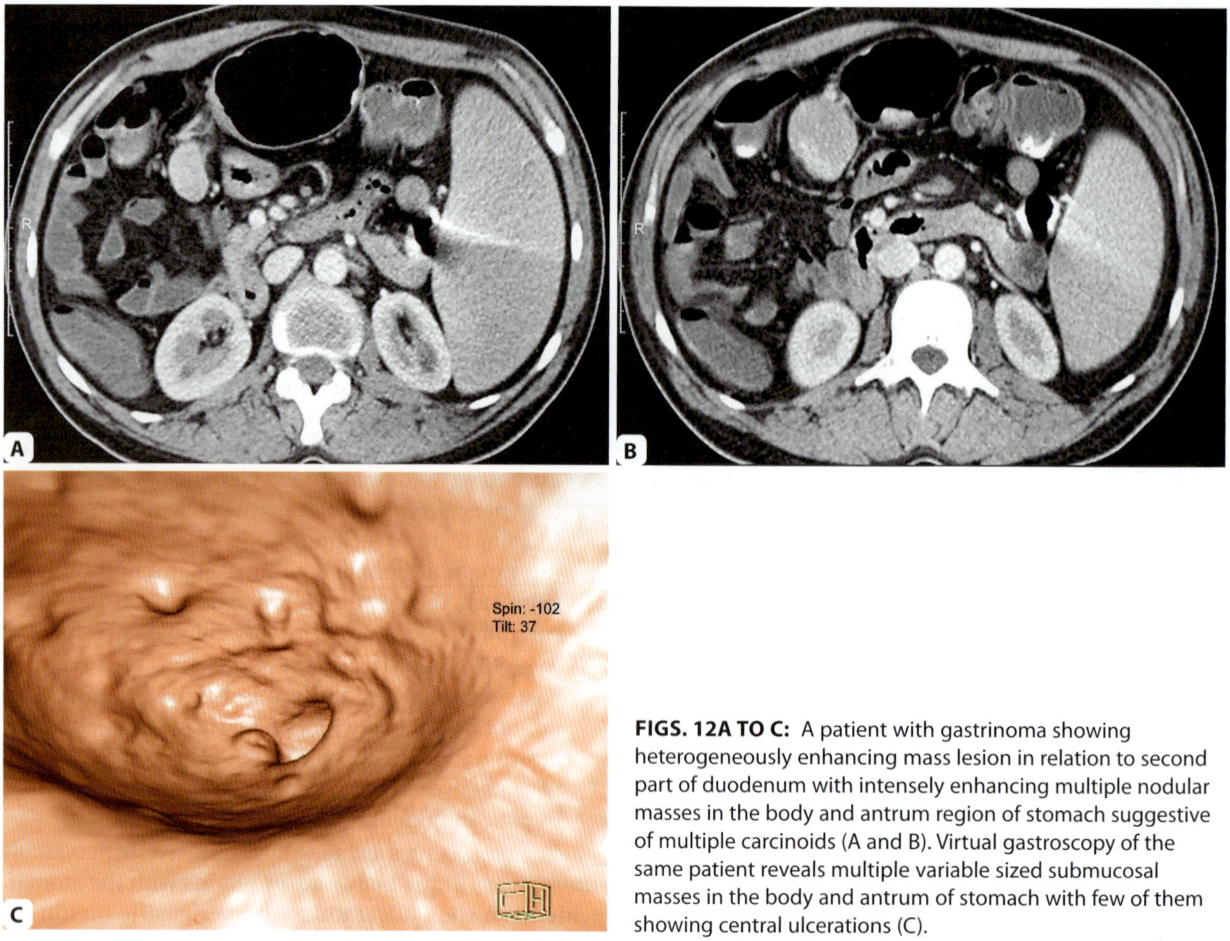

FIGS. 12A TO C: A patient with gastrinoma showing heterogeneously enhancing mass lesion in relation to second part of duodenum with intensely enhancing multiple nodular masses in the body and antrum region of stomach suggestive of multiple carcinoids (A and B). Virtual gastroscopy of the same patient reveals multiple variable sized submucosal masses in the body and antrum of stomach with few of them showing central ulcerations (C).

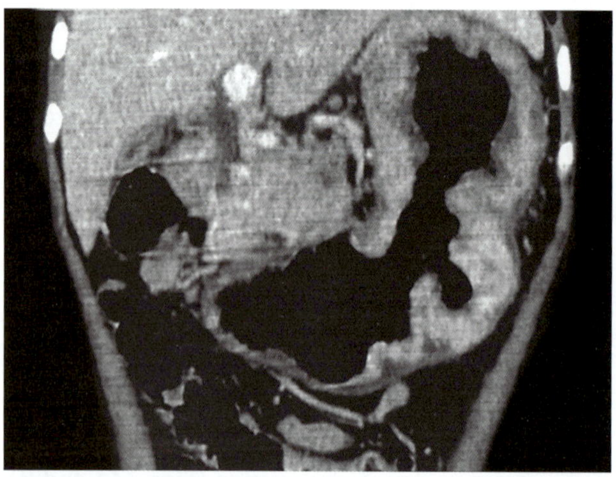

FIG. 13: Gastric carcinoid (type III)—CECT coronal reformat of another patient reveals diffuse mural thickening with irregular polypoidal lesions in the fundus and body of the stomach. There is a large heterogeneously enhancing mass lesion seen in the region of head of the pancreas.

(CECT: contrast-enhanced computed tomography)

stromal tumor (GIST, most common), non-GIST sarcomas, lipomas, leiomyomas, schwannomas, glomus tumors, hemangiomas, inflammatory fibroid polyps, inflammatory myofibroblastic tumors (IMTs) and plexiform fibromyxomas. Mesenchymal tumors are usually well circumscribed with intact overlying mucosa and can be endoluminal, exophytic, or mixed. Immunohistochemical stains are useful for characterization of certain mesenchymal tumors, c-KIT (CD-117) or DOG1 is used to confirm GIST, desmin for leiomyoma, and S-100 protein schwannoma. IMTs are seen as spindle cell tumors with intratumoral plasma cells and immunoreactivity to anaplastic lymphoma kinase (ALK).

Gastrointestinal Stromal Tumor

Gastrointestinal stromal tumor is the most common mesenchymal neoplasm that can be found throughout the GIT with 60–70% of the tumors affecting the stomach.[38] Majority of these lesions are benign with 10–30% of the lesions being aggressive. Before the immunohistochemical tests were available, GISTs were considered to be leiomyomas but c-KIT (CD-117) and DOG-1 immunoreactivity helps

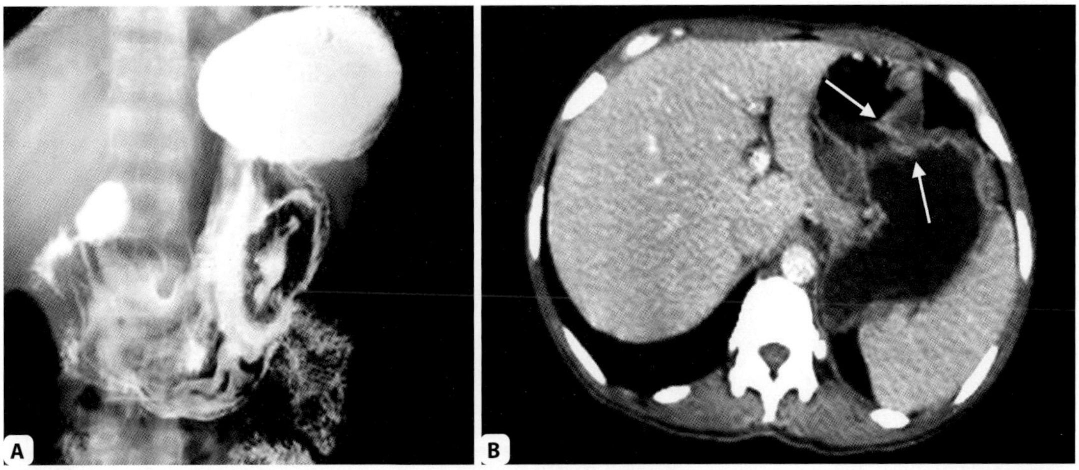

FIGS. 14A AND B: (A) Target/Bull's eye lesion—DCBM reveals a large filling defect in body of stomach with central pooling of barium; (B) CECT shows focal thickening of stomach wall in the region of body with central ulceration in a patient with submucosal metastasis from melanoma.

(CECT: contrast-enhanced computed tomography; DCBM: double-contrast barium meal study)

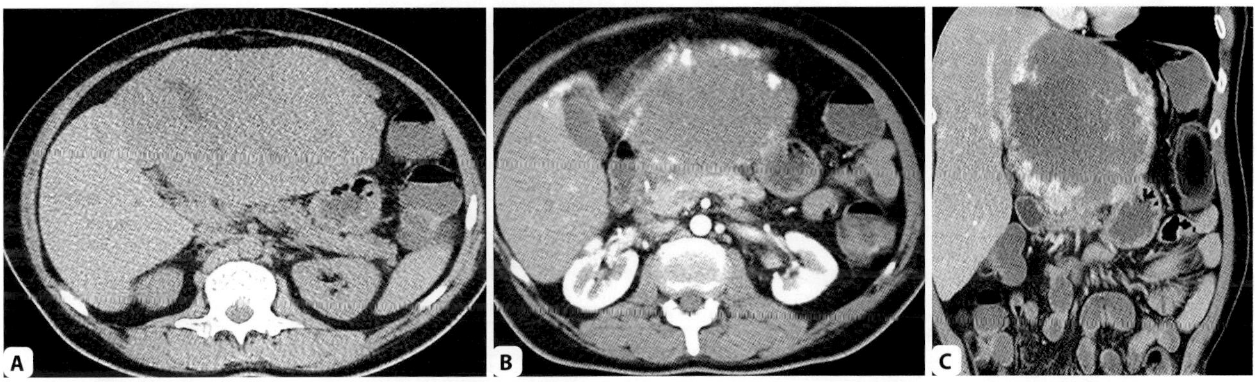

FIGS. 15A TO C: Noncontrast axial, CECT axial and coronal images reveal a large lobulated exophytic soft-tissue mass lesion along the lesser curvature of the stomach with heterogeneous enhancement and nonenhancing central hypodense areas symptoms of necrosis in a case of gastric GIST.

(CECT: contrast-enhanced computed tomography; GIST: gastrointestinal stromal tumor)

to differentiate GIST from other neoplasms. 5% cases of GIST, however, do not show CD-117 immunoreactivity and rather harbor mutations for platelet-derived growth factor receptor-α (*PDGFR*-α) gene.[39]

They arise from pacemaker interstitial cells of Cajal normally present in myenteric plexus, which are responsible for peristalsis.[40] Because they arise from the deep muscularis propria, GISTs frequently have an exophytic or intramural pattern of growth. Endoluminal tumors although less common, if present, have features of intramural masses like smoothly circumscribed masses forming obtuse or right angles with the gastric wall.[41] Pressure necrosis can cause focal mucosal ulcerations in lesions larger than 2 cm which appears as "bull's eye" lesion on double contrast barium study.

Clinical manifestations of the GIST depend on their size and location. Small lesions are discovered incidentally. Ulcerated lesions are usually present with bleed in form of hematemesis, melena, or iron-deficiency anemia.[42] Larger masses are usually present with abdominal pain and early satiety. However, because of predominantly exophytic nature of tumors, many of these patients remain asymptomatic until the tumors become quite large.[41]

Gastrointestinal stromal tumors are commonly found in the gastric body and antrum. The typical CT appearance of small tumors is often homogeneous whereas large tumors are heterogeneously enhancing, lobulated, hypervascular exophytic mass with mucosal ulceration, central necrosis, hemorrhage, cavitation, and areas of cystic degeneration[40] **(Figs. 15 and 16)**. Ulcerations and fistulization can be seen as air and oral contrast within the lesion. 5–10% of the cases can show calcification. The following imaging features favor the diagnosis of malignant GIST: size of the lesion >5 cm, necrosis, mesenteric or contiguous organ infiltration and metastasis.[43,44] Rarely clumps of calcification can be seen. Nearly half of the patients present with metastasis in the advanced stages when the tumor has invaded the adjacent organs such as colon, diaphragm, and pancreas

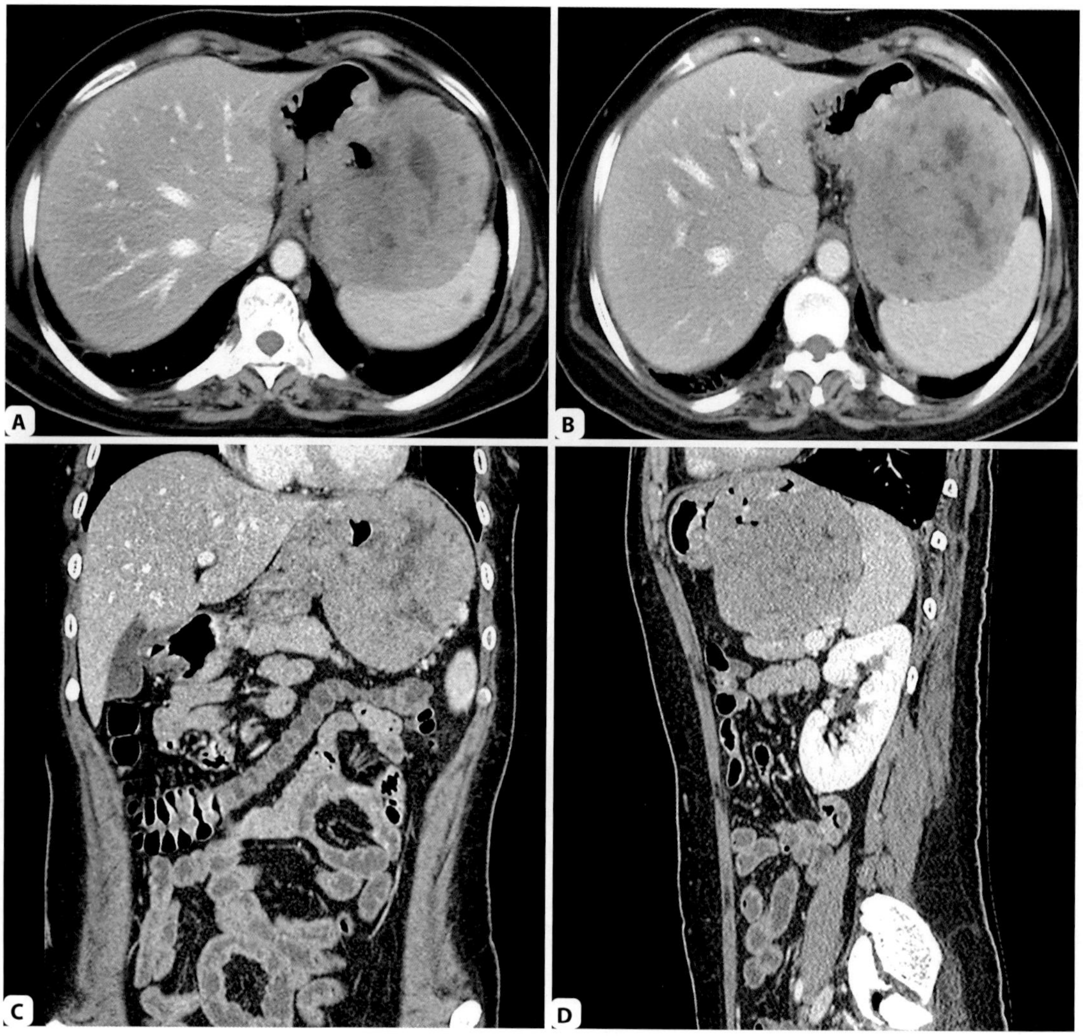

FIGS. 16A TO D: CECT axial (A and B) and coronal (C) and sagittal (D) images show a well-defined, heterogeneously enhancing exophytic lesion arising from the greatest curvature of stomach with hypo-enhancing necrotic areas within, with crescent-shaped internal air-fluid levels in a case of gastric GIST.

(CECT: contrast-enhanced computed tomography; GIST: gastrointestinal stromal tumor)

with deposits predominantly seen in liver and peritoneum. Nodal metastasis is infrequent in GISTs.[45]

Differential diagnosis for GIST includes neural tumors such as schwannomas, true leiomyomas, and small type 3 solitary carcinoid tumors. Immunoreactivity to c-KIT or DOG1 (discovered on GIST-1), however, can confirm the diagnosis. Other tumors showing intramural growth like gastric adenocarcinoma or lymphoma can mimic a GIST. However, lymphadenopathy is rare for GISTs. Submucosal metastases to the stomach from melanoma or breast cancer can manifest as bull's-eye lesions, they can be solitary, however, usually they are multiple.[41]

Gastrointestinal stromal tumors smaller than 2 cm are generally considered benign with a very low risk of recurrence. However, no GIST can truly be labeled benign.[46] A definitive diagnosis is particularly important because advanced GIST can be treated with Imatinib, which is a tyrosine kinase inhibitor and is associated with a remarkable response and a prolonged survival.[47,48] On treatment, GISTs typically become homogeneous and hypoattenuating from heterogeneously hyperattenuating lesions, with disappearance of enhancing tumor nodules and tumor vessels in the early posttreatment period with imatinib. Myxoid degeneration is seen and occasional areas of hemorrhage and necrosis can be noted within the healing tumor which can paradoxically increase the size of tumor. However, with overall reduction in tumor enhancement this does not indicate tumor progression. The term *cystic change* is usually avoided while patient is under treatment with imatinib. Development of a nodule within the treated tumor is unique to GISTs and indicates recurrence regardless of changes in tumor size.[49] Imatinib therapy can be associated with fluid overload and ascites, pleural effusion, pericardial effusion, and subcutaneous edema may be seen on imaging. Therefore, presence of new ascites should not be interpreted as peritoneal disease in such patients.

Leiomyoma and Nongastrointestinal Stromal Tumor Sarcoma

Leiomyomas are well circumscribed intramural tumors usually arising from the region of the gastric cardia. The true leiomyomas are rare benign tumors of the stomach and are negative for c-KIT and strongly and diffusely positive for desmin and smooth muscle actin on immunohistochemistry. On CT, leiomyomas appear as homogeneous, low-attenuation masses with an endoluminal growth pattern.[50-52] They may show central ulceration if > 2 cm in size and can mimic GIST and schwannoma.

Non-GIST sarcomas include liposarcomas, leiomyosarcomas, and unclassified sarcomas. They are seen as large, aggressive masses with heterogeneous enhancement, and areas of necrosis **(Figs. 17A to C)**. Endoscopically, the tumor appears as a smooth, submucosal mass over which the mucosal folds are stretched and effaced. Leiomyosarcomas can undergo hematogenous spread to the liver and lungs.[53]

Nerve Sheath Tumors (Schwannoma)

These tumors arise from the myenteric plexus in the muscularis propria and comprise 4% of all benign gastric neoplasms.[54] They are submucosal, slow-growing exophytic tumors which are mostly asymptomatic and are usually diagnosed incidentally on cross-sectional imaging or on endoscopy.[55] Carney's triad is associated with gastric neurogenic tumors along with pulmonary chondromas and extra-adrenal paragangliomas. Schwannomas arising from the gastric body can have an exophytic or intramural growth, may be asymptomatic or present with pain, bleeding or obstruction, if large.[56]

On CT scans, they appear as submucosal masses (with or without ulceration) that may be indistinguishable from other mesenchymal tumors. Gastric schwannomas are usually homogeneous and low-attenuation masses. Hemorrhage, ulceration, calcification, and cystic changes are rare unlike in schwannomas at other places and this feature helps in distinguishing them from the most heterogeneous GISTs. Contrast enhancement is variable. They usually show minimal enhancement on arterial phase but show delayed enhancement on equilibrium phase.[41]

Glomus Tumors

Neuromyoarterial receptors or glomus bodies are composed of modified smooth muscle cells and glomus tumors account for 2% of benign gastric tumors and arise from muscularis propria in nearly in all cases.[57] They may be asymptomatic or present with pain, hematemesis, or melena.

They are usually seen in the gastric antrum as hypervascular lesions.[57] These tumors are also soft tumors like lipomas and on barium studies they can change in size and shape. However, on CT, strong arterial enhancement with persistent enhancement on delayed films differentiate these from lipomas. The differentials for gastric glomus tumors include GIST, carcinoid, lipoma, metastasis, and ectopic pancreas. Hemangioma may also be considered as a differential due to the peripheral nodular pattern of enhancement with delayed fill in.[51,57]

Hemangioma

Hemangioma is an extremely rare solitary vascular gastric tumor accounting for approximately 1.7% of benign gastric lesions.[58] They are formed by a collection of dilated vessels

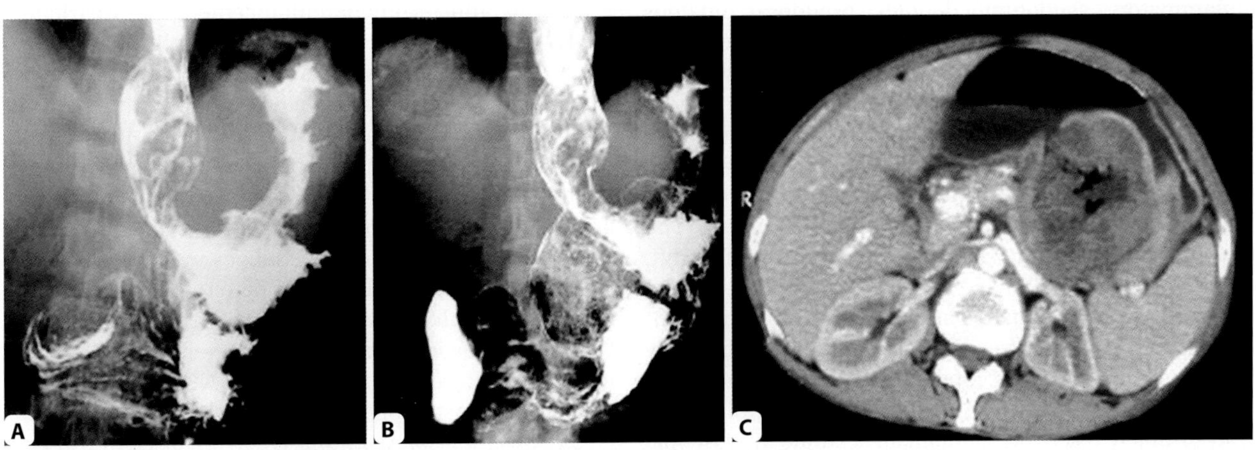

FIGS. 17A TO C: (A and B) DCBM shows a large exoendophytic mass lesion indenting the gastric fundus with irregular barium pooling within, in a patient with leiomyosarcoma; (C) CECT of the same patient reveals large soft-tissue mass showing central necrosis and air lucency suggesting communication with the gastric lumen.

(CECT: contrast-enhanced computed tomography; DCBM: double-contrast barium meal study)

due to endothelial cell proliferation with concomitant pericytic hyperplasia or abnormal pericyte division. It is found to be associated with number of syndromes such as Klippel–Trénaunay syndrome, Maffucci syndrome, blue rubber-bleb nevus syndrome, or Osler–Rendu–Weber disease. They are mostly seen in children and gradually involute with age. However, due to the possibility of massive GI bleed, they are usually resected. They are seen as submucosal masses on endoscopy and show avid enhancement on CT scans or MRI. Phleboliths, if seen in the lesion, are considered pathognomonic.

Gastric Lipoma

Gastric lipomas are solitary submucosal lesions usually detected incidentally in asymptomatic patients. They are composed of mature fat cells surrounded by fibrous capsule.[59] Small tumors are asymptomatic although, larger tumors can present with abdominal pain and bleeding due to ulceration of overlying mucosa. Infrequently, they can develop into pedunculated lesions which can intermittently prolapse through the pylorus and cause obstruction.[49]

The most common location of gastric lipomas is the gastric antrum. They appear as smooth submucosal masses on fluoroscopy; however, they can show central ulceration. The size and shape of the lipoma can vary with peristalsis.[49] On CT, they appear as solitary, submucosal, and well-demarcated lesions with homogeneous fat attenuation. Occasionally, linear strands of soft tissue at the base or mild adjacent gastric wall thickening may be present. On CT images, attenuation values of –70 to –120 HU are diagnostic of a lipoma.[59] Rarely, they can present with complications such as ulceration, intussusception, and hemorrhage and may show soft-tissue density attenuation rather than that of fat.[60]

Inflammatory Myofibroblastic Tumor

The term "inflammatory myofibroblastic tumor" or inflammatory pseudotumor denotes a pseudosarcomatous inflammatory lesion that contains spindle cells, myofibroblasts, plasma cells, lymphocytes, and histiocytes which can frequently be a benign lesion or have a more aggressive behavior with propensity of local recurrence and a low rate of metastasis. The pathogenesis of IMT remains unclear, although various allergic, immunologic, and infectious mechanisms have been postulated. The myofibroblastic tumor cells often show reactivity for ALK. ALK-negative IMFTs have been associated with older patient's age at presentation and can manifest with distant metastases.[61] In most cases, IMT features mimic malignancy on upper flexible endoscopy and radiological imaging, therefore, most IMT cases require surgical exploration and complete resection to obtain an accurate microscopic diagnosis.

It is seen mostly in children or young adults. It occurs in the soft tissue of children and young adults and lungs are the most commonly affected site. It is rare in abdomen, but when present, it is seen along terminal ileum or greater curvature of stomach.[62]

On CT, IMTs appear as enhancing, aggressive intramural masses,[63] which can invade through the gastric wall into the peritoneal cavity or nearby organs. They can also have ulcerations and calcifications at occasions.[64] GIST, solitary fibrous tumor, and schwannomas hence make the differentials because of similar appearances on CT imaging.

INFLAMMATORY AND INFECTIOUS CONDITIONS

A variety of inflammatory conditions can affect the stomach with *gastritis* being the most common condition. *Gastritis* includes several entities that are associated with inflammation in the gastric mucosa. The use of nonsteroidal anti-inflammatory drugs (NSAIDs) is thought to account for approximately 50% of the cases, other etiologies include infection, alcohol abuse, steroids and Crohn disease. Previously barium studies played an important role in the detection of ulceration and deformities consequent to it such as small ulcers, large giant ulcers associated with use of NSAIDs and hour-glass deformities of stomach. Antrum is the most common site as seen on CT, the proximal half of stomach or even the entire stomach may also be involved. Thickened gastric folds are visualized on CT with maintained mural stratification due to presence of mucosal hyperemia with submucosal edema **(Figs. 18A and B)**. Occasionally, circumferential wall thickening or a polypoid or lobulated morphology may be seen which can mimic malignancy. Gastric or peptic ulcer disease (PUD) is associated with the use of NSAIDs, *H. pylori* infection and cigarette smoking. With the high spatial and temporal resolution of MDCT, the detection of uncomplicated PUD has improved. Direct signs on CT include disruption of the normal mucosal enhancement or focal luminal outpouching while low-attenuation wall thickening, mucosal hyperenhancement and gastric fold thickening are nonspecific findings. Complications of PUD include bleeding, most commonly from the left gastric artery and CT angiography plays an important role in its evaluation. Intraluminal contrast extravasation helps to confirm and localize the site of bleeding. Presence of oral contrast outside the gastric lumen and pneumoperitoneum are suggestive of perforation which is a life-threatening complication. Inflammatory changes in adjacent fat and soft tissues including liver and pancreas can be seen in patients with ulcerous penetration without perforation. With advances in medical management of PUD, fistula formation is rare. Imprudent use of NSAIDs can lead to formation of gastrocolic fistula.[65]

Zollinger–Ellison syndrome (ZES) is caused by a gastrin secreting tumor that causes increased secretion of gastric acid and can present with PUD. 20–60% of these cases are associated with MEN1. Imaging features on CT include marked thickening of gastric rugal folds with thickened

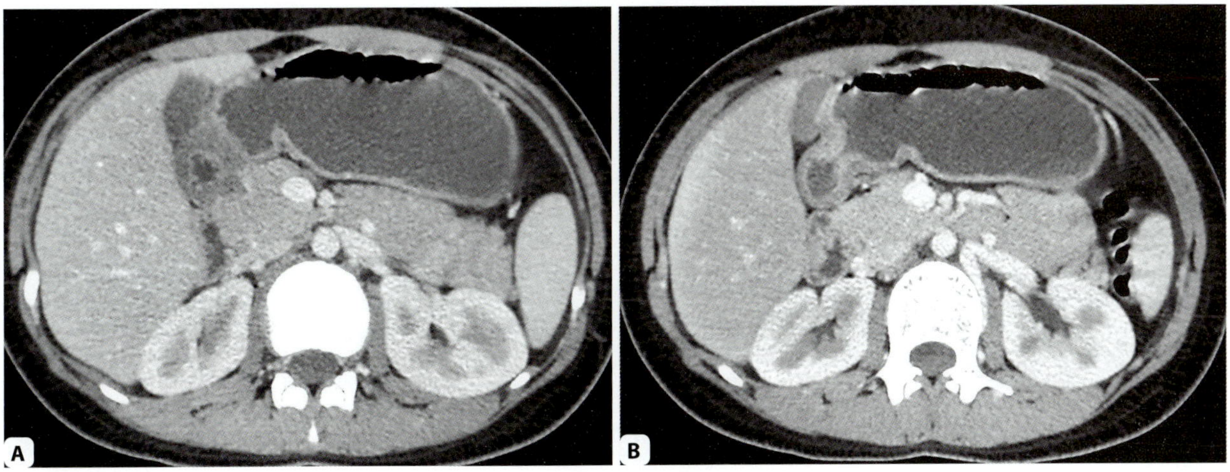

FIGS. 18A AND B: CECT axial images show circumferential, enhancing mural thickening of the pylorus and first part of duodenum with maintained mural stratification suggestive of inflammatory thickening—gastritis.
(CECT: contrast-enhanced computed tomography)

folds in the esophagus, duodenum, and jejunum. Multiple ulcers, hypervascular pancreaticoduodenal tumor, and liver metastases may be seen.

Ménétrier's disease (hypoproteinemic hypertrophic gastropathy) is a rare condition with massive foveolar hyperplasia leading to enlarged gastric folds. Patients present with hypochlorhydria and hypoproteinemia. On CT, diffuse enlargement of rugal folds is seen in the region of the gastric fundus and body with relative sparing of the antrum.

Gastric anisakiasis is a parasitic infection caused by anisakid nematodes (worms). It usually results from ingestion of raw or undercooked seafood. Imaging findings include diffuse mural thickening with severe submucosal edema and mild perigastric inflammation. Anisakiasis may be indistinguishable from other causes of gastritis at imaging but the presence of severe submucosal edema can suggest the diagnosis. The treatment consists of endoscopic extraction of live larvae.

VASCULAR CONDITIONS

Gastric varices are a common cause of UGI bleed in cirrhotic patients. Primary vascular etiologies are rare causes of GI bleed in noncirrhotic patients. Gastric varices result from reversal of flow in the gastric fundal venous plexus. Portal hypertension is a progressive complication of hepatic cirrhosis and 5–33% of patients develop gastric varices. Gastric varices may also be seen in patients with splenic vein thrombosis consequent to pancreatitis that leads to localized portal hypertension. On CT, gastric varices are seen as multiple dilated tubular contrast-filled vessels coursing along the lesser curvature of the stomach and in most cases contiguous with esophageal varices **(Figs. 19A and B)**. CT also shows communication of the varices and other collateral vessels.[65]

Gastric arteriovenous malformation is a rare cause of UGI bleed. Gastric AVMs may be seen in patients with Osler–Weber–Rendu disease (hereditary hemorrhagic telangiectasia). On CT angiography, AVMs appear as a tangle of vessels along the gastric wall with early opacification of draining veins in the arterial phase.[65]

Gastric aneurysm or pseudoaneurysm is most commonly seen in patients with pancreatitis, other etiologies include trauma, recent intervention, or surgery or connective tissue disorders. The left gastric artery is most commonly involved. These are seen as a well-defined, round or oval mass that enhances with the same intensity as the abdominal aorta. The aneurysm may be partially thrombosed and show an eccentric nonenhancing component.

EMERGENCY CONDITIONS AFFECTING THE STOMACH

Emphysematous gastritis results from infection caused by gas forming organisms gaining access to deeper tissue layers following a gastric mucosal injury. Patients present with a toxic clinical picture and this condition is associated with a high mortality. The common organisms involved include hemolytic *Streptococci, Clostridia welchi, Escherichia coli,* and *Staphylococcus aureus*. Predisposing factors include alcohol, intake of toxic or corrosive agents, trauma, ulcer disease, and necrotizing enterocolitis. Gastric infarction may progress to emphysematous gastritis.

Gastric emphysema or *gastric pneumatosis* results from disruption of gastric mucosa with dissection of air into the gastric wall. Predisposing factors include conditions associated with increased intragastric pressure such as gastric outlet obstruction, recent instrumentation (postgastroscopy), severe vomiting, steroid use, chemotherapy, chronic obstructive pulmonary disease (COPD), vascular

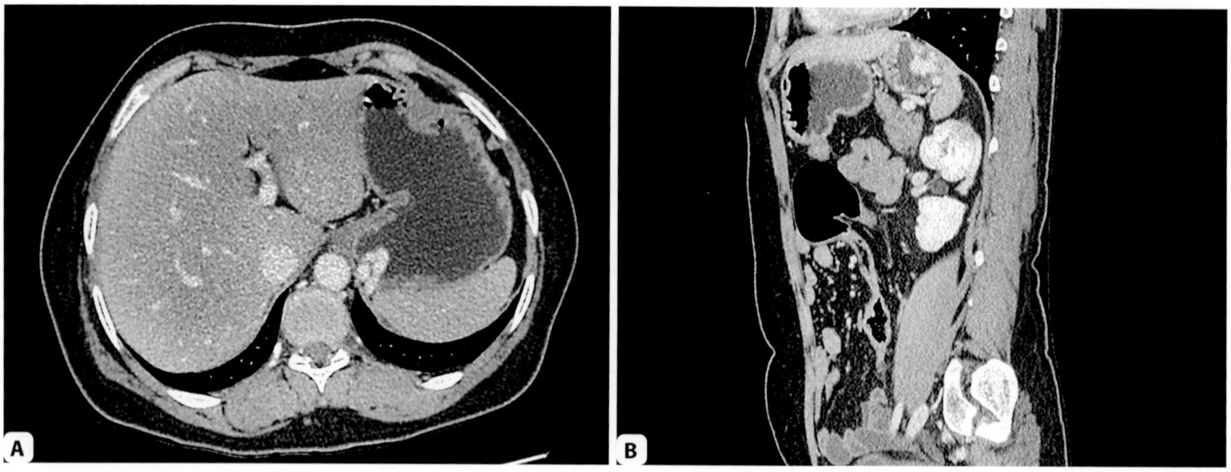

FIGS. 19A AND B: CECT axial (A) and sagittal (B) images show dilated, tortuous vessels within the gastric walls, predominantly along the greater curvature, suggestive of gastric varices.
(CECT: contrast-enhanced computed tomography)

occlusion, volvulus or it may be idiopathic. These patients are usually asymptomatic with a benign clinical course and spontaneous resolution.

On CT, both the conditions can show distended stomach with focal intramural gas or diffuse gas conforming to the stomach contour. Presence of gastric wall thickening, hypoenhancement, perigastric edema and/or inflammatory stranding suggests emphysematous gastritis. Portal venous gas may be seen in late stages of emphysematous gastritis.

Bezoar is an intraluminal mass that results from the accumulation of undigested or inedible ingested material. The common forms include trichobezoar (Rapunzel syndrome) and phytobezoar. Less frequently occurring forms include lactobezoar (accumulation of milk protein) and pharmacobezoar (accumulation of medications). Trichobezoar results from chronic ingestion of hair in patients with psychiatric illness while phytobezoar is seen in patients with decreased gastric motility. Other predisposing factors include poor mastication, altered anatomy, and prior gastric surgery. On CT, a bezoar appears as an inhomogeneous mottled mass which can cause gastric outlet obstruction resulting in gastric distension.[66] Small bezoars may displace gastric contents **(Fig. 20)**.

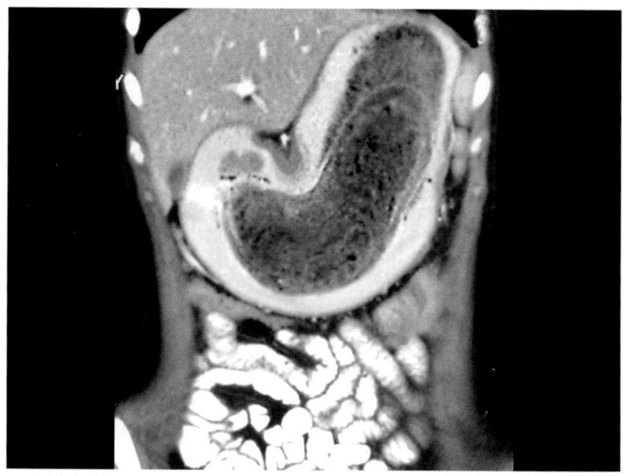

FIG. 20: CECT image in the coronal plane shows heterogenous hypodense contents within the gastric lumen, showing mottled gas shadows suggestive of bezoar.
(CECT: contrast-enhanced computed tomography)

Gastric volvulus is a condition where the stomach twists > 180° upon itself, creating a closed loop obstruction associated with a large defect in the diaphragm that allows part or all of the stomach to herniate into the chest cavity. Conditions that predispose to gastric volvulus include post-traumatic diaphragmatic hernia and paraesophageal hernia. There are two types of gastric volvulus depending upon the axis of rotation: organoaxial and mesenteroaxial. Organoaxial volvulus is more common and results from rotation of the stomach along its long axis resulting in anterosuperior displacement of the antrum and posteroinferior displacement of the fundus with the greatest curvature lying superior to the lesser curvature **(Figs. 21A to C)**. Mesenteroaxial volvulus results from rotation of the stomach along its short axis and the antrum is displaced above the GEJ. Imaging findings on CT include herniation of a large part of the stomach above the diaphragm with differential air-filled levels and a transition point. The presence of obstruction with failure of passage of oral contrast into the small bowel suggests a volvulus than an abnormal lie of the stomach. Other imaging findings may include gastric wall thickening, adjacent fluid, and fat stranding and pneumatosis.[65]

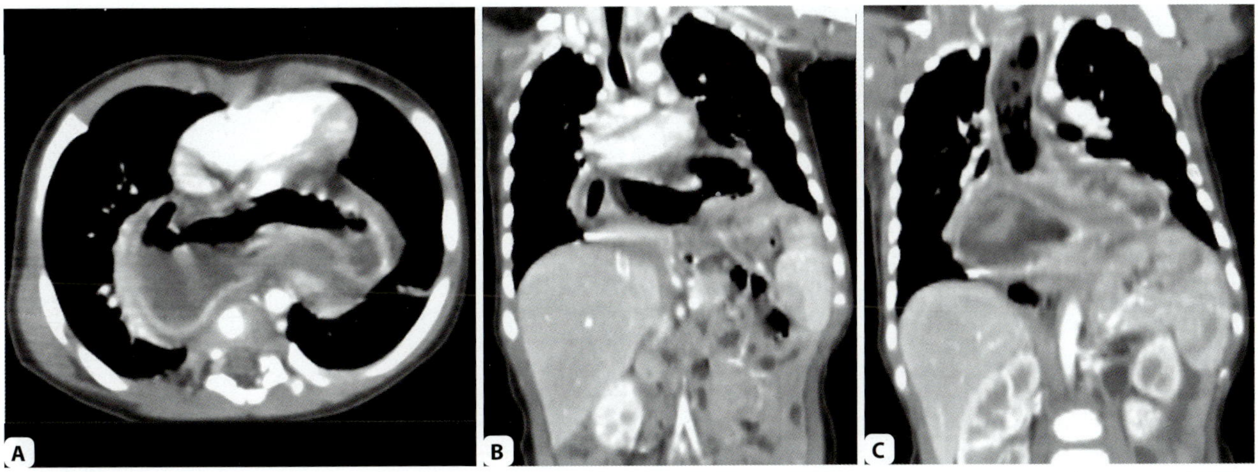

FIGS. 21A TO C: CECT images in the axial (A) and coronal (B and C) planes reveal herniation of the gastroesophageal junction and stomach into the thorax along with rotation of the stomach along its long axis suggestive of organoaxial volvulus.

(CECT: contrast-enhanced computed tomography)

OTHER GASTRIC LESIONS

Hiatus Hernia

Hiatus hernia is the herniation of abdominal organs and structures from the abdominal cavity into the thoracic cavity through the esophageal hiatus. The most common content of hiatus hernia is the stomach. Hiatus hernia is divided into four types.

- *Type 1*: Sliding hiatal hernia
- *Type 2*: Paraesophageal hiatal hernia
- *Type 3*: Mixed type
- *Type 4*: Mixed type with herniation of other viscera

The risk factors affecting the development of hiatus hernia include obesity, old age, trauma, pregnancy, or inherited diaphragmatic weakness. Patients with hiatus hernia may present with dysphagia, symptoms of reflux, chest pain, abdominal pain, or shortness of breath. Cross-sectional imaging modalities such as CT and MRI have replaced ultrasound and fluoroscopic examination in the diagnosis of hiatus hernia. Accurate diagnosis helps in appropriate management and surgical decision making. Type 1 or sliding hiatal hernia is the most common, accounting for approximately 95% of cases with extension of the GEJ toward the mediastinum and widening of the esophageal hiatus to 3–4 cm (normal limit is 1.5 cm). The gastric fundus may also be displaced above the diaphragm. In type 2 or paraesophageal type of hiatal hernia the GEJ is in normal position with fundus of the stomach herniating into the thorax. Type 3 refers to the herniation of the GEJ along with a large portion of the stomach which is usually rotated. Large paraesophageal hernias with most of the stomach in the thorax are at an increased risk of complications which include volvulus, obstruction, and ischemia.

Ectopic Pancreatic Rests

This is also known as heterotopic, accessory, or aberrant pancreas and is defined as pancreatic tissue lacking anatomic and vascular continuity with the main body of the gland. These lesions are most commonly found incidentally in asymptomatic patients mainly along the greatest curvature of prepyloric region of stomach and duodenum. Some patients present with abdominal pain, GI bleeding, and obstruction due to complications like pancreatitis, pseudocyst, insulinoma, and pancreatic cancer.[67]

Ectopic pancreas may manifest as a submucosal mass in the stomach or duodenum and may easily be misinterpreted as another submucosal tumor such as GIST or leiomyoma. They can appear as well-defined submucosal masses on either single- or double-contrast barium studies and can even have central umbilication and rarely barium may even be seen to enter into rudimentary ductal system. However, the typical location (prepyloric antrum and duodenum), endoluminal growth pattern, ill-defined border, prominent enhancement of overlying mucosa, and a long diameter/short diameter ratio of > 1.4 are considered significant CT features for differentiating ectopic pancreas from other tumors.[68]

Magnetic resonance imaging is diagnostic, as ectopic pancreas follows pancreatic signal and enhancement pattern on all sequences.[69] Usually, these lesions are flat (LD/SD > 1.4); however, they can acquire ovoid form and protrude endoluminally after intraglandular cyst formation. Small cystic areas within the mass represent dilated anomalous ducts.[37]

Gastric Duplication Cyst

Duplication of the alimentary tract is a rare congenital anomaly with the gastric duplication cysts (GDCs)

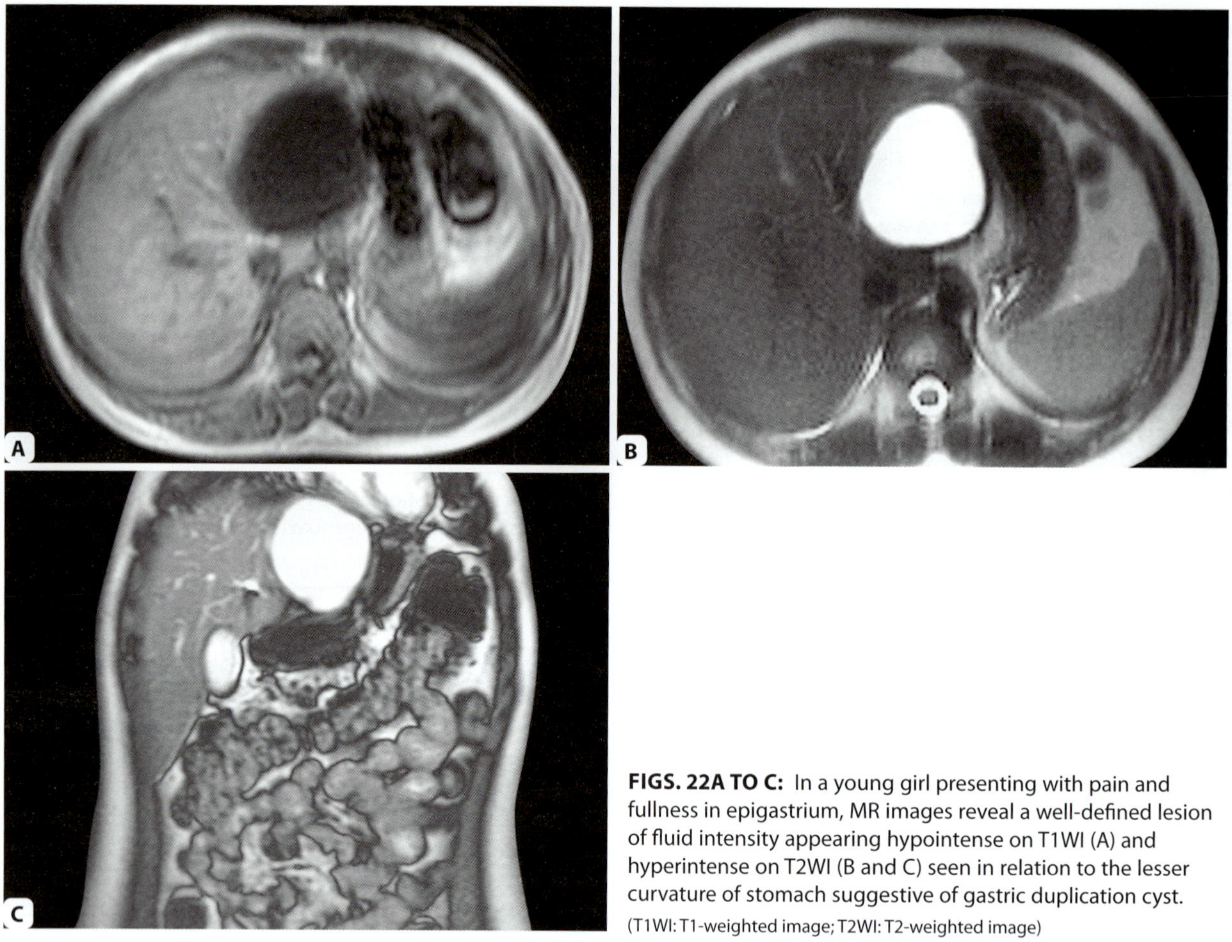

FIGS. 22A TO C: In a young girl presenting with pain and fullness in epigastrium, MR images reveal a well-defined lesion of fluid intensity appearing hypointense on T1WI (A) and hyperintense on T2WI (B and C) seen in relation to the lesser curvature of stomach suggestive of gastric duplication cyst.
(T1WI: T1-weighted image; T2WI: T2-weighted image)

being rarest, representing only 4% of all alimentary tract duplications. The common age of presentation being the first decade with approximately 67% manifest within the first year of life.[70] Classically, barium studies show an intramural filling defect indenting the gastric contour. Typical NCCT appearance is a spheric to ovoid nonenhancing cystic lesion in close approximation to greater curvature. Occasionally, marginal calcifications may be present. Contrast-enhanced CT scan typically demonstrates a thick-walled cystic lesion with enhancement of the inner lining. They follow fluid signal intensity on MR sequences, appearing hyperintense on T2-weighted images and hypointense on T1-weighted images **(Figs. 22A to C)**. EUS can further add to the diagnosis by demonstrating an echogenic internal mucosal layer and a hypoechoic intermediate muscular layer making the diagnosis of GDC highly likely.

The essential criteria for diagnosis of a GDC includes—contiguity of the cyst wall with that of the stomach; smooth muscles in the cyst wall, which is continuous with the muscle of the stomach; and lining of the cyst wall by either gastric epithelium or any other type of gut mucosa.[71]

Majority of gastric duplications are cystic (80%) and do not communicate with lumen of the stomach. Few of them are tubular and may show some communication. It is defined as tubular when the lumen is contiguous with the stomach lumen and cystic when the lumen is not contiguous.

Because most of the duplication cysts occur along the greatest curvature of the stomach, they can potentially compress the adjacent organs such as pancreas, kidney, spleen, and adrenal gland, and hence lesions arising from these organs become the differential diagnosis of duplication cysts.

As with the native gastric mucosa, the cyst lining may undergo erosions, ulceration, bleeding, and regenerative changes. In noncommunicating cysts, pressure necrosis of the mucosa may be seen due to increased fluid production. These changes may lead to bleeding into the cyst or perforation into the peritoneal cavity. Duplication cysts have the potential for neoplastic transformation especially by production of oncofetal antigens which raises the problem of a precancerous condition in long-standing cases.

POSTOPERATIVE IMAGING OF THE STOMACH

Traditionally, gastric surgery was primarily performed to address conditions such as gastric or duodenal ulcer

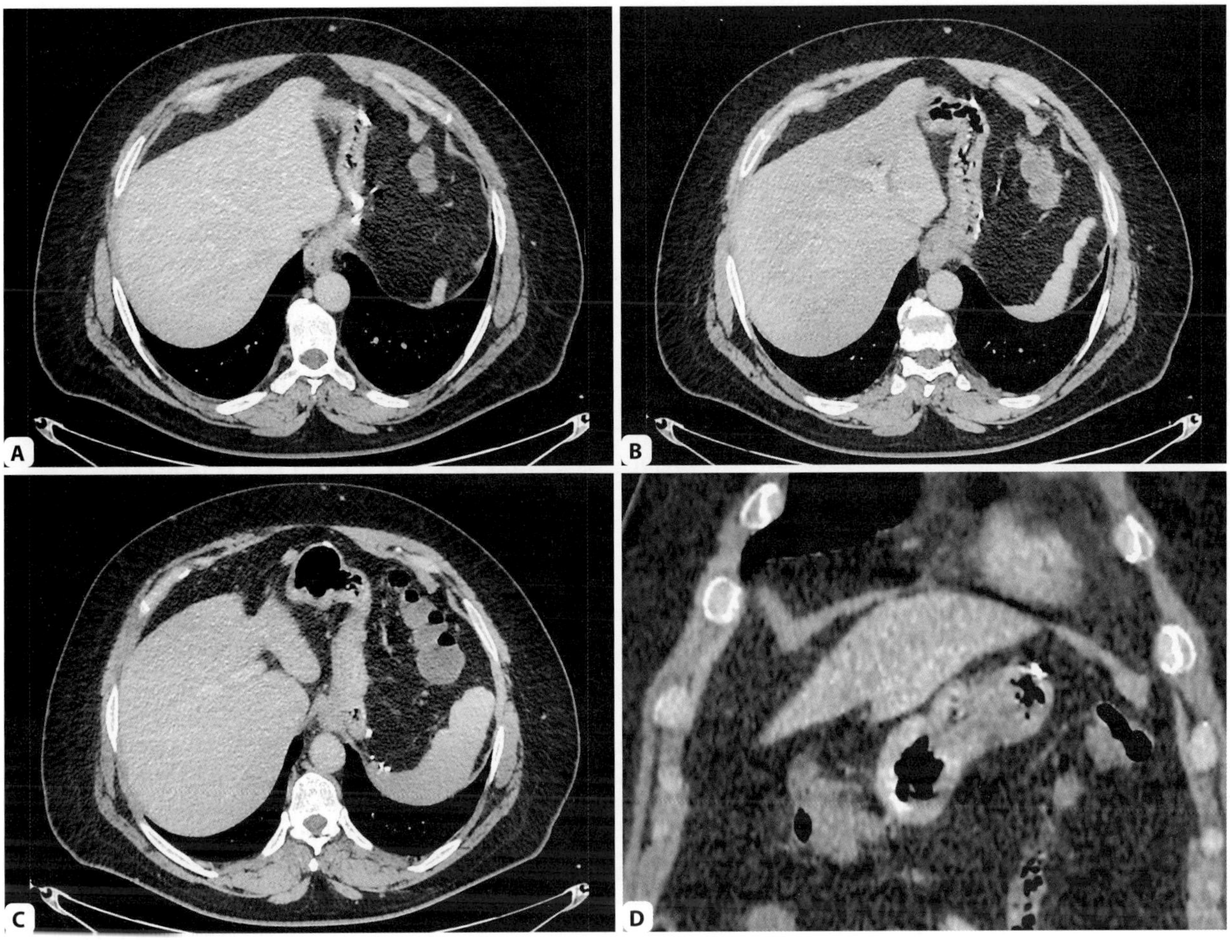

FIGS. 23A TO D: CECT images in the axial (A to C) and coronal (D) plane in a patient who underwent laparoscopic sleeve gastrectomy reveal tubular gastric sleeve with surgical staples along the greater curvature of the stomach.

(CECT: contrast-enhanced computed tomography)

refractory to medical treatment or resectable malignancies of the stomach. However, in contemporary practice, a large number of gastric surgeries are performed for morbid obesity, particularly gastric bypass procedures. For gastric cancer, surgical resection remains the definitive treatment option, with tumor depth and lymph node involvement being critical predictors of recurrence. The term "stump cancer" refers to malignancy in the gastric remnant occurring 15–25 years postgastrectomy, often following surgery for benign conditions like gastric ulcer. Postgastrectomy follow-up typically involves CT scans, which are effective in detecting recurrent cancer or metastasis. In gastric bypass patients, CT is commonly used to assess anastomotic sites during follow-up.

Roux-en-Y gastric bypass, laparoscopic adjustable gastric banding and laparoscopic sleeve gastrectomy **(Figs. 23A to D)** are commonly performed surgical procedures for obesity. Fluoroscopic UGI examination with water soluble contrast and abdominal CT are useful to detect leaks after gastric bypass. Barium studies are useful to diagnose anastomotic strictures. "Marginal" ulceration, occurring at or near suture lines, is frequently seen in patients who have undergone gastrojejunostomy or Roux-en-Y gastric bypass. CT scans are valuable in investigating postgastric surgery complications such as stomal stenosis, bleeding, or perforation in patients presenting with symptoms such as obstruction, pain, or bleeding. Gastric banding, another popular bariatric procedure, involves creating a small gastric pouch using an adjustable band near the GEJ. Complications such as band slippage can increase the risk of obstruction or volvulus. Proper positioning of the gastric band, assessed through features like the alignment of its anterior and posterior aspects and the angle between the spine and band axis, is best evaluated using topograms or coronal images. Data analysis in patients undergoing laparoscopic sleeve gastrectomy has shown that MDCT-calculated resected stomach volume (preoperative volume minus reconstructed sleeve volume) correlates well with early postoperative weight loss. Complications that can occur following laparoscopic sleeve gastrectomy include gastric leaks, gastric strictures, gastric outlet obstruction, gastric dilatation, and gastroesophageal reflux.

DUODENUM

The duodenum, a curved hollow organ situated at the L1–3 vertebrae level, coils in a C-shape anterior to the vertebral column, closely associated with the pancreatic head. Comprising four segments, it begins at the duodenal bulb which extends from the pylorus. The first part (D1) lies anterior to the common bile duct, portal vein, and gastroduodenal artery, superior to the pancreatic head, and posterior to the gallbladder and liver. Following this, the descending (D2) segment commences at the superior duodenal flexure, reaching its end at the inferior duodenal flexure. It lies anterior to the right kidney, ureter, and adrenal gland, and medial to the ascending colon and hepatic flexure, the pancreatic head resides medially. The major and minor duodenal papillae are situated on the medial wall of the second part of duodenum. Subsequently, the third part (horizontal, D3) originates from the inferior duodenal flexure, traversing transversely to the left, crossing the vertebral column. The right psoas muscle, aorta, and inferior vena cava lie posteriorly, while the small bowel mesentery root lies anteriorly. Finally, the ascending (D4) portion ascends and then curves anteriorly, terminating at the duodenojejunal flexure, continuing as the jejunum. The left psoas muscle and the aorta are situated posterior to D4 while the stomach is positioned superiorly.

Arterial supply is provided by the right gastric and right gastroepiploic arteries in the duodenal cap (first 2.5 cm), the superior pancreaticoduodenal artery from remaining D1 to mid-D2, and the inferior pancreaticoduodenal artery from mid-D2 to the ligament of Treitz. Venous drainage occurs through the prepyloric vein in the duodenal cap and superior and inferior pancreaticoduodenal veins in the remaining duodenum. Duodenal nodes drain distally to superior mesenteric nodes and proximally to celiac nodes.

Initially, the duodenum is intraperitoneal for the first 2–3 cm and then it transitions to a retroperitoneal location (anterior pararenal space). Due to its unique positioning and proximity to neighboring organs, the duodenum is susceptible to involvement in various primary and secondary processes. Previously, barium studies and hypotonic duodenography played an important role in evaluation of duodenal pathologies. With advent of endoscopy and cross-sectional imaging, their role has been relegated to past. Endoscopy plays an important role in duodenal evaluation, especially in depicting the mucosa and obtaining tissue for histopathological diagnosis. Cross-sectional imaging modalities have been increasingly effective in staging duodenal lesions, some of which are incidentally detected.[72] **Table 3** lists the various pathological conditions that can affect the duodenum.

TUMORS OF THE DUODENUM

Malignant Tumors

Adenocarcinoma

Adenocarcinoma is the most common malignant tumor of the duodenum accounting for approximately 85% of all primary duodenal malignant tumors. It is commonly seen in the sixth and seventh decades with a male predominance. Most of the cases are sporadic, although an association with FAP, Peutz–Jeghers syndrome, and Crohn disease has been reported. Patients present with abdominal pain, weight loss, jaundice, duodenal obstruction and upper GI bleeding. On barium upper GI series, it may be seen as an annular constricting wall thickening or a polypoid or ulcerative mass **(Figs. 24A to C)**. "Apple-core" lesions are a classical finding.

Imaging features on cross-sectional imaging include soft-tissue polypoid mass, concentric or asymmetric soft-tissue attenuation thickening, annular narrowing with irregular borders or an ulcerated infiltrating mass. The mass shows delayed enhancement due to the presence of significant fibrous component. It most commonly arises from the periampullary region and rarely involves

TABLE 3: Duodenal pathological conditions.

Infectious and inflammatory	Malignant	Benign	Traumatic and vascular	Anatomic and miscellaneous
Tuberculosis	Adenocarcinoma	Gastrointestinal stromal tumor (GIST)	Hematoma	Bulging papilla
Peptic ulcer disease	Lymphoma	Gangliocytic paraganglioma	Aortoenteric fistula	Heterotopic pancreas
Pancreatic pseudocyst in wall	Neuroendocrine tumor	Hamartomatous polyp	Superior mesenteric artery (SMA) syndrome	Intussusception
Paraduodenal or groove pancreatitis	Leiomyosarcoma	Lipoma	Henoch–Schönlein purpura	Duplication cyst
Crohn disease		Villous adenoma		Duodenal diverticula
Bouveret syndrome		Schwannoma		Pancreatic divisum
Zollinger–Ellison syndrome				Extension of gastric bezoar

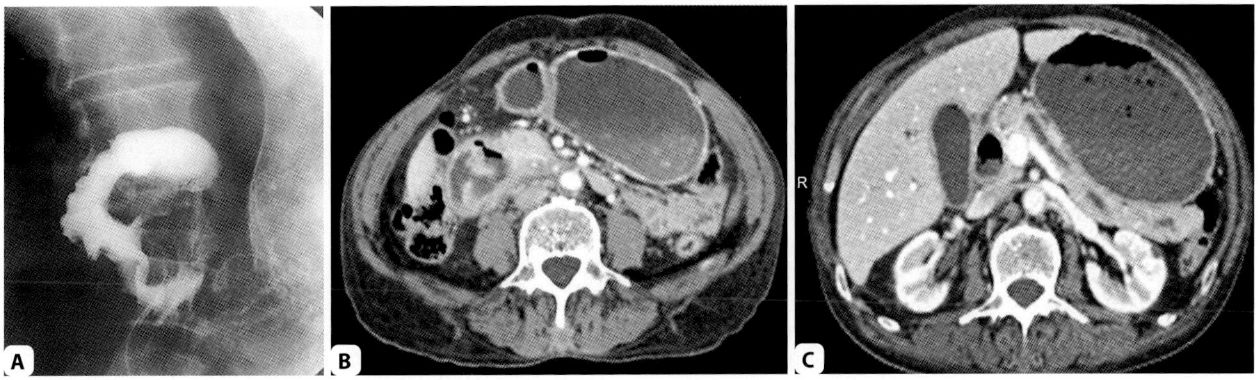

FIGS. 24A TO C: Duodenal adenocarcinoma—(A) Single contrast upper gastrointestinal (GI) barium study reveals irregular luminal narrowing along second part of duodenum. Axial CECT images (B and C) reveal circumferential enhancing mural thickening of the second part of the duodenum with luminal narrowing and obstruction as evident by distended stomach with residual contents. The main pancreatic duct also appears to be dilated.

(CECT: contrast-enhanced computed tomography)

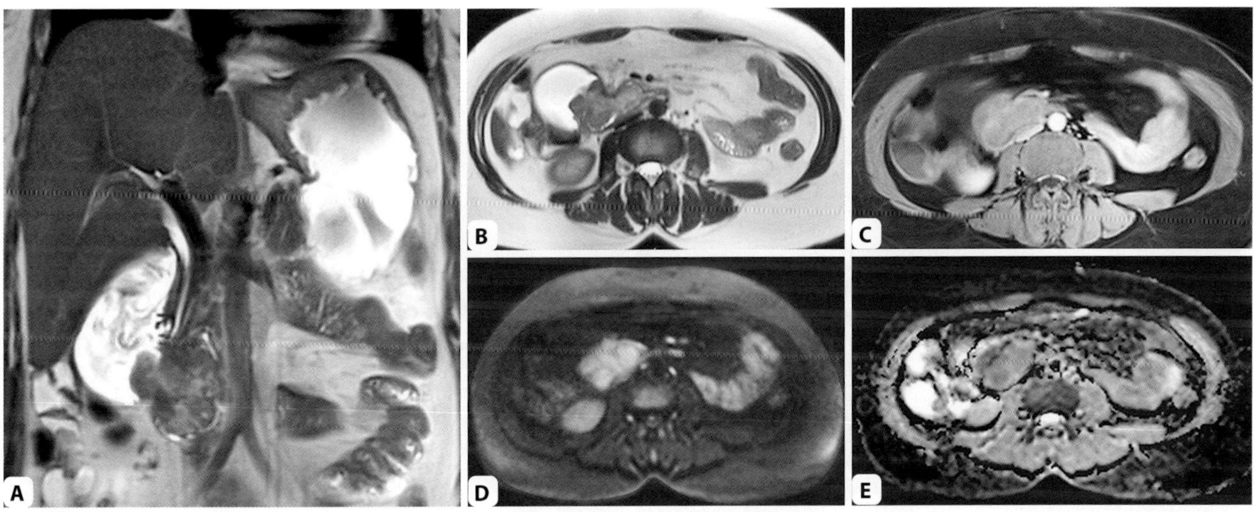

FIGS. 25A TO E: In an elderly male patient presenting with weight loss, vomiting and signs of gastric outlet obstruction, T2WI coronal (A) and axial (B) images show an iso- to hypointense lesion involving second and third parts of duodenum causing upstream dilatation of the stomach. The lesion shows diffusion restriction (D and E) along with postcontrast enhancement (C). Histopathological examination revealed adenocarcinoma.

(T2WI: T2-weighted image)

the bulb **(Figs. 25A to E)**. Duodenal adenocarcinoma involves a short segment of the bowel and causes upstream obstruction which is in contrast to lymphoma which does not result in obstruction. Obstruction to the common bile duct may be caused by lesions involving the second part of the duodenum. Locoregional lymphadenopathy is frequent at the time of diagnosis and 5–40% of the patients have distant metastases or peritoneal seeding at the time of presentation.[72]

Lymphoma

Although primary lymphoma of the duodenum is rare, the duodenum may be involved in systemic lymphoma. Primary intestinal lymphoma is usually non-Hodgkin T-cell type and originates from the lymphatic tissue of the lamina propria. Lymphoma is most commonly seen in the sixth decade of life. On barium upper GI series, thickened or effaced mucosal folds, with narrowed, normal, or dilated lumen may be seen. Imaging features on CT include a mural polypoid lesion or a large necrotic infiltrating mass with moderate and homogeneous enhancement. Other features include aneurysmal luminal dilatation, diffuse lymph node enlargement, and splenomegaly. Obstruction is usually not a feature of lymphomas. Primary lymphoma of the duodenum is curable by surgery in only 40% of patients and unresectable cases of lymphoma requires radiotherapy and chemotherapy. Surgery in such cases is being used only to treat complications such has bleeding from high-grade lesions.

Neuroendocrine Tumors

Neuroendocrine tumors of the duodenum account for approximately 3% of all GI neuroendocrine tumors. They mostly arise from the first or second part of the duodenum. 62% are gastrinomas which arise from the gastrin-producing G cells, these may be sporadic or associated with MEN1. 21% are somatostatinomas which arise from D cells, they are seen in the periampullary region and are strongly associated with MEN1. Other types such as carcinoid tumors and nonfunctional NETs are less frequent.

On imaging, majority of the lesions (>80%) present as an intraluminal polyp or mural mass while few may be associated with wall thickening or an exophytic growth pattern **(Figs. 26A to D)**. These tumors show early arterial enhancement with delayed washout. Nodal and distant metastases are uncommon. Locoregional hyperenhancing lymph nodes may be seen.

Secondary Involvement and Metastases

Secondary involvement of duodenum by malignant process in adjacent viscera, like pancreas is fairly common and it is often not possible to distinguish a primary tumor of duodenum from a tumor of pancreas involving duodenum.[73]

Metastases to the duodenum can also occur and can present as filling defect with central ulceration and necrosis leading to classical "bull's eye" or "target" appearance. They are seen with metastasis from malignant melanoma **(Fig. 27)** and in patients with Kaposi's sarcoma.

Benign Tumors

Duodenal Polyps

Duodenal polyps smaller than 2 cm are typically benign and asymptomatic. Other than polyps found in polyposis syndrome, duodenal polyps are solitary. Multiple

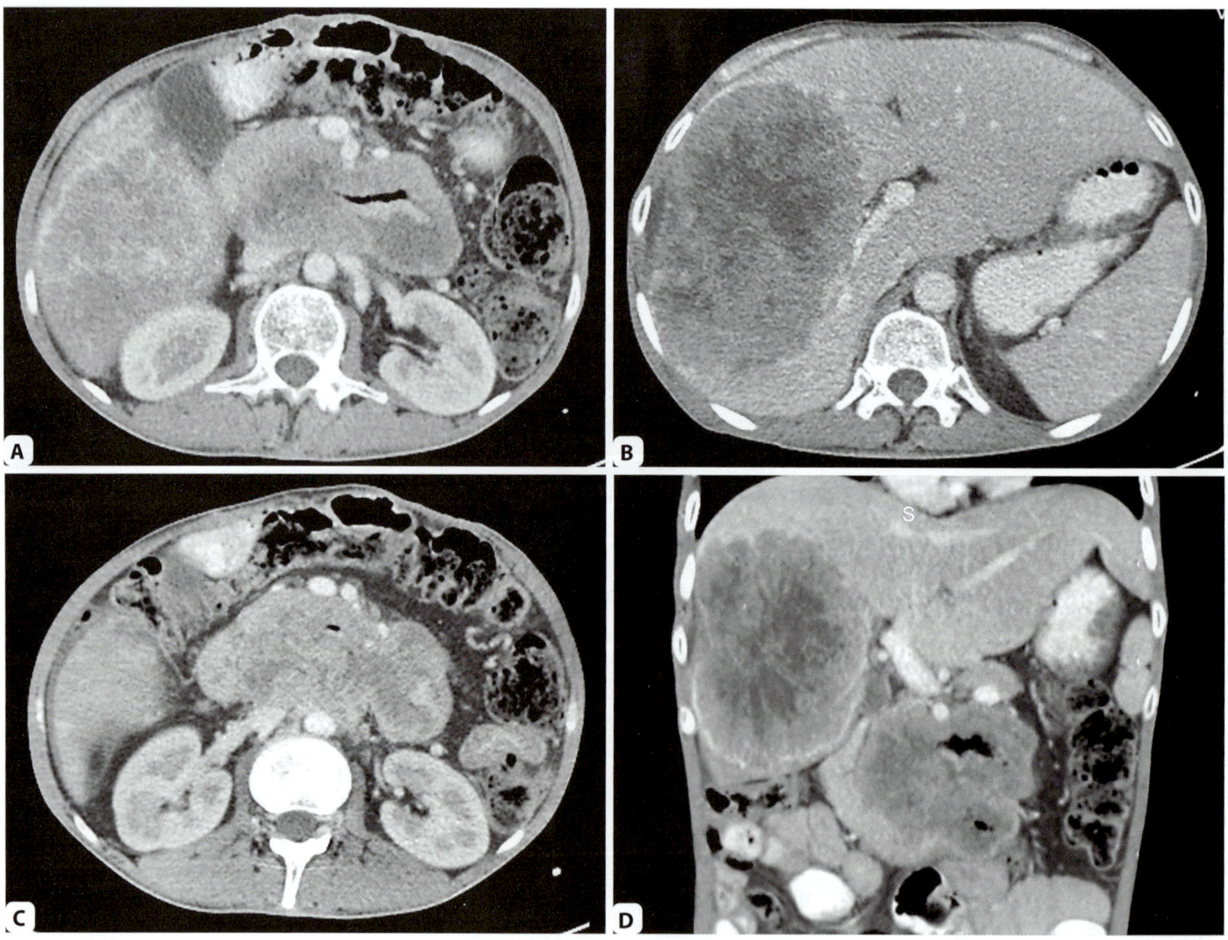

FIGS. 26A TO D: Malignant neuroendocrine tumor of duodenum—CECT images in the axial (A to C) and coronal (D) plane reveal a large, heterogeneous mass lesion arising from the second and third part of the duodenum with evidence of ulceration, the mesenteric vessels are displaced anteriorly. A large heterogeneously hypodense lesion is seen in right lobe of liver suggestive of metastasis.

(CECT: contrast-enhanced computed tomography)

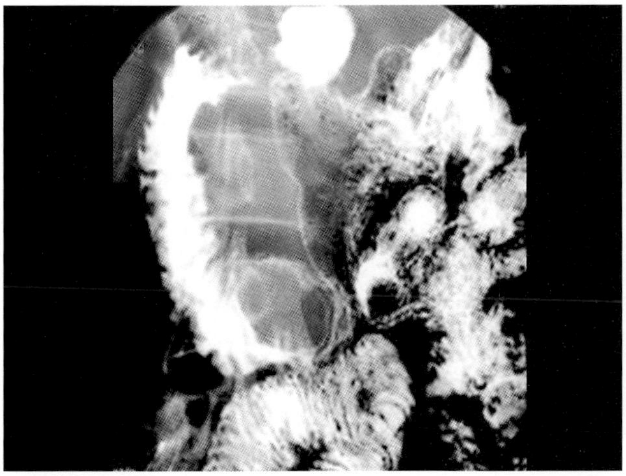

FIG. 27: Single-contrast barium study showing large submucosal filling defect on en-face view in the third part of duodenum in a patient with malignant melanoma suggestive of metastasis.

polyps can be seen in Peutz–Jeghers syndrome, familial polyposis, Gardner syndrome, and juvenile polyposis. The most common epithelial polyps in the duodenum are adenomatous and appear in the sixth decade of life. They are classified as tubular, tubulovillous or villous according to their growth pattern. Villous adenomas exhibit a characteristic "cauliflower" or "soap bubble" appearance on barium studies, caused by the trapping of barium in the crevices between the multiple frond-like projections of the tumor **(Figs. 28A and B)**. As villous adenomas have malignant potential they should be resected, other adenomas are resected when they are symptomatic. CT has poor sensitivity for ampullary adenomas, detecting < 50%.[74] On CECT, ampullary adenomas are seen as smooth, frondlike, flat or lobulated filling defects in the duodenal lumen, as an enhancing mass with smooth margins or as a bulging and enhancing papilla. The role of CT is to detect features that suggest malignant change such as ulceration, vascular invasion, lymph nodal enlargement, or metastases.

Brenner's gland hamartoma is a rare benign tumor that occurs in the proximal duodenum and appears as one or more submucosal or sessile polyps.

Gastrointestinal Stromal Tumor

Less than 5% of GISTs are found in the duodenum. They arise from the interstitial cells of Cajal or their precursors along the muscular wall of the GIT. These tumors are positive for C-KIT at immunohistochemistry. Duodenal GISTs are mostly seen in the sixth decade of life. Although most GISTs exhibit benign clinical behavior, small bowel lesions are more likely to be malignant. Imaging reveals a large well-circumscribed mass with a heterogeneously enhancing pattern. The mass may show necrotic areas, ulceration, and central cavitation. An extraluminal growth pattern is commonly seen and therefore obstruction is rare **(Figs. 29A to C)**.

Duodenal Lipoma

Lipomas of the GIT are most commonly seen in the colon, ileum, and jejunum with duodenal lipomas being rare. They occur in the submucosal plane of the second part of duodenum but can extend into deeper planes through the wall. Most cases are asymptomatic and diagnosed incidentally. If larger than 4 cm they can cause bleeding or intussusception. On CT, a duodenal lipoma is seen as a well-circumscribed nodule with attenuation between –60 and –120 HU **(Fig. 30)**. On MRI, it follows the signal intensity of fat on all sequences.

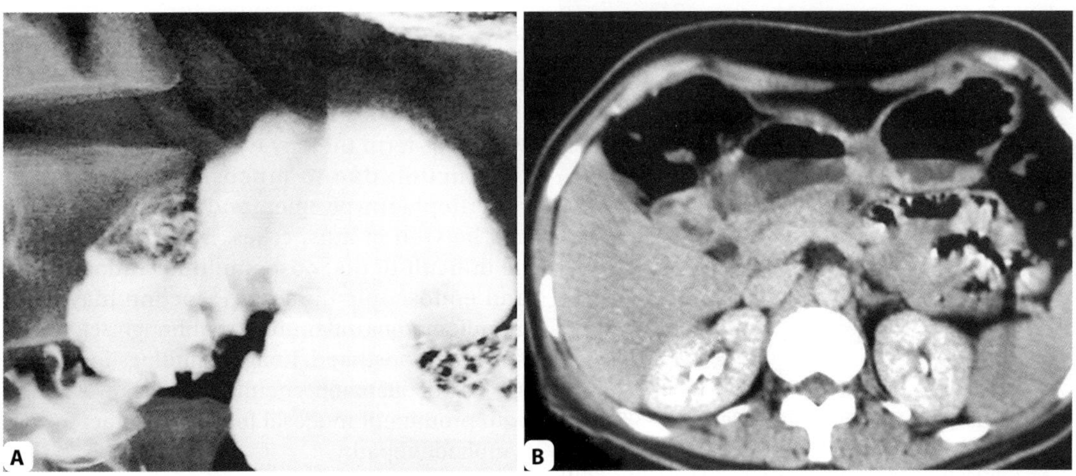

FIGS. 28A AND B: Villous adenoma—polypoidal filling defect along the lateral wall of duodenal bulb characteristic "cauliflower" or "soap bubble" appearance on barium studies, caused by the trapping of barium in the crevices between the multiple frond-like projections of the tumor (A). CECT axial section (B) reveals heterogeneously enhancing polypoidal mass lesion in first part of duodenum with nonenhancing fluid-filled hypodense linear areas symptoms of crevices between fronds with tracking of fluid in it.

(CECT: contrast-enhanced computed tomography)

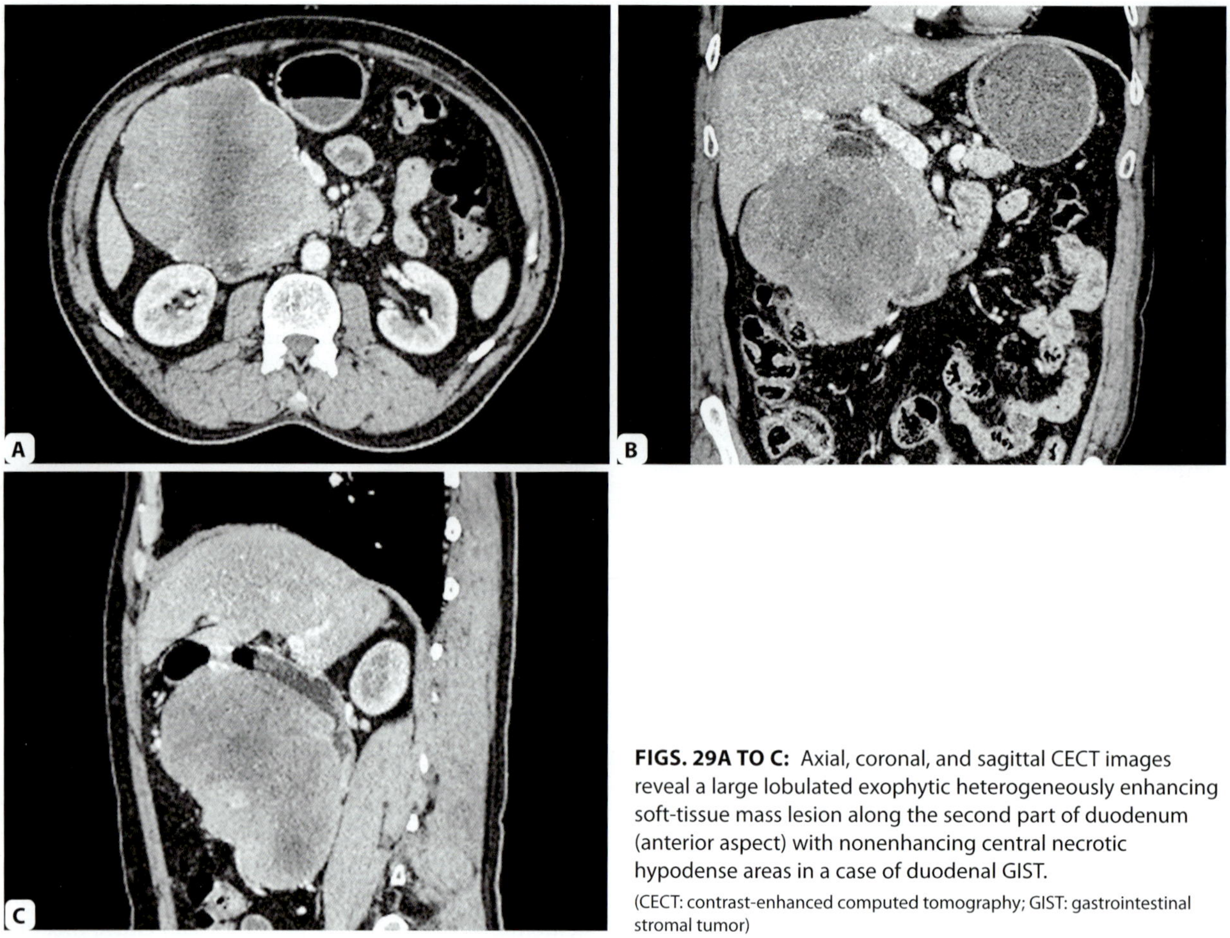

FIGS. 29A TO C: Axial, coronal, and sagittal CECT images reveal a large lobulated exophytic heterogeneously enhancing soft-tissue mass lesion along the second part of duodenum (anterior aspect) with nonenhancing central necrotic hypodense areas in a case of duodenal GIST.

(CECT: contrast-enhanced computed tomography; GIST: gastrointestinal stromal tumor)

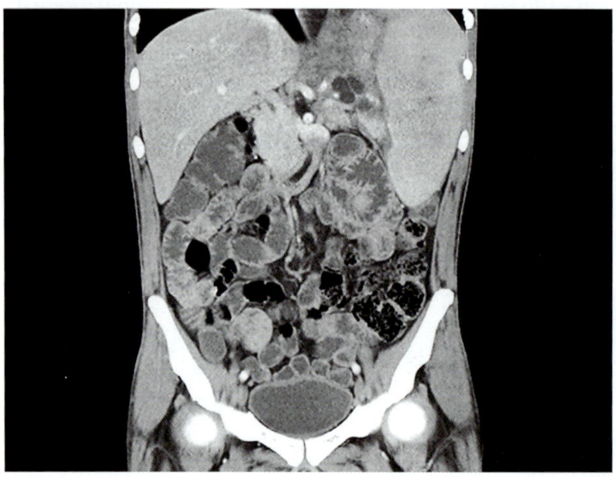

FIG. 30: CECT image in the coronal plane reveals a well-defined, nonenhancing, submucosal hypodense lesion of fat attenuation seen along the third part of duodenum extending into the fourth part suggestive of lipoma.

(CECT: contrast-enhanced computed tomography)

INFECTIOUS AND INFLAMMATORY CONDITIONS

Duodenal Tuberculosis

Duodenal tuberculosis can be seen in individuals living in endemic locations, those with underlying PUD and with long-term therapy with H2 blockers. Gastric outlet obstruction due to mucosal ulcerations, muscular hypertrophic involvement and extrinsic lymphadenopathy can be seen in most cases. Duodenal tuberculosis can be difficult to diagnose, multiple endoscopic biopsies, and endoscopic mucosal resection may demonstrate granulomatous inflammation although acid-fast bacilli are rarely demonstrated. Imaging findings include segmental stenosis or dilatation, circumferential bowel wall thickening with prominent mucosal folds, sinus tract formation, and lymphadenopathy.

Crohn Disease

Duodenal involvement is seen in 0.5–4% cases of Crohn disease. It is usually seen in the third and fourth decades with no significant sex predilection. Although any segment of the duodenum can be affected, the fourth part is the most common location, usually in association with strictures of the proximal jejunum. Most patients have involvement of the terminal ileum or large intestine at presentation. Imaging findings include duodenal wall thickening, stenosis with mucosal enhancement, fat stranding, and formation of fistulas. The complications of Crohn disease include strictures, gastric outlet obstruction, acute or chronic pancreatitis and malignancy resulting from long-standing obstruction.

Peptic Ulcer Disease

Peptic ulcer disease affects about 10% of the world population. The risk factors include *H. pylori*, NSAIDs, corticosteroid use, physiologic stress, inflammatory bowel disease, Zollinger–Ellison syndrome, and smoking and alcohol consumption. Previously, barium studies played an important role in detection of ulceration and deformities consequent to it thereof like trifoliate or clover leaf-like deformity of first part of duodenum (duodenal bulb). The indirect imaging signs on CT include mural thickening, per duodenal fat stranding and adjacent lymphadenopathy. Direct signs include discontinuity of the mucosal hyperenhancement, luminal outpouching, and contiguous extramural gas.

Pancreatic Pseudocyst in Duodenal Wall

Pancreatic pseudocyst in duodenal wall is defined as a fluid collection that develops at least 4 weeks after an episode of interstitial edematous pancreatitis. The symptoms of this condition include abdominal pain, gastric outlet obstruction, bilious vomiting, and jaundice. Imaging features include homogeneous fluid collection along the duodenal wall, narrowing of the bowel lumen, gastric outlet obstruction, and dilatation of the bile duct.[72]

Paraduodenal Pancreatitis

Paraduodenal pancreatitis is defined as focal chronic pancreatitis centered in the pancreaticoduodenal groove, that is between the pancreatic head and duodenum. The risk factors include male sex, age between 40 and 50 years, and history of alcohol addiction. The theories behind its pathogenesis include presence of heterotopic pancreatic rests in the medial duodenal wall, disturbed pancreatic secretion through Santorini duct and functional or anatomic changes of the minor papilla.

Imaging findings include a solid and cystic mass centered at the pancreaticoduodenal groove, medial duodenal wall thickening, absence of biliary dilatation or significant pancreatic parenchymal atrophy and a displacement of the common bile duct and gastroduodenal artery rather than encasement **(Figs. 31A to D)**.[72]

Cholecystoduodenal Fistula

Bouveret syndrome is characterized by gastric outlet obstruction secondary to an impacted gallstone that reaches the duodenum through a bilioenteric fistula usually from the gallbladder to duodenum. It results from chronic inflammation and adherence between the biliary system and the duodenum with secondary wall ischemia and wall perforation. Patients present with epigastric pain, nausea, and vomiting. Cholecystoduodenal fistula may be difficult to diagnose endoscopically if the stone is highly embedded in mucosa and suboptimally visualized. Imaging features include bowel obstruction, pneumobilia, and ectopic gallstone.

TRAUMATIC AND VASCULAR CONDITIONS

Hematoma

Duodenum is the most common site of intramural hematoma in the GIT. The causes include blunt trauma to the abdomen, coagulopathy and anticoagulant therapy, hematologic conditions (lymphoma, leukemia, and myeloma), vasculitis, and pancreatitis. The third part of the duodenum which is horizontal and the duodenojejunal flexure are more prone to abrupt avulsion due to a lack of mesentery and fixation by the Treitz ligament, respectively. Duodenal hematoma is associated with a high morbidity and mortality due to hypovolemic shock. Imaging findings on CECT include high-density collection in the duodenal wall, hemoperitoneum, paraduodenal gas foci, leakage of oral contrast agent, and surrounding fat stranding.

Aortoenteric Fistula

Aortoenteric fistula may be primary or secondary. Primary aortoenteric fistula is rare and is associated with a preexisting aortic aneurysm, usually a mycotic aneurysm. Secondary aortoenteric fistula are more common with an annual incidence of 0.6–2% as there has been an increase in these kinds of surgery. These are related to complications of aortic reconstructive surgery, most commonly a delayed complication after open abdominal aortic aneurysm repair or aortobifemoral bypass. It usually affects the duodenum with the third and fourth parts being the most common locations. CT is the mainstay of diagnosis. The direct signs of aortoenteric fistula include the presence of vascular contrast inside the bowel lumen, ectopic gas adjacent, and within the aorta and visualization of the fistulous tract itself. Indirect signs include duodenum wall thickening, disruption of the aortic fat cover, retroperitoneal hematoma, and increased perigraft soft tissue.[72]

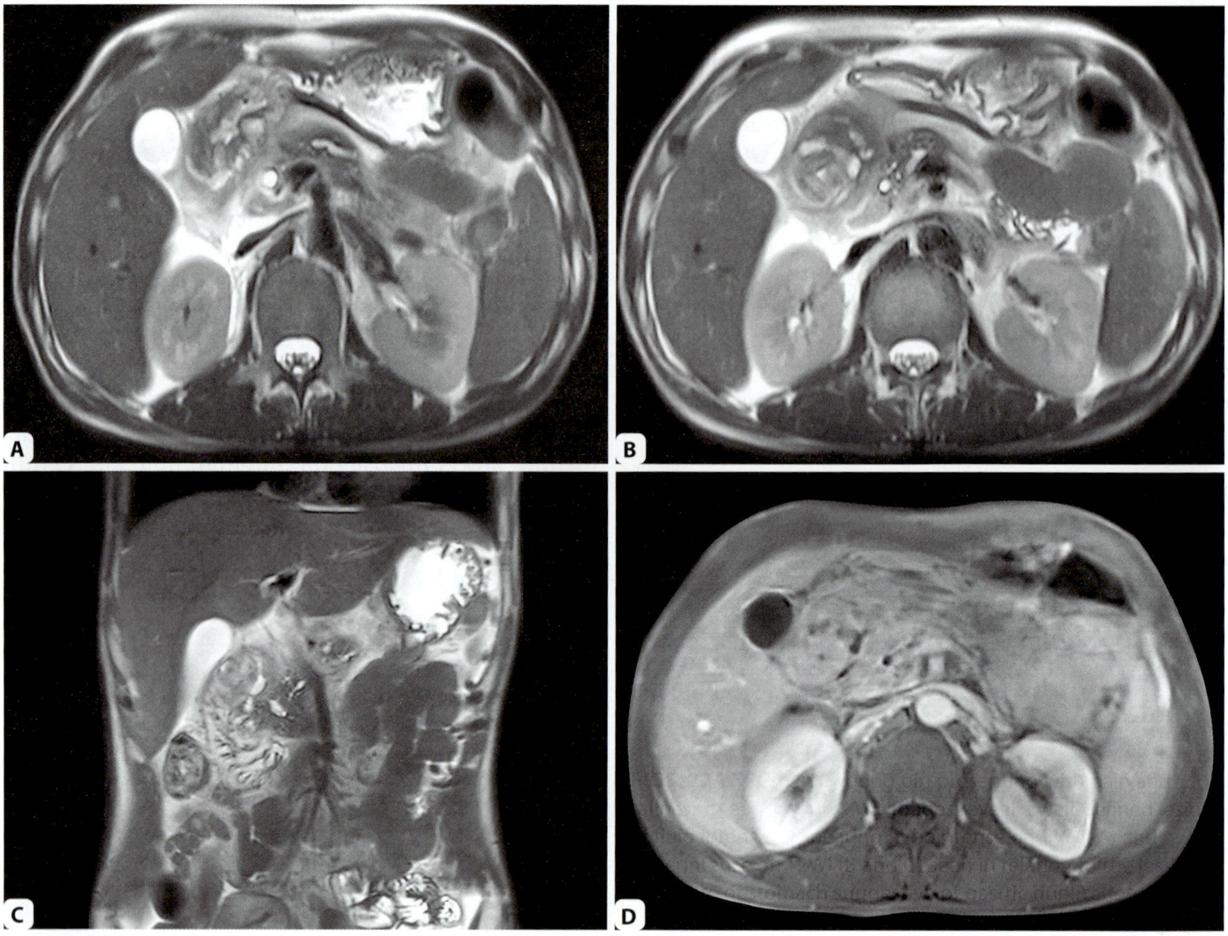

FIGS. 31A TO D: T2W axial (A and B) and coronal (C) MR images reveal subtle heterogeneous soft tissue in the pancreaticoduodenal groove with enhancement on postgadolinium T1WFS image (D), thickening of the walls of duodenum along with presence of intramural cystic lesions. Dilatation of main pancreatic duct is noted. Findings are suggestive of paraduodenal pancreatitis.
(T1WFS: T1-weighted fat saturation; T2W: T2-weighted image)

Superior Mesenteric Artery Syndrome

Superior mesenteric artery syndrome is a rare cause of high-intestinal obstruction, caused by extrinsic compression of third part of duodenum, due to narrowing of the normal angle between the aorta and the superior mesenteric artery. Patients are usually young females, with conditions associated with rapid and severe weight loss, resulting in a loss of retroperitoneal fat. Patients present with postprandial or intermittent abdominal pain, vomiting, nausea, and anorexia.

On barium UGI series, there may be strong to-and-fro peristalsis and stomach and duodenal dilatation proximal to a vertical extrinsic impression at the level of third part of duodenum, during a symptomatic episode. A change in posture can cause relief of obstruction.

The measurement of the distance between the aorta and the superior mesenteric artery can be measured on CT angiography or MR angiography. Normally, the aortomesenteric angle and aortomesenteric distance are 28–65° and 10–34 mm, respectively. In SMA syndrome, both parameters are reduced, with values of 6–15° and 2–8 mm, respectively.[72] Focal duodenal narrowing with upstream dilatation can be seen.

ANATOMIC CONDITIONS

Duodenal Diverticula

Duodenal extramural diverticula are often incidental findings in patients, typically resulting from mucosal prolapse or the prolapse of the entire duodenal wall. They are commonly located on the inner aspect of second part of duodenum, adjacent to the ampulla of Vater. While they are benign, duodenal diverticula may lead to serious complications such as perforation, duodenal fistulas, intra-abdominal abscesses, and sepsis.

On UGI studies, they appear as barium-filled pouch-like projections beyond the normal lumen, distinguishable from ulcers by the visualization of mucosal folds entering the neck of the diverticulum and changes in appearance with peristalsis. CT scans typically reveal fluid and/or gas-filled collections in a characteristic location, communicating with the duodenal lumen **(Figs. 32A to C)**. However, a duodenal diverticulum entirely filled with fluid may mimic a cystic neoplasm or pseudocyst originating from the pancreas. In rare instances, periampullary diverticula can lead to bile duct obstruction, resulting in jaundice, cholangitis, and/or pancreatitis, a condition known as Lemmel syndrome.

Bulging Papilla

A bulging papilla may be caused by benign or malignant causes. The benign causes include inflammatory conditions such as passage of biliary stones, pancreatitis, or cholangitis. Malignant causes include periampullary neoplasm or intraductal mucinous papillary neoplasm. Imaging findings include an enlarged and hyperenhancing duodenal major papilla, edematous thickening at the ampulla of Vater and homogeneous or a target like stratification enhancement at CT and MRI.

Ectopic Pancreas

Ectopic pancreas is defined as abnormally located pancreatic tissue with its own ductal system, with no vascular, neural, or anatomic contact with the normal gland. It is the most common heterotopia within the GI system and is incidentally seen on CT scan or autopsy. The most common locations are the duodenum (28%), stomach (26%), and jejunum (16%). It usually occurs in the submucosa (75%), but can also be present within the muscularis propria or the serosa.

On barium UGI series, a characteristic appearance is that of a central small collection of barium inside an umbilicated nodule in the duodenal submucosa. On CT, it is seen as a mass in the duodenal wall with enhancement pattern similar to that of pancreatic parenchyma. GIST and leiomyoma should be differentiated from this entity as they all share a submucosal origin. A flat shape, lobulated contour, and endoluminal growth are suggestive of ectopic pancreas. MRCP may show the presence of ducts within the tissue, a finding that is pathognomonic for ectopic pancreas.

A broad spectrum of gastric and duodenal diseases, spanning from inflammatory conditions to neoplasms, can be observed on various imaging modalities. These findings may range from innocuous incidental discoveries to serious clinical situations involving bleeding, obstruction, or perforation, underscoring the importance of recognizing their radiological appearance to guide proper management. Cross-sectional imaging modalities have been increasingly useful in diagnosis of various conditions affecting the stomach and duodenum. **Flowcharts 1 and 2 and Box 2** present a diagnostic approach to gastric pathological conditions and **Box 3** presents an approach to duodenal pathological conditions.

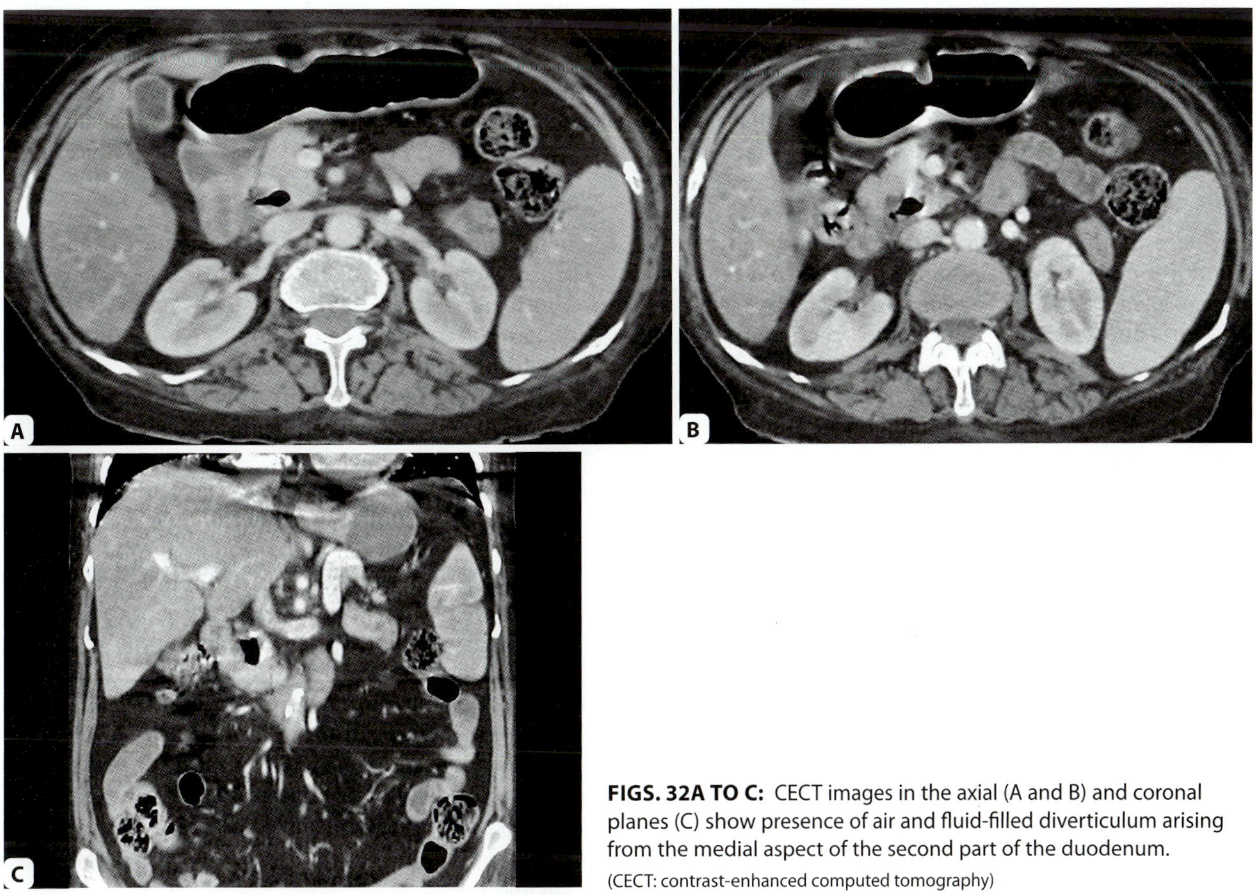

FIGS. 32A TO C: CECT images in the axial (A and B) and coronal planes (C) show presence of air and fluid-filled diverticulum arising from the medial aspect of the second part of the duodenum.
(CECT: contrast-enhanced computed tomography)

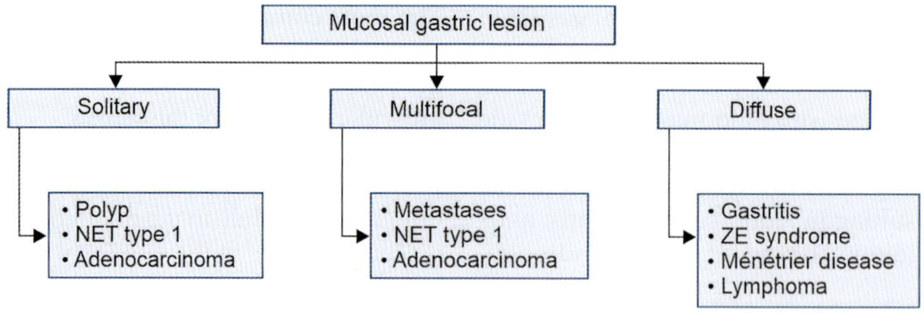

FLOWCHART 1: Approach to gastric mucosal lesion.

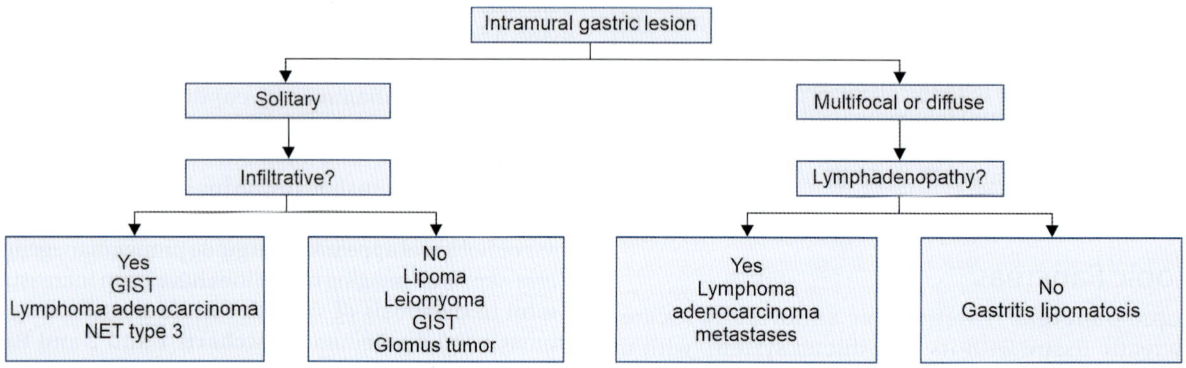

FLOWCHART 2: Approach to intramural gastric lesion.
(GIST: gastrointestinal stromal tumor)

BOX 2 Thickened gastric folds.

Barium/CT: >10 mm (12 mm in distal antrum)

EUS: >4 mm

Look for:

- Fold thickness
- Mural architecture preservation
- Superficial/deep layer thickening
- Ascites
- Lymphadenopathy

Ménétrier disease: Smooth thickened folds typically in proximal stomach, dilution of barium

Polyposis: Polyps and extra-gastrointestinal manifestations

Carcinoma: Loss of mural stratification, heterogeneously enhancing irregular mural thickening, gastric obstruction, perigastric infiltration/fat standing and adenopathy

Lymphoma: Preserved perigastric fat planes, no luminal obstruction, bulky adenopathy, multifocal

(EUS: endoscopic ultrasound)

BOX 3 Approach to duodenal pathological conditions based on imaging features.

- *Presence of fat*: Lipoma
- *Targetoid appearance*: Crohn disease, intussusception, Henoch–Schönlein purpura
- *Hyperenhancing lesions*: Zollinger–Ellison syndrome, neuroendocrine tumors, GIST, paraganglioma, and ectopic pancreatic rests
- *Lesions with soft-tissue attenuation*: Adenocarcinoma, lymphoma, polyp, Schwannoma, hematoma, tuberculosis, and bulging papilla
- *Presence of gas or fluid*: Peptic ulcer disease, pancreatic pseudocyst, and duplication cyst
- *Presence of upstream dilatation*: SMA syndrome
- *Presence of tethering*: Aortoenteric fistula

REFERENCES

1. Vikram R, Balachandran A, Bhosale PR, Tamm EP, Marcal LP, Charnsangavej C. Pancreas: peritoneal reflections, ligamentous connections, and pathways of disease spread. Radiographics. 2009;29(02):e34.
2. Young JJ, Pahwa A, Patel M, Jude CM, Nguyen M, Deshmukh M, et al. Ligaments and lymphatic pathways in gastric adenocarcinoma. Radiographics. 2019;39(03):668-89.
3. Grainger and Allison's Diagnostic Radiology—A Textbook of Medical Imaging, 7th edition. United Kingdom: Churchill Livingstone; 2020.
4. Carmack SW, Genta RM, Graham DY, Lauwers GY. Management of gastric polyps: a pathology-based guide for gastroenterologists. Nat Rev Gastroenterol Hepatol. 2009;6:331-41.

5. Stolte M, Sticht T, Eidt S, Ebert D, Finkenzeller G. Frequency, location, and age and sex distribution of various types of gastric polyp. Endoscopy. 1994;26(8):659-65.
6. Chandrasekhara V, Ginsberg GG. Endoscopic management of gastrointestinal stromal tumors. Curr Gastroenterol Rep. 2011;13(6):532-9.
7. Shand AG, Taylor AC, Banerjee M, Lessels A, Coia J, Clark C, et al. Gastric fundic gland polyps in south-east Scotland: absence of adenomatous polyposis coli gene mutations and a strikingly low prevalence of *Helicobacter pylori* infection. J Gastroenterol Hepatol. 2002;17(11):1161-4.
8. Goddard AF, Badreldin R, Pritchard DM, Walker MM, Warren B. The management of gastric polyps. Gut. 2010;59(9):1270-6.
9. el-Zimaity HM, Jackson FW, Graham DY. Fundic gland polyps developing during omeprazole therapy. Am J Gastroenterol. 1997;92(10):1858-60.
10. Bianchi LK, Burke CA, Bennett AE, Lopez R, Hasson H, Church JM. Fundic gland polyp dysplasia is common in familial adenomatous polyposis. Clin Gastroenterol Hepatol. 2008;6(2):180-5.
11. Abraham SC, Singh VK, Yardley JH, Wu TT. Hyperplastic polyps of the stomach: associations with histologic patterns of gastritis and gastric atrophy. Am J Surg Pathol. 2001;25(4):500-7.
12. Ohkusa T, Miwa H, Hojo M, Kumagai J, Tanizawa T, Asaoka D, et al. Endoscopic, histological and serologic findings of gastric hyperplastic polyps after eradication of *Helicobacter pylori*: comparison between responder and non-responder cases. Digestion. 2003;68(2-3):57-62.
13. Dirschmid K, Platz-Baudin C, Stolte M. Why is the hyperplastic polyp a marker for the precancerous condition of the gastric mucosa? Virchows Arch. 2006;448(1):80-4.
14. Ginsberg GG, Al-Kawas FH, Fleischer DE, Reilly HF, Benjamin SB. Gastric polyps: relationship of size and histology to cancer risk. Am J Gastroenterol. 1996;91(4):714-7.
15. Schmitz JM, Stolte M. Gastric polyps as precancerous lesions. Gastrointest Endosc Clin N Am. 1997;7(1):29-46.
16. Rugge M, Nitti D, Farinati F, di Mario F, Genta RM. Non-invasive neoplasia of the stomach. Eur J Gastroenterol Hepatol. 2005;17:1191-6.
17. Calva D, Howe JR. Hamartomatous polyposis syndromes. Surg Clin North Am. 2008;88(4):779-817.
18. Beggs AD, Latchford AR, Vasen HF, Moslein G, Alonso A, Aretz S, et al. Peutz-Jeghers syndrome: a systematic review and recommendations for management. Gut. 2010;59(7):975-86.
19. Rubesin SE, Levine MS, Laufer I. Double-contrast upper gastrointestinal radiography: a pattern approach for disease of the stomach. Radiology. 2008;246:33-48.
20. Bray F, Ferlay J, Soerjomataram I, Siegel RL, Torre LA, Jemal A. Global cancer statistics 2018: GLOBOCAN estimates of incidence and mortality worldwide for 36 cancers in 185 countries. CA Cancer J Clin. 2018;68(06):394-424.
21. Collaborators GBDSC GBD 2017 Stomach Cancer Collaborators. The global, regional, and national burden of stomach cancer in 195 countries, 1990-2017: a systematic analysis for the Global Burden of Disease study 2017. Lancet Gastroenterol Hepatol. 2020;5(01):42-54.
22. Lauren P. The two histological main types of gastric carcinoma: diffuse and so-called intestinal-type carcinoma. An attempt at a histo-clinical classification. Acta Pathol Microbiol Scand. 1965;64:31-49.
23. López Sala P, Leturia Etxeberria M, Inchausti Iguíñiz E, Astiazaran Rodríguez A, Aguirre Oteiza MI, Zubizarreta Etxaniz M. Gastric adenocarcinoma: A review of the TNM classification system and ways of spreading. Radiologia (Engl Ed). 2023;65(1):66-80.
24. Japanese Gastric Cancer Association. Japanese Classification of Gastric Carcinoma—2nd English Edition. Gastric Cancer. 1998;1(01):10-24.
25. Sobin L, Wittekind C. UICC TNM Classification of Malignant Tumours, 6th edition. New York: Wiley; 2002.
26. Brennan MF. Current status of surgery for gastric cancer: a review. Gastric Cancer. 2005;8(02):64-70.
27. Muhammad A, Rochita R, Mohamed E, Raghunandan V. Imaging of Gastric Carcinoma. Part One: Diagnosis and Staging. J Gastrointest Abdomin Radiol. 2021.
28. Teresa G, Cesare M, Giuseppe M, Michele R, Maria R, Vittorio B, et al. Imaging in Gastric Cancer: Current Practice and Future Perspectives. Diagnostics. 2023.
29. Isaacson PG. Gastrointestinal lymphomas of T and B-cell types. Mod Pathol. 1999;12:151-8.
30. Dawson IM, Cornes JS, Morson BC. Primary malignant tumors of the intestinal tract. Br J Surg. 1961;49:80-9.
31. Rohatiner A, d'Amore F, Coiffier B, Crowther D, Gospodarowicz M, Isaacson P, et al. Report on a workshop convened to discuss the pathological and staging classifications of gastrointestinal tract lymphoma. Ann Oncol. 1994;5:397-400.
32. Yoo CC, Levine MS, Furth EE, Salhany KE, Rubesin SE, Laufer I, et al. Gastric mucosa associated lymphoid tissue lymphoma: radiographic findings in six patients. Radiology. 1998;208:239-43.
33. Isaacson PG. Recent developments in our understanding of gastric lymphoma. Am J Surg Pathol. 1996;20(Suppl l):S1-7.
34. Miller FH, Kochman ML, Talamonti MS, Ghahremani GG, Gore RM. Gastric cancer: radiologic staging. Radiol Clin North Am. 1997;35:331-49.
35. Ciftci AO, Tanyel FC, Kotiloglu E, Hicsonmez A. Gastric lymphoma causing gastric outlet obstruction. J Pediatr Surg. 1996;31:1424-6.
36. Levy AD, Sobin LH. Gastrointestinal Carcinoids: Imaging Features with Clinicopathologic Comparison. Radio Graphics. 2007;27:237-57.
37. Virmani V, Khandelwal A, Sethi V, Hill MF, Fasih N, Kielar A. Neoplastic stomach lesions and their mimickers: spectrum of imaging manifestations. Cancer Imaging. 2012;12:269-78.
38. Gong J, Kang W, Zhu J, Xu J. CT and MR imaging of gastrointestinal stromal tumor of stomach: a pictorial review. Quant Imaging Med Surg. 2012;2(4):274-9.
39. Heinrich MC, Corless CL, Duensing A, McGreevey L, Chen CJ, Joseph N, et al. PDGFRA activating mutations in gastrointestinal stromal tumors. Science. 2003;299(5607): 708-10.
40. Lee NK, Kim S, Kim GH, Jeon TY, Kim DH, Jang HJ, et al. Hypervascular subepithelial gastrointestinal masses: CT-pathologic correlation. Radiographics. 2010;30:1915-34.
41. Kang HC, Menias CO, Gaballah AH, Shroff S, Taggart MW, Garg N, et al. Beyond the GIST: Mesenchymal Tumors of the Stomach. Radiographics. 2013;33:1673-90.
42. Levy AD, Remotti HE, Thompson WM, Sobin LH, Miettinen M. Gastrointestinal stromal tumors: radiologic features with pathologic correlation. Radiographics. 2003;23(2):283-304.

43. Salamah AB, Prokop M, Uffmann M, Pokieser P, Teleky B, Lechner G. Dedicated Multidetector CT of the Stomach: Spectrum of Diseases. Radiographics. 2003;23:625-44.
44. Kim HC, Lee JM, Kim KW, Park SH, Kim SH, Lee JY, et al. Gastrointestinal stromal tumors of the stomach: CT findings and prediction of malignancy. AJR Am J Roentgenol. 2004;183:893-8.
45. DeMatteo RP, Lewis JJ, Leung D, Mudan SS, Woodruff JM, Brennan MF. Two hundred gastrointestinal stromal tumors: recurrence patterns and prognostic factors for survival. Ann Surg. 2000;231(1):51-8.
46. Demetri GD, Benjamin R, Blanke CD, Choi H, Corless C, DeMatteo RP, et al. NCCN task force report: optimal management of patients with gastrointestinal stromal tumors (GIST)—expansion and update of NCCN clinical practice guidelines. J Natl Compr Cancer Netw. 2004;2:S1-S26.
47. Joensuu H, Roberts PJ, Sarlomo-Rikala M, Andersson LC, Tervahartiala P, Tuveson D, et al. Effect of the tyrosine kinase inhibitor STI571 in a patient with a metastatic gastrointestinal stromal tumor. N Engl J Med. 2001;344:1052-6.
48. Blanke C, Joensuu H, Demetri G, Heinrich M, Roberts P, Eisenberg B et al. Long-term follow up of advanced gastrointestinal stromal tumor (GIST) patients treated with imatinib mesylate (abstr). In: Proceedings of the 2004 Gastrointestinal Cancers Symposium: Current Status and Future Directions for Prevention and Management. Alexandria, Va: American Society of Clinical Oncology; 2004. p. 43.
49. Hong X, Choi H, Loyer EM, Benjamin RS, Trent JC, Charnsangavej C. Gastrointestinal Stromal Tumor: Role of CT in Diagnosis and in Response Evaluation and Surveillance after Treatment with Imatinib. Radiographics. 2006;26:481-95.
50. Miettinen M, Lasota J. Gastrointestinal stromal tumors: definition, clinical, histological, immunohistochemical, and molecular genetic features and differential diagnosis. Virchows Arch. 2001;438(1):1-12.
51. Hur BY, Kim SH, Choi JY, Rha SE, Lee MW, Kim SY, et al. Gastroduodenal glomus tumors: differentiation from other subepithelial lesions based on dynamic contrast-enhanced CT findings. AJR Am J Roentgenol. 2011;197(6):1351-9.
52. Lee MJ, Lim JS, Kwon JE, Kim H, Hyung WJ, Park MS, et al. Gastric true leiomyoma: computed tomographic findings and pathological correlation. J Comput Assist Tomogr. 2007;31(2):204-8.
53. Chappuis CW, Divincenti FC, Cohn I Jr. Villous tumors of the duodenum. Ann Surg. 1989;209:593-9.
54. Park SO, Han JK, Kirn TK, Lee JW, Kim SH, Kim YI, et al. Unusual gastric tumors: radiologic pathologic correlation. Radiographics. 1999;19:1435-46.
55. Raber MH, CMPZ des Plantes, Vink R, Vink R, Klaase JM. Gastric schwannoma presenting as an incidentaloma on CT-scan and MRI. Gastroenterol Res. 2010;3(6):276-80.
56. Hong HS, Ha HK, Won HJ, Byun JH, Shin YM, Kim AY, et al. Gastric schwannomas: radiological features with endoscopic and pathological correlation. Clin Radiol. 2008;63(5):536-42.
57. Miettinen M, Paal E, Lasota J, Sobin LH. Gastrointestinal glomus tumors: a clinicopathologic, immunohistochemical, and molecular genetic study of 32 cases. Am J Surg Pathol. 2002;26(3):301-11.
58. Levy AD, Abbott RM, Rohrmann CA Jr, Frazier AA, Kende A. Gastrointestinal hemangiomas: imaging findings with pathologic correlation in pediatric and adult patients. AJR Am J Roentgenol. 2001;177(5):1073-81.
59. Thompson WM, Kende AI, Levy AD. Imaging characteristics of gastric lipomas in 16 adult and pediatric patients. AJR Am J Roentgenol. 2003;181(4):981-5.
60. Ferrozzi F, Tognini G, Bova D, Pavone P. Lipomatous tumors of the stomach: CT findings and differential diagnosis. J Comput Assist Tomogr. 2000;24:854-8.
61. Coffin CM, Hornick JL, Fletcher CD. Inflammatory myofibroblastic tumor: comparison of clinicopathologic, histologic, and immunohistochemical features including ALK expression in atypical and aggressive cases. Am J Surg Pathol. 2007;31(4):509-20.
62. Bjelovic M, Micev M, Spica B, Babic T, Gunjic D, Djuric A, et al. Primary inflammatory myofibroblastic tumor of the stomach in an adult woman: a case report and review of the literature. World J Surg Oncol. 2013;11:35.
63. Karnak I, Senocak ME, Ciftci AO, Cağlar M, Bingöl-Koloğlu M, Tanyel FC, et al. Inflammatory myofibroblastic tumor in children: diagnosis and treatment. J Pediatr Surg. 2001;36(6):908-12.
64. Narla LD, Newman B, Spottswood SS, Narla S, Kolli R. Inflammatory pseudotumor. Radiographics. 2003;23:719-29.
65. Zulfiqar M, Shetty A, Shetty V, Menias C. CT Imaging of Non-Neoplastic and Neoplastic Benign Gastric Disease. Curr Prob Diagn Radiol. 2018;48:75-96.
66. Nagpal P, Prakash A, Pradhan G, Vidholia A, Nagpal N, Saboo S, et al. MDCT Imaging of the Stomach: Advances and Applications. Br j radiol. 2017;90(1069):20160412.
67. Grendell JH, Ermak TH. Anatomy, histology, embryology, and developmental anomalies of the pancreas. In: Feldman M, Friedman LS, Brandt LJ (Eds). Sleisenger and Fordtran's gastrointestinal and liver disease. Philadelphia, PA: Saunders; 1998. pp. 761-71.
68. Kim JY, Lee JM, Kim KW, Park HS, Choi Y, Kim SH, et al. Ectopic Pancreas: CT Findings with Emphasis on Differentiation from Small Gastrointestinal Stromal Tumor and Leiomyoma. Radiology. 2009;252(1):92-100.
69. Okuhata Y, Maebayashi T, Furuhashi S, Abe K, Takahashi M, Kanamori N, et al. Characteristics of ectopic pancreas in dynamic gadolinium-enhanced MRI. Abdom Imaging. 2008;35:85-7.
70. Singh JP, Rajdeo H, Bhuta K, Savino JA. Gastric Duplication Cyst: Two Case Reports and Review of the Literature. Case Rep Surg. 2013;2013:605059.
71. Horne G, Ming-Lum C, Kirkpatrick AW, Parker RL. High-grade neuroendocrine carcinoma arising in a gastric duplication cyst: a case report with literature review. Int J Surg Pathol. 2007;15(2):187-91.
72. Terra C, Ramos-Andrade D, Sá-Marques I, Brito J, Caseiro-Alves F, Curvo-Semedo L. Duodenal imaging on the spotlight: from A to Z. Insights Imaging. 2021;12(1):94.
73. Winfield RD, Hochwald SN, Vogel SB, Hemming AW, Liu C, Cance WG, et al. Presentation and management of gastrointestinal stromal tumors of the duodenum. Am Surg. 2006;72(8):719-22; discussion 722-3.
74. Domenech-Ximenos B, Juanpere S, Serra I, Codina J, Maroto A. Duodenal tumors on cross-sectional imaging with emphasis on multidetector computed tomography: a pictorial review. Diagn Interv Radiol. 2020;26(3):193-9.

CHAPTER

3

Devasenathipathy Kandasamy, Manisha Jana, Ankita Aggarwal

Ulceroconstrictive Diseases of the Gut

INTRODUCTION

Imaging in ulceroconstrictive lesions of the gut has seen a paradigm change over the last few decades. While earlier conventional imaging studies relied predominantly on the luminal distension and opacification of the bowel lumen using positive oral contrast, newer modalities like CT and MRI are capable of providing information on both intraluminal and extrinsic abnormalities. CT enterography (CTE) and magnetic resonance enterography (MRE) are unique imaging techniques having the combined advantages of both CT/MRI and enterography.

PLAIN RADIOGRAPH

The role of plain radiographs has diminished to a great extent because of the wider availability of cross-sectional modalities. They are useful only in a patient with acute or subacute intestinal obstruction when they are often the first-line modality. An erect abdominal radiograph can provide valuable information regarding the level and severity of bowel obstruction, and the presence of pneumoperitoneum; although an erect chest radiograph is the best method to detect the latter. Enteroliths can be seen sometimes proximal to the site of obstruction and the presence of calcified lymph nodes can point toward the diagnosis of tuberculosis (TB). The drawback of this study is that it is often not helpful in detecting the etiology of obstruction. It plays no role in purely ulcerative disease entities.

BARIUM STUDIES

Barium meal follow-through (BMFT) was the most widely used imaging technique for the evaluation of small bowel until a few years ago. Constrictive lesions of the small bowel presenting as small bowel obstruction remain a challenge in diagnosis as a large part of the small bowel is not accessible by endoscopy. With the advent of better modalities such as multidetector computed tomography (MDCT) and MRI, the importance of BMFT has declined. BMFT, along with colonic evaluation by barium enema, can give valuable information regarding both small and large bowel obstructive lesions.[1] It is the best imaging technique to evaluate the mucosal details of small and large bowel. There are many classical signs described for TB and Crohn's disease (CD) on barium studies, and they are good at demonstrating bowel narrowing, dilatation, mucosal ulcerations, kinking and clumping of bowel loops, and fistulae **(Figs. 1 and 2)**. They are one of the few imaging techniques capable of studying bowel motility, which is an important parameter in bowel imaging. The evaluation of lesions in the ileum and cecum can be further enhanced by peroral pneumocolon (i.e., insufflation of air through the rectum).[2] Peroral pneumocolon can also provide valuable information regarding colonic pathologies.

Single contrast BMFT is usually performed with barium suspension having 66% w/v barium. With the technological advances in the field of fluoroscopic techniques, coupled with their wide availability and low radiation burden; most often the procedure is performed under fluoroscopic guidance nowadays. The major drawback in the evaluation of intestinal strictures by BMFT is the differentiation of a true stricture from a transient peristaltic contraction. To alleviate this drawback, enteroclysis (small bowel enema) came into practice; wherein the small bowel lumen is distended through a nasojejunal tube using diluted barium. Enteroclysis yielded superior mucosal details compared to BMFT. Also, as the distension of the bowel lumen was controlled and the luminal distension was visualized in real-time; this technique was superior to BMFT in the detection of subtle intestinal strictures. However, this technique

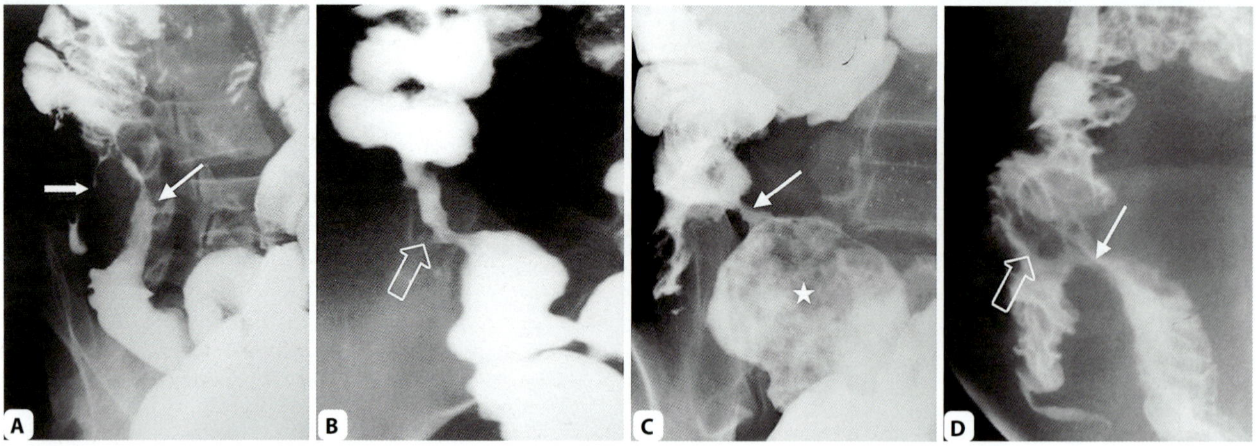

FIGS. 1A TO D: Ileocecal tuberculosis (TB) on barium studies. Barium meal follow-through (BMFT) image (A) shows narrowing and mild mucosal irregularity (thin arrow) in the terminal ileum (string sign) with associated contracted cecum (thick arrow). BMFT image (B) of another patient shows narrowing of the terminal ileum which is emptying directly into the ascending colon (outlined arrow) with nonvisualization of the cecum (Stierlin's sign). BMFT image (C) in a different patient shows fibrotic stricture in the terminal ileum (thin arrow) with proximal dilatation (star) and contracted cecum. BMFT image (D) of another patient shows mild gaping (thin arrow) and filling defect (outlined arrow) in the region of the ileocecal valve (Fleischner's sign) due to edema of the valve.

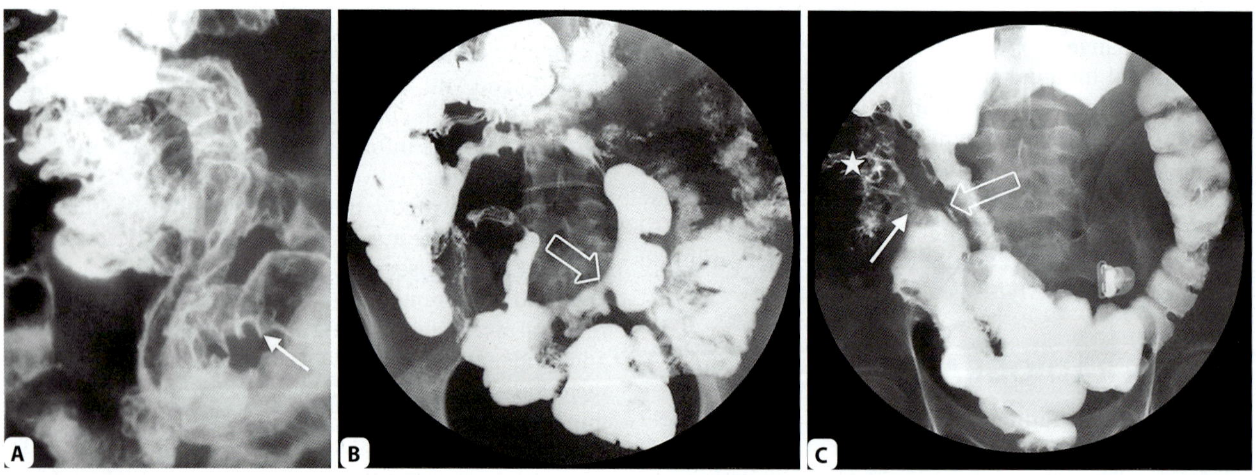

FIGS. 2A TO C: Crohn's disease (CD) involving the small bowel. Barium meal follow-through (BMFT) (A) shows mucosal irregularity in the terminal ileum and rose thorn ulcers (thin arrow). BMFT in another patient with CD (B) shows multiple strictures in the distal ileum, shortening of the mesenteric border, and pseudosacculations in the antimesenteric border (outlined arrow). BMFT image (C) in a patient with CD showing narrowing of terminal ileum (thin arrow) with proximal dilatation, irregularity, and narrowing of the cecum (star). In one of the ileal loops, there is a thin longitudinal extraluminal barium (outlined arrow) seen paralleling the bowel loop (double tracking) which is due to the presence of deep fissures in the bowel wall in CD.

entails ionizing radiation to the patient and the yield is also poor when compared with CTE or MRE. Hence, barium studies should be used only if CT or MRE is unavailable.

Single-contrast barium enema and double-contrast barium enema (DCBE) are two other important barium studies. While single-contrast barium enema is adequate for delineating the strictures in the large bowel; DCBE is preferable in cases of suspected mucosal lesions such as in ulcerative colitis (UC). However, colonoscopy is the primary modality of choice in the evaluation of patients with UC, and imaging is not commonly performed for their evaluation.

CONTRAST-ENHANCED CT AND CT ENTEROCLYSIS/CT ENTEROGRAPHY

Contrast-enhanced CT (CECT) is the workhorse of imaging in suspected intestinal strictures. With the advent of fast MDCT scanners, CT can provide crucial information regarding mural/extraluminal findings in bowel pathology. CT enteroclysis combines the benefits of the two imaging modalities; good luminal distension similar to a conventional enteroclysis and visualization of extraluminal/transmural pathologies similar to CECT.[3] CTE is an imaging technique wherein the luminal distension

TABLE 1: Computed tomography enterography protocol.

Preparation	6 hours fasting
Oral contrast	Water + mannitol (300 mL of 20% mannitol in 1,500 mL water)
Antiperistaltic agent (optional but preferred)	20–40 mg hyoscine butylbromide given IV
Technique	450 mL at 60 minutes before scanning 450 mL at 40 minutes before scanning 225 mL at 20 minutes before scanning 225 mL at 10 minutes before scanning 250–300 mL on the table just before scanning (plain water)

of the small bowel is achieved without a nasojejunal tube; hence, ameliorating patient discomfort arising from intubation. In this procedure, either diluted mannitol/ polyethylene glycol (PEG) solution is used as a neutral oral contrast agent to distend the bowel loops. There are various protocols described for CTE in literature aimed at adequate bowel distension during scanning. The protocol given below is followed in our institute **(Table 1)**. CTE is a very sensitive tool in the diagnosis of inflammatory small bowel diseases; comparable to capsule endoscopy.[4-6] Another important role of CTE is to rule out any strictures in the small bowel; before a capsule endoscopy; to avoid capsule impaction/retention.[6] The usage of ionizing radiation is an important drawback of CTE which limits its utility in follow-up imaging. The radiation dose of a standard CTE study is around 1-4 mSv.[7,8] Radiation dose can be minimized by optimizing the scan parameters and using new techniques such as iterative reconstruction methods.

Chest CT has an important role to play in the screening of inflammatory bowel disease (IBD) patients for whom treatment with biological agents is planned. The purpose of a CT chest is to detect the features of latent or active TB which can flare up after the immunosuppressant biological therapy which carries significant mortality.[9,10] Pleural thickening, fibrosis, nodules with or without calcifications, and calcified mediastinal or hilar lymph nodes are the features of latent TB on the chest CT. Patients even with latent TB would receive isoniazid prophylaxis before starting them on biological therapy. Another utility of chest CT is detecting concomitant involvement of the chest in patients with abdominal TB which can occur in up to 25% of patients.[11]

MRI/MRE

Although CECT can provide a lot of diagnostic information in intestinal strictures, it comes with a high radiation burden; more so in patients with IBDs who need repeated imaging.[12] MRI has the advantage of superior soft tissue contrast resolution, multiplanar imaging capability and lack of any ionizing radiation. MRI has the unique advantage of evaluating multiple paradigms such as T1 and T2 characteristics, diffusion restriction, and pattern of contrast enhancement. In addition, new ultrafast sequences (true FISP cine MR) have made the real-time evaluation of the small bowel possible; which is crucial for differentiating a stricture from a peristaltic contraction. MRE has all the inherent advantages of CTE; with the additional benefit of being able to differentiate a fibrotic stricture from an active one. Diffusion-weighted MRI (DW-MRI) is also being increasingly used in cases of IBDs.[13-16] The active lesions tend to show restriction of diffusion (hyperintense signal on high b-value images). Diffusion-weighted imaging (DWI) can be an effective alternative to intravenous contrast in the evaluation of lesion activity in IBDs in patients in whom gadolinium-based contrast is contraindicated. Commonly used intraluminal contrast in MRE is diluted mannitol, which can act as a biphasic contrast agent. On the T2-weighted (T2W) images, it causes high-signal intensity within the lumen and the bowel wall is seen as a hypointense structure. On postcontrast T1-weighted (T1W) images, it serves as a "negative" contrast agent and helps in better delineation of the wall enhancement against a dark lumen. The formulation of oral contrast and the timing of giving aliquots for MRE is the same as the CTE protocol **(Table 1)**.[17]

ULTRASONOGRAPHY AND CONTRAST-ENHANCED ULTRASONOGRAPHY

Ultrasound (US) has a limited role in the initial evaluation of intestinal obstruction, owing to gaseous abdominal distension, which makes ultrasonographic visualization of bowel loops difficult. However, in cases of abdominal TB or IBDs where the disease has been localized by other imaging modalities (such as CT or MRI), US is a useful tool for follow-up evaluation. CT is associated with radiation burden, and MRI evaluation in children often needs sedation or general anesthesia. High-resolution US is an emerging technique to evaluate bowel disorders, and it is very sensitive in detecting bowel wall abnormalities in the terminal ileum and ileocecal junction region. The spatial resolution of high-resolution US is better than CTE or MRE, and it can show wall thickening, dilated segments of the bowel loop, and bowel motility in real-time. An increase in bowel and mesenteric vascularity can be detected on Doppler, which is considered a marker for disease activity in CD. Wide availability, repeatability, and lack of radiation have made US an attractive technique in the evaluation of ulceroconstrictive bowel diseases. US is very sensitive to detecting abnormalities in the terminal ileum; however, for the evaluation of proximal small bowel loops, the accuracy falls. Various studies across the globe have shown sonographic sensitivity and specificity for the diagnosis of CD ranging from 75 to 94% and 67 to 100%, respectively.[18,19]

Contrast-enhanced ultrasonography (CEUS) is a recent advancement that has been evaluated and recommended in the evaluation of disease activity in IBDs, distinguishing fibrous from inflammatory strictures, abscesses, and fistula.[20,21] It utilizes a special contrast agent such as sulfur hexafluoride microbubbles which is given intravenously to look for areas of abnormal enhancement. It can be used even in patients with renal impairment as the mode of excretion is via pulmonary route. Lack of expertise and limited availability of hardware and software for CEUS and contrast agents are the current limitations. The cine loops of CEUS can be processed using software, and various quantifiable perfusion parameters can be obtained by placing region of interest (ROI) markers.

ABDOMINAL TUBERCULOSIS

Tuberculosis is one of the leading causes of death killing around 1.5 million people worldwide in 2014 and India constitutes 23% of all TB cases which is the highest in the world.[22] Abdominal TB constitutes about 17% of all inpatients admitted with the diagnosis of TB.[23] Intestine is the sixth most common of all the extrapulmonary sites involved by TB.[24] TB is caused by *Mycobacterium tuberculosis* and abdominal TB generally includes the involvement of the gastrointestinal (GI) tract, lymph nodes, peritoneum, and solid visceral organs of the abdomen.

Gastrointestinal Tuberculosis

Gastrointestinal tuberculosis (GI TB) can present either with symptoms related to the bowel like abdominal pain, vomiting, diarrhea, and abdominal distension, or systemic symptoms like fever, loss of appetite, and weight.[25] The above symptoms of GI TB are not specific and can be seen in patients with CD. The role of imaging in differentiating GI TB and CD will be dealt with later in this chapter. Apart from diagnosis, imaging is also useful in guiding fine needle aspiration cytology (FNAC) or biopsy in patients where the diagnosis is uncertain on imaging alone. TB can involve any part of the GI tract, but the ileocecal region is most commonly involved (50–90%).[26,27] The other less commonly involved areas are ascending colon, jejunum, rest of the colon, rectum, duodenum, anal canal, esophagus, and stomach in that order.[28,29]

Small Bowel Tuberculosis

The ileocecal region is by far the most common site for small bowel TB. There are various reasons hypothesized for this predilection which are as follows:

- Physiological stasis leading to longer contact
- Closer contact with tubercle bacilli
- The ileum is rich in lymphoid tissue
- Relatively neutral pH promotes bacterial growth

Ileocecal TB has three morphological types—(1) *ulcerative* (60%), (2) *hypertrophic* (10%), and (3) *ulcerohypertrophic* (30%). Ulcerative type is more common in immunocompromised individuals and hypertrophic type is more common in immunocompetent individuals. The ulcerohypertrophic form can closely mimic malignancy because of its morphology. The caseation necrosis occurring in the submucosal lymphoid tissue causes mucosal ulcerations whereas extensive inflammation and fibrosis in reaction to the bacilli leads to thickening in the hypertrophic type.

Before the advent of new cross-sectional techniques such as CTE and MRE, barium studies used to be the imaging modality of choice in suspected patients with intestinal tuberculosis (ITB) because of its unsurpassed ability to show mucosal abnormalities. There are various signs on barium studies described in the different stages of GI TB **(Figs. 1A to D)**. Spasm, hypermotility, mucosal edema, and edema of the ileocecal valve are the earliest signs of ileocecal TB. Fleischner or inverted umbrella sign which is due to the thickening of the ileocecal valve with narrowing of the terminal ileum is considered to be characteristic of ileocecal TB.[30] Stierlin's sign is due to the rapid emptying of barium into the cecum because of mucosal irritability **(Figs. 1A to D)**. As the disease progresses, there will be fibrosis and shortening of the involved bowel segment and napkin ring stenosis. This is called a string sign showing persistent narrowing of the barium column in the area of stenosis **(Figs. 1A to D)**. Cecum is pulled out of the right iliac fossa which is often referred to as pulled up cecum **(Figs. 3A to C)**. This also leads to contraction of the cecum which can appear conical on imaging. Because of the cranial migration of the cecum, there is an alteration in the angle between the terminal ileum and colon. The terminal ileum may appear hanging down and stretched from the contracted cecum called goose-neck deformity.

High-resolution US can also show changes in GI TB in the form of abnormal wall thickening (>3 mm in distended state and >5 mm in collapsed state), inflammation in the surrounding mesentery, and enlarged lymph nodes which may have calcification and necrosis. Bowel wall thickening is a nonspecific finding that can be seen in CD, lymphoma, amebiasis, and carcinoma. However, TB commonly affects the ileocecal junction and often the cecum is pulled up because of fibrosis. Ultrasonography (USG) is optimal for the evaluation of ileocecal region wall thickening. However, USG is not sensitive enough to detect abnormalities in more proximal small bowel loops because of its inability to evaluate the entire length of the bowel.

Contrast-enhanced CT is better than USG to detect and characterize small bowel TB which can show the bowel wall thickening, mesenteric changes, and adenopathy **(Fig. 4)**. The necrosis in the nodes is better detected on CECT. Though it is not sensitive enough to detect early mucosal changes, it can comprehensively evaluate most of the other features of abdominal TB such as peritoneal and solid organ involvement. CTE is a relatively new technique that is considered superior to conventional CECT in the evaluation of mucosal abnormalities and the detection

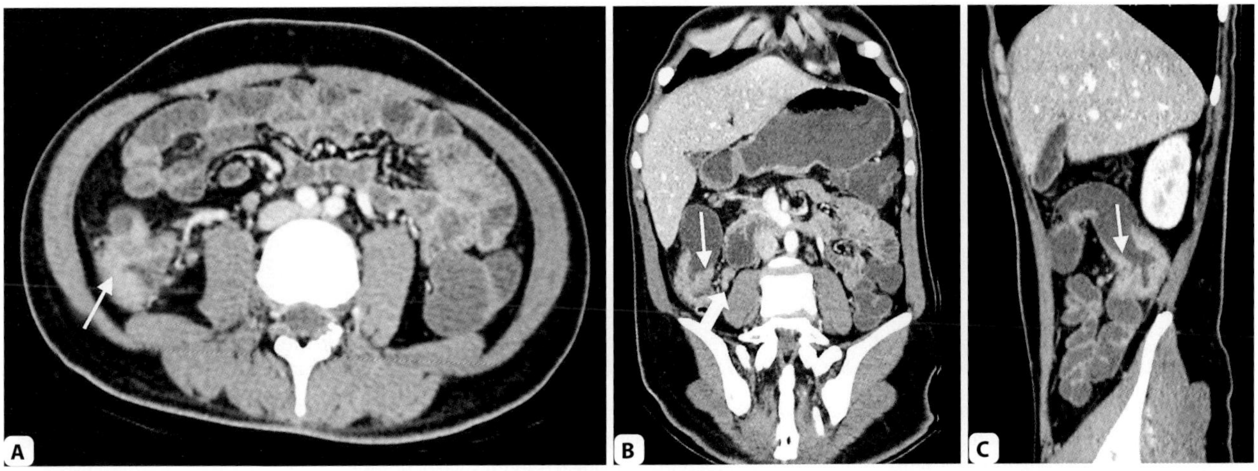

FIGS. 3A TO C: Pulled up cecum. Axial CTE image (A), oblique MPR (B), and sagittal MPR (C) showing wall thickening and abnormal enhancement involving the cecum (thin arrow) with few enlarged regional lymph nodes (thick arrow). The cecum is contracted and has migrated cranially to the right lumbar region suggestive of pulled-up cecum in a patient with ileocecal TB.

(CTE: computed tomography enterography; MPR: multiplanar reformation; TB: tuberculosis)

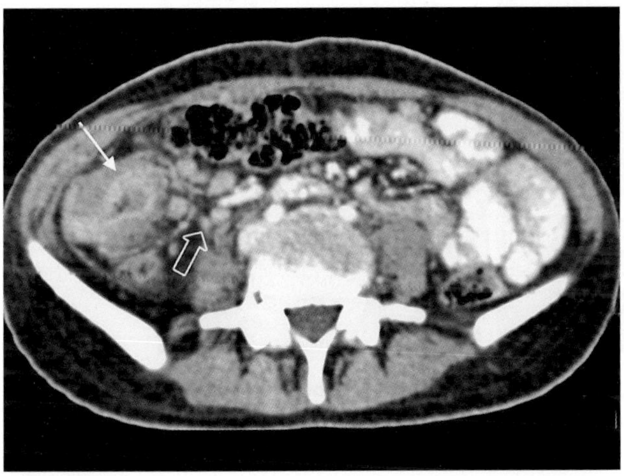

FIG. 4: Ileocecal TB. Axial CECT image showing circumferential wall thickening involving the cecum (thin arrow) with surrounding fat stranding and enlarged lymph nodes (outlined arrow). The above features are suggestive of TB.

(CECT: contrast-enhanced computed tomography; TB: tuberculosis)

of subtle wall thickening and narrowing of the lumen. In the early stage, CTE may show nonspecific inflammatory changes in the form of stratified wall thickening in the distal ileum, ileocecal junction, and cecum which can later progress to more severe homogeneous wall thickening and narrowing leading to obstruction **(Figs. 5 and 6)**. It can also show clumping of bowel loops, adhesions, mesenteric changes, and occasionally cocoon formation in which varying lengths of bowel loops are encapsulated by a thick fibrotic membrane **(Figs. 7A to C)**. Because of superior contrast resolution, MRI or MRE can also be used to show the features of GI TB. Sometimes the inflammatory changes in the bowel wall and the surrounding mesentery are better seen on MRI as compared to CT and the tubercular lesions are usually hypointense on T1W images and hyperintense on T2W images **(Figs. 8A to D)**. MRE may show wall thickening, lymphadenopathy, ascites, peritoneal thickening, and other associated extraluminal findings. It also shows a good correlation with BMFT studies in detecting wall thickening and has the advantage of being a radiation-free one-stop-shop technique.[31] Most of these findings are common to GI TB and CD making the diagnosis difficult. There are imaging features that can help in this differentiation to a certain extent, and they are discussed later in this chapter.

Colonic and Anorectal TB

Colon is the second most common site of involvement in GI TB and isolated colonic involvement occurs in about 9% of patients.[32] Cecum is the most common site followed by ascending colon. Colonic involvement usually presents with chronic pain in the abdomen, rectal bleeding, and alterations in bowel habits. On imaging, colonic involvement presents as short or long segment thickening of the wall, ulcerations which are usually circumferential, and strictures with or without proximal dilatation. Occasionally, it can present with inflammatory polyps, bowel perforation, or fistula formation. There may be other sites of involvement in the abdomen that can support the diagnosis. Barium enema can show early mucosal abnormalities, ulcerations, spasms, and stricture but is seldom used. A strictured area is seen as smooth narrowing producing an hourglass configuration as opposed to carcinoma colon which produces an apple core configuration. Colonic TB can closely resemble CD, UC, colonic carcinoma, and amebic colitis.

Rarely, TB can involve the rectum and anal canal which can present as proctitis, strictures, fistula, ischiorectal fossa abscess, perianal fissures, and warty growths. These findings

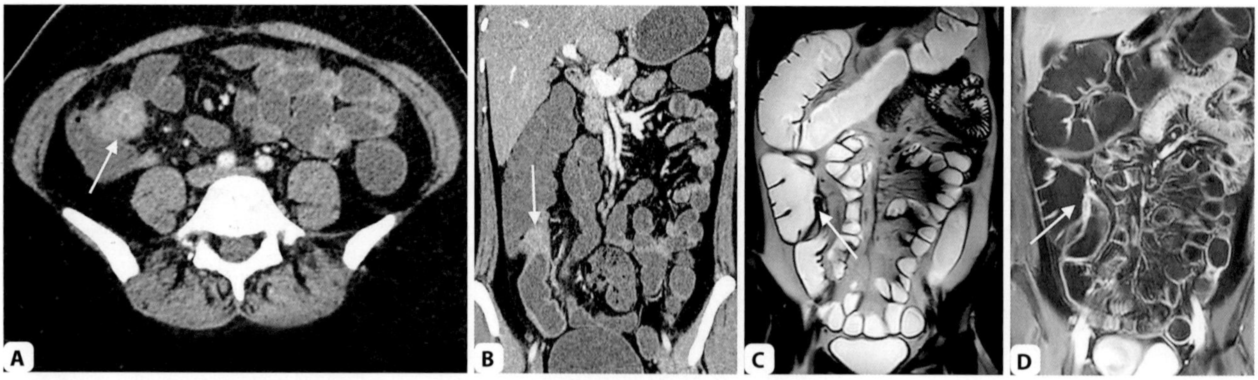

FIGS. 5A TO D: Fibrotic stricture in TB. CTE images (A and B) and MRE images (C and D) show circumferential wall thickening involving the terminal ileum and ileocecal junction (thin arrow) causing mild proximal obstruction. The wall thickening is hypointense on the T2-weighted image (C) and shows homogeneous enhancement on the postcontrast image (D) suggestive of fibrosis.

(CTE: computed tomography enterography; MRE: magnetic resonance enterography; TB: tuberculosis)

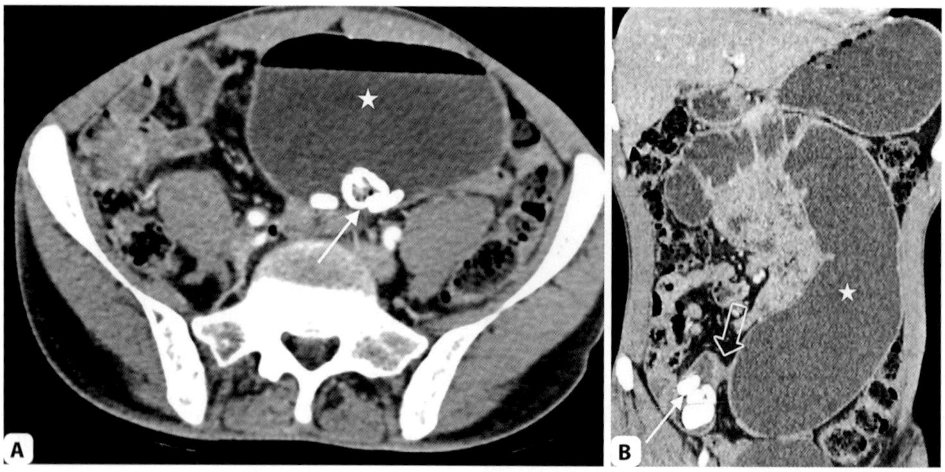

FIGS. 6A AND B: Small bowel obstruction with enteroliths. Axial CECT image (A) and coronal MPR (B) show a short segment ileal stricture (outlined arrow). There is marked proximal dilatation of the small bowel with an air-fluid level (star) suggestive of small bowel obstruction. Also noted is the presence of multiple enteroliths (thin arrow).

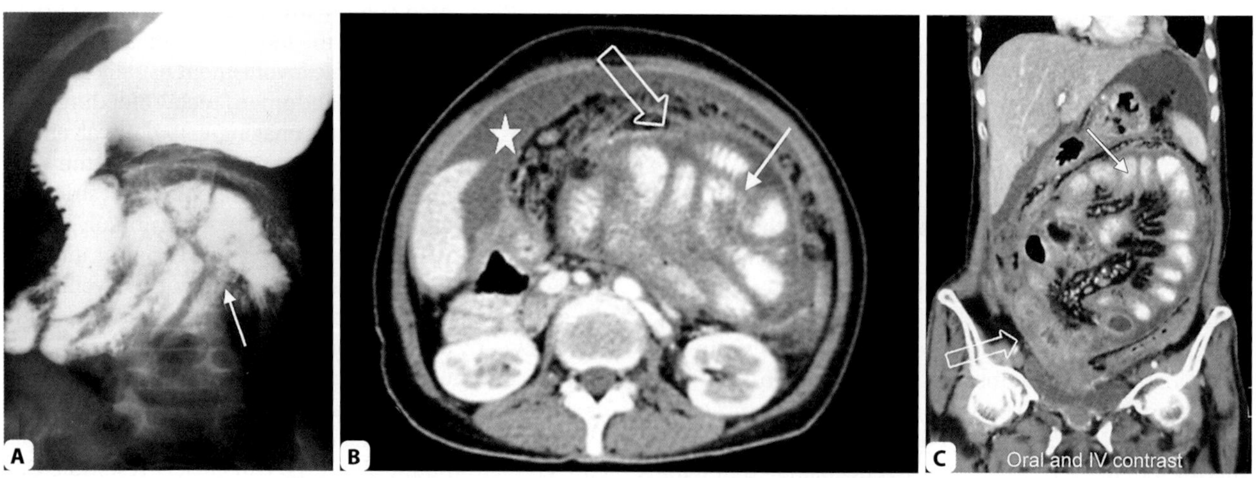

FIGS. 7A TO C: Sclerosing encapsulating peritonitis. Barium meal follow-through (BMFT) (A) shows clumping and fixed position of the dilated small bowel loops (thin arrow) in the central abdomen. Axial CECT (B) and coronal MPR (C) images show clumped dilated proximal jejunal loops which are encapsulated by a thick membrane (outlined arrow) all around suggestive of sclerosing encapsulating peritonitis (cocoon formation). There is associated loculated ascites (star) seen.

(CECT: contrast-enhanced computed tomography; MPR: multiplanar reformation)

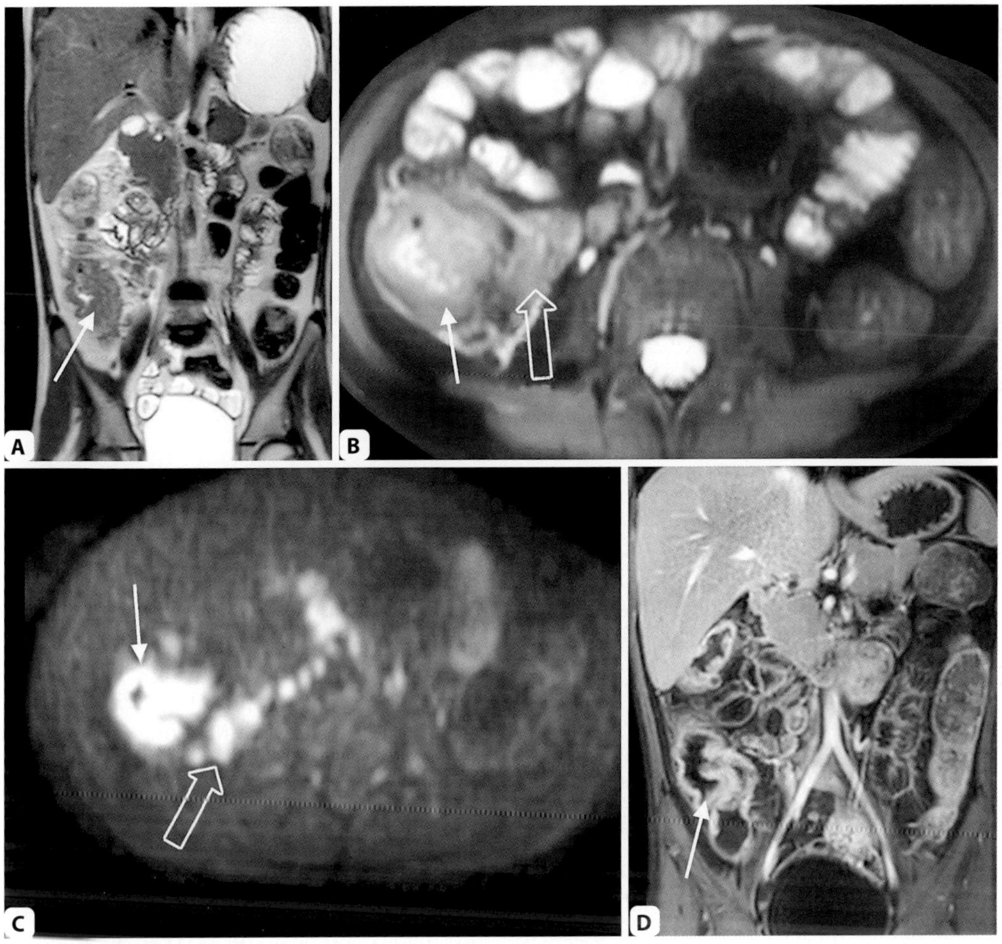

FIGS. 8A TO D: Ileocecal TB. MRE T2-weighted images (A and B) show wall thickening which is hyperintense involving the ileocecal region (thin arrow) with enlarged regional lymph nodes (outlined arrow). The wall thickening shows diffusion restriction on diffusion-weighted b-800 image (C) and hyperenhancement on post-gadolinium image (D) suggestive of active disease.
(MRE: magnetic resonance enterography; TB: tuberculosis)

are not specific to TB because they can occur in CD as well. Circumferential wall thickening because of tuberculous involvement can resemble carcinoma rectum. In doubtful cases, sampling should be done to confirm the diagnosis.

Duodenal Tuberculosis

It constitutes only about 2% of all GI TB and duodenum can be involved either by an extrinsic or intrinsic process.[33] Duodenum may be compressed or involved secondarily due to adjacent lymphadenopathy in which case barium studies can show widening of the C-loop of the duodenum and smooth narrowing. Primary involvement can manifest either as an ulcerative or hyperplastic form which can be seen in barium studies as ulcers, polyps, fistula formation, and narrowing of lumen. CT may show thickening of the duodenal wall commonly involving the second and the third part, which may be associated with stricture and proximal dilatation **(Figs. 9A to C)**.[34] Duodenal TB can mimic CD, lymphoma, and carcinoma and it is usually difficult to differentiate them. Biopsy is confirmatory for the diagnosis.

Gastric Tuberculosis

Stomach involvement by TB is exceedingly rare because of the lack of lymphoid tissue in the stomach, acidic environment, and rapid emptying of gastric contents. Usually, the spread of infection is via the hematogenous route or secondary to adjacent involved lymph nodes. Symptoms are very nonspecific like epigastric discomfort, vomiting, and weight loss which can be seen in other diseases. Imaging features are usually nonspecific and depend on the nature of involvement. They are usually focal and commonly involve the antropyloric region of the stomach. The ulcerative type can present with an ulcer which can be seen in barium studies as a benign ulcer whereas the hypertrophic type can present with gross wall thickening which can mimic carcinoma or lymphoma. Stricture due to fibrosis can also be seen in the antropyloric

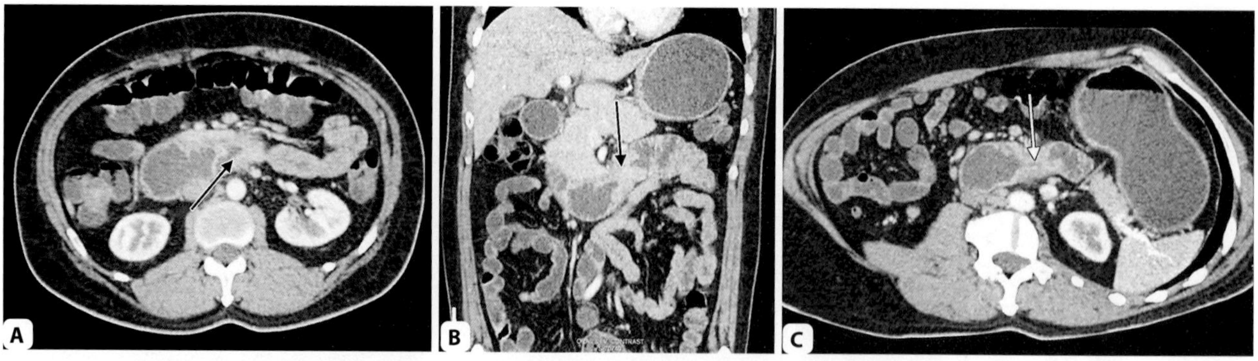

FIGS. 9A TO C: Duodenal TB. Axial CTE image (A) coronal MPR (B) and curved MPR (C) of a patient who presented with vague abdominal pain and weight loss showing irregular thickening and narrowing of the third part of the duodenum (thin arrow). Endoscopic biopsy revealed caseating granulomas and the patient responded to ATT.

(ATT: antitubercular treatment; CTE: computed tomography enterography; MPR: multiplanar reformation; TB: tuberculosis)

region which can mimic CD. Occasionally, the entire stomach may be involved showing diffuse wall thickening and contracted stomach giving an appearance of linitis plastica. Diagnosis is usually confirmed on biopsy since the imaging features are not conclusive.

Esophageal Tuberculosis

Esophageal TB is a rare entity and it is usually secondary to adjacent mediastinal or pulmonary involvement. Tuberculous involvement of adjacent lymph nodes or vertebral bodies can spread to the esophagus, which is the most common mode of spread.[33] Patients usually present with odynophagia, hematemesis, and chest pain. Because of the proximity with the lymph nodes, the middle third of the esophagus is the commonly involved site. Barium studies can show subtle findings such as ulcerations and mucosal irregularity. In advanced stages, it may show stricture, traction diverticulum, and sinus formation. Occasionally, there can be fistulous communication with the tracheobronchial tree. CT scan is more reliable in showing the extraluminal findings and associated mediastinal and lung disease. It can closely mimic carcinoma esophagus because of which endoscopic sampling is necessary in almost all cases.

Extraintestinal Tuberculosis of the Abdomen

Extraintestinal manifestation of TB can often be seen as associated findings in patients with GI TB. The salient features of extraintestinal TB will be covered briefly in this chapter.

Peritoneal Tuberculosis

The peritoneum is the most common location in the abdomen for involvement by TB; however, isolated involvement is relatively rare.[35] Most of the time it occurs in association with other sites of involvement. The involvement of peritoneum, mesentery, and omentum are grouped under peritoneal TB. The spread of infection is either from rupture of involved lymph nodes or direct extension across the bowel wall. Peritoneal involvement manifests as thickening of the peritoneum (2–6 mm) with or without associated nodules. On USG, the peritoneal thickening is seen as hypoechoic lesions and on CECT it is seen as smooth or nodular peritoneal thickening and enhancement. Contrast MRI may show the same features better mainly because of its superior contrast resolution and DW-MRI can also delineate this well. Ascites which can be either free or loculated is also a manifestation of peritoneal TB which can be seen in around 30–100% of patients.[36] USG is very sensitive in detecting ascites and also characterizing its nature. It is superior to CT in showing the septations and debris within the fluid. Usually, high-density ascites is seen in TB, but the density of ascites can range from water attenuation to high attenuation, depending on the amount of fibrin content and cellular debris.[37] Apart from characterizing ascites, imaging can also help in guiding the aspiration of ascitic fluid for biochemical analysis. Tuberculous ascites usually shows low serum-ascites albumin gradient (SAAG <1.1 g/dL) and elevated levels of adenosine deaminase (ADA) and lymphocytes. There are three types of peritoneal involvement based on the amount of ascites and associated features **(Figs. 10A to C)**:

1. Wet type—most common type, gross free, or loculated ascites.
2. Fibrotic-fixed type—less common, with matted bowel loops, mesenteric masses, and loculated ascites.
3. Dry-plastic type—rare, nodular dense fibrotic reaction of peritoneum.

Sclerosing encapsulating peritonitis (SEP) or cocoon is another manifestation of peritoneal TB in which a part or entire bowel loop or abdominal viscera is encapsulated by a fibrocollagenous membrane.[38] Barium studies may show clumping of bowel loops with or without obstructive features and CT scan shows the membrane itself as a thick enhancing structure around the bowel loops **(Figs. 7A to C)**. The other causes of SEP are chronic ambulatory peritoneal dialysis, ventriculoperitoneal shunts, sarcoidosis, GI malignancies, etc.

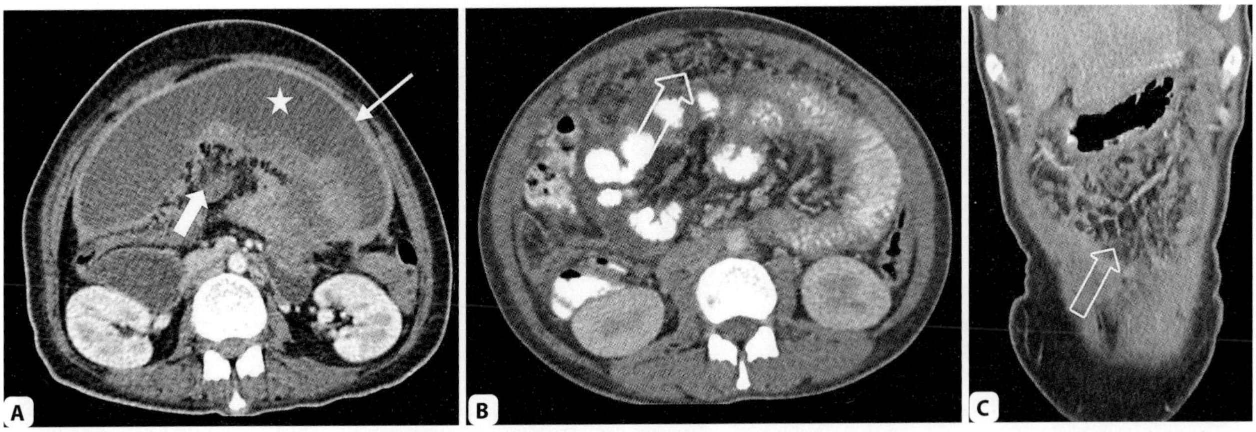

FIGS. 10A TO C: Peritoneal TB. Axial CECT image of the abdomen showing loculated ascites (star) with smoothly thickened enhancing peritoneal lining (thin arrow) and associated omental thickening (thick arrow). The above features are suggestive of a wet type of peritoneal TB. CECT images of the abdomen in a different patient (B and C) show minimal ascites and omental thickening giving a smudged appearance (outlined arrow) suggestive of a fibrotic fixed type of peritoneal TB.

(CECT: contrast-enhanced computed tomography; TB: tuberculosis)

Mesentery is frequently involved in TB and the appearance on imaging may be mild fat stranding, thickening, nodularity, diffuse infiltration, or abscess formation.[35] Like mesentery, omental involvement may also show various imaging features. It may show a smudged, nodular thickening or caking of which a smudged appearance is the most common type of involvement in TB **(Figs. 10A to C)**. Omental caking is a nonspecific finding and can be seen more commonly in peritoneal carcinomatosis.[35] CT scan is the preferred modality to evaluate the omental involvement and recently DW-MRI is also being evaluated in omental pathologies.[39]

Lymph Node Tuberculosis

Mesenteric, omental, peripancreatic, periportal, and upper retroperitoneal lymph nodes are commonly involved in TB **(Figs. 11 and 12)**. It is because these nodes are the regional draining sites for small bowel loops and proximal colon which are the common areas of involvement by TB.[37,40] The appearance of lymph nodes on imaging may vary depending on the stage of the disease. Enlarged lymph node with peripheral enhancement and central necrosis is the most common type of appearance and is relatively specific for TB **(Figs. 11 and 12)**. However, central necrosis can be seen in malignancies, aggressive lymphoma, and Whipple's disease.[40,41] Other less common appearances are homogeneous, heterogeneous, or nonenhancement of the involved node. The nodes in TB tend to be matted and conglomerated because of periadenitis. Multiple normal-sized lymph nodes can also be a manifestation of TB, however not specific to TB. During the healing process, the nodes can become smaller in size and become calcified. Enlargement of nodes, necrosis, and calcification can be seen on both USG and CECT scan of which CT can provide a comprehensive evaluation of the disease. Both can be used to guide sampling from the abnormal lymph nodes when imaging features are not conclusive. Enlarged nodes are seen as T1 hypointense and T2 hyperintense lesions on MRI. Necrosis and liquefaction in the center are seen as T2 hyperintensity within the node.

Visceral Solid Organ Tuberculosis

Visceral organs, such as the liver, spleen, and pancreas can be involved by TB and the usual route of spread is hematogeneous.

Hepatosplenic Tuberculosis

Hepatosplenic TB usually occurs as a part of miliary TB and it is found in 80–100% of patients with miliary TB according to an autopsy series.[42] However, diagnosis on antemortem imaging is quite unusual. Hepatosplenic TB can manifest as micronodular or macronodular type **(Figs. 11A to C)**. In the micronodular type, the lesions are tiny and often they are less than the resolving ability of routine imaging. Diffuse enlargement of the liver and spleen may be the only manifestation of this type. Sometimes, with high-resolution USG images, these micronodular lesions can be visualized as hypoechoic lesions. In this regard, USG is superior to CT scan. Other differential diagnoses for this type are sarcoidosis, metastasis, fungal infection, and lymphoma. In the macronodular type, lesions are usually 1–3 cm in size and they are seen as hypoechoic lesions on USG and hypoenhancing lesions on CECT **(Figs. 11 and 12)**. These nodular lesions are hypointense on T1W scans and hyperintense on T2W scans. DWI can also help in detecting these lesions as they show restriction of diffusion. To start with these lesions may be solid and as the disease progresses they become liquefied and the imaging appearance changes accordingly. They get calcified during the healing phase and in patients with compromised immunity, the lesions can progress in size and can become an abscess.

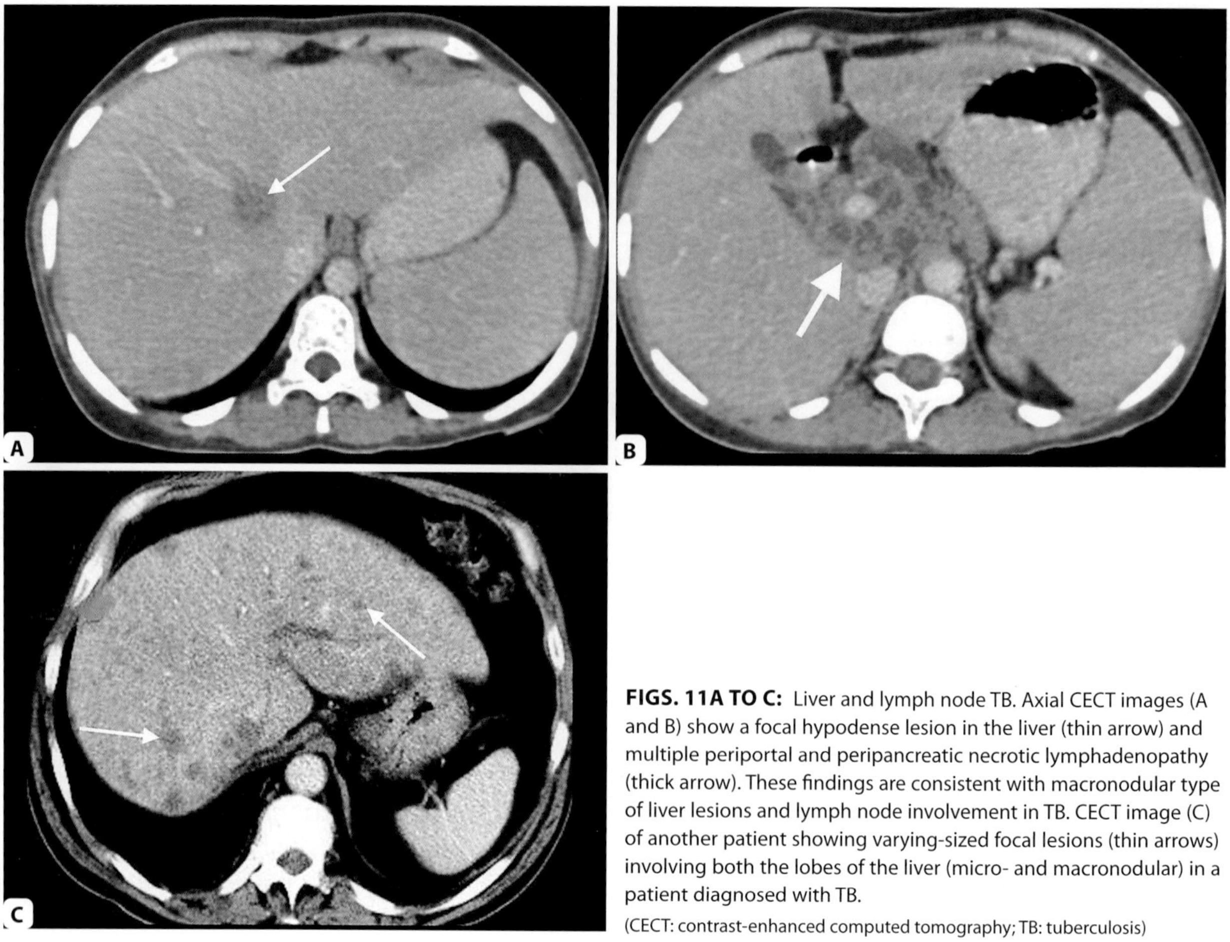

FIGS. 11A TO C: Liver and lymph node TB. Axial CECT images (A and B) show a focal hypodense lesion in the liver (thin arrow) and multiple periportal and peripancreatic necrotic lymphadenopathy (thick arrow). These findings are consistent with macronodular type of liver lesions and lymph node involvement in TB. CECT image (C) of another patient showing varying-sized focal lesions (thin arrows) involving both the lobes of the liver (micro- and macronodular) in a patient diagnosed with TB.

(CECT: contrast-enhanced computed tomography; TB: tuberculosis)

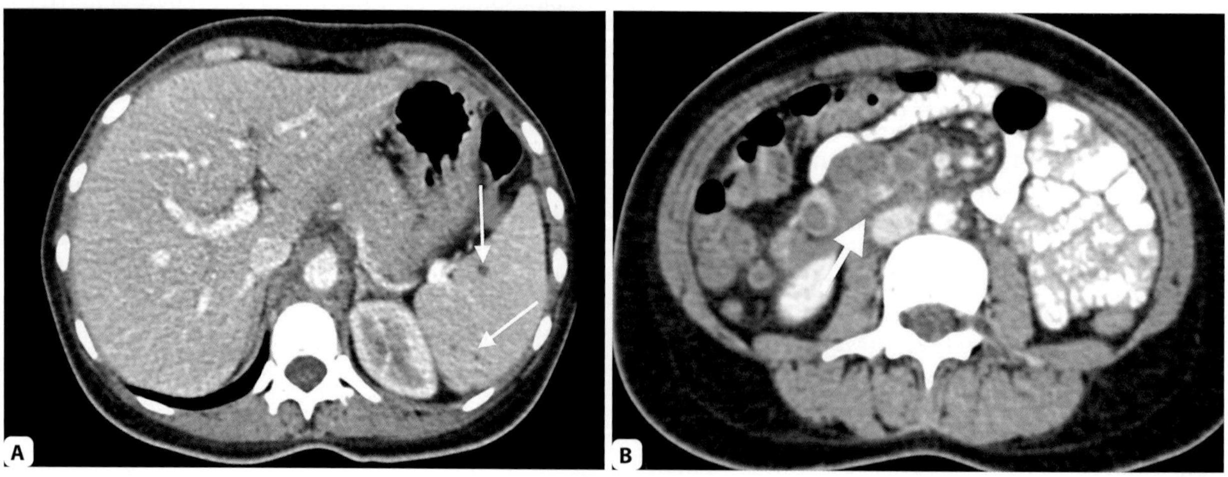

FIGS. 12A AND B: Splenic and lymph node TB. Axial CECT images of the abdomen show multiple hypodense lesions in the spleen (thin arrows) and multiple enlarged mesenteric lymph nodes which show peripheral enhancement and central necrosis (thick arrow). This patient responded to ATT confirming the diagnosis.

(ATT: antitubercular treatment; CECT: contrast-enhanced computed tomography; TB: tuberculosis)

Pancreatic Tuberculosis

Pancreatic TB is very rare and only a few cases are reported in the literature. It is thought to be because of the pancreatic juice which protects the pancreas from the tubercle bacilli.[43] The most common site of involvement is the head of the pancreas. There are three types of patterns described which are diffuse, focal, and multifocal. Lesions can be seen as heterogeneously hypoechoic on USG and heterogeneously hypodense mass lesions on CT scan. Calcification can also be seen in some lesions which can be used to differentiate from pancreatic carcinoma. There may be enlarged lymph nodes with necrosis seen in the vicinity of the pancreas. None of these features are diagnostic for TB and it is usually difficult to differentiate tuberculous lesions from carcinoma pancreas or other inflammatory mass lesions. Most often the diagnosis is apparent only after sampling or after surgical resection. Sampling is usually done under endoscopic US guidance. However, recently there have been efforts to differentiate these lesions using CT pancreatic perfusion.[43] There is a limited role of MRI in these patients and it can be used to differentiate it from cystic neoplasms of the pancreas.

INFLAMMATORY BOWEL DISEASE

Inflammatory bowel disease comprises a group of bowel disorders characterized by idiopathic chronic inflammation of the bowel. It includes mainly CD and UC. Majority of the time, based on the clinical and imaging features, it is possible to classify these disorders into one of these two entities. However, in a small subset, it is not possible to categorize them accurately and they are grouped as indeterminate colitis or IBD unclassified. There is another entity called microscopic colitis which is distinctly different from CD and UC and can present with chronic watery diarrhea.[44] Microscopic colitis which includes collagenous colitis and lymphocytic colitis usually has a normal appearance on colonoscopy and imaging. Inflammation can only be seen on microscopy, hence the name microscopic colitis.

Crohn's Disease

Earlier CD was considered to be a disease of the West and thought to be uncommon in India. Only a few cases were reported in the past from India and this was because the clinical and imaging features of CD closely resemble TB which is endemic in this region. Diagnosing CD with reasonable certainty was difficult under those circumstances. However, in recent years, the improvement in sanitation standards coupled with a better understanding of disease and advancements in the field of imaging have led to an increase in the detection of CD.[45] The true incidence of CD in India is still not clear because of the sparsity of data.

Crohn's disease is a transmural granulomatous inflammatory process of the bowel wall characterized by a waxing and waning course and discontinuous involvement of the bowel, which can be complicated by fistulae and abscesses. It can affect any part of the GI tract, from the oral cavity to the anus, often involving multiple discontinuous segments. Small intestine involvement is seen in 70% of cases, most commonly at the terminal ileum and colonic involvement can be seen in up to 50% of which exclusive colonic involvement is seen in 15–20% of patients.[46] Patients present with pain in the abdomen, diarrhea, low-grade fever, and easy fatigability. Fecal calprotectin is a reliable marker of bowel inflammation but is nonspecific as far as the etiology of inflammation is concerned and can be elevated in GI TB also.

Imaging is an integral part of the evaluation for CD and it provides vital luminal and extraluminal information. Often imaging can differentiate active inflammatory CD from fibrostenotic CD which is one of the main aims of imaging in these patients apart from diagnosis and evaluating the extent of the disease and its complications. The above differentiation is of paramount importance because the management of these two stages is very different. Active CD is managed by medical treatment whereas fibrostenotic CD may need surgical management.

Many attempts have been made to standardize the classification and scoring of the severity of the disease. Montreal classification is one of these which is widely used in clinical practice and research to describe the disease phenotype in CD **(Table 2)**.[47] It describes the type, extent, and behavior of disease and studies have proven the reliability of the classification.[48-50] Crohn's disease activity index (CDAI) is another widely used tool for scoring the disease severity which can be used to prognosticate CD and is useful in the follow-up of these patients.[51,52] A score of <150 is considered as remission of disease and a score of >450 is considered as severe disease.

TABLE 2: Montreal classification of Crohn's disease.

Age at diagnosis (A)	
A1	16 years or younger
A2	17–40 years
A3	>40 years
Location (L)	
L1	Terminal ileum
L2	Colon
L3	Ileocolon
L4	Upper gastrointestinal
Behavior (B)	
p—modifier for perianal disease, added as a suffix to B	
B1	Nonstricturing, nonpenetrating
B2	Stricturing
B3	Penetrating

Imaging Features of Crohn's Disease

Imaging features of CD vary with the stage of the disease process and the associated complications.

Double-contrast barium enteroclysis was the imaging modality of choice before the emergence of cross-sectional modalities such as CTE and MRE. It is the best modality to show the aphthous ulcers seen in the active phase of the disease as a punctate collection of barium with surrounding radiolucent halo due to mucosal edema. When the disease progresses, the ulcers coalesce and form deep linear ulceration separating the edematous mucosa **(Figs. 2A to C)**. This is seen in barium studies as cobble-stoning. Later, the mesenteric border shortens due to fibrosis with the formation of pseudosacculation along the antimesenteric border **(Figs. 2A to C)**. Stenosis of the bowel loop with or without proximal dilatation and complications like bowel fistulization or contained perforation can also be seen on barium studies. Despite the ability of double-contrast barium to show the mucosal changes in great detail, the extraluminal changes of CD are not well evaluated for which the cross-sectional modalities are better. In current practice, barium studies are not routinely done for the diagnosis or follow-up of CD. It may be done for a few niche indications such as demonstration of aphthous ulcers, cobble-stoning of mucosa, and fistula formation.[53] The Ideal imaging modality for the evaluation of CD is CTE or MRE and the diagnostic performance of both modalities is comparable for the detection of CD.[54-56] The choice between the two techniques depends largely on the local availability of equipment and expertise and a few other clinical considerations. The radiation hazard involved in CTE and the ability of MRE to differentiate active and fibrotic disease tilts the balance toward MRE in appropriate clinical scenarios. When CD is suspected in a child or a patient is being evaluated for response to treatment or follow-up imaging or there is suspicion of fistula, MRE is better than CTE. However, when CD is suspected in an elderly patient or clinical suspicion of CD is low or a diagnosis other than CD is suspected, CTE may be preferred over MRE because it is faster, reliable, relatively resistant to artifacts, and gives consistent image quality.

Thickening of Bowel Wall

Bowel wall thickening is the most common finding in patients with CD **(Figs. 13 and 14)**. It is usually eccentric and asymmetrical, preferentially affecting the mesenteric border, most commonly involving the terminal ileum and the ileocecal junction.[4] This preferential involvement of the mesenteric border is a specific feature of CD.[57] Sometimes the involvement can be circumferential. Often in CD, the degree of involvement of the ileum is more than that of the cecum.[58] Thickening of the bowel wall is a nonspecific finding that can occur in both active inflammatory and fibrostenotic diseases. In a distended bowel, a wall thickness of >3 mm is abnormal. Single-shot fast spin-echo (FSE) or postcontrast sequence on MRE is the optimal sequences to look for wall thickening. This finding has high sensitivity and specificity in the range of 83–91% and 86–100%, respectively.[59] Wall thickening may reduce during the remission phase but, usually, there will be some residual thickening compared to the normal segment. One pitfall of this finding is that the bowel wall may look thick when the bowel is collapsed. One should be careful not to label collapsed bowel loops as wall thickening.

Submucosal Edema

Submucosal edema leads to wall thickening and is usually seen as a hypodense area on CTE and a hyperintense area on T2W sequence with or without fat suppression **(Figs. 13 to 15)**. Submucosal edema is a sign of active disease.

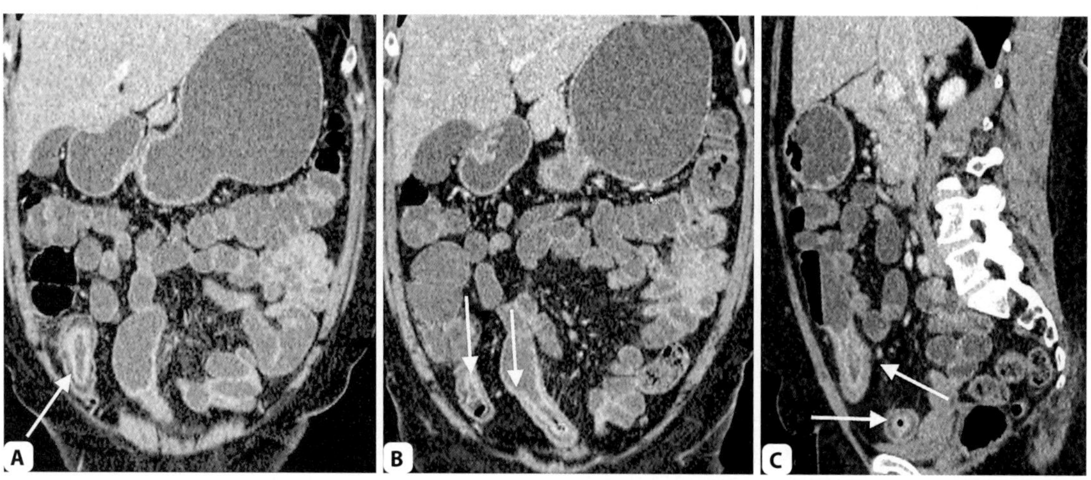

FIGS. 13A TO C: Stratified wall enhancement in active CD. Coronal CTE images (A and B) and sagittal MPR (C) show thickening and stratified wall enhancement involving the ileal loops (thin arrow) which is a sign of active inflammatory stage of CD.

(CD: Crohn's disease; CTE: computed tomography enterography; MPR: multiplanar reformation)

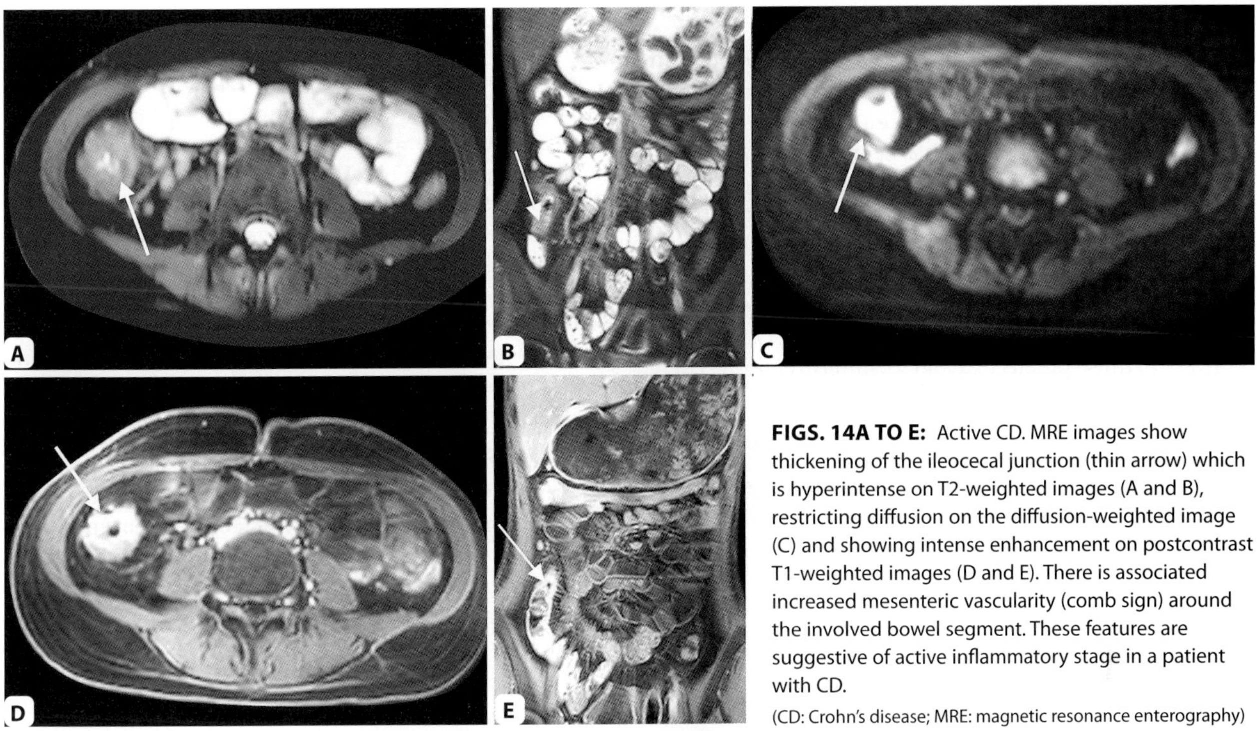

FIGS. 14A TO E: Active CD. MRE images show thickening of the ileocecal junction (thin arrow) which is hyperintense on T2-weighted images (A and B), restricting diffusion on the diffusion-weighted image (C) and showing intense enhancement on postcontrast T1-weighted images (D and E). There is associated increased mesenteric vascularity (comb sign) around the involved bowel segment. These features are suggestive of active inflammatory stage in a patient with CD.
(CD: Crohn's disease; MRE: magnetic resonance enterography)

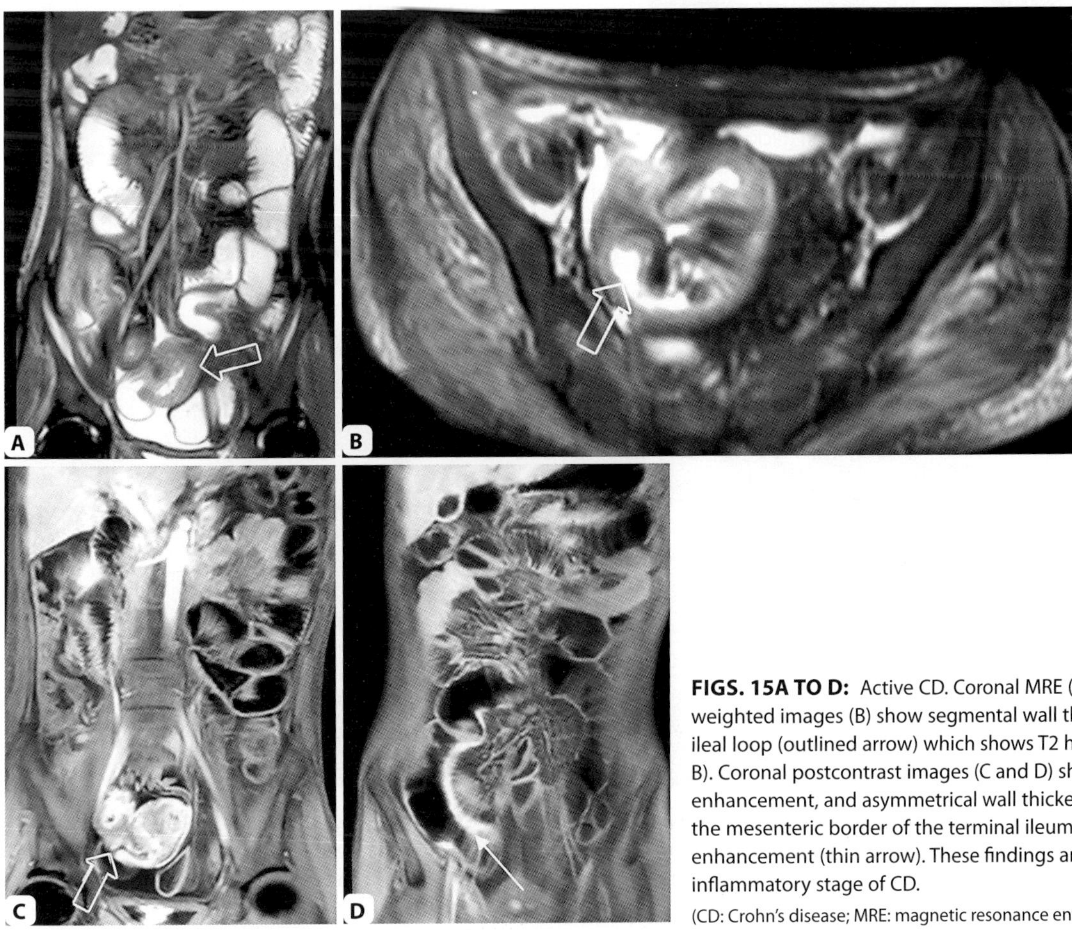

FIGS. 15A TO D: Active CD. Coronal MRE (A) and axial T2-weighted images (B) show segmental wall thickening of a pelvic ileal loop (outlined arrow) which shows T2 hyperintensity (A and B). Coronal postcontrast images (C and D) show stratified mural enhancement, and asymmetrical wall thickening involving the mesenteric border of the terminal ileum with intense enhancement (thin arrow). These findings are typical for active inflammatory stage of CD.
(CD: Crohn's disease; MRE: magnetic resonance enterography)

Bowel Wall Contrast Enhancement

Contrast enhancement of the involved segment can occur both in active inflammatory disease and in the fibrostenotic phase. It is considered to be the earliest and the most sensitive sign for active CD.[60] It has been shown to correlate with the level of inflammation in histopathology. At the same time, absence of abnormal enhancement almost excludes disease activity in CD.[61] Potential pitfalls in contrast enhancement are that the normal jejunal enhancement is more than ileal enhancement and collapsed bowel loops can show apparent increased enhancement. One should be aware of these pitfalls to avoid misinterpretation. There are two types of enhancement patterns described in CD—(1) stratified and (2) homogeneous enhancement. Of the above types, stratified bowel wall enhancement (target-like) is specific for the active inflammatory phase **(Figs. 13 and 15)**. Homogeneous enhancement is suggestive of the fibrotic phase **(Figs. 16 and 17)**. It is also known that often fibrosis and active inflammation can coexist and can present as varying features on imaging **(Figs. 18A to C)**. One promising alternative for contrast enhancement is DWI in which the hyperintensity on trace images corresponds with active inflammation **(Fig. 14)**.[62] This technique is useful in patients where contrast cannot be administered for reasons like deranged renal parameters.

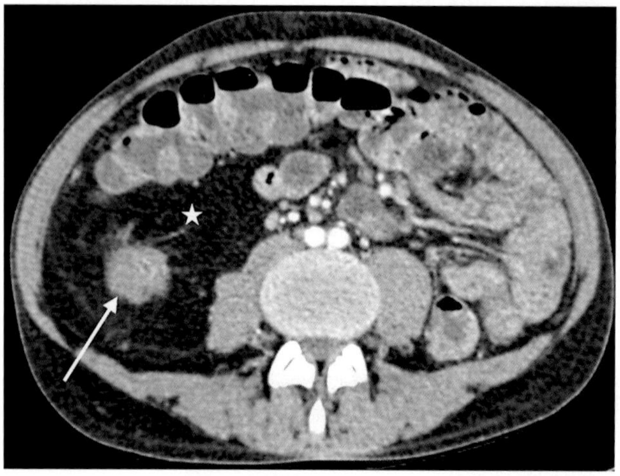

FIG. 16: Fat proliferation. Axial CTE image showing thickening of ascending colon (thin arrow) with surrounding fat proliferation (star). Minimal enhancement of the involved segment coupled with fat proliferation is suggestive of chronic fibrotic stage of CD.
(CD: Crohn's disease; CTE: computed tomography enterography)

Submucosal Fat Infiltration

In patients with chronic inflammation, there can be fat deposition in the submucosa which can appear markedly hypodense on CTE and lose signal on fat-saturated sequences on MRE.[63,64] Although it is a nonspecific sign, the presence of submucosal fat infiltration in CD suggests chronicity.

Skip Lesions

This is defined as multifocal areas of involvement with normal healthy bowel in between. It is considered an important sign to differentiate CD from other infective processes like TB but is not very specific.

Stricture

A stricture is defined as a combination of the narrowed lumen, thickened wall, and prestenotic dilatation of the bowel (> 3 cm).[65] Bowel narrowing in CD can be because of active inflammation leading to spasm or due to chronic

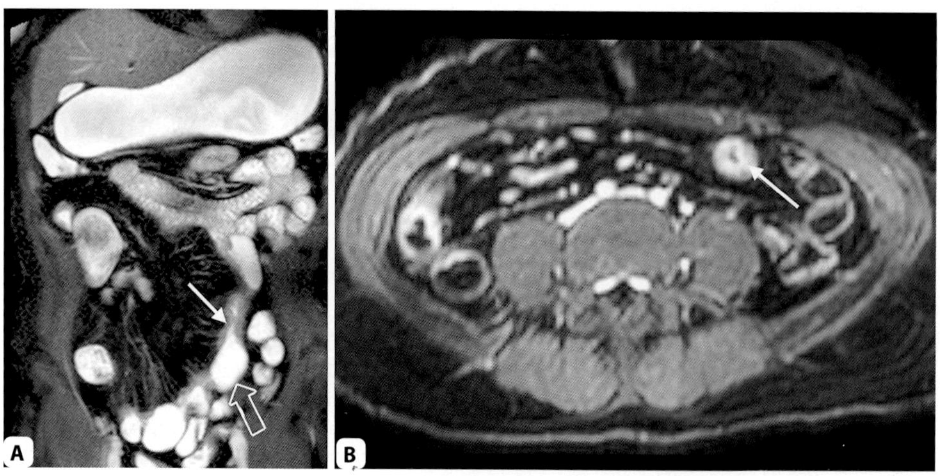

FIGS. 17A AND B: Pseudosacculations in fibrotic CD. Coronal T2-weighted image (A) of MRE study showing wall thickening and multiple segments of luminal narrowing involving the ileal loops (thin arrow). There are multiple pseudosacculations seen in the antimesenteric border (outlined arrow). Axial postcontrast T1-weighted image (B) shows homogeneous wall enhancement of the involved loop. The above imaging features are characteristic of fibrostenotic stage of CD.
(CD: Crohn's disease; MRE: magnetic resonance enterography)

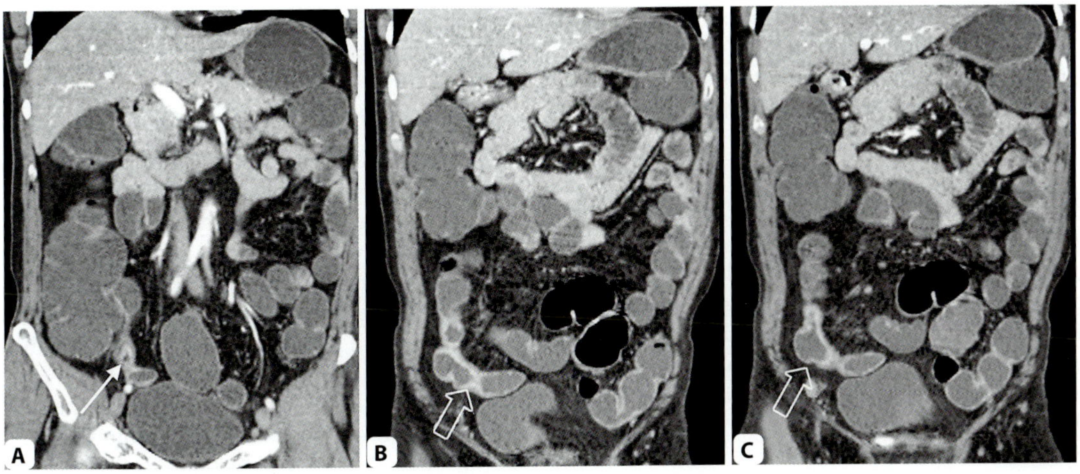

FIGS. 18A TO C: Coexisting active and chronic CD. Coronal CTE images (A to C) showing hyperenhancement with mural stratification (thin arrow) and pseudosacculation involving the antimesenteric border of distal ileum (outlined arrow). Mural stratification is a sign of active inflammatory stage whereas pseudosacculation is a sign of chronic CD.

(CD: Crohn's disease; CTE: computed tomography enterography)

TABLE 3: Definition for a naïve small bowel stricture on USG, CTE, and MRE.[65]

Appropriate criteria	
Luminal diameter	Reduced by at least 50%, compared to normal adjacent well-distended bowel loop
Bowel wall thickening	Wall thickness of >25% in the maximally thickened area in a well-distended lumen, compared to normal adjacent bowel loop
Prestenotic dilatation	Diameter > 3 cm
Uncertain	
Luminal diameter	<1 cm in a well-distended lumen
Bowel wall thickening	>3 mm in a well-distended lumen, compared to a normal adjacent bowel loop
Prestenotic dilatation	>20% compared to a normal adjacent bowel loop

(CTE: CT enterography; MRE: MR enterography; USG: ultrasonography)

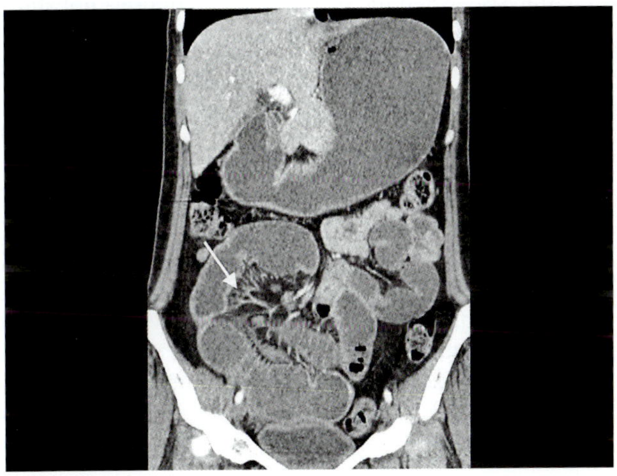

FIG. 19: Comb sign in active CD. Coronal CTE image showing a segment of dilated ileal loop with increased mesenteric vascularity (comb sign) (thin arrow) in a patient with CD. The presence of comb sign is a marker of active inflammatory stage of CD.

(CD: Crohn's disease; CTE: computed tomography enterography)

fibrostenosing disease. This differentiation can sometimes be difficult based on imaging because of overlapping features. The presence of stratified enhancement, wall edema, and ulcerations favor active inflammation whereas homogeneous enhancement, T2 dark mural signal intensity, and marked prestenotic dilatation of bowel loops indicate a chronic process. Almost 50% of patients with CD develop strictures in the future. The consensus statement published in 2018 elaborates on the criteria for strictures (both appropriate and uncertain) which is given in **Table 3**.

Comb Sign

Comb sign is a manifestation of prominent vasa recta due to an increase in vascularity in the mesentery. It is regarded as one of the specific signs of active inflammation **(Figs. 14 and 19)**. This is best seen on TruFISP (BTFE) and postcontrast sequences.

Mesenteric Edema

It is due to inflammation and resultant edema in the mesentery secondary to bowel wall inflammation. It is also considered as a sign of active inflammation. It is seen as increased attenuation on CTE (mesenteric fat stranding) and increased intensity on fat-saturated T2W sequences. In severe cases, minimal free fluid can also be seen.

Ulcerations

Ulcerations which are considered a sign of active disease are sometimes seen on imaging especially on MRE when the loops are adequately distended **(Fig. 20)**. It may be seen as irregularity of the wall or thin linear hyperintensity extending into the wall. In a recent study, using high-resolution MRE images, the sensitivity in detecting the mucosal features is in the range of 69–99% for superficial ulcers and 94–99% for deep ulcers.[66]

Abnormal Motility

Abnormal bowel motility is a known feature of active CD and sometimes it can be the early sign of disease. It can be classified into different patterns as follows:[67]

- Paralysis—when the involved segment does not show peristalsis
- Hypomotility—when the involved segment shows decreased motility
- Hypermotility—when the involved segment shows increased motility
- Intraluminal pendular movement—inefficient to-and-fro movement of bowel content.

The movement of the involved bowel loop is compared with the surrounding normal loops for any abnormality. If there is any abnormal movement of a segment, it has to be carefully studied in the other sequences on MRE to confirm the abnormality. Cine MRI which can be done as a part of MRE is the best way to evaluate bowel motility and it is found to increase the detection rate of lesions compared to standard MRE sequences.[67]

Abscesses, Sinuses, and Fistulae

Abscesses, sinuses, and fistulae developing in a patient with CD are considered major complications and are also signs of the penetrating phenotype of the disease. Abscesses are seen as hypodense lesions on CTE and hyperintense on T2W sequences on MRE with the wall showing post-contrast enhancement. Sinuses and fistulae are seen as linear enhancing structures beyond the confines of the bowel loop on CTE and MRE. In CD, there can be blind sinuses extending from the bowel wall or enteroenteric, enterocolonic, enterovesical, enterocutaneous, or perianal fistula. A stellate or clover leaf configuration of bowel loops (star sign) which are adherent to each other is suggestive of enteroenteric fistula **(Fig. 21)**. The diagnosis of this entity has a bearing on management and may be an indication for initiating treatment with a biological agent like infliximab. The sensitivity and specificity of CTE and MRE in detecting sinuses and fistulas is around between 83 and 100%, respectively.[64] However, MRE performs better in the diagnosis and evaluation of the extent of perianal fistulae in relation to the internal and external sphincters **(Figs. 22A to D)**.[68,69]

Fibrosis

Recognizing fibrosis on imaging is crucial for the management of stricturing CD because those patients are often considered for balloon dilatation or surgery as they are unlikely to benefit from medical therapy.[70] Fibrosis is a result of chronic inflammation which has a nonspecific appearance on CTE. MRE has an edge over CTE in this regard as fibrosis manifests as hypointensity on both T1

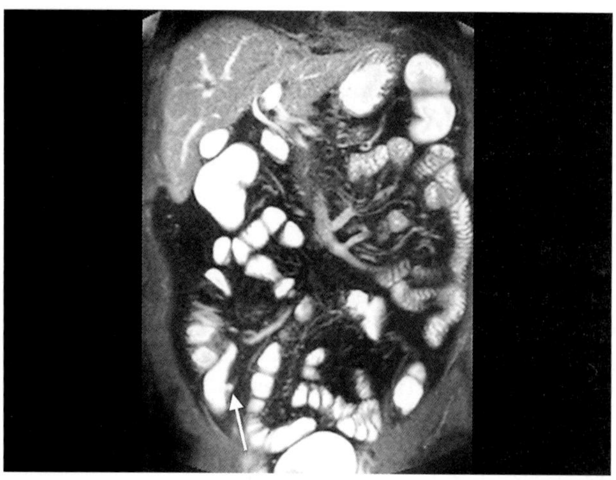

FIG. 20: Deep ulcer on CD. T2-weighted coronal image of MRE showing hyperintense outpouching (thin arrow) in the distal ileal loop suggestive of deep ulceration in a patient with CD.
(CD: Crohn's disease; MRE: magnetic resonance enterography)

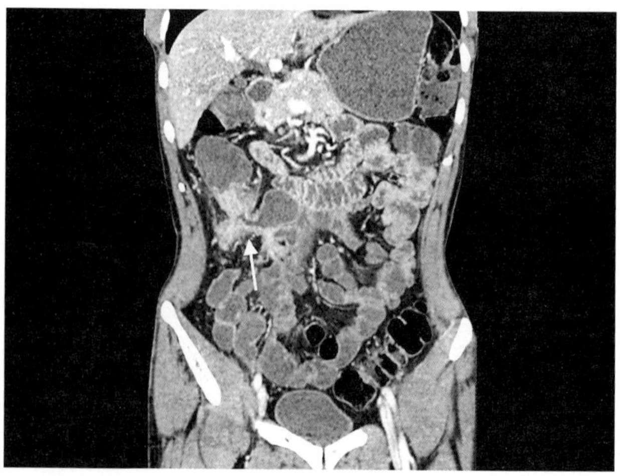

FIG. 21: Fistulizing stage of CD. Coronal CTE image showing abnormal thickening, distorted stellate configuration, and communication between the small bowel loop and the ascending colon (thin arrow) suggestive of enterocolic fistula.
(CD: Crohn's disease; CTE: computed tomography enterography)

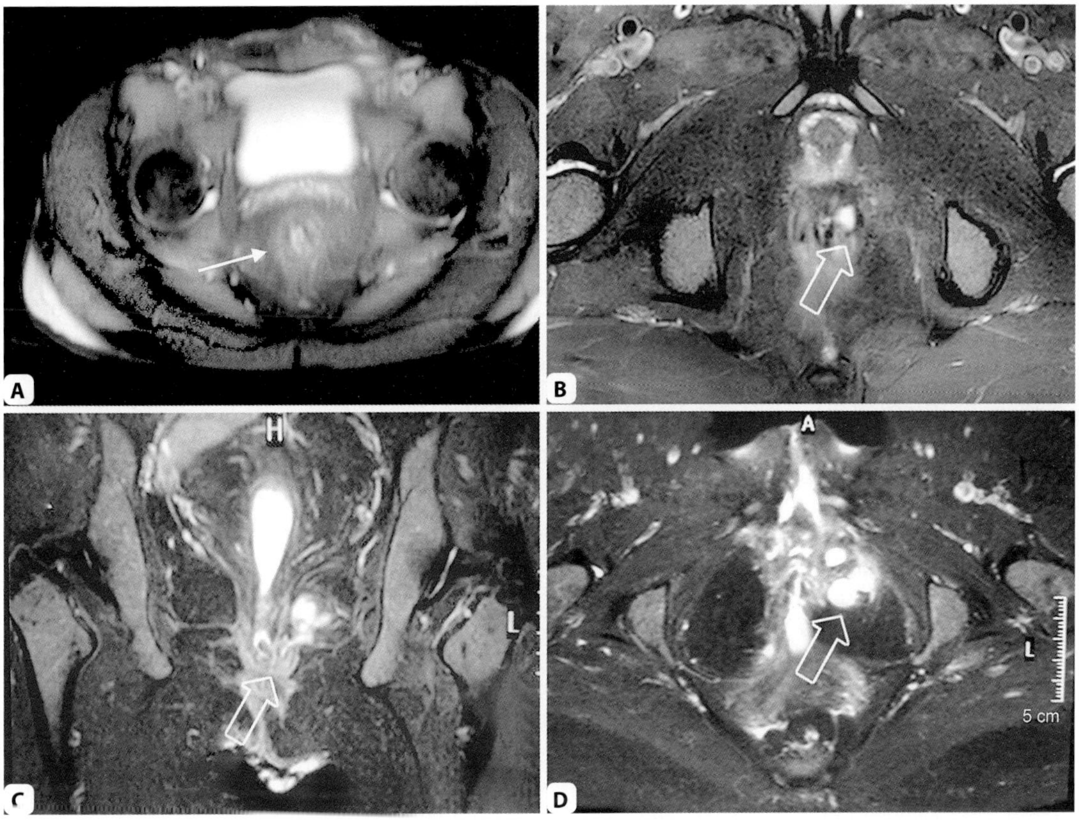

FIGS. 22A TO D: Perianal fistulas. T2-weighted MR images (A and B) of a patient with rectal involvement by CD (thin arrow) showing a small fistulous tract (outlined arrow) arising from the anal canal. T2-weighted images (C and D) of a different patient showing a more complex fistulous tract and collections (outlined arrow) in the left ischioanal fossa. The presence of a fistula or sinus tract is a marker of active inflammatory stage in CD.

(CD: Crohn's disease; MR: magnetic resonance)

and T2W images and shows progressive homogeneous enhancement in the delayed phase **(Figs. 16 to 18)**.

Pseudodiverticulum Formation

This sign is a result of asymmetrical fibrosis and shortening of the mesenteric border leading to apparent sacculations along the antimesenteric border. It is usually seen in chronic CD and associated with other features of chronic disease **(Figs. 2, 17, and 18)**.

Fibrofatty Proliferation

It is seen in long-standing CD as a result of chronic inflammation in bowel loops. It is seen as increased fat surrounding the involved bowel loops on all imaging modalities **(Fig. 16)**. This is a nonspecific finding and may be seen in any cause of chronic inflammation.

Reactive Lymphadenopathy

In India, enlarged regional lymph nodes with bowel wall thickening occur more commonly in TB. However, enlarged lymph nodes can occur in patients with CD also. However, lymph nodes in CD are usually <1 cm in size. Necrotic lymph nodes are seen in TB and are a reliable differentiating feature. Mesenteric lymphadenopathy in CD is a nonspecific finding that can occur in both active and inactive diseases. There is some evidence that the increased degree of nodal enhancement favors active disease in CD.[71]

Most of the features of CD described above are almost similar to CTE and MRE. These findings are described in **Table 4**.[72] Abnormalities such as submucosal edema, submucosal fat infiltration, and fibrosis may appear as nonspecific hypoattenuation on CTE whereas they are more accurately characterized on MRE. The imaging features and their significance in differentiating active from fibrotic disease are listed in **Table 5**.

Extraintestinal Manifestations and Complications of Crohn's Disease

Crohn's disease can have multiple extraintestinal manifestations, some of which can have management implications. Sacroiliitis, primary sclerosing cholangitis, ankylosing spondylitis, avascular necrosis, pancreatitis, cholelithiasis, nephrolithiasis, and acute or chronic mesenteric thrombosis are a few of the manifestations that can be diagnosed on CTE and MRE.[57] Other manifestations that can be associated with CD are deep venous thrombosis, pulmonary embolism, uveitis, pyoderma gangrenosum, erythema nodosum, and a variety of other autoimmune diseases. CD can occasionally present with intestinal obstruction and bowel perforation. In long-standing CD, there is an increase in the risk of small bowel and colorectal malignancies depending on the site of the disease. Also, there is a weak association with the development of lymphoma in long-standing disease apart from other nonbowel malignancies.[73,74] It is difficult to differentiate inflammatory thickening from a neoplastic one on imaging. Endoscopy is the first-line modality to detect malignancies developing in CD. However, features like asymmetric mural thickening >1.5 cm, a focal loss of wall stratification, and locoregional adenopathy should raise a suspicion of malignancy.[75]

TABLE 4: Imaging findings associated with inflammation in Crohn's disease.

Imaging finding	Description
Segmental mural hyperenhancement	Increased attenuation/signal intensity of bowel as compared to adjacent normal bowel segment
Intramural edema	The gray attenuation layer of the water halo sign in CT represents edema in submucosa; hyperintense signal from fat-saturated T2-weighted scan in MRI
Ulcerations	Small focal breaks in the intraluminal surface of the bowel wall with focal extension of air
Fistulae	Extraenteric tract with or without internal air or fluid. Including simple/complex fistulae, sinus tract, and perianal fistulae
Inflammatory mass	Ill-defined mass-like lesion of mixed fat and/or soft tissue attenuation/signal intensity usually associated with penetrating disease such as complex fistulae
Abscess	Mesenteric/peritoneal/perianal fluid collection with rim enhancement with or without internal air
Perienteric edema/inflammation	Increased attenuation (CT) or high T2 signal (MR) in mesenteric fat adjacent to abnormal bowel loops
Comb sign	Engorged vessels that supply an inflamed bowel loop
Fibrofatty proliferation	Increased fat adjacent to or around the abnormal bowel, displacing bowel loops; usually along mesenteric border, but can be circumferential

Scoring systems

There are multiple signs of active inflammation in IBD described in the literature, based on which various scoring systems have been devised both on endoscopy and imaging. These scoring systems help to measure, monitor, grade, and prognosticate the disease activity in CD. One such scoring system based on MRI is the magnetic resonance index of activity (MaRIA) score, which correlates well with the endoscopic scoring system.[76] However, as this is time-consuming, a simplified version was released in 2020.[77] Other scoring systems, such as the London, Nancy, and Clermont scores are also used.

Magnetic resonance index of activity score includes mural thickening, mural edema, mucosal ulceration, and perienteric fat stranding.[78] The London score is also a simplified score based on similar features. The other two scoring systems, Nancy and Clermont are based on DWI. DWI has well-known applications in the abdomen with the advantage of no requirement of exogenous contrast, being radiation-free, and also being a fast sequence. The Nancy scoring system incorporates a qualitative assessment of DWI along with other five features, i.e., rapid gadolinium enhancement, differentiation between the mucosa-submucosa complex and the muscularis propria, bowel wall thickening, edema, and the presence of ulceration.16 The Clermont system is a quantitative assessment of DWI wherein apparent diffusion coefficient (ADC) values are used.[79]

NEWER TECHNIQUES TO DIFFERENTIATE INFLAMMATORY VERSUS FIBROTIC STRICTURES

Magnetization Transfer

In IBD, chronic inflammation leads to fibrosis and finally stricture formation. Inflammation and fibrosis

TABLE 5: Imaging features to differentiate active inflammatory from fibrostenotic disease in Crohn's disease (CD).

Active disease	Fibrotic stage	Nonspecific
• Submucosal edema • Early hyperenhancement • Stratified enhancement of the wall • Comb sign • Mesenteric edema • Ulcerations • Abnormal motility • Abscesses, sinuses, and fistulas	• Late progressive and homogeneous wall enhancement • Submucosal fatty infiltration • Fibrosis • Pseudodiverticulum • Fibrofatty proliferation	• Bowel wall thickening • Skip lesions • Bowel stenosis • Reactive lymphadenopathy

coexist in variable ratios, depending on the stage of the disease. The narrowing of the lumen caused by predominant inflammatory changes usually gets reversed with anti-inflammatory and immunosuppressant treatment. However, once it progresses to fibrotic stricture, definitive management in the form of endoscopic or surgical release is essential to relieve the symptoms. Almost 30% of the patients with IBD will develop fibrotic strictures in about 10 years.[85] Noninvasive diagnosis of the type of stricture remains a challenge and various new techniques are being investigated to make the distinction between inflammatory and fibrotic strictures.

Magnetization transfer (MT) MRI is a potential sequence that not only detects but also grades the severity of fibrosis in inflammatory strictures. The coexistence of active inflammation at the time of scanning does not alter the findings.[86] This is very useful for guiding the appropriate management as well as for monitoring the response to the treatment. Normalized MT ratios are calculated which increase with the increasing grade of fibrosis. Hence, the highest value of approximately 0.88 is seen in severe fibrotic strictures whereas the value of approximately 0.51 is seen in purely inflammatory strictures.[86] A cut-off value of 0.71 is suggested to differentiate moderate-to-severe fibrosis from mild fibrosis with a sensitivity of 84.42% and a specificity of 90%.[86]

Conventional MR sequences are not sufficient to make this differentiation. Multiphasic MRI is somewhat helpful in differentiating severe from mild-grade fibrosis based on delayed enhancement. DWI also shows potential in differentiating fibrotic versus inflammatory strictures; however, no statistical difference is seen in ADC value in various grades of fibrosis. Positron emission tomography is another potential investigation that can differentiate fibrotic disease from active disease; however, the amount of radiation exposure along with the high cost precludes its repeated use.

Delayed Enhancement

Active inflammation in the bowel tends to show stratified mural hyperenhancement, ulcerations, and blurred margins on contrast-enhanced MRI. Fibrotic stricture on the other hand shows uniform delayed enhancement at 7 minutes. This technique is utilized to assess the degree of underlying fibrosis.[80]

Visceral Fat to Subcutaneous Ratio

Accumulation of mesenteric fat and fat wrapping of the bowel is one of the early signs of CD. High visceral fat (VF) is a sign of complex CD and is associated with higher rates of stenosis, fistulae and higher postoperative recurrence.[81,82] The latest literature has also observed a direct correlation between the degree of fibrosis in the bowel wall and the VF ratio to the subcutaneous fat (SF). The higher the ratio, more is the degree of fibrosis. Also, the ratio of stenosis to dilatation has been inversely related to the degree of fibrosis. With a cut-off of VF/SF volume ratio of 0.880, the sensitivity and specificity to distinguish severe from moderate fibrosis were observed to be 76.9% and 68.6%, respectively.[83] This feature is also useful in excluding the diagnosis of ITB. High VF and high VF/SF with a cut-off of 0.63 is suggested to differentiate CD from ITB with a sensitivity of 82% and specificity of 81%.[84]

Magnetic Resonance Elastography

This is another new technique that can quantitatively assess the amount of fibrosis in the bowel wall. This is similar to the technique used for hepatic fibrosis. A separate hardware is required to generate the propagating shear waves which bring about micromovements in the local environment. These movements can further be analyzed by phase-contrast sequence which generates stiffness maps. One of the studies by Avila et al. obtained bowel stiffness ≥ 3.57 kPa having a fair accuracy for predicting the occurrence of clinical event, with a sensitivity of 81%, and a specificity of 82%.[87]

T1 Mapping

T1 mapping is a new technique that has shown positive results in preclinical studies. Quantitative T1 mapping is based on the tissue's intrinsic longitudinal magnetization relaxation time and increases with increasing extracellular water.[72] In a preliminary study, the T1 value of none-to-mild fibrotic bowel walls was seen to be lower than that of moderate-to-severe ones.[88]

IMAGING FEATURES TO DIFFERENTIATE INTESTINAL TB FROM CD

Intestinal tuberculosis and CD have many features in common and their differentiation is difficult. This poses a greater problem in countries like India where TB is endemic. There is no single test that can reliably differentiate ITB from CD. Hence a combination of clinical, endoscopic, imaging, histopathology, and biochemical features should be used. Sometimes follow-up imaging and even a trial of antituberculous therapy may be required to differentiate them. Imaging is an important tool that is used routinely and the common imaging features used to differentiate both entities are summarized in **Table 6**.

ULCERATIVE COLITIS

Ulcerative colitis is characterized by superficial inflammation involving the colon. The colonic involvement in UC is symmetric and contiguous. Rectum is involved in almost all cases with varying lengths of proximal colonic involvement sometimes involving the entire colon (pancolitis).[89] Occasionally, the terminal ileum can be affected and

TABLE 6: Imaging features to differentiate GI TB and CD.

Imaging features	Intestinal tuberculosis	CD
Site of involvement	Cecum more than ileum	Ileum more than cecum
Length of involvement	Shorter segment	Longer segment
Multiple site involvement	Uncommon	Common
Skip lesions	Rare	Common
Type of wall enhancement	Homogeneous	Stratified
Mural stratification of wall	Rare	Common
Perianal fistula	Uncommon	Common
Mesenteric abscess	Very rare	Relatively common
Bowel fistulas	Rare	Relatively common
Strictures	Concentric	Eccentric with sacculations
Enteroliths	More common	Less common
Increased mesenteric vascularity	Uncommon	Common
Fibrofatty proliferation	Uncommon	Common
Mesenteric nodes	Large and necrotic	Small and homogeneous
Omental involvement	Often seen	Rare
Ascites	Frequent	Uncommon
Solid organ involvement	Relatively common	Very rare

(CD: Crohn's disease; GI TB: gastrointestinal tuberculosis)

Source: Modified and reproduced with permission from Sharma R et al. (2016).[58]

becomes edematous and dilated when the entire colon is involved and is called backwash ileitis. UC is well evaluated with colonoscopy and imaging is seldom used.

The earliest finding of UC on imaging is seen on DCBE as a diffuse granular appearance of the mucosa because of inflammation and edema. This leads to the thickening of the wall and haustral folds. As the disease progresses to the submucosa, collar button ulcers develop. Collar button ulcers are not specific to UC because they can occur in other inflammatory diseases. In chronic disease, the colon shows narrowing and shortening and loses its haustral folds appearing featureless which is referred to as a lead pipe sign **(Figs. 23A and B)**.[90] When the mucosa gets denuded, residual mucosal mounds can develop into inflammatory pseudopolyps. Severe cases can be associated with backwash ileitis which may be seen as a fixed and patulous ileocecal valve with a dilated terminal ileum and granular appearance of mucosa. Because of chronic inflammation, there may be increased presacral fat. However, barium enema is seldom used as colonoscopy is far superior and accurate. One of the dreaded complications of UC is toxic megacolon which manifests as colonic dilatation of >6 cm, thinning of wall, and loss of haustrations. Plain radiography is usually diagnostic and barium studies are generally contraindicated because of the risk of perforation.

Computed tomography scan shows the extraluminal changes of UC such as localized perforation and abscess. CT is not sensitive in showing the early mucosal changes

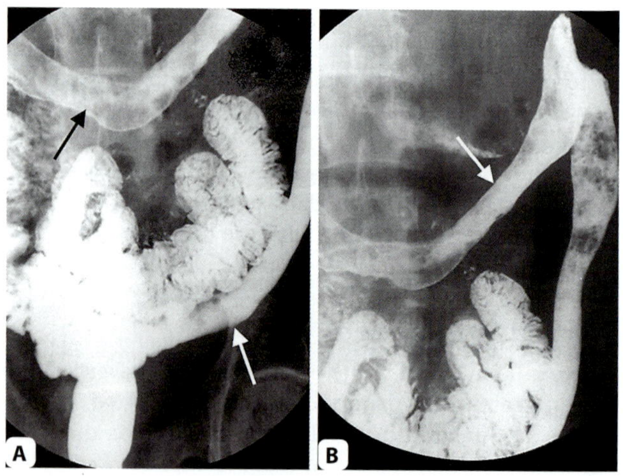

FIGS. 23A AND B: Lead pipe sign in chronic ulcerative colitis (UC). Barium study images (A and B) of a patient with UC showing diffuse luminal narrowing and loss of haustrations (thin arrow) involving the entire colon without any skip areas. This featureless appearance of the colon in chronic UC is known as a lead pipe sign.

of UC. Inflamed bowel shows thickening and may show mural stratification. In the chronic stage, there may be narrowing of the colon, alteration of the haustral pattern, and submucosal fat infiltration which can also be seen on CT. Narrowing of the colon is usually because of benign strictures; however, if there is asymmetry or eccentric thickening with focal loss of mural stratification, malignancy developing in UC should be suspected. The overall risk of developing malignancy in UC is 3.7% and in CD is around 2.9%.[91,92] Pericolonic fat proliferation is much better seen on CT scans rather than on conventional modalities.[89,90] Pericolonic fatty proliferation or creeping fat around the colon occurs more frequently in CD as compared to UC.[93,94] MRI is not routinely used for the evaluation of UC but it can show most of the features that are seen on CT scans. USG is an emerging technique for bowel evaluation that can show bowel wall thickening and mural stratification. The USG is particularly useful in the initial evaluation and in the assessment of treatment response in cases of acute severe UC where repeated colonoscopies or CT scans are not possible. In a recent study, USG has been useful in predicting the treatment response. Bowel wall thickening >6 mm in acute severe UC warrants early initiation of salvage therapy instead of corticosteroids.[95]

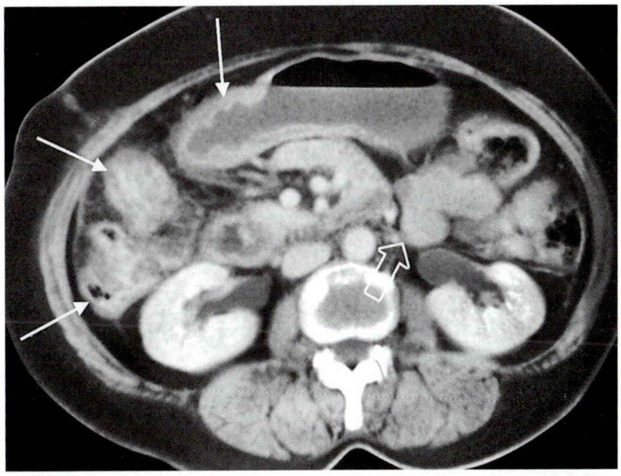

FIG. 24: Acute radiation enteritis. Axial contrast-enhanced CT (CECT) image of a patient who received radiotherapy for carcinoma gallbladder showing thickening of bowel loops with mural stratification and surrounding fat stranding (thin arrow) which are confined to the irradiated area. The bowel loops outside the irradiated area (outlined arrow) appear normal. These features are typical for acute radiation enteritis.

MISCELLANEOUS DISEASES

This category includes radiation enteritis, nonsteroidal anti-inflammatory drug (NSAID) enteropathy, eosinophilic enteritis, etc., which will be discussed in brief.

Radiation Enteritis

Radiation enteritis occurs as a result of the toxic effects of radiation (usually >3,000 cGy) on the bowel wall and the vasculature. Radiation effects can be acute, subacute, or chronic depending on the time of onset of manifestations after radiation therapy. The acute stage occurs within 2 months whereas subacute and chronic stages occur after 2 and 12 months, respectively. In the acute phase, imaging may show spasm and edema of the involved bowel loops which can mimic other inflammatory conditions.[96] However, in radiation enteritis, the involvement is limited to the irradiated area **(Fig. 24)**. In the chronic stage, there may be wall thickening, narrowing, ulceration, and fat proliferation around the bowel. The history of radiation and the area of involvement is the key to differentiating from other inflammatory diseases.

Nonsteroidal Anti-inflammatory Drugs Enteropathy

Nonsteroidal anti-inflammatory drugs are one of the most commonly prescribed drugs worldwide. They cause alterations in the protective mechanism of the gut by affecting prostaglandin synthesis. It can affect the esophagus, stomach, and small bowel and cause local complications. In the esophagus and stomach, it can cause multiple tiny mucosal erosions which may be seen on barium studies as a focal collection of barium with a surrounding halo due to edema around.[97,98] In the small bowel, it can cause focal ulcers with associated wall edema in the acute phase. When the disease progresses to a chronic phase it can lead to ulcers and circumferential strictures which are typically thin short segment or annular and membrane-like (mucosal diaphragm). They can cause bowel obstruction and lead to proximal bowel dilatation. Mucosal diaphragms are not specific to NSAID enteropathy because they can occur in other inflammatory diseases like CD.[97]

Eosinophilic Gastroenteritis

Eosinophilic gastroenteritis is a relatively uncommon entity that is characterized by patchy or diffuse infiltration of eosinophils in the bowel wall.[99] Majority of these patients have peripheral eosinophilia. Clinical features are nonspecific such as pain abdomen, vomiting, or diarrhea. Gastric antrum is the most common site of involvement; however, it can also affect the duodenum and small bowel. It leads to mucosal fold thickening and submucosal infiltration which can be visualized on barium studies and CT scans. As the clinical and imaging features are nonspecific, the index of suspicion should be high to diagnose this condition, and the presence of peripheral eosinophilia is an important indicator.

Opioid Enteropathy

After alcohol and tobacco, opium is the third most common substance of abuse in India. In places where opioid addiction is rampant, cases of enteric strictures have been found in patients having a history of long-term opioid addiction (6–20 years). They usually have a short segment and multifocal strictures in the small bowel with superficial ulceration and variable enhancement.[100] Pyloric strictures may also be present. The pathogenesis behind the development of strictures has been attributed to reduced intestinal motility, high resting muscle tone, inflammation, and ischemia of the bowel.[101] The most common site of involvement is the proximal small bowel (duodenum and jejunum) unlike TB or CD which has a predilection for the terminal ileum or ileocecal region. They usually do not respond to anti-inflammatory drugs. Endoscopic balloon dilatation is attempted and if fails, then surgical management is the mainstay of treatment.

Chronic Enteropathy Associated with *SLCO2A1* Gene Mutation

It is a recently recognized, rare, chronic enteropathy associated with loss of functional mutation of the *SLCO2A1* gene. Most commonly, it affects adolescents or middle-aged females. Patients often present with pain abdomen associated with anemia and hypoalbuminemia. The small bowel is the preferential site of involvement especially the ileum with less predilection for large bowel. It is similar to CD at presentation, hence often confused with the latter. Only when the patient does not respond to treatment for CD, suspicion for this diagnosis should be raised and a genetic workup should be done for its evaluation. On imaging, multiple long segment strictures (10–85 mm) that can vary in number (1–10) can be seen. Inflammatory bowel thickening was observed with layered enhancement without any perienteric inflammation. Close differential diagnoses of this entity are CD and cryptogenic multifocal ulcerous stenosing enteritis (CMUSE).[102] Perienteric inflammation changes would be observed in CD which is not a prominent feature of chronic enteropathy associated with *SLCO2A1* gene (CEAS).

Postischemic Strictures

Postischemic strictures develop after a few weeks to months of the ischemic event. Radiologically, these are usually of moderate to long length and develop usually in watershed areas (especially at splenic flexure in the colon). The most common site of occurrence is the ileum followed by the jejunum and colon. They appear as a concentrically thickened segment of the bowel, which is generally solitary and shows mucosal hyperenhancement in the portal phase than the arterial phase with prominent vasa recta.[103]

Vasculitis Involving the Gut

Intestinal vasculitis is rare and an often overlooked entity due to its nonspecific presentation and imaging findings. A combination of intestinal ischemia along with extraintestinal involvement in the form of vascular changes may help to clinch the diagnosis. Imaging findings of intestinal involvement include segmental involvement of the bowel with circumferential mural thickening, abnormal enhancement (mild mural enhancement in the arterial phase which intensifies in the portovenous phase), and submucosal edema. Usually, a long-segment of the gut is involved. The abnormal mural enhancement with poor intimal enhancement gives a classical "double ring" appearance on the black blood MRI sequence. Vascular involvement may be in the form of abnormal wall thickening, enhancement, aneurysmal dilatation, luminal stenosis, or transmural calcification.[104] The vasculitis which involves the bowel includes Henoch-Schönlein purpura, polyarteritis nodosa, lupus vasculitis, and microscopic polyangiitis among others. The response to corticosteroids further helps in confirming the diagnosis.

Role of Artificial Intelligence

Artificial intelligence (AI), as in other fields, has shown great potential in the evaluation of ulceroconstrictive diseases of the gut. Its utility begins right from the data collection, its holistic evaluation along with genetic markers, calculation of severity scores, construction of prediction models, response assessment after treatment, and neoplasia surveillance. The strength of AI primarily lies in its capability to evaluate large complex data in a very short time.

By automation, there will be a reduction in interobserver variability, quantification of bowel features can be done and the scoring can be done more objectively. One of the studies by Ryan et al. compared the results of a radiologist picking up stricture sites versus an AI algorithm detecting strictures based on maximum bowel wall thickness, maximum bowel dilatation, minimum lumen diameter, and the presence of a stricture. They found no statistically significant difference in the observations made by the algorithm and radiologist.[105] Even quantitative assessment of bowel fibrosis has been attempted by radiomics.[106] Radiomics, a machine learning technique, involves the computer-based extraction of a large number of high-dimensional features from images and detects disease characteristics that are not visible to radiologists.

CONCLUSION

In India where TB is endemic, it is often difficult to differentiate ITB from CD only on the basis of clinical features. Imaging is an integral part of the management of these patients and it can help in differentiating these two entities. A judicious combination of clinical, imaging, endoscopic, and histological features should be used. There are other mimics of IBD and it is important to be aware of these entities. Imaging also has an important role in the follow-up of these patients to look for complications and assess their response to therapy. Hence, the radiologist must be aware of the imaging features to correctly diagnose these diseases and avoid mismanagement.

REFERENCES

1. Maglinte DDT, Kelvin FM, O'Connor K, Lappas JC, Chernish SM. Current status of small bowel radiography. Abdom Imaging. 1996;21(3):247-57.
2. Nijhawan S, Kumpawat S, Mallikarjun P, Bansal RP, Singla D, Ashdhir P, et al. Barium meal follow through with pneumocolon: Screening test for chronic bowel pain. World J Gastroenterol. 2008;14(43):6694-8.
3. Bender GN, Timmons JH, Williard WC, Carter J. Computed tomographic enteroclysis: one methodology. Invest Radiol. 1996;31(1):43-9.
4. Paulsen SR, Huprich JE, Fletcher JG, Booya F, Young BM, Fidler JL, et al. CT enterography as a diagnostic tool in evaluating small bowel disorders: review of clinical experience with over 700 cases 1. Radiographics. 2006;26(3):641-57.
5. Solem CA, Loftus EV, Fletcher JG, Baron TH, Gostout CJ, Petersen BT, et al. Small-bowel imaging in Crohn's disease: a prospective, blinded, 4-way comparison trial. Gastrointest Endosc. 2008;68(2):255-66.
6. Ha AS, Levine MS, Rubesin SE, Laufer I, Herlinger H. Radiographic Examination of the Small Bowel: Survey of Practice Patterns in the United States 1. Radiology. 2004;231(2):407-12.
7. Ilangovan R, Burling D, George A, Gupta A, Marshall M, Taylor SA. CT enterography: review of technique and practical tips. Br J Radiol. 2012;85(1015):876-86.
8. Mettler FA, Huda W, Yoshizumi TT, Mahesh M. Effective Doses in Radiology and Diagnostic Nuclear Medicine: A Catalog. Radiology. 2008;248(1):254-63.
9. Keane J, Gershon S, Wise RP, Mirabile-Levens E, Kasznica J, Schwieterman WD, et al. Tuberculosis associated with infliximab, a tumor necrosis factor alpha-neutralizing agent. N Engl J Med. 2001;345(15):1098-104.
10. Kedia S, Sharma R, Makharia G, Ahuja V, Desai D, Kandasamy D, et al. Indian guidelines on imaging of the small intestine in Crohn's disease: A joint Indian Society of Gastroenterology and Indian Radiology and Imaging Association consensus statement. Indian J Radiol Imaging. 2019;29(2):111-32.
11. Debi U, Ravisankar V, Prasad KK, Sinha SK, Sharma AK. Abdominal tuberculosis of the gastrointestinal tract: Revisited. World J Gastroenterol. 2014;20(40):14831-40.
12. Makanyanga JC, Taylor SA. Current and future role of MR enterography in the management of Crohn disease. Am J Roentgenol. 2013;201(1):56-64.
13. Kiryu S, Dodanuki K, Takao H, Watanabe M, Inoue Y, Takazoe M, et al. Free-breathing diffusion-weighted imaging for the assessment of inflammatory activity in Crohn's disease. J Magn Reson Imaging. 2009;29(4):880-6.
14. Oto A, Zhu F, Kulkarni K, Karczmar GS, Turner JR, Rubin D. Evaluation of diffusion-weighted MR imaging for detection of bowel inflammation in patients with Crohn's disease. Acad Radiol. 2009;16(5):597-603.
15. Oto A, Kayhan A, Williams JT, Fan X, Yun L, Arkani S, et al. Active Crohn's disease in the small bowel: evaluation by diffusion weighted imaging and quantitative dynamic contrast enhanced MR imaging. J Magn Reson Imaging. 2011;33(3):615-24.
16. Oussalah A, Laurent V, Bruot O, Bressenot A, Bigard MA, Régent D, et al. Diffusion-weighted magnetic resonance without bowel preparation for detecting colonic inflammation in inflammatory bowel disease. Gut. 2010;59(8):1056-65.
17. Chatterji M, Fidler JL, Taylor SA, Anupindi SA, Yeh BM, Guglielmo FF. State of the Art MR Enterography Technique. Top Magn Reson Imaging. 2021;30(1):3-11.
18. Chiorean L, Schreiber-Dietrich D, Braden B, Cui XW, Buchhorn R, Chang JM, et al. Ultrasonographic imaging of inflammatory bowel disease in pediatric patients. World J Gastroenterol. 2015;21(17):5231-41.
19. Levine A, Koletzko S, Turner D, Escher JC, Cucchiara S, De Ridder L, et al. ESPGHAN revised porto criteria for the diagnosis of inflammatory bowel disease in children and adolescents. J Pediatr Gastroenterol Nutr. 2014;58(6):795-806.
20. Dietrich CF, Cui XW, Schreiber-Dietrich DG, Ignee A. EFSUMB guidelines 2011: comments and illustrations. Ultraschall Med Eur J Ultrasound. 2012;33(S 01):S11-21.
21. Dietrich CF. Comments and illustrations regarding the guidelines and good clinical practice recommendations for contrast-enhanced ultrasound (CEUS)–update 2008. Ultraschall Med-Eur J Ultrasound. 2008;29(S 04):188-202.
22. WHO. (2015). Global tuberculosis report 2015. [online] Available from https://iris.who.int/bitstream/handle/10665/191102/9789241565059_eng.pdf?sequence=1 [Last accessed June, 2024].
23. Sircar S, Taneja VA, Kansra U. Epidemiology and clinical presentation of abdominal tuberculosis—a retrospective study. J Indian Med Assoc. 1996;94(9):342-4.
24. Marshall JB. Tuberculosis of the gastrointestinal tract and peritoneum. Am J Gastroenterol. 1993;88(7):989-99.
25. Sood R. Diagnosis of abdominal tuberculosis: role of imaging. J Indian Acad Clin Med. 2001;2(3):169-77.
26. Sharma MP, Bhatia V. Abdominal tuberculosis. Indian J Med Res. 2004;120(4):305-15.
27. Balthazar EJ, Gordon R, Hulnick D. Ileocecal tuberculosis: CT and radiologic evaluation. Am J Roentgenol. 1990;154(3):499-503.
28. Gulati MS, Sarma D, Paul SB. CT appearances in abdominal tuberculosis. A pictorial essay. Clin Imaging. 1999;23(1):51-9.
29. Ramesh J, Banait GS, Ormerod LP. Abdominal tuberculosis in a district general hospital: a retrospective review of 86 cases. QJM. 2008;101(3):189-95.
30. Carrera GF, Young S, Lewicki AM. Intestinal tuberculosis. Abdom Imaging. 1976;1(1):147-55.
31. Krishna S, Kalra N, Singh P, Kochhar R, Gupta R, Singh R, et al. Small-Bowel Tuberculosis: A Comparative Study of MR Enterography and Small-Bowel Follow-Through. Am J Roentgenol. 2016;207(3):571-7.
32. Thoeni RF, Margulis AR. Gastrointestinal tuberculosis. Semin Roentgenol. 1979;14(4):283-94.
33. Chong VH, Lim KS. Gastrointestinal tuberculosis. Singapore Med J. 2009;50(6):638-45; quiz 646.
34. Chavhan GE, Ramakantan R. Duodenal tuberculosis: radiological features on barium studies and their clinical correlation in 28 cases. J Postgrad Med. 2003;49(3):214-7.
35. da Rocha EL, Pedrassa BC, Bormann RL, Kierszenbaum ML, Torres LR, D'Ippolito G. Abdominal tuberculosis: a radiological review with emphasis on computed tomography

and magnetic resonance imaging findings. Radiol Bras. 2015;48(3):181-91.
36. Akhan O, Pringot J. Imaging of abdominal tuberculosis. Eur Radiol. 2002;12(2):312-23.
37. Leder RA, Low VH. Tuberculosis of the abdomen. Radiol Clin North Am. 1995;33(4):691-705.
38. Jayant M, Kaushik R. Abdominal cocoon in a young man. World J Emerg Med. 2014;5(3):234-6.
39. Foti PV, Attinà G, Spadola S, Caltabiano R, Farina R, Palmucci S, et al. MR imaging of ovarian masses: classification and differential diagnosis. Insights Imaging. 2015;7(1):21-41.
40. Yang ZG, Min PQ, Sone S, He ZY, Liao ZY, Zhou XP, et al. Tuberculosis versus lymphomas in the abdominal lymph nodes: evaluation with contrast-enhanced CT. Am J Roentgenol. 1999;172(3):619-23.
41. Li DK, Rennie CS. Case Report Abdominal Computed Tomography in Whipple's Disease. J Comput Assist Tomogr. 1981;5(2):249-52.
42. Brauner M, Buffard MD, Jeantils V, Legrand I, Gotheil C. Sonography and computed tomography of macroscopic tuberculosis of the liver. J Clin Ultrasound. 1989;17(8):563-8.
43. Yadav AK, Nadrajah J, Kandasamy D, Sharma R, Gamanagatti S, Garg PK. Volume perfusion computed tomography as an aid to diagnosis of pancreatic tuberculosis. Trop Gastroenterol. 2015;35(4):264-6.
44. Bohr J, Wickbom A, Hegedus A, Nyhlin N, Hultgren Hörnquist E, Tysk C. Diagnosis and management of microscopic colitis: current perspectives. Clin Exp Gastroenterol. 2014;7:273-84.
45. Makharia GK. Rising incidence and prevalence of Crohn's disease in Asia: Is it apparent or real? J Gastroenterol Hepatol. 2006;21(6):929-31.
46. Yacoub JH, Oto A. New magnetic resonance imaging modalities for Crohn disease. Magn Reson Imaging Clin N Am. 2014;22(1):35-50.
47. Silverberg MS, Satsangi J, Ahmad T, Arnott IDR, Bernstein CN, Brant SR, et al. Toward an integrated clinical, molecular and serological classification of inflammatory bowel disease: report of a Working Party of the 2005 Montreal World Congress of Gastroenterology. Can J Gastroenterol. 2005;19 Suppl A:5A-36A.
48. Spekhorst LM, Visschedijk MC, Alberts R, Festen EA, van der Wouden EJ, Dijkstra G, et al. Performance of the Montreal classification for inflammatory bowel diseases. World J Gastroenterol. 2014;20(41):15374-81.
49. Dassopoulos T, Nguyen GC, Bitton A, Bromfield GP, Schumm LP, Wu Y, et al. Assessment of reliability and validity of IBD phenotyping within the National Institutes of Diabetes and Digestive and Kidney Diseases (NIDDK) IBD Genetics Consortium (IBDGC). Inflamm Bowel Dis. 2007;13(8):975-83.
50. Krishnaprasad K, Andrews JM, Lawrance IC, Florin T, Gearry RB, Leong RWL, et al. Inter-observer agreement for Crohn's disease sub-phenotypes using the Montreal Classification: How good are we? A multi-centre Australasian study. J Crohns Colitis. 2012;6(3):287-93.
51. Best WR, Becktel JM, Singleton JW, Kern F. Development of a Crohn's disease activity index. National Cooperative Crohn's Disease Study. Gastroenterology. 1976;70(3):439-44.
52. Peyrin-Biroulet L, Panés J, Sandborn WJ, Vermeire S, Danese S, Feagan BG, et al. Defining Disease Severity in Inflammatory Bowel Diseases: Current and Future Directions. Clin Gastroenterol Hepatol. 2016;14(3):348-54.e17.
53. Marshak RH. Granulomatous Disease of the Intestinal Tract (Crohn's Disease) 1: Annual Oration in Honor of Benjamin H. Orndoff, MD, 1881–1971. Radiology. 1975;114(1):3-22.
54. Grand DJ, Beland MD, Machan JT, Mayo-Smith WW. Detection of Crohn's disease: comparison of CT and MR enterography without anti-peristaltic agents performed on the same day. Eur J Radiol. 2012;81(8):1735-41.
55. Lee SS, Kim AY, Yang SK, Chung JW, Kim SY, Park SH, et al. Crohn disease of the small bowel: comparison of CT enterography, MR enterography, and small-bowel follow-through as diagnostic techniques. Radiology. 2009;251(3):751-61.
56. Siddiki HA, Fidler JL, Fletcher JG, Burton SS, Huprich JE, Hough DM, et al. Prospective comparison of state-of-the-art MR enterography and CT enterography in small-bowel Crohn's disease. Am J Roentgenol. 2009;193(1):113-21.
57. Bruining DH, Zimmermann EM, Loftus Jr EV, Sandborn WJ, Sauer CG, Strong SA, et al. Consensus recommendations for evaluation, interpretation, and utilization of computed tomography and magnetic resonance enterography in patients with small bowel Crohn's disease. Gastroenterology. 2018;154(4):1172-94.
58. Sharma R, Madhusudhan KS, Ahuja V. Intestinal tuberculosis versus Crohn's disease: Clinical and radiological recommendations. Indian J Radiol Imaging. 2016;26(2):161-72.
59. Constantino CPL, Rodrigues RS, Neto JAO, Marchiori E, Araujo ALE, de Mello Perez R, et al. Computed Tomography and Magnetic Resonance Enterography Findings in Crohn's Disease: What Does the Clinician Need to Know From the Radiologist? Can Assoc Radiol J. 2014;65(1):42-51.
60. Fidler JL, Guimaraes L, Einstein DM. MR Imaging of the Small Bowel 1. Radiographics. 2009;29(6):1811-25.
61. Lawrance IC. Correlation of MRI-determined small bowel Crohn's disease categories with medical response and surgical pathology. World J Gastroenterol. 2009;15(27):3367-75.
62. Buisson A, Joubert A, Montoriol PF, Ines DD, Hordonneau C, Pereira B, et al. Diffusion-weighted magnetic resonance imaging for detecting and assessing ileal inflammation in Crohn's disease. Aliment Pharmacol Ther. 2013;37(5):537-45.
63. Elsayes KM, Al-Hawary MM, Jagdish J, Ganesh HS, Platt JF. CT Enterography: Principles, Trends, and Interpretation of Findings 1. Radiographics. 2010;30(7):1955-70.
64. Sinha R, Verma R, Verma S, Rajesh A. MR enterography of Crohn disease: part 2, imaging and pathologic findings. Am J Roentgenol. 2011;197(1):80-5.
65. Rieder F, Bettenworth D, Ma C, Parker CE, Williamson LA, Nelson SA, et al. An expert consensus to standardise definitions, diagnosis and treatment targets for anti-fibrotic stricture therapies in Crohn's disease. Aliment Pharmacol Ther. 2018;48(3):347-57.
66. Sinha R, Murphy P, Sanders S, Ramachandran I, Hawker P, Rawat S, et al. Diagnostic accuracy of high-resolution MR enterography in Crohn's disease: comparison with surgical and pathological specimen. Clin Radiol. 2013;68(9):917-27.
67. Froehlich JM, Waldherr C, Stoupis C, Erturk SM, Patak MA. MR motility imaging in Crohn's disease improves lesion detection compared with standard MR imaging. Eur Radiol. 2010;20(8):1945-51.

68. Haggett PJ, Moore NR, Shearman JD, Travis SP, Jewell DP, Mortensen NJ. Pelvic and perineal complications of Crohn's disease: assessment using magnetic resonance imaging. Gut. 1995;36(3):407-10.
69. Halligan S, Buchanan G. MR imaging of fistula-in-ano. Eur J Radiol. 2003;47(2):98-107.
70. Van Assche G, Dignass A, Reinisch W, van der Woude CJ, Sturm A, De Vos M, et al. The second European evidence-based Consensus on the diagnosis and management of Crohn's disease: Special situations. J Crohns Colitis. 2010;4(1):63-101.
71. Gourtsoyianni S, Papanikolaou N, Amanakis E, Bourikas L, Roussomoustakaki M, Grammatikakis J, et al. Crohn's disease lymphadenopathy: MR imaging findings. Eur J Radiol. 2009;69(3):425-8.
72. Wang Y di, Zhang RN, Mao R, Li XH. Inflammatory bowel disease cross-sectional imaging: What's new? United Eur Gastroenterol J. 2022;10(10):1179-93.
73. Carchman E. Crohn's Disease and the Risk of Cancer. Clin Colon Rectal Surg. 2019;32(4):305-13.
74. Peyrin-Biroulet L, Loftus EV, Colombel JF, Sandborn WJ. Long-term complications, extraintestinal manifestations, and mortality in adult Crohn's disease in population-based cohorts. Inflamm Bowel Dis. 2011;17(1):471-8.
75. Furfaro F, Buono AD, Sicuso C, Allocca M, D'Amico F, Zilli A, et al. Carcinomas in inflammatory bowel disease: a narrative review on diagnostic imaging techniques. Chin Clin Oncol. 2022;11(3):22.
76. Rimola J, Rodríguez S, García-Bosch O, Ordás I, Ayala E, Aceituno M, et al. Magnetic resonance for assessment of disease activity and severity in ileocolonic Crohn's disease. Gut. 2009;58(8):1113-20.
77. Roseira J, Ventosa AR, de Sousa HT, Brito J. The new simplified MARIA score applies beyond clinical trials: A suitable clinical practice tool for Crohn's disease that parallels a simple endoscopic index and fecal calprotectin. United Eur Gastroenterol J. 2020;8(10):1208-16.
78. Ordás I, Rimola J, Alfaro I, Rodríguez S, Castro-Poceiro J, Ramírez-Morros A, et al. Development and Validation of a Simplified Magnetic Resonance Index of Activity for Crohn's Disease. Gastroenterology. 2019;157(2):432-9.e1.
79. D'Amico F, Chateau T, Laurent V, Danese S, Peyrin-Biroulet L. Which MRI Score and Technique Should Be Used for Assessing Crohn's Disease Activity? J Clin Med. 2020;9(6):1691.
80. Allocca M, Fiorino G, Bonifacio C, Furfaro F, Gilardi D, Argollo M, et al. Comparative Accuracy of Bowel Ultrasound Versus Magnetic Resonance Enterography in Combination With Colonoscopy in Assessing Crohn's Disease and Guiding Clinical Decision-making. J Crohns Colitis. 2018;12(11): 1280-7.
81. Kedia S, Madhusudhan KS, Sharma R, Bopanna S, Yadav DP, Goyal S, et al. Combination of increased visceral fat and long segment involvement: Development and validation of an updated imaging marker for differentiating Crohn's disease from intestinal tuberculosis. J Gastroenterol Hepatol. 2018;33(6):1234-41.
82. Erhayiem B, Dhingsa R, Hawkey CJ, Subramanian V. Ratio of visceral to subcutaneous fat area is a biomarker of complicated Crohn's disease. Clin Gastroenterol Hepatol. 2011;9(8):684-7.e1.
83. Yuan G, He Y, Cao QH, Tang MM, Xie ZL, Qiu Y, et al. Visceral adipose volume is correlated with surgical tissue fibrosis in Crohn's disease of the small bowel. Gastroenterol Rep. 2022;10:goac044.
84. Yadav DP, Madhusudhan KS, Kedia S, Sharma R, Pratap Mouli V, Bopanna S, et al. Development and validation of visceral fat quantification as a surrogate marker for differentiation of Crohn's disease and intestinal tuberculosis. J Gastroenterol Hepatol. 2017;32(2):420-6.
85. Rieder F, Fiocchi C, Rogler G. Mechanisms, Management, and Treatment of Fibrosis in Patients With Inflammatory Bowel Diseases. Gastroenterology. 2017;152(2):340-50.e6.
86. Li XH, Mao R, Huang SY, Sun CH, Cao QH, Fang ZN, et al. Characterization of Degree of Intestinal Fibrosis in Patients with Crohn Disease by Using Magnetization Transfer MR Imaging. Radiology. 2018;287(2):494-503.
87. Avila F, Caron B, Hossu G, Ambarki K, Kannengiesser S, Odille F, et al. Magnetic Resonance Elastography for Assessing Fibrosis in Patients with Crohn's Disease: A Pilot Study. Dig Dis Sci. 2022;67(9):4518-24.
88. Lu B, Lin J, Du J, He S, Cao Q, Huang L, et al. Native T1 Mapping and Magnetization Transfer Imaging in Grading Bowel Fibrosis in Crohn's Disease: A Comparative Animal Study. Biosensors. 2021;11(9):302.
89. Roggeveen MJ, Tismenetsky M, Shapiro R. Best cases from the AFIP: Ulcerative colitis. Radiogr Rev Publ Radiol Soc N Am Inc. 2006;26(3):947-51.
90. Gore RM, Balthazar EJ, Ghahremani GG, Miller FH. CT features of ulcerative colitis and Crohn's disease. Am J Roentgenol. 1996;167(1):3-15.
91. Canavan C, Abrams KR, Mayberry J. Meta-analysis: colorectal and small bowel cancer risk in patients with Crohn's disease. Aliment Pharmacol Ther. 2006;23(8):1097-104.
92. Eaden JA, Abrams KR, Mayberry JF. The risk of colorectal cancer in ulcerative colitis: a meta-analysis. Gut. 2001; 48(4):526-35.
93. Deepak P, Bruining DH. Radiographical evaluation of ulcerative colitis. Gastroenterol Rep. 2014;2(3):169-77.
94. Parente F, Greco S, Molteni M, Anderloni A, Bianchi Porro G. Imaging inflammatory bowel disease using bowel ultrasound. Eur J Gastroenterol Hepatol. 2005;17(3):283-91.
95. Bezzio C, Vernero M, Ribaldone DG, Manes G, Saibeni S. Insights into the role of gastrointestinal ultrasound in ulcerative colitis. Ther Adv Gastroenterol. 2021;14:17562848211051456.
96. Addley HC, Vargas HA, Moyle PL, Crawford R, Sala E. Pelvic imaging following chemotherapy and radiation therapy for gynecologic malignancies. Radiogr Rev Publ Radiol Soc N Am Inc. 2010;30(7):1843-56.
97. McGettigan MJ, Menias CO, Gao ZJ, Mellnick VM, Hara AK. Imaging of Drug-induced Complications in the Gastrointestinal System. Radiogr Rev Publ Radiol Soc N Am Inc. 2016;36(1):71-87.
98. Frye JM, Hansel SL, Dolan SG, Fidler JL, Song LMWK, Barlow JM, et al. NSAID enteropathy: appearance at CT and MR enterography in the age of multi-modality imaging and treatment. Abdom Imaging. 2015;40(5):1011-25.
99. Baig MA, Qadir A, Rasheed J. A review of eosinophilic gastroenteritis. J Natl Med Assoc. 2006;98(10):1616-9.

100. Joshi A, Falodia S, Kumar N, Solanki RL. Small intestine strictures in opium addicts: An unrecognized cause of intestinal obstruction. Indian J Gastroenterol. 2018;37(2):169-73.
101. Mahajan R, Gupta Y, Singh A, Dhiman P, Midha V, Kakkar C, et al. Clinical profile and outcomes of opioid abuse gastroenteropathy: an underdiagnosed disease entity. Intest Res. 2020;18(2):238-44.
102. Jeong B, Park SH, Ye BD, Kim J, Yang SK. A Novel Chronic Enteropathy Associated with *SLCO2A1* Gene Mutation: Enterography Findings in a Multicenter Korean Registry. Korean J Radiol. 2023;24(4):305-12.
103. Kim JS, Kim HJ, Hong SM, Park SH, Lee JS, Kim AY, et al. Post-Ischemic Bowel Stricture: CT Features in Eight Cases. Korean J Radiol. 2017;18(6):936-45.
104. Amouei M, Momtazmanesh S, Kavosi H, Davarpanah AH, Shirkhoda A, Radmard AR. Imaging of intestinal vasculitis focusing on MR and CT enterography: a two-way street between radiologic findings and clinical data. Insights Imaging. 2022;13:143.
105. Stidham RW, Enchakalody B, Waljee AK, Higgins PDR, Wang SC, Su GL, et al. Assessing Small Bowel Stricturing and Morphology in Crohn's Disease Using Semi-automated Image Analysis. Inflamm Bowel Dis. 2020;26(5):734-42.
106. Li X, Liang D, Meng J, Zhou J, Chen Z, Huang S, et al. Development and Validation of a Novel Computed-Tomography Enterography Radiomic Approach for Characterization of Intestinal Fibrosis in Crohn's Disease. Gastroenterology. 2021;160(7):2303-16.e11.

CHAPTER 4

Rashmi Dixit, Gaurav Shanker Pradhan, Anju Garg

Tumors of the Small Bowel and Appendix

INTRODUCTION

The first part of this chapter deals with small bowel tumors while tumors of the appendix are dealt with in the second part.

SMALL BOWEL TUMORS

Tumors of the small bowel both benign and malignant are quite uncommon, this despite the fact the small bowel constitutes about 75% of the total length of the gastrointestinal (GI) tract and 90% of its mucosal surface. It also lies between two areas of high cancer risk, i.e., the colon and the stomach yet only about 3–5% of all GI tumors and <2% of all GI malignancies arise in the small bowel.[1-3] However, with advances in endoscopy and imaging, an increasing number of small bowel tumors is being diagnosed.

About 40 different histologic types of tumors have been described in the small bowel. Although over two-thirds of lesions found at autopsy are benign, most symptomatic lesions and those detected at surgery tend to be malignant.[1] The major tumors are listed in **Box 1**.

BOX 1 Small bowel tumors.

- *Epithelial*:
  - Adenoma
  - Carcinoma
  - Others
- *Neuroendocrine tumors/carcinoid*
- *Nonepithelial/Mesenchymal*:
  - Lipoma
  - Leiomyoma
  - Hemangioma/Lymphangioma
  - Gastrointestinal stromal tumors (GISTs)
  - Leiomyosarcoma
  - Kaposi's sarcoma
  - Others
- *Lymphoid tissue*: Lymphomas
- *Neurogenic*:
  - Neurofibroma
  - Schwannoma
- *Secondary tumors/metastasis*

SMALL BOWEL CARCINOGENESIS: PATHOGENESIS

The exact reason for the low incidence of malignancy in the small intestine is not certain but several theories have been proposed including liquid contents of the small bowel causing less mucosal irritation, relatively rapid transit, lower bacterial load in small bowel and high levels of immunoglobulin A (IgA) due to increased lymphoid tissue.[1,4]

Certain syndromes or conditions are associated with increased incidence of specific histologic types of small intestine tumors, e.g., Peutz-Jeghers syndrome (PJS), familial adenomatous polyposis (FAP), Lynch syndrome, and Gardner syndrome predispose to adenoma and adenocarcinoma and von Recklinghausen's disease or neurofibromatosis to gastrointestinal stromal tumors (GISTs). Gardner syndrome also predisposes to multiple desmoid tumors.[1,4]

DIAGNOSTIC TECHNIQUES

The clinical presentation of most small bowel tumors is nonspecific. The diagnosis is further challenged by lack of easy endoscopic access and relative rarity of disease leading to low index of suspicion. The various techniques available to evaluate the small intestine tumors are—conventional small bowel follow through examination, conventional enteroclysis, ultrasound, CT, and MR (including CT and MR enterography and enteroclysis) and endoscopic techniques such as capsule endoscopy and push enteroscopy. Noninvasive imaging techniques are generally preferred before more invasive and expensive endoscopic techniques are used.[5,6]

With the widespread use of CT enterography barium meal follow through and conventional enteroclysis are rarely performed these days because although they provide good mucosal detail, little information on mural and extramural extent of tumor is garnered.

Ultrasound is often the first investigation performed in nonspecific abdominal complaints and it may detect a bowel mass. A malignant mass can be seen as asymmetric wall thickening, "target lesion" or pseudokidney lesion. Occasionally a large mass where the organ of origin is not clear may be seen, like in GISTs. Increased vascularity may be evident on color Doppler. Contrast-enhanced ultrasound has also been used in bowel masses especially for follow-up of treated GISTs. Associated findings such as nodal involvement and ascites can also be seen.[7] Endoscopic ultrasound can be used for detection of small tumors and guided endoscopic biopsy.

Conventional CT has relatively low sensitivity for small tumors, however, CT/MR enterography has a sensitivity of 85–95%.[4,8,9] CT enterography is the current standard practice given with the excellent sensitivity to detect even small tumors due to superior tumor to background contrast enhancement owing to the use of neutral oral contrast. MR has superior soft-tissue contrast but due to its higher cost, lower spatial resolution as compared to CT and artifacts due to bowel motion MR enteroclysis/enterography is generally not used as a first-line investigation. However, MR of the GI tract is gaining clinical acceptance especially when radiation dose due to repeat examinations is a concern. Diffusion-weighted imaging (DWI) and cine sequences or MR fluoroscopy are also useful.[1,4]

Ultrasound and CT may also be used to guide percutaneous biopsy or needle aspiration.

Fludeoxyglucose F18-positron emission tomography/computed tomography (18F-FDG-PET/CT) may be useful in patients with adenocarcinoma, lymphomas, and sarcomas, mainly for staging. PET-CT with octreotide analogs is useful in detection and staging of neuroendocrine tumors (NETs) (carcinoids).[4]

Hybrid PET-MRI has very limited availability as yet but appears to hold promise for evaluation of GI malignancy. It combines the high contrast and spatial resolution of MR with the high sensitivity of PET allowing for improved staging and restaging of disease status after treatment.[10]

Among the endoscopic techniques capsule endoscopy can screen the entire small bowel and has higher sensitivity to detect tumors and polyps than push enteroscopy which evaluates only the first 120 cm of the small bowel beyond the ligament of Treitz. However, some lesions may be missed due to poor bowel preparation, orientation of camera away from lesion and rapid or delayed small bowel transit. It is also not very accurate in exact localization and size estimation and is contraindicated in patients with bowel stricture, intestinal obstruction, swallowing, and motility disorders.[4,5]

Balloon enteroscopy allows evaluation of the entire small bowel. Double balloon enteroscopy (DBE) has a sensitivity of about 86% in detecting small bowel tumors which is comparable with capsule endoscopy.[4,5] All endoscopic methods are limited in the evaluation submucosal and mural lesions unless combined with endoscopic ultrasound.

BENIGN TUMORS AND POLYPS

Adenoma

Adenomas represent the most common benign tumor of the small intestine. Histologically, these can be tubular, villous, or tubulovillous. Although adenomas are benign, they are considered premalignant. Large size and villous component are associated with an increased risk of malignant transformation. They occur as pedunculated or sessile polypoid lesions, usually 2–3 cm in size. They may act as a lead point for intussusception.[11,12]

Adenomas are difficult to appreciate on routine CT or MR but may be seen on CT/MR enteroclysis or enterography. On CT enteroclysis, they are seen as well-defined soft-tissue lesions with moderate enhancement on postcontrast images with a clear fat plane around the lesion **(Figs. 1A and B)**.[13,14] On MR enteroclysis, adenomas are seen as homogeneously enhancing intraluminal masses on fat-saturated postcontrast T1-weighted (T1W) images, while on T2-weighted (T2W) images they appear as low-signal intensity intraluminal masses. Generally, there is no proximal dilatation.[15,16]

Inflammatory fibroid polyps, also known as "Vanek's tumors," are an important differential diagnosis which are predominantly located in the ileum and represent rare non-neoplastic pseudotumors submucosal lesions of uncertain etiology. They can be sessile or pedunculated polypoid lesions. Histologically, inflammatory fibroid polyps (IFPs) consist of mass of loose fibrous connective tissue, with presence of inflammatory infiltrate consisting of large number of eosinophils. On CT, a well-defined, smooth, homogeneous, low attenuation, nonenhancing, or hypoenhancing polypoid mass is seen **(Figs. 2A to C)**.[17]

Multiple adenomas can be found in hereditary polyposis syndromes. A major risk factor is familial adenomatous polyposis (FAP) where 80% patients develop duodenal adenomas. Patients frequently develop jejunal and ileal polyps also.[4]

Treatment includes endoscopic resection for pedunculated tumors and surgical removal of large sessile tumors.[1,4]

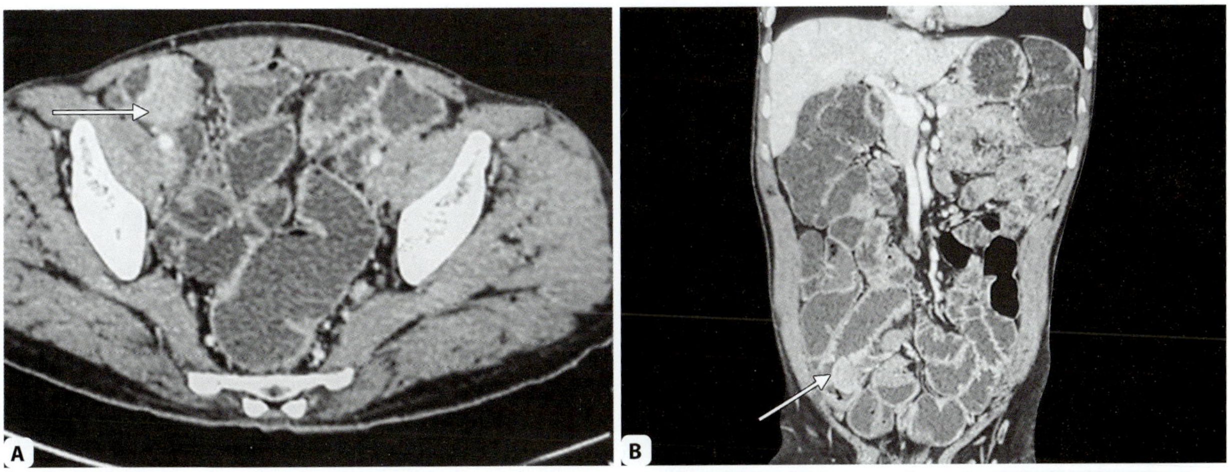

FIGS. 1A AND B: Small bowel adenoma: Axial (A) and coronal (B) CT enteroclysis images reveal a sessile polypoid moderately enhancing mass lesion in the ileum (arrows) with normal surrounding fat planes suggestive of an adenoma.

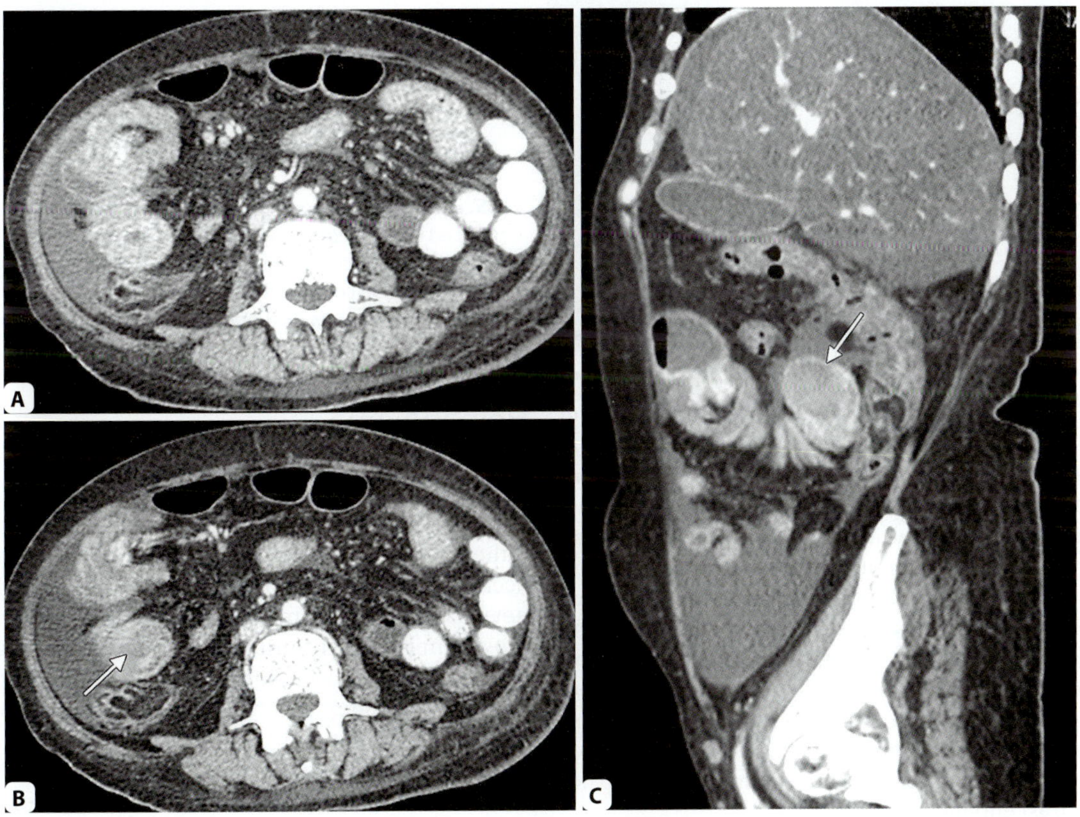

FIGS. 2A TO C: Inflammatory fibroid polyp: Axial (A and B) and sagittal (C) Contrast-enhanced computed tomography (CECT) images show free fluid in the right paracolic region and telescoping of proximal ileum into a distal ileal loop along with a sleeve of mesenteric fat and vessels consistent with ileo-ileal intussusception. A well-defined poorly enhancing hypodense polyp is seen at the apex (arrow in B and C) which was proven to be an inflammatory fibroid polyp on histopathological examination.

Lipoma

Lipomas account for 15–20% of all small intestinal neoplasms. The small bowel is the most common site in the GI tract after the colon and within the small bowel ileum is the most common location. The vast majority of these are sessile or pedunculated submucosal tumors that are composed of mature adipose tissue. About 5–10% may be subserosal. Usually, they are solitary but occasionally may be multiple. Small lesions are mostly asymptomatic whereas larger lesions may produce intussusception, rarely surface ulceration may occur leading to GI bleed.[13,16,18]

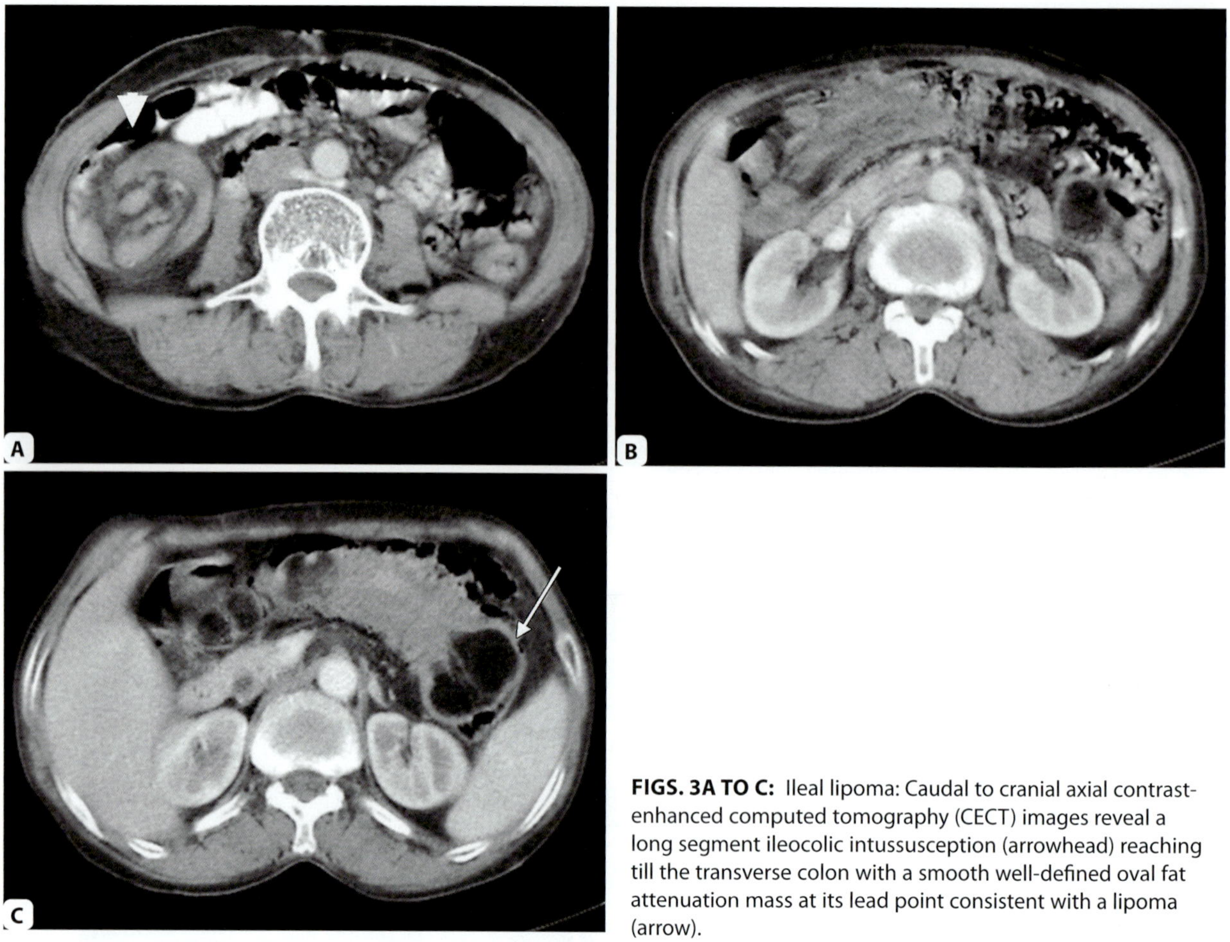

FIGS. 3A TO C: Ileal lipoma: Caudal to cranial axial contrast-enhanced computed tomography (CECT) images reveal a long segment ileocolic intussusception (arrowhead) reaching till the transverse colon with a smooth well-defined oval fat attenuation mass at its lead point consistent with a lipoma (arrow).

On CT, lipomas are seen as a low-density fat attenuation masses (between -60 and -120 HU) in the wall of the small intestine **(Figs. 3A to C)**. No contrast enhancement or nonfatty elements are seen, however, sometimes few linear strands of soft-tissue attenuation may be seen at the base corresponding to prominent fibrovascular septae on histopathology. Such tumors may at times show surface ulceration and must not be mistaken for liposarcoma—the septae being presumably enlarged due to inflammation associated with the ulcer.[18] On MR enterography, they are seen as well-circumscribed masses which are bright on T1W, match the signal on intraabdominal fat on T2W images with signal suppression on fat-saturated images and do not show contrast enhancement.[16]

Leiomyoma

True leiomyomas of the small intestine are extremely rare most lesions previously diagnosed as leiomyomas may actually represent GISTs. They can be seen as round or crescentic predominantly submucosal masses showing homogeneous enhancement on CT or MRI and are virtually impossible to distinguish from small GISTs on imaging. Occasionally, intraluminal polyp or extraluminal masses may be seen.[1,13]

Hemangioma

Small bowel hemangiomas are rare most often situated in the jejunal submucosa and can be sessile, pedunculated or infiltrative. Most lesions represent venous malformations rather than true tumors (hemangioma). Some cases can occur in association with syndromes like blue rubber bleb nevus and Klippel-Trenaunay syndrome. In contrast to most other benign tumors, most are symptomatic and commonly produce manifest or occult GI bleed. Other symptoms include pain, obstruction due to intussusception, and rarely perforation.[1,13]

On contrast-enhanced CT enterography, they can be seen as intensely enhancing lesion with or without phleboliths. Progressive enhancement may be seen with multiphase CT.[19,20] On MR, they are T1 hypointense, markedly hyperintense on T2W images with no loss of signal on fat-saturated images. Nodular enhancement has been reported in the arterial phase and homogeneous enhancement in the delayed phase.[16]

Neurogenic Tumor

Neurogenic tumors are relatively rare arising from the intramural neural plexus. Most often these are nonplexiform neurofibromas occurring as well-defined subserosal masses on the antimesenteric border, difficult to detect on contrast examinations. They can be multiple especially in patients with neurofibromatosis. Occasionally, they are submucosal when it is difficult to distinguish them from other submucosal masses on imaging. Schwannomas usually occur as solitary masses. Plexiform neurofibromas can also involve the small bowel.[13]

POLYPOSIS SYNDROMES INVOLVING THE SMALL BOWEL

Polyps arising in the small bowel can be hamartomatous, hyperplastic, adenomatous, or inflammatory in nature. Multiple polyps should raise the suspicion of a polyposis syndrome—the important ones being—Peutz-Jeghers syndrome (PJS); FAP generalized juvenile polyposis; and Cronkhite-Canada syndrome. These disorders are characterized by the presence of multiple polyps affecting all or parts of the GI tract. They are distinguished by the way they can be inherited, location, associated extraintestinal symptoms, and the microscopic appearance of the polyps.

Peutz–Jeghers Syndrome

Peutz-Jeghers syndrome is a rare autosomal dominant syndrome but has incomplete penetrance.[1,11] It is associated with mutation of *STK-11* tumor suppression gene resulting in hamartomas throughout the GI tract. The characteristic feature of PJS polyp is the smooth muscle core arising from muscularis mucosae extending into the polyp. The polyps are most common in the small bowel and less so in the stomach and colon. They tend to be multiple and vary in size and shape. These can be sessile or pedunculated and produce intraluminal filling defects.[1,11,21]

The polyps, being firm, are especially prone to intussusception and may cause bleeding as well **(Figs. 4A to D)**. Although the polyps of PJS, being hamartomatous, are benign, the syndrome is associated with a definitely increased risk of small bowel adenocarcinoma. It is not clear whether this arises from the polyp or from coexisting adenomas. PJS is associated also with 10- to 18-fold increase in GI cancers.[1,11]

In patients presenting with multiple polyps, the presence of multiple colorectal polyps and duodenal polyps (adenomas) favors the diagnosis of FAP while the presence of small number of large polyps in the distal duodenum and jejunum favors PJS.[1,11] Other associated findings which help to clinch the diagnosis of PJS include pigmented lesions on the buccal mucosa, lips, and on the skin especially hands and feet.[1,21]

Management of these polyps may be done by enteroscopic clearance. Intestinal resection is limited to the necessary minimum when required. The primary aim of polyp removal is to prevent intussusception.[1]

Cowden's Disease[4,21]

Cowden's disease consists of gastric, small bowel, and colonic hamartomas and facial trichilemmomas.

Familial Adenomatous Polyposis[1,4,21]

Familial adenomatous polyposis is an inherited and autosomal dominant syndrome characterized by the presence of multiple adenomatous polyps in the colon, 80% of patients can also have adenomas involving the small intestine most common in the duodenum. Extraintestinal manifestation of FAP includes osteomas of mandible, long bones and skull, thyroid malignancy, adrenal adenoma/carcinoma, central nervous system (CNS) tumors (particularly medulloblastoma) and desmoid tumors.

Turcot syndrome and Gardner syndrome are also associated with multiple adenomatous small bowel polyps.

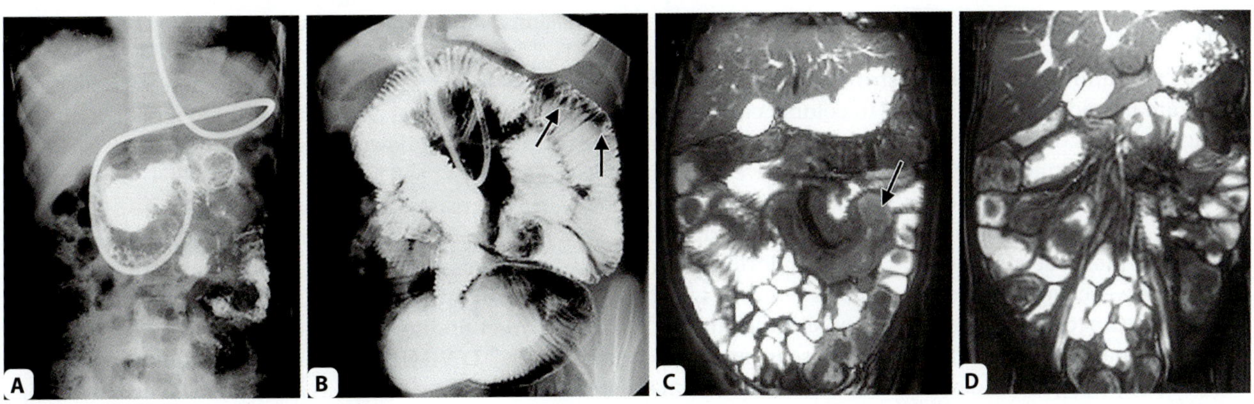

FIGS. 4A TO D: Peutz–Jegher's syndrome: Barium enteroclysis (A and B) in a patient with mucocutaneous pigmentation demonstrates multiple round to oval filling defects in the jejunum with jejuno-jejunal intussusception producing a coiled spring appearance in A. Coronal T2W (C and D) MR enteroclysis images of the same patient reveal multiple round to oval T2 iso- to hypointense polyps in the jejunum. Jejunojejunal intussusception due to a polyp acting as a lead point is also well seen (arrow).

Cronkhite–Canada Syndrome[21]

It is an acquired syndrome characterized by several intestinal polyps of the inflammatory type, hyperpigmentation, dystrophy of nails, alopecia, and diarrhea. The onset is usually after 40 years. The polyps are most commonly found in the small intestine and are generally not considered premalignant. The patient's main problem is usually malabsorption and protein loss.

Juvenile Polyposis[22]

Juvenile polyps are most often seen within first 10 years of life. The term juvenile, however, refers to the histology of the lesion and not the age of onset. Solitary lesions occur in the colon commonly presenting with bleeding per rectum. Juvenile polyposis is an autosomal dominant condition with multiple, i.e., > 5 polyps throughout the colon (juvenile polyposis coli) but polyps can occur anywhere in the GI tract (generalized juvenile polyposis) usually presenting in adolescence or late childhood. The familial variety may be associated with an increased risk of GI cancer most often colonic.

MALIGNANT TUMORS

Adenocarcinoma

Adenocarcinoma of the small intestine is somewhat less common in Asia and developing countries than the western world where it accounts for 30–50% of small bowel malignancies. It occurs usually in the sixth to seventh decade and is slightly more common in males than females.[1,23]

The duodenum and proximal jejunum are the most sites for adenocarcinoma, the jejunum accounting for about 30% cases of adenocarcinoma small bowel (generally within 30 cm of ligament of Treitz) and the duodenum for 50%. Ileal involvement is seen only in 20% cases and is more common in patients with Crohn's disease.[1,14,24]

Etiopathogenesis

Risk factors and geographical distribution for the small bowel are considered to be similar to colonic carcinoma. An increased risk of small bowel adenocarcinoma has been reported in colorectal cancer survivors. It is believed that an adenoma carcinoma sequence occurs in the small bowel as well. The presence of adenoma whether single or multiple is considered the most important risk factor for development of small bowel cancer. Syndromes such as FAP, PJS, Lynch syndrome, Cowden's disease, Gardner's syndrome,[1,24,25] and inflammatory disorders like Crohn's disease and celiac disease also predispose to development of adenocarcinoma. Some studies have shown an association with alcohol consumption, high animal fat intake, consumption of red meat and salt cured or smoked meat. Some urological procedures like ileal conduit of ileocystoplasty also increase the risk of adenocarcinoma.[1,24,25]

Clinical Presentation

Small bowel adenocarcinomas tend to become symptomatic later than the lesions located in the duodenum. The clinical features are nonspecific and include nausea, vomiting, pain abdomen, small bowel obstruction, weight loss and GI bleed which may be occult. The nonspecific nature of clinical symptoms and uncommon nature of disease results in diagnostic delay.[1,26] Misinterpretation of radiological studies can also cause diagnostic delay.[1,26] As a result most lesions are already metastatic by the time they are diagnosed. Small intestinal mucosa, unlike the large bowel, contains lymphatics which extend till the luminal surface and invasion of mucosal tumors into these lymphatics may be responsible for early tendency to metastases.[1] A significant proportion of patients may present acutely with obstruction, massive GI bleed or perforation.[1,24,26]

Imaging Features

On barium studies, adenocarcinoma produces a short segment circumferential narrowing with mucosal irregularity and ulceration. The lesions tend to have overhanging margins—the so-called "apple core" lesion **(Figs. 5A to D)**. These strictures have a fixed unchanging character on compression and with advanced lesions bowel obstruction is common.[11,26]

On CT/MR enterography, moderate wall-thickening resulting in short segment annular narrowing with abrupt overhanging edges is seen. Annular lesions are more common in the distal small bowel while polypoid lesions are more common in the duodenum. The high-grade stenosis may result in proximal small bowel obstruction.[4,14,24] On T2W MR images, the mass may show a heterogeneous signal. Moderate postcontrast enhancement which is often heterogeneous may be seen on CT or MR.[27] Marked diffusion restriction has been also reported on DW-MRI.[28] Occasionally, the lesions can be large and bulky mimicking lymphoma or GISTs,[26-28] but bowel obstruction is unusual in lymphoma or GISTs. The features favoring an adenocarcinoma include a short segment, solitary, stricturing lesion more common in the proximal small bowel with infiltration of perivisceral fat **(Figs. 6A to D)**.[16,26,27] The tumors are also FDG-avid and can be seen as increased activity on PET-CT.[29]

With advanced lesions invasion of mesentery and adjacent organs may occur. Retroperitoneal and mesenteric lymphadenopathy, hepatic, and peritoneal metastases are the other findings that may be seen on cross-sectional imaging.[26-28] DW-MRI is useful for detection of even small peritoneal metastases seen as nodular or linear areas of high signal on DW imaging which may be more easily seen with background suppression.[30-32]

The key imaging findings are summarized in **Box 2**.

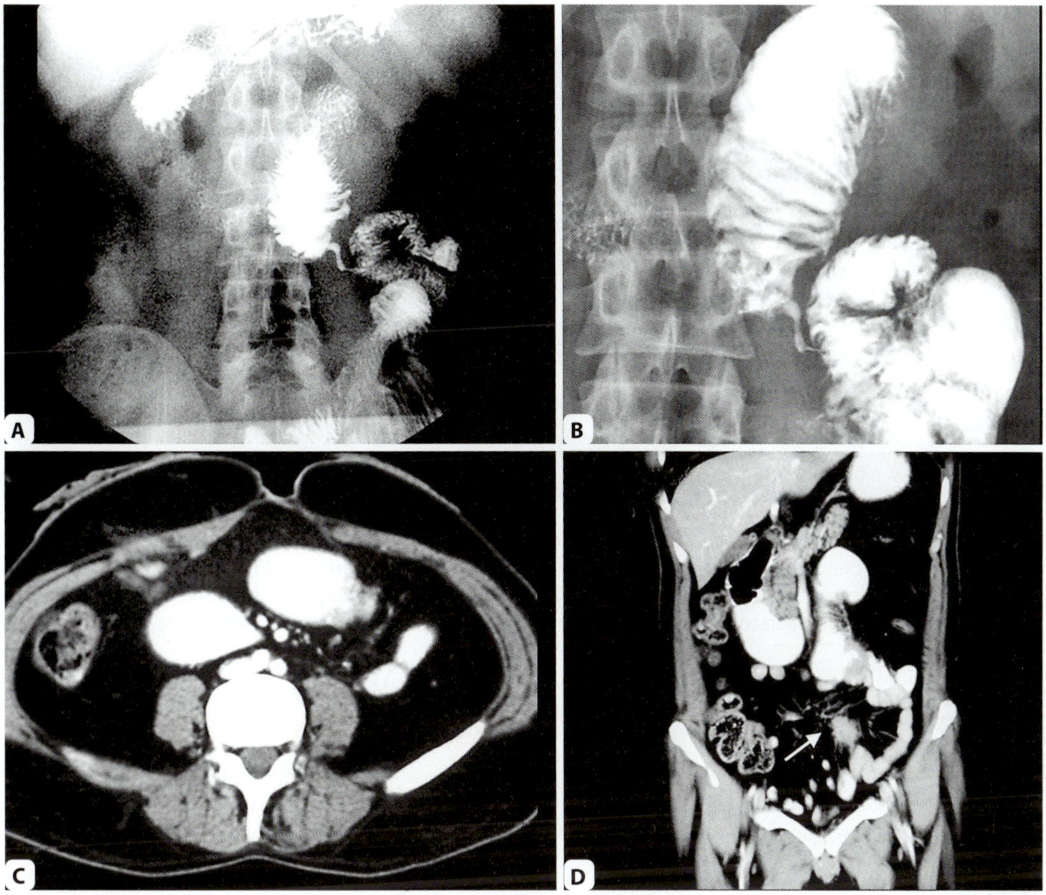

FIGS. 5A TO D: *Adenocarcinoma jejunum*: Barium meal follow through examination (A and B) showing a short segment tight stricture in the proximal jejunum with shouldering and mucosal irregularity—better appreciated on the magnified image (B). Axial and coronal contrast-enhanced computed tomography (CECT) images (C and D) of the same patient depict homogeneously enhancing moderate wall thickening causing significant luminal narrowing with abrupt overhanging edges. Mesenteric lymphadenopathy is noted (arrow). Perivisceral fat appears normal.

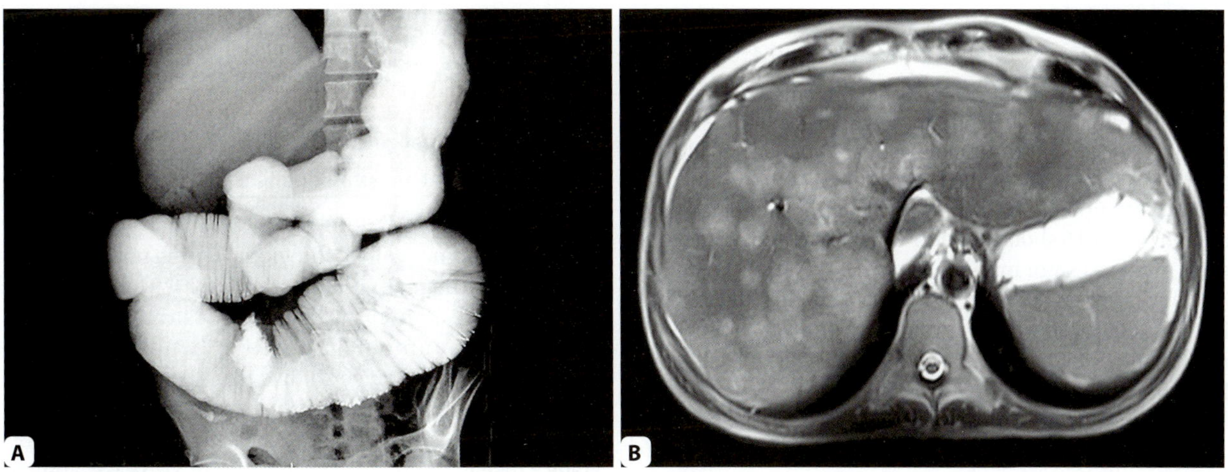

FIGS. 6A TO D: *Continued*

Continued

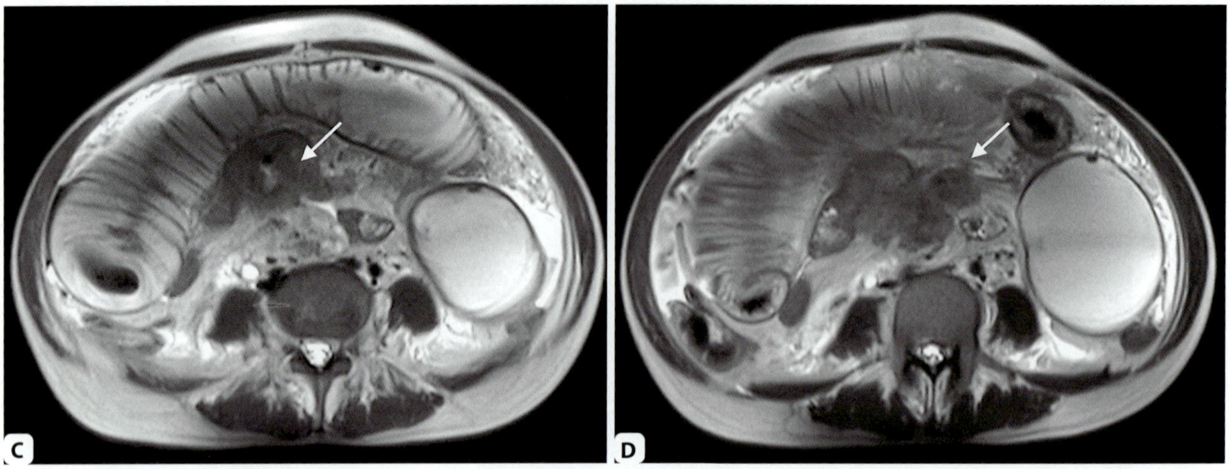

FIGS. 6A TO D: *Adenocarcinoma jejunum with hepatic metastases*: Barium meal follow through (A) reveals abrupt irregular narrowing of the jejunum producing complete obstruction and proximal dilatation. Cranial to caudal axial T2-weighted magnetic resonance (T2W MR) images. (B to D) depict moderate circumferential mural thickening of the jejunum in the same region with resultant marked luminal compromise (arrow in C) and adjacent lymphadenopathy (arrow in D). Multiple hepatic metastases and ascites are also noted.

BOX 2 Adenocarcinoma small bowel: Key imaging findings.

- *Site*: Duodenum and proximal jejunum
- *Barium*: Short segment stricture with shouldered margins
- *CT/MRI*: Focal moderate wall thickening with overhanging margins
- Polypoid mass
- Heterogeneous moderate enhancement
- Associated findings
- Perilesional fat infiltration
- Lymphadenopathy
- Small bowel obstruction common

Staging and Prognosis

Once the diagnosis of small bowel adenocarcinoma is established, a staging of thoraco-abdominopelvic CT to search for metastasis is recommended. Upper GI endoscopy and colonoscopy may also be done to look for predisposing genetic disease such as polyposis syndromes. Baseline plasma carcinoembryonic antigen (CEA) and carbohydrate antigen (CA) 19.9 should be done in advanced disease as the levels of these tumor markers have prognostic significance. Since most patients have advanced disease by the time diagnosis is made the prognosis is generally poor. Ileal or jejunal lesions have a slightly better prognosis than duodenal lesions.[1,24]

TNM staging system[33] is used to stage adenocarcinoma small intestine given in **Table 1**.

TABLE 1: TNM staging of small bowel adenocarcinoma.

T stage	
T1S	Tumor limited to epithelium or carcinoma in situ
T1	Tumor invades lamina propria submucosa or muscularis mucosa
T2	Tumor extends into the muscularis propria
T3	Tumor invades into subserosa or into nonperitonealized perimuscular tissue (mysentery or retroperitoneum) surrounding the small bowel
T4	Tumor invades into adjacent organs or extends through visceral peritoneum
N stage	
N0	No lymph node involvement
N1	Metastases in one to two regional lymph nodes
N2	Metastases in three or more regional lymph nodes
M stage	
M0	No distant metastases
M1	Distant metastases present

Treatment

Though surgical resection is the primary and the only potentially curative treatment option, very few cases are resectable at the time of diagnosis. Complete resection of the primary tumor with locoregional lymph node dissection is essential. The main prognostic factor for localized small bowel adenocarcinoma is lymph node invasion.

Also, the number of positive lymph nodes have prognostic value in stage III disease.[24]

If following surgery, the disease is found to be stage 0 or 1, and no adjuvant treatment is recommended. For stage 2 disease with pT4 tumor or stage 3 disease, adjuvant treatment is recommended. No standard adjuvant regimen has been defined to date due to lack of randomized controlled trials. Generally, a chemotherapy regimen similar to that for colorectal cancer[34] is followed. Patients with advanced disease may be treated by chemotherapy or radiotherapy for palliation. Radiotherapy being mainly used for duodenal lesions. Stenting of the bowel strictures can also be done as a palliative measure.[24]

NEUROENDOCRINE TUMORS (NETS)

Carcinoid tumors were originally described by Langhans and Lubarsch,[35,36] but Oberndorfer, in 1907, was the first to use the term carcinoid or "Karzinoide" meaning "carcinoma like".[37] This is because these tumors displayed less aggressive growth than seen with most other GI carcinomas.[38] The current preferred nomenclature for these tumors is neuroendocrine tumors. NETs are relatively rare neoplasms arising from Amine Precursor Uptake and Decarboxylation (APUD) cells of the diffuse endocrine system.[39] These cells have a number of antigens that are common with nerve elements too (neuroendocrine markers) hence the term neuroendocrine is used for these cell types and tumors.[40,41] There are several types of diffuse endocrine cells in the GI tract such as "Gastrin" or G cells, D cell (somatostatin producing cell), enterochromaffin or EC cell, etc. They represent the largest number of neuroendocrine cells in the body, therefore, the GI tract is the most common site of NETs accounting for 60–70% cases.[39]

Small bowel NETs account for 26–30% of all GI NETs. Ileum is the most common site, the usual location being within 60 cm of ileocecal valve.[39-44] They are multiple in 30–40% of patients and occur most frequently between the fifth and seventh decades. Some studies report a slightly higher incidence in males, others report equal incidence in males and females. Rarely NETs can arise in a Meckel's diverticulum.[41,45] Small bowel NETs are generally sporadic. Those associated with MEN-I are mostly foregut carcinoids while patients with NF-1 typically have periampullary carcinoids.[42,43]

A second primary malignancy (synchronous/metachronous) may present in GI NETs. This is most frequent in the small intestinal NETs occurring in about 29% cases. GI adenocarcinomas are the most commonly associated malignancy, others being prostate, breast, bronchus, and bladder malignancies.[39,45]

Pathological Features

Majority of the jejunal and ileal NETs arise from the EC cells in the crypts of Lieberkühn also called Kulchitsky cells. They are submucosal tumors which may produce intramural masses or protrude into the lumen forming polypoid nodules with occasional focal ulceration of the overlying mucosa. These nodules can cause intussusception. Primary intestinal tumors are usually small—generally not > 3.5 cm but have already invaded the muscularis propria at the time of diagnosis in most cases, forming tumor masses in the subserosa of the intestine extending into the adjacent mesentery. Local release of serotonin and other vasoactive substances as well as the pattern of growth described above results in desmoplasia, which is most marked in the submucosa and adjacent mesentery. In addition, mesenteric vessels close to the tumor as well as those far away may be thickened with focal occlusions or stenosis due to the vasoactive substances released or vascular invasion.[45]

Conventional argentaffin and argyrophil silver-staining techniques can be used to identify the tumor cells as EC cells. Immunohistochemical markers for serotonin, substance P, and other tachykinins have also been used. These tumors are also strongly positive for general endocrine markers such as chromogranin A, neuron-specific enolase and synaptophysin.[41,45]

Many pathologic classification systems have been proposed for carcinoid/NET. Based on their location and embryologic origin, they were traditionally classified as foregut, midgut, and hindgut[39,45] to emphasize clinicopathologic difference between these groups. However, this did not explain the heterogeneity in their biologic behavior following which the World Health Organization (WHO) classification was developed in 2000. Currently the WHO 2019 classification is used. This classification is given in **Table 2**.

Tumors previously referred to as carcinoids essentially represent well-differentiated NETs while poorly differentiated tumors are referred to as neuroendocrine carcinomas (NECs). A new category of *mixed neuroendocrine and non-neuroendocrine neoplasms* (*MiNEN*) has been introduced, where each component represents > 30% of the tumor cells. Both components of the tumor are graded separately.[46]

Molecular Genetics

In recent years, genetic studies have shown that GI NECs commonly show TP53 and RB1 mutations, like pancreatic and pulmonary NECs, but these are absent in NETs. On the other hand, well-differentiated NETs show *MEN1, DAXX,* and *ATRX* mutations. Some studies also suggest

TABLE 2: World Health Organization 2019 classification and grading of neuroendocrine tumors (NETs).

NET type	Tumor classification
NET, grade I	Well-differentiated, low-grade, mitotic count < 2/HPF, Ki-67, index < 3%
NET, grade II	Well-differentiated, intermediate-grade mitotic count 2–20/HPF, Ki-67, index 3–20%
NET, grade III	Well-differentiated, high-grade, mitotic count > 20/HPF, Ki-67 > 20%, small cell features
NEC, large cell (LCNEC)	Poorly differentiated, high-grade,* mitotic count > 20/HPF, Ki-67 > 20%, large cell features
NEC small cell (SCNEC)	Poorly differentiated, high-grade,* mitotic count > 20/HPF, Ki-67 >,20%, small cell features
MiNEN	Well/Poorly differentiated, variable grade, mitotic count, and Ki-67 index

*Poorly differentiated NECs are considered high grade by default.

(HPF: high power field; Ki-67 index refers to the % of cells which are positive for Ki-67—a marker for cell proliferation; MiNEN: mixed neuroendocrine and nonneuroendocrine neoplasms; NEC: neuroendocrine carcinoma)

that epigenetic mutations, like global hypomethylation, could have an important role in tumorigenesis of small bowel NETs. As high as 70–80% small bowel NETs are epigenetically dysregulated and this may have therapeutic implications as epigenetic changes may be reversible, hence be possible targets for treatment in the future.[46,47]

Cytogenetics/immunohistochemistry (IHC) may also help in localizing an unknown primary. If the metastatic tumor is positive for transcription factor CDX-2 then the primary is likely to be in the midgut whereas positive paired box gene 6 (PAX6) and/or insulin gene enhancer-binding protein (ISL1) staining suggests a pancreatic primary.[16,46,47]

Clinical Features

Many patients are asymptomatic because of the slow-growing nature of these tumors. Symptoms may be related to the primary tumor, mesenteric involvement, or metastatic disease. A long history of crampy abdominal pain, weight loss, fatigue or diarrhea and small bowel obstruction and very rarely obscure GI bleed may be seen.[45]

Carcinoid syndrome is seen in about 17–30% of patients with small bowel NETs. Patients with ileal NETs who have extensive hepatic metastases are most likely to develop carcinoid syndrome due to vasoactive substance such as serotonin, kallikrein, bradykinin, and prostaglandins, produced by the tumor, entering systemic circulation without metabolic degradation, which normally occurs in the liver. The classic carcinoid syndrome consists of cutaneous flushing, diarrhea, abdominal pain, wheezing due to bronchospasm, palpitations, and low blood pressure. This can be precipitated by alcohol, cheese, chocolate, exercise or emotional stress.[39,45] About 75% of patients with carcinoid syndrome develop carcinoid heart syndrome, i.e., right-sided valvular fibrosis and fibrosis of right cardiac chambers. Inactivation of the bioactive peptides in the lungs is thought to be responsible for left-sided sparing.[39,45]

Laboratory tests that are useful in establishing the diagnosis of small bowel NETs/carcinoid include 24 hours urinary 5-hydroxyindoleacetic acid (5-HIAA) a serotonin breakdown product which is elevated in 75% of midgut carcinoids and serum chromogranin A which is elevated in 80–90% of all GI carcinoids (foregut, midgut, and hindgut). The latter is also used to assess response to therapy.[39,45] In patients who have clinical features of carcinoid syndrome, echocardiography is indicated to detect carcinoid heart disease which is an independent poor prognostic factor.

Imaging

While conventional abdominal CT has very low sensitivity for detection of small (<2 cm) lesions, multiphase helical CT with neural oral contrast, i.e., CT enterography improves detection of smaller lesions because of improved tumor to background contrast. The scan acquisition must be done earlier than usual, i.e., in the late arterial phase.[47,48] Small ileal NETs may be seen as solitary or multiple hyperenhancing polyps, plaque-like lesions or carpet lesions.[39,49]

Transmural extension of the tumor and associated mesenteric involvement and fibrosis is seen in 50–75% cases of midgut NETs with median size of 3 cm.[50,51] On CT, it is seen as a focal soft-tissue mass adjacent to mural thickening in the bowel. Deposits of NETs in the mesentery produce masses which are commonly spiculated and produce mesenteric retraction due to fibrosis. These masses may be much larger than the primary tumor and completely obscure it. Fine stippled or bulky and dense calcification may be seen in 40–70% of these.[45,50] Associated fibrosis angulates and kinks the involved intestine producing "hair pin" bends—well appreciated on both axial images and multiplanar reconstructions **(Figs. 7A to E)**. It can also produce a "spoke wheel" or "sunburst" pattern of radiating mesenteric vessels.[45] Occasionally, signs of bowel ischemia are evident. Retroperitoneal or mesenteric lymphadenopathy and associated retroperitoneal fibrosis can result in ureteric obstruction.[52-54]

On MR enterography NETs may be seen as solitary or multiple nodular masses or nodular fold thickening appearing isointense to muscle on T1W images and isointense to mildly hyperintense on T2W images with intense contrast enhancement with mesenteric extension resulting in stretching, and angulation of small bowel loops. The mesenteric mass itself is isointense on both T1W and T2W images due to fibrosis. Calcification though not as well seen as on CT may be seen as signal voids.[16,54]

Hepatic metastases are common and are best seen on arterial phase CT or MRI since they are generally hypervascular.[54] Occasionally, they can be necrotic and may calcify. On ultrasound, liver metastases may be hyperechoic. Contrast-enhanced ultrasound may help in improving sensitivity of ultrasound from 68 to 99%. MR has a higher sensitivity for detection of liver metastases than CT, USG, or somatostatin receptor scintigraphy (SRS).[54]

Other less common sites of metastases include bones, lungs, peritoneal cavity, and ovary.[39] Rarely, diffuse mesenteric or peritoneal disease can occur producing miliary peritoneal implants, large masses, and mesenteric caking or ascites.[45,53]

Nuclear medicine/functional studies in GI NETs help in staging the disease, detect additional sites of involvement before surgery and detect unknown primary in patients presenting with metastases. SRS is performed using radiolabeled synthetic somatostatin analog ^{111}I octreotide because NETs express somatostatin receptors especially subtypes 2 and 5, but it is rarely performed these days with the advent of PET-CT. ^{68}Ga labeled DOTATOC/DOTANOC/DOTATATE PET-CT (which are octreotide derivatives) is currently the technique of choice. It has higher sensitivity for tumor burden than SRS ranging from 93 to 97%.[45,55,56]

Fludeoxyglucose F18-positron emission tomography/computed tomography is not useful in diagnosing typical low-grade NETs because of the low glycolytic rate but has a role in prognostication of poorly differentiated tumors. The tumors that are ^{18}F-FDG PET/CT avid have a poorer prognosis and more rapid disease progression than those with negative uptake.[57-59]

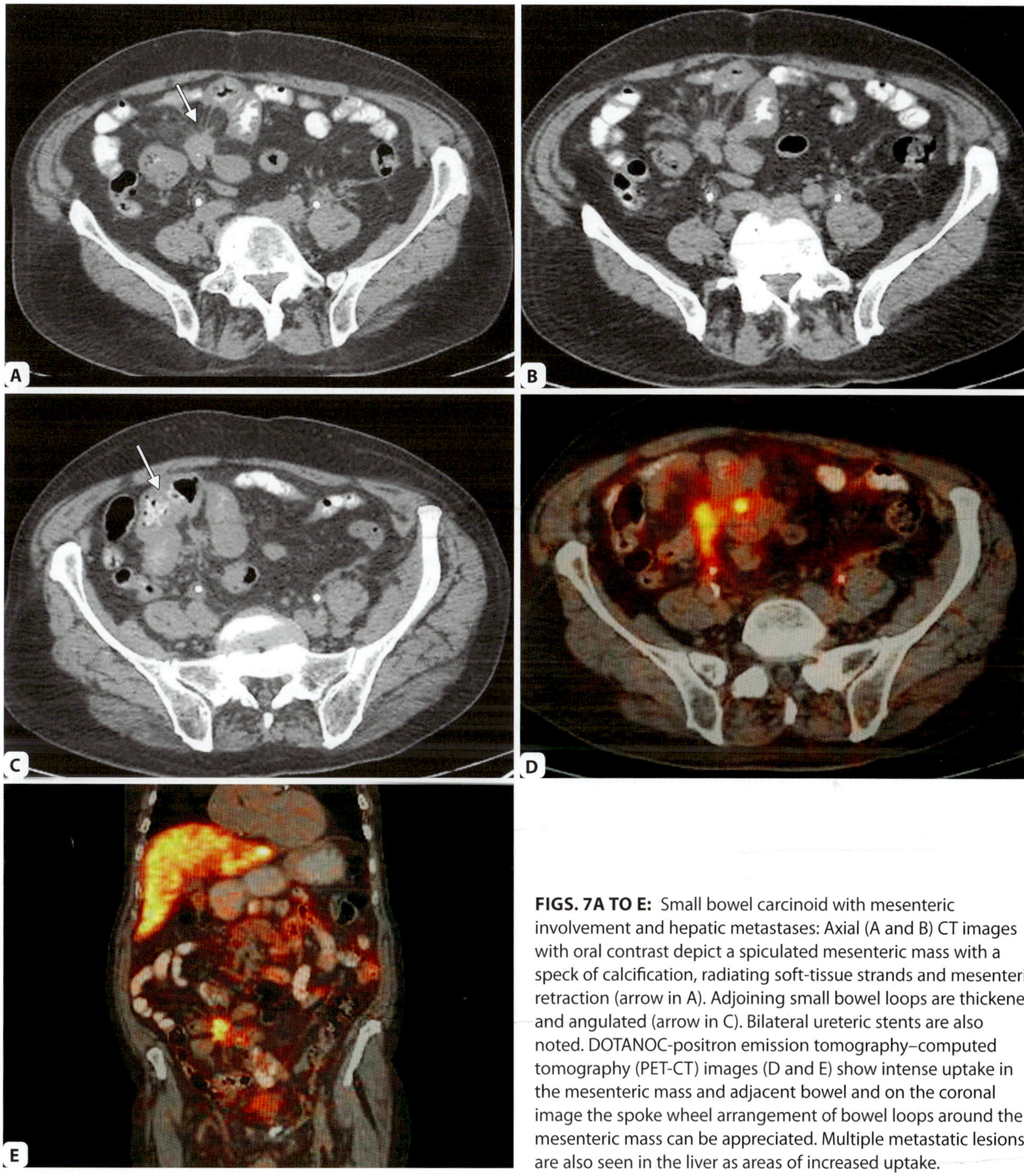

FIGS. 7A TO E: Small bowel carcinoid with mesenteric involvement and hepatic metastases: Axial (A and B) CT images with oral contrast depict a spiculated mesenteric mass with a speck of calcification, radiating soft-tissue strands and mesenteric retraction (arrow in A). Adjoining small bowel loops are thickened and angulated (arrow in C). Bilateral ureteric stents are also noted. DOTANOC-positron emission tomography–computed tomography (PET-CT) images (D and E) show intense uptake in the mesenteric mass and adjacent bowel and on the coronal image the spoke wheel arrangement of bowel loops around the mesenteric mass can be appreciated. Multiple metastatic lesions are also seen in the liver as areas of increased uptake.

Differential Diagnosis

The differential diagnosis of small primary tumors includes GIST, adenoma, or leiomyoma. Other lesions that need to be distinguished from NETs include lymphoma, adenocarcinoma, metastases, GIST, and Kaposi's sarcoma. Presence of fibrosis and angulation of bowel loops is characteristic of NETs; however, it can occur with mesenteric extension of adenocarcinoma or metastases. DOTANOC-PET-CT can be extremely useful when the diagnosis is not clear.

The mesenteric mass of carcinoid tumor may mimic sclerosing mesenteritis and it can be very difficult to distinguish these conditions preoperatively. The soft-tissue mass in sclerosing mesenteritis may envelop the mesenteric vessels with collateral vessel formation; however, the fat around the mesenteric vessels is preserved, the so-called "fat ring sign" unlike in NETs.[16]

Box 3 summarizes the important imaging findings in NETs.

BOX 3 NET key imaging findings.

- Site-distal ileum
- Intensely enhancing polypoid mass/bowel wall thickening
- Mesenteric mass with calcification and desmoplasia (spiculation)
- Mesenteric retraction
- Angulated or hair pin small bowel loops
- DOTANOC-PET avid

(NET: neuroendocrine tumor; PET: positron emission tomography)

Treatment and Prognosis

Treatment depends on the extent of disease, symptomatology, and receptor status. Localized small bowel NETs are treated surgically by removing the involved bowel and affected nodes. The entire bowel must be examined at surgery to rule out multiple lesions. Prophylactic cholecystectomy is recommended when treatment with somatostatin analogs is planned as these drugs cause impairment of gallbladder function with gallstones formation and cholecystitis. Even in patients with unresectable disease debulking may be carried out for symptomatic relief. Precautions to prevent a carcinoid crisis such as octreotide infusion may be desirable before surgery.[47]

A multidisciplinary approach is required in patients with metastases. DOTANOC/DOTATOC-PET should be done if treatment with somatostatin analogs (octreotide/lanreotide/vapreotide) is planned to determine receptor status. Somatostatin analog injections help to provide symptomatic relief in patients with carcinoid syndrome. They are also thought to inhibit the growth of tumors, hence have an important role in the treatment of carcinoid tumors with positive receptor status. Polypeptide receptor radionuclide therapy (PRRT) with ^{111}In, ^{90}Y, or ^{177}Lu labeled octreotide analogs represents another alternative therapy in receptor positive disease. It uses a radioisotope conjugated to a somatostatin receptor analog for selective delivery of isotope to tumor cells.

For limited liver metastases complete resection should ideally be done with curative intent. The various treatment options for extensive hepatic metastases include radiofrequency ablation (RFA), arterial embolization, chemotherapy, and PRRT. Tyrosine kinase inhibitors (TKIs) and vascular endothelial growth factor (VEGF) monoclonal antibodies are also being evaluated.[39]

Carcinoid syndrome which is refractory to other management may be managed with tryptophan hydroxylase inhibitor telotristat. NECs arising from the small bowel are extremely rare, and platinum-based chemotherapy regimens-cisplatin/carboplatin are used.[46,47]

Although NETs have a less aggressive growth pattern than adenocarcinoma, the 5-year survival rate for small bowel NETs is about 54%. If complete surgical resection can be performed, the survival rate improves greatly approaching 75%. The 5-year survival rate for patients with liver metastases in patients with few liver metastases (<5) is similar to those without metastasis and much better than in those with extensive hepatic metastases.[47,54]

GASTROINTESTINAL STROMAL TUMORS

Gastrointestinal stromal tumors (GISTs) are the most common nonepithelial or mesenchymal tumor of the GI tract. The term was first used by Mazur and Clark.[60,61] Prior to 1983, these tumors were variably referred to as smooth muscle tumors; leiomyomas, leiomyosarcomas, and leiomyoblastomas. However, they are distinct from true smooth muscle or neural tumors and are thought to arise from the interstitial cells of Cajal (intestinal pacemaker cells).

Clinical Features

The exact prevalence of GISTs is difficult to ascertain; however, it is estimated that there are about 5,000–10,000 new cases every year.[62] Most patients are over 50 years at the time of diagnosis and there is no definite sex predilection. Ethnicity, race, occupation, or geographic location have no association with GISTs.

The clinical presentation is extremely variable and depends on the size and location of tumors. Small GISTs may be discovered incidentally during radiological evaluation or surgery for another condition. Nausea, vomiting, abdominal pain, distention, palpable abdominal mass, and feeling of satiety may occur with large masses.[63,64] GI bleeding from mucosal ulceration is a common manifestation of symptomatic GISTs. This may be in the form of hematemesis melena or anemia due to occult bleed.[64]

Pathological Features

GISTs can arise all along the GI tract, the stomach being the most frequent site followed by the small intestine. Any part of the small intestine can be involved. The esophagus is the only site in the GI tract where leiomyomas are more common than GISTs accounting for 75% of mesenchymal esophageal tumors. Rarely, they can arise primarily in the omentum, mesentery, and retroperitoneum.[64]

Macroscopically, these tumors are well-circumscribed masses without a true capsule, size varying from few mm to over 30 cm. On gross pathology, cut surface is pink, tan, or gray in color. Larger lesions can show focal areas of hemorrhage cystic degeneration and necrosis. GISTs arise from the interstitial cells of Cajal in the outer muscular layer or muscularis propria of the GI tract. They can grow endophytically into the intestinal lumen, be completely intramural, or be exophytic or show a combination of growth patterns. Exophytic and mixed patterns are common in the small bowel often producing large masses arising from the intestinal wall and projecting into the abdominal cavity. Mucosal ulceration may be seen in a significant number of lesions as a component of the tumor extends to the mucosal surface.[64,65]

Histologically, these can be spindle cell, epithelioid cell, or mixed cell types. No GIST can be unequivocally labeled benign although lesions < 2 cm in size have a very low risk of recurrence and are mostly considered benign. Small bowel GISTs in general have a more aggressive course than gastric tumors.

Molecular Genetics and Immunohistochemistry

GISTs show gain of function mutations in *KIT* or *PDGFRA* genes which are receptor tyrosine kinases. These mutations are found in various gene regions, including exons 8, 9, 11, 13, 14, 15, and 17. It has been observed that *KIT* exon 13 and exon 17 mutant GISTs are more frequently seen in the small bowel, and usually have spindle-cell morphology.[63] Classically, *PDGFRA*-mutated GISTs are commonly located in the stomach and show an epithelioid pattern on histology.

A minority of GISTs have no *KIT* or *PDGFRA* mutations and are known as "wild type" gastrointestinal stromal tumors (WT-GISTs). The WT-GISTs are further divided into succinate dehydrogenase (SDH)-deficient and SDH competent according to SDHB-IHC expression. The tumors seen in patients with neurofibromatosis are of the SDH competent WT-GISTs type and have a low malignant potential.[63] These patients almost exclusively have multiple small intestinal GISTs. SDH-deficient WT-GISTs are a feature of Carney's triad consisting of epithelioid GIST with paraganglioma and pulmonary chondroma with female predominance. All three of these do not necessarily occur at the same time. Other syndromes associated with GISTs include Carney–Stratakis syndrome characterized by GISTs and paraganglioma. Patients with these syndromes are younger tend to have multiple gastric GISTs.[63,64]

On immunohistochemistry GISTs express CD117 which is a tyrosine kinase growth factor receptor and is the result of c-KIT gene expression. Most GISTs are CD34 positive also. Immunoreactivity to *KIT* helps to differentiate GISTs from true smooth muscle tumors.[60-62] A small percentage that are KIT negative express discovered on GIST-1 (DOG1), a calcium-activated chloride channel protein.

Imaging Appearances

Although plain radiographs have no role in the diagnosis of GISTs they may reveal a soft-tissue haze due to the mass. Rarely, irregular gas collections may be seen when the masses are cavitating with presence of air in the cavity.[65]

Ultrasound can detect large masses which appear heterogeneous due to areas of necrosis; however, it may be difficult to identify the exact organ of origin **(Fig. 8)**.[65]

On barium studies, due to a large extraluminal component these masses exhibit mass effect on the affected segment of intestine. A cavity or fistula communicating with the intestinal lumen hence filling with barium may be seen and rarely aneurysmal dilatation can be seen **(Figs. 9A to C)**. Small lesions may produce submucosal masses indistinguishable from other benign submucosal lesions, sometimes mucosal irregularity due to ulceration can be seen.[64]

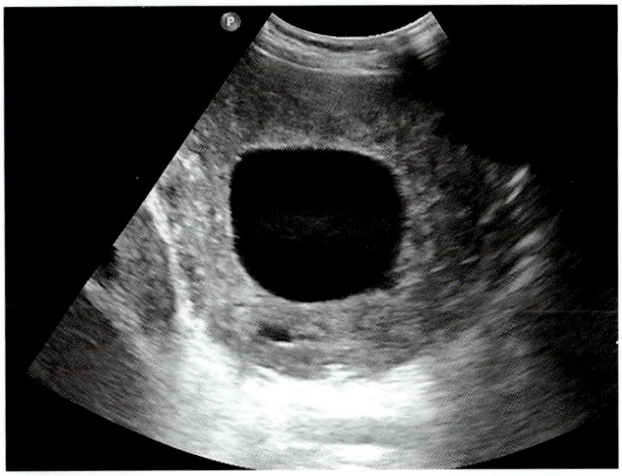

FIG. 8: Gastrointestinal stromal tumor (GIST): Gray-scale ultrasound image reveals a large heterogeneous mass with a central area cavitation in a patient with GIST.

Computed tomography is the mainstay for diagnosis and staging. The entire tumor including the mural, extramural, and luminal component is well-delineated on CT. In many cases, the bulk of the tumor is extraserosal making it difficult to determine its origin from small bowel. The appearances and enhancement patterns are variable including hypervascular, intermediate, and delayed enhancement pattern. It has been reported by some authors that the degree of enhancement of GISTs in the venous phase gradually increases from the duodenum to the ileum. Most large lesions tend to be heterogeneous due to necrosis, hemorrhage, or cystic degeneration and show inhomogeneous patchy enhancement following contrast administration **(Figs. 10A to C)**. Small GISTs (< 5 cm) usually produce homogeneous, hyperenhancing, submucosal, or endoluminal polypoid masses with washout. Calcification is rarely seen. The vascular supply is well-demonstrated on CTA using MIP or curved planar reconstructions. A prominent "early draining vein" (i.e., venous return, in the arterial phase) is common in small bowel GISTs and can be helpful to determine the tumor origin as well. Usually, the tumors displace adjacent organs but with advanced disease direct invasion of adjacent structures may be seen. Rarely, the tumors may appear predominantly cystic and may be misdiagnosed as pseudocysts.[60,62,64,65]

Nearly 50% of patients with GISTs present with metastasis. Liver and peritoneal metastases are the most common occurring due to hematogenous spread and peritoneal seeding, respectively **(Figs. 11A and B)**. Less common sites of metastasis include lung, pleura, and soft-tissue. Lymph node metastases are distinctly uncommon. Dual-phase contrast-enhanced computed tomography

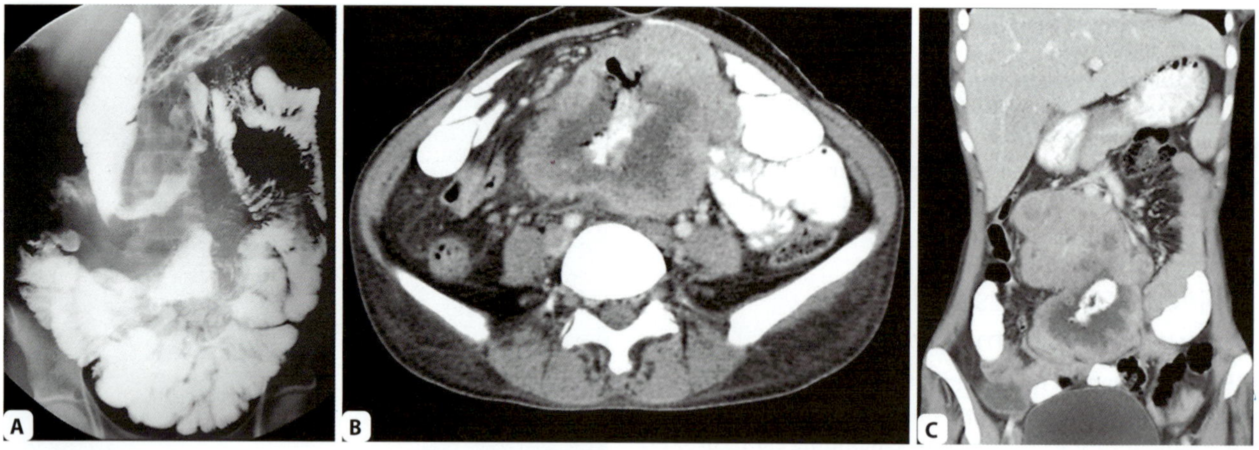

FIGS. 9A TO C: Gastrointestinal stromal tumor-ileum (A to C): Barium meal follow through examination (A) shows a soft-tissue haze in the central abdomen displacing the small bowel loops. A large irregular extraluminal collection of barium is noted within the mass suggesting cavitation and fistulization. Axial and coronal contrast-enhanced computed tomography (CECT) images (B and C) of the same patient reveal a large heterogeneously enhancing lobulated mass. An area of cavitation showing air foci and oral contrast is seen in the mass due to cavitation and fistula formation. Note the absence of any lymphadenopathy, ascites, or bowel obstruction.

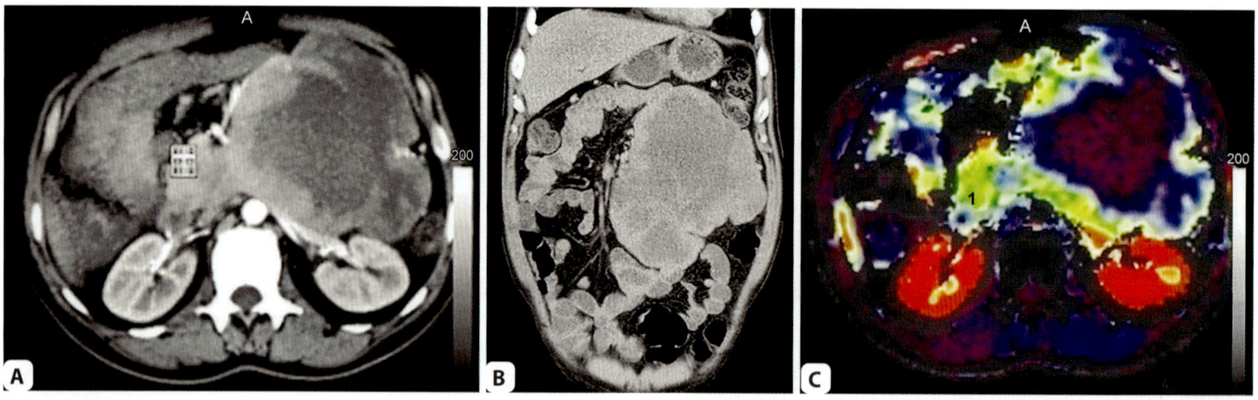

FIGS. 10A TO C: Gastrointestinal stromal tumor (GIST)-jejunum: Axial and coronal (A and B) contrast-enhanced computed tomography (CECT) images depict a large mass in close proximity to the jejunum with heterogeneous predominantly peripheral enhancement. Increased blood flow to this area is also confirmed on the perfusion CT blood flow map (C) seen as blue and green areas at the periphery. Note the lobulated but relatively smooth outer margin of the lesion with no evidence of mesenteric fat stranding or lymphadenopathy. On surgery, a large jejunal GIST was resected.

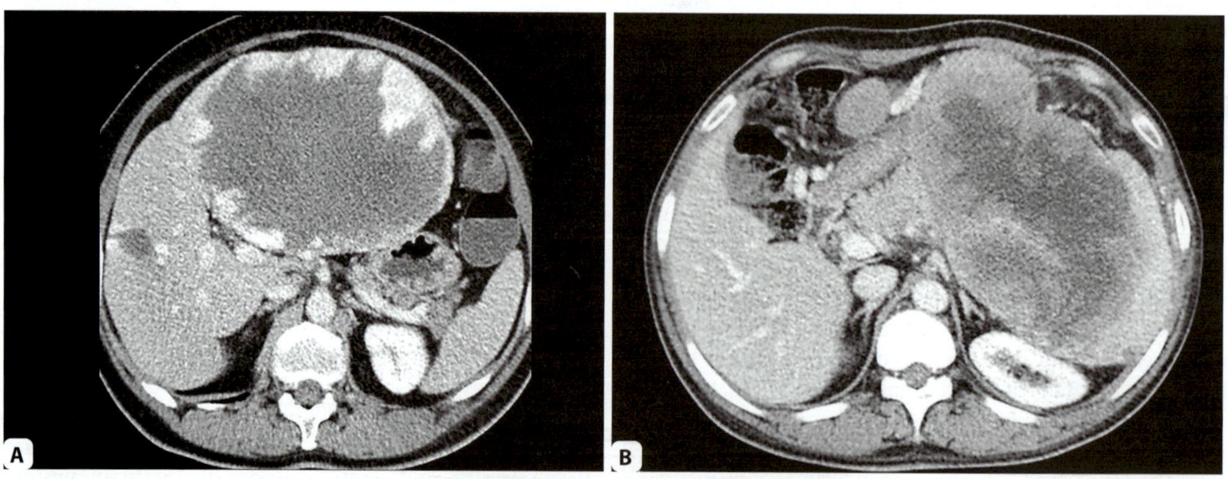

FIGS. 11A AND B: Gastrointestinal stromal tumor (GIST) with hepatic metastases: Metastasis to the left lobe liver in a patient with GIST shows hypodense mass with multiple peripheral solid enhancing nodules on contrast-enhanced computed tomography (CECT). Also note the smaller lesion in the right lobe showing a similar appearance.

(CECT) is recommended especially for hepatic metastases as they may be hypervascular and not visible on portal phase imaging.[60,66]

Magnetic resonance is indicated for evaluation of liver lesions indeterminate at CT, when CT is contraindicated and for surgical planning of rectal GISTs. The MR appearances depend on the size, degree of necrosis, and hemorrhage. The most common appearance is an exophytic bulky mass. Sometimes a protruding intraluminal mass or bidirectional growth pattern relative to the intestinal wall may be seen. The solid areas of the tumor are low signal on T1W images, high signal on T2W images, and show enhancement after contrast administration. Areas of hemorrhage show variable signal intensity depending on the age of hemorrhage. Mesenteric masses in the case of GISTs tend to be smooth, without any spiculation.[16] DWI may reveal restricted diffusion with low apparent diffusion coefficient (ADC) values **(Figs. 12A to F)**.[67]

Fludeoxyglucose F18-positron emission tomography/ computed tomography is also a highly sensitive technique for detection and staging of GISTs but a small number of lesions are not FDG avid.[60]

The imaging findings are summarized in **Box 4**.

Complications

Gastrointestinal bleeding is the most common complication of GISTs because they are frequently associated with mucosal ulceration. This can result in fistula, rupture, and perforation in large tumors. Fistula formation can be visualized as surface irregularity or crevices with a tract containing gas or fluid reaching the small bowel lumen. Reactive lymphadenopathy may be seen in such cases. Rupture can produce an intraperitoneal abscess or hemoperitoneum.

Gastrointestinal stromal tumors may occasionally cause small bowel obstruction due to intussusception, narrowing of the intestinal lumen or torsion involving the small bowel and mesentery which is seen in large exophytic GISTs.[65]

Staging and Prognosis

Contrast-enhanced computed tomography of the abdomen and pelvis is the imaging technique of choice for staging and follow-up. FDG-PET-CT/MRI is especially useful when early detection of tumor response to molecular targeted therapy is to be done. A TNM staging system for GISTs has been developed by the American Joint Committee on Cancer (AJCC) and takes into account the location of the tumor

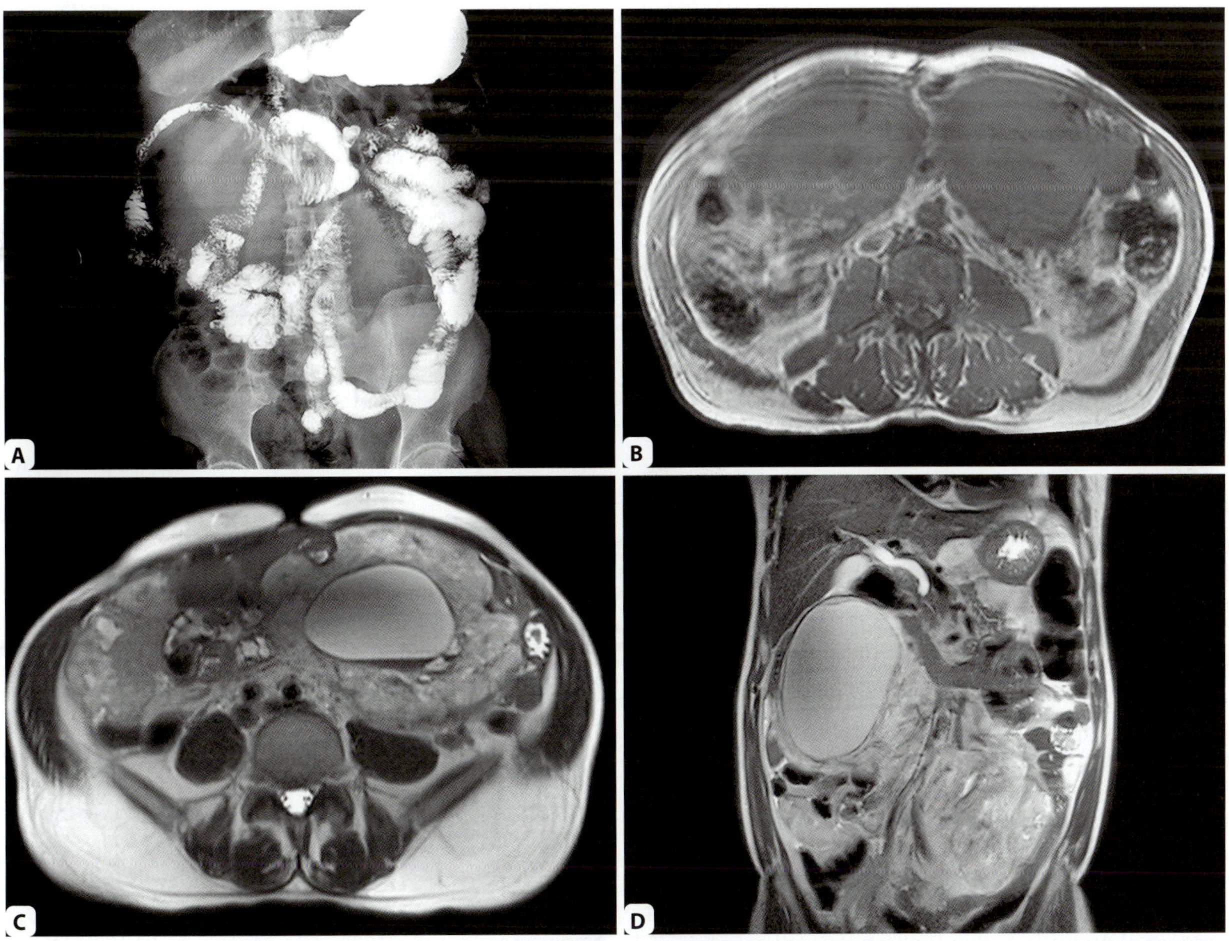

FIGS. 12A TO F: *Continued*

Continued

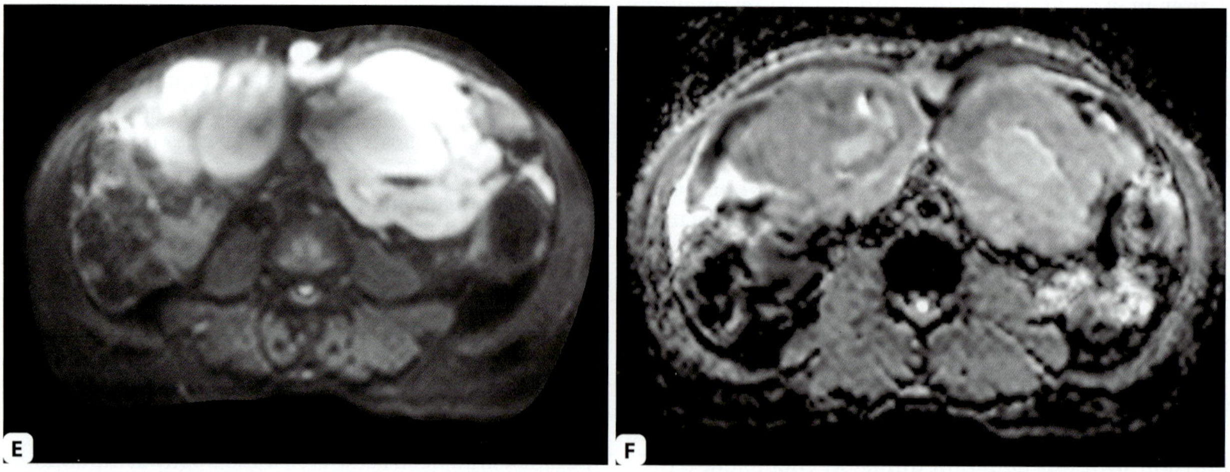

FIGS. 12A TO F: Gastrointestinal stromal tumor: Barium meal follow through examination (A) reveals evidence of extrinsic compression and displacement of small bowel loop around soft-tissue masses. T1-weighted (T1W) (B) and T2-weighted (T2W) axial and coronal MR images (C and D) reveal T1W iso and T2W heterogeneously hyperintense masses in the mesentery in close proximity to the small bowel loops. A central area of cystic degeneration with fluid–fluid levels is seen in one of the lesions. (B) On diffusion-weighted imaging (DWI) and apparent diffusion coefficient (ADC) maps (E and F); there is evidence of restricted diffusion in the peripheral solid component appearing bright on DWI and dark on ADC maps. Note absence of lymphadenopathy or small bowel obstruction.

BOX 4 Gastrointestinal stromal tumor (GIST) key imaging findings.

- Site–stomach followed by small bowel
- Bulky exophytic heterogenous mass
- Moderate heterogeneous enhancement
- Smooth lobulated outline
- Internal gas, cavitation, and fistulization
- Lymphadenopathy is distinctly uncommon
- Usually, there is no obstruction

(gastric/extragastric) and the mitotic rate besides the tumor size nodal and metastatic status .

Several criteria have been proposed to prognosticate GISTs. The term "benign" and "malignant" are not applied any longer since all GISTs have some potential to behave in a malignant fashion.[63] Risk of recurrence is dependent on tumor size, mitotic index, and site (i.e., location in GI tract). Nongastric location is associated with poorer prognosis than gastric lesions. Modified National Institutes of Health (NIH) criteria have stratified tumors into risk categories depending on risk of recurrence. For any location, tumors < 2 cm in size with a mitotic count < 5/50 HPF are categorized as very low risk while tumors > 10 cm (any mitotic rate) or those with mitotic rate > 10/50 HPF (any size) are classified as high-risk. For extra-gastric GISTs, even tumors < 5 cm with mitotic index > 5 or between 5 and 10 cm and ≤ 5 mitotic index are considered high risk. Presence of rupture whether spontaneous or iatrogenic and male sex are independent adverse prognostic features.[63]

Certain "critical mutations" in *KIT* are found in patients with an increased risk of recurrence but are not a part of the above-mentioned prognostication system.[63]

Imaging may also provide some clues to the aggressiveness of GISTs. In general, malignant tumors tend to be larger than benign lesions and are more necrotic show greater enhancement and may show prominent peritumoral vessels. Tumor size over 10 cm has been reported as a strong predictor of a malignant GIST. Local invasion and metastases obviously indicate malignancy. It has also been reported that on dual-energy CT, a greater spectral curve slope and higher normalized iodine concentration indicate high-risk GISTs. maximum standardized uptake value (SUV_{max}) on PET-CT has also been suggested as a complementary tool to predict the malignant potential of GISTs. In recent years, Radiomics research groups have tried to estimate histopathological risk and gene mutations using CT data.[63,66,68]

Pediatric Gastrointestinal Stromal Tumors

Gastrointestinal stromal tumors are extremely rare in pediatric patients. They are WT, SDH-deficient GISTs, and can be isolated or associated with syndromes like Carney's triad and Carney–Stratakis syndrome. Pediatric patients have gastric lesions which tend to be multicentric can show lymph node metastases, but are slow growing with a very good prognosis despite metastases.[63]

Treatment

Management of GISTs requires a multidisciplinary approach. Tumors 2 cm or more in size should be surgically resected. The management of lesions that are < 2 cm in size and discovered incidentally is controversial and endoscopic monitoring every 6–12 months may be done. The recommended standard treatment for localized tumors is complete surgical resection with an intact pseudocapsule and with macroscopic clear resection margin of a centimeter. Lymph node dissection is generally not required unless lymph nodes are evident clinically. A preoperative biopsy is not required when the primary lesion is considered to be likely GIST radiologically and surgically resectable. A biopsy is, however, required when the radiological diagnosis is questionable and/or for locally advanced disease to be put on neoadjuvant therapy. A biopsy is preferred over fine-needle aspiration to allow a definitive histological and molecular diagnosis. Endoscopic ultrasound-guided biopsy is the preferred technique for localized disease. US-/CT-guided percutaneous biopsy may be done only if the aforementioned option is not feasible with care to avoid tumor spill or rupture.[63]

Although smaller tumors may be laparoscopically resected (if expertise is available) following the principles of oncologic surgery it is not recommended for large tumors due to higher risk of tumor rupture which has a very high-risk of recurrence. If the risk of relapse is substantial, the patient is put on adjuvant imatinib, a tyrosine kinase inhibitor (TKI) adjuvant treatment, close monitoring of treatment response is carried out during the treatment. Imatinib is also the standard treatment for inoperable and metastatic lesions. Ideally, molecular profiling is recommended before initiation of adjuvant imatinib as some mutations are associated with TKI resistance. This is known as "primary resistance". In some patients despite a good initial response or stable disease on imatinib, tumor progression occurs after 12–36 months in one or more lesions. This is referred to as "secondary resistance" and is usually due to secondary acquired mutations in the KIT kinase domain. In case of confirmed nonresponse and disease progression or rarely intolerance to imatinib, a second-line TKI sunitinib may be used. Other drugs being tried include regorafenib, sorafenib, ripretinib, avapritinib, etc.[63]

Response Evaluation and Surveillance

Surveillance is required for all cases as recurrence occurs in many patients even after complete resection, median time to recurrence being approximately 2 years. Generally, recurrent disease first occurs in the liver or peritoneum. Response evaluation to adjuvant imatinib treatment is done on CT especially when ^{18}F-FDG-PET-CT/MRI is not available and is generally done at 3 months.

Traditional response evaluation criteria in solid tumors (RECIST) criteria based assessment of tumor size are insensitive in evaluating response to TKI as decrease in tumor size may take several months. Good response to imatinib is seen as lesions becoming homogeneous, hypoattenuating or hypodense, disappearance of enhancing nodules, and tumor vessels. These changes represent a favorable effect even in the absence of anatomic decrease in size. Consistent similar signal changes on MRI should also be considered as tumor response.[63] Choi et al. proposed CT response criteria which take into account both the tumor size and density. A complete disappearance of lesion with no new lesions is considered complete response while a 10% decrease in diameter or 15% decrease in density with no new lesions is required for partial response.[69]

A paradoxical increase in tumor size may occur during treatment. This does not imply tumor progression in the absence of enhancing nodules. It may be caused by myxoid degeneration or hemorrhage. Hemorrhage may also produce an increase in tumor attenuation complicating the CT-based assessment further. Sometimes intratumoral hemorrhage may be significant, producing possible decrease in hemoglobin levels in the first 4–8 weeks of imatinib therapy.[60] At times even the appearance of new lesions in the liver may be due to their becoming more apparent with decrease in density rather than true lesions.[60,63] Imatinib therapy may result in fluid retention which is the most common side effect. This may be seen as ascites, pleural effusion, pericardial effusion, or subcutaneous edema **(Figs. 13A and B)**. Hence, the presence of these on CT should not interpreted as new peritoneal disease.

Criteria for true disease progression include development of new lesions, increase in tumor size with new or enhancing nodules development of new lesions at previous site of disease, and finally development enhancing nodules in hypoattenuating treated tumor even without increase in tumor size which is a typical pattern of progression seen in GIST **(Figs. 14A and B)**.[63]

Fludeoxyglucose F18-positron emission tomography is extremely sensitive to detect early tumor response. A good response in the form of marked decrease in FDG uptake may be seen within 24 hours after a single dose. This may be very useful to identify early nonresponders. Response criteria using SUV_{max} on FDG-PET/CT have also been developed by some societies. Even in patients showing a paradoxical increase in size on conventional CT due to hemorrhage or myxoid degeneration FDG-PET/CT can show no increase in metabolic activity resolving the dilemma.[60,63] Other techniques that have been used include contrast-enhanced ultrasound, perfusion CT, dual-energy CT, and DW-MRI. On contrast-enhanced ultrasound, tumor response is seen as decreased tumor contrast uptake as early as day 5 or 7. Perfusion CT has also been used to both prognosticate response to treatment and monitor treatment response with decrease in perfusion parameters such as blood flow and blood volume occurring with good response.[70,71] Dual-energy CT using iodine quantification has also shown excellent results being able to distinguish between hemorrhage and enhancement. Using DW-MRI some authors have reported that ADC values correlate closely with SUV parameters derived from PET-CT.

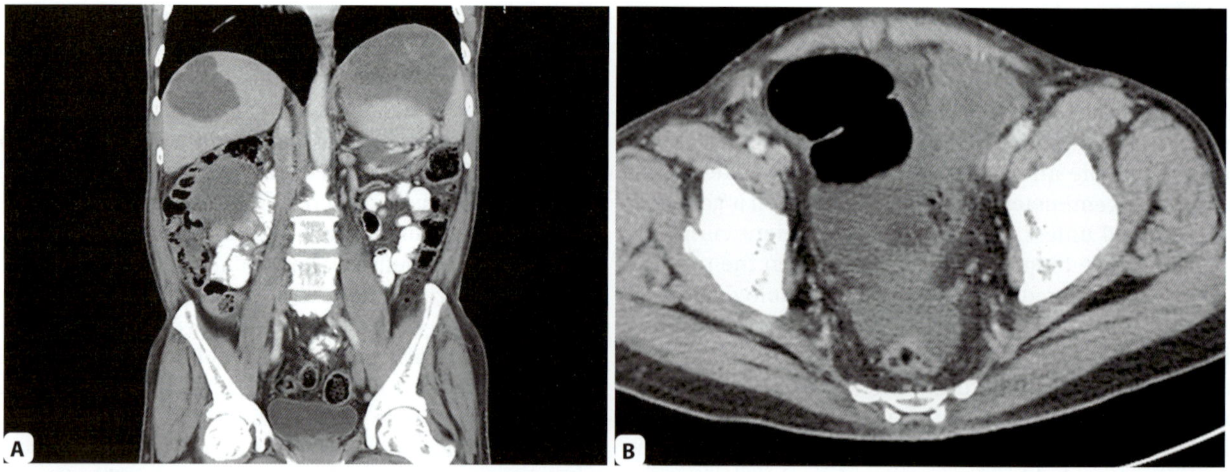

FIGS. 13A AND B: Gastrointestinal stromal tumor (GIST) on imatinib therapy: Coronal and axial contrast-enhanced computed tomography (CECT) images of a patient with hepatic and peritoneal metastases from GIST on imatinib reveal markedly hypodense lesions with no enhancing nodules consistent with a favorable response. Note the presence of free fluid in the pelvis due to fluid retention.

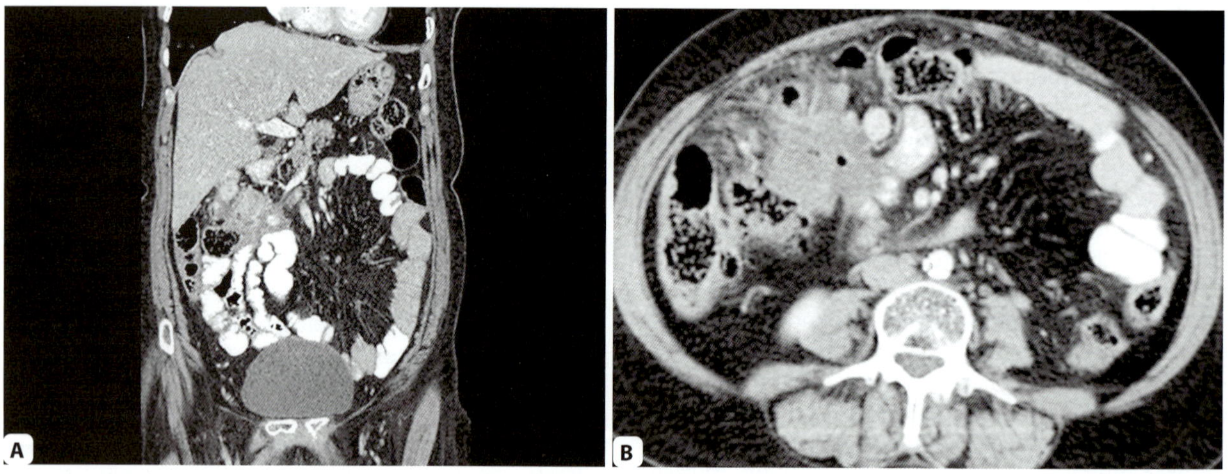

FIGS. 14A AND B: Recurrent jejunal gastrointestinal stromal tumor: Coronal and axial contrast-enhanced computed tomography (CECT) images of an operated case of jejunal gastrointestinal stromal tumor showing a heterogeneously enhancing recurrent mass with irregular and spiculated margins at the site of previous disease involving the jejunum and adjacent transverse colon.

LYMPHOMA

Gastrointestinal tract is the most common site for extranodal non-Hodgkin's lymphoma (NHL) since the lymphoid tissue occurring in the mucosa, lamina propria, and submucosa forms the largest collection of lymphocytes compared to any other immune organ in the body. Most GI tract lymphoid tissue is referred to as mucosa associated lymphoid tissue.[72-74]

Involvement of the GI tract can be primary or secondary to generalized disease. Primary GI NHL constitutes 10–15% of all NHLs and 30–40% of extranodal lymphomas. These generally involve only a single site. The criteria described by Dawson et al.[75] are used to define primary GI disease. These are:

- Predominant involvement of GI tract with lymph node involvement restricted to primary drainage area
- No palpable lymph nodes
- No liver or spleen involvement
- Normal chest radiograph, i.e., no mediastinal lymphadenopathy
- Normal peripheral white blood cell count

Although this definition was developed before the availability of cross-sectional imaging, it is still applicable.[72] Some authors, however, advocate a more liberal definition of primary GI lymphoma as lymphomas that predominantly involve the GI tract presenting with GI symptoms notwithstanding the presence or absence of lymph node involvement.[76,77]

Secondary GI tract involvement in generalized disease is much more frequent since lymphomas commonly arise in retroperitoneal and mesenteric lymph nodes. At autopsy, GI involvement has been reported in up to 50% cases although this may not be clinically evident.[75]

The primary form when diagnosed sufficiently early has a much better progress than systemic lymphoma with GI involvement. However, in advanced cases, it may be difficult to distinguish between primary and secondary involvement clinically, radiologically, and even pathologically.[78]

Etiopathogenesis and Classification

The incidence of NHL is reportedly increasing due to increasing incidence of human immunodeficiency virus (HIV) infection and a variety of environmental factors.[78] Risk factors that have been identified in the pathogenesis of small bowel lymphoma include HIV infection, celiac disease, inflammatory bowel disease, and immunosuppression after solid organ transplantation. The risk of lymphoma is 45–100 times in patients who have received allograft or marrow transplants. These tumors are commonly associated with Ebstein–Barr virus (EBV) infection and referred to as EBV-related posttransplant lymphoproliferative disorder.[78] GI tract involvement is seen in one-fourth to one-third of patients with acquired immunodeficiency syndrome (AIDS) and involvement of stomach, small and large bowel has been reported with an almost equal frequency.[72,78]

Peak incidence is in the sixth decade of life with a slight male predilection of 3:2, a small peak is also noted around 10 years. Although uncommon in childhood, lymphomas constitute the most common GI tumor in children.[78] Small bowel involvement represents about one-third of the cases of GI lymphoma and is the second most common site after the stomach. It is a common malignant tumor of the small bowel constituting about 20% of all malignant lesions. The distal ileum is the most common site likely due to the abundant lymphoid follicles in this region.[72,76,78]

The recent WHO classification of lymphomas has categorized lymphomas immunophenotypically into two major types—B-cell lineage (including Hodgkin's lymphoma) and T-cell or NK (natural killer) cell lineage.[72] The various types under these two categories that may involve the small bowel are given in **Table 3**.

TABLE 3: Classification of small bowel/gastrointestinal lymphoma.

B-cell	T-cell/NK cell
Diffuse large B-cell lymphoma (DLBCL)	Enteropathy associated T-cell lymphoma (EATL)
Extranodal marginal zone B-cell lymphoma (ENMZL) or (Malt lymphoma)	Type I and II (EATL)
Mantle cell lymphoma (MCL)	
Follicular lymphoma	
Burkitt lymphoma	
Hodgkin's lymphoma	

(NK: natural killer)

Most small bowel lymphomas like other GI lymphomas are NHLs of the B-cell lineage. Although any histological subtype can occur diffuse large B-cell lymphoma (DLBCL) is the most common type of GI lymphoma in adults. Extranodal marginal zone B-cell lymphoma (ENMZL), so named because it arises from the marginal zone of Peyer's patches, is found predominantly in the stomach but does occur in the small and large intestine also. ENMZL also referred to marginal zone lymphoma of mucosa associated lymphoid tissue (MALT lymphoma).[76] Immunoproliferative small intestinal disease (IPSID), also known as α-chain disease is a subtype of extranodal marginal zone B-cell lymphoma found in the small bowel. It is thought to occur as a result of combination of genetic risk factors and chronic infection by *Campylobacter jejuni.* It affects young adults with almost equal sex incidence and is associated with poor socioeconomic status. Patients may show α-heavy chain immunoglobulins in the serum. Infiltration of the bowel wall by plasma cells leads to protein losing enteropathy. It can transform to high-grade Mediterranean lymphoma. This condition is common in the Middle East, far east, and Mediterranean region.[78] Mantle cell lymphoma (MCL) produces multiple lymphomatous polyposis first described by Cornes in 1961.[79] Burkitt's lymphoma is a highly aggressive B-cell lymphoma.[78]

T-cell lymphomas of the small bowel represent about 10–20% of primary intestinal lymphomas. Though a variety of T-cell lymphomas may involve the small bowel, most of these are enteropathy associated T-cell lymphomas (EATL) occurring in refractory celiac disease (RCD).[72] These usually manifest over 60 years and are more common in men. Besides NHL, celiac disease is also a risk factor for small bowel adenocarcinoma, esophageal carcinoma, and melanoma.[73]

The WHO has classified enteropathy associated T-cell lymphoma or EATL as type I which is strongly associated with celiac disease and accounts for 80–90% of cases of EATL. Type II EATL is also referred to as monomorphic CD56 +ve intestinal lymphoma which is not related to celiac disease although enteropathy like changes may be found on histology. Type I generally involves the jejunum and proximal ileum as the jejunum is the site where most villous damage and inflammation occur.[72,73,80]

Clinical Presentation

Clinical features of small bowel lymphoma are nonspecific. Patients may present with malaise, pain abdomen, weight loss, fever, lump abdomen, chronic diarrhea, and occasionally GI bleed and small bowel perforation.[72]

Imaging

Conventional small bowel follows through series or enteroclysis is rarely performed these days but is useful to show small polypoid lesions. On ultrasound, these tumors produce hypoechoic circumferential or asymmetric bowel wall thickening. Aneurysmal dilatation or intussusception may also be appreciated **(Figs. 15A and B)**.[78]

Computed tomography especially enterography is useful both for initial diagnosis, staging and in the follow-up after surgery or chemotherapy. MR enterography provides similar information.[81]

Traditionally described radiological patterns[72,73,81] that are evident on barium studies and a well-performed CT or CT/MR enterography are:

- Infiltrating form
- Polypoid form/multiple nodules
- Endoexoenteric form with excavation and fistulization
- Mesenteric invasive form

Infiltrative Form

Circumferential infiltration of the bowel wall by lymphoma causes bowel wall thickening and subsequently distortion or effacement of folds. On barium studies, submucosal infiltration by tumor causes loss or effacement of mucosal folds to produce a smooth featureless appearance. The bowel lumen is generally not narrowed, in fact it may be dilated, referred to as "aneurysmal or pseudoaneurysmal dilatation". This implies a localized nonobstructive dilatation of bowel lumen with diameter >4 cm in areas of bowel wall thickening and is seen in about 31% of small bowel lymphoma. The underlying cause is the loss of bowel wall tone due to infiltration of submucosal myenteric plexus and muscularis propria by tumor **(Figs. 16A to C)**.[72,81]

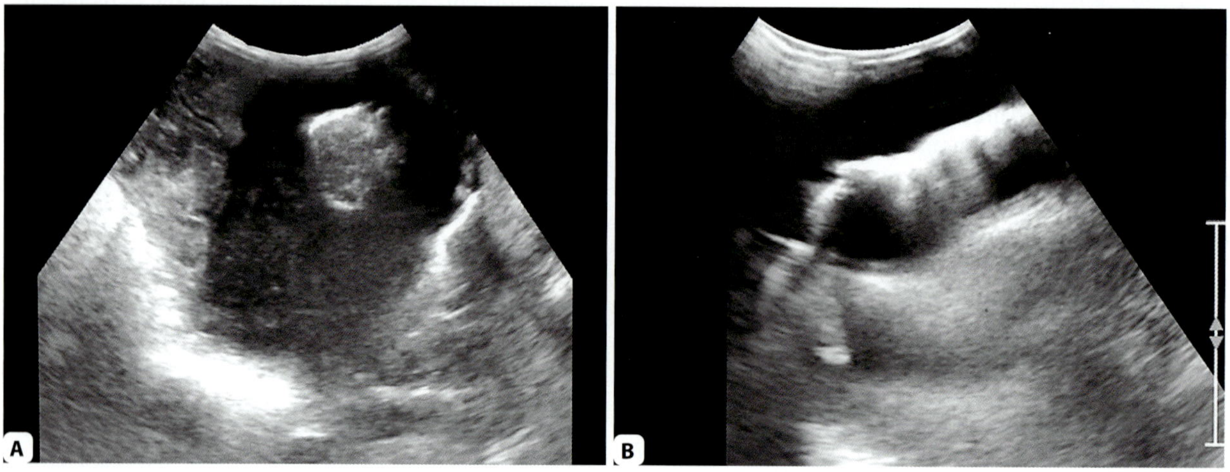

FIGS. 15A AND B: Lymphoma small bowel: Transverse and longitudinal ultrasound images reveal marked homogenously hypoechoic bowel wall thickening with the dilated hyperechoic lumen in the center.

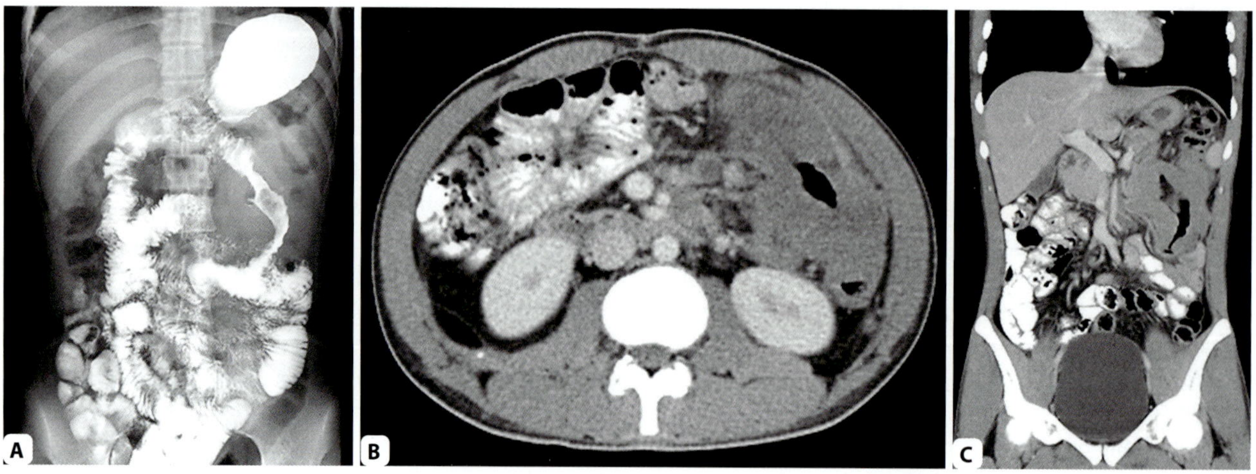

FIGS. 16A TO C: Lymphoma jejunum: Barium meal follow through examination (A) reveals an abnormal proximal jejunal loop showing a featureless appearance, fold thickening is noted along its proximal and distal aspect with separation of bowel loops due to the marked wall thickening which is appreciated on the axial and coronal CT images (B and C). The wall thickening is iso to hypodense to skeletal muscle with minimal enhancement typical of lymphoma. Note the presence of mesenteric lymphadenopathy, absence of any obstructive features with aneurysmal dilatation of lumen. Radiological features consistent with an infiltrative variety of lymphoma.

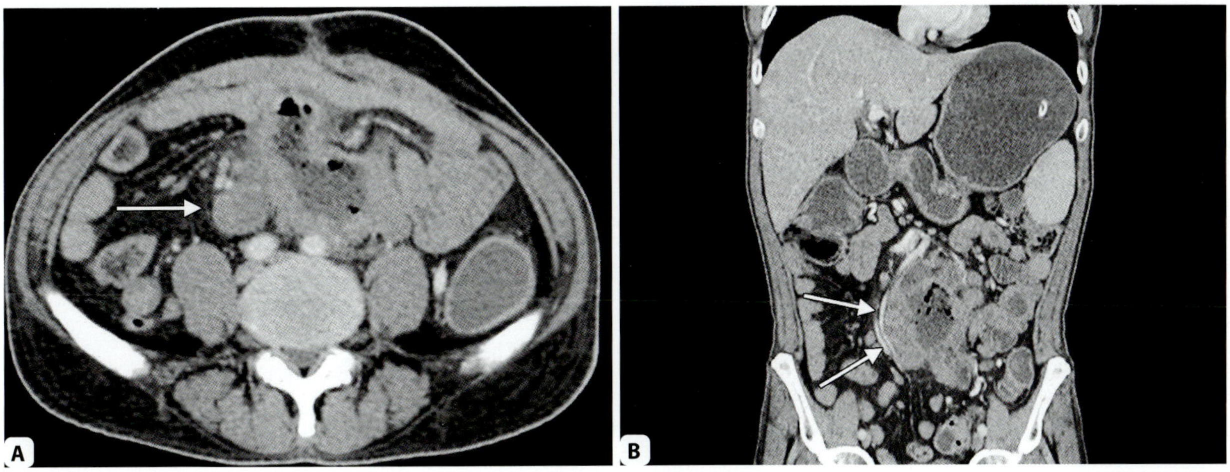

FIGS. 17A AND B: Lymphoma ileum: Axial and coronal contrast-enhanced computed tomography (CECT) images reveal hypodense mildly enhancing wall thickening involving the ileum with aneurysmal dilatation of the lumen of the involved segment. Adjacent lymphadenopathy is also noted (arrow). The mesenteric vessels (arrows) are displaced by the mass but not encased or narrowed.

On CT or MR, there is marked homogeneous circumferential thickening of bowel wall with diameter > 2 cm, generally involving a long segment of bowel. The mural thickening results in separation of bowel loops which can also be appreciated on barium studies. The bowel wall attenuation is lower than or equal to muscle attenuation on CT **(Figs. 17A and B)**. On MR, the wall tends to be isointense on T1W and mildly hyperintense on T2W. These lesions tend to show homogeneous enhancement which is generally less than that in other malignant tumors.[15,16] One study has reported lower ADC values in small bowel lymphoma compared with adenocarcinoma.[67,82]

This variety of lymphoma can generally be distinguished from carcinoma. The longer length of involvement, lack of luminal narrowing or the presence of aneurysmal dilatation, absence of obstructive features, and a smooth mural contour with bulky mesenteric adenopathy favor the diagnosis of lymphoma. Obstruction is less common than with other tumors because NHL does not evoke a desmoplastic reaction. Although aneurysmal dilatation is considered a characteristic feature of lymphoma, it can be seen with GISTs, metastatic disease, and rarely adenocarcinoma.[72,73]

Polypoid Form

This form produces multiple or solitary polypoid filling defects ranging from few mm to 4 cm in the small bowel. A polypoid lesion that is large enough may produce homogeneous polypoid nodule protruding into the lumen on CT or MR.[78] The polypoid lesions may act as a lead point for intussusception.[73] The differential diagnosis of multiple/solitary polypoid lesions includes intestinal polyposis syndromes, GISTs, lipomas, adenomas, or metastases. A positive family history (though not always present), presentation during childhood or early adulthood more widespread involvement, and characteristic extraintestinal findings may help to establish the diagnosis of polyposis syndromes.[72] Metastases are generally larger, more randomly distributed and may produce submucosal masses, "bull's eye" or target lesions with central ulceration with pooling of contrast.[73]

Endoexoenteric Form

This form is associated with bowel wall thickening, a large lymphomatous mass showing exocentric growth and deep ulceration. There may be formation of sinus tracts to mesentery with resultant sterile abscesses or fistulization to other abdominal viscera.[73] CT reveals gross wall thickening, large cavitating mass with extraluminal contrast extending into the cavity which commonly shows fluid and debris.[73,83] Similar findings may be found with cavitating GISTs and occasionally metastatic melanoma.[73]

Mesenteric Invasive Form

This produces bowel wall thickening with tethered and angulated folds contiguous with bulky mesentric mass. This is the variety most commonly associated with obstruction. On CT/MR, a "sandwich appearance" may be seen with mesenteric vessels forming the middle of the sandwich and surrounding conglomerate nodal/intestinal masses forming the outer layers **(Figs. 18A to C)**.[72,83]

Box 5 summarizes the most common imaging appearances of lymphoma.

Radiological Appearances of Some Specific Lymphoma Types

Hodgkin's variety of B-cell lymphoma rarely involves the bowel with only isolated case reports being available. This may produce a stenotic mass as it produces fibrosis unlike NHL.[72]

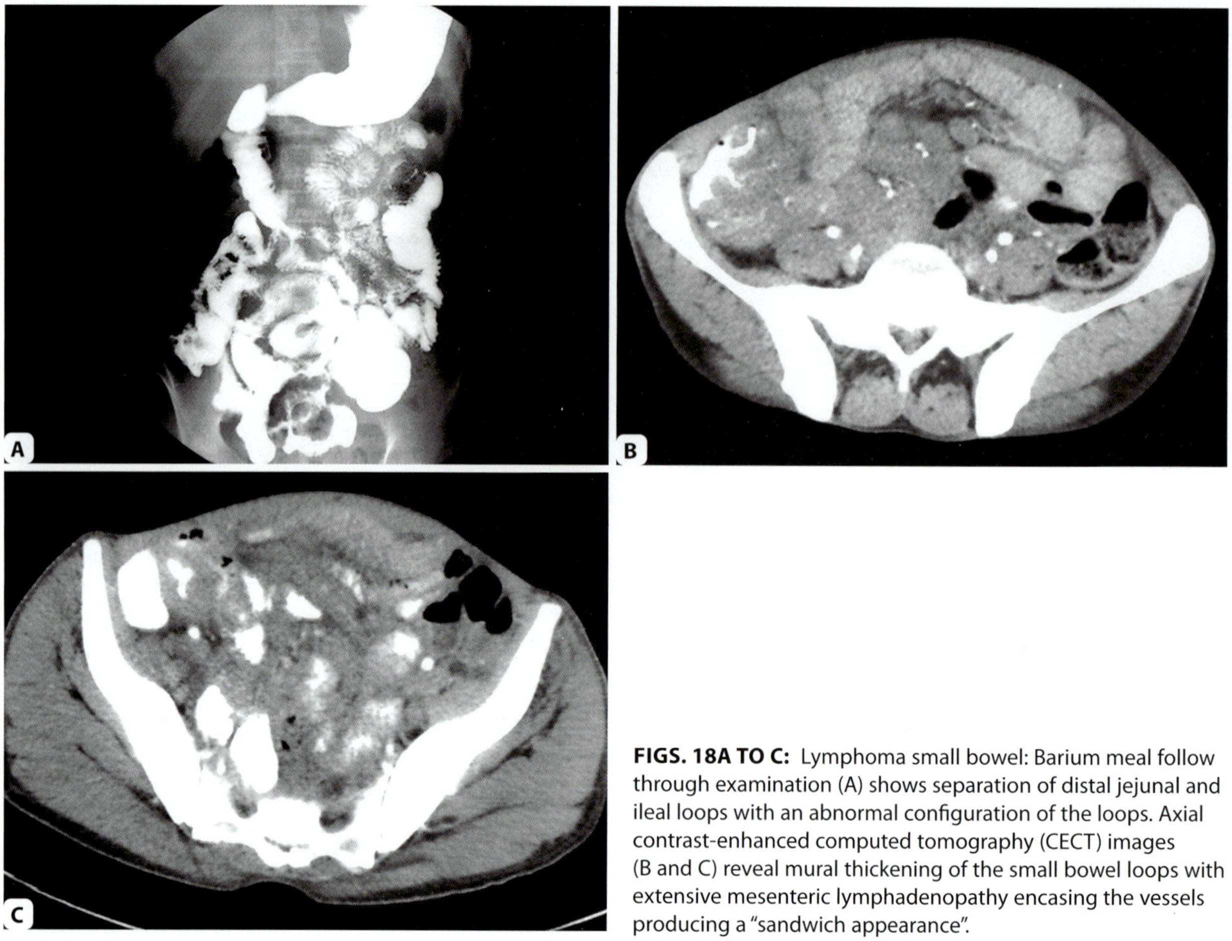

FIGS. 18A TO C: Lymphoma small bowel: Barium meal follow through examination (A) shows separation of distal jejunal and ileal loops with an abnormal configuration of the loops. Axial contrast-enhanced computed tomography (CECT) images (B and C) reveal mural thickening of the small bowel loops with extensive mesenteric lymphadenopathy encasing the vessels producing a "sandwich appearance".

BOX 5 Lymphoma key imaging findings.

- *Site*: Terminal ileum
- Long-segment involvement
- *Barium*: Fold thickening/featureless appearance, aneurysmal dilatation
- *CT/MR*: Marked homogeneous hypodense/hypoattenuating wall thickening
- Minimal enhancement
- Smooth mural contour
- Associated findings
- Bulky adenopathy
- Bowel obstruction distinctly uncommon

T-cell lymphoma on barium studies, especially enteroclysis, may depict thickened nodular folds with ulceration and stricture formation usually in the jejunum, but it can be multifocal. On CT/MR, there may be only mild-to-moderate wall thickening **(Figs. 19A and B)**. Associated lymphadenopathy and infiltration of mesenteric fat may also be seen. Perforation is much more common in this variety of lymphoma and is believed to be due to angiocentric growth of lymphoid cells with infiltration of vessel walls producing vascular occlusion and ischemic necrosis. It has been reported that perforation may be present in 16–33% of patient with types I and II EATL, respectively.[73] Laparotomy may be required in as many as 50% patients for complications such as hemorrhage, perforation, or obstruction.[72] This variety of lymphoma needs to be distinguished from other complications of celiac disease like chronic jejunoileitis (CJI) and RCD. CJI is a rare complication difficult to distinguish and considered by some to represent a low-grade enteropathy-associated T-cell lymphoma. Findings of effacement of jejunal folds, small bowel wall thickening, intussusception, infiltration of mesenteric fat, lymphadenopathy, and splenic atrophy have been reported on CT and MR in RCD. FDG-PET has an important role in distinguishing between RCD and EATL as 86–100% of EATL lymphomas show increased uptake. The 5-year survival for T-cell lymphomas at 25% is much worse than the 75% survival rate for B-cell lymphomas.[72,73]

Burkitt's Lymphoma

The endemic variety of Burkitt's lymphoma is associated with EBV infection and commonly involves the head and neck region. Other variants include sporadic variety and that associated with HIV infection (the immunodeficiency associated variant). It is a very rapidly growing tumor,

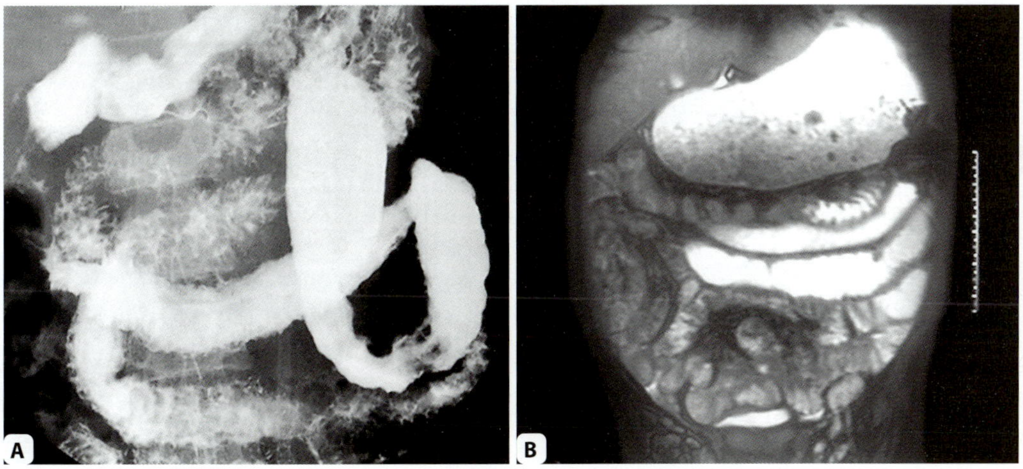

FIGS. 19A AND B: T-cell lymphoma jejunum: Barium enteroclysis (A) reveals nodular fold thickening in the jejunum with dilated featureless segment of jejunum in a patient with symptoms of malabsorption. Coronal T2-weighted magnetic resonance (T2W MR) enteroclysis image (B) shows only mild wall thickening of the involved segments.

commonly occurring in children and usually affects the terminal ileum or ileocecal region in sporadic cases. Less commonly it may involve the stomach or colon. Peak age of occurrence is 11 years. The genetic defects identified include translocation and deregulation of *c-Myc* gene on chromosome 8. On histology, a typical "starry sky appearance" is seen due to macrophage containing cellular debris lying scattered within dense sheets of lymphoid cells.[76,77]

Barium studies may show markedly thickened valvulae conniventes while grossly thickened bowel wall due to infiltration by tumor is seen on CT. There may be associated aneurysmal dilatation and intussusception with the thickened walls serving as the lead point. Diffuse lymphadenopathy, infiltration of the mesentery, and peritoneum with peritoneal carcinomatosis may be seen. These tumors show high FDG uptake on initial scans due to their rapidly prolife-rating nature which reverts to normal following treatment **(Figs. 20A to F)**.

Endemic Burkitt's lymphoma is very chemosensitive and 5-year survival rates exceed 90% in children with localized disease. Sporadic and immunodeficiency associated Burkitt's are less sensitive to chemotherapy but 50–70% overall survival rate may be seen in adults after intensive chemotherapy.

Although radiological features of lymphoma are not specific to various pathological types, some radiologic pathologic correlation does exist[76] and is summarized in **Table 4**.

Staging and Prognostication

Staging and response assessment systems in lymphoma have evolved over time owing to the introduction of radiation therapy, CT, and FDG-PET/CT. 18F-FDG-PET/CT along with a CECT has been recommended as a staging tool for all FDG avid lymphomas. For the non-FDG avid varieties, a CECT is recommended. FDG-PET/CT is also an excellent tool to evaluate early response after treatment before morphological changes become apparent allowing treatment modification, and to distinguish necrotic residual mass often seen on CT from tumor persistence which is FDG-avid.[84]

Lymphomas comprise an extremely heterogeneous group of tumors hence their metabolic activity and glucose uptake are variable with low-grade NHLs showing lower glucose uptake than aggressive lesions. Low-grade follicular lymphomas and indolent extranodal marginal zone B-cell lymphoma (ENMZL) may show very low FDG uptake making it difficult to detect primary lesions. On the other hand, DLBCL, MCL, EATL, Burkitt's lymphoma, and Hodgkin's disease are FDG avid. However, studies suggest that most low-grade lymphomas can also be accurately staged with PET/CT.[84,85] In some studies, a cut-off value of SUV_{max} at 10 reportedly had 71% sensitivity and 81% specificity in differentiating aggressive and indolent lymphomas.[84,85]

Whole body of diffusion-weighted MRI (WB-DWMRI) has also been evaluated as a tool to stage and follow-up GI lymphoma with reports suggesting comparable diagnostic value as FDG-PET-CT.[82,86]

Lugano staging[87,88] developed at a workshop in Lugano, Switzerland is a modification of the original Ann Arbor staging designed for the staging of primary GI lymphomas depicted in **Box 6**.

The Paris staging system[89,90] proposed by the European Gastrointestinal Lymphoma Study (EGILS) group is summarized in **Table 5**. The major advantage of this staging system is its ability to record the depth of tumor infiltration, specific lymphoma spread, and extent of nodal involvement.

The prognosis of NHL is better than that of adenocarcinoma as it remains confined to the bowel wall for a long time and because more effective chemotherapy is available.

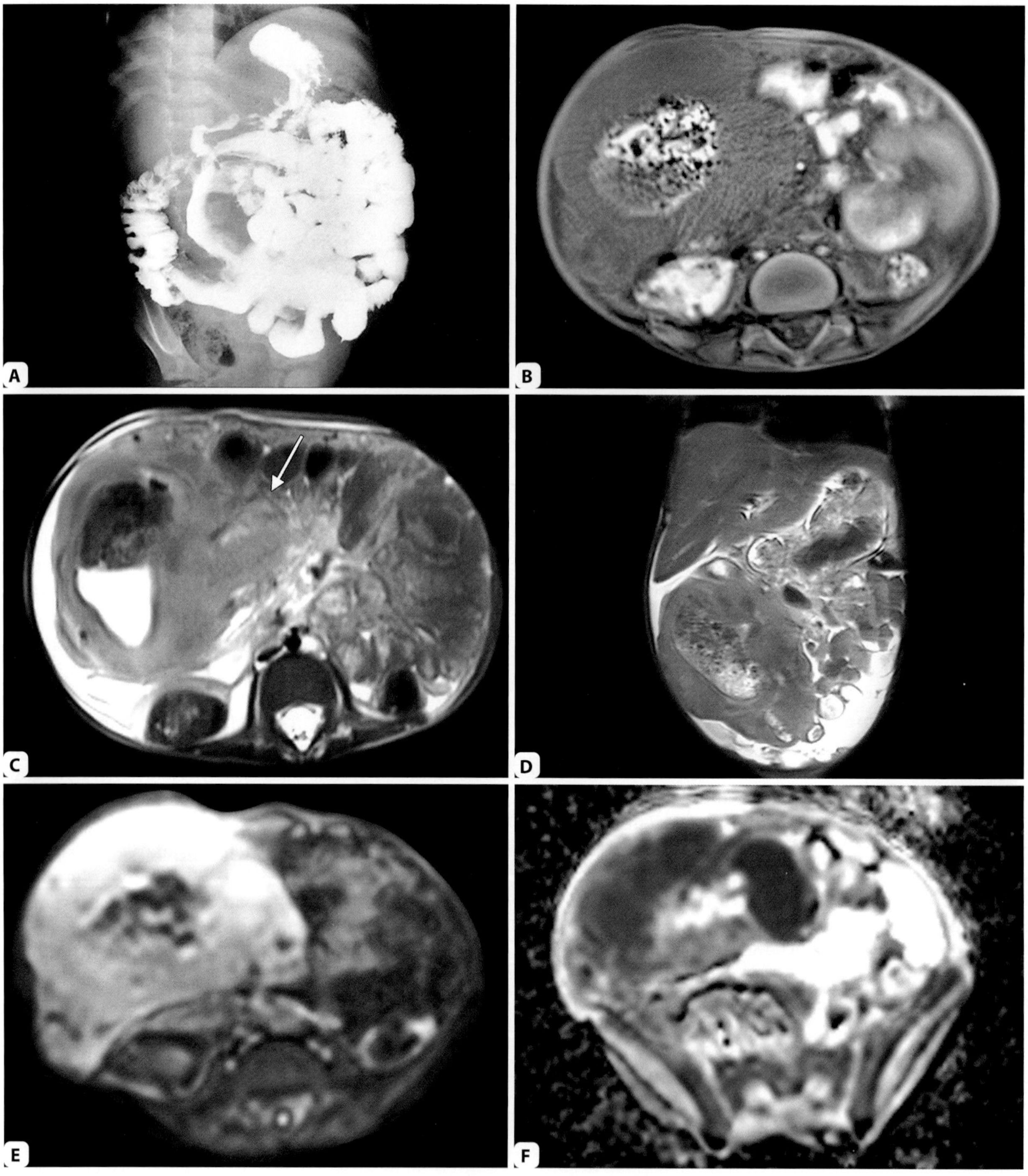

FIGS. 20A TO F: Burkitt's lymphoma: Barium meal follow through examination (A) of an 11-year-old boy presenting with a rapidly enlarging abdominal lump reveals long-segment effacement of mucosal folds resulting in a smooth featureless appearance of the distal ileum along with luminal dilatation. The presence of a significant extraluminal component is suggested by the surrounding soft-tissue haze and displacement of bowel loops. T1-weighted (T1W) axial (B), T2-weighted (T2W) axial and coronal (C and D) depict marked wall thickening of the terminal ileum appearing hypointense on T1W images, mildly hyperintense on T2W images with evidence of diffusion restriction seen as bright signal on the diffusion-weighted imaging (DWI) (E) and hypointense signal on apparent diffusion coefficient (ADC) (F). Note the presence of ascites and adjacent lymphadenopathy (arrow).

TABLE 4: Radiologic findings in various pathologic types of small bowel lymphoma.

Radiologic findings	Likely lymphoma type
1. Marked homogeneous nonobstructive bowel wall thickening, aneurysmal dilatation and bulky lymph nodes Site-distal ileum FDG-PET avid	DLBCL
2. *Barium*: Multiple small polyps *CT*: Polyps/nonobstructive bowel wall thickening and lymph nodes *Site-distal ileum, colon, and rectum*: Curvilinear areas of FDG-PET uptake	MCL Occasionally, ENMZL (more often in stomach/colon)
3. Circumferential/asymmetric wall thickening polypoid mass FDG-PET avidity variable	MCL, ENMZL
4. Nodular fold thickening site -proximal jejunum, entire small bowel in young adult males from middle east	IPSID
5. Tiny polyps/fold thickening in jejunum FDG PET—unreliable	Follicular lymphoma
6. Bulky terminal ileal/ileocecal disease in a child, rapidly progressive Strongly FDG-PET avid	Burkitt's lymphoma
7. *Barium nodular fold thickening, ulceration CT*: Long-segment eccentric circumferential mild wall thickening perforation in up to 50% Associated features of celiac disease Site-proximal jejunum FDG-PET–avid	EATL

(DLBCL: diffuse large B-cell lymphoma; EATL: enteropathy-associated T-cell lymphoma; ENMZL: extranodal marginal zone B-cell lymphoma; IPSID: immunoproliferative small intestinal disease)

BOX 6 Lugano classification for gastrointestinal lymphoma.

- *Stage I*: Tumor confined to gastrointestinal tract, single primary or multiple noncontiguous lesions
- *Stage II*: Tumor extends into the abdominal cavity from primary gastrointestinal site
- *Stage II1*: Local nodal involvement
- *Stage II2*: Distant nodal involvement
- *Stage IIE*: Penetration of serosa to involve adjacent organ or tissue
- *Stage III*: no stage III in this system
- *Stage IV*: Disseminated extranodal involvement or gastrointestinal tract lesion with supradiaphragmatic nodal involvement (CME lymphoma—12)
- Specify site of involvement, e.g., IIE pancreas. If both nodal and adjacent organ involvement—both subscript 1 or 2 and E is used, e.g., II2E (pancreas)

Note: Local/regional nodes: jejunum/ileum: mesenteric nodes and, for the terminal ileum only, the ileocolic and posterior cecal nodes.

TABLE 5: Paris staging system for primary gastrointestinal lymphomas (TNMB).

Stage	Gastrointestinal lymphomas
TX	Lymphoma extent not specified
T0	No evidence of lymphoma
T1	Lymphoma confined to the mucosa/submucosa
T1m	Lymphoma confined to the mucosa
T1sm	Lymphoma confined to the submucosa
T2	Lymphoma infiltrates muscularis propria or subserosa
T3	Lymphoma penetrates serosa (visceral peritoneum) without invasion of adjacent structures
T4	Lymphoma invades adjacent structures or organs
NX	Involvement of lymph nodes not assessed
N0	No evidence of lymph nodes involvement
N1	Involvement of regional lymph nodes
N2	Involvement of intra-abdominal lymph nodes beyond the regional area
N3	Spread to extra-abdominal lymph nodes
MX	Dissemination of lymphoma not assessed
M0	No evidence of extranodal dissemination
M1	Noncontinuous involvement of separate site in gastrointestinal tract (e.g., stomach and rectum)
M2	Noncontinuous involvement of other tissues (e.g., peritoneum and pleura) or organs (e.g., tonsils, parotid gland, ocular, adnexa, lung, liver, spleen, kidney, breast, etc.)
BX	Involvement of bone marrow not assessed
B0	No evidence of bone marrow involvement
B1	Lymphomatous infiltration of bone marrow
TNM	*Clinical staging*: Status of tumor, node, metastasis, and bone marrow
$_p$TNMB	*Histopathological staging*: Status of tumor, node metastasis, and bone marrow
pN	The histopathological examination will ordinarily include six or more lymph nodes

The adverse risk factors for GI lymphoma include advanced stage, involvement of para-aortic nodes, large tumor bulk, serosal penetration, and intestinal rather than gastric origin. Other poor prognostic factors include advanced age of patient and higher grade of lymphoma.[78,81]

Treatment

Treatment[83] usually consists of a combination of chemotherapy, surgery, and radiotherapy.

B-cell Lymphoma

Anthracycline based chemotherapy is the mainstay in the treatment of intestinal DLBCL. Primary surgery may be required at times to establish the diagnosis, reduce tumor bulk, to manage complications from perforation, obstruction and for staging. Radiotherapy may be used when there is bulky residual disease or only partial resection has been possible.

Immunoproliferative small intestinal disease is initially treated with tetracycline and metronidazole. A wait and watch policy may be adopted for lower grades of lymphoma like follicular lymphoma.

T-cell Lymphoma

Owing to its rarity the treatment of primary T-cell lymphoma is not well-defined. A gluten-free diet helps to reduce the risk of lymphoma in celiac disease. Primary surgery along with chemotherapy is generally recommended due to the risk of perforation, hemorrhage, and obstruction. However, following surgery initiation of chemotherapy is usually delayed because of postoperative infection and the difficulty in healing due to malnutrition.

KAPOSI'S SARCOMA

Kaposi's sarcoma is a tumor commonly associated with AIDS. It is a low-grade systemic vascular neoplasm involving skin in the form of pigmented cutaneous lesions, internal organs, and lymph nodes. In AIDS-associated Kaposi' sarcoma, early involvement of intestine and lymph nodes is seen. Lesions of Kaposi's sarcoma tend to be multiple and are generally seen as elevated submucosal nodules in the jejunum and ileum. Small bowel folds may be diffusely thickened. The lesions generally show mild heterogeneous enhancement. Associated retroperitoneal and mesenteric lymphadenopathy is common. Differentiation from lymphoma may be very difficult although Kaposi's sarcoma is more focal and nodular.[15,16]

LEIOMYOSARCOMA

True leiomyosarcomas of the small bowel arise from the smooth muscle of the small bowel wall or blood vessels and are very rare accounting for < 15% of primary intestinal malignant tumors. Usually, these are solitary being situated in the jejunum and ileum and most commonly in Meckel's diverticulum. The growth pattern is mainly slow extraluminal growth resulting in late presentation. Usually, tumors exceed 5 cm in size at presentation.[14,16]

On barium studies, a predominantly extrinsic lesion with barium-filled cavitation may be seen. On CT/MR, they produce large heterogeneous masses with area of necrosis and cystic degeneration with rim enhancement. There can be associated cavitation or fistulization **(Figs. 21A to C)**. Liver and peritoneal metastasis may also be seen which tend to be large with peripheral rim enhancement due to central necrosis. On imaging these cannot be distinguished from GIST.[1,14,16]

METASTATIC NEOPLASMS

Secondary metastatic involvement of the small bowel is more common than primary and may account for nearly half of all small bowel tumors.[1] The major pathways for metastatic spread are hematogenous, direct extension, intraperitoneal seeding and lymphatic.[1] Tumors from the stomach, colon, ovary, and uterus spread to the small bowel either by direct invasion or intraperitoneal spread while hematogenous metastases are seen in carcinoma breast, lung, and melanoma.

The extraintestinal malignancy with the greatest propensity to metastasize to the bowel is melanoma. Small bowel is the most frequent site involved in the GI tract owing to its rich blood supply. The vasa recti form a rich submucosal plexus on the antimesenteric border of the small bowel, hence hematogenous metastatic deposits occur on the antimesenteric border. Hematogenous metastasis may produce solitary or multiple submucosal nodules on barium studies with or without central ulceration—"the bulls' eye" appearance. On CT or MR, these produce a short segment wall thickening or focal mass with contrast enhancement and at times may mimic primary neoplasm **(Figs. 22A to D)**.[1,14,16,28]

Intraperitoneal metastases most commonly arise from the colon or ovary. Transperitoneal seedling follows the circulatory pathway of peritoneal fluid. This fluid after flowing over the mesenteric recesses settles at the termination of small bowel mesentery in the ileocecal region. Therefore, transperitoneal metastases occur at the mesenteric border. They produce small contrast-enhancing nodules along the serosal surface with disease progression they can encase the small bowel and cause obstruction. Gadolinium enhanced fat saturated MR has been shown to be more sensitive than CT to detect small tumor nodules **(Figs. 23A and B)**.[1,30,32]

Infiltration from advanced colonic, ovarian, pancreatic or biliary neoplasms can also involve the small bowel **(Figs. 24A to C)**.

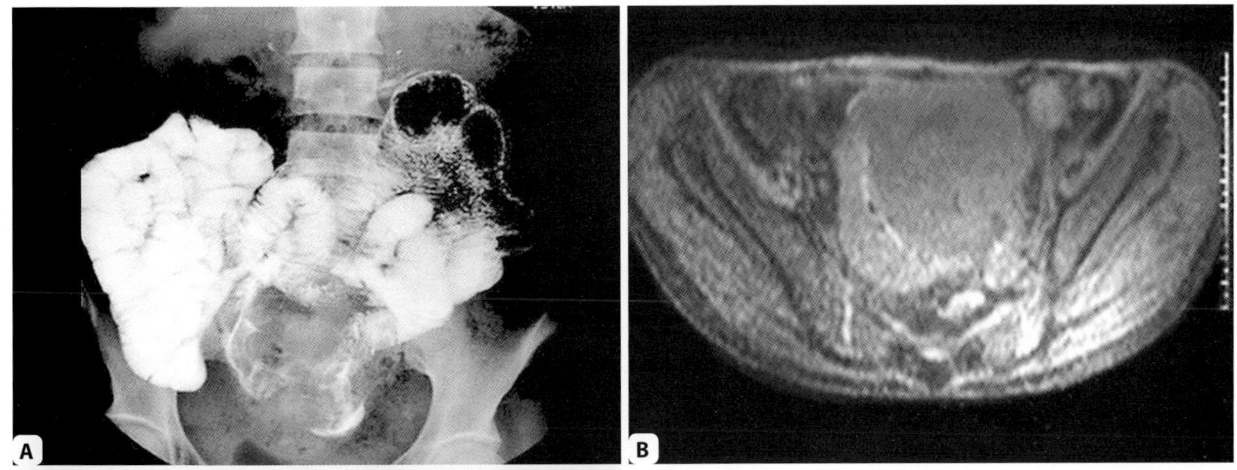

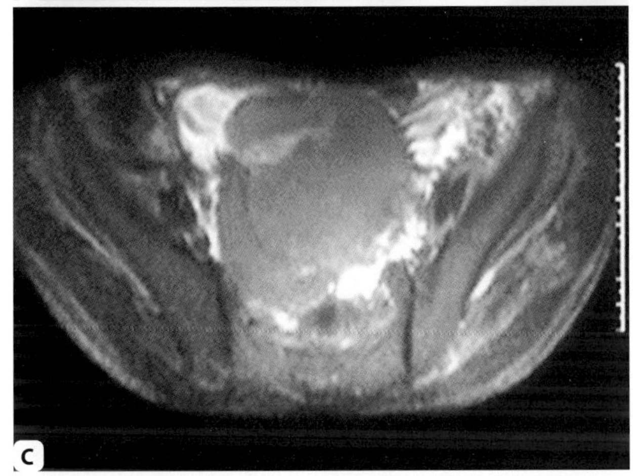

FIGS. 21A TO C: Leiomyosarcoma jejunum: Barium enteroclysis (A) depicts mucosal irregularity and ulceration in the distal jejunum with associated a soft-tissue mass as evidenced by displacement of adjacent small bowel loops. Axial T1-weighted (T1W) fat saturated (B) and T2-weighted (T2W) magnetic resonance (MR) (C) images reveal the large soft-tissue mass responsible for the barium findings. Histopathology revealed findings suggestive of leiomyosarcoma.

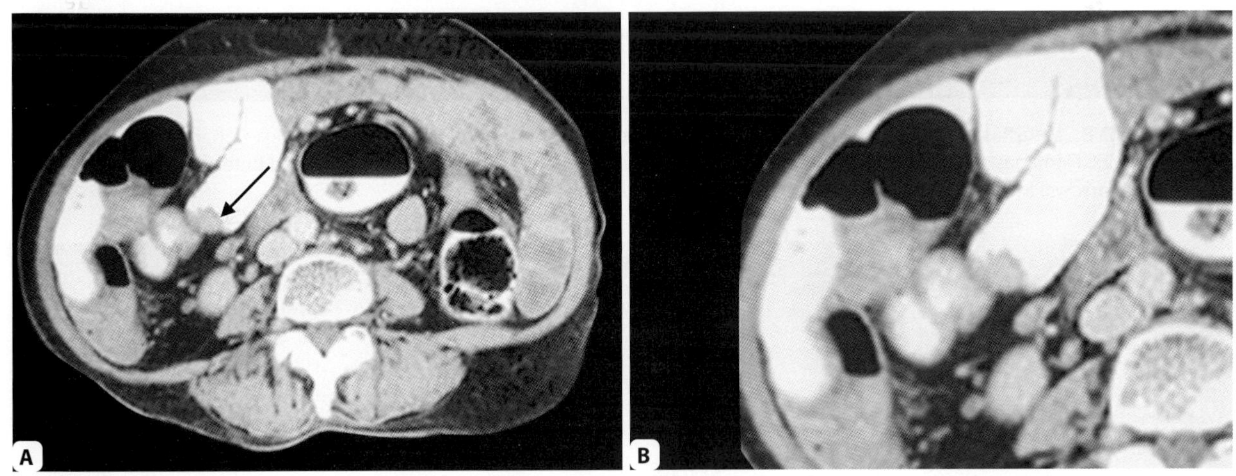

FIGS. 22A TO D: *Continued*

Continued

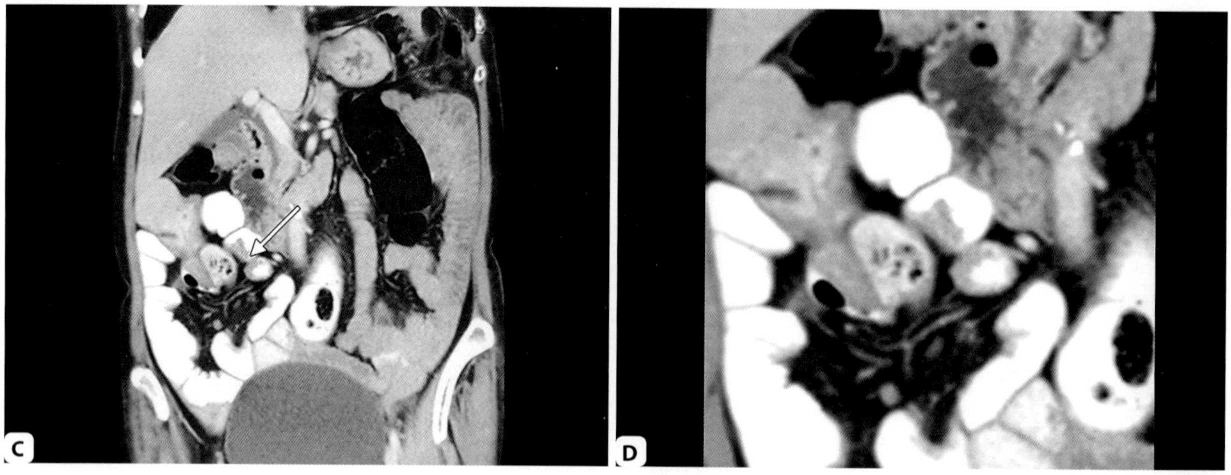

FIGS. 22A TO D: Metastases small bowel: Axial and coronal contrast-enhanced computed tomography (CECT) images (A to D) in a patient of melanoma with hematogenous metastases reveal a focal polypoid intraluminal mass and wall thickening in the jejunum better seen on the magnified images (B and D) with mild dilatation of the loops.

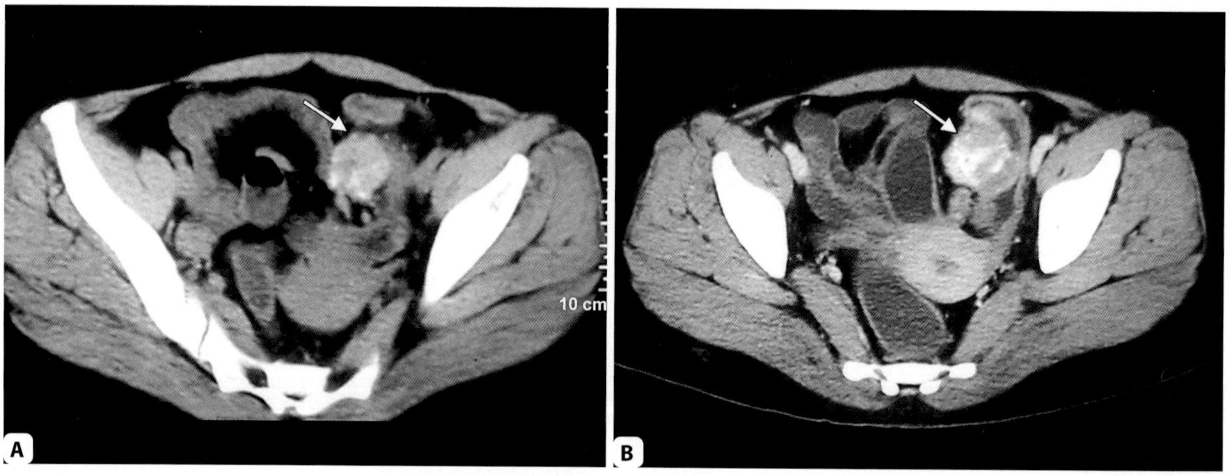

FIGS. 23A AND B: Metastases small bowel: Axial noncontrast computed tomography (NCCT) and contrast-enhanced computed tomography (CECT) images show a serosal deposit on an ileal loop in the pelvis showing calcification and heterogeneous enhancement (arrows) in an operated case of adenocarcinoma carcinoma ascending colon.

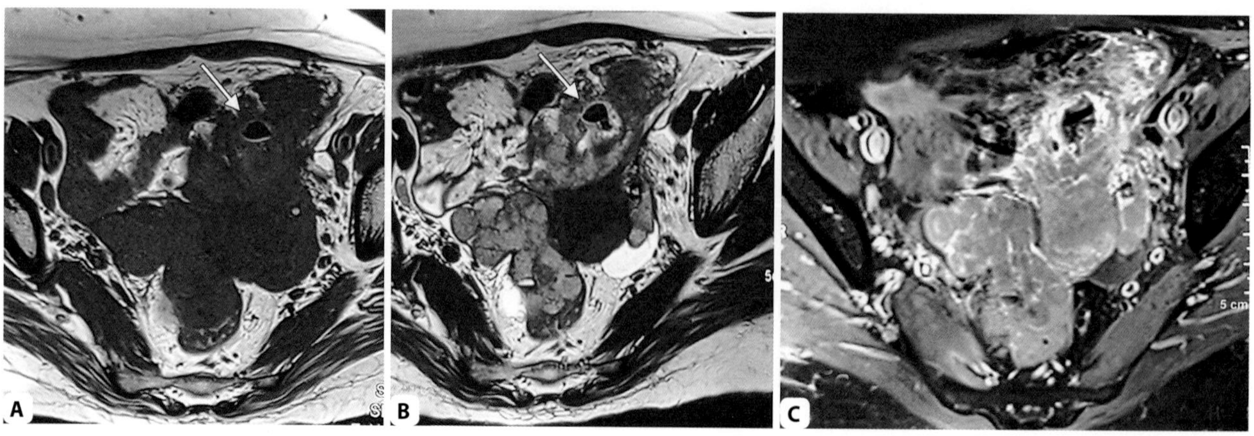

FIGS. 24A TO C: Secondary small bowel involvement: T1-weighted (T1W) (A), T2-weighted (T2W) (B) and postcontrast axial images (C) in a case of carcinoma right ovary reveals a large irregularly marginated heterogeneous mass lesion encasing and involving an ileal loop seen as an air-fluid level (arrows). Deposits are also noted in the right adnexal region and pouch of Douglas.

Non-neoplastic Mimics of Small Bowel Tumors

Non-neoplastic lesions that may mimic tumors include small bowel diverticulitis, intramural hematoma; Meckel's diverticulitis and occasionally localized lymphangiectasia. In the Indian context even atypical tubercular small bowel involvement can be a cause for confusion. Diverticulitis may simulate masses with oval lesions containing air, fluid/mottled densities, and adjacent fat standing due to inflammation. An intramural hematoma is typically associated with a history of anticoagulation, trauma, or vasculitis, with hyperattenuating wall thickening which can be marked and associated with luminal narrowing. It resolves spontaneously on subsequent imaging. Focal hypoattenuating wall thickening is seen in lymphangiectasia.

APPENDICEAL NEOPLASMS

Neoplasms of the appendix are seen in around 1% of appendectomy specimens. Acute appendicitis is the most common clinical presentation, reported more frequently in NETs than epithelial neoplasms.

The most common neoplasms are tabulated in **Box 7**.

EPITHELIAL NEOPLASMS

These tumors occur in middle age to older adults and are more often detected on imaging than NETs due to their larger size. Serum tumor markers—CA 125, CA 19.9, and CEA are elevated in most patients with advanced disease whether mucinous or nonmucinous. When initially elevated they are used for monitoring treatment response.

BOX 7 Primary tumors of the appendix.

- *Epithelial tumors (enterocyte)*:
  - Mucinous neoplasms:
    - Adenoma
    - LAMN
    - HAMN
    - Mucinous adenocarcinoma
  - Nonmucinous adenocarcinoma
  - Goblet cell carcinoma (goblet cells)
- *NETs (EC cells)*:
  - Classic
  - Tubular
- *Lymphoma (lymphoid tissue)*
- *Others*:
  - GIST
  - Nerve sheath tumors
  - Desmoid
  - Smooth muscle tumors
  - Kaposi sarcoma

(GIST: gastrointestinal stromal tumor; HAMN: high-grade appendiceal mucinous neoplasm; LAMN: low-grade appendiceal mucinous neoplasm; NET: neuroendocrine tumor)

Mucinous Epithelial Neoplasms

Mucinous epithelial neoplasms are categorized into four types by the international oncology group depending on the degree of cytologic atypia and degree of infiltration, i.e., adenoma, low-grade appendiceal mucinous neoplasm (LAMN), high-grade appendiceal mucinous neoplasm (HAMN), and mucinous adenocarcinoma.

All mucinous neoplasms whether low grade or high grade can cause pseudomyxoma peritonei (PMP) which is considered a malignant disease. PMP has a separate histologic classification as: acellular mucin, low grade, high grade, and lastly high grade with signet ring cells.

Imaging

An appendiceal mucocele, especially that measuring >2 cm in diameter, is the most frequent imaging finding of mucinous tumors. A smaller mucocele may represent a nonneoplastic simple mucous retention cyst due to luminal obstruction. On US, a mucocele is seen as an elliptical cystic structure with variable echogenicity in the right iliac fossa with an occasional *onion peel* appearance and mural calcification. On CT, an appendix distended with low attenuation material is seen **(Figs. 25A to D)**. Asymmetric wall thickening, mural nodularity, and septae may help to distinguish from malignant benign mucoceles. Periappendiceal stranding and free fluid may be seen in both scenarios.

Careful search for extramural mucin should be done in all cases, which indicates the development of PMP. This may be initially localized to the periappendiceal space. Spread subsequently occurs along the normal flow of peritoneal fluid with low attenuation deposits occurring in the pelvis, paracolic gutters, perihepatic space, omentum, and bowel. Extensive disease can be distributed throughout the peritoneal cavity producing large volume ascites. Associated scalloping of surfaces of solid abdominal organs is characteristic and represents a combination of mass effect as well as parenchyma invasion **(Figs. 26A and B)**. These mucinous deposits can show calcific foci and may result in bowel obstruction. It is said an appendiceal mucinous tumor is almost invariably the cause of PMP, though uncommonly it may arise from tumors of the ovary, colon, pancreas, and urachus. Hence, even when mucinous ovarian neoplasms are seen in patients with PMP, a careful search for an appendiceal neoplasm should be done.

Tumor implants >5 cm in size on the small bowel, adjoining mesentery extensive disease in the upper abdomen and presence of ureteric obstruction suggest high-grade disease and a poor prognosis. MRI with DWI, use of fat saturation, and delayed postcontrast imaging is an excellent technique for disease detection. DWI, especially, can help to differentiate between cellular

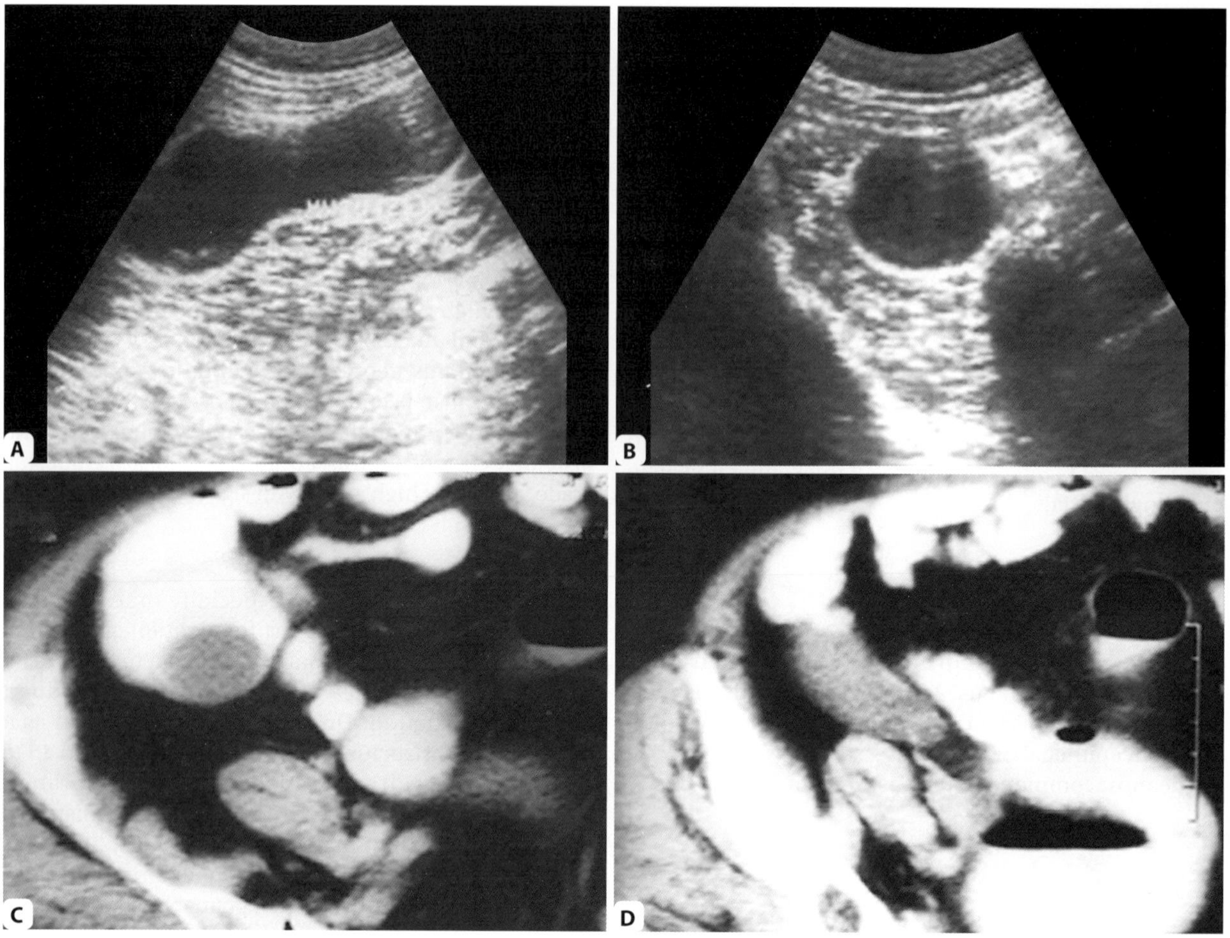

FIGS. 25A TO D: Mucocele of the appendix. (A and B) Axial and longitudinal views on sonography show a well-defined, thin-walled, tubular, fluid-filled mass in the right iliac fossa; (C and D) Axial contrast-enhanced computed tomography (CECT) scans show the mucocele invaginating into base of cecum. No wall thickening or nodularity is noted.

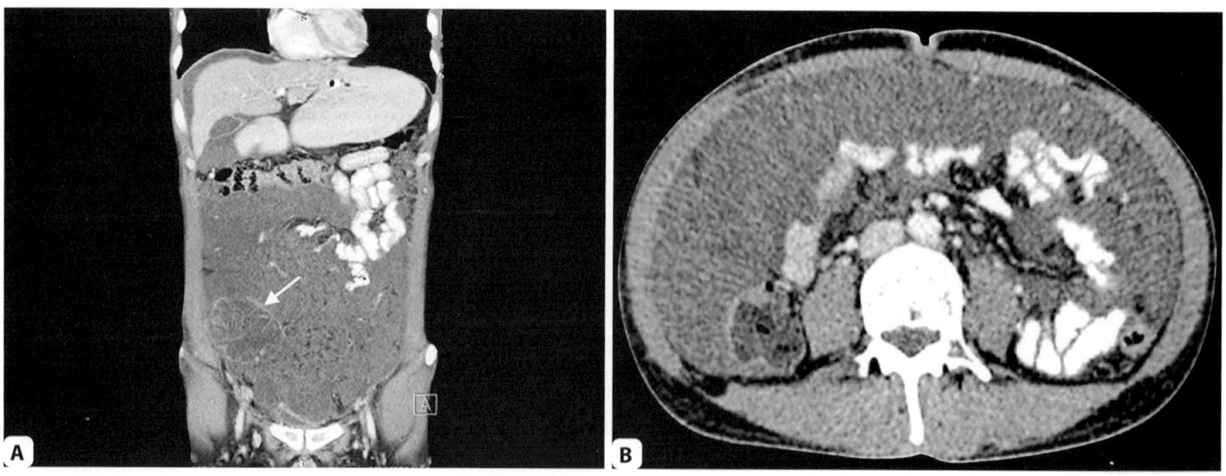

FIGS. 26A AND B: Pseudomyxoma peritonei from mucinous adenocarcinoma of the appendix manifesting as increasing abdominal girth in a 48-year-old man. Coronal (A) and axial (B) contrast-enhanced computed tomography (CECT) scan show a multiloculated mass in the right iliac fossa (arrow in A) with displacement and distortion of the bowel caused by diffuse intraperitoneal locules of pseudomyxoma peritonei which appears denser than simple fluid.

implants and acellular mucin. PET-CT, because of its low sensitivity, is not routinely used.

The staging system for appendiceal mucinous adenocarcinoma is different from colonic adenocarcinoma due to differences in prognosis and natural history. The TNM stage takes into account the histologic grade besides other components usually included in TNM staging. Detailed TNM staging is not discussed here; however, certain pertinent facts include—periappendiceal mucin constitutes T4 disease, while the presence of mucin beyond this area indicates metastatic disease (M1a).

Treatment and Prognosis

Treatment of appendiceal mucinous neoplasms depends on histologic type, TNM stage, and peritoneal disease. Adenomas and LAMN confined to the appendix are managed by appendectomy. LAMN with nodes, HAMN or adenocarcinoma without peritoneal dissemination require right hemicolectomy with lymph node dissection besides appendectomy. The treatment option for patients with peritoneal spread—whether cytoreductive surgery (CRS) or hyperthermic intraperitoneal chemotherapy (HIPEC) is decided based on laparoscopic extent of peritoneal disease and histologic characteristics of the primary and peritoneal disease. CRS aims at surgical resection of all visible tumor (>2.5 mm) while HIPEC involves intraperitoneal infusion of chemotherapeutic agents at 42°C immediately after cytoreductive surgery. The lymph node status has little impact on the outcome of patients with peritoneal disease treated with CRS or HIPEC. Extraperitoneal metastatic disease is generally considered a contraindication to surgery with curative intent. Other absolute contraindications for CRS with HIPEC include biliary obstruction and multiple small bowel obstructions, while a foreshortened mesentery is a relative contraindication.

Recurrence of mucinous adenocarcinoma is common and morbidity and mortality are generally due to PMP and associated complications.

Nonmucinous or Colonic Type Neoplasms[91,92]

These tumors have the same histologic features as those of colonic neoplasms and share the same classification, i.e., adenomas, polyps, and adenocarcinoma. They are less common than their mucinous counterparts accounting for 10–30% of epithelial neoplasms. They most frequently present as acute appendicitis due to luminal obstruction usually around the sixth decade and do not produce mucoceles.

On imaging a soft-tissue mass or focal wall thickening should be carefully looked for. Periappendiceal fat stranding may represent changes of acute appendicitis or tumor infiltration. Direct infiltration of adjacent organs, regional and distant lymphadenopathy, and visceral metastases should raise the possibility of nonmucinous adenocarcinoma. Peritoneum, liver, ovary, and lungs are the most common sites of spread.

Limited data is available, hence staging and management of these tumors follows that of colonic carcinoma.

Goblet Cell Adenocarcinoma[91,92]

Goblet cell tumors (GCTs) are infiltrative tumors that arise from goblet cells in the epithelium and show an overwhelming predilection for the appendix. On histology, they show components of both adenocarcinoma and carcinoid and are referred to in previous literature as "Goblet cell carcinoid". A higher proportion of the former component indicates a poorer prognosis. They may be mucinous or nonmucinous and imaging features are similar to adenocarcinoma.

Localized disease is treated with hemicolectomy while nodal involvement requires adjuvant chemotherapy. CRS and HIPEC are indicated for metastasis limited to peritoneal cavity only.

Goblet cell tumor has a better prognosis than adenocarcinoma but long-term surveillance should be done.

NEUROENDOCRINE TUMORS[91,92]

Neuroendocrine tumors of the appendix are detected in 0.3–0.9% of appendectomy specimens making them the most common appendiceal neoplasms. They are generally seen around the fourth decade, more often in females. Around 75% of these occur at the apex while 25% occur at the base, the latter may present with acute appendicitis.

Due to their small size (mean diameter—1 cm) they are often not seen on imaging, and detected in postoperative appendectomy specimens. When seen on CT, hyperenhancing nodular mucosal thickening and at times calcification may be evident. The latter can be misdiagnosed as an appendicolith. A mesenteric mass, similar to small bowel NETs, may also be seen. Lymphadenopathy and metastatic diseases are rare being evident in < 10% of cases. Tumors that are < 2 cm in size are unlikely to have either lymphadenopathy or metastatic disease, whereas larger tumors may show the same in up to a third of cases.

In patients in whom a NET over 2 cm in size is discovered in the postoperative specimen, cross-sectional imaging of abdomen and pelvis should be done. The same is true if resection margins are positive or there is associated carcinoid syndrome or metastatic disease. In the presence of carcinoid syndrome a chest CT, chromogranin A and urinary 5-HIAA are also recommended. DOTANOC PET-CT is useful like in small bowel NETs.

Grading of these tumors is done based on the WHO 2019 classification (see **Box 2**) while the TNM classification takes into account tumor size and depth of invasion.

Tumors < 1 cm are treated with simple appendectomy while those larger than 2 cm require right hemicolectomy and lymphadenectomy. The treatment of tumors between these two groups is variable.

Follow-up with physical examination and CGA levels and cross-sectional imaging at 3–12 months is recommended for tumors larger than 2 cm. Annual surveillance is then recommended by some up to 10 years. Octreotide analogs can be used in patients with metastatic disease and carcinoid syndrome.

APPENDICEAL LYMPHOMA

Primary appendiceal lymphoma is extremely rare and is seen as diffuse, marked wall thickening with preserved shape and sometimes aneurysmal dilatation. Secondary involvement may be seen with regional lymphadenopathy and bowel involvement.

Treatment of primary disease is surgery with chemotherapy or radiotherapy, if needed.

DIFFERENTIAL DIAGNOSIS

Since appendiceal tumors may present with acute appendicitis, it is important to carefully search for findings such as irregular, nodular wall thickening presence of a solid mass or infiltration which could suggest an associated neoplasm especially in older individuals. Other findings which should raise the suspicion of a co-existing mucocele in acute appendicitis are outer appendiceal diameter of over 15 mm, cystic appendiceal dilatation, luminal diameter over 13 mm and mural calcification.

CONCLUSION

Small bowel and appendiceal tumors are rare neoplasms, this combined with the nonspecific presentation and the relative difficulty in evaluation makes early diagnosis of these lesions difficult. Despite advances in endoscopy, the radiologist continues to play a key role in their diagnosis. The imaging features of various small bowel tumors may overlap with each other, however, recognition of certain characteristic features on imaging studies may help to narrow the differential. The imaging findings of appendiceal neoplasms may be mimic those of acute appendicitis and hence may be overlooked on cross-sectional imaging. The radiologist therefore needs to be fully conversant with the imaging features of small bowel and appendiceal tumors and consider these as a differential diagnosis in the appropriate clinical and radiologic context to avoid delay in diagnosis.

REFERENCES

1. Xynopoulos D, Mihas AA, Paraskevas E, Dimitroulopoulos D, Heuman DM, Mihas AA. Small bowel tumors. Ann Gastroenterol. 2002;15(1):18-35.
2. Martin RG. Malignant tumors of the small intestine. Surg Clin N Am. 1986;66:779-85.
3. Neugut AI, Jacobson JS, Suh S, Mukherjee R, Arber N. The epidemiology of cancer of the small bowel. Cancer Epidemiol Biomarkers Prev. 1999;7:243-51.
4. Pourmand K, Itzkowitz SH. Small Bowel Neoplasms and Polyps Current Gastroenterology Reports. 2016;18:23.
5. Hara AK, Leighton JA, Sharma VK, Height RI, Fleischer DE. Imaging of Small Bowel Disease: Comparison of Capsule Endoscopy, Standard Endoscopy, Barium Examination and CT. Radiographics. 2005;25:697-718.
6. Nolan DJ, Traill ZC. The current role of barium examination of the small intestine. Clin Radiol. 1997;52:809-20.
7. Wale A, Pilcher J. Current Role of Ultrasound in Small Bowel Imaging. Semin Ultrasound CT MR. 2016;37(4):301-12.
8. Pilleul F, Penigaud M, Milot L, Saurin JC, Chayvialle JA, Valette PJ. Possible small-bowel neoplasms: contrast-enhanced and water-enhanced multidetector CT enteroclysis. Radiology. 2006;241(3):796-801.
9. Pappalardo G, Gualdi G, Nunziale A, Masselli G, Floriani I, Casciani E. Impact of magnetic resonance in the preoperative staging and the surgical planning for treating small bowel neoplasms. Surg Today. 2013;43(6):613-9.
10. Goh V, Prezzi D, Mallia A, Bashir U, Stirling JJ, John J, et al. Positron Emission Tomography/Magnentic Resonance Imaging of Gastrointestinal Cancers: Seminars in Ultrasound CT and MRI. 2016;37(4):352-7.
11. Levine MS, Rubesin SE, Laufer I. Pattern Approach for Diseases of Mesenteric Small Bowel on Barium Studies. Radiology. 2008;249(2):445-60.
12. Rubesin SE. Simplified approach to differential diagnosis of small bowel abnormalities. Radiol Clin North Am. 2003;41:343-64.
13. Lappas JC, Maglinte DD, Sandrasegaran K. Benign tumors of the small-bowel. In: Gore R, Levine M (Eds). Textbook of gastrointestinal radiology, 3rd edition. Philadelphia, PA: Saunders Elsevier; 2008. pp. 845-51.
14. Sailer J, Zacherl J, Schimaa W. MDCT of small bowel tumors. Cancer Imaging. 2007;7(1):224-33.
15. Masselli G, Polettini E, Casciani E, Bertini L, Vecchioli A, Gualdi G. Small-bowel neoplasm: prospective evaluation of MR enteroclysis. Radiology. 2009;251:743-50.
16. Masselli G, Colaiacomo MC, Marcelli G, et al. MRI of the small-bowel: how to differentiate primary neoplasms and mimickers. British J Radiol. 2012;85(1014):824-37.
17. CY Lee, MK Yuen. Inflammatory fibroid polyps causing intussusception in adult patients: Two case reports and review of literature focusing on radiological features. Hong Kong J Radiol. 2014;17:271-6.
18. Thompson WM. Imaging and Findings of Lipomas of the Gastrointestinal Tract. Am J Roentgenol. 2005;184:1163-71.
19. Corsi A, Ingegnoli A, Abelli P, De Chiara F, Mancini C, Cavestro GM, et al. Imaging of a small bowel cavernous hemangioma: report of a case with emphasis on the use of computed tomography and enteroclysis. Acta Biomed. 2007;78(2):139-43.
20. Huprich JE, Barlow JM, Hansel SL, Alexander JA, Fidler JL. Multiphase CT Enterography Evaluation of Small-Bowel Vascular Lesions. Am J Roentgenol. 2013;201:65-72.
21. Buck JL, Harned RK. Polyposis syndromes. In: Gore RM, Levine MS (Eds). Textbook of Gastrointestinal Radiology, 2nd edition. Philadelphia, Pa: Saunders; 2000. pp. 1075-88.

22. Durno CA. Colonic polyps in children and adolescents. Can J Gastroenterol. 2007;21(4):233-9.
23. Brucher BL, Roder JD, Fink U, Stein HJ, Busch R, Siewert JR. Prognostic factors in resected primary small bowel tumors. Dig Surg. 1998;15:42-51.
24. Aparicio T, Zaanan A, Svrcek M, Laurent-Puig P, Carrere N, Manfredi S, et al. Small bowel adenocarcinoma: epidemiology, risk factors, diagnosis and treatment. Dig Liver Dis. 2014;46:97-104.
25. Negri E, Bosetti C, La Vecchia C, Fioretti F, Conti E, Franceschi S. Risk factors for adenocarcinoma of the small intestine. Cancer. 1999;82:171-4.
26. Maglinte DD, Lappas JC, Sandrasegaran K. Malignant Tumors of the small bowel. In: Gore R, Levine M (Eds). Textbook of Gastrointestinal Radiology, 3rd edition. Philadelphia, PA: Saunders Elsevier; 2008. pp. 853-69.
27. Masselli G, Gualdi G. Evaluation of small bowel tumors: MR enteroclysis: Abdm Imaging. 2010;35:23-30.
28. Faggian A, Fracella MR, D'Alesio G, Alabiso ME, Berritto D, Feragalli B, et al. Small-Bowel Neoplasms: Role of MRI Enteroclysis. Gastroenterol Res Pract. 2016:Article ID 9686815, 6 pages.
29. Cronin CG, Scott J, Kambadakone A, Catalano OA, Sahani D, Blake MA, et al. Utility of positron emission tomography/CT in the evaluation of small bowel pathology. Br J Radiol. 2012;85(1017):1211-21.
30. Sinha R, Rajiah P, Ramachandran I, Sanders S, Murphy PD. Diffusion-weighted MR imaging of the gastrointestinal tract: technique, indications, and imaging findings. Radiographics. 2013;33(3):655-76.
31. Kyriazi S, Collins DJ, Morgan VA, Giles SL, deSouza NM. Diffusion-weighted imaging of peritoneal disease for non-invasive staging of advanced ovarian cancer. Radiographics. 2010;30(5):1269-85.
32. Low RN, Sebrechts CP, Barone RM, Muller W. Diffusion-weighted MRI of peritoneal tumors: comparison with conventional MRI and surgical and histopathologic findings—a feasibility study. AJR. 2009;193(2):461-70.
33. Sobin LH, Gospodarowicz MK, Wittekind C. TNM classification of malignant tumors, 7th edition. United States: Wiley Blackwell; 2009. pp. 153-9.
34. Cunningham D, Atkin W, Lenz HJ, Lynch HT, Minsky B, Nordlinger B, et al. Colorectal cancer. Lancet. 2010;375(9719):1030-47.
35. Langhans T. Ubereinendrusenpolypimileum. Virchow Archiv Pathol Anatom Phys Klin Med. 1867;38:559-60.
36. Lubarsch O. Ueber den primaren krebs des ileum nebst bemerkungen uber das gleichzeitige vorkommen von krebs and tuberculose. Virchow Archiv Pathol Anatom Phys Klin Med. 1888;111:280-317.
37. Oberndorfer S. Karzinoide tumoren des dunndarms. Frankf Z Pathol. 1907;9:425-9.
38. Yao JC, Hassan M, Phan A, Dagohoy C, Leary C, Mares JE, et al. One hundred years after "carcinoid": epidemiology of and prognostic factors for neuroendocrine tumors in 35,825 cases in the United States. J Clin Oncol. 2008;26:3063-72.
39. Ganeshan D, Bhosale P, Yang T, Kundra V. Imaging features of carcinoid tumor of gastrointestinal tract. Am J Roentgenol. 2013;201(4):773-86.
40. Rindi G, Bordi C. Highlights of the biology of endocrine tumors of the gut and pancreas. Endocr Relat Cancer. 2003;10:427-36.
41. Chang S, Choi D, Jin Lee S, Jae Lee W, Park M, Sang Won Kim, et al. Neuroendocrine Neoplasms of the Gastrointestinal Tract: Classification, Pathologic Basis, and Imaging Features. Radiographics. 2007;27:1667-79.
42. Williams GT. Endocrine tumors of the gastrointestinal tract-selected topics. Histopathology. 2007;50(1):30-41.
43. Duh QY, Hybarger CP, Geist R, Gamsu G, Goodman PC, Gooding GA, et al. Carcinoids associated with multiple endocrine neoplasia syndromes. Am J Surg. 1987;154(1):142-8.
44. Karatzas G, Kouraklis G, Karayiannakis A, Patapis P, Givalos N, Kaperonis E. Ampullary carcinoid and jejunal stromal tumor associated with von Recklinghausen's disease presenting as gastrointestinal bleeding and jaundice. Eur J Surg Oncol. 2000;26(4):428-9.
45. Levy AD, Sobin LH. Gastrointestinal Carcinoids: Imaging Features with Clinicopathologic Comparison. Radiographics. 2007;27:237-57.
46. Popa O, Taban SM, Pantea S, Plopeanu AD, Barna RA, Cornianu M, et al. The new WHO classification of gastrointestinal neuro-endocrine tumors and immunohistochemical expression of somatostatin receptor 2 and 5. Exp Ther Med. 2021;22(4):1179.
47. Tran CG, Sherman SK, Howe JR. Small Bowel Neuroendocrine Tumors. Curr Probl Surg. 2020;57(12):100823.
48. Horton KM, Kamel I, Hofmann L, Fishman EK. Carcinoid tumors of the small bowel: a multitechnique imaging approach. AJR. 2004;182:559-67.
49. Paulsen SR, Huprich JE, Fletcher JG, Booya F, Young BM, Fidler JL, et al. CT enterography as a diagnostic tool in evaluating small bowel disorders: review of clinical experience with over 700 cases. Radiographics. 2006;26:641-57, discussion 657-62.
50. Woodard PK, Feldman JM, Paine SS, Baker ME. Midgut carcinoid tumors: CT findings and biochemical profiles. J Comput Assist Tomogr. 1995;19:400-5.
51. Bader TR, Semelka RC, Chiu VC, Armao DM, Woosley JT. MRI of carcinoid tumors: spectrum of appearances in the gastrointestinal tract and liver. J Magn Reson Imaging. 2001;14:261-9.
52. Pantongrag-Brown L, Buetow PC, Carr NJ, Lichtenstein JE, Buck JL. Calcification and fibrosis in mesenteric carcinoid tumor: CT findings and pathologic correlation. Am J Roentgenol. 1995;164:387-91.
53. Maglinte DDT, Herlinger H. Small bowel neoplasms. In: Herlinger H, Maglinte DDT, Birnbaum BA (Eds). Clinical imaging of the small intestine, 2nd edition. New York, NY: Springer; 1999. pp. 377-438.
54. Reznek RH. CT/MRI of neuroendocrine tumors. Cancer Imaging. 2006;6(Spec No A):S163-S177.
55. Hofman MS, Lau WF, Hicks RJ. Somatostatin receptor imaging with 68Ga DOTATATE PET/CT: clinical utility, normal patterns, pearls, and pitfalls in interpretation. Radiographics. 2015;35(2):500-16.
56. Pelage JP, Soyer P, Boudiaf M, Brocheriou-Spelle I, Dufresne AC, Coumbaras J, et al. Carcinoid tumors of the abdomen: CT features. Abdom Imaging. 1999;24(3):240-5.
57. Adams S, Baum R, Rink T, Schumm-Drager PM, Usadel KH, Hor G. Limited value of fluorine-18 fluorodeoxyglucose positron emission tomography for the imaging of neuroendocrine tumors. Eur J Nucl Med. 1998;25:79-83.
58. Binderup T, Knigge U, Loft A, Mortensen J, Pfeifer A, Federspiel B, et al. Functional imaging of neuroendocrine

tumors: a head-to-head comparison of somatostatin receptor scintigraphy, 123I-MIBG scintigraphy, and 18F-FDG PET. J Nucl Med. 2010;51:704-12.
59. Zalom ML, Waxman AD, Yu R, Lee J, Ih G, Wolin EM. Metabolic and receptor imaging in patients with neuroendocrine tumors: comparison of fludeoxyglucose-positron emission tomography and computed tomography with indium in 111 pentetreotide. Endocr Pract. 2009;15:521-7.
60. Hong X, Choi H, Loyer EM, Benjamin RS, Trent JC, Charnsangavej C. Gastrointestinal stromal tumor: Role of CT in diagnosis and in response evaluation and surveillance after treatment with Imatinib. Radiographics. 2006;26:481-95.
61. Mazur MT, Clark HB. Gastric stromal tumors: reappraisal of histogenesis. Am J Surg Pathol. 1983;7:507-19.
62. Sripathi S, Rajagopal KV, Srivastava RK, Ayachit A. CT Features, Mimics and Atypical Presentations of Gastrointestinal Stromal Tumor (GIST). Indian J Radiol Imaging. 2011;21(3):176-81.
63. Serrano C, Martín-Broto J, Asencio-Pascual JM, López-Guerrero JA, Rubió-Casadevall J, Bagué S, et al. 2023 GEIS Guidelines for gastrointestinal stromal tumors. Adv Med Oncol. 2023;15:17588359231192388.
64. Levy D, Remotti HE, Thompson WM, Sobin LH, Miettinen M. Gastrointestinal stromal tumors: radiologic features with pathologic correlation. Radiographics. 2003;23(2):283-304.
65. Inoue A, Ota S, Yamasaki M, Batsaikhan B, Furukawa A, Watanabe Y. Gastrointestinal stromal tumors: a comprehensive radiological review. Jpn J Radiol. 2022;40(11):1105-20.
66. Jasti R, Carucci LR. Small Bowel Neoplasms: A Pictorial Review. Radiographics. 2020;40(4):1020-38.
67. Afifi AH, Ela AM, Albanna A. Feasibility of diffusion weighted MRI in evaluation of different small bowel pathology. Egypt j radiol nucl med. 2015;46:459-69.
68. Meyer M, Hohenberger P, Overhoff D, Bartsch A, Henzler T, Haubenreisser H, et al. Dual-energy CT vital iodine tumor burden for response assessment in patients with metastatic GIST undergoing TKI therapy: comparison with standard CT and FDG PET/CT criteria. AJR Am J Roentgenol. 2022;218(4):659-69.
69. Fletcher CD, Berman JJ, Corless C, Gorstein F, Lasota J, Longley BJ, et al. Diagnosis of gastrointestinal stromal tumors: a consensus approach. Int J Surg Pathol. 2002;10:81-9.
70. Choi H, Charnsangavej C, de Castro Faria S, Tamm EP, Benjamin RS, Johnson MM, et al. CT evaluation of the response of gastrointestinal stromal tumors after imatinib mesylate treatment: a quantitative analysis correlated with FDG PET findings. AJR Am J Roentgenol. 2004;183:1619-28.
71. Schlemmer M, Sourbron SP, Schinwald N, Nikolaou K, Becker CR, Reiser MF, et al. Perfusion patterns of metastatic gastrointestinal stromal tumor lesions under specific molecular therapy. Eur J Radiol. 2011;77:312-8.
72. Lassau N, Lamuraglia M, Chami L, Leclère J, Bonvalot S, Terrier P, et al. Gastrointestinal stromal tumors treated with imatinib: monitoring response with contrast-enhanced sonography. AJR Am J Roentgenol. 2006;187:1267-73.
73. Gollub MJ. Imaging of Gastrointestinal Lymphoma. Radiol Clin N Am. 2008;46:287-312.
74. Lewis RB, Mehrotra AK, Rodríguez P, Manning MA, Levine MS. From the Radiologic Pathology Archives: Gastrointestinal Lymphoma: Radiologic and Pathologic Findings: Radiographics. 2014;34:1934-53.
75. Levine MS, Rubesin SE, Pantongrag-Brown L, Buck JL, Herlinger H. Non-Hodgkin's lymphoma of the gastrointestinal tract: radiographic findings. AJR Am J Roentgenol. 1997;168(1):165-72.
76. Dawson I, Cornes J, Morson B. Primary malignant lymphoid tumors of the intestinal tract. Report of 37 cases with a study of factors influencing prognosis. Br J Surg. 1961;49:80-9.
77. Manning MA, Somwaru AS, Mehrotra AK, Levine MS. Gastrointestinal lymphoma: radiologic-pathologic correlation. Radiol Clin North Am. 2016:54(4):765-84.
78. Krol AD, le Cessie S, Snijder S, Kluin-Nelemans JC, Kluin PM, Noordijk EM. Primary extranodal non-Hodgkin's lymphoma: the impact of alternative definitions tested in the Comprehensive Centre West population-based NHL registry. Ann Oncol. 2003;14(1):131-9.
79. Ghai S, Pattison J, Ghai S, O'Malley ME, Khalili K, Stephens S. Primary gastrointestinal lymphoma: spectrum of imaging findings with pathologic correlation. Radiographics. 2007;27: 1371-88.
80. Cornes JS. Multiple lymphomatous polyposis of the gastrointestinal tract. Cancer. 1961;14:249-57.
81. Catassi C, Bearzi I, Holmes GKT. Association of celiac disease and intestinal lymphomas and other cancers. Gastroenterology. 2005;128:S79-86.
82. Lo Re G, Federica V, Midiri F, Picone D, La Tona G, Galia M, et al. Radiological Features of Gastrointestinal Lymphoma. Gastroenterology Research and Practice. 2016;2016: 2498143.
83. Mayerhoefer ME, Karanikas G, Kletter K, Prosch H, Kiesewetter B, Skrabs C, et al. Evaluation of Diffusion-Weighted MRI for Pretherapeutic Assessment and Staging of Lymphoma: Results of a Prospective Study in 140 Patients. Clin Cancer Res. 2014;20(11):2984-93.
84. Ghimire P, Wu GY, Zhu L. Primary gastrointestinal lymphoma. World J Gastroenterol. 2011;17(6):697-707.
85. Allen-Auerbach M, de Vos S, Czernin J. The impact of fluorodeoxyglucose-positron emission tomography in primary staging and patient management in lymphoma patients. Radiol Clin N Am. 2008;46:199-211.
86. Schoder H, Noy A, Gonen M, et al. Intensity of 18 fluorodeoxyglucose uptake in positron emission tomography distinguishes between indolent and aggressive non-Hodgkin's lymphoma. J Clin Oncol. 2005;23(21):4643-51.
87. Stecco A, Buemi F, Quagliozzi M, Lombardi M, Santagostino A, Saccheti GM, et al. Staging of primary abdominal lymphoma: comparison of whole-body MRI with diffusion-weighted imaging and 18F-FDG-PET/CT. Gastroenterol res pract. 2015;article ID: 104794, 8 pages.
88. Musshoff K. Clinical staging classification of non-Hodgkin's lymphomas. Strahlentherapie. 1977;153(4):218-21.
89. Rohatiner A, d'Amore F, Coiffier B, Crowther D, Gospodarowicz M, Isaacson P, et al. Report on a workshop convened to discuss the pathological and staging classifications of gastrointestinal tract lymphomas. Ann Oncol. 1994;5(5): 397-400.
90. Ruskoné-Fourmestraux A, Dragosics B, Morgner A, Wotherspoon A, De Jong D. Paris staging system for primary gastrointestinal lymphomas. Gut. 2003;52(6):912-3.
91. Brassil M, Lee R, O'Neill D, Woods G, Moloney BM, Dunne R, et al. Appendiceal tumours—A correlation of CT features and histopathological diagnosis. J Med Imaging Radiat Oncol. 2022;66(1):92-101.
92. Leonards LM, Pahwa A, Patel MK, Petersen J, Nguyen MJ, Jude CM. Neoplasms of the Appendix: Pictorial Review with Clinical and Pathologic Correlation. Radiographics. 2017;37(4): 1059-83.

CHAPTER **5**

Ajay Gulati, Naveen Kalra, Mandeep Kang, Mahesh Prakash

Colorectal Tumors

INTRODUCTION

Colorectal tumors can be broadly classified as epithelial lesions, which include adenoma and adenocarcinoma; and nonepithelial or mesenchymal lesions, which include lipoma, leiomyoma, gastrointestinal stromal tumor (GIST), leiomyosarcoma, and Kaposi's sarcoma. Other tumors are lymphoma, metastases, and nonneoplastic benign polyps such as hyperplastic and hamartomatous polyps. In this chapter, there will be an overview of various imaging techniques and spectrum of imaging findings in colorectal malignancies. A subsection is also included with emphasis to the staging and management of rectal malignancies.

EPIDEMIOLOGY

Colorectal cancer ranks as the third common cause of cancer globally and is the second most common cause of cancer related mortality.[1,2] The prevalence of colon cancer varies throughout the world with high incidences reported in developed countries of the western world, and relatively lower incidence in South America, Africa, and Asia.[3,4] Colon cancer is more frequently seen in economically affluent population, who have western lifestyle practices with more consumption of dietary fat, meat, alcohol, and lower intake of dietary fiber with sedentary lifestyles.[5] The incidence of colorectal cancer rises beyond 40 years of age with 90% of these cases reported in patients above 50 years.[6] Nearly half of the colonic malignancies occur in rectosigmoid and these can be visualized using flexible sigmoidoscope.[7] Rectal malignancies alone comprise nearly one-third of the entire colorectal cancers.

RISK FACTORS

There are multiple risk factors which are associated with colorectal cancer. Primarily, these include dietary and lifestyle factors, hereditary factors, inflammatory bowel disease (IBD), and some other miscellaneous causes.

Many lifestyle practices contribute to the increasing rates of incidence of colorectal cancer such as a high intake of fat and processed meats with low intake of fiber-rich diet.[8] Obesity coupled with physical inactivity, excessive tobacco, and alcohol consumption are other important predisposing factors contributing to higher rates. There is some protective effect by certain dietary antioxidant supplements, calcium, selenium, and vitamins such as A, C E, which may inhibit the carcinogenesis and reduce the occurrence of colon cancer.[9]

Prior cholecystectomy has been reported to increase the risk of developing right-sided colonic malignancy in females by 1.5 times.[10] Prior ureterosigmoidostomy following cystectomy also poses risk for developing adenocarcinoma at the site of anastomosis.

Occupational and environmental risk factors include exposure to asbestos, oils, printing materials, halogens, metal fumes, organic solvents, paint, and dyes.

Radiation-induced colorectal cancers may develop in rectum and sigmoid colon in patients who have received prior radiation treatment for malignancies of cervix, bladder, and prostate.

Hereditary factors have also been associated with increased risk of colorectal cancers.[3] Hereditary nonpolyposis colorectal cancer (HNPCC) or Lynch syndrome is the most common hereditary syndrome associated with nearly 4–6% of all colorectal malignancies. It has an autosomal dominant pattern of inheritance and may be associated with increased risk of some other gynecological and gastrointestinal malignancies. Right-sided colon cancer occurring in younger age group is the hallmark of Lynch syndrome. Colon cancers associated with Lynch syndrome have a better prognosis than other colorectal cancer varieties.[9]

Familial adenomatous polyposis (FAP) is another genetic syndrome which commonly presents with multiple precancerous polyps which tend to grow with increasing age. If prophylactic colostomy is not performed in these patients, colorectal cancer generally always develops in them.

In juvenile polyposis coli, there are higher chances of colorectal malignancy (dysplasia and adenocarcinoma) seen in up to 20% of patients.[9] Screening should be performed periodically in patients with Cronkhite–Canada syndrome, in which there are multiple juvenile polyps within the entire gastrointestinal tract excluding the esophagus. These can eventually undergo malignant transformation to overt malignancies.

Colon cancer in ulcerative colitis is uncommon, occurs in patients with pancolitis, and constitutes about 1% of cancers. Patients with background chronic IBD have a twofold increased risk of colorectal cancer. The activity of the disease, however, does not directly correlate with the increased risk. The mean age of presentation in these patients is 40–45 years.[9]

In Crohn's disease, the chronic inflammation will facilitate carcinogenesis in combination with underlying genetic factors. Most malignancies develop in the chronically inflamed segments and in segments having strictures and fistulae. The predisposition to develop malignancy depends upon the duration and extent of the disease, younger age of diagnosis of primary disease, degree of inflammation, and prior family history. Multifocal malignancies may develop which are frequently diagnosed late since they cannot be confidently distinguished from the benign strictures.[9]

PATHOGENESIS

Most colorectal cancers tend to develop in the adenomatous polyps.[11] Adenomas >1 cm in size have a higher risk of malignant transformation. The gradual transition from benign adenoma to cancer usually takes 7–10 years. This adenoma-carcinoma sequence suggests that colon cancer is potentially preventable if polyps lesions >1 cm are detected and removed. This stresses the importance of screening programs for colonic cancer.

In patients with background IBD, carcinoma evolves through a sequence of inflammation, dysplasia followed by carcinoma.

The malignant potential of an adenomatous polyp has four main determinants. These include size, associated stalk, villous texture, and severity of cellular dedifferentiation/dysplasia.[9] Sessile polyps pose greater risk for cancer (>50%) than the pedunculated polyps. Polyps with a more marked cellular atypia and dysplasia are more likely to become malignant.

CLINICAL FEATURES

Colorectal cancer is a slow-growing malignancy with most early-stage patients being symptomatic, and these may be detected during routine screening. Symptomatic colorectal cancers usually present with bleeding which may range from occult blood in the stool, to passage of frank blood per rectum or development of iron deficiency anemia. The symptoms depend upon the size and location of the tumor. Right-sided colonic malignancies usually resent later with large masses before becoming symptomatic due to more capacious state of the right-sided colon complemented by more fluid-like contents. On the other hand, the clinical presentation in sigmoid cancers is generally earlier since it is the narrowest segment of colon and the cancer frequently causes obstruction to the passage of solid fecal matter. They often present with obstructive symptoms and may have crampy abdominal pain or per rectal bleeding. A feeling of incomplete bowel evacuation, persistent diarrhea or constipation should raise suspicion of colorectal carcinoma in patients older than 40 years. Unexplained weight loss and iron deficiency anemia are some of the other common although nonspecific clinical features. Patients with colorectal carcinoma usually have a normal physical examination. Sometimes, there may be a palpable lump or clinical features of intestinal obstruction. Among the laboratory investigations, carcinoembryonic antigen (CEA) which is a serum biomarker is a widely available tool, which is used in routine clinical practice. CEA is a sensitive marker for colorectal cancer, although it is nonspecific and may be elevated in various other malignancies such as medullary thyroid cancer, breast cancer, and mucinous ovarian cancer. Although not specific, the elevated levels of serum CEA correlate with the cancer stage and tumor size.

PATHOLOGY

The gross morphology of the colorectal adenocarcinoma generally depends upon its location. Large and bulky polypoidal masses are commonly seen in the right-sided colon. These may overgrow their vascular supply and undergo necrosis. Tumors occurring in the transverse and descending colon are generally more invasive in nature and are frequently ulcerated, infiltrative and have a large intramural component. Distal colonic and rectal tumors are also infiltrative and exhibit annular constricting or "napkin-ring" appearance. These tumors frequently are more aggressive in nature. In patients with IBD, colon cancers may be scirrhous, plaque-like or finely nodular.[12]

Malignancies of the large bowel are predominantly adenocarcinoma. Mucinous/colloid carcinomas are seen in the setting of IBD and hereditary nonpolyposis-related carcinoma in early age and tend to have worse prognosis. These comprise 10–15% of the cancers and have lakes of mucin in which there is a scattered collection of tumor cells with signet-ring cells. Calcification may occur in these tumors. Tumors that arise at the anorectal junction include squamous cell carcinoma, transitional cell carcinoma, cloacogenic carcinoma, and melanocarcinoma[9] which account for <5% of malignant large bowel tumors. Other uncommon neoplasms include primary lymphomas, carcinoids, leiomyosarcoma, and metastatic lesions to the bowel.

ROUTE OF SPREAD

There are various routes of tumor dissemination after it becomes invasive in nature:

- *Direct extension*: Direct invasion may happen along the tissue layers which provide the path of least resistance. As peritoneum represents a potential barrier, contiguous spread to adjoining intraperitoneal organs is rare. After invading the visceral peritoneum, the tumor can spread to stomach, omentum, small bowel, spleen, another segment of colon, bladder, uterus, fallopian tubes, and ovaries. Retroperitoneal tumor may involve kidneys, ureters, pancreas, and posterior abdominal musculature. Rectal carcinoma after breaching the Waldeyer's fascia may invade the sacral plexus, sacrum, and coccyx.[13] These may also extend to the internal iliac vessels and obturator muscles posterolaterally, and involve the bladder, seminal vesicles, prostate, vagina, and cervix anteriorly after compromising the fascia of Denonvillier's.
- *Lymphatic spread*: This is seen after the invasion of muscularis through submucosal lymphatics. Intramural spread of colorectal malignancy is through the submucosal, muscular, and subserosal lymphatic channels. Usually, the epiploic and the paracolic group of lymph nodes are the first sites of involvement. The intermediate lymph nodes (all present along vascular branches) and the principal lymph nodes (at the origin of the colonic vessels) get involved as the disease progresses. The prognosis worsens when multiple lymph nodes are involved.
- *Hematogenous metastases*: This may be the route of spread once the colorectal malignancy infiltrates the capillary network present in lamina propria. It primarily happens through the tributaries of portal vein, resulting in liver being the most common site. The distal part of rectum has venous drainage through the tributaries of internal iliac vein, which subsequently drain into the inferior vena cava. Batson's vertebral venous plexus is another path of hematogenous spread. In 20–40% colorectal carcinoma patients, liver is the only organ with metastasis. Pulmonary metastases are seen in 20% of patients. Other uncommon sites include adrenals, bones, kidneys, pancreas, spleen, and central nervous system.
- *Peritoneal seeding*: Intraperitoneal seeding may occur during operation because of breach in serosa. The anterior wall of rectosigmoid junction is the site of metastatic seedling. Eventually, both the parietal and the visceral surfaces of peritoneum become involved causing malignant ascites.
- *Intraluminal implantation*: The tumor spillage within the lumen during surgery is the likely cause for implantation, metastases, and recurrence at anastomotic sites.[14] Anastomotic recurrences may also happen secondary to partial excision of the primary tumor or a metachronous tumor.

STAGING

Staging of colorectal cancer has evolved over many years. The Astler and Coller modification of the Dukes classification is commonly employed to stage colonic neoplasm.

In this method, the staging is as follows:

A: Tumor limited to mucosa
B1: Tumor extending into, but not through, the muscularis propria
B2: Tumor penetrating the bowel wall, but without any lymph nodes
C: Tumor with regional lymph nodes. This is subclassified into C1, where the primary tumor is within the bowel wall and C2, where the primary tumor has spread beyond the bowel wall.

Turn ball introduced an additional staging category in 1967 as stage D in which stage D1, included fixed cancers that invaded adjoining organs and stage D2, where distant metastases were present.

Currently, the American Joint Committee on Cancer (AJCC) and Union for International Cancer Control (UICC) advocate staging by TNM ("Tumor", "Nodes", "Metastasis") classification (with recent update in 8th edition).[15]

Primary Tumor (T)

Tx: Primary tumor cannot be assessed
T0: No evidence of primary tumor
Tis: Carcinoma in situ
T1: Tumor invades submucosa
T2: Tumor invades muscularis propria
T3: Tumor extending through the muscularis propria into subserosa or nonperitonealized pericolic or perirectal tissue
T4: Tumor directly invades other organs or structures
T4a: Tumor penetrating visceral peritoneum
T4b: Tumor directly invading or adhering to other organs or structures

Regional Lymph Node (N)

Nx: Regional lymph nodes cannot be assessed
N0: No regional nodal metastasis
N1: 1–3 pericolic or perirectal lymph nodes involved
N1a: One lymph node metastases
N1b: 2–3 lymph nodes metastases
N2: Metastasis in four or more pericolic or perirectal lymph nodes
N2a: 4–6 regional nodal metastases
N2b: More than or equal to seven nodal metastases

Distant Metastasis (M)

M1: There is distant lymph node metastasis
M1a: Metastasis is limited to one organ or site (e.g., liver, lung, ovary, and extraregional lymph node metastases)
M1b: Metastasis in more than one organ or site[1]
M1c: Peritoneal metastases with or without metastasis of other organs.[1]

Stage Grouping

Stage 0	Tis	N0	M0
I	T1-2	N0	M0
IIA	T3	N0	M0
IIB	T4a	N0	M0
IIC	T4b	N0	M0
IIIA	T1-2	N1/N1c	M0
	T1	N2a	M0
IIIB	T3-T4a	N1/N1c	M0
	T2-3	N2a	M0
	T1-2	N2b	M0
IIIC	T4a	N2a	M0
	T3-4a	N2b	
	T4b	N1-2	
IVA	Any T	Any N	M1a

Source: AJCC Cancer staging Manual, 8th edition. Springer international publishing, 2017.

In the present era, there has been a growing interest to classify the colorectal cancer (CRC) molecularly using the expression of immunohistochemistry (IHC) antibodies that would in turn facilitate in deciding on the appropriate targeted therapy. In this context, four consensus molecular subtypes (CMS 1–4) were introduced in 2005, based on different molecular characteristics and epithelial-mesenchymal transition (EMT). Like in other malignancies, the future of CRC management aims at taking all therapeutic decisions based on the molecular diagnostic tests. This would in turn lead to improved stratification of patients, above the limitations of standard staging systems, in constant search for more validated prognostic biomarkers thereby improving patient outcomes.

ROLE OF RADIOLOGY

Radiology plays a pivotal role in surveillance for colorectal cancer. The primary objective of imaging studies in patients of colorectal cancer is to provide the surgeon and the oncologist with comprehensive and accurate evaluation of the primary tumor, local staging, and presence of any distant metastasis, detection of any synchronous lesions, and identification of any clinically occult complications. Imaging is also playing a crucial role in posttreatment setting by enabling detection of any residual or recurrent disease, local or distant metastatic lesions, and presence of any metachronous cancers.[16]

Screening for Colorectal Cancer

The American Cancer Society in its recent revision of guidelines for screening advise that regular screening for colorectal cancer should start at the age of 45 years for people with average risk instead of 50 years which was the earlier recommendation by most of the societies.[17]

In 2017, the US Multi-Society Task Force on Colorectal Cancer revised the recommendations for screening and classified the screening tests into three tiers, based upon the level of effectiveness:[18]

- *Tier 1 tests* consist of:
  - Colonoscopy every 10 years
  - Annual fecal immunochemical test (FIT)
- *Tier 2 tests* consist of:
  - CT colonography every 5 years
  - FIT—fecal DNA every 3 years
  - Flexible sigmoidoscopy every 5–10 years
- *Tier 3 tests* consist of:
  - Capsule colonoscopy every 5 years

Fecal occult blood test (FOBT) is readily available and cost-effective screening test for colorectal malignancy. Colorectal cancers often bleed intermittently and the lost blood in the stool gets converted to hematin. The hemoccult test is the most widely used and is technically based on the guaiac reaction. However, it is believed that a polyp must be >2 cm in size before it regularly bleeds. The reported sensitivity rates are <50% and nearly 90% of polyps may be missed by FOBT.[19] Newer screening methods are now available which include fecal immunochemical test (FIT). FIT employs the use of antibodies to discern the presence of blood in the stool. Recommendations advocate that the FIT should replace the traditional guaiac-based FOBT due to its improved diagnostic performance.[20]

Flexible sigmoidoscopy is an endoscopic procedure which can evaluate the rectal and the distal sigmoid mucosa and can easily diagnose polyps and cancer in these locations. The main limitation being that even significant lesions in the rest of the colon beyond the reach of sigmoidoscope would not be detected. It is an outpatient procedure which is generally safe and well-tolerated without the requirement of any sedation, although it is expensive and may have rare complications like bleeding or perforation.

Double-contrast barium enema (DCBE) is a widely available, inexpensive, and simple test. In a study comparing the effectiveness of DCBE in comparison to colonoscopy, sensitivity of DCBE for detecting polyps smaller than 0.5 cm was only 32%, for polyps 0.6–1 cm, was 53% and for polyps >1 cm was 48%.[21]

Colonoscopy is one of the most sensitive tests for colorectal screening as it can directly visualize the colonic mucosa with exquisite detail with benefit of taking biopsies from suspicious areas in the same sitting. Optical colonoscopy is generally regarded as the reference standard for determining sensitivities of other investigative techniques of the colon. However, in a study with review of tandem or back-to-back colonoscopies, an average of 21% of adenomas was not detected.[22] 26% of these were 1–5 mm and 2% of them were 10 mm or more in size. The limitations include technical blind spots behind the folds and around the flexures which may be difficult to visualize. The examination may be incomplete in some situations due to technical reasons. Colonoscopy being invasive also has potential risk of colonic perforation or bleeding in 1:500 examinations with reported mortality rate of 1:5,000 examinations.

Virtual colonoscopy is a novel noninvasive technique wherein a three-dimensional endoluminal image is generated after processing data acquired by multidetector helical CT using dedicated postprocessing softwares. In a study by National CT Colonography Trial which was conducted across 15 study centers on 2,600 asymptomatic participants, it was found that CT colonography had 90% sensitivity and 86% specificity for detection of polyps measuring 10 mm or more in size.[23] Thus, it was concluded that virtual colonoscopy has good diagnostic performance in detection of lesions >1 cm which are actually the more clinically significant lesions. The entire colon is evaluated by virtual colonoscopy which may sometimes not be feasible with optical colonoscopy in markedly stricturing lesions. However, patients with significant lesions detected by CT colonography must also get optical colonoscopy done. The reported complications with this technique are rare (0.08%).

DIAGNOSTIC MODALITIES

Imaging modalities available are plain abdominal radiographs, barium enema, and ultrasound (US) including endoluminal and Doppler US, CT/CT colonography, MRI/MR colonography (MRC), and angiography.

Plain Radiographs

There is only limited utility of radiographs in the present modern era and may depict complications of advanced colorectal malignancy like obstruction or colonic perforation. Dilatation of bowel loops in cases of obstructing lesions, thumb printing in cases of ischemic colitis proximal to any obstructing lesions, and free intraperitoneal air in cases of perforation are some of the other findings which may be detected on plain films. Calcification within the malignant lesions or bulky hepatic metastases may sometimes be evident. With advanced malignancies, bony destruction with associated soft tissue mass may sometimes be seen due to osseous metastasis. Lung metastases may also be seen on the chest skiagram.

Barium Enema

Barium enema is a radiological investigation which gives a panoramic view of the entire colon and has the ability to identify and determine the extent of any colonic lesions. It is reasonably accurate, minimally invasive procedure that is cost-effective and rated high in terms of safety, convenience, and acceptance by patients, and does not require sedation. Complications are extremely uncommon. DCBE has a 20% more sensitivity than single-contrast barium enema for detection of polyps <1 cm in size.[24] However, this difference in the diagnostic performance of the two types of barium enema is not in context of detection of colorectal carcinoma. The reported sensitivity of barium enema is 90–95% for the detection of significant (>1 cm) sized polyps and cancer.[25] The most important prerequisite for an optimal barium examination is thorough bowel preparation with selection of an appropriate technique, strict quality control during the study and careful interpretation of radiographs. The technique for bowel preparation primarily includes combination of dietary manipulation along with oral cathartics and cleansing enema based on institutional preferences. About 10–40% of colonic cancers may be missed on initial barium enemas due to inadequate bowel preparartion.[26,27] Fecal matter within the lumen can mimic or mask underlying polyps and cancer. The single-contrast barium enema is simpler in concept than the double-contrast examination, but requires meticulous technique. The selection of particular type of barium enema to be performed will depend on the indication for the examination, sensitivity for detecting specific diseases, age, and general condition of the patient.

The DCBE gives better visualization of mucosal surface with improved detection of smaller lesions. It requires frequent turning of the patient for proper mucosal coating; therefore, the patient should be relatively active for a technically successful examination. It is an ideal technique in patients who are older than 40 years, who have prior personal or family history of colonic polyps, cancer or IBD, and a positive FOBT.

Single-contrast barium enema is a relatively simpler and quick procedure and does not require rigorous maneuvers. Therefore, it is indicated in patients who are elderly, debilitated or even obtunded and in those patients where barium study is indicated for evaluation of anastomotic integrity in postoperative patients; or exclusion of obstruction, fistula, or diverticulitis. Young patients with low likelihood of colon disease may also be candidates for single-contrast study. One of the most important technical considerations is the density of the barium sulfate or water-soluble contrast which generally may be 20% weight/volume (w/v). Manual palpation or mechanical compression of the colon during the examination and spot radiographs of the various segments are critical in detecting small polypoidal lesions. Postevacuation radiographs may be performed at the end of the examination in certain situations. Optimized technique protocol should be followed during the examination with careful fluoroscopy and obtaining views of different colonic segments in specific positions performed for obtaining optimal results. Additional spot radiographs of questionable lesions should be obtained when needed.

Meticulous review and interpretation of the barium enema spots at the control station is needed to avoid diagnostic errors due to associated fecal matter, air bubbles, and diverticulae. False-negative errors may be caused by perceptive lapses, technical issues, interpretation errors, or combination of all these factors. Accuracy of DCBE for evaluation of colorectal polyps is dependent on the size of the colonic polyps and the location of the lesion. As stated earlier, the sensitivity of DCBE is poor for polyps under 5 mm, improving for polyps measuring 5–9 mm and is best for diagnosing polyps over 1 cm.

Complications of barium enema are uncommon. Many of these can be potentially prevented by meticulous technique and careful review of the indications to identify patients who are at increased risk. The reported rates of perforation during barium enema are 1:25,00–1:12,500 and rare mortality in 1:50,000.[28,29] In the event of a biopsy performed through a rigid scope, enema should be deferred for 2 weeks due to risk of perforation. Most researchers, however, believe that enema can be safely performed on the same day in patients where a superficial biopsy is performed through a flexible sigmoidoscope or colonoscope, but it should be deferred for 5–7 days after deep biopsy (involving muscularis propria) or polypectomy. Allergic reactions to barium, transient bacteremia, cardiac arrhythmias, barium impaction, dehydration, and inadvertent misplacement of the enema tip into vaginal vault are other complications which may also be encountered. Despite the risk of transient bacteremia, there is no recommendation to administer prophylactic antibiotics.

Colorectal malignancies have a wide spectrum of morphological appearances on imaging. The mucosal surface can be seen en face, either in the barium pool or in the air contrast. The normal mucosa is smooth whereas abnormal mucosa may have a granular, finely nodular or ulcerated surface. Early carcinoma is usually seen as a sessile polypoid mass. The primary role of various imaging modalities in screening for early malignancies is primarily aimed at detection of small polyps. There are two common types of colonic polyps, hyperplastic and adenomatous. Hyperplastic polyps have no malignant potential. Small polypoidal carcinomas may have a smooth outline and be radiographically in distinguishable from benign tumors **(Figs. 1 and 2)**. Barium enema cannot however accurately determine the benign or malignant nature of polypoid lesions in the size range of 0.5–3 cm. Whenever polyps >1 cm in size are detected, they must be removed by colonoscopic polypectomy followed by histological examination.

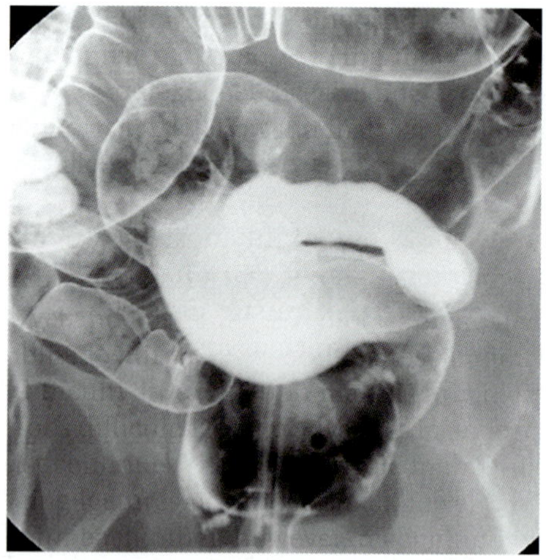

FIG. 1: Double-contrast barium enema (DCBE) showing a solitary, small, smooth polypoid lesion in the sigmoid colon which was malignant on histopathology.

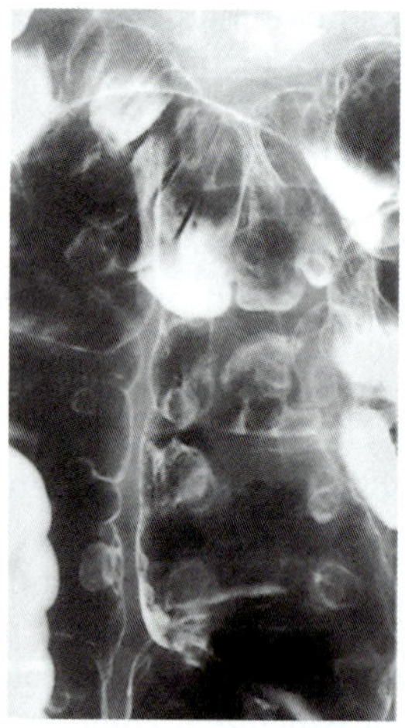

FIG. 2: Double-contrast barium enema (DCBE) performed in a patient with familial adenomatous polyposis showing multiple polyps in the colon.

Pedunculated polyps are best demonstrated on erect or lateral decubitus views of the colon. Those arising from the nondependent wall of the colon give the appearance of "Mexican hat" sign[30] where the central ring represents the stalk with the outer ring representing the head of polyp. Changing in position of the patient will show the stalk in profile and confirm the diagnosis.

Sessile polyps may have variable appearance ranging from small, smooth polypoidal lesions to more bulky and lobulated masses which form acute angles with the adjacent colonic wall. When viewed enface, these appear as filling defects in the thin barium pool if present in the dependent wall and etched in white when seen on nondependent surface. However, they may be potentially missed if excess of high-density barium is present in the lumen, obscuring the lesion. In the oblique projections, sessile polyps show "Bowler hat" sign,[31] with the dome representing the head of polyp and brim representing base of the polyp. Although the "Bowler hat" sign can also be seen in a diverticulum, the direction of the dome helps to distinguish a polyp from a diverticulum. The key imaging feature to distinguish between these entities is that when the dome points away from the axis of the bowel, the lesion is a diverticulum contrary to the dome pointing toward the lumen of the bowel in a polyp.

The assessment of malignancy in the polyps is based on certain radiological criteria which include sessile versus pedunculated morphology, size and number of polyps, basal indentation, and surface contour. A size criterion of 1 cm is regarded as threshold for increased cancer risk in a polyp. Pedunculation is generally regarded as a sign for benignity, if stalk length >2 cm, it is usually not associated with malignant infiltration into the adjoining wall. Smooth basal indentation is primarily attributed to the geometric factors between the junction of the base and underlying colonic surface and can be seen in both benign and the malignant lesions. Presence of basal indentation is most predictive of malignant infiltration when it is prominent and irregular in larger-sized polyps. The smooth surface contour is generally unreliable in distinguishing benign from malignant polyps. Lesions that have an irregular, "soap bubbly" surface generally have villous elements and show malignant degeneration in at least 50% of lesions.[32,33] The majority of colonic adenomas are tubular adenomas. These have varying degrees of villous change which tends to increase as the size of polyp increases. The villous adenomas on the other hand have a frond-like surface. The risk of malignant transformation is related to the proportion of villous change in an adenoma. As the barium gets entrapped in the frond-like protrusions which go hand in hand with the villous change, the surface of the polyp assumes a "soap bubbly" or a "lacy" pattern. The term "carpet lesion" has also been used for flat lobulated lesion that manifest due to an alteration in surface texture of the bowel. These are also spectrum of tubular adenomas with varying degrees of villous change.

Once a polyp is detected, there is a 3.5% risk of having synchronous cancer and a 20% chance of another polyp.[34] Therefore, the remainder of the colon should be meticulously examined to search for other lesions.

Advanced colorectal cancers have various morphological types. These include polypoidal, annular, scirrhous, and flat lesions. The polypoidal lesions project within the lumen and have an irregular outline **(Figs. 3A to D)**. They may

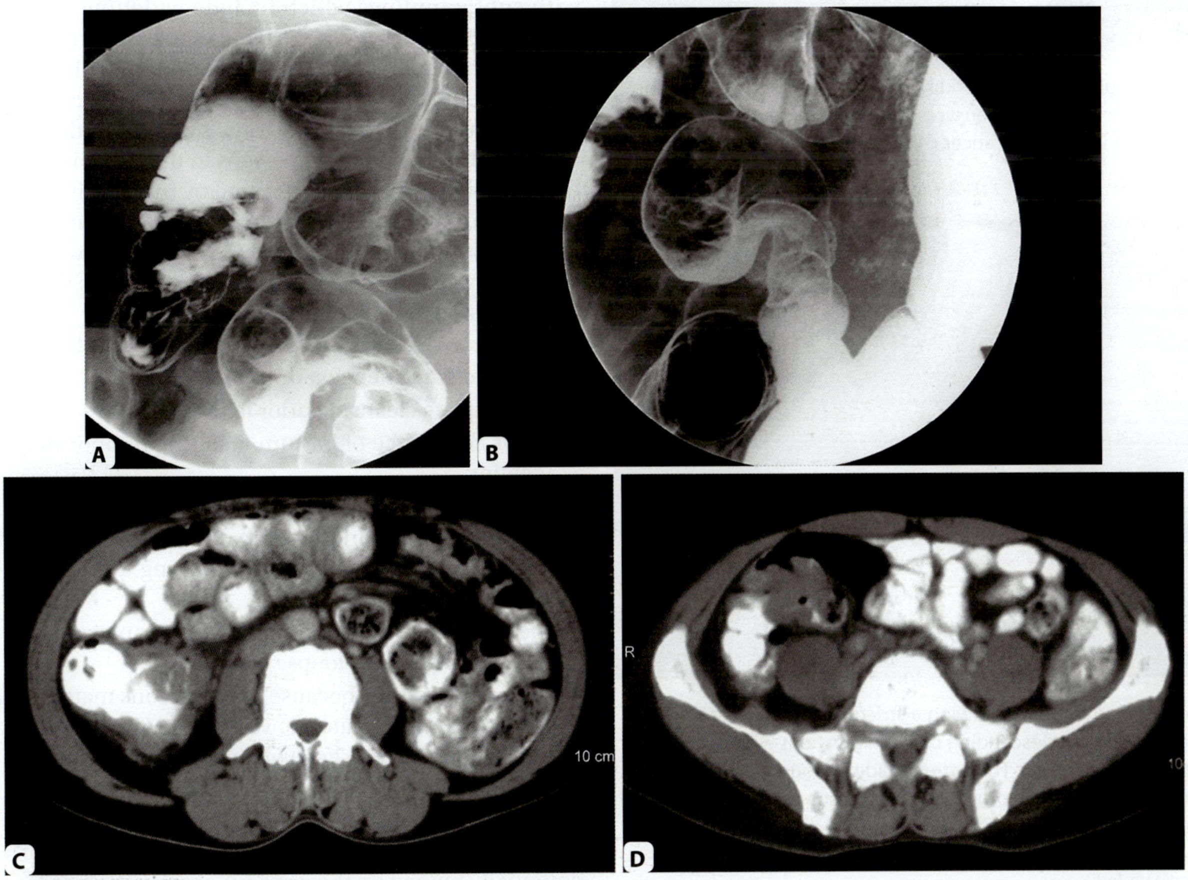

FIGS. 3A TO D: Double-contrast barium enema (DCBE) showing synchronous cancers in the ascending colon (A) and sigmoid colon (B). There is a short-segment stricture in the ascending colon with a polypoidal component protruding into the colon. The sigmoid colon also shows a segment of narrowing. Axial contrast-enhanced CT (CECT) sections in the same patient showing circumferential mural thickening with a polypoidal component in the ascending colon (C). A similar lesion is also seen in the sigmoid colon with presence of ulcerations (D).

present with bowel obstruction or intussusception in some cases. Annular cancers are generally shorter in length with abrupt transition between the normal and tumor mucosa **(Figs. 4 and 5)**. The mucosa is destroyed and there may be heaped up edges or ulceration. Focal spastic areas may cause confusion on DCBE but the diagnostic peril to look for is that mucosal folds will remain intact within the area of the spasm. The differential considerations in annular colonic narrowing include presence of adhesions, inflammation, diverticulitis, endometriosis, postradiation changes, and metastatic lesions in addition to primary adenocarcinoma. Semiannular or "saddle" tumor involves only a portion of the wall and results in asymmetry of bowel lumen. Enface, these tumors will show overlapping lines with an abnormal orientation on double-contrast studies. Scirrhous tumor present with marked mural thickening and smooth strictures with submucosal and muscular invasion. Flat lesions are uncommon and are seen in long-standing ulcerative colitis, these may present as abnormal lines on DCBE.

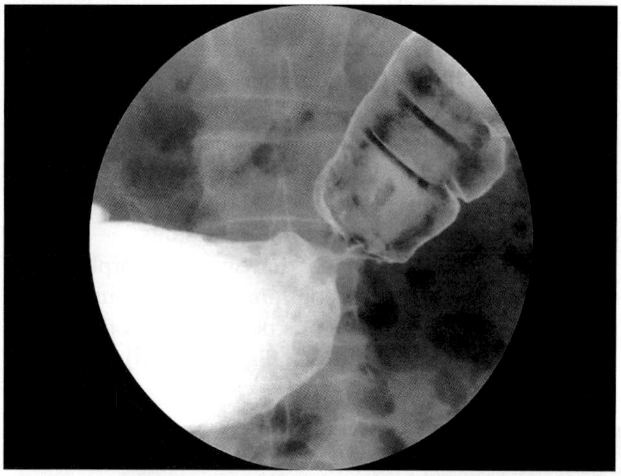

FIG. 4: Double-contrast barium enema (DCBE) showing a short annular stricture in the transverse colon with mucosal irregularity in a patient with colon cancer.

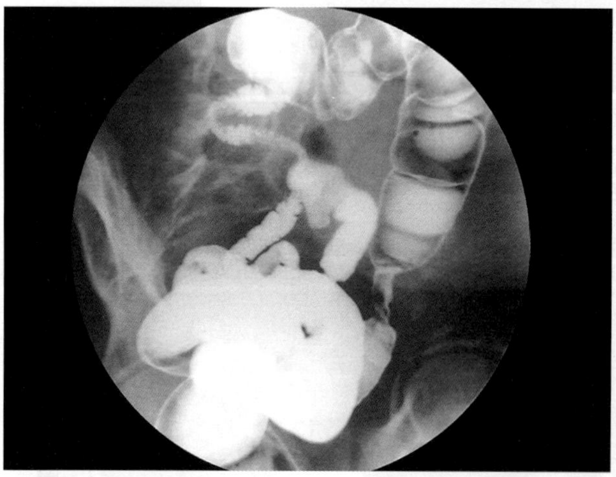

FIG. 5: Barium enema showing a stricture with mucosal irregularity in the descending colon in a patient with metachronous cancer. The patient had previous history of right hemicolectomy and ileotransverse anastomosis for carcinoma of ascending colon.

Courtesy: Professor B Nagi, Department of Gastroenterology, PGIMER, Chandigarh, India.

Problem Areas in Barium Studies

Distal rectum: The tip of the catheter in the rectum can itself mask plaque like or polypoidal lesions. Large internal hemorrhoids may mimic carcinoma, which appear on DCBE as thickened lobulated folds extending 3 cm or less from the anal verge or as cluster of small submucosal nodules in the rectum. On the other hand, low-lying rectal cancers spreading submucosally may mimic hemorrhoids, but asymmetry of lesion and extent of rectal involvement favor the diagnosis of malignancy.

Ileocecal valve: Tumors in this location may present with subtle findings which include widening, splaying, straightening, or asymmetric lobulation of the valve. These findings may sometimes be missed on initial observation if not carefully looked for. Associated diverticulitis may also obscure underlying lesions. In cases of diagnostic uncertainty with equivocal lesions in the sigmoid colon, a "sigmoid flush" may be performed by introducing a small amount of low-density barium into the rectum to help identify polypoidal lesions as filling defects within the thin barium pool.[35] Some of the common errors in barium interpretation may be due to:

- Failure to detect small filling defects in a pool of barium
- Insufficient distension or overdistension
- Incomplete cleansing prior to the study
- Poor adherence of barium resulting in poor mucosal coating
- Failure to detect synchronous lesions in presence of one lesion. Satisfaction of search or distraction by finding one lesion may result in overlooking a synchronous lesion.
- Lesions may be obscured by the haustral folds or overlapping bowel loops.
- Perceptive errors, because of extraneous material such as fecal matter, anatomic variation such as redundant bowel loops or presence of diverticulae.

As most colorectal carcinomas are slow-growing, it is assumed that if a carcinoma is detected within 3 years of a previous normal barium enema study, the tumor was potentially missed on the previous examination.[25,36,37]

Ultrasound

Ultrasound has a growing role in the evaluation of gastrointestinal diseases due to its ready availability, noninvasive nature, and better patient's acceptance. Recent technological advancements in the last decade have led to improved diagnostic accuracy and better characterization of bowel pathologies. The sonographic appearance depends not only upon the inherent anatomic characteristics of segment assessed but also upon the intraluminal contents and distension. The bowel may be collapsed, containing only a small amount of mucus (the mucus pattern), or may contain gas/air (gas pattern) or liquid contents (fluid pattern). The mucus pattern is seen as a classical target with a highly reflective core of mucus. Large bowel often produces a more complex pattern, because of presence of mild fluid and gas even in the fasting state. Sometimes, colonic contents are reflective with distal shadowing due to fecal material. In case of colorectal malignancy, bowel wall thickening may be visualized by US resulting in a target or "pseudokidney" configuration **(Figs. 6A to C)**. Normal bowel wall thickness in the nondistended state is 5 mm and up to 3 mm in the distended state. When the bowel wall is thickened, the mucus pattern changes to a thickened, sometimes irregular "halo" of bowel wall, with highly reflective irregular center giving a "pseudokidney" sign.[37] This sign is nonspecific but strongly favors bowel pathology. The site of the involved bowel must be inferred from the position of the lesion in the abdomen. In inflammatory/infective pathologies, mural thickening is regular, long segmental with preserved stratification. However, in neoplastic states, thickening is irregular, segmental with loss of mural stratification. A notable exception is lymphoma in which the mural stratification is also generally preserved. The diagnostic performance of transabdominal US is improved by retrograde instillation of fluid into the colon. This procedure known as "sonocolonography" enables an accurate evaluation of the colonic lumen along with the colonic wall and pericolonic tissues. According to a study done by Bernd,[38] the sensitivity of this technique in the detection of colonic carcinomas was 94% and the specificity was 100%. US screening of abdomen helps to detect hepatic metastasis and associated retroperitoneal lymph nodes in advanced cases of malignancy. US also helps to guide fine needle aspiration and core biopsy of lesions for histological diagnosis.

Endorectal ultrasound (ERUS): Evaluation of rectum with an endosonic probe was first performed by Wilde and Reed in 1956.[37] The procedure is performed with an endorectally placed, rotating, and high-frequency transducer. If technically feasible, the transducer should be passed proximal to the visualized tumor for adequate assessment of mural involvement. With the modern high-frequency transducers, the five layers of the rectal wall can be well delineated as layers of alternating echogenicity allowing for accurate assessment of depth of invasion in early rectal tumors. The innermost ring is hyperechoic and represents the interface of the probe with mucosa. The second ring is hypoechoic and is due to the muscularis mucosa. The third ring is hyperechoic and represents submucosa. The fourth ring is again hypoechoic and is formed by the muscularis propria. The fifth ring is hyperechoic and is due to the mesorectal fat or in areas of peritoneal reflection by the serosa and fat. Rectal carcinoma on US commonly presents as hypoechoic mass with irregular borders interrupting the normal five-layer wall pattern. Most guidelines regard ERUS as the most sensitive modality for staging early rectal cancers and differentiating between T1 and T2 disease. The accuracy of ERUS in staging of colorectal carcinoma is variably reported from 88 to 95%. Most of the errors are secondary to overestimation of depth of invasion possibly as a result of coexisting inflammation.[39] Tumor confined to the muscularis mucosa can be differentiated from tumor extending into the perirectal fat with invasion of adjacent structures and metastatic involvement of perirectal lymph nodes **(Figs. 7A and B)**.

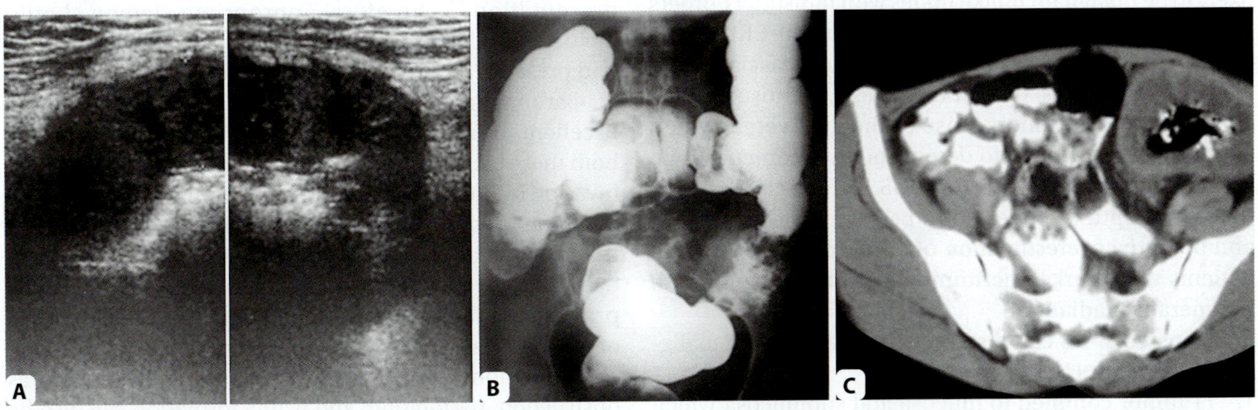

FIGS. 6A TO C: (A) Ultrasound of the lump in the left iliac fossa shows thickened bowel wall with highly reflective center consistent with "pseudokidney" sign; (B) Barium enema in the same patient shows a mass-like lesion with deep ulcerations in the region of descending colon; (C) Axial contrast-enhanced (CECT) section shows concentric mural thickening with ulcerations in the same segment.

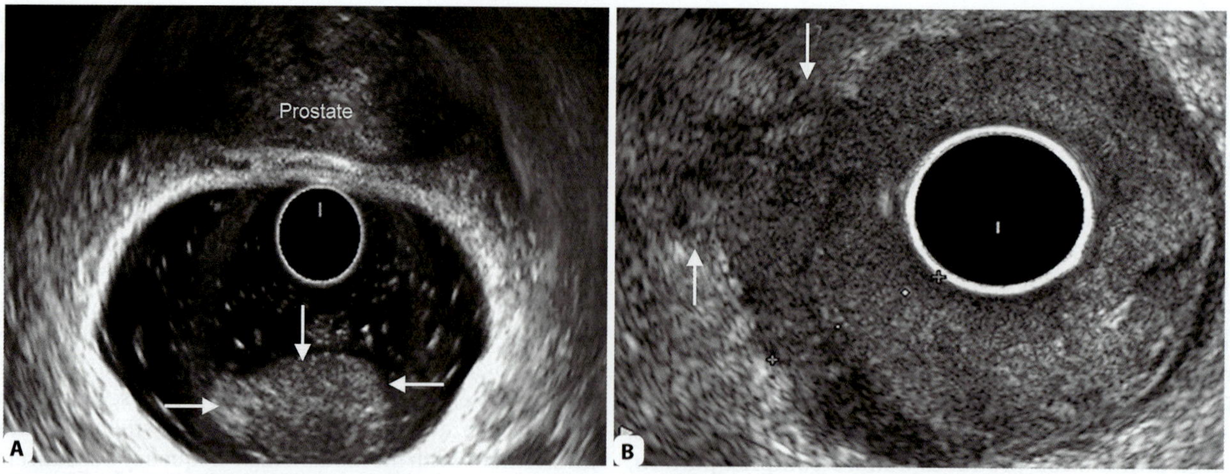

FIGS. 7A AND B: (A) Endorectal ultrasound (ERUS) with radial echo endoscope shows polypoidal lesion (white arrows) with muscularis propria seen intact all around suggestive of T1 lesion; (B) ERUS with radial echo endoscope shows involvement of all layers of rectum with infiltration of serosa and adjacent perirectal tissue (arrows) suggestive of T4 lesion.
Courtesy: Dr Surinder Rana, Department of Gastroenterology, PGIMER, Chandigarh, India.

ERUS may also help in differentiating benign villous adenomas from those with focal areas of invasive carcinoma. Glaser et al.[40] reported that benign villous adenoma appears hyperechoic and areas of invasive carcinoma appear hypoechoic. The presence of invasive carcinoma within a villous adenoma is determined by the involvement of the muscularis propria.[41] ERUS, however, cannot reliably visualize the mesorectal fascia and thus may not be as accurate as MRI in locally advanced rectal cancers.

ERUS can detect perirectal lymph nodes as small as 5 mm in size; however, assessment for nodal metastases is less accurate than tumor depth. In fact, studies evaluating nodal metastasis based on the size criteria have shown rather low accuracy rates. Nodal echo texture and morphology are most often used criteria for predicting involvement. Nodes which have sharply demarcated borders with inhomogeneous hypoechoic pattern are more likely to be malignant unlike nodes with indistinct borders and a hyperechoic pattern. Limitations of ERUS is in evaluating lymph nodes outside mesorectal fascia, lateral pelvic lymph nodes, distant metastasis, stenosing rectal carcinomas, and tumors close to the anal verge, which are technically difficult to detect and may sometimes be missed. Other limitations of ERUS include the inability to assess depth of penetration beyond the colonic wall and potential overestimation of tumor measurements in patients with marked peritumoral inflammation or with preoperative radiation.[37]

Transrectal US can distinguish three stages of malignancy based on TNM classification:

1. T1 tumor confined to mucosa and submucosa which does not interrupt the middle echogenic ring.
2. T2 tumor confined to rectal wall in which the outermost echogenic interface is intact.
3. T3 tumor which penetrates the perirectal fat and leads to disruption of outermost echogenic ring.

Doppler US may complement the US imaging by showing increased color flow, increased diastolic flow within tumor with low resistance waveform, as tumor vessels lack smooth muscle layer, thus offering little resistance **(Figs. 8A to E)**. A cut-off value of peak systolic velocity (PSV) >25 cm/s is used to differentiate T3 and T4 tumors from T1 and T2 tumors and a PSV of >20 cm/s in lymph nodes is classified as malignant.

Computed Tomography

The primary aim of computerized tomography in evaluation of colorectal carcinoma is for preoperative staging, to assess any postoperative complications, and for the detection of tumor recurrence. It is estimated that up to 25% of patients with colorectal cancer have metastases at the time of initial presentation.[42] Therefore, appropriate staging should include both local staging of primary colorectal neoplasm and presence of any distant metastases.

Barium studies and colonoscopy/sigmoidoscopy provide excellent visualization of the mucosal surface. However, both these techniques do not determine the depth of mural invasion by the tumor or presence of any metastatic disease. Accurate preoperative staging is vital to individualize the treatment strategy, assess risk of disease recurrence, and determine overall prognosis. In colonic cancer, CT is the primary modality for locoregional staging, identification of any enlarged lymph nodes or distant metastatic disease. Complications of primary colonic malignancies such as obstruction, perforation, and fistula formation can also be readily visualized with CT. However, local staging of rectal cancers is primarily by MRI with CT being more commonly used for detection of any distant spread.

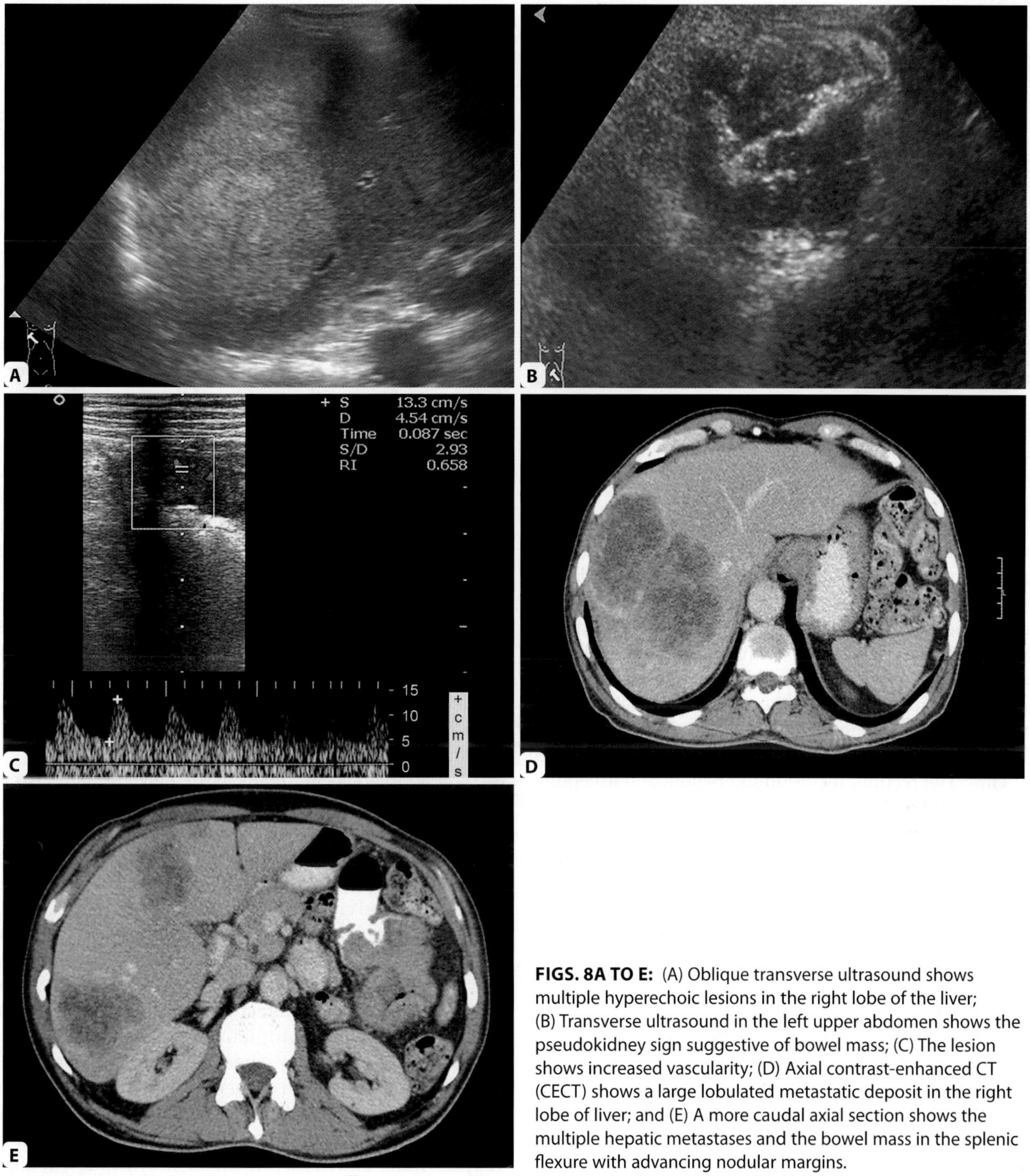

FIGS. 8A TO E: (A) Oblique transverse ultrasound shows multiple hyperechoic lesions in the right lobe of the liver; (B) Transverse ultrasound in the left upper abdomen shows the pseudokidney sign suggestive of bowel mass; (C) The lesion shows increased vascularity; (D) Axial contrast-enhanced CT (CECT) shows a large lobulated metastatic deposit in the right lobe of liver; and (E) A more caudal axial section shows the multiple hepatic metastases and the bowel mass in the splenic flexure with advancing nodular margins.

The accuracy of CT for colonic evaluation can be improved by additional techniques including adequate cleansing of colon, administration of IV spasmolytics, distension of the colon with either air, carbon dioxide (CT colonography) or neutral luminal contrast agents, and by reconstructing thinner sections to improve the quality of multiplanar reformats **(Fig. 9)**. The optimal protocol is acquisition in the portal venous phase. The addition of hepatic arterial phase routinely has not been shown to improve the sensitivity of distant metastasis, even though it may aid in improving the specificity of hepatic metastasis in some cases.[43] A rectal enema may be given to adequately delineate the lesions in the recto-sigmoid and descending colon. Recent technological developments like dual-energy spectral CT allow for more reliable depiction of subtle contrast enhancement based on iodine uptake thereby improving the detection and overall staging.

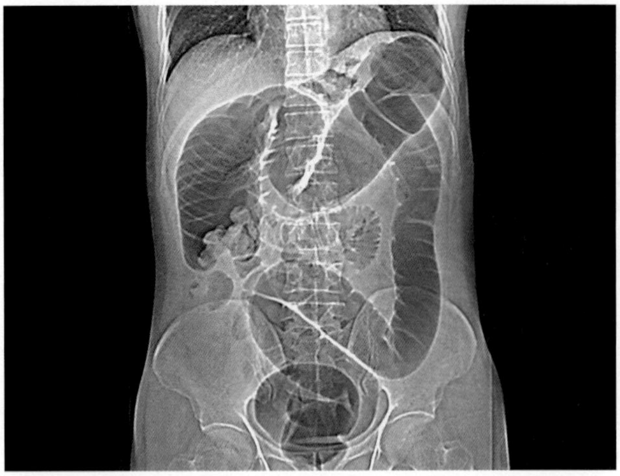

FIG. 9: Tomogram obtained before acquiring data for CT colonography shows the polypoidal mass lesion in the cecum. The rest of the colon is well distended with air.

The normal wall thickness of the colon varies depending on state of distension. In a well-distended state, it measures up to 3 mm. Often, it may be difficult to measure the true wall thickness because of contracted or collapsed state, associated fecal or fluid contents, redundancy of segments, and wall thickness of up to 6 mm and in the distal colon and even up to 8 mm may still be considered normal in totally contracted states. On the other hand, wall thickness measuring 5 mm should be considered as thickened if the colonic segment is distended with luminal width of >2 cm.[44] The rectum, rectosigmoid region, and ascending and descending segments of the colon are relatively fixed structures and therefore, more easily assessed by routine CT. However, lesions in the flexures and transverse colon are relatively less suited to examination by CT because of peristalsis and diaphragmatic excursions make these segments more difficult to assess. These limitations have partially been overcome with the advent of fast helical CT scanners.

The primary tumor is identified as focal or circumferential mural thickening or more frequently appears as a discrete mass. The mural thickening is usually asymmetric with loss of mural stratification and associated with shouldering of borders. Occasionally, an intraluminal polypoid mass without wall thickening is seen. Sometimes, CT with rectal contrast can show a typical "napkin ring" appearance of annular constricting malignancy and plaque-like lesion. Large masses may undergo necrosis and appear as soft tissue masses with internal areas of low attenuation. CT scan can enable detection of the mucinous variant of tumors, which characteristically show markedly hypoattenuating areas with heterogeneous contrast enhancement.[45] Mucinous tumors may sometimes contain calcification; however, this occurs more often in hepatic metastasis than in the primary tumor. In rectal and sigmoid cancers, the asymmetric nodular mural thickening may sometimes mimic diverticulitis, especially if there is infiltration of the tumors into the pericolic fat. However, identification of fluid in root of sigmoid mesentery and prominence of adjoining mesenteric vasculature favors the diagnosis of diverticulitis; on the other hand associated pericolic lymph nodes raise the suspicion of colon cancer. Pericolic lymph nodes adjacent to a thickened segment of colon are much more commonly seen with colonic malignancy than in cases of diverticulitis. Mural thickening can sometimes be concentric and appear symmetric and then it becomes extremely challenging to radiologically differentiate malignant from benign etiologies.

The pericolonic and perirectal fat on CT appears uniformly hypodense without any soft tissue stranding. Thickening of the perirectal fascia produces the "halo sign" which is seen with extension of tumor into perirectal fat. Extramural spread should be suspected whenever a focal mass deforms the contour of the outer colonic wall with an advancing nodular margin and may be associated with or without pericolonic soft tissue stranding **(Figs. 10 and 11)**. Extracolonic spread of malignancy may also be suggested by the loss of fat planes between the colon and adjoining muscles like levator ani, obturator internus, piriformis, coccygeus, and gluteus. It is however important to remember that the loss of fat planes on imaging is a nonspecific sign and may also be secondary to cachexia or vascular/lymphatic congestion, and therefore care must be taken to interpret it with caution.[46] However, definite invasion is present when the tumor extends directly into adjacent muscles with obliteration of fat planes along with focal enlargement of the muscle or presence of an intramuscular mass.

Spread to adjacent organs in the pelvis should also be interpreted with caution and diagnosed only if a major portion of that viscera is enveloped or if an obvious mass involves that contiguous organ **(Figs. 12A and B)**. Primary or recurrent colonic cancers can infiltrate the adjacent small bowel loops and colonic segments, seminal vesicles, sciatic nerve, prostate, bladder, uterus, and ovaries and also cause hydronephrosis by obstructing the ureters. Fistula between the colon and adjoining viscera such as bladder can be demonstrated by either direct visualization of the fistulous tract especially on multiplanar reformats or presence of associated secondary signs such as of air within the bladder. Fistulization can occur into the uterovaginal areas, ischiorectal fossa, or adjacent small bowel loops. Colonic cancers can also cause adjoining bony destruction which may be minor and more evident on bony window settings or may present with dominant extraosseous soft tissue mass in more advanced cases.

Regional lymph nodes are the most common metastatic site in colorectal carcinoma. CT however cannot reliably distinguish benign from malignant lymphadenopathy, especially in smaller-sized nodes. Metastatic foci may harbor in normal-sized lymph nodes (<1 cm), on the contrary reactive inflammatory lymph nodes may often be larger than 1 cm resulting in false-positive assessment of nodal disease. Till date, there are no validated and accurate radiologic criteria for diagnosing lymph node involvement in colon cancer. Many researchers have

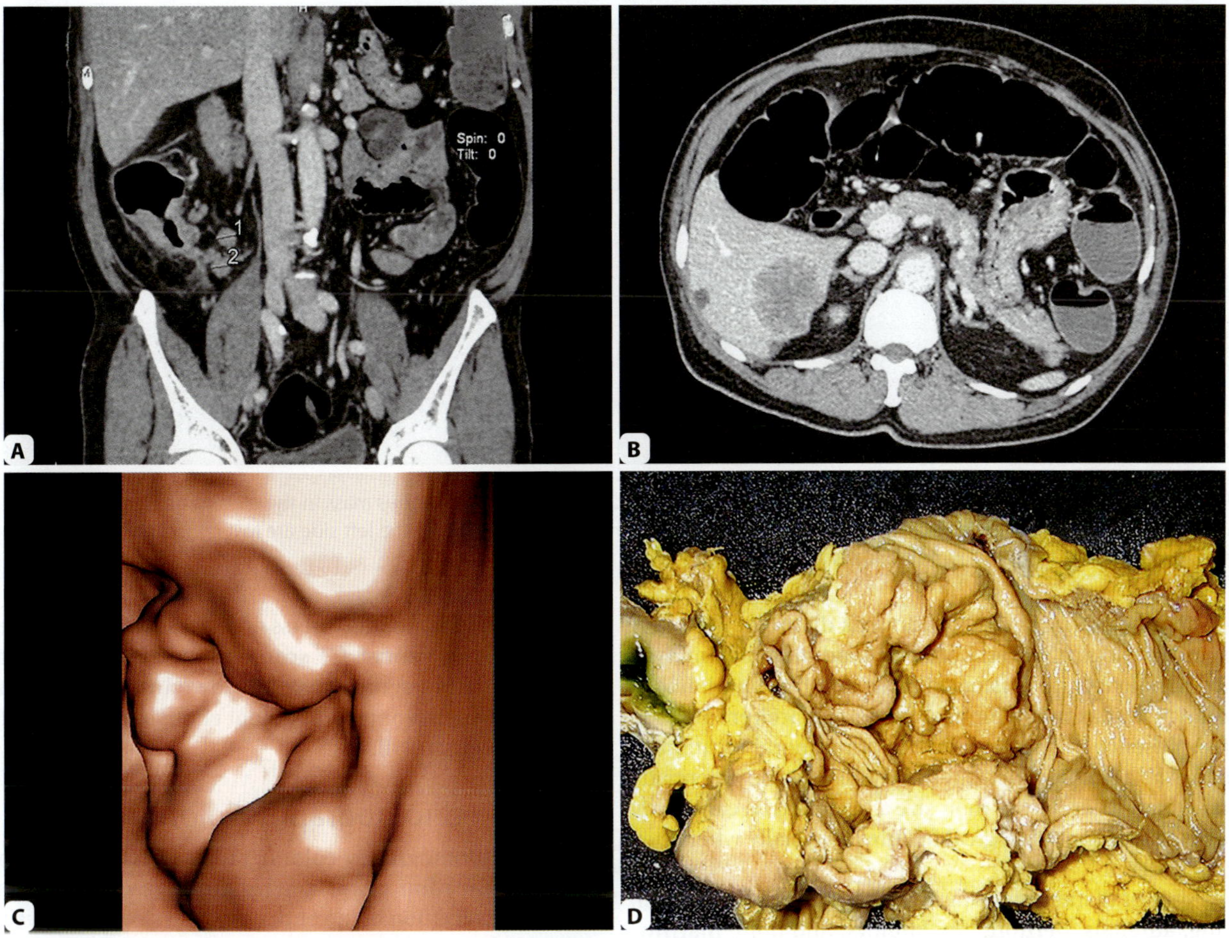

FIGS. 10A TO D: (A) Coronal MPR image shows concentric mural thickening with a polypoidal component in the cecum. Pericolonic stranding and multiple enlarged pericolonic lymph nodes are also seen; (B) Axial CECT section of the upper abdomen shows hypodense lesions in segment VI of liver suggestive of metastases; (C) CT colonoscopy endoluminal image shows the intraluminal irregular polypoidal growth; and (D) Gross photograph of the ulceroproliferative growth involving the cecum which appears to be infiltrating up to the serosal fat.

(CECT: contrast-enhanced CT; MPR: multi-planar reconstruction)

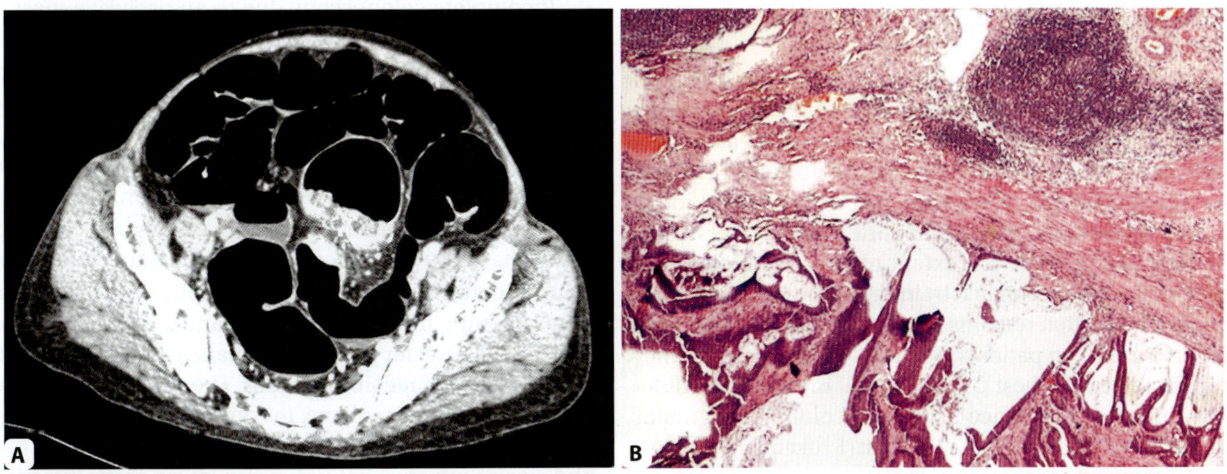

FIGS. 11A AND B: (A) Contrast-enhanced CT colonography (CE-CTC) image shows heterogeneously enhancing rectosigmoid growth with pericolonic stranding, CT stage: T3; (B) Representative microphotograph of this T3 tumor showing infiltration through the muscularis propria into the subserosa consistent with stage T3 (H&E, ×250).

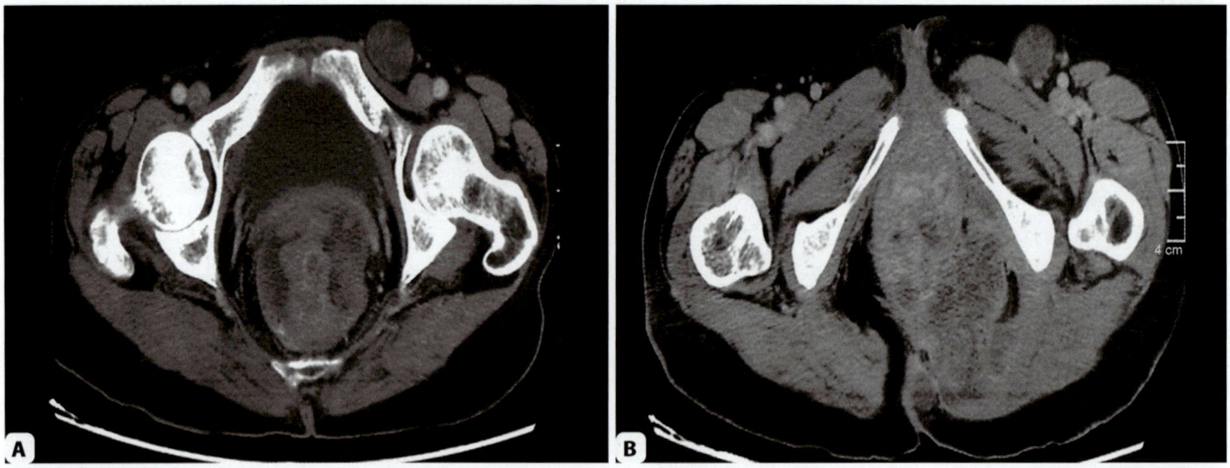

FIGS. 12A AND B: Axial contrast-enhanced CT (CECT) sections show a large heterogeneous mass in the rectum obliterating the lumen. The planes of the mass with the vagina, lateral pelvic wall and gluteal muscles on the left side are lost consistently with invasion. A large left inguinal lymph node is also seen.

used size criteria, such as short axis diameter > 10 mm or morphological criteria of ill-defined margins, internal heterogeneity, and clusters of three or more lymph nodes to favor nodal involvement. Some researchers believe that presence of lymph nodes, in peritumoral location or along the adjoining mesenteric vessels, may be potentially malignant regardless of their size and should be cautiously reviewed for morphological features especially when they are clustered.[47]

Sites of distant metastasis generally include the liver, lung, adrenals, peritoneum, kidneys, and bone marrow. The liver is the most common site for hematogenous metastasis. On noncontrast CT, hepatic metastases usually appear as discrete, hypodense lesions of variable sizes, and foci of calcification may be seen with metastatic mucinous adenocarcinoma. On CECT, these may remain hypoattenuating compared to the background liver on dynamic contrast-enhanced phases. More typically they show hypodense necrotic center with progressively enhancing rim producing classic "target appearance" on multiphasic scans.

Peritoneal carcinomatosis results from spread of tumor over peritoneal surfaces and is seen on CT as enhancing linear or nodular peritoneal thickening often associated with ascites. Common sites for peritoneal implants include omentum, mesentery, surface of bowel loops, pouch of Douglas, paracolic gutter, and undersurface of diaphragm. However, extent of peritoneal disease is frequently underestimated by imaging and early peritoneal involvement often remains undetected until a laparotomy is performed.[48] In patients with disseminated malignancy, careful review of chest CT may reveal metastatic nodules. In women with advanced stages of colonic malignancy, bilateral ovarian masses may be seen (Krukenberg's tumor).

Computed tomography is fairly accurate in staging patients with advanced malignancy. Pitfalls, however, occur in interpretation in patients with less advanced tumors. Associated perforation/ulceration of colonic cancer may result in an inflammatory mass or abscess which obscures the underlying cancer. CT scan obtained in postsurgical or postradiation setting may be viewed with caution as associated edema or posttreatment changes may simulate residual/recurrent disease.

Computed Tomography Colonography

Computed tomography colonography (CTC) is an innovative application of surface rendering technique that entails visualization of the entire colon as an alternative to optical colonoscopy for screening and diagnostic purposes **(Figs. 13A to D)**. It was in 1994 that Vining and Gelfand from Bowman Gray University introduced CT colonography and exhibited the first CT colonography fly-through video at the annual meeting of the Society of Gastrointestinal Radiologists.[49]

The accepted indications for CT colonography are as follows:

- Incomplete colonoscopy due to an occlusive mass or stricture preventing examination of the proximal colon.
- Incomplete colonoscopy due to colonic tortuosity, adhesions, severe diverticular disease, or patient intolerance of colonoscopy.
- Inability to perform colonoscopy due to requirement for anticoagulant therapy or risks of sedation.
- Patients who adamantly refuse to undergo colonoscopy but have a strong indication for diagnostic colonoscopy.

Computed tomography colonography is under analysis as a screening tool for colorectal cancer as it is relatively safe and has greater patient acceptance as compared with other available screening methods. The contraindication for CT colonography are allergy to contrast, suspected colonic perforation, acute colonic infection (acute diverticulitis and severe infective colitis), acute lower gastrointestinal bleeding, complete colonic obstruction, very recent colonic surgery (<1 week), medically unstable patients, and refusal to undergo colonic preparation.

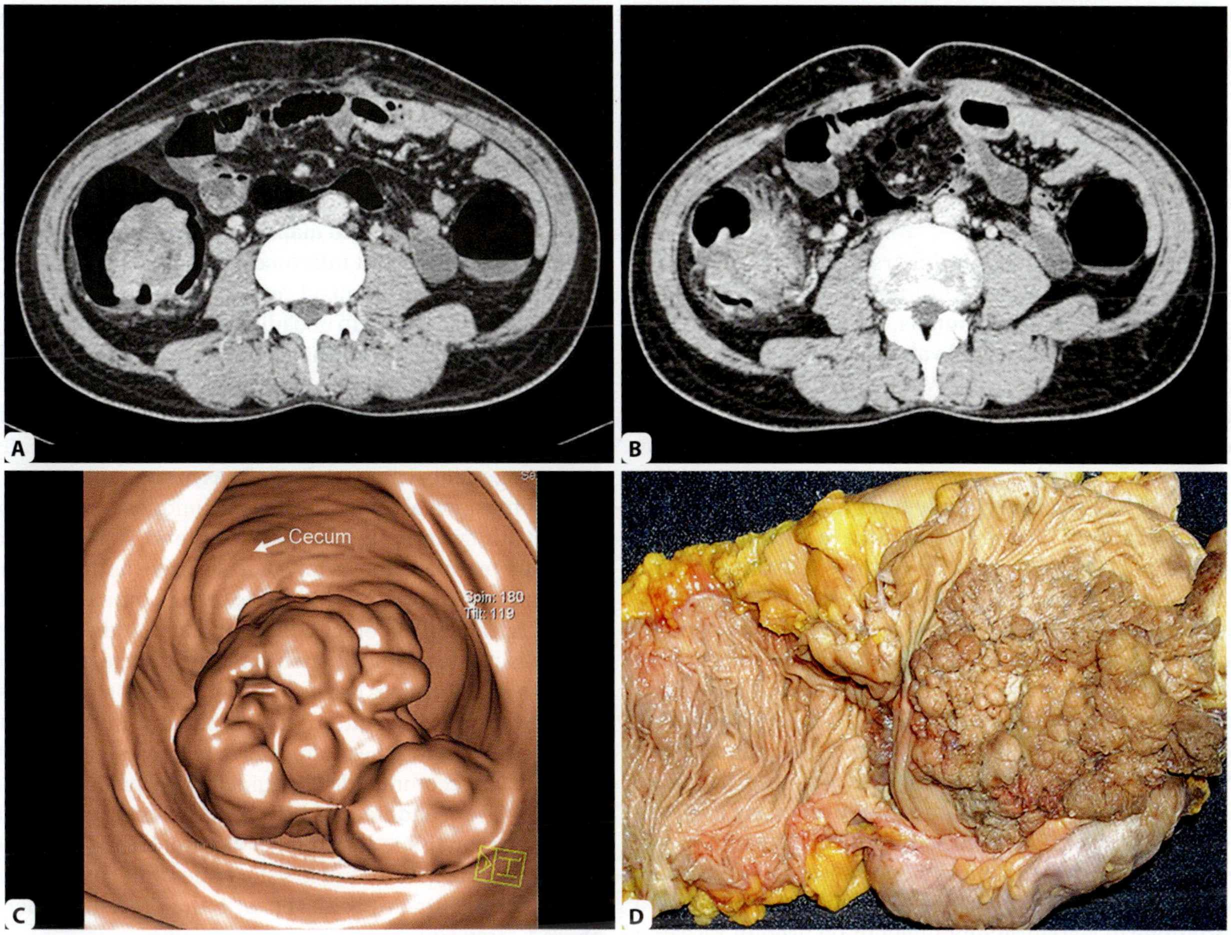

FIGS. 13A TO D: (A and B) Axial contrast-enhanced CT colonography (CECTC) images show presence of polypoidal cecal growth with classical pericolonic stranding and lymph nodes—CT stage: T3N2M0. Surgical stage: T3N2M0. Histological stage: T3N0M0; (C) CT colonographic image of the same patient showing a polypoidal intraluminal cecal mass; and (D) Gross photograph showing a proliferative tumor almost completely filling up the cecal lumen.

The basic technique for a successful CT colonography involves adequate colonic cleansing and optimal distension of colon followed by image acquisition with multidetector computed tomography (MDCT), and postprocessing of acquired data using dedicated CT colonography softwares to readily detect clinically relevant polyps. Robust colonic preparation is crucial for accurate polyp detection and involves both cleansing and tagging. For "wet preparation" polyethylene glycol is used; while for "dry preparation", phosphosoda is used. Optimal colonic distension is critical for increasing the polyp conspicuity. This is generally distinct from maximal distension, because patient's comfort and safety must be given due diligence for more wider acceptance and clinical usage. This can be achieved by using room air or carbon dioxide. Colonic perforation is rarely seen (0.059–0.08%).[50] Advanced age and underlying colonic pathology are the risk factors for colonic perforation. Air can be administered easily, is available at no cost, but is less well tolerated than carbon dioxide as it is not absorbed by the colonic mucosa. Carbon dioxide, on the other hand, is gradually absorbed by the colonic wall, resulting in diminished discomfort to the patient **(Fig. 14)**.

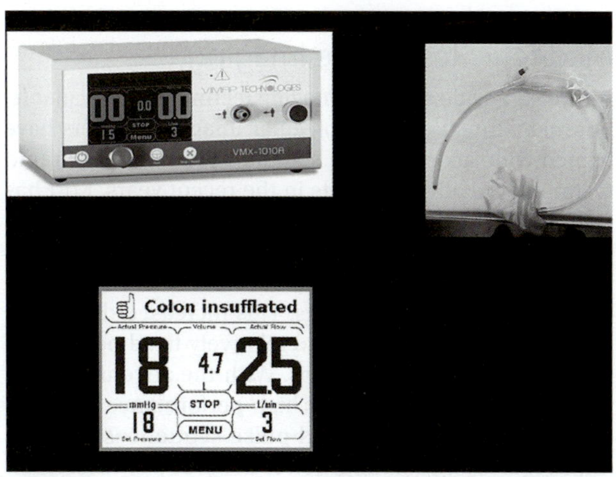

FIG. 14: CO_2 insufflation pump, insufflation tube catheter, and the final message on the pump when the colon is completely insufflated.

Image acquisition is done after colonic insufflations in supine and prone positions on a helical CT scanner using low-dose technique. The radiation dose is about half of the dose of a barium enema.[50] Intravenous contrast improves detection of medium-sized polyps (6–9 mm), especially in a suboptimally prepared colon.[51] After acquiring supine and prone scans, various software packages are used to display images. Both 2D and 3D (endoluminal) visualization modes should be used for detection of polyp, although the latter is much easier and more effective for low-prevalence screening.

There are various mimickers of polyps which are potential pitfalls of CT colonography. These include adherent fecal matter, lipomas, inverted appendicular stump, prominent ileocecal valve, inverted diverticulum, and bulbous colonic folds. While some of these are due to technical reasons on account of inadequate colon preparation or distension, others are due to perceptive errors.

In the first published study from India, the sensitivity and specificity of CT colonography have been reported to be 65% and 77%, respectively for lesions 1–5 mm; 97% and 83%, respectively for lesions 6–9 mm; and 100% and 100%, respectively for lesions 10 mm or larger.[52] CT colonography scores over optical colonoscopy as it provides information about extracolonic findings. The incidence of significant extracolonic findings ranges from 6.8 to 21%.[50] A reporting system for CT colonography has been devised by the Working Group on Virtual Colonoscopy and has been termed "C-RADS" or CT colonography reporting and data system which has been revised in 2023.[53] The aim of this reporting system is to achieve standardization of reporting which allows more consistent and reliable communication and uniform classification of data to be used in research studies. The advances in CT colonography include fluid and fecal tagging to achieve "prepless" studies by digital bowel cleansing using subtraction techniques. Computer-aided detection (CAD) software and novel 3D views that slice open and flatten the colonic wall have been developed.

Magnetic Resonance Imaging

Although a wide range of imaging techniques is available, not many functional or molecular imaging markers have gained wide acceptance in standard practice. With rapid technological advancements in the recent years, MRI has established itself as a standard imaging modality in the diagnostic armamentarium for evaluation of rectosigmoid malignancies where it performs more accurately than the rest of the colonic tumors. This increased diagnostic performance is mainly due to relatively fixed position of the rectosigmoid in the pelvis. With the advent of latest advanced MR techniques with high-performance gradients and faster and more refined pulse sequences, there is improved resolution and better accuracy of MR which guides in taking appropriate management decisions.

Rectal Cancer Assessment

Magnetic resonance imaging serves an integral role in clinical evaluation and preoperative management of colorectal cancer, and has become the fundamental diagnostic technique for the early detection and accurate local staging of primary malignancy. It facilitates the detection of important prognostic signs, which aids in taking appropriate management decisions. In patients of rectal cancer, it helps in appropriate risk stratification with low-risk patients being considered for upfront surgery where MR provides a road map to the surgeons for the best surgical approach; and intermediate to high-risk patients with more locally advanced rectal cancers (LARCs) who are generally subjected to neoadjuvant chemoradiotherapy (CRT) for potential downstaging prior to any surgery later if feasible. In posttreatment setting, MRI helps in evaluating the response to treatment and restaging. MR also helps in early recognition of local recurrence which is especially useful in patients who are clinically asymptomatic.

Optimization of MR acquisition techniques and protocol along with systematic interpretation and standardized reporting template allows for more accurate and reproducible interpretations, which fosters better communication with surgical and oncology colleagues in multidisciplinary team discussions for all such patients. There are some controversial practices like bowel preparation or endorectal filling which are based on individual and institutional preferences and may be performed in select cases; however, these are not recommended by guidelines of major scientific societies. Use of endorectal MRI with its potential advantage of superior soft tissue resolution is also not endorsed by the guidelines due to cost and logistic issues and comparable diagnostic accuracies achieved with the present modern phased-array coils of MRI.[4]

The standard workhorse MRI sequence in rectal cancers includes high-resolution two-dimensional (2D) T2-weighted fast spin-echo (FSE) sequence which offers the best resolution for accurate assessment of the depth of tumor invasion, prediction of infiltration of mesorectal fascia, adjacent pelvic visceral, and lymph node involvement. The sagittal plane is the first sequence to be performed which identifies the tumor; and it is used for guiding the planning of oblique axial images. The axial images should be acquired with correct angulation perpendicular to the long axis of the tumor to correctly identify its margins and avoid any partial volume effects thereby aiding in accurate T staging.[54] The coronal images are generally planned parallel to the major axis of the anal canal, particularly in lower rectal tumors. This is the most useful plane for assessment of the tumor infiltration into anal sphincteric complex and levator ani muscle.[55] Correct angulation is important as incorrect plane obliquity may cause blurring of the outline of muscularis propria, which may result in errors in T staging and impact consequent management decisions.

Diffusion-weighted imaging (DWI) is another sequence now being increasingly adopted as a part of routine protocol in most institutions. DWI should be acquired with similar angulation as T2-weighted images with high b-values > 800 s/mm^2 and calculation of quantitative parameters in the form of apparent diffusion coefficient (ADC) maps.

The value of DWI for primary tumor staging is limited, although may be helpful in directing attention to the radiologist to small tumors or in presence of loaded fecal matter within the lumen. DWI helps in easy detection of lymph nodes owing to the high cellular density of lymphoid tissue. The usefulness of visual assessment of DWI for characterization of nodes is however less apparent with potential risk of nodal over staging. There is increasing evidence in literature which shows that DWI is especially useful in posttreatment setting to assess the response to treatment and detect residual/recurrent disease. In the recent years, there has been increasing interest in the utility of quantitative DWI parameters being employed as a prognostic imaging biomarker to assess and predict clinical response.[56] The routine use of DWI for restaging of rectal cancer is also recently advocated by expert consensus guidelines of the European Society of Gastrointestinal and Abdominal Radiology (ESGAR).[57]

Another optional sequence is T1-weighted FSE sequence of the entire pelvis which aides in detection of common iliac and lower retroperitoneal lymph nodes especially in the setting of mucinous/signet-cell carcinomas where the T2 signal intensity of the primary malignancy approaches close to mesorectal fat. It is also useful adjunct in evaluation of bony lesions and other incidental genitourinary lesions.

Postcontrast T1-weighted sequence is generally not a part of routine protocol for primary staging as various studies have shown that addition of post-gadolinium sequence to the standard high-resolution T2-weighted sequences does not improve the diagnostic accuracy of local staging. However, some researchers believe that when MR is performed for response assessment/restaging, intravenous contrast may help in more confident detection of residual/ recurrent tumors which will generally shows heterogeneous enhancement.[58]

For primary staging of rectal tumors, MRI can accurately describe the exact location of the tumor, its morphology, T stage, status of infiltration of anal sphincter complex, relation of tumor to the mesorectal fascia with prediction of circumferential resection margin (CRM) status, extramural vascular invasion (EMVI), and N category, all of which should be clearly documented in a standardized reporting template. Mucinous and signet-cell carcinomas have characteristic morphology with variably hyperintense signal on T2-weighted image as compared to the more intermediate signal of adenocarcinomas.[59] This distinction and identification of mucinous variant is clinically relevant since mucinous tumors tend to have worse prognosis and generally respond poorly to neoadjuvant treatment regimens **(Figs. 15A and B)**. Although the standard definition is primarily histologic, it has been argued that mucinous tumors may be more efficiently identified on T2-weighted MR sequence than on biopsy with the imaging criteria being >50% hyperintense signal areas within the bulk of the tumor.[59,60] The signet-ring cell carcinomas on MRI typically manifest as diffuse long-segmental mural thickening with submucosal infiltrative pattern of growth resulting in "target" appearance on the axial sections. "Diffuse infiltration of the mesorectal fat" is another frequent feature of signet-cell tumors **(Figs. 16A to C)**.[61]

The accuracy of MR for the assessment of T stage is variably reported in literature ranging from 66 to 94% with histopathology being the reference standard.[62,63] The invasion of the tumor through the muscularis propria into the surrounding mesorectum can be well-recognized as an interruption of the hypointense muscularis with nodular extension of tumor signal beyond the rectal wall into the mesorectal fat **(Figs. 17A to C)**. MRI can reliably visualize the infiltration of the tumor into the mesorectal fascia with high degree of accuracy **(Figs. 18A and B)**. The primary diagnostic challenge is however in differentiating between T2 and early T3, and this distinction is particularly important in low rectal tumors considering the anatomic tapering of mesorectal fat inferiorly and proximity to the

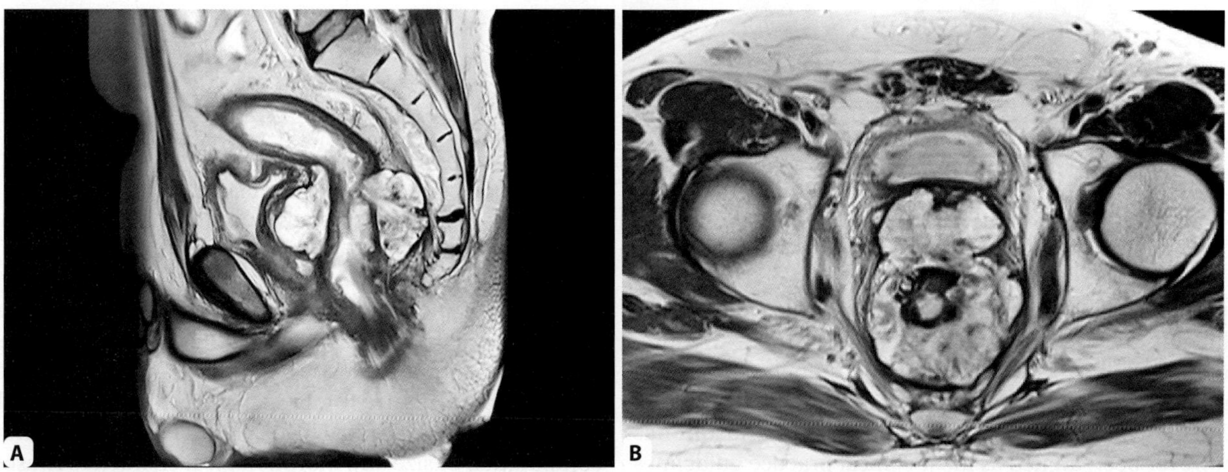

FIGS. 15A AND B: Sagittal and axial T2-weighted MR sections showing bulky mucinous tumor with distinct bright signal characteristic of mucinous histology. Mucinous tumors contain >50% of stromal mucin.

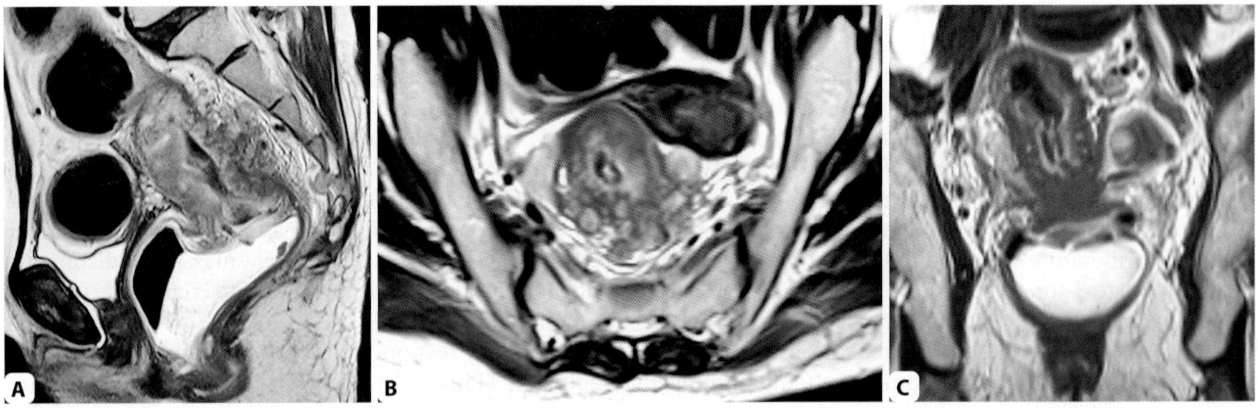

FIGS. 16A TO C: Sagittal, axial, and coronal T2-weighted sections showing diffuse long-segmental mural thickening involving mid and upper rectum with T2 intermediate to hyperintense signal, and infiltrative pattern of growth and associated adenopathy.

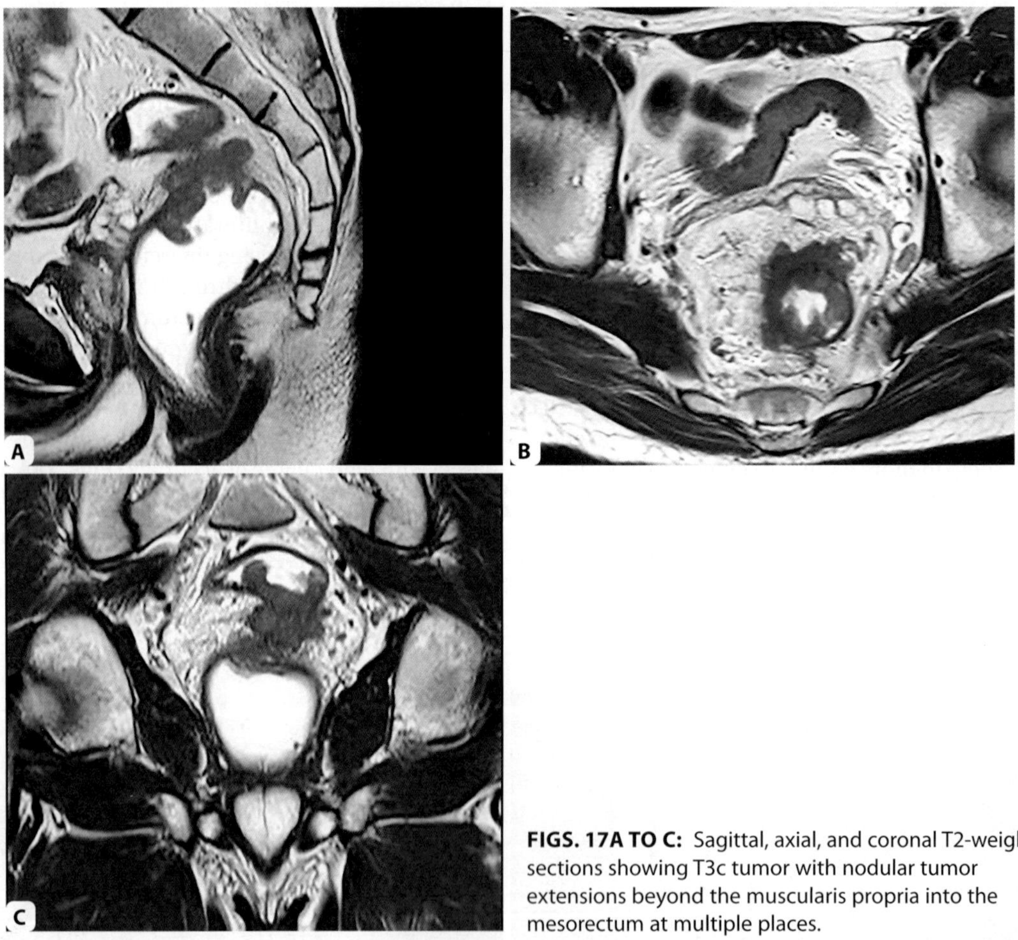

FIGS. 17A TO C: Sagittal, axial, and coronal T2-weighted sections showing T3c tumor with nodular tumor extensions beyond the muscularis propria into the mesorectum at multiple places.

sphincteric complex and the levator ani muscle. It can be difficult to clearly differentiate between true extramural infiltration in early T3 tumors from desmoplastic reaction in T1-2 tumors which can result in potential over staging.[64] The clinical relevance of this imaging conundrum has however been argued as most clinical practice guidelines stratify early T3 tumors with <5 mm extramural infiltration (cT3ab) in the same low-risk group as the T1-T2 tumors for management perspective.

Nodal staging still remains challenging for radiologists as lymph nodal assessment by MRI has a relatively lower accuracy as compared to the determination of the T stage. MRI cannot recognize tumor foci in normal-sized lymph nodes. Prediction of nodal involvement is improved when combination of size and morphological characters is used to characterize these lymph nodes. The morphology and signal intensity are in fact regarded as better predictors and more reliable than the size alone.[65] The presence,

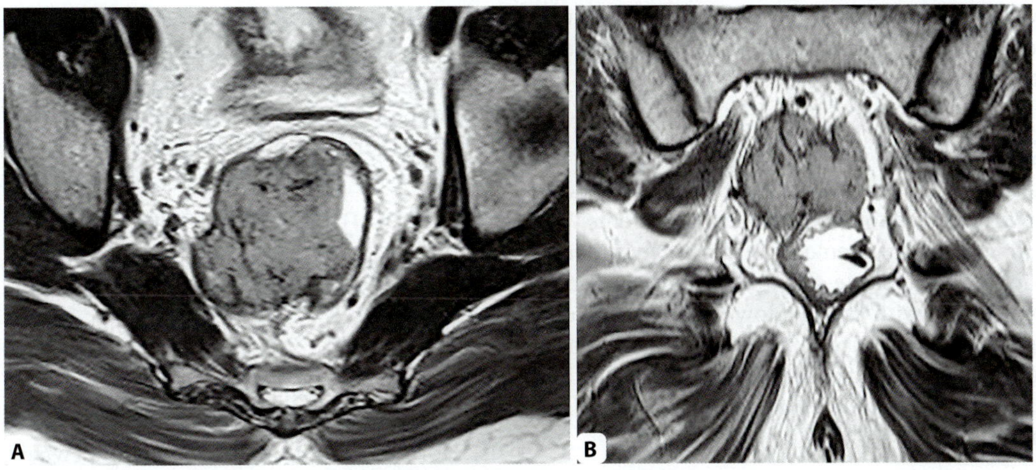

FIGS. 18A AND B: Axial and Coronal T2-weighted sections showing T3d mesorectal fascia (MRF) + with broad nodular tumor extension on the right side reaching up to the MRF (compare the intermediate signal intensity of the tumor in this case which was adenocarcinoma on histology to the bright signal of the mucinous tumor in patient shown in Figure 15).

number, and precise location of any suspicious lymph nodes must be diligently documented. Depiction of tumor in normal-sized lymph nodes is currently being explored in research studies by use of additional novel contrast agents directed at imaging nodal metastasis. From management perspective, most current clinical guidelines consider node-positive disease as high-risk feature and advocate using neoadjuvant chemoradiation in these patients, regardless of the T stage. Extramesorectal (or lateral pelvic) lymph nodes are more important from treatment perspective as these are not routinely dissected in "standard total mesorectal excision (TME)". These need to be carefully looked for and documented as it may alter the surgical procedure or lead to additional boost radiation treatment in their location to optimize the oncological treatment results.

Magnetic resonance imaging can accurately identify extramural vascular invasion (EMVI), which is another important prognostic marker even when the normal vascular outline is completely replaced by the tumor. There is vascular expansion with irregularity or nodular margins and intermediate signal intensity in the vessel lumen corresponding to the signal of the primary tumor. This may be challenging to report by the pathologists since the vascular structure may be destroyed and replaced by the tumor.[79]

Liver and other visceral metastases are as well demonstrated on MR as on helical CT. All extrahepatic sites must be carefully evaluated to assess for any metastatic lesions. Assessment for peritoneal carcinomatosis remains challenging owing to complex peritoneal anatomy. Traditionally, MDCT is regarded as the more versatile tool and better than conventional MR techniques. However, with advances in MR technology and protocols, MRI is now considered comparable with MDCT in the detection of peritoneal deposits (>1 cm). The fat-suppressed and delayed gadolinium-enhanced sequences coupled with use of water-soluble luminal contrast agents have resulted in more improved sensitivities exceeding those of CT in some studies. Peritoneal deposits generally tend to enhance slowly after administering gadolinium and appear most conspicuous on delayed sequence obtained after 5 minutes. MRI is regarded superior to CT for depiction of subtle osseous metastases. MRI is superior to CT at distinguishing between fibrosis and recurrent cancer and could eliminate the need for biopsies.

Magnetic Resonance Colonography

Magnetic resonance colonography (MRC) is another noninvasive technique for evaluation of the entire colon and is primarily based on the acquisition of MR datasets which optimize the visualization of the large bowel. Data collection is mainly performed with breath-hold scans. As with CT colonography, sufficient distension of the bowel is the key prerequisite to optimize the examination which can be achieved by water, barium, room air, or CO_2. Spasmolytics are given intravenously before rectal filling. Patient preparation involves administering cathartics and enemas based on institutional protocols. 2D and/or 3D fast imaging with steady state precession (FISP) is a useful sequence for MRC. 3D T1-weighted images are also acquired before and after administration of gadolinium intravenously. A T1-weighted 2D FLASH (fast low-angle shot) sequence is acquired in the axial plane for evaluation of adjacent abdominal organs. Similar to the technique in CT colonography, patients are imaged in both supine and prone positions. Axial, MPR, and "fly-through" images are then analyzed on workstations in both antegrade and retrograde directions. MRC has been reported to have 100% sensitivity for lesions larger than 10 mm and 89% for lesions 5–10 mm in size.[67] However, most polyps smaller than 5 mm were not detected by MRC.

Magnetic resonance colonography has evolved as an alternative technique over CT colonography with some distinct advantages including the lack of ionizing radiation, superior soft tissue resolution, and the use of safer intravenous contrast agents. Some limitations include higher susceptibility to motion artifacts, longer examination time, limited availability, and cost concerns.

Arteriography

Arteriography has only limited value in colonic cancers. Its application is restricted to the evaluation of patients with acute bleeding of apparent colonic origin for therapeutic embolization. The bleeding site may be indentified in patients presenting with chronic low-grade blood loss. Arteriography with chemoembolization or radiofrequency/ microwave ablation is also used for treating metastatic liver deposits in patients with colonic malignancies, who are not surgical candidates.

Immunoscintigraphy

Labeled anti-carcinoembryonic antigen (anti-CEA) monoclonal antibodies (MoAbs) have been used as in vivo tumor localizing agents. Primary adenocarcinoma of colon and metastatic foci are seen as areas of increased radioactivity (hot spots). Depending on the size of tumor necrosis, liver metastases may appear as areas of intense, absent, or intermediate uptake. The reported sensitivity of MoAb staging of colorectal cancer is 65–86% with specificity for detection of primary tumor, local recurrence, and distant metastasis varying from 77 to 92%.[68]

Positron Emission Tomography

Fluorodeoxyglucose positron emission tomography/ computed tomography (FDG PET/CT) is an advanced imaging technique which is increasingly being used in the comprehensive assessment of colorectal cancers. PET is the most sensitive modality which may be used for excluding any occult hepatic or extrahepatic metastases in patients of colorectal carcinoma who are otherwise candidates for surgery. Another clinically useful application of PET/ CT over routine conventional imaging is in assessment of early therapy response in patients receiving neoadjuvant therapy for rectal cancer. Another frequent indication is in evaluating patients with suspected recurrent disease who have rising CEA levels[69] **(Figs. 19 and 20)**. Dedicated oncology centers are using PET/CT data for

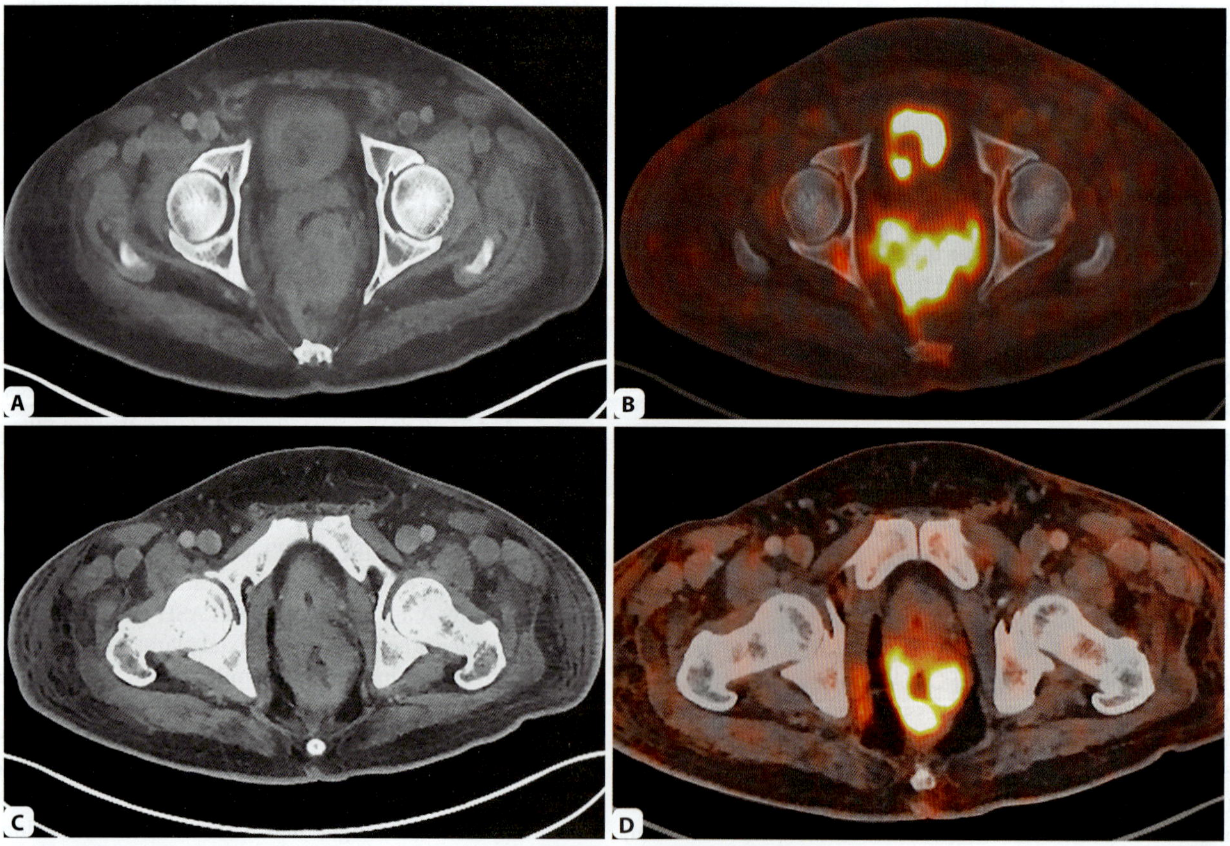

FIGS. 19A TO D: (A and B) Axial CT and PET/CT fused images showing FDG-avid rectal malignancy with small FDG-avid osteolytic lesion in posterior pillar of right acetabulum confirming the osseous metastasis which was missed on conventional CT. (C and D) Axial CT and PET/CT fused images in a different patient showing FDG-avid lower rectal malignancy with small FDG-avid deposits in right obturator internus muscle not detected on routine CT.

(FDG: fluorodeoxyglucose; PET/CT: positron emission tomography/computed tomography)

Courtesy: Dr Rajender Kumar, Department of Nuclear Medicine, PGIMER, Chandigarh, India.

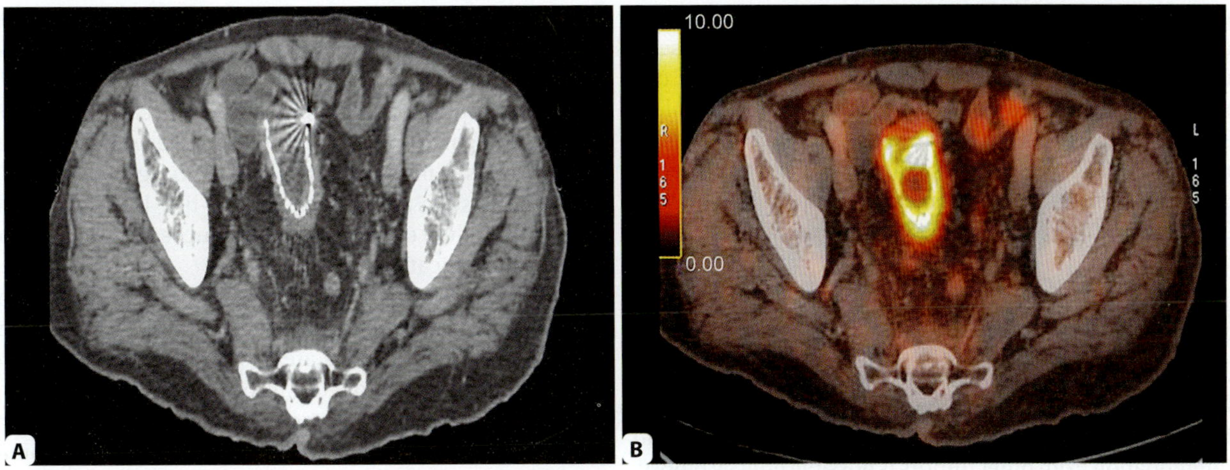

FIGS. 20A AND B: Axial CT (A) and positron emission tomography/computed tomography (PET/CT) fusion image (B) in a patient postchemoradiation and postcolonic stent showing recurrent rectosigmoid thickening and locoregional lymph node. The bowel wall thickening showed more tracer uptake than the lymph node.

Courtesy: Professor BR Mittal, Department of Nuclear Medicine, PGIMER, Chandigarh, India.

the determination of target volumes in place of traditional CT for planning and optimization of radiation treatments. Limitations of PET include poor sensitivity in detecting colon lesions ≤10 mm in diameter and reduced tracer uptake by mucinous tumors. Another limitation of PET is its limited ability to distinguish between chronic infection and tumor because both of them may be show increased FDG uptake. Nonspecific PET findings can result in negative impact on patient care in up to 9% patients.[70]

RECENT ADVANCES

These include PET/CT colonography and CT perfusion imaging for colorectal tumors. PET/CT colonography involves the combination of 18F-FDG PET with CT colonography and has distinct advantage of combining both anatomic and metabolic information in a single study. It has been used both for staging of colon cancer and for screening purposes.[71,72] PET/CT colonography is recommended in patients with obstructing colorectal malignancies where scope cannot be negotiated beyond the site of obstruction. The standard uptake value of malignant tumors has been reported to be between 4 and 20 with a mean of 9.[72]

Tumor perfusion of rectal cancer has been measured with first-pass perfusion CT. Rectal cancers show higher blood flow (BF) and shorter mean transit time (MTT) compared with those of normal rectum. After chemotherapy and radiotherapy, responders show significant reduction in BF and increase in MTT.[73,74] Significant difference in baseline BF and MTT is seen between responders and nonresponders. Another study by Ippolito D et al. concluded that dynamic contrast-enhanced MR (CEMR) perfusion analysis is a complementary diagnostic technique for identifying vascularity patterns of tumor tissue in local advanced rectal cancer and is a useful marker in evaluation of treatment response.[75]

AMERICAN COLLEGE OF RADIOLOGY RECOMMENDATIONS FOR COLORECTAL CANCER STAGING

The latest recommendations of the American College of Radiology (ACR) are based on the concept that for colon cancer, the value of imaging for locoregional staging (T and N stage) is of questionable utility. This is because neoadjuvant therapy has not shown any added survival benefit over surgery alone and the standard surgical approach is radical resection. On the other hand, for rectal cancer, the surgical options are much more diverse and are dependent on the involvement or sparing of sphincteric complex, CRM, and the peritoneal reflection. Neoadjuvant chemotherapy and radiation, in addition to surgical resection have shown benefit in reducing local recurrences and improve survival rates. Hence, there is a justifiable need for more precise and accurate preoperative staging in patients of rectal cancer.

As per the revised ACR appropriateness criteria[76] of 2021, MRI pelvis without and with IV contrast and US pelvis (transrectal) are usually most appropriate modalities for locoregional staging of primary rectal cancer. TRUS has been the reference standard for T-stage evaluation of rectal carcinoma. Although TRUS performs better than MRI for T1 tumors, comparable for T2 and T3, it may be less accurate in characterizing locally advanced T4 tumors with a tendency to understage. CT chest with IV contrast and MRI abdomen with IV contrast or CT chest abdomen pelvis with IV contrast are usually appropriate for assessment of distant metastasis in the initial imaging of colorectal cancer. Locoregional staging is not routinely required for colon cancer. The most common sites of metastatic involvement are liver and lungs. Accurate depiction of number, size, and distribution is the primary goal of colon cancer staging. Multiphase CECT or contrast-enhanced MRI with optimization of technique is best suited for diagnosing liver metastases. MRI is more accurate in the setting of fatty liver and following neoadjuvant therapy. Because of limited sensitivity of MRI for lung nodules, a chest CT can be utilized in addition to abdominal MRI for complete staging. Although there is some evidence to support the use of PET/CT in the local staging of patients with rectal carcinoma, the more common clinical application of PET/CT is in identifying nodal and distant metastases.

OTHER EPITHELIAL TUMORS OF COLON

Squamous cell carcinomas are rare except in the rectum. Radiographic appearance is similar to adenocarcinoma and differentiation from other tumors is possible only by biopsy. Cloacogenic carcinomas arise from transitional cloacogenic remnants of the anorectal junction. Radiographically the lesions are plaque-like and have a smooth or finely irregular surface. In profile, the borders form a tapered obtuse angle with the bowel wall. Ulceration is usually present. Since the lesions lie in the distal rectal areas, the catheter tip may completely obscure the lesion.

Carcinoid tumors present as submucosal lesions. The most common sites of colonic carcinoids are the rectum and cecum. They are seen as round and well-circumscribed masses **(Figs. 21A and B)**. Invasion of the bowel wall by tumor mass produces intense desmoplastic reaction and proliferation of fibrous tissue, resulting in contraction and kinking of the large bowel. Carcinoid tumors located in cecum and ascending colon are indistinguishable from adenocarcinoma on imaging.

NONEPITHELIAL TUMORS OF COLON

Mesoderm sarcomas of the large bowel are uncommon. They have a predilection for the rectal region. The lesions are usually rounded and lobulated but may be pedunculated. The tumors may grow extramurally and when the overlying mucosa ulcerates, necrosis, and cystic cavitations can develop. Kaposi's sarcoma can involve any part of the gastrointestinal tract and presents as typical extramucosal mass or masses. On imaging, Kaposi's sarcoma is seen as a flat or plaque-like lesion, a small polypoid nodule or a polypoid submucosal lesion with or without umbilication.

Gastrointestinal stromal tumors (GISTs) arise from the interstitial cells of Cajal and express CD34. Only 1% of all gastrointestinal tumors are of stromal origin and these are least commonly located in the colon. Small tumors are seen as sessile or pedunculated polyps. Large tumors may be seen as cavitating masses with a large extraluminal component or as submucosal masses with or without central ulceration **(Fig. 22)**. These lesions may mimic colonic lymphoma or carcinoma.

Colonic lipomas are uncommon benign tumors. Most lipomas are found in the right colon. About two-thirds of these tumors are pedunculated. On barium enema, they are seen as smooth sessile or polypoidal lesions with a pedicle. Some of these lipomas may be lead points of intussusceptions. When this occurs, the lipomas may ulcerate and undergo fat necrosis resulting in CT attenuation more than fat. They are then confused with an intussuscepting carcinoma **(Figs. 23A to C)**.

Lymphoma of the colon is rare. The colon is the third most common primary site of lymphoma involving the gastrointestinal tract after stomach and the small bowel. As a primary lesion, lymphoma accounts for only 0.5% of all malignant tumors. Secondary involvement by lymphoma is usually multicentric **(Figs. 24A and B)**. The radiographic pattern may be localized or diffuse. In the localized form, the lesion is seen either as a polypoid mass that protrudes into the colonic lumen or as a constricting lesion that simulates an annular carcinoma. In the diffuse form, multiple small

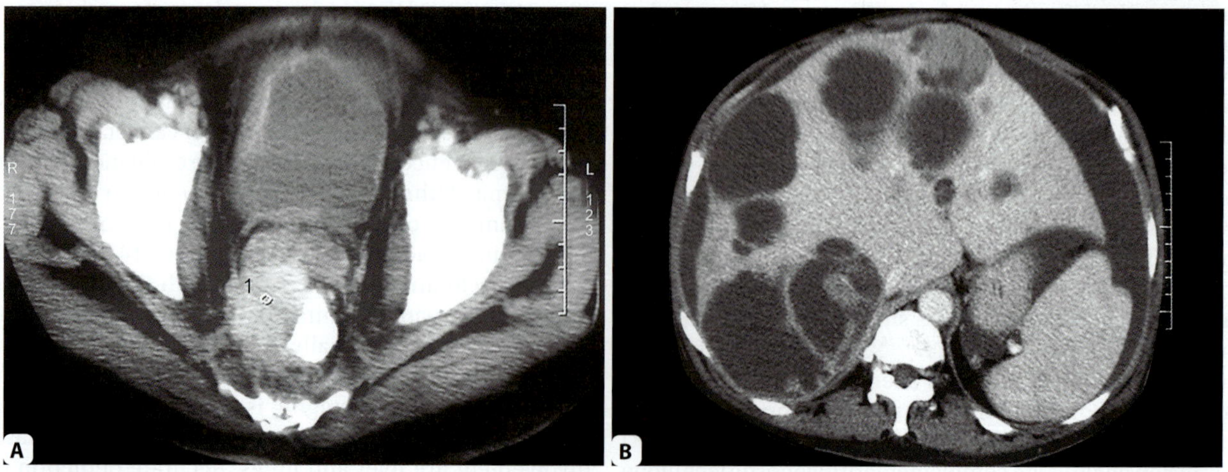

FIGS. 21A AND B: Axial contrast-enhanced computed tomography (CECT) showing a well-defined mass lesion along the right lateral wall of the rectum (A) with multiple cystic lesions in the liver (B) some of which are showing solid component in a patient with biopsy-proven carcinoid.

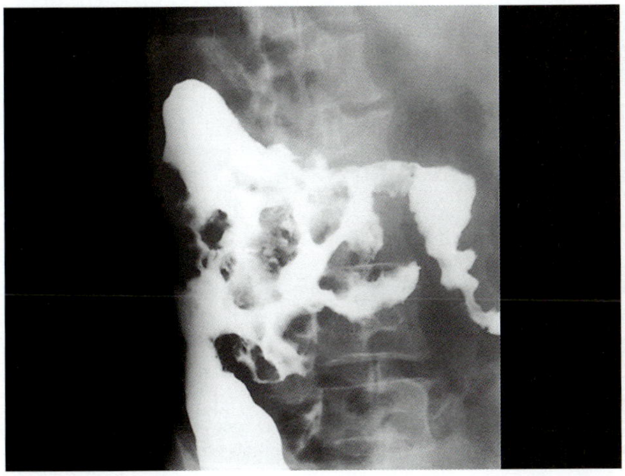

FIG. 22: Barium enema shows a large cavitatory mass lesion in the hepatic flexure with presence of deep ulcerations in a patient with leiomyosarcoma.

Courtesy: Professor B Nagi, Department of Gastroenterology, PGIMER, Chandigarh, India.

nodular lesions are seen. The defects are submucosal in origin with intact overlying mucosa. When lymphoma involves the mesentery, large masses may cause extensive compression on the colon.

SECONDARY TUMORS OF COLON

Tumors that commonly metastasize to colon include stomach, breast, pancreas, and gynecologic pelvic malignancies. Infiltration of the colon by secondary tumors produces thickening of the colonic wall and mucosal folds. The classic radiographic appearances include indentations, spiculation, angulation, narrowing, displacement, and fixation. Lymphogenous spread of tumors to the colon is characterized by the involvement of long segments, variable narrowing, and loss of haustral markings. When metastases occur by the hematogenous route, as in melanoma, lesions present as smoothly marginated submucosal masses.

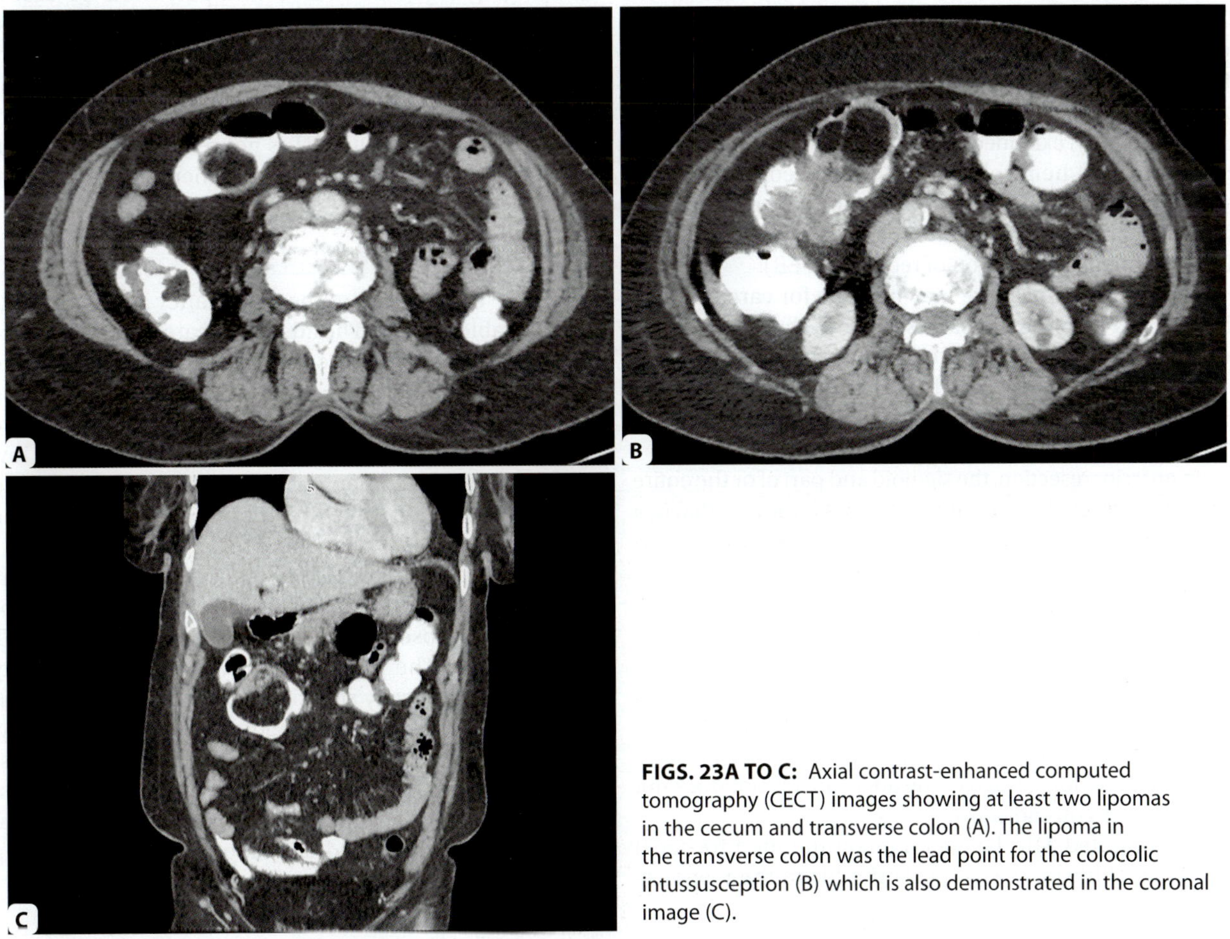

FIGS. 23A TO C: Axial contrast-enhanced computed tomography (CECT) images showing at least two lipomas in the cecum and transverse colon (A). The lipoma in the transverse colon was the lead point for the colocolic intussusception (B) which is also demonstrated in the coronal image (C).

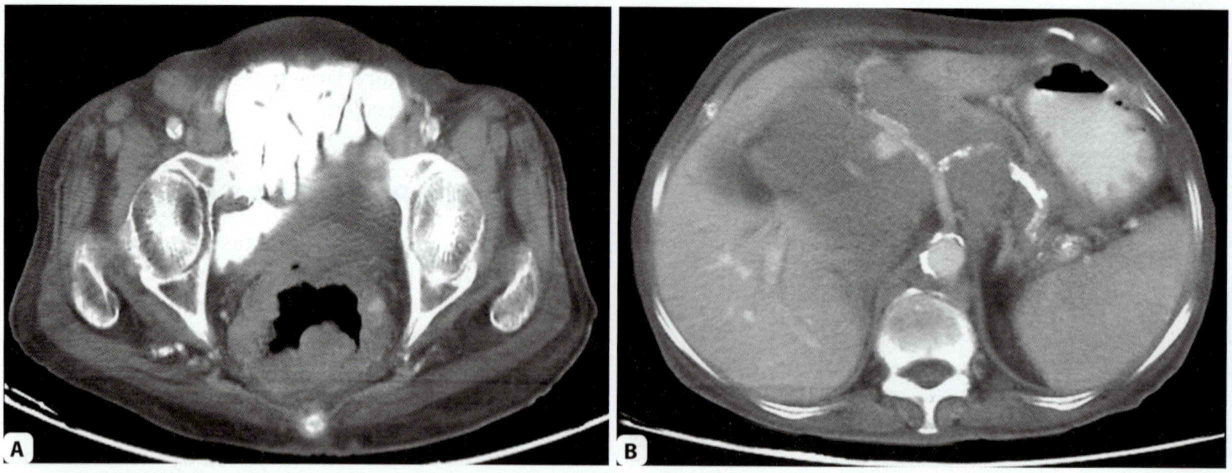

FIGS. 24A AND B: Axial contrast-enhanced computed tomography (CECT) sections show concentric nodular mural thickening of the rectum (A) with conglomerate lymph nodal mass encasing the celiac trunk (B) in a patient with disseminated lymphoma.

POSTOPERATIVE COLON AND RECURRENT CANCER

The radiologist should be aware of the various surgical techniques and postoperative anatomy for assessing the therapeutic response and for diagnosing tumor recurrence. In addition to the usual surgical resections, such as right hemicolectomy, extended right hemicolectomy, transverse colectomy, left hemicolectomy, sigmoid colectomy, the radiologist will come across more complex procedures, such as Hartmann's procedure, anterior resection, and abdominoperineal excision of rectum (APER).

Hartmann's procedure may be done for carcinoma of the sigmoid colon. It entails resection of the sigmoid and formation of the left-sided end colostomy. The rectum and distal sigmoid are closed off to form a rectal stump or Hartmann's pouch which is reattached to the colon within 3–6 months of the primary surgery.

In anterior resection, the sigmoid and part of or the entire rectum, is resected. If the entire rectum is removed, that is, a low anterior resection is done, then a coloanal anastomosis is made. In case the entire rectum is not removed, a colorectal anastomosis is made. A temporary defunctioning stoma is usually made in cases of anterior resection.

Abdominoperineal excision of rectum involves resection of the anus, rectum, and part of the distal sigmoid colon through incisions made in the abdomen and perineum. This procedure is done for cancer of the distal third of rectum or anal canal and for salvage of the anal cancer that does not respond to chemoradiation.

T2-weighted MRI has been recommended for local restaging. Diffusion-weighted MRI adds to the response evaluation after chemoradiation **(Figs. 25A to E)**.[77,78] However, characterization of metastatic lymph nodes is challenging. Dynamic CEMR and perfusion CT assess the residual or recurrent tumor by showing contrast enhancement. The role of PET/CT is controversial. There are studies which show that irradiated rectal mucosa may show increased FDG uptake resulting in false-positive data.[78,80] Therefore, FDG PET is not recommended within the first 4 weeks after completion of chemoradiation.

CONCLUSION

Colorectal cancer is a unique malignancy as it represents a preventable disease. The adenoma-carcinoma sequence reiterates the need for screening for polyps which are precursors of colorectal cancer. Screening is of immense importance in countries which have high prevalence of colorectal cancer. Though this malignancy has a low prevalence in the Indian subcontinent, it is expected to increase as more people are adopting Western lifestyle and dietary habits.

Imaging plays a key role in the screening program as well as for detection and staging of colorectal cancer. For screening purpose, the radiological options include CT colonography. The high sensitivity of CT colonography for detecting clinically significant polyps >1 cm has been possible due to the spectacular advances in CT technology. Endoscopic sonography, CT, and MRI are the primary cross-sectional techniques used for staging of colorectal cancer. Of these modalities, MRI is preferred for the locoregional staging of rectal cancer and CECT is preferred for the staging of colorectal metastases.

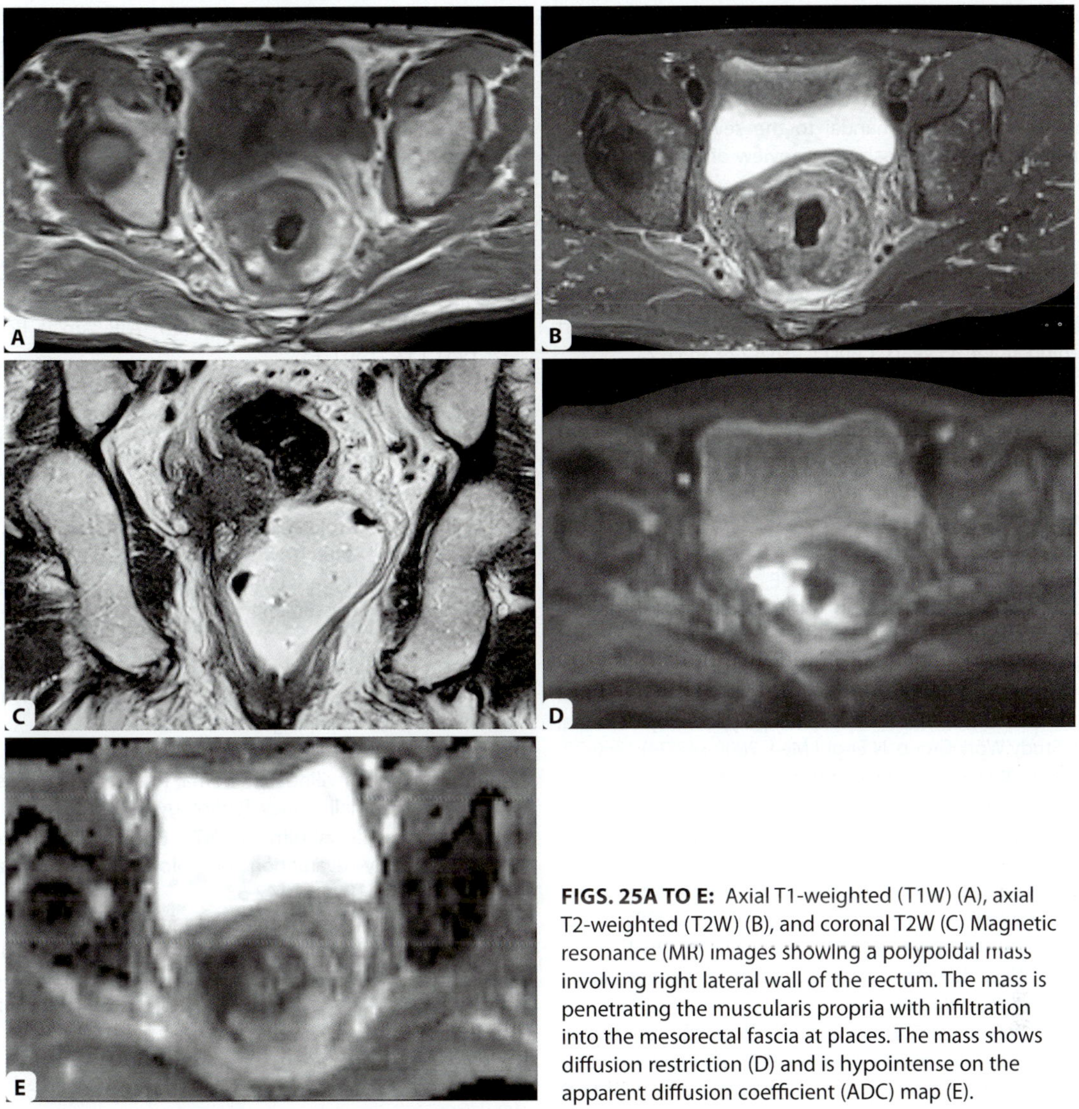

FIGS. 25A TO E: Axial T1-weighted (T1W) (A), axial T2-weighted (T2W) (B), and coronal T2W (C) Magnetic resonance (MR) images showing a polypoidal mass involving right lateral wall of the rectum. The mass is penetrating the muscularis propria with infiltration into the mesorectal fascia at places. The mass shows diffusion restriction (D) and is hypointense on the apparent diffusion coefficient (ADC) map (E).

REFERENCES

1. Jemal A, Siegel R, Ward E, Murray T, Xu J, Thun MJ. Cancer statistics, 2007. CA Cancer J Clin. 2007;57:43-66.
2. Ferlay J, Soerjomataram I, Dikshit R, Eser S, Mathers C, Rebelo M, et al. Cancer incidence and mortality worldwide: sources, methods and major patterns in GLOBOCAN 2012. Int J Cancer. 2015;136(5):E359-86.
3. Theoni RF, Lauferl. Polyp sand carcinoma of the colon. In: Gore RM, Levine MS (Eds). Textbook of Gastrointestinal Radiology. Philadelphia: WB Saunders; 2008. pp. 1121-66.
4. Horvat N, Carlos Tavares Rocha C, Clemente Oliveira B, Petkovska I, Gollub MJ. MRI of Rectal Cancer: Tumor Staging, Imaging Techniques, and Management. Radiographics. 2019;39(2):367-87.
5. Potter JD, Slattery ML, Bostick RM, Gapstur SM. Colon cancer: a review of the epidemiology. Epidemiol Rev. 1993;15(2):499-545.
6. Fleshner P, Slater G, Aufses AH Jr. Age and sex distribution of patients with colorectal cancer. Dis Colon Rectum. 1989;32(2):107-11.
7. Bond JH. Colonic tumors. Endoscopy.1998;30:150-7.
8. Kritchevsky D. Colorectal cancer: the role of dietary fat and caloric restriction. Mutat Res. 1993;290(1):63-70.
9. Gore RM. Colorectal cancer. Clinical and pathologic features. Radiol Clin North Am. 1997;35(2):403-29.
10. McFarlane MJ, Welch KE. Gallstones, cholecystectomy, and colorectal cancer. Am J Gastroenterol. 1993;88(12):1994-9.
11. Lane N, Fenglio CM. The adenoma-carcinoma sequence in the stomach and colon: I. Observation on the adenoma asprecurs or to ordinary large bowel carcinoma. Gastrointest Radiol. 1976;1:111-9.
12. Lev R, Lee M. Colorectal carcinoma: Pathology. In: Rustgi AK (Ed). Gastrointestinal Cancers: Biology, Diagnosis, and Therapy. Philadelphia: Lippincott-Raven; 1995. pp. 379-98.
13. Gore RM, Meyers MA. Pathways of abdominal and pelvic disease spread. In: Gore RM, Levine MS, Laufer I (Eds). Textbook of Gastrointestinal Radiology. Philadelphia: WB Saunders; 1994. pp. 2352-66.

14. Turnbull RB. The no-touch isolation technique of resection. JAMA.1975;231:1181-5.
15. Tong GJ, Zhang GY, Liu J, Zheng ZZ, Chen Y, Niu PP, et al. Comparison of the eighth version of the American Joint Committee on Cancer manual to the seventh version for colorectal cancer: A retrospective review of our data. World J Clin Oncol. 2018;9:148-61.
16. Silva AC, Hara AK, Leighton JA, Heppell JP. CT colonography with intravenous contrast material: varied appearance of colorectal carcinoma. Radiographics. 2005;25:1321-34.
17. American Cancer Society updates its colorectal cancer screening guideline: New recommendation is to start screening at age 45 years. Cancer. 2018;124:3631-2.
18. Rex DK, Boland CR, Dominitz JA, Giardiello FM, Johnson DA, Kaltenbach T, et al. Colorectal Cancer Screening: Recommendations for Physicians and Patients from the U.S. Multi-Society Task Force on Colorectal Cancer. Am J Gastroenterol. 2017;112(7):1016-30.
19. McMahon PM, Gazelle GS. The case for colorectal screening. Sem Roentgenol. 2000;35:325-32.
20. Young GP, Symonds EL, Allison JE, Cole SR, Fraser CG, Halloran SP, et al. Advances in Fecal Occult Blood Tests: the FIT revolution. Dig Dis Sci. 2015;60:609-22.
21. Winawer SJ, Stewart ET, Zauber AG, Bond JH, Ansel H, Waye JD, et al. A comparison of colonoscopy and double-contrast barium enema for surveillance after polypectomy. National Polyp Study Work Group. N Engl J Med. 2000;342(24):1766-72.
22. van Rijn JC, Reitsma JB, Stoker J, Bossuyt PM, van Deventer SJ, Dekker E. Polyp miss rate determined by tandem colonoscopy: a systematic review. Am J Gastroenterol. 2006;101(2):343-50.
23. Johnson CD, Chen MH, Toledano AY, Heiken JP, Dachman A, Kuo MD, et al. Accuracy of CT colonography for detection of large adenomas and cancers. N Engl J Med. 2008;359(12): 1207-17. Erratum in: N Engl J Med. 2008;359(26):2853.
24. Gelfand DW. Colorectal cancer: Screening strategies. Radiol Clin North Am. 1997;35:431-8.
25. Brady AP, Stevenson GW, Stevenson I. Colorectal cancer over looked at barium enema examination and colonoscopy: A continuing perceptual problem. Radiology. 1994;192:373-8.
26. Ott DJ, Gelfand DW. How to improve the efficacy of the barium enema examination. AJR Am J Roentgenol. 1993;160(3): 491-5.
27. Ott DJ, Gelfand DW, Ramquist NA. Causes of error in gastrointestinal radiology. II. Barium enema examination. Gastrointest Radiol. 1980;5(2):99-105.
28. Gelfand DW, Ott DJ. Cost-effective screening for colorectal cancer. The radiologist's view. Primary Care Cancer. 1992;12: 11-3.
29. Stevenson GW. Normal anatomy and technique of examination of the colon: Barium, CT and MRI. In: Freeny PC, Stevenson GW (Eds). Margulis and Burhenne's Alimentary Tract Radiology. St Louis: Mosby and Company; 1994. p.692.
30. Laufer I, Kressel HY. Principles of double contrast diagnosis. In: LauferI, Levine MS (Eds). Double-contrast Gastrointestinal Radiology. Philadelphia: WB Saunders; 1992. pp. 9-54.
31. Youker JE, Welin S. Differentiation of true polypoid tumors of the colon from extraneous material: A new Roentgen sign. Radiology. 1985;84:610-5.
32. Buetow PC, Buck JL, Carr NJ, Pantongrag-Brown L. From the archives of the AFIP. Colorectal adenocarcinoma: radiologic-pathologic correlation. Radiographics. 1995;15(1):127-46; quiz 148-9. Erratum in: Radiographics. 1995;15(3):640.
33. Delamarre J, Descombes P, Marti R, Rémond A, Trinez G. Villous tumors of the colon and rectum: double-contrast study of 47 cases. Gastrointest Radiol. 1980;5(1):69-73.
34. Bond JH. Polyp guideline: Diagnosis, treatment, and surveillance for patients with non familal colorectal polyps. Ann Intern Med. 1993;119:836-43.
35. Lappas JC, Maglinte DD, Kopecky KK, Cockerill EM, Lehman GA. Diverticular disease: imaging with post-double-contrast sigmoid flush. Radiology. 1988;168(1):35-7.
36. Kelvin FM, Gardiner R, Vas W, Stevenson GW. Colorectal carcinoma missed on double contrast barium enema study: a problem in perception. AJR Am J Roentgenol. 1981;137(2):307-13.
37. Dubbins PA. The small bowel and colon. In: Cosgrove DO, Meire HB, Dewbury KC (Eds). Abdominal and General Ultrasound. New York: Churchill Livingstone; 1993. pp. 765-76.
38. Bernd L. Diagnosis of large bowel tumors by colonic sonography. Lancet. 1990;20:144-6.
39. Puli SR, Bechtold ML, Reddy JB, Choudhary A, Antillon MR, Brugge WR. How good is endoscopic ultrasound in differentiating various T stages of rectal cancer? Meta-analysis and systematic review. Ann Surg Oncol. 2009;16: 254-65.
40. Glaser F, Schalg P, Harfarth C. Endorectal Ultrasonography for the assessment of invasion of rectal tumors and lymph node involvement. Br J Surg. 1990;77:883-7.
41. Hulsmans FH, Tio TL, Mathus-Vliegen EM, Bosma A, Tytgat GN. Colorectal villous adenoma: transrectal US in screening for invasive malignancy. Radiology. 1992;185(1):193-6.
42. Scharling ES, Wolfman NT, Bechtold RE. Computed tomography evaluation of colorectal carcinoma. Semin Roentgenol.1996;31:142-53.
43. Tan CH, Iyer R. Use of computed tomography in the management of colorectal cancer. World J Radiol. 2010;2:151-8.
44. Wiesner W, Mortelé KJ, Ji H, Ros PR. Normal colonic wall thickness at CT and its relation to colonic distension. J Comput Assist Tomogr. 2002;26:102-6.
45. Li ZH, You DY, Gao DP, Yang GJ, Dong XX, Zhang DF, et al. Role of CT scan in differentiating the type of colorectal cancer. Onco Targets Ther. 2017;10:2297-303.
46. Kalra N, Suri S, Gupta R, Natarajan SK, Khandelwal N, Wig JD, et al. MDCT in the staging of gallbladder carcinoma. AJR Am J Roentgenol. 2006;186:758-66.
47. Hong EK, Landolfi F, Castagnoli F, Park SJ, Boot J, Van den Berg J, et al. CT for lymph node staging of Colon cancer: not only size but also location and number of lymph node count. Abdom Radiol (NY). 2021;46:4096-105.
48. Klaver YL, Lemmens VE, Nienhuijs SW, Luyer MD, de Hingh IH. Peritoneal carcinomatosis of colorectal origin: Incidence, prognosis, and treatment options. World J Gastroenterol. 2012;18:5489-94.
49. Vining DJ, Gelfand DW. Non-invasive colonoscopy using helical CT scanning, 3D reconstruction and virtual reality. Presented in the syllabus of the 23rd annual meeting. Maui (Hawaii): Society of Gastrointestinal Radiologists; 1994.
50. Summerton S, Little E, Cappell MS. CT colonography: Current status and future promise. Gastroenterol Clin N Am. 2008;37:161-89.
51. Bhatia A, Saxena AK, Kalra N, Sodhi KS, Thapa BR, Rao KL, et al. Intravenous contrast enhanced computed tomography colonoscopy in children with suspected colonic polyps. Eur J Radiol. 2013;82(6):905-12.

52. Kalra N, Suri S, Bhasin DK, Sinha SK, Saravanan N, Kour T, et al. Comparison of multidetector computed tomographic colonography and conventional colonoscopy for detection of colorectal polyps and cancer. Indian J Gastroenterol. 2006;25(5):229-32.
53. Yee J, Dachman A, Kim DH, Kobi M, Laghi A, McFarland E, et al. CT Colonography Reporting and Data System (C-RADS): Version 2023 Update. Radiology. 2024;310(1):e232007.
54. La Tegola L, Guglielmi G. The Role of MRI in Rectal Cancer: An Updated Review. Curr Radiol Rep. 2020;8(10).
55. Congedo A, Mallardi D, Danti G, De Muzio F, Granata V, Miele V. An Updated Review on Imaging and Staging of Anal Cancer-Not Just Rectal Cancer. Tomography. 2023;9: 1694-710.
56. Schurink NW, Lambregts DMJ, Beets-Tan RGH. Diffusion-weighted imaging in rectal cancer: current applications and future perspectives. Br J Radiol. 2019;92(1096):20180655.
57. Beets-Tan RGH, Lambregts DMJ, Maas M, Bipat S, Barbaro B, Curvo-Semedo L, et al. Magnetic resonance imaging for clinical management of rectal cancer: Updated recommendations from the 2016 European society of gastrointestinal and abdominal radiology (ESGAR) consensus meeting. Eur Radiol. 2018;28:1465-75.
58. Vliegen RF, Beets GL, von Meyenfeldt MF, Kessels AG, Lemaire EE, van Engelshoven JM, et al. Rectal cancer: MR imaging in local staging--is gadolinium-based contrast material helpful? Radiology. 2005;234(1):179-88.
59. Wnorowski AM, Menias CO, Pickhardt PJ, Kim DH, Hara AK, Lubner MG. Mucin-containing rectal carcinomas: overview of unique clinical and imaging features. AJR Am J Roentgenol. 2019;213:26-34.
60. Yu S, Chand M, Tait D, Brown G. Magnetic resonance imaging defined mucinous rectal carcinoma is an independent imaging biomarker for poor prognosis and poor response to preoperative chemoradiotherapy. Eur J Cancer. 2014;50: 920-7.
61. Suthar M, Baheti AD, Ankathi SK, Choudhari A, Haria PD, Engineer R, et al. MRI features of signet ring rectal cancer. Abdom Radiol (NY). 2021;46:5536-49.
62. Videhult P, Smedh K, Lundin P, Kraaz W. Magnetic resonance imaging for preoperative staging of rectal cancer in clinical practice: high accuracy in predicting circumferential margin with clinical benefit. Colorectal Dis. 2007;9:412-9.
63. Brown G, Radcliffe AG, Newcombe RG, Dallimore NS, Bourne MW, Williams GT. Preoperative assessment of prognostic factors in rectal cancer using high-resolution magnetic resonance imaging. Br J Surg. 2003;90(3):355-64.
64. Santiago I, Figueiredo N, Parés O, Matos C. MRI of rectal cancer-relevant anatomy and staging key points. Insights Imaging. 2020;11(1):100.
65. Brown G, Richards CJ, Bourne MW, Newcombe RG, Radcliffe AG, Dallimore NS, et al. Morphologic predictors of lymph node status in rectal cancer with use of high-spatial-resolution MR imaging with histopathologic comparison. Radiology. 2003;227:371-7.
66. Srisajjakul S, Prapaisilp P, Bangchokdee S. Pitfalls in MRI of rectal cancer: What radiologists need to know and avoid. Clin Imaging. 2018;50:130-40.
67. Ajaj W, Pelster G, Treichel U, Vogt FM, Debatin JF, Ruehm SG, et al. Dark lumen magnetic resonance colonography: comparison with conventional colonoscopy for the detection of colorectal pathology. Gut. 2003;52(12):1738-43.
68. Britton KE, Granowska M. The diagnostic role of radio labeled antibodies. In: Murrary IPS, EIIPJ (Eds). Nuclear Medicine in Clinical Diagnosis and Treatment. Edinburgh; Churchill Living Stone; 1998. pp. 871-92.
69. Agarwal A, Marcus C, Xiao J, Nene P, Kachnic LA, Subramaniam RM. FDG PET/CT in the management of colorectal and anal cancers. AJR Am J Roentgenol. 2014;203:1109-19.
70. Ramos E, Valls C, Martinez L, Lladó L, Torras J, Ruiz S, et al. Preoperative staging of patients with liver metastases of colorectal carcinoma. Does PET/CT really add something to multidetector CT? Ann Surg Oncol. 2011;18(9):2654-61.
71. Kinner S, Antoch G, Bockisch A, Veit-Haibach P. Whole-body PET/CT-colonography: a possible new concept for colorectal cancer staging. Abdom Imaging. 2007;32(5):606-12.
72. Gollub MJ, Akhurst T, Markowitz AJ, Weiser MR, Guillem JG, Smith LM, et al. Combined CT colonography and 18F-FDG PET of colon polyps: potential technique for selective detection of cancer and precancerous lesions. AJR Am J Roentgenol. 2007;188(1):130-8.
73. Sahani DV, Kalva SP, Hamberg LM, Hahn PF, Willett CG, Saini S, et al. Assessing tumor perfusion and treatment response in rectal cancer with multisection CT: initial observations. Radiology. 2005;234(3):785-92.
74. Bellomi M, Petralia G, Sonzogni A, Zampino MG, Rocca A. CT perfusion for the monitoring of neoadjuvant chemotherapy and radiation therapy in rectal carcinoma: initial experience. Radiology. 2007;244(2):486-93.
75. Ippolito D, Drago SG, Pecorelli A, Maino C, Querques G, Mariani I, et al. Role of dynamic perfusion magnetic resonance imaging in patients with local advanced rectal cancer. World J Gastroenterol. 2020;26:2657-68.
76. Expert Panel on Gastrointestinal Imaging; Korngold EK, Moreno C, Kim DH, Fowler KJ, Cash BD, et al. ACR Appropriateness Criteria® Staging of Colorectal Cancer: 2021 Update. J Am Coll Radiol. 2022;19(5S):S208-S222.
77. Sun YS, Zhang XP, Tang L, Ji JF, Gu J, Cai Y, et al. Locally advanced rectal carcinoma treated with preoperative chemotherapy and radiation therapy: preliminary analysis of diffusion-weighted MR imaging for early detection of tumor histopathologic downstaging. Radiology. 2010;254(1):170-8.
78. Hein PA, Kremser C, Judmaier W, Griebel J, Pfeiffer KP, Kreczy A, et al. Diffusion-weighted magnetic resonance imaging for monitoring diffusion changes in rectal carcinoma during combined, preoperative chemoradiation: preliminary results of a prospective study. Eur J Radiol. 2003;45(3):214-22.
79. Konski A, Li T, Sigurdson E, Cohen SJ, Small W Jr, Spies S, et al. Use of molecular imaging to predict clinical outcome in patients with rectal cancer after preoperative chemotherapy and radiation. Int J Radiat Oncol Biol Phys. 2009;74(1):55-9.
80. Kalff V, Ware R, Heriot A, Chao M, Drummond E, Hicks RJ. Radiation changes do not interfere with postchemoradiation restaging of patients with rectal cancer by FDG PET/CT before curative surgical therapy. Int J Radiat Oncol Biol Phys. 2009;74(1):60-6.

CHAPTER 6

Ajay Gulati, Naveen Kalra, Arun Sharma, Mandeep Kang

Imaging of Ischemic Bowel Diseases

INTRODUCTION

Ischemic bowel disease occurs due to impaired arterial supply and/or venous drainage of splanchnic circulation, resulting in ischemic injury and altered bowel metabolism. Ischemic bowel disease presents as a complex spectrum of disorders with variable imaging manifestations depending upon time of onset, duration, severity of ischemic insult; the segment and length of bowel involved; vessels affected and status of collateral circulation. Ischemia may be stratified, on the basis of symptom time frame as acute or chronic; and may be arterial or venous in origin. Ischemia may involve the small bowel, large bowel, or both segments resulting in *mesenteric ischemia*, *colonic ischemia,* and *ischemic enterocolitis,* respectively. Variability in the above factors not only affects the clinical scenario, but also influences the management options, outcome, and prognosis. Despite major technological advancements in the recent era, the diagnosis is still often challenging in this uncommon disease due to its vague clinical symptomatology, and often subtle or nonspecific imaging findings.

Bowel ischemia has numerous causes and variable presentations. Frequently patients complain of nonspecific symptoms. The classic triad of *abdominal pain, pyrexia, and frank blood in stool* is elicited only in less than one-third of the patients. Majority of the patients present with vague clinical symptoms including diarrhea, vomiting, bloating, and abdominal discomfort.[1] If there are clinical signs of peritonitis like rebound tenderness, rigidity, and guarding on physical examination, it usually indicates irreversible infarction and is an ominous prognostic indicator.[2] Laboratory workup is often nonspecific and time consuming. Unlike acute myocardial insults, there are no reliable and validated serum biomarkers of mesentric ischemia. The serum lactate values may often be normal in the early course and mistakenly reassuring. Radiologists should be wary of the fact that serum lactate levels are not specific for diagnosis of acute mesenteric ischemia (AMI) but should be used more for prognostication since elevated levels correlate well with ensuing transmural necrosis. In the present modern era with advancements in imaging techniques, radiologists have a pivotal role in evaluating bowel ischemia by making an early and accurate diagnosis and help in treatment planning along with providing vital prognostic information as they are able to characterize and delineate the disease process. Therefore, knowledge and familiarity of the varied imaging appearances of intestinal ischemia will certainly aid radiologists in prompt and confident recognition of this potentially lethal condition.

ANATOMY OF SPLANCHNIC CIRCULATION

Knowledge of the mesenteric vascular anatomy is mandatory to understand and evaluate bowel ischemia; knowing the normal mesenteric vessels and common anatomic variants is helpful in angiogram assessment and planning appropriate endovascular treatment. Splanchnic circulation consists of arterial supply and their collateral system; and venous drainage alternatively called portal venous system.

Arterial Supply

There are three major arterial trunks which arise anteriorly from aorta, namely *celiac axis, superior mesenteric artery (SMA), and inferior mesenteric artery (IMA).* These provide arterial supply to intra-abdominal viscera.

Celiac Axis

Celiac axis originates from the aorta at the level of T12 vertebra, supplies foregut derivatives such as liver, pancreas, spleen, and bowel from stomach to second part of duodenum by branching into *common hepatic artery,*

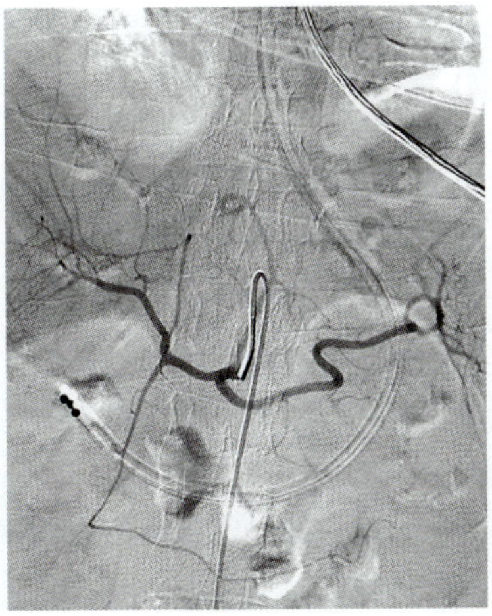

FIG. 1: Conventional angiography [digital subtraction angiography (DSA)] run of celiac axis trunk with its branches.

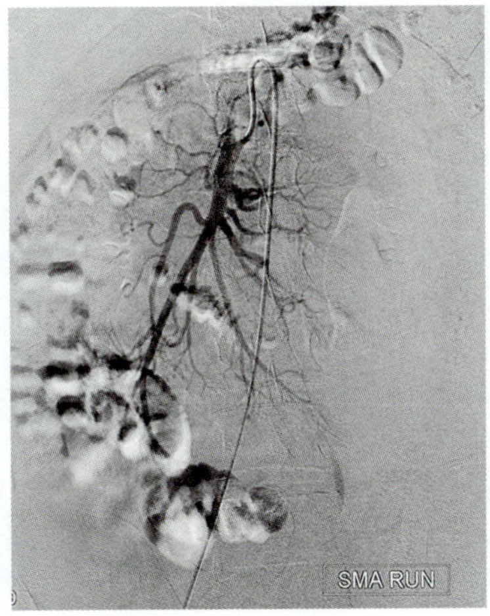

FIG. 2: Digital subtraction angiography (DSA) run showing superior mesenteric artery and its branches.

left gastric artery, and splenic artery. The common hepatic artery divides into gastroduodenal artery and continues as proper hepatic artery. The gastroduodenal artery further branches into the right gastroepiploic artery and anterior and posterior superior pancreaticoduodenal arteries. The splenic artery branches into the left gastroepiploic artery and pancreatic artery **(Fig. 1)**.

Superior Mesenteric Artery

The SMA serves as the predominant source of blood supply to the small bowel and originates from the aorta at L1 vertebral level. It supplies the midgut derivatives, from the second part of duodenum till middle third of transverse colon. The major vascular branches include the anterior and posterior inferior pancreaticoduodenal arteries, middle colic artery, right colic artery, ileocolic artery, and numerous jejunal and ileal branches. All these branches contribute to form multiple anastomotic vascular arcades, from which the straight vessels known as vasa recta arise and supply the jejunal and ileal walls **(Fig. 2)**.

Inferior Mesenteric Artery

Inferior mesenteric artery originates from anterior aspect of aorta at L3/L4 vertebral body level and supplies the hindgut derivatives from the level of distal one-third of transverse colon till the proximal rectum. Major branches include the left colic artery, sigmoidal artery and superior rectal artery; the mid and distal rectum is supplied by the branches of anterior division of internal iliac artery **(Fig. 3)**.

Collateral Systems

Abundant collateral pathways exist between major mesenteric arterial trunks and their branches which can provide adequate perfusion to the bowel in patients with critical vascular stenosis or obstruction. These extensive

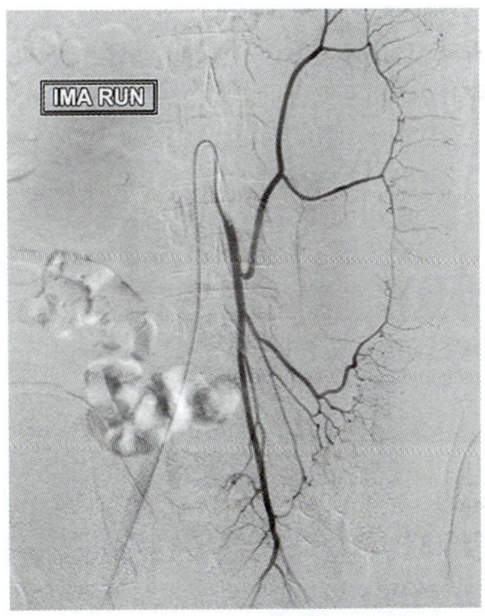

FIG. 3: Digital subtraction angiography (DSA) run showing inferior mesenteric artery (IMA) and its branches.

collateral vessels are more conspicuous in the stomach, duodenum and rectum thereby accounting for inherent resistance of these areas to develop ischemia. The important collateral circuits include:
- Pancreaticoduodenal arcade connecting celiac axis to SMA
- Marginal artery of Drummond
- Central anastomotic artery
- Arc of Riolan (a.k.a. the "meandering mesenteric artery") are the potential conduits connecting SMA with the IMA **(Figs. 4A and B)**. Meandering artery connecting the proximal middle colic artery of SMA with the proximal left colic artery of IMA may be visualized angiographically in presence of superior or IMA occlusive pathology; hence, it is essential to determine the direction of blood flow within this artery before dissecting any of the major mesenteric arteries.[1,3]

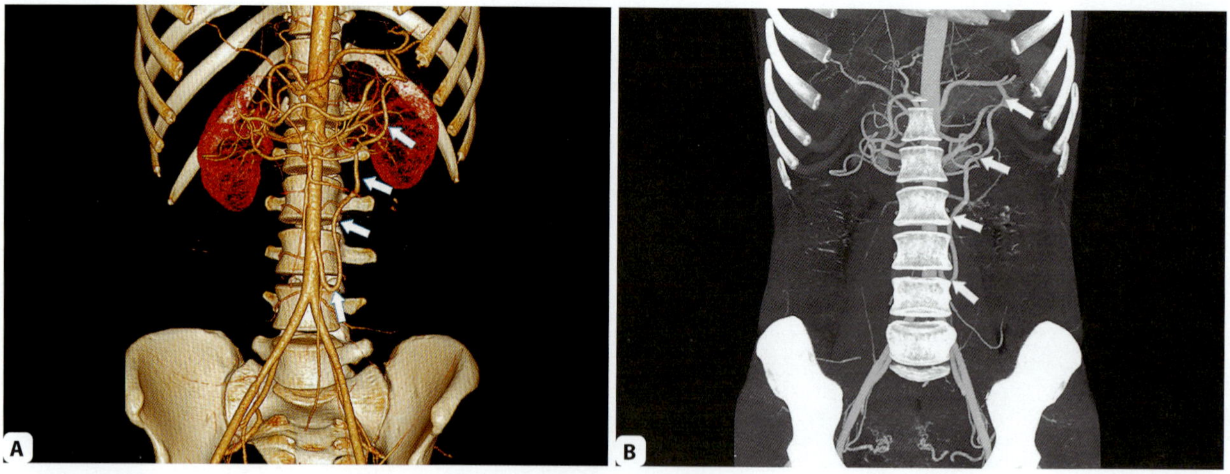

FIGS. 4A AND B: Coronal CT images [volume rendered and maximum intensity projection (MIP)] showing proximal superior mesenteric artery (SMA) obstruction with arc of Riolan (arrows) reconstituting distal SMA and its branches.

Portal Venous System

The small bowel and colon are drained by superior and inferior mesenteric veins (SMV and IMV). The latter drains into the splenic vein, which joins the SMV to form the main portal vein.

ETIOLOGY

Ischemic bowel disease is classified depending on the time of presentation, anatomic segment of bowel involved and etiopathogenesis of disease **(Table 1)**.

PATHOPHYSIOLOGY OF ISCHEMIC BOWEL DISEASE

Mesenteric ischemia is a dynamic process that generally evolves over time. Ischemic injury deprives nutrition and oxygen supply which is necessary for cellular metabolism and their intactness. In the early phase of ischemia, collateral vessels are recruited after major vessel occlusion due to arterial pressure drop distal to the occlusion and provide alternate pathway to maintain the viability of the bowel. However, after a critical period of time, persistence of ischemia causes development of vasoconstriction, thereby increasing the arterial pressure and hampering the collateral blood flow.

The precise time frame of transition from ischemia to infarction is unknown and depends on the acuteness and severity of vascular obstruction and the status of collateral vessels. Persistent arterial obstruction causes vasospasm with subsequent loss of cellular integrity, whereas venous ischemia causes blood column stasis with edema and subsequently reduced arterial blood flow causing mucosal cellular detachment. Thus, recognizing the early manifestations of ischemia is extremely important for better outcomes.

TABLE 1: Bowel ischemia types and etiology.[4]

A. Mesenteric ischemia • Acute MI (95%):	
- Arterial occlusion (60–85%)	• Embolic • Thrombotic • Dissection/Transection • Vasculitis • *Other causes*: Adhesions, volvulus, and internal hernias • Closed loop obstruction
- Venous occlusion (5–15%)	• Thrombophilia and hypercoagulable states • Portal hypertension • Recent surgery
- Nonocclusive mesenteric ischemia (NOMI) (20–30%)	• Hospitalized critically ill patients • Systemic hypoperfusion and shock • Drugs (*Digitalis/Ergot*/cocaine)
• Chronic MI (5%)	• Atherosclerotic disease • Fibromuscular dysplasia and vasculitides • Arterial hyperplasia
B. Colonic ischemia	• Nonocclusive causes such as hypotension and vasculitides • Occlusive causes
C. Ischemic enterocolitis	• Vasculitides • Iatrogenic/Traumatic vascular injury

If the initial ischemic insult is relieved early, the reversibly injured mucosa typically recovers completely without sequelae, but if reperfusion is delayed, the restored perfusion to the ischemic segment can further accentuate the cellular damage termed reperfusion injury

TABLE 2: Radiopathological correlation of CT findings in ischemic bowel disease.

Pathologic events	CT imaging correlation
• Early vasodilatation • Vasoconstriction	• Wall hyperdensity (in both arterial and venous phase) • Absence/reduced bowel wall enhancement
Increased vascular permeability	• Bowel wall thickening • Bowel luminal dilatation
Mucosal cellular necrosis and microflora proliferation	• Pneumatosis intestinalis • Mesenteric/portal venous gas
Transmural bowel necrosis and bowel perforation	• Pneumoperitoneum • Retropneumoperitoneum • Ascites

as the leukocytes in the blood release free radicals and interleukins. With prolonged ischemic insult, the eventual outcome in both types of vascular obstruction is transmural infarction. Bacterial translocation can further potentiate the existing inflammatory changes resulting in bowel gangrene, perforation peritonitis, and sepsis with multiorgan failure in its natural course. It is essential to understand, differentiate and define the nature of vascular obstructive pathology radiologically as the prognosis in these two types of vascular obstruction differs significantly with reported mortality rate of 89% in the arterial occlusion and 11% in the venous obstruction.[5,6]

Understanding the pathophysiology of ischemic bowel disease is important for the proper interpretation of CT as the radiological findings correlate with extent of disease process as shown in **Table 2.**[6] The acute bowel ischemia is dynamic pathophysiologically and includes three stages according to the degree of bowel wall involved; further super infection of the involved segment facilitates ensuing necrosis and subsequent perforation.[1] The early radiological changes seen on CT is secondary to vasodilatation, which is manifested as diffuse wall hyperdensity on both arterial and venous phases. This implies that ischemia has yet not progressed to advanced stage and is possibly reversible, if treated expediently. If ischemia persists and is severe enough, it leads to vasoconstriction thereby hampering the collateral flow, which manifests as reduced bowel wall enhancement. Persistence of ischemia leads to necrosis of the bowel wall causing proliferation and migration of microbial flora into the bowel wall resulting in pneumatosis intestinalis, air in mesenteric, and portal vein and their branches. Subsequently, more advanced cases result in bowel perforation causing pneumoperitoneum, retropneumoperitoneum, and ascites.[6]

Stage 1	Stage 2	Stage 3
• Pathology limited to mucosa only • Reversible	Pathology extends to submucosa and muscularis propria	• Transmural involvement • Highest mortality

ACUTE MESENTERIC ISCHEMIA

Acute mesenteric ischemia is an uncommon abdominal emergency accounting for less than 1 in 1,000 hospital admissions, which may be potentially life-threatening if not treated expediently. The reported mortality rates are variable depending upon how early is the diagnosis made and intervention performed and may be as high as ~60–90%, representing the extreme sensitivity of the small intestine to reduced blood supply.[6,7] AMI results from occlusive and nonocclusive vascular causes and is further subclassified into arterial, venous, or both categories depending upon the type of vessels involved. Understanding the pathophysiology of bowel changes aids in better understanding of the corresponding radiological findings thereby improving the accuracy of diagnosis and planning appropriate treatment.

The common clinical presentation of AMI is "excruciating abdominal pain which is poorly localized and out of proportion to the physical examination". The proposed hypothesis for the pain being disproportionate to the clinical examination findings is that ischemia begins from the mucosa and gradually progresses to transmural state which is why the initial severe pain is without corroborative physical examination findings.[8]

Superior Mesenteric Artery Thromboembolism

The SMA is particularly susceptible arterial trunk involved by the thromboembolic events due to its high-flow rate and inherent anatomic factors including wide caliber and narrow take-off angle at its origin. Mesenteric emboli commonly originate from the left atrium in pre-existing cardiovascular comorbidities such as atrial fibrillation, myocardial infarction, in global heart failure or may be aortic in origin. Most commonly emboli lodge in the SMA in the initial ~3–10 cm from its origin and are typically seen distal to the origin of the middle colic artery. Synchronous emboli can be visualized in other extraintestinal organs (such as spleen and kidneys) in >20% of patients.[2]

Mesenteric arterial thrombosis on the other hand is almost always seen in underlying pre-existing atherosclerotic vascular disease. Other uncommon etiologies of thrombosis include fibromuscular dysplasia, median arcuate ligament syndrome, vasculitis, arterial dissection or aneurysm **(Figs. 5A to C)**. Thrombotic occlusion commonly involves the ostia of major mesenteric vessels which generally result in long segments of bowel being involved and commonly have worst outcomes than the embolic type.[9] Embolic event related ischemic patients generally present acutely, whereas thrombotic patients present more subacutely due to antecedent partially occluding atherosclerotic plaques causing collateral development. This group of patients may present as mesenteric angina secondary to chronic mesenteric ischemia or may present acutely due to superimposed thrombus in background of atherosclerotic disease causing ambient radiological features.

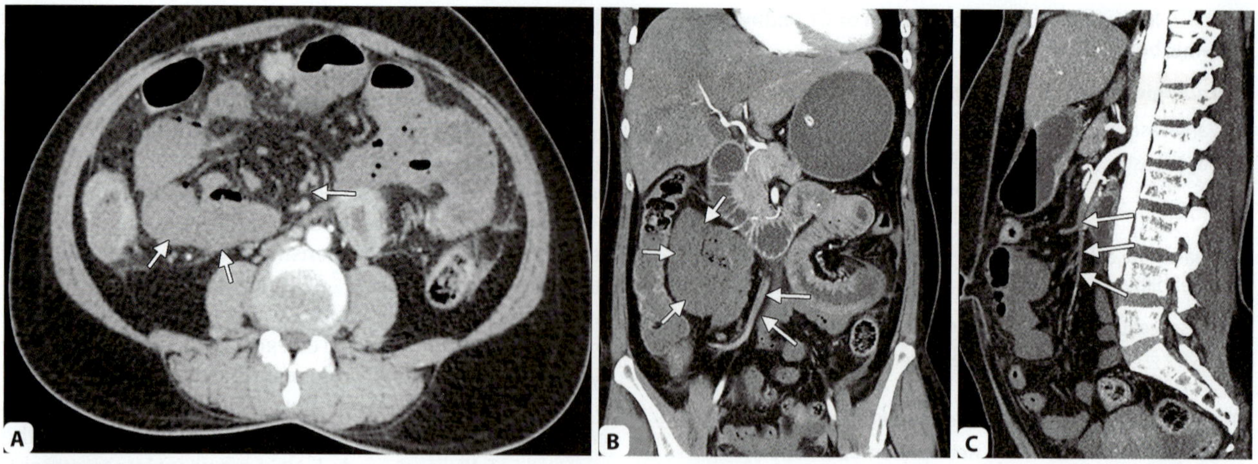

FIGS. 5A TO C: Axial, coronal, sagittal reconstructed CT images showing complete occlusion of the superior mesenteric artery (long arrows) with nonenhancing proximal small bowel loops in the right side of abdomen (short arrows).

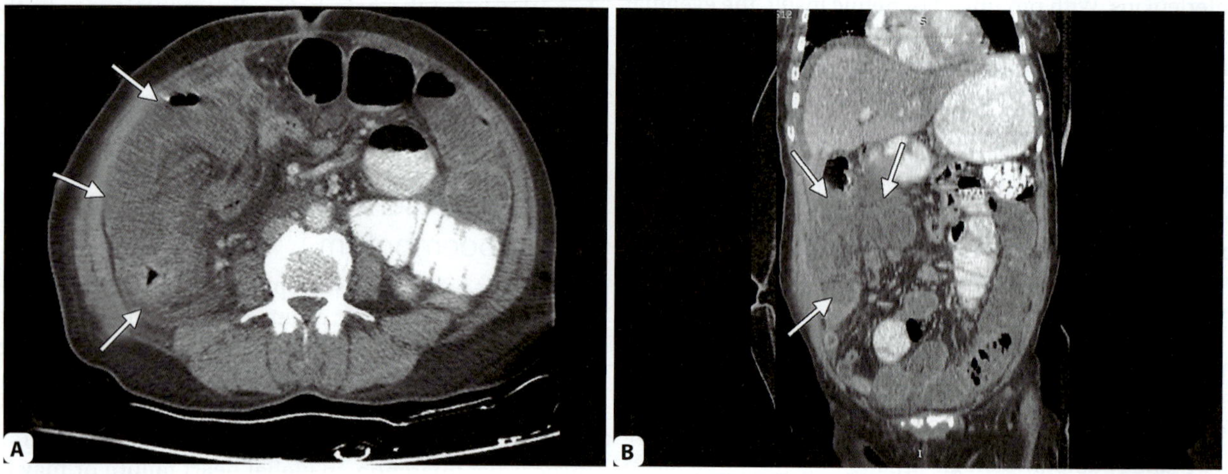

FIGS. 6A AND B: Venous ischemia secondary to closed loop (arrows) obstruction in the right upper quadrant with engorgement of vessels and fluid in the mesentery with thickened bowel wall.

Venous Mesenteric Ischemia

Less commonly venous occlusion causes mesenteric ischemia and accounts for 5–15% of all cases of bowel ischemia. Venous occlusive ischemic disease is most frequently encountered in relatively younger patients with mortality rate of ~10–40%.[5] Closed loop obstruction is the most common cause for venous bowel ischemia **(Figs. 6A and B)**.[6] Venous thrombosis may also be seen in patients with hypercoagulable hematological disorders, vasculitides, and less frequently in pregnancy, oral contraceptive pill (OCP) consumption and underlying inflammatory conditions like systemic lupus erythematosus (SLE).[1] Nearly 60% of these patients have remote history of deep vein thrombosis or pulmonary embolus.[10]

Nonocclusive Mesenteric Ischemia

Nonocclusive mesenteric ischemia (NOMI) is seen commonly in patients admitted in critical care units and is multifactorial in etiology, comprising 20–30% of all cases of ischemic disease. Due to its uncertain etiology and compromised host status, mortality rates are generally high ranging from 30 to 90%. Shock bowel injury is generally seen with hypotensive and low cardiac output states with no definite vascular occlusion. Systemic hypotension provokes autoregulation and homeostasis, preserving the coronary and cerebral vascular supply at the expense of the splanchnic and peripheral circulation causing mesenteric hypoperfusion.

Any form of shock, renal failure with overly dialysis, and vasoconstrictor drugs (catecholamines, digitalis, and diuretics) are other common risk factors of NOMI.[1,11]

Imaging Modalities

Acute mesenteric ischemia patients generally present with vague and nonspecific clinical features and it is challenging to accurately diagnose this condition early, since the delay in the management will reflect in worse prognosis and higher mortality rates.

Plain radiographs have traditionally been considered as an initial investigation in patients presenting with acute abdomen, but because of their limited role and low diagnostic yield, their use is debated in current clinical practice. The findings on X-rays are generally nonspecific and may demonstrate dilated bowel loops, or thumb printing in early ischemic phase and may show pneumatosis, portal venous gas, and pneumoperitoneum in advanced ischemic stage.[6] The sensitivity is significantly low and normal radiograph does not exclude ischemic bowel disease **(Fig. 7)**.[8,11]

Ultrasonography (USG) is another common modality used in assessment of patients presenting acutely and its role is mainly to exclude other potential etiologies of acute abdomen. The diagnostic yield in patients with mesenteric ischemia is limited and more often suboptimal due to gaseous distension of bowel loops causing technical difficulty in evaluation of mesenteric vasculature. It can be used to monitor the peristaltic activity of bowel or the ascitic fluid mainly in patients of NOMI.[8]

In the present modern era with significant technological advancements, multidetector CT (MDCT) is the imaging modality of choice for evaluating patients with clinical suspicion of ischemic bowel disease. It has nearly replaced conventional angiography for diagnostic purposes and aids in making early and accurate diagnosis, as well as excluding other alternative pathologies.[4] In patients with ischemia, CT examination can help in understanding the pathophysiology to confidently diagnose and characterize arterial versus venous occlusive disease, can grade the severity of ischemia, help in planning accurate treatment, and also provide vital prognostic information. A systematic approach of interpreting the CT angiography (CTA) will ensure comprehensive assessment of the bowel wall, mesenteric vasculature and surrounding mesentery which are essential for not only improved detection but also estimation of the grade and extent of ischemia.[9,12]

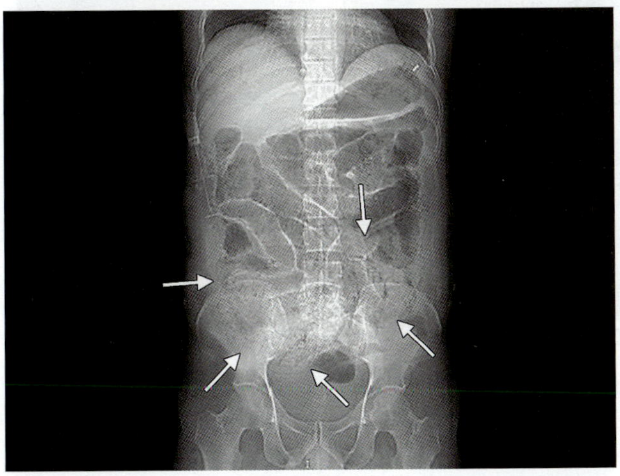

FIG. 7: Abdominal radiograph showing dilated bowel loops with pneumatosis intestinalis (arrows).

Technical Aspects

The study protocol consists of biphasic CT abdomen with an arterial phase (35–40 seconds) performed for evaluating the arterial stenosis and occlusions, and venous phase (65–70 seconds) for assessing the mesenteric venous system and various abdominal viscera for changes of ischemia. Nonenhanced CT has been shown to be of benefit in some studies in literature as it can better evaluate the submucosal hemorrhage, hyperdense clots, and also provide baseline attenuation of the bowel.[1,4] However, results of some studies have suggested that nonenhanced CT does not improve the accuracy of diagnosis and adds to more radiation burden and timeliness and therefore may not be performed routinely.[13,14] Acquiring separate noncontrast scan therefore, remains contentious issue and may be practiced based on individual preferences.

Pearl: Biphasic protocol with acquisition of both arterial and portal venous phases is the standard protocol in all patients with suspected ischemia and arterial phase should not be excluded from the examination in order to achieve dose reduction. This biphasic imaging protocol maintains high sensitivity (96–100%) and specificity (94–100%) for the diagnosis of AMI.[15,16] CTA is also the preferred imaging modality in patients with renal impairment as benefit of an early and precise diagnosis outweighs the potential risk of contrast-induced nephropathy.

The role of oral contrast is controversial in literature and preference is individualistic. In patients presenting acutely, CT is obtained only with IV contrast, to expedite the study, although these cases may be technically difficult to evaluate due to inadequate distension of the bowel loops. In patients presenting with more subacute features, neutral oral contrast is generally preferred by most radiologists as it helps in better assessment of the mural status and also improves the visualization of vascular tree by various postprocessing techniques.[1] Present generation MDCT scanners allow volumetric data acquisition which can be further postprocessed by various dedicated computer softwares on workstations. Multiplanar reconstruction (MPR) and 3D reconstructions help in better anatomical and vascular evaluation and increase the confidence of radiologist in making an accurate diagnosis.[6] Masking the bowel enhancement pattern and interference with 3D reconstruction is a major drawback of administration of positive oral contrast agents and is therefore not generally recommended.[10]

Dual-energy CT (DECT) is a recent advancement in the CT technology which increases the accuracy and sensitivity for diagnosis of AMI. The generation of iodine selective and low keV monoenergetic images using dedicated postprocessing softwares accentuates the conspicuity of differential enhancement between ischemic and normally perfused bowel in comparison to routine CT.[17] Virtual noncontrast images generated from DECT data can help to delineate the hyperdense hemorrhage within the bowel wall and obviate the requirement of acquiring true noncontrast scan thereby potentially reducing the radiation dose. DECT can also improve the evaluation of the mesenteric vasculature as it is feasible to artificially increase the contrast signal intensity using low keV images in comparison to routine 120 kVp images and simulate arterial phase enhancement from the portal venous phase scans.[10] DECT with iodine overlay technique may be useful in detecting subtle bowel wall enhancement to differentiate ischemia from infective/inflammatory bowel wall thickening.[18]

Vascular Findings

Computed tomography angiographic abnormalities are commonly the initial imaging sign identified in the setting of AMI. CTA should be the first step in imaging approach as it guides the treatment planning by stratification of patients to those who would benefit from prior conventional angiography as opposed to those who require to undergo emergency surgery.[10,19] CTA and its dedicated reconstruction techniques such as curved MPR, maximum intensity projection (MIP), tissue transition projection (TTP), and vessel probe (VP) are more specific and often demonstrate arterial occlusions as filling defect within the vessel lumen with/without associated collateral formation **(Figs. 8A and B)**.[6] Similarly, venous thrombosis is identified as central filling defect with mural rim enhancement.[20] An investigative pitfall to remember is that although MIP images facilitate quick overview of mesenteric vessels, but these can potentially underestimate the amount of clot burden as any contrast adjacent to the thrombus will be projected as the brightest pixel in the volume of tissue reconstructed, and could mask the underlying clot. Therefore, correlation with corresponding thin section axial and multiplanar images is always essential for accurate assessment of the clot burden.[10]

Nonvascular Computed Tomography Findings of Bowel Ischemia

Regardless of the etiology, a spectrum of imaging findings is seen in bowel ischemia which represent the obstructive state traits and correlate with the underlying pathophysiologic state of the disease. The CT examination may reveal dilated and thickened bowel loops associated with mesenteric stranding and ascites in initial stages of AMI, whereas pneumatoses, pneumoperitoneum, and portal and mesenteric venous gas signify advanced stages of the spectrum **(Figs. 9A and B)**.

Few patterns of traits may aid in differentiating occlusive and nonocclusive causes **(Table 3)**. Arterial occlusion generally causes paper thin bowel wall with absent enhancement or hypoattenuation **(Figs. 10A to D)**; whereas venous occlusive disease results in markedly thickened edematous bowel wall, mesenteric fat stranding, and marked luminal dilatation even in the early stages. Similar changes are however seen in advanced cases of ischemia which have progressed to transmural necrosis. Distinguishing CT imaging features of arterial and venous ischemia are enumerated in **Table 4**.[1,21]

Bowel Wall Thickening

Circumferential edematous mural thickening is one of the most sensitive imaging signs of ischemia, although the specificity is limited, it can be seen with a wide variety of other causes like infectious or inflammatory diseases.[2] Intramural hemorrhage or edema in the bowel wall can cause mural thickening, which is manifested as hyperattenuation or hypoattenuation of the thickened wall. The presence and grade of bowel wall thickening however correlates poorly with the severity of ischemia, and many

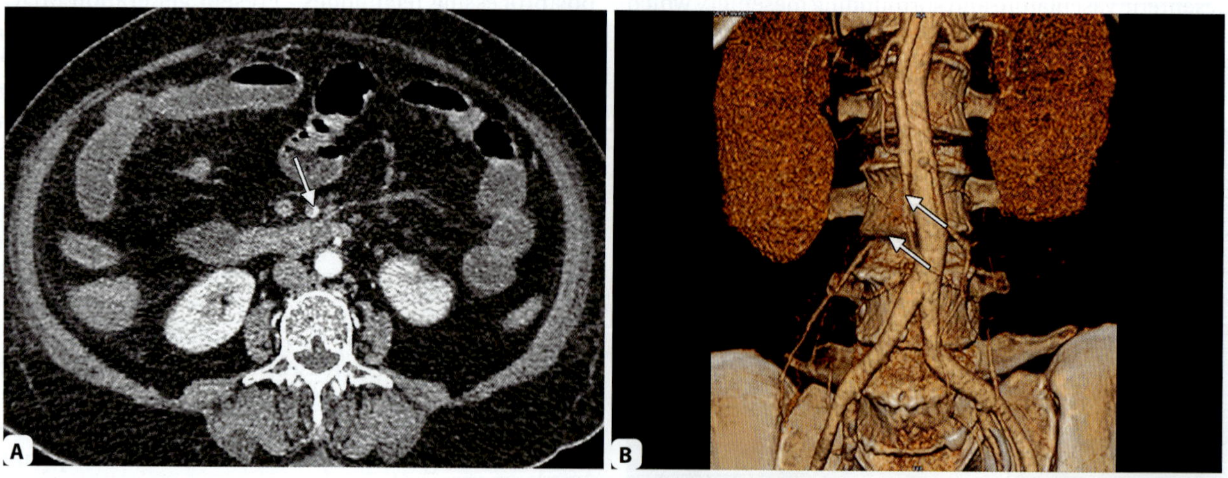

FIGS. 8A AND B: Axial and volume-rendered (VR) CT images showing occlusion of the branch of superior mesenteric artery (long arrows).

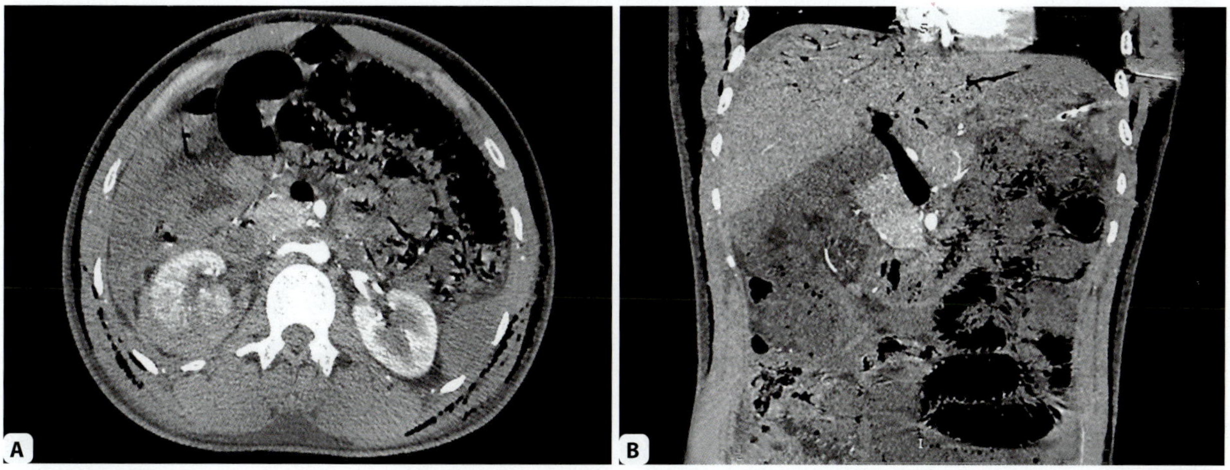

FIGS. 9A AND B: Patient of blunt trauma abdomen. Axial and coronal reconstructed CT images showing extensive pneumatosis, air in the mesenteric/portal venous branches, and hemoperitoneum. Note is made of right renal contusion with perinephric hematoma.

TABLE 3: Clinical and CT features of mesenteric ischemia.[1]

Features	Arterial occlusive ischemia	Venous occlusive ischemia	Nonocclusive mesenteric ischemia
Time of onset	Acute, chronic, and acute on chronic	Acute or chronic	Acute or chronic
Predisposing conditions	Atrial fibrillation, recent myocardial infarction, atherosclerosis, aortic dissection, and vasculitis, drugs such as ergotamine and cocaine	Closed loop bowel obstruction and strangulation, hypercoagulable disorders, portal hypertension, pregnancy, malignancy, and oral contraceptive pills (OCPs)	Hypotension and shock, vasculitis, and vasoconstricting drugs
Bowel wall status	May be thin in acute state or may be thickened with associated inflammation and edema	Edematous, markedly thickened bowel wall	Thickened bowel wall
Bowel wall enhancement	Depending on state of reperfusion, may nonenhance before reperfusion, and may hyperenhance in reperfused state **(Figs. 10A and B)**	Target sign with significant mucosal hyperenhancement **(Figs. 11A and B)**	Reduced enhancement
Mesenteric vasculature	Arterial stenosis/occlusion, aneurysm, and dissection	Venous thrombosis	Nonspecific with pruning of distal mesenteric vascular branches
Mesentery	Fat stranding with fluid in advanced stages	Significant fat stranding and fluid in early stages	Variable

cases of arterial ischemia show thinning of the wall due to destruction of the intramural nerves causing subsequent loss of muscular tone. This has been termed as classic "paper-thin wall" in arterial AMI and may be challenging sign to prospectively recognize. Wall thickening is more significant in venous ischemia, where thickness typically measures 8–9 mm and may be even >15 mm.[10]

Bowel Wall Enhancement

The mural enhancement can have varied patterns in bowel ischemia and may be increased, reduced, or absent in patients with AMI. Reduced or absent enhancement is an early and very specific finding of arterial hypoperfusion which may sometimes be subtle and hence should be carefully looked for. Comparison with normal perfused bowel segments which act as internal reference will assist and improve the identification of reduced enhancement (refer **Figs. 5A and B**). Paradoxically, hyperenhancement in AMI which generally implies viable state of the bowel is seen with venous obstruction (secondary to vascular congestion), NOMI, in arterial occlusion (after reperfusion) and in cases of bowel obstruction with strangulation.[10] A trilaminar appearance with "target" or "halo" sign has also been described **(Figs. 11A and B)** with hypoenhancing submucosa sandwiched between hyperenhancing mucosa and muscularis propria/serosa although this imaging sign may also been seen in other etiologies like infective/inflammatory diseases, radiation enteritis, acute graft versus host disease in addition to ischemia.[10]

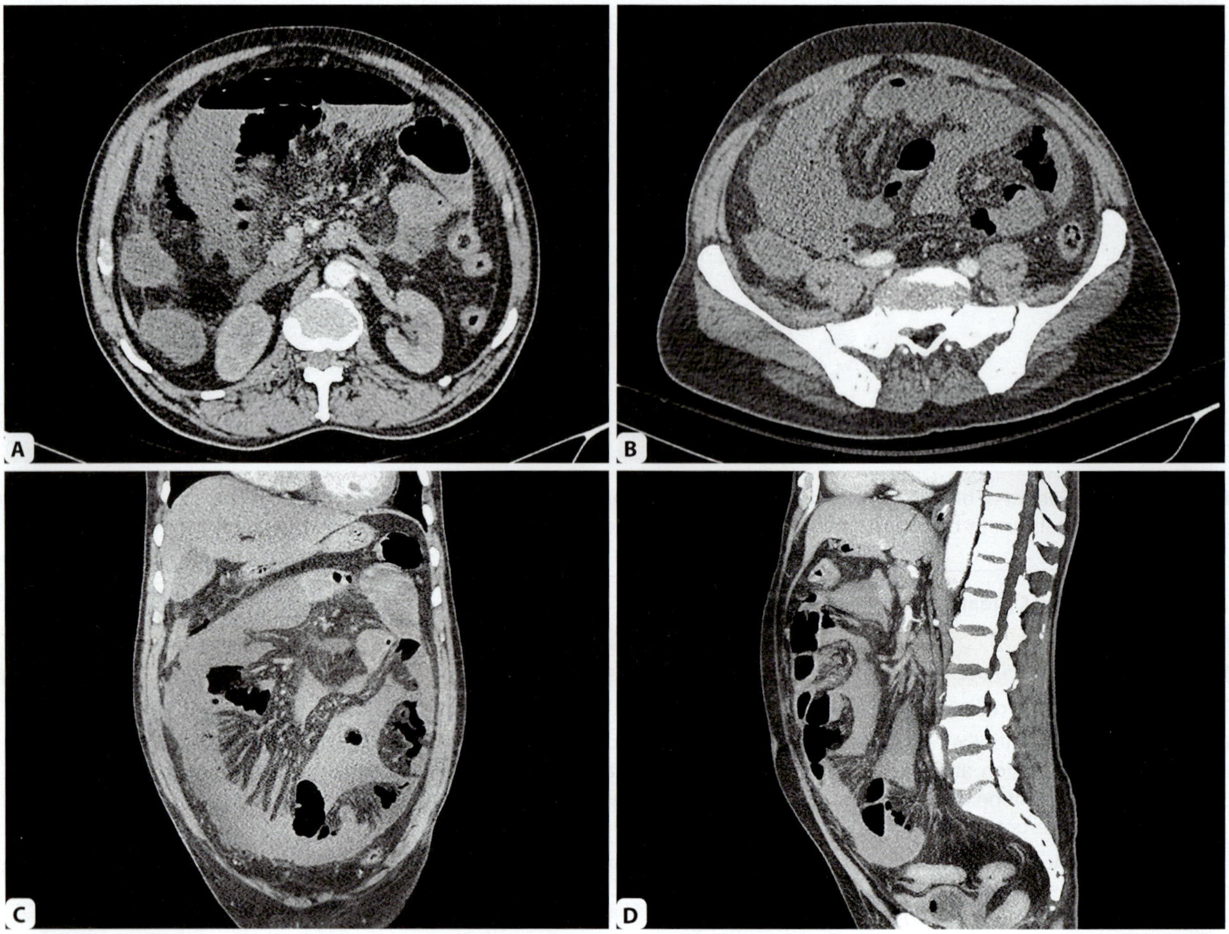

FIGS. 10A TO D: Axial, coronal, sagittal reconstructed CT images showing occlusion of the superior mesenteric artery (SMA) with papery thin nonenhancing small bowel loops with pneumatosis and mesenteric air pockets. The bowel loops appear indistinct from adjacent gross intraperitoneal fluid.

TABLE 4: CT imaging features to differentiate arterial and venous occlusive ischemia.[10]

Arterial occlusion	Venous occlusion
SMA thrombosis	SMV thrombosis
No/subtle bowel wall enhancement	Hypo/Hyperdense bowel wall
Thinned out bowel wall	Significantly thickened bowel wall
Mucosal nonenhancement	Mucosal hyperenhancement
Bowel dilatation after transmural infarction	Dilated bowel lumen without infarction
Late mesenteric stranding, hemorrhage or edema	Marked early mesenteric fat stranding and hemorrhage

Note: Advanced cases of both arterial and venous ischemia show similar imaging manifestations such as air in mesenteric and portal venous system, pneumoperitoneum and retropneumoperitoneum.

(SMA: superior mesenteric artery; SMV: superior mesenteric vein)

Bowel Lumen Dilatation

Another common but nonspecific finding is dilatation of the bowel with associated air-fluid levels which is more commonly seen in ischemia associated with bowel obstruction as compared to occlusive causes of ischemia. In the setting of bowel ischemia, the proposed pathophysiology is aperistalsis and hypotonia, which may be reactionary to ischemia or due to destruction of the intramural musculature and nerves. As dilatation of bowel is so common with other pathologies, its main utility is to draw attention to the involved segment of bowel which may then be assessed for other more specific imaging signs of ischemia.[10]

Mesenteric Changes and Ascites

Mesenteric findings such as fat stranding along with mesenteric fluid can be present adjacent to the affected

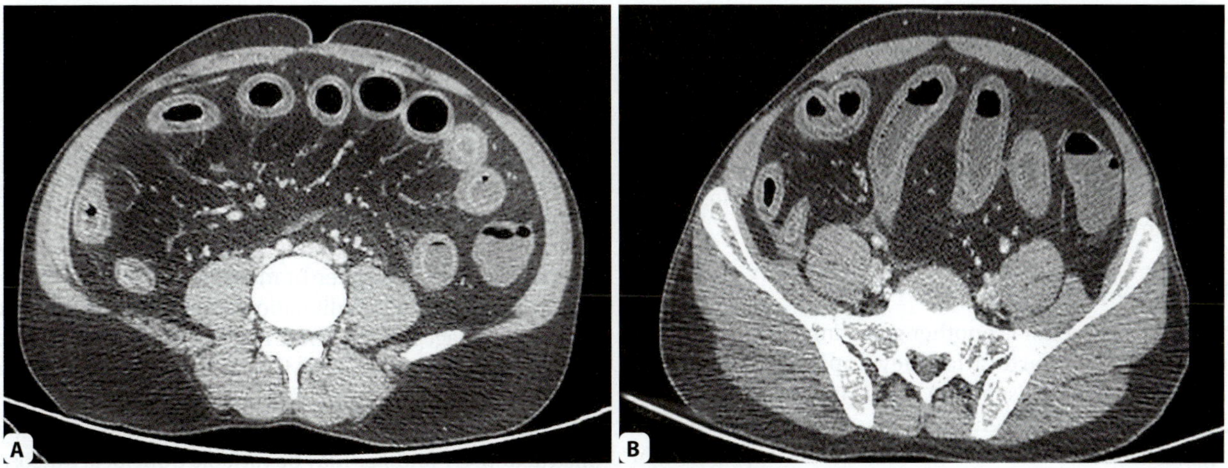

FIGS. 11A AND B: Axial CT images showing characteristic target sign with mucosal and serosal hyperenhancement in a patient of venous ischemia.

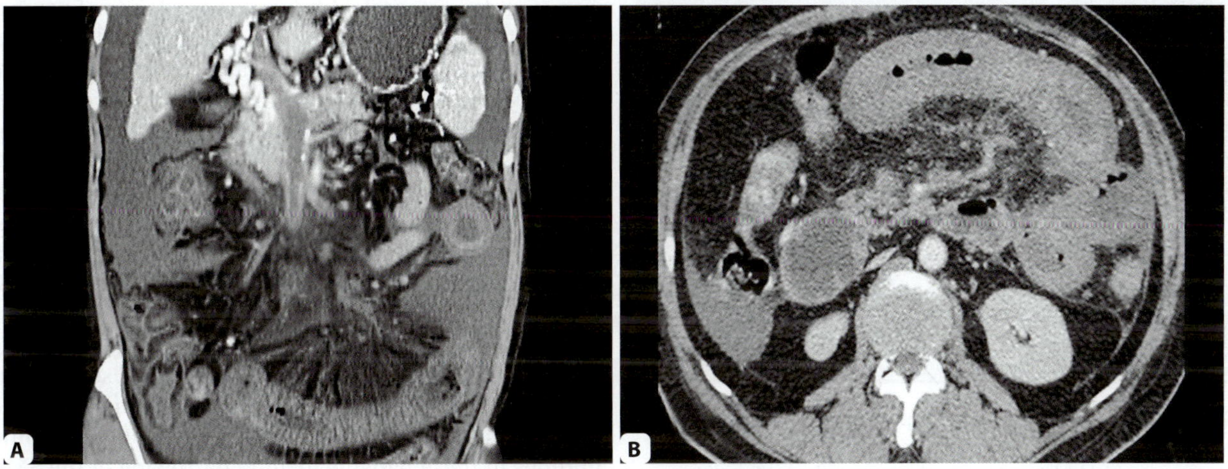

FIGS. 12A AND B: (A) Coronal CT image showing splenoportal thrombosis with thickened bowel loops and engorgement of mesenteric vessels suggestive of early venous ischemia; (B) Another patient of venous ischemia showing markedly thickened bowel wall with mesenteric changes.

bowel segments of ischemia. Mesenteric fluid in a patient with bowel obstruction may raise the consideration of ensuing ischemia. These findings are however often nonspecific similar to bowel dilatation and may frequently be seen in other entities. They can serve to direct attention of the radiologist to nearby bowel loops to look for more specific signs of bowel ischemia. These changes are more commonly seen with venous thrombosis **(Figs. 12A and B)** and are uncommon early in the course of acute arterial ischemia, where they generally appear after reperfusion, or when transmural infarction and/or intestinal perforation ensues.[10]

Pneumatosis Intestinalis

Advanced stages of ischemia secondary to any underlying etiology may ultimately result in pneumatosis intestinalis, which is an ominous sign in the setting of bowel ischemia.[10] On recognizing pneumatosis, radiologists are generally hurriedly tempted to make a diagnosis of ischemia; however, it is important to emphasize that pneumatosis intestinalis should not be considered as a diagnosis but more as an imaging sign that can be visualized not only in ischemic bowel disease but also in some other benign conditions.[22] When detected in combination with portomesenteric gas, the specificity for diagnosis of bowel ischemia is close to 100% **(Figs. 9A and B)**.[1,2]

Pneumatosis cystoides intestinalis is an uncommon benign condition that typically affects the large bowel and is characterized by presence of numerous gas-filled bubble-like cysts in the submucosa and subserosa of the bowel wall.[9] These cysts appear more circular and grape-like clusters on CT and these patients are often clinically asymptomatic.

Another interpretive pitfall is "pseudopneumatosis" when intraluminal gas bubbles get trapped between the wall and the intraluminal fluid that can radiologically simulate pneumatosis **(Fig. 13)**. Pseudopneumatosis is commonly seen in right-sided colon and may be differentiated from pneumatosis by absence of such gas bubbles in the antidependent location of the bowel.[9] Knowledge and awareness of these imaging pitfalls and their differentiating key findings may improve the accuracy of diagnosis and prevent misdiagnosis of bowel ischemia.[9]

Ancillary Findings

Pneumoperitoneum is another grave imaging sign which suggests bowel perforation developing secondary to advanced stages of ischemia and is identified in 21% of AMI patients; it has high specificity of 94–97%.[10] Visceral organ infarcts may also be encountered in patients of ischemia, particularly in those with embolic states or nonocclusive pathophysiology.[10]

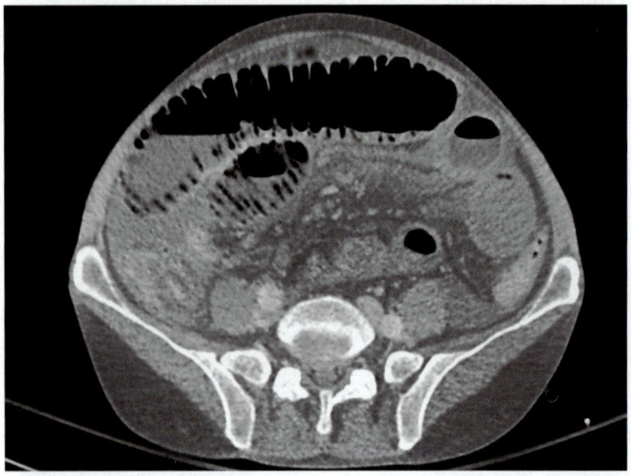

FIG. 13: Pseudopneumatosis: Interpretive pitfall of diagnosing pneumatosis in bowel ischemia is pseudopneumatosis which is seen as gas bubbles get trapped between the wall and the intraluminal fluid within the dilated pelvic ileal loops. Such gas bubbles are typically absent in the antidependent location of the bowel.

Nonocclusive Mesenteric Ischemia (NOMI)

Computed tomography features of NOMI are overlapping with other inflammatory or infectious conditions involving the bowel, which makes it challenging to diagnose this condition. CTA may depict narrowing of the mesenteric arteries to their first-order branches and beaded appearance with focal areas of dilatation and narrowing (termed "string of sausages" sign). These features are better depicted with the multiplanar and MIP reformats. Specifically, reduced caliber of SMA has been reported in literature.[9]

Bowel ischemia in NOMI happens secondary to inflow obstruction. CT findings may be variable from focal mucosal damage in watershed areas to the damage of entire bowel. Small bowel loops generally show mural thickening with hyperenhancement.[1] The changes are typically discontinuous and segmental with intervening loops of normal bowel. Usually, there is normal appearing colon. Similar to arterial occlusive MI, the bowel wall in NOMI can become thinner in the advanced stages of ischemia. However, after reperfusion, it is generally thicker with a target or halo sign or shows hyperenhancement.

There are associated infarcts seen in the spleen, liver, and kidneys with NOMI secondary to hypoperfusion. Ancillary features like reduced caliber of inferior vena cava and abdominal aorta may be identified along with hyperenhancement of the adrenal glands and kidneys as part of CT hypoperfusion complex.[9,23] Clinical setting is generally integral to this diagnosis and digital subtraction angiography (DSA) may be performed as an adjunctive tool in cases of diagnostic dilemma. The angiographic findings in these patients include narrowing of the SMA branches with associated irregularities, spasm of mesenteric arcades, and reduced filling of the intramural vessels **(Figs. 14A to C)**.[23]

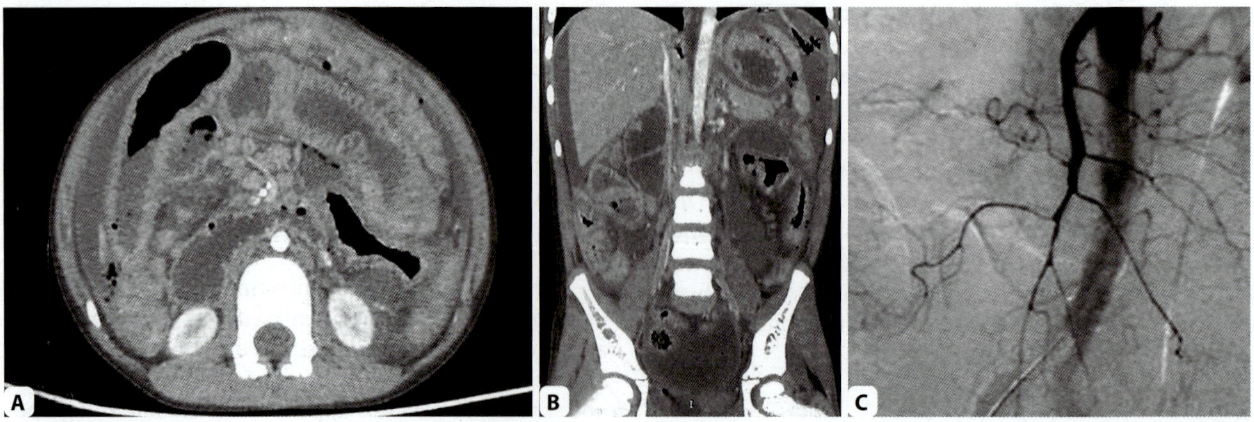

FIGS. 14A TO C: Patient of cardiogenic shock, CT axial (A) and coronal (B) section showing reduced caliber of abdominal aorta with chinked IVC and showing diffuse concentric mural thickening involving bowel loops with ascites. DSA (C) SMA run showing reduced caliber and paucity of the distal branches with pruning.

(DSA: digital subtraction angiography; IVC: inferior vena cava; SMA: superior mesenteric artery)

Conventional catheter angiography (DSA) has historically been the reference standard for the evaluation and treatment of arterial thromboembolism. However, with rapid advancements in field of technology, CTA has supplanted catheter angiography as the first-line imaging technique for all suspected cases of AMI and catheter angiography has gradually transitioned to complementary adjunctive role in cases where diagnosis is uncertain or equivocal on CT. Assessment of the distal vascular occlusion and catheter-directed interventions may be performed in suitably selected patients. In the current practice, DSA is mainly performed with intent of therapeutic purposes for performing interventions such as thrombolysis, aspiration of thrombus, or vasodilatory medication administration in patients where diagnosis has already been made on CT.[24]

Magnetic resonance (MR) is another advanced modality which has been employed in patients with mesenteric ischemia. Its role in acute presentations is generally not advocated due to long imaging duration and critical status of such patients.[23] Also magnetic resonance angiography (MRA) is tailored mainly for assessment of ostia and proximal segments of mesenteric vessels and has only limited role in diagnosing stenotic involvement of distal vessels as well as NOMI. Patients with subacute/chronic features may be assessed by gadolinium-enhanced MRA which can provide accurate assessment of the mesenteric vasculature comparable to CT evaluation. Experimental studies have shown that MR techniques may be able to differentiate between acutely ischemic and infarcted segments based on signal changes on T2-weighted sequence and postcontrast enhancement images.[25]

American College of Radiology (ACR) has formulated guidelines for various radiological modalities aiding in systematic, appropriate, and timely evaluation of suspected AMI **(Table 5)**.[19]

Management of Acute Mesenteric Ischemia

Immediately prompt treatment is instituted after establishing diagnosis of AMI. Treatment aims at revascularization of the mesenteric vessels to prevent further bowel ischemia. Early medical supportive management includes fluid resuscitation, nasogastric/orogastric tube decompression, and anticoagulation. Broad-spectrum antibiotics must be started and due diligence must be taken to avoid vasoconstrictive drug administration, especially in nonocclusive mesenteric ischemic patients. Urgent bowel reperfusion is critical for good clinical outcomes and requires a focused multidisciplinary approach of interventional radiologists, vascular surgeons, and critical care unit who need to work collaboratively in their resuscitation efforts and individualizing the treatment. The emphasis of treatment has shifted from surgical intervention to endovascular therapy in recent years. The present clinical practice guidelines, however, do not provide precise information on the optimal timing for revascularization. On literature review, a study has shown that a "period of 48 hours from the presentation may be taken as the golden period" for providing appropriate management, beyond which the mortality rates in these patients increase dramatically.[26]

However, sadly 30 day mortality rates in patients with AMI remain high despite emergency endovascular revascularization/along with stenting of the SMA. Since there is nonavailability of robust prognostic markers for predicting clinical outcomes and guiding management options toward alternative treatments, some researchers have advocated immediate revascularization endovascularly followed by surgical exploration for ischemic bowel in all such patients.[27]

TABLE 5: ACR appropriateness criteria for imaging suspected acute ischemic bowel disease.[19]

Radiologic modality	Appropriateness category	Remarks	Relative radiation level
CTA abdomen with IV contrast	Usually appropriate	• Fast, noninvasive • First step in imaging approach	+++
CT abdomen and pelvis with IV contrast	May be appropriate	Lack of arterial phase may cause suboptimal evaluation of mesenteric arteries compared to CTA	+++
Arteriography abdomen	May be appropriate (disagreement)	Diagnosis and treatment in single procedure	+++
MRA abdomen and pelvis without and with IV contrast	May be appropriate (disagreement)	• Long examination, may delay treatment options in acute settings • Limited benefits in distal thromboembolism and NOMI	0
Radiography/US duplex Doppler	May be appropriate	Low diagnostic yield	++/0
CT abdomen without and with IV contrast	Usually not appropriate		++++
CT and MR abdomen without IV contrast	Usually not appropriate		+++/0

(ACR: American College of Radiology; CTA: CT angiography; IV: intravenous; MRA: magnetic resonance angiography; NOMI: nonocclusive mesenteric ischemia)

Nonetheless, if peritoneal signs are present and in patients who have clinical signs of significant hypovolemia or hypotension, emergency laparotomy is recommended. The aim of surgical intervention is to restore the perfusion of ischemic bowel by immediate surgical embolectomy or bypass, the resection of all nonviable segments, and intraoperative meticulous bowel assessment for the preservation of all viable bowel. Embolectomy and angioplasty are the currently accepted standard of care treatment for SMA emboli. The patients with thrombotic occlusion of the SMA involving the origin will generally require a bypass procedure. Single-vessel revascularization (SMA) will usually suffice in the acute setting. Patients with NOMI or venous thrombosis typically do not require vascular repair. Anticoagulation should be started in all such patients prior to the surgical procedure.[8] A second look laparotomy may also be required after emergency surgery in some cases owing to vasospasm of normal vascular tree, inadequate resection of ischemic segment, doubtful perfusion of bowel segments, or if the condition of the patient fails to stabilize.[28] Flowmetry with fluorescein dye are currently accepted standard of clinical care for intraoperative determination of viable status of bowel. Fluorescein is frequently used to identify perfusion during open surgery using a Woods Lamp or laparoscopically using an endoscope with appropriate filters.

Catheter-guided therapies are performed on patients without frank imaging and clinical features suggestive of gangrene/bowel necrosis; these may be either aspiration embolectomy or catheter-guided thrombolysis using rt-PA or urokinase. If atherosclerotic changes are noted in the vessel wall, this procedure can be electively followed by a percutaneous transluminal angioplasty (PTA) with or without stenting. PTA with stent placement is more effective in immediate and long-term vessel patency than PTA alone as stents offer additional structural support to the vessel wall leading to lesser repeat interventions.[29] Endovascular techniques have led to a decrease in surgery-related complications including decreased amount of bowel resected leading to lower incidence of short bowel syndrome, lesser incidence of systemic complications, and reduced mortality.[19] On review of literature for comparison of clinical outcomes between surgical and endovascular treatment options, several observational studies and meta-analyses have shown superiority for endovascular therapy as compared to open surgery in terms of reduced bowel resection rates and lower 30-day mortality rates. Retrograde open mesenteric stenting (ROMS) is another emerging hybrid technique which may be utilized in cases of AMI if facilities exist. This procedure includes performing laparotomy which is simultaneously coupled with retrograde endovascular revascularization of the SMA. Theoretically, if technical feasibility and infrastructure for such hybrid procedures are available, ROMS may be a promising treatment option for such patients who require laparotomies.[8]

Acute NOMI can be treated in the same sitting in which diagnostic catheter angiography is done for confirmation of diagnosis. The typical treatment consists of administration of intra-arterial vasodilators such as papaverine, nitroglycerin, or glucagon. Intravenous high-dose prostaglandin E1 is equally effective in management if transarterial catheterization is not feasible. However, these vasodilator drugs can lead to systemic hypotension which must be taken care during the procedure.[19]

The mainstay of treatment of venous mesenteric ischemia is by systemic anticoagulation. Long-term maintenance therapy on anticoagulants has a higher chance of recanalization of occluded veins and lower incidence of recurrence. One of its complications can be bleeding in the gangrenous bowel; however, this should not prevent or delay in administration of the systemic anticoagulant and bleeding has to be managed if it occurs. Transhepatic or transjugular cannulation of the SMV and thrombolysis with or without thrombectomy needs to be considered in acute or subacute venous occlusion based on the severity to prevent bowel infarction. Adjunct transjugular intrahepatic portosystemic shunt (TIPS) can be created to improve the outflow of the venous system.[19]

CHRONIC MESENTERIC ISCHEMIA

Chronic mesenteric ischemia is an uncommon condition which generally affects elderly population often with widespread atherosclerosis. It is more prevalent in patients with major risk factors for atherosclerosis, such as hypertension, hyperlipidemia, and history of smoking. The diagnosis is often late in its course as at least two of the three major mesenteric vascular trunks should have significant luminal narrowing before developing symptoms **(Figs. 15A to E)**.[30] Central clue for making the diagnosis of chronic mesenteric ischemia is not only the presence of significant vascular stenosis, but also prominent and tortuous collateral conduits between the mesenteric trunks which maintain the bowel viability. Frequently patients with this condition will be elderly, fragile females who experience postprandial abdominal pain, develop fear of food, and often avoid meals resulting in chronic weight loss.[31,32] Widespread atherosclerosis of the abdominal vasculature is the most frequent etiology for chronic mesenteric ischemia, other uncommon conditions, such as vasculitis, radiation vasculopathy, and fibromuscular dysplasia also cause chronic mesenteric ischemia **(Figs. 16A and B)**.[30,33]

Imaging Modalities

Noninvasive imaging modalities, such as US, CTA, MRI/MRA are employed for the evaluation. Angiography has its role in further evaluation of equivocal diagnosis or if endovascular treatment is contemplated.[24] According to ACR appropriateness criteria for evaluation of chronic mesenteric ischemia, the preference of the imaging modalities is discussed in the **Table 6**.

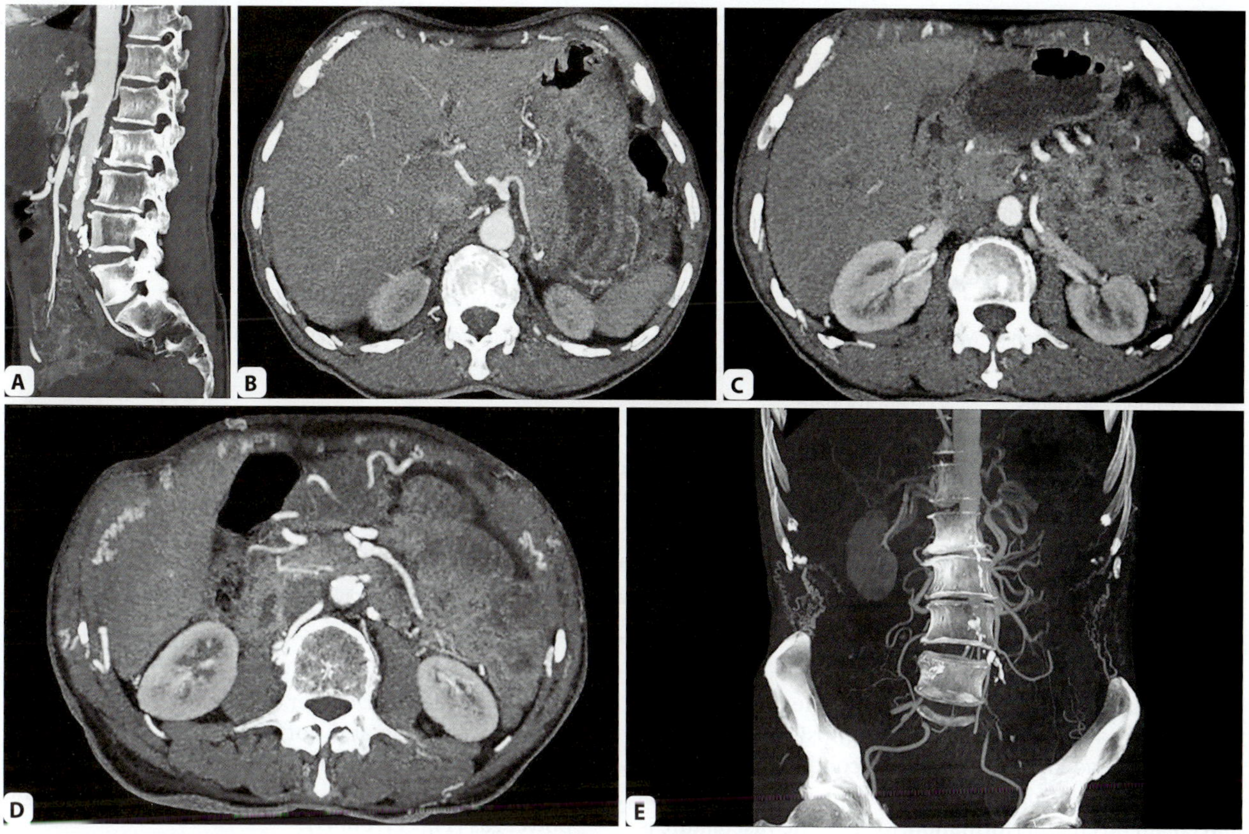

FIGS. 15A TO E: Patient of chronic mesenteric ischemia. Sagittal, axial, and coronal reconstructed CT images showing atherosclerotic changes with hemodynamically significant stenosis in the proximal celiac trunk, SMA, and IMA. Multiple mesenteric and abdominal wall collaterals are identified.

(IMA: inferior mesenteric artery; SMA: superior mesenteric artery)

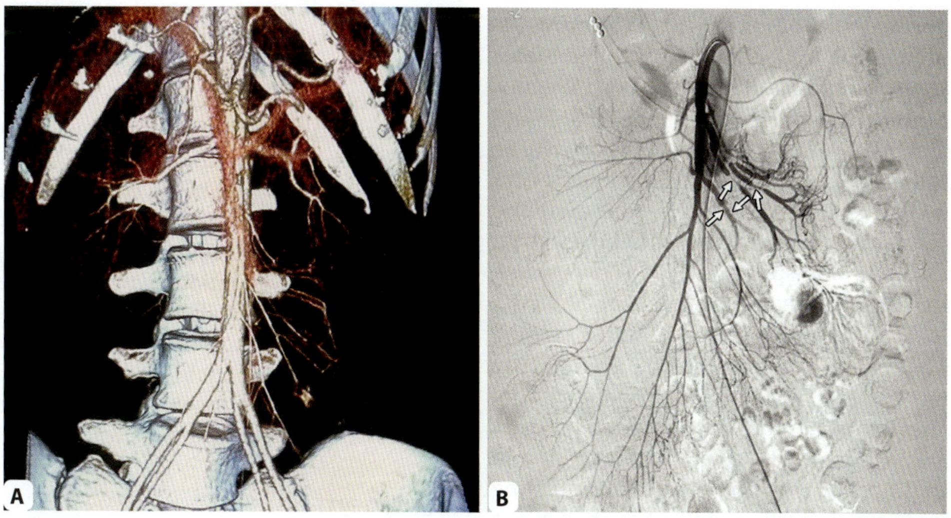

FIGS. 16A AND B: Patient of vasculitis with mesenteric angina. Volume-rendered CT image showing subtle irregularity in the branches of SMA. DSA showing SMA run confirming the irregularities and multifocal narrowing in the branches of SMA.

(DSA: digital subtraction angiography; SMA: superior mesenteric artery)

TABLE 6: ACR appropriateness criteria to evaluate chronic mesenteric ischemia.[15]

Radiologic modality	Appropriateness category	Remarks	Relative radiation level
CTA abdomen and pelvis with IV contrast	Usually appropriate	Best accuracy and inter-reader agreement for grading severity of stenosis	+++
MRA abdomen and pelvis without and with IV contrast	Usually appropriate	• Increasingly accurate in assessment of stenosis of proximal mesenteric vessels, particularly celiac artery and SMA • Limited role in distal thromboembolism and NOMI	+++
Arteriography abdomen	May be appropriate (disagreement)	Presently transitioned to more complementary role to CTA as the first line technique	+++
CT abdomen and pelvis with IV contrast	May be appropriate		+++
MRA abdomen and pelvis without IV contrast	May be appropriate	MRA without contrast may be used in some case scenarios, assessment of smaller distal vessels may be suboptimal	0
US abdomen	May be appropriate	Useful initial screening tool for chronic MI	0

(ACR: American College of Radiology; CTA: CT angiography; MI: myocardial infarction; MRA: magnetic resonance angiography; NOMI: nonocclusive mesenteric ischemia; SMA: superior mesenteric artery)

Computed tomography and CTA is the primary diagnostic tool as it allows accurate diagnosis and excludes other alternative causes of the clinical condition. CTA allows confident depiction of vascular tree with occlusions/stenosis and collateral channel formation. Mesenteric vasculature is better demonstrated by 3D imaging techniques and other postprocessing tools available in the modern workstations.

Summary of ACR Recommendations

- Computed tomography angiography abdomen with pelvis using iodinated contrast or MRA abdomen/pelvis performed without and with IV contrast is recommended as the initial imaging test in patients with clinical suspicion of chronic mesenteric ischemia.
- Computed tomography angiography abdomen and pelvis performed with IV contrast has been shown to be the most accurate modality with excellent inter-reader agreement while grading the severity of mesenteric vascular stenosis when compared to MRA and USG with reported sensitivity and specificity of 95–100% while using catheter angiography as the reference standard.[29]
- Duplex USG is another promising initial screening modality which has an important role in nonacute presentations. Sonography along with color and spectral Doppler correlation can detect hemodynamically significant stenosis in proximal celiac artery (CA) and SMA. It should preferably be performed in fasting state in order to avoid or reduce bowel gas shadows as visualizing the mesenteric vessels may be technically challenging. The peak systolic velocity measurements of >275 cm/s and >200 cm/s in SMA and celiac trunk respectively are reliable indicators of 70% or more stenosis in the fasting state.[20,34] Comparison of pre- and postprandial peak systolic velocity may also suggest vascular occlusion. Doppler USG also allows assessment of the mesenteric and portal veins which may show absence of color filling in venous thrombosis; however, it is operator dependent and often limited by overlying bowel gas **(Fig. 17A to D)**.

Magnetic resonance angiography has also been shown to have comparable accuracy to CTA for evaluation of stenosis in the mesenteric vessels. Noncontrast sequences (time-of-flight and phase contrast) are employed in patients with renal function derangement in addition to the benefit of being radiation-free modality. In chronic mesenteric ischemia, insufficient collateral channels may fail to meet with the metabolic demands of bowel with decreased blood oxygenation in SMV or artery other mesenteric veins. This deranged physiology can also be assessed through MR perfusion techniques coupled with food challenge. Cine contrast phase imaging and MR oximetry can evaluate SMV flow and blood oxygenation respectively.[35] Decrease in superior mesenteric venous flow in phase contrast imaging and reduction in superior mesenteric venous blood oxygenation level with resultant T2 value reduction after food challenge is noted with symptomatic chronic mesenteric ischemic patients.[35] However, lengthy acquisition time and inability to accurately evaluate the narrower caliber of vessels like IMA and other smaller branches are limitations in practice.

Treatment

Considering the individual patient anatomical factors and comorbities; lifestyle changes with surgery or endovascular treatment are advised, for alleviation of symptoms and to halt the progression of chronic mesenteric ischemia into more acute events.[24,36,37] Angioplasty and vascular stenting of the affected segment are the endovascular

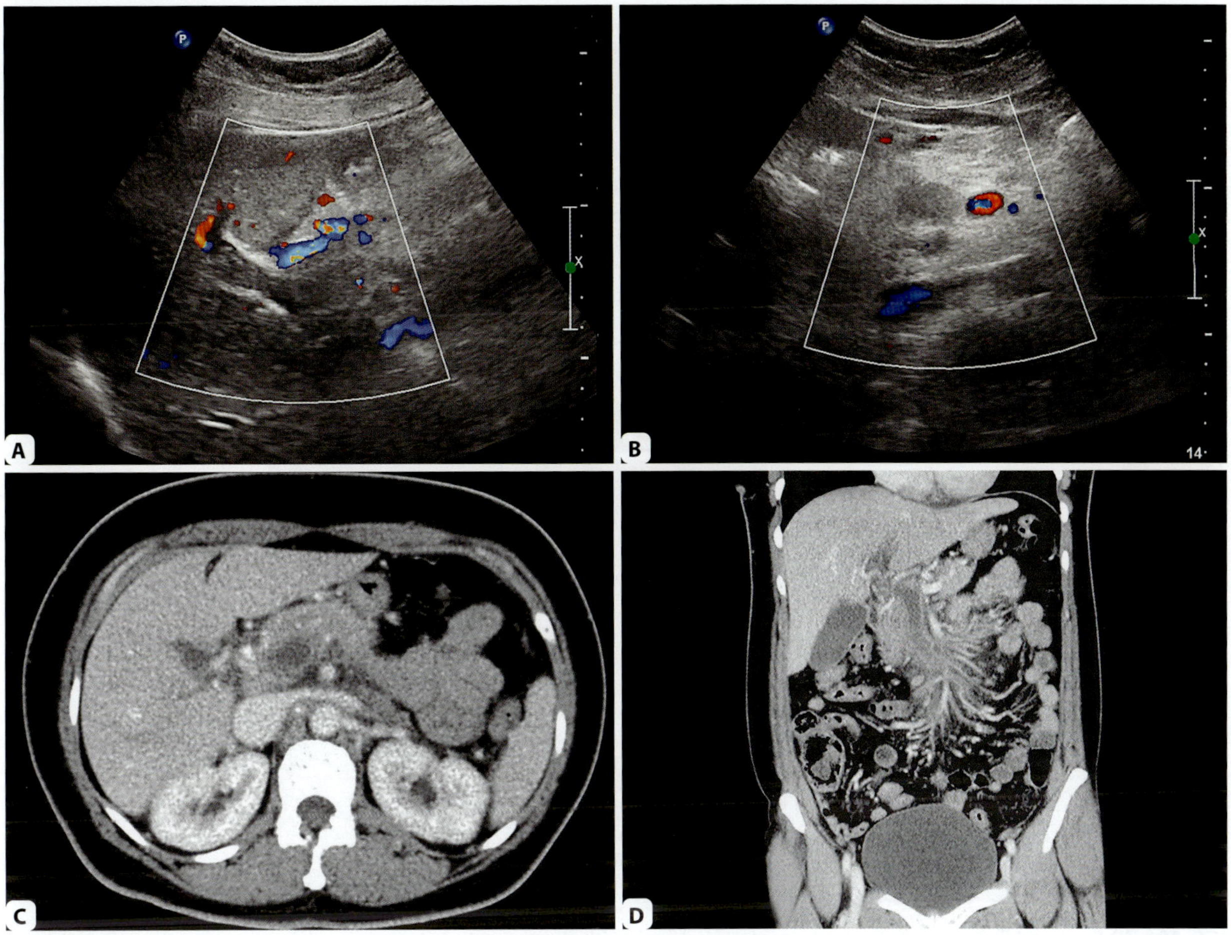

FIGS. 17A TO D: Doppler ultrasound Images: (A and B) Showing dilated superior mesenteric artery (SMV) and portal vein with no color filling suggestive of thrombosis; (C and D) Axial and coronal images confirming SMV and portal venous thrombosis.

procedures performed on affected vessels with high initial technical success rates of >90% **(Figs. 18A to F)**. However, recurrent stenosis is not uncommon and reintervention is recommended **(Figs. 19A to F)**.[37-40] Endarterectomy, vascular bypass, and arterial reimplantation are the surgically available options for treating chronic mesenteric ischemia.[36] Revascularization of single vessel (usually SMA) is sufficient with long-term patency rate of 70–93%, despite multivessel involvement.[36]

COLONIC ISCHEMIA

Colonic ischemia is regarded as the most frequently encountered form of bowel ischemia, usually seen in seventh decade of life, and is the second most common cause of lower gastrointestinal bleeding.[41] Based upon the location, it may be classified as right-sided or left-sided ischemic colitis. Underlying pathophysiologic changes are due to altered circulation, failing in meeting colonic metabolic demands. Most cases are caused by sudden transient hemodynamic alterations (systemic hypoperfusion states, aortic procedures, dialysis, etc). However, the exact underlying cause is only infrequently identified and the supplying colonic vascular arteries (arising from SMA or IMA) are usually patent. Only 25% of patients are attributed to vascular occlusion,[42] which is almost always related with impairment of the arterial supply rather than of the venous outflow.

Vascular compromise can cause evolution of pathophysiologic changes in colon and may be seen sequentially as mucosal/submucosal damage, reversible colitis, ulcerative changes, stricture formation, and gangrenous changes.[23,42] Patients usually present with mild lower abdominal pain and bloody diarrhea.[43] Watershed areas of colon such as Griffith's point at the splenic flexure and Sudeck's point in the sigmoid colon are more prone for ischemic changes.[44]

Diagnosis

Radiographic changes depend upon the underlying pathophysiology and severity of bowel necrosis. Plain abdominal radiographic features can vary from normal study to very severe damage resulting in pneumo-/retropneumoperitoneum. Other features such as nonspecific

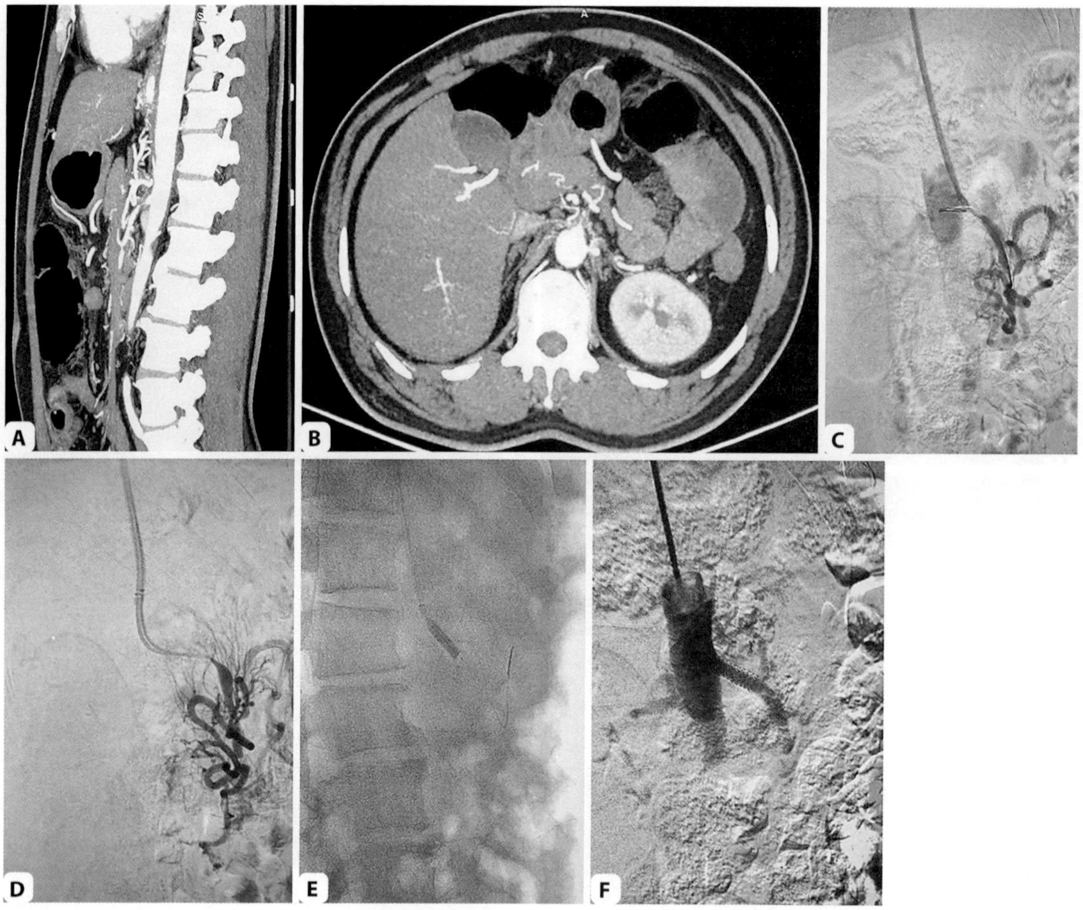

FIGS. 18A TO F: (A and B) Patient of chronic mesenteric ischemia with short segment stenosis involving superior mesenteric artery (SMA) and celiac axis; (C to F) Digital subtraction angiography (DSA) performed with balloon dilatation and placement of metallic stent in proximal SMA caused significant relief of symptoms.

ileus, thumb printing, transverse ridging, and ahaustration may be observed, occasionally pneumatosis or portal venous gas may be identified due to transmural bowel necrosis.[45,46]

Barium examination features vary with stage and degree of ischemic damage. Serial changes in the barium study characteristics is the hallmark feature of colonic ischemia.[47-49] Features observed on barium studies may include thumb printing (most common), transverse ridging, spasm, ulceration, intramural barium, and stricture formation.[45] USG also demonstrates nonspecific bowel wall thickening and diminished color flow in involved bowel segment.[34]

Contrast-enhanced computed tomography (CECT) in the present era is the first imaging technique performed for diagnosing ischemic colitis which usually tends to involve a specific segment of colon. This is contrary to the infective/inflammatory etiology which may be patchy or diffuse and generally shows nonsegmental colonic involvement. Most common bowel segment affected is left colon; CT features in colonic ischemia are similar to those seen in small bowel ischemia include mural thickening, reduced or lack of enhancement, target/double halo sign, luminal dilatation pneumatosis intestinalis, portal venous gas, peritoneal fluid, or pneumoperitoneum. Limitations of CT evaluation is lack of specificity and difficult assessment of the bowel wall thickening secondary to inadequate bowel distension.[43] Also in colonic ischemia, initial imaging features cannot be utilized for definite prognostication.

Colonoscopic evaluation is regarded as the diagnostic test of choice for suspected colonic ischemia due to its excellent sensitivity. The specific location and patchy segmental involvement of the colon are features which may favor the diagnosis. Recent evidence supports that suspected clinical diagnosis should be confirmed by performing careful colonoscopy (CS) and biopsy whenever feasible, even if this being considered relatively unsafe in the acute phases.[50] Guidelines from the American College of Gastroenterology (ACG) recommend CT as the imaging modality of choice which should be done within the initial few hours of admission.[51] Colonoscopy is recommended within 48 hours to detect the bowel alterations and exclude other differential diagnosis.[52] Favier classification is widely utilized by clinicians to make the diagnosis, to ascertain prognosis, and to decide surgical intervention.[53,54]

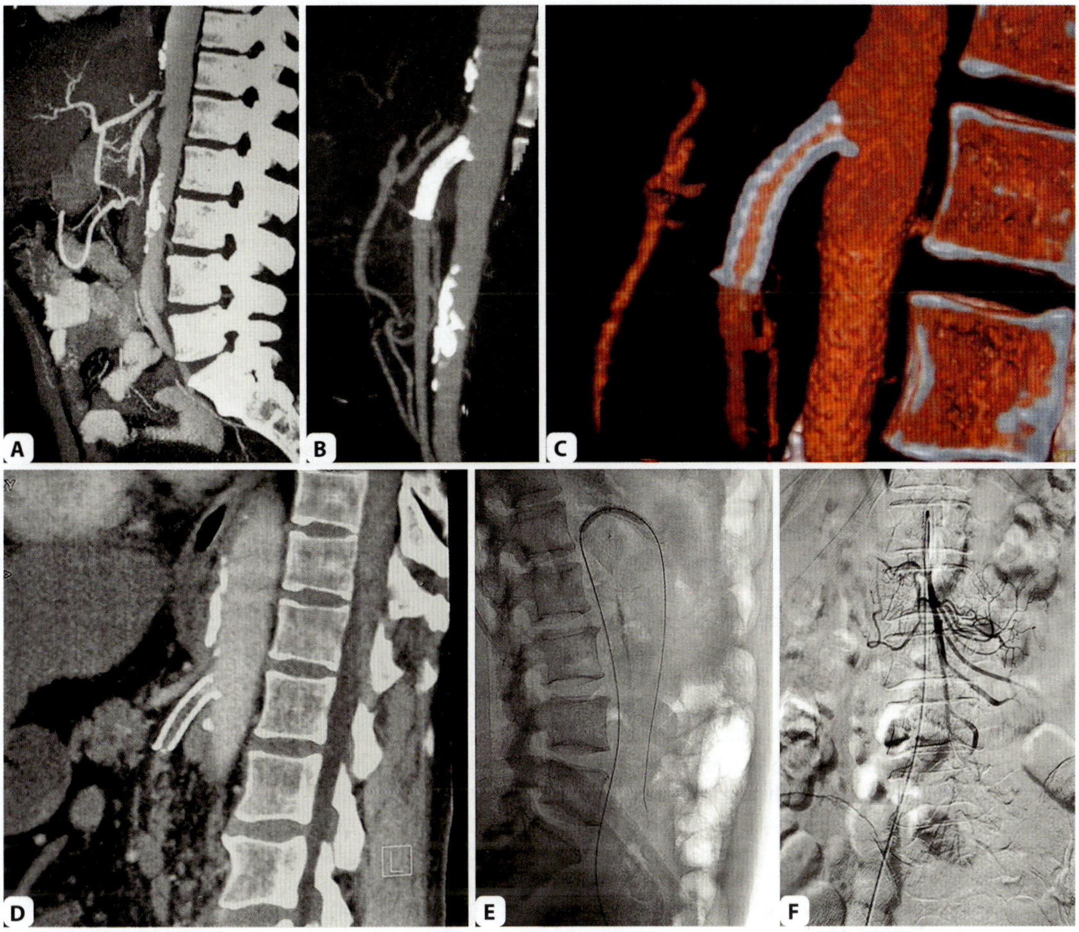

FIGS. 19A TO F: (A) Patient of chronic mesenteric ischemia with short segment stenosis involving proximal celiac trunk and superior mesenteric artery (SMA); (B and C) Metallic stenting performed in proximal SMA with good distal opacification; (D) Relapse of symptoms with CT repeated after 7 months showed in stent thrombosis with poor distal flow; (E and F) Reintervention with balloon dilatation performed across the stent with restored flow in the distal SMA and relief of symptoms.

Treatment

Correction of hypovolemia and treating primary cause is the primary goal. Medical management consists of gastric rest, fluid and electrolyte management, administration of broad-spectrum antibiotics, and prophylaxis against venous thromboembolism. Resection of ischemic bowel with/without bowel anastomosis and/or cholecystectomy is the surgical management available for suitable patients.[43]

REFERENCES

1. Dhatt HS, Behr SC, Miracle A, Wang ZJ, Yeh BM. Radiological evaluation of bowel ischemia. Radiol clin N Am. 2015; 53: 1241-54.
2. Olson MC, Fletcher JG, Nagpal P, Froemming AT, Khandelwal A. Mesenteric ischemia: what the radiologist needs to know. Cardiovasc Diagn Ther. 2019;9(Suppl 1):S74-S87.
3. Gourley EJ, Gering SA. The meandering mesenteric artery: a historic review and surgical implications. Dis Colon Rectum. 2005;48:996-1000.
4. Upponi S, Harvey JJ, Uberoi R, Ganeshan A. The role of radiology in the diagnosis and treatment of mesenteric ischemia. Postgrad Med J. 2013;89:165-72.
5. Nakamura Y, Kondo S, Narita K, Maeda S, Fonseca D, Honda Y, et al. Understanding CT imaging findings based on the underlying pathophysiology in patients with small bowel ischemia. Jpn J Radiol. 2023;41:353-66.
6. Moschetta M, Telegrafo M, Rella L, Stabile Ianora AA, Angelelli G. Multi-detector CT features of acute intestinal ischemia and their prognostic correlations. World J Radiol. 2014;6:130-8.
7. Brandt LJ, Fuerstadt P. Intestestinal ischemia. In: Feldman M, Friedman LS, Lawrence J. Brandt LJ (Eds). Sleisenger and Fordtran's Gastrointestinal and Liver Disease, 10th edition. Philadelphia, PA: Elsevier; 2015. pp. 2076-101.
8. Bala M, Catena F, Kashuk J, De Simone B, Gomes CA, Weber D, et al. Acute mesenteric ischemia: updated guidelines of the World Society of Emergency Surgery. World J Emerg Surg. 2022:19;17:54.

9. Fitzpatrick LA, Rivers-Bowerman MD, Thipphavong S, Clarke SE, Rowe JA, Costa AF. Pearls, Pitfalls, and Conditions that Mimic Mesenteric Ischemia at CT. Radiographics. 2020; 40:545-61.
10. Yu H, Kirkpatrick IDC. An Update on Acute Mesenteric Ischemia. Can Assoc Radiol J. 2023;74:160-71.
11. Oliva IB, Davarpanah AH, Rybicki FJ, Desjardins B, Flamm SD, Francois CJ, et al. ACR Appropriateness Criteria® imaging of mesenteric ischemia. Abdom Imaging. 2013;38:714-9.
12. Furukawa A, Kanasaki S, Kono N, Wakamiya M, Tanaka T, Takahashi M, et al. CT diagnosis of acute mesenteric ischemia from various causes. AJR. 2009;192:408-16.
13. Aschoff AJ, Stuber G, Becker BW, Hoffmann MH, Schmitz BL, Schelzig H, et al. Evaluation of acute mesenteric ischemia: accuracy of biphasic mesenteric multi-detector CT angiography. Abdom Imaging. 2009;34(3):345-57.
14. Barmase M, Kang M, Wig J, Kochhar R, Gupta R, Khandelwal N. Role of multidetector CT angiography in the evaluation of suspected mesenteric ischemia. Eur J Radiol. 2011;80:e582-7.
15. Kirkpatrick IDC, Kroeker MA, Greenberg HM. Biphasic CT with mesenteric CT angiography in the evaluation of acute mesenteric ischemia: initial experience. Radiology. 2003;229: 91-8.
16. Yikilmaz A, Karahan OI, Senol S, Tuna IS, Akyildiz HY. Value of multislice computed tomography in the diagnosis of acute mesenteric ischemia. Eur J Radiol. 2011;80:297-302.
17. Navas-Campo R, Moreno-Caballero L, Ezponda Casajús A, Muñoz DI. Acute mesenteric ischemia: a review of the main imaging techniques and signs. Radiologia (Engl Ed). 2020;62:336-48.
18. Fulwadhva UP, Wortman JR, Sodickson AD. Use of dual energy CT and iodine maps in evaluation of bowel disease. RadioGraphics. 2016; 36:393-406.
19. Expert Panels on Vascular Imaging and Gastrointestinal Imaging:; Ginsburg M, Obara P, Lambert DL, Hanley M, Steigner ML, et al. ACR Appropriateness Criteria® Imaging of Mesenteric Ischemia. J Am Coll Radiol. 2018;15(11S): S332-40.
20. Bradbury MS, Kavanagh PV, Bechtold RE, Chen MY, Ott DJ, Regan JD, et al. Mesenteric venous thrombosis: diagnosis and noninvasive imaging. Radiographics. 2002;22(3):527-41.
21. Raman SP, Fishman EK. Computed tomography angiography of the small bowel and mesentery. Radiol Clin N Am. 2016;54:87-100.
22. Wang JH, Furlan A, Kaya D, Goshima S, Tublin M, Bae KT. Pneumatosis intestinalis versus pseudo-pneumatosis: review of CT findings and differentiation. Insights Imaging. 2011;2:85-92.
23. Gore RM, Thakrar KH, Mehta UK, Berlin J, Yaghmai V, Newmark GM, et al. Clinical imaging, clinical gastroenterology and hepatology. 2008;6:849-58.
24. Walker TG. Mesenteric ischemia. Semin Intervent Radiol. 2009;26(3):175-83.
25. Wilkerson DK, Mezrich R, Drake C, Sebok D, Zatina MA. Magnetic resonance imaging of acute occlusive intestinal ischaemia. J Vasc Surg. 1990;11:567-71.
26. Zargar I, Robanni I, Shah O, Gojwari T, Rasool R, Choh N, et al. Imaging Evaluation of Mesenteric Ischemia: Is There a Golden Period for This Entity? Galician Med J. 2022;29:E202212.
27. Estler A, Estler E, Feng YS, Seith F, Wießmeier M, Archid R, et al. Treatment of Acute Mesenteric Ischemia: Individual Challenges for Interventional Radiologists and Abdominal Surgeons. J Pers Med. 2022:27;13:55.
28. Klar E, Rahmanian PB, Bucker A, Hauenstein K, Jauch KW, Luther B. Acute mesenteric ischemia: a vascular emergency. Dtsch Arztebl Int. 2012;109:249-56.
29. Landis MS, Rajan DK, Simons ME, Hayeems EB, Kachura JR, Sniderman KW. Percutaneous management of chronic mesenteric ischemia: outcomes after intervention. J Vasc Interv Radiol. 2005;16:1319-25.
30. Hohenwalter EJ. Chronic mesenteric ischemia: diagnosis and treatment. Semin Intervent Radiol. 2009;26(4):345-51.
31. Ujiki M, Kibbe MR. Mesenteric ischemia. Perspect Vasc Surg Endovasc Ther. 2005;17:309-18.
32. Kougias P, El Sayed HF, Zhou W, Lin PH. Management of chronic mesenteric ischemia. The role of endovascular therapy. J Endovasc Ther. 2007;14:395-405.
33. Sreenarasimhaiah J. Chronic mesenteric ischemia. Best Pract Res Clin Gastroenterol. 2005;19:283-95.
34. Reginelli A, Genovese E, Cappabianca S, Iacobellis F, Berritto D, Fonio P, et al. Intestinal Ischemia: US-CT findings correlations. Crit Ultrasound J. 2013;5 Suppl 1(Suppl 1):S7.
35. Chow LC, Chan FP, Li KCP. A comprehensive approach to MR imaging of mesenteric ischemia. Abdom Imaging. 2002;27:507-16.
36. Schaefer PJ, Schaefer FKW, Mueller-Huelsbeck S, Jahnke T. Chronic mesenteric ischemia: stenting of mesenteric arteries. Abdom Imaging. 2007;32:304-9.
37. Atkins MD, Kwolek CJ, LaMuraglia GM, Brewster DC, Chung TK, Cambria RP. Surgical revascularization versus endovascular therapy for chronic mesenteric ischemia: a comparative experience. J Vasc Surg. 2007;45:1162-71.
38. Sharafuddin MJ, Olson CH, Sun S, Kresowik TF, Corson JD. Endovascular treatment of celiac and mesenteric arteries stenoses: applications and results. J Vasc Surg. 2003;38:692-8.
39. Matsumoto AH, Angle JF, Spinosa DJ, Hagspiel.KD, Cage DL, Leung DA, et al. Percutaneous transluminal angioplasty and stenting in the treatment of chronic mesenteric ischemia: results and longterm followup. J Am Coll Surg. 2002;194(1 Suppl):S22-31.
40. Sarac TP, Altinel O, Kashyap V, Bena J, Lyden S, Sruvastava S, et al. Endovascular treatment of stenotic and occluded visceral arteries for chronic mesenteric ischemia. J Vasc Surg. 2008;47(3):485-91.
41. Paterno F, Longo WE. The etiology and pathogenesis of vascular disorders of the intestine. Radiol Clin North Am. 2008;46:877-85.
42. Balthazar EJ, Yen BC, Gordon RB. Ischemic colitis. Radiology. 1999;211:381-8.
43. Moszkowicz D, Mariani A, Trésallet C, Menegaux F. Ischemic colitis: the ABCs of diagnosis and surgical management. J Visc Surg. 2013;150:19-28.
44. Rogers AI, David S. Intestinal blood flow and diseases of vascular impairment. In: Haubrich WS, Schaffner F, Berk JE (Eds). Gastroenterology, 5th edition. Philadelphia, PA: Saunders; 1995. pp. 1212-34.
45. Parfitt JR, Driman DK. Pathological effects of drugs on the gastrointestinal tract: A review. Hum Pathol. 2007;38:527-36.
46. Wittenberg J, Athanasoulis CA, Williams LF Jr, Paredes S, O'Sullivan P, Brown B. Ischemic colitis. Radiology and pathophysiology. Am J Roentgenol Radium Ther Nucl Med. 1975;123(2):287-300.

47. Gore RM, Calenoff L, Rogers LF. Roentgenographic manifestations of ischemic colitis. JAMA. 1979;241:1171-3.
48. Iida M, Matsui T, Fuchigami T, Iwashita A, Yao T, Fujishima M. Ischemic colitis: serial changes in double contrast barium enema examinations. Radiology. 1986;159:337-41.
49. Greenberg HM, Goldberg HI, Axel L. Colonic"urticaria" pattern due to early ischemia. Gastrointest Radiol. 1981;6:145-9.
50. Iacobellis F, Narese D, Berritto D, Brillantino A, Di Serafino M, Guerrini S, et al. Large Bowel Ischemia/Infarction: How to Recognize It and Make Differential Diagnosis? A Review. Diagnostics (Basel). 2021;11(6):998.
51. Trotter JM, Hunt L, Peter MB. Ischaemic colitis. BMJ. 2016;355: i6600.
52. Brandt LJ, Feuerstadt P, Longstreth GF, Boley SJ. ACG clinical guideline: Epidemiology, risk factors, patterns of presentation, diagnosis, and management of colon ischemia (CI). Am J Gastroenterol. 2015;110:18-44.
53. Favier C, Bonneau HP, Tran Minh V, Devic J. Endoscopic diagnosis of regressive ischemic colitis. Endoscopic, histologic and arteriographic correlations. Nouv Presse Med. 1976;5:77-9.
54. Beppu K, Osada T, Nagahara A, Matsumoto K, Shibuya T, Sakamoto N, et al. Relationship between endoscopic findings and clinical severity in ischemic colitis. Intern Med. 2011;50:2263-7.

CHAPTER 7

Shivanand Gamanagatti, Devasenathipathy Kandasamy, Stuti Chandola

Gastrointestinal Hemorrhage: Imaging and Interventions

INTRODUCTION

The term "gastrointestinal (GI) hemorrhage" (GIH) refers to bleeding within any part of the alimentary tract, extending from the esophagus to anal canal. It is a potential medical emergency requiring prompt assessment for localization of source and subsequent management.[1,2] GIH can be acute and chronic/recurrent at presentation. The treatment is based on a multidisciplinary approach with significant contributions from both diagnostic and interventional radiology. Imaging plays a crucial role in site identification, ascertaining a definite or probable etiology, and providing minimally invasive approaches for bleeding cessation.[2,3] This chapter reviews the role of imaging in diagnosis and provides a brief overview of the image-guided interventions in GIH.

TERMINOLOGIES AND CLASSIFICATION

Awareness of the proper terminology for the types of GIH is essential for effective communication. The glossary of these terms is reviewed in **Table 1**. The ligament of Treitz at the duodenojejunal flexure serves as a major landmark dividing GIH into upper (proximal) and lower (source distal to ligament). Upper GI hemorrhage (UGIH) is more frequent as compared to lower GI hemorrhage (LGIH), with an annual incidence rate varying from 50 to 120 per 100,000 as compared to 20.5–27 per 100,000 for LGIH.[4-6] The recent consensus recommendations from American College of Gastroenterology (ACG) and Society of Abdominal Radiology (SAR) define LGIH as bleeding distal to ileocecal valve.[2] Mid-GI or small bowel bleeding is a unique entity accounting for 5–10% of GIH and often manifests as obscure

TABLE 1: Common terminology utilized in gastrointestinal (GI) hemorrhage.

Term	Description
Upper GI hemorrhage (UGIH)	Bleed source proximal to the ligament of Treitz (from esophagus to duodenum)
Lower GI hemorrhage (LGIH)	Bleed source distal to the ligament of Treitz (including rectum and anal canal)
Mid-GI hemorrhage	Bleed source from small bowel distal to ampulla and proximal to ileocecal valve; also known as *small bowel bleeding*
Suspected small bowel hemorrhage	GI bleeding in which no bleeding source is identified after performing both upper GI endoscopy and colonoscopy
Obscure GI hemorrhage	• GI bleeding in which no bleeding source is identified even after complete evaluation of the entire GI tract, including advanced endoscopic techniques • Can further be overt or occult depending on whether clinically evidence of bleeding is visible or not • Overt GI bleed—symptoms such as hematemesis, hematochezia, or melena • Occult GI bleed—not visible clinically, detected as positive fecal occult blood test result or iron deficiency anemia
Massive GI hemorrhage	GI bleeding with associated hemodynamic instability and symptoms of shock (e.g., hypotension with systolic blood pressure < 90 mm Hg, tachycardia) or bleeding requiring transfusion of >4 units of packed red blood cells (RBCs) within 24 hours

GIH, with the source remaining unknown even after complete endoscopic and imaging GI evaluation.[1,2] Obscure GIH can further be categorized into overt and occult based upon the manifestation of symptoms **(Table 1)**.[1,2]

CLINICAL PRESENTATION

Patients with UGIH complain of hematemesis (coffee-colored vomiting) or melena (black tarry stools). Melena is consequent to degeneration of the blood by gastric and intestinal enzymes and requires a considerable amount of time within the intestinal tract.[7] LGIH patients present with fresh blood in stools, also known as hematochezia. Occasionally however, blood from upper GI source may reach the rectum rapidly due to its purgative properties, consequently manifesting as hematochezia. On the other hand, right colonic bleeding may also manifest as melena due to slow colonic transit. Symptom-based categorization of GIH is therefore not universal and may deceive the clinician. Hence, all patients with GIH are evaluated with both upper GI endoscopy (UGIE) and lower GI endoscopy until a source is identified.[8] Massive GIH is characterized by GI bleed which causes hemodynamic instability and symptoms of shock or which requires transfusion of >4 units of packed red blood cells (RBCs) within 24 hours.[1] Patients with chronic or recurrent GIH present with anemia. They may be asymptomatic if hemorrhage is <100 mL/day.

ETIOLOGIES

A multitude of causes present as GI bleeding and can broadly manifest due to abnormality at arterial, venous, or capillary level. Identification of specific risk factors entails the cause to be ascertained without imaging as well. **Table 2** enumerates the various common causes and risk factors of GIH. It is essential to note that 11–15% of patients with suspected LGIH have a source in the upper GI tract (GIT).[1]

EVALUATION AND ALGORITHMIC APPROACH

After presentation, all patients with suspected GIH are investigated with endoscopy, which remains the initial diagnostic procedure of choice **(Flowchart 1)**. This assessment includes a UGIE and colonoscopy for UGIH and LGIH, respectively.

Endoscopic evaluation carries dual benefits of detection of bleeding source and allowing management in the same sitting. Direct visualization allows lesion sampling whenever needed as well. Commonly administered endoscopic treatment options include placing clips and bands, injections of alcohol and epinephrine, and thermal ablative procedures such as electrocoagulation and laser ablations. In case endoscopic treatment fails, placing metallic clips as a marker close to bleeding source may be of assistance during further procedures such as computed

TABLE 2: Etiologies and risk factors of gastrointestinal hemorrhage.

Causes	Risk factors and specific comments
Upper gastrointestinal hemorrhage	
PUD	• Most common cause of GIH • *Helicobacter pylori* infection; NSAID, anticoagulant, or low-dose aspirin use; physiologic stress; Zollinger–Ellison syndrome
Varices and portal hypertensive gastropathy	• Most common cause of GIH in a cirrhotic patient • Cirrhosis, portal hypertension, portal vein thrombosis
Esophagitis	Gastroesophageal reflux disease, medications (e.g., erythromycin or NSAIDs), infections (e.g., herpes simplex virus or cytomegalovirus)
Gastritis and duodenitis	Same as PUD
Mallory–Weis tear	Vomiting or retching, often related to heavy alcohol consumption
Neoplasms	Unexplained weight loss, change in bowel habits, anemia
Vascular malformations/lesions—angioectasia, Dieulafoy's lesions, arteriovenous malformation, GAVE	Risk factors for angioectasia—advanced age, presence of multiple angioectasias elsewhere, aortic stenosis, left ventricular assist device, end-stage renal disease
Iatrogenic and postoperative	Aortic surgery (aortoenteric fistula), gastric surgeries, use of NSAIDs
Hemosuccus pancreaticus	Chronic pancreatitis, necrotizing pancreatitis, pseudocysts, pancreatic neoplasms
Lower gastrointestinal hemorrhage	
Colitis and ulceration	• Infection (enteric, amoebic, and tubercular), nonspecific ulcers (contribute to 30% of cases LGIH in India) • History of inflammatory bowel disease
Diverticular disease	Painless hematochezia, advanced age, hypertension
Angioectasia	Same as above
Hemorrhoids	Advanced age, constipation, increased abdominal pressure
Colonic ischemia	Hypotension, advanced age, embolic disease, recent high-risk surgery
Neoplasms	Same as above
Iatrogenic and postoperative	Polypectomy, aortic surgery (aortoenteric fistula), colonic surgeries, NSAIDs

(GAVE: gastric antral vascular ectasia; GIH: gastrointestinal hemorrhage; LGIH: lower GIH; NSAIDs: nonsteroidal anti-inflammatory drugs; PUD: peptic ulcer disease)

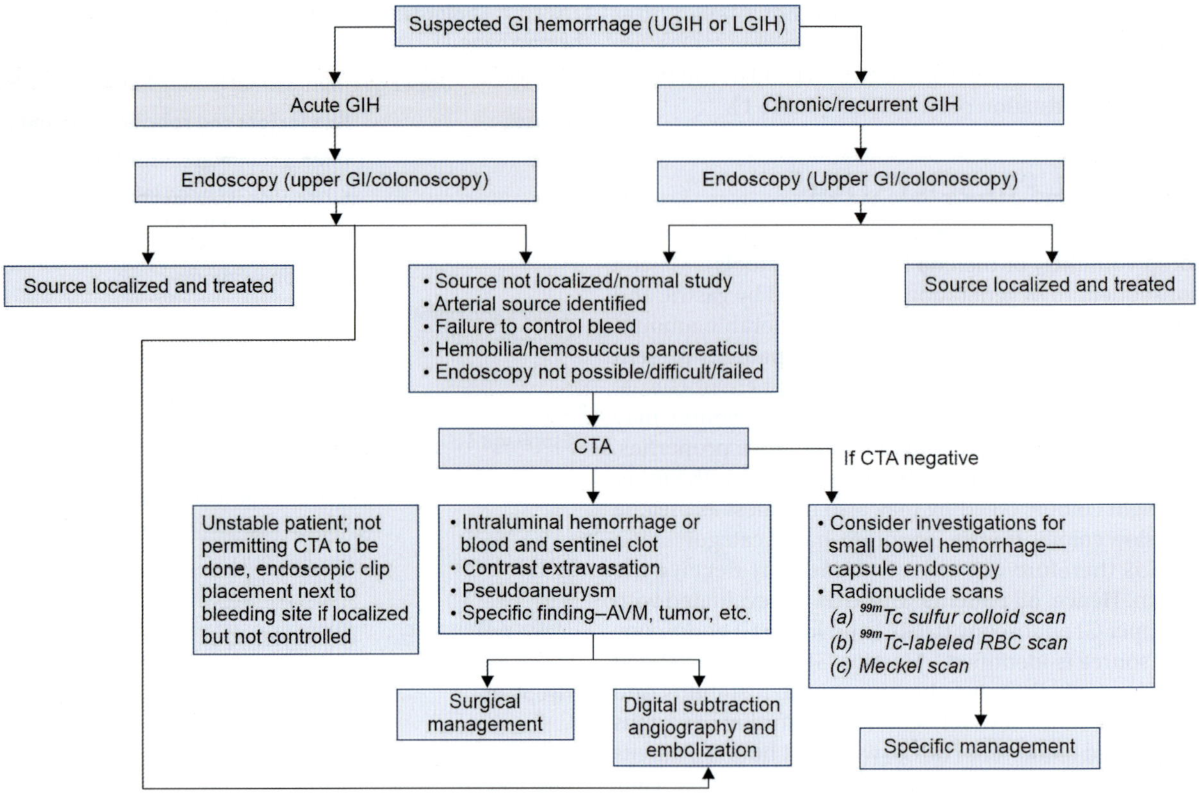

FLOWCHART 1: Algorithmic approach in a patient with suspected GI hemorrhage.

(AVM: arteriovenous malformation; CTA: computed tomography angiography; GI: gastrointestinal; GIH: GI hemorrhage; LGIH: lower GIH; RBC: red blood cell; UGIH: upper GIH)

tomography (CT) angiography (CTA) and digital subtraction angiography (DSA) and the same should be communicated to the gastroenterologist.

Upper GI endoscopy in particular has a high sensitivity and specificity in UGIH evaluation, approaching 98% and 100%, respectively,[8,9] as compared to colonoscopy, which has a variable diagnostic accuracy ranging from 45% to 90%.[8]

Endoscopy is, however, not without limitations. Endoscopic evaluation requires patient cooperation, hence may be difficult in sick patients. Blood in GIT may obscure the bleeding source due to which treatment may not be possible. Colonoscopy additionally requires bowel preparation for adequate assessment. Despite these drawbacks, it is still the first line of investigation as many of the lesions responsible for GIH may not be seen on imaging.

Few additional investigations are available for GIH where no bleeding source is identified after performing both UGIE and colonoscopy. Double-balloon enteroscopy carries a diagnostic accuracy of 40–80% for evaluating small bowel GIH.[9] Wireless capsule endoscopy is another noninvasive technique for obscure and chronic GIH and carries a diagnostic yield of 49%.[10] However, it is mainly reserved for chronic and intermittent GIH as it is a lengthy procedure and requires patient preparation. Another major risk is retention of capsule consequent to an intestinal stricture which would warrant surgical removal.[11]

A patient who has failed the initial endoscopic management is subjected to imaging. **Flowchart 1** provides an overview of algorithmic approach in a patient with GIH.

IMAGING MODALITIES

A myriad of imaging modalities are available for evaluation of GIH, of which three are routinely utilized—CTA, DSA, and radionuclide scans. Clinical presentation and suspicion are two major factors determining selection amongst these investigations. The timing of imaging is additionally vital in improving detection rates as bleeding is usually intermittent. It is essential to realize that imaging may not be required in a substantial proportion of patients where endoscopic diagnosis and management has been sufficient. Another caveat is that imaging may be negative in about 14% cases of UGIH and 20% of LGIH.[12] It is therefore important to carefully define the indications for imaging **(Flowchart 1)**.

Computed Tomography Angiography

Computed tomography angiography is the workhorse modality for radiological assessment of GI bleed due to its high spatial resolution and ability to detect bleeding rate as low as 0.1 mL/min.[2,13,14] The sensitivity, specificity, and diagnostic accuracy of CTA in the detection and localization of GIH approaches 90%, 92%, and 94–95%, respectively.[2,15]

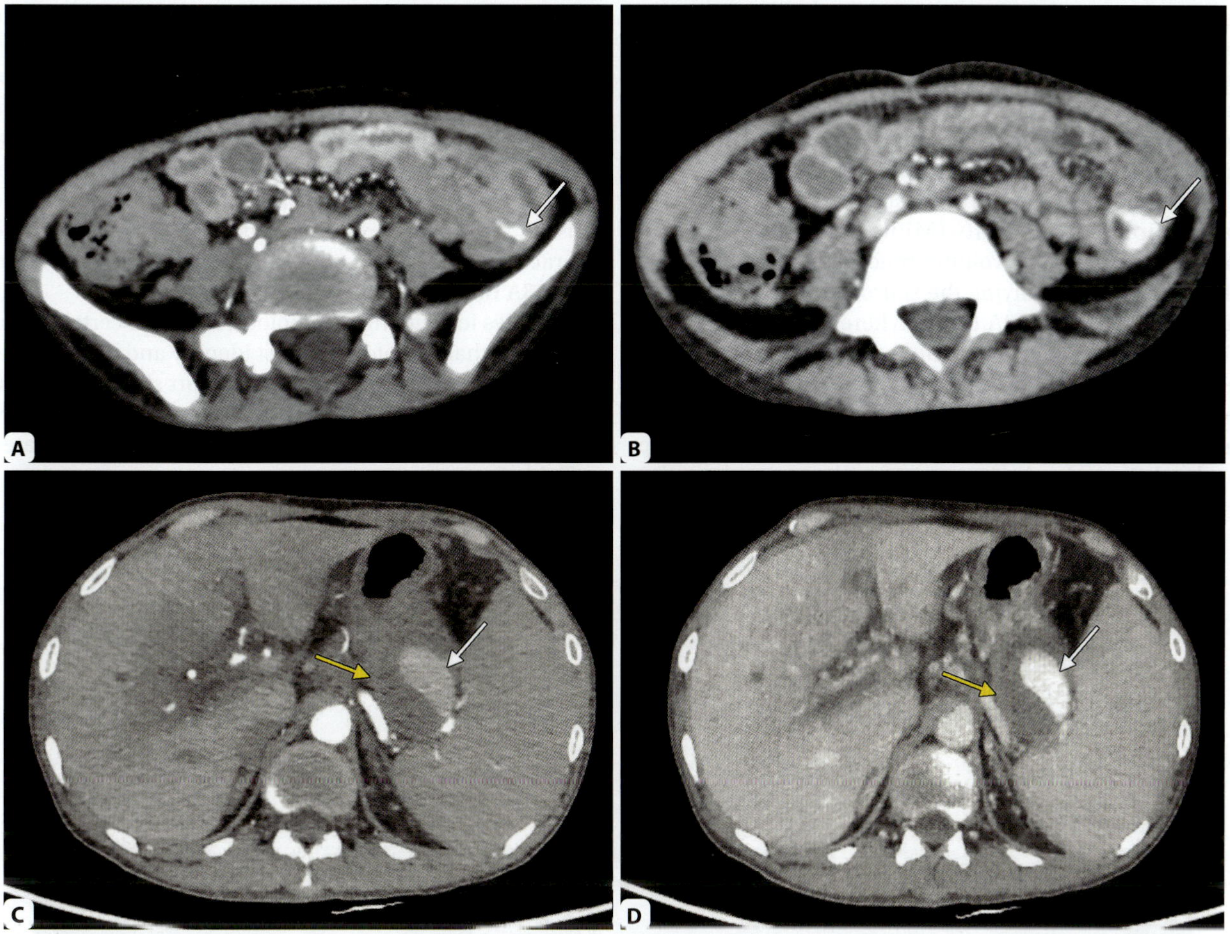

FIGS. 1A TO D: Imaging features of gastrointestinal hemorrhage (GIH) on computed tomography (CT) angiography (CTA): (A and B) Contrast extravasation: Axial CT images in arterial (A) and portal venous phases (B) demonstrate active bleed in the form of contrast extravasation within the descending colon, which appears during the arterial phase (arrow, A) and changes size, shape, and attenuation in the portal venous phase (arrow, B). (C and D) Pseudoaneurysm: Axial CT images in arterial (C) and portal venous phases (D) in a patient with chronic pancreatitis show a focal contrast-filled outpouching (white arrows, C and D) along the splenic artery at hilum which follows the aortic attenuation, however, shows similar size and shape in portal venous phase. Associated perianeurysmal hematoma (yellow arrows, C and D) is also appreciated.

CTA additionally can be prognostic by identifying the extravasated volume which can affect the transfusion requirement and hemostatic therapy.[2]

Computed tomography angiography is performed with different aims in different types of GIH. The major objective in acute or overt GIH remains delineation of the exact source (intraluminal bleed vs. pseudoaneurysm or contrast extravasation) along with cause **(Figs. 1A to D)**. In contrast to this, delineating the etiology is of prime importance when dealing with chronic or occult GIH.

Protocol

Different protocols are adopted for overt and occult GIH due to variability in goals. In acute GI bleeding, a multiphasic protocol is advocated universally with acquisition of a noncontrast CT (NCCT) phase and arterial and venous phases.[2] The noncontrast phase can be omitted on dual energy scanners. About 100–125 mL (1.5 mL/kg) of high-concentration iodinated contrast media (i.e., 350–375 mg/mL) is injected intravenously at a rate of 4–5 mL/s. Oral contrast is not recommended due to the following reasons: (1) Delay in scanning during which transient or intermittent bleeding may cease; (2) oral contrast administration increases the aspiration risk during sedation or anesthesia, thereby precluding or delaying subsequent urgent interventions; (3) positive oral contrast material masks intraluminal contrast extravasation due to similar attenuation; and (4) neutral oral contrast material may dilute contrast extravasation, leading to difficulty in identification.[1] Both phases should cover from the dome of diaphragms to femoral lesser trochanter. Automated bolus tracking is utilized with regions of interest in abdominal aorta at mid-liver level with a trigger attenuation of 150 HU. A late arterial phase should be obtained 10–15 seconds after aortic bolus trigger, i.e., at about 25–30 seconds from the beginning of contrast injection.[1,2] This is followed by venous phase acquisition (60–70 seconds post beginning of injection). An additional "enteric" phase, acquired at 50 seconds after injection begins, may also be acquired for demonstrating peak bowel enhancement; few inflammatory conditions and neuroendocrine tumors are more conspicuous on this phase.[2]

The acquired data is reconstructed with generation of multiplanar reformats (MPR), maximum intensity projection (MIP), and volume-rendered images (VRT), as these assist in identifying the source of bleeding and the feeding artery **(Figs. 2A to D)**. Wherever dual-energy CT (DECT) is available, virtual noncontrast reconstructions eliminate the need for true noncontrast images, thereby reducing the total CT radiation dose.[16] Additionally, monoenergetic images (40–60 keV), iodine density map, and color overlay images may facilitate the detection of active extravasation by increasing the conspicuity of iodinated contrast material.[1,3,14]

Whenever a small bowel source is suspected, CT enterography should be performed with neutral oral contrast, either as a single-phase examination or as a multiphase exam with both arterial and venous phases.[1,2] While single-phase studies are sufficient for inflammatory conditions and masses, multiphase examinations improve detection and characterization of vascular lesions such as angioectasias **(Figs. 3A to D)**.[2]

Besides identifying the etiology, there are certain signs and terms that radiologists must identify and differentiate for effective communication. The report should incorporate whether there are signs of active bleeding and if there is an associated etiology **(Figs. 1 to 4)**. These are tabulated in **Table 3**.

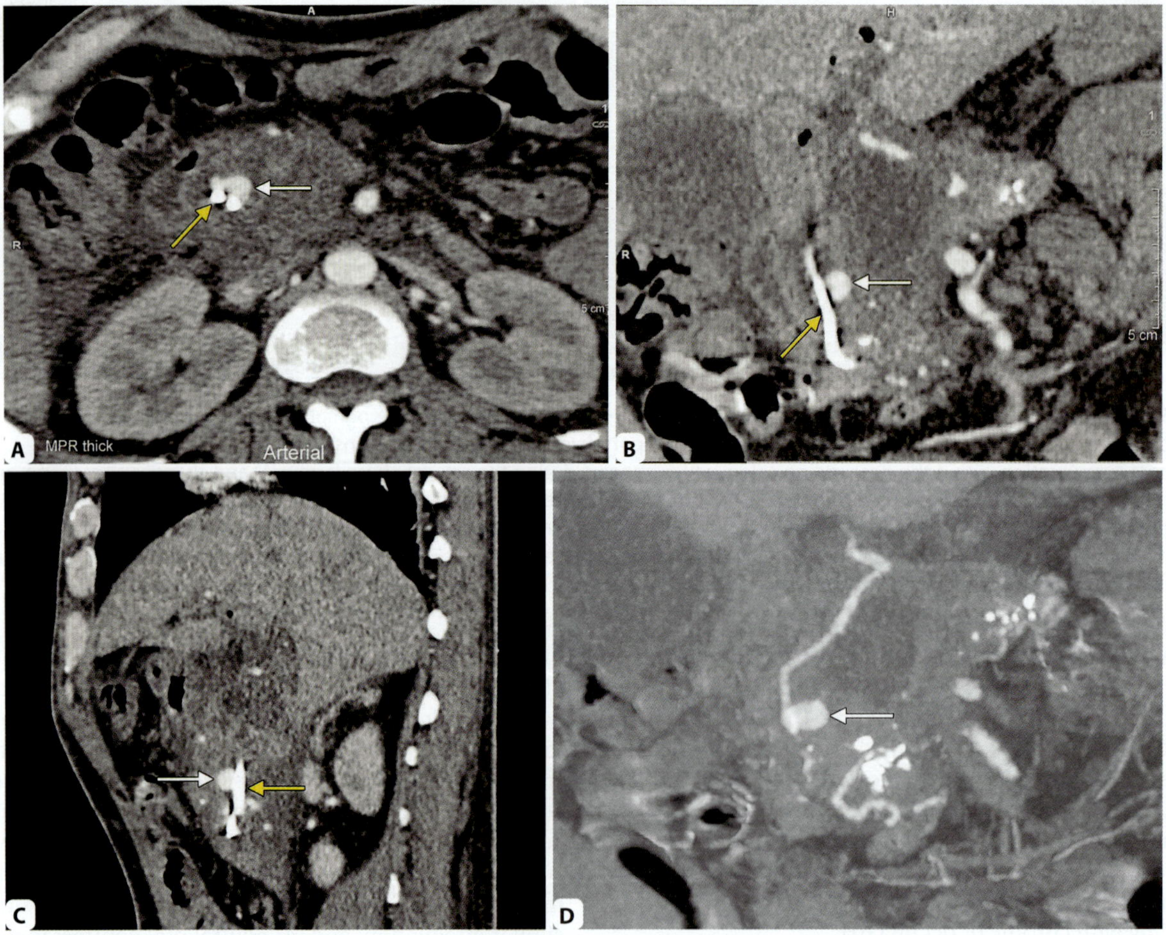

FIGS. 2A TO D: Pseudoaneurysm arising from the GDA in a patient of chronic calcific pancreatitis who developed lower CBD obstruction and underwent PTBD procedure post failure of ERCP. The patient complained of melena and bleeding from the PTBD drain after 2 days. Axial (A), Coronal (B), Sagittal (C) Multiplanar images show a blob of contrast attenuation (white arrows, A to C) adjacent to the ring biliary catheter (yellow arrow, A to C) suggestive of a pseudoaneurysm. Curved maximum intensity projection image (D) shows the pseudoaneurysm along the GDA course (arrow, D).

(CBD: common bile duct; ERCP: endoscopic retrograde cholangiopancreatography; GDA: gastroduodenal artery; PTBD: percutaneous transhepatic biliary drainage)

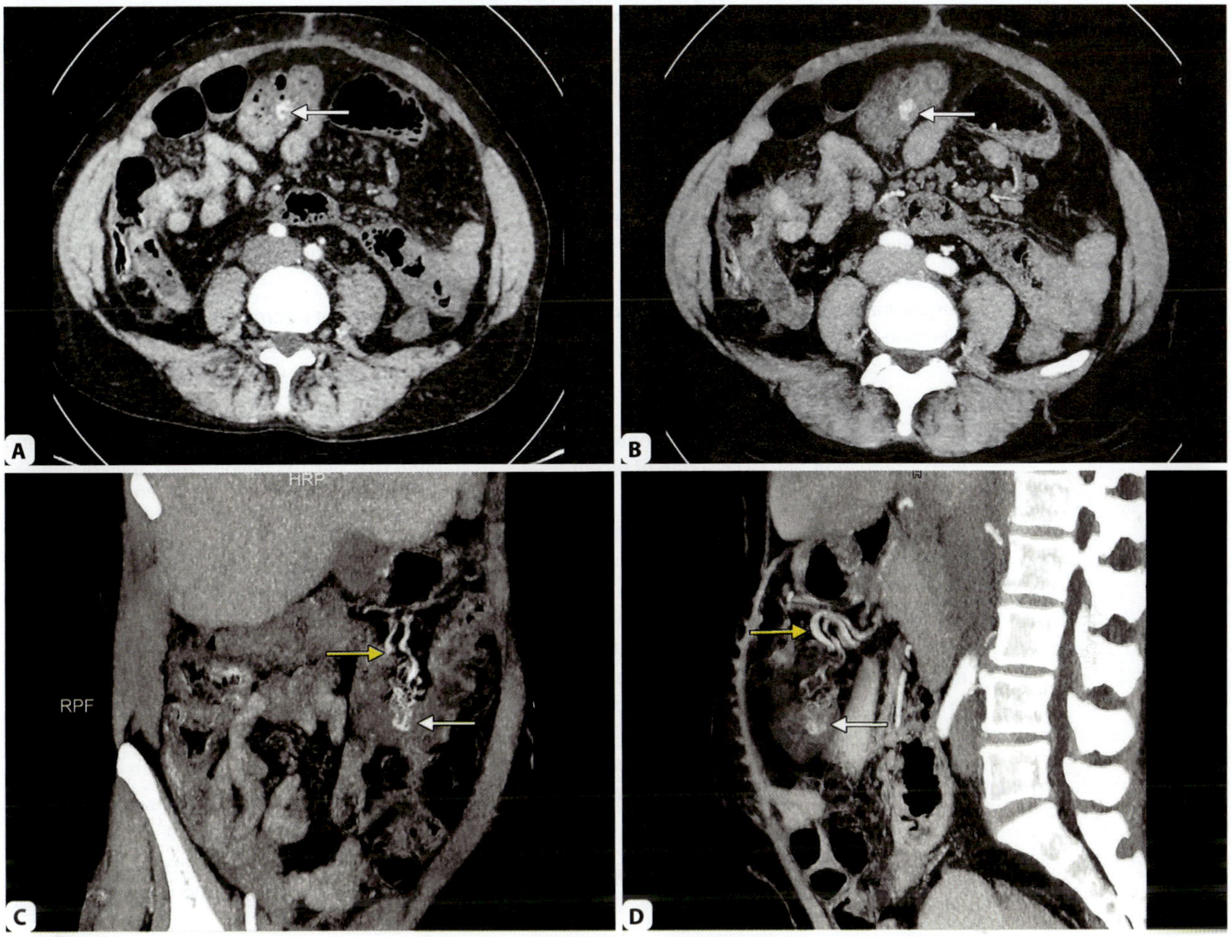

FIGS. 3A TO D: Angioectasia in an elderly lady who presented with recurrent melena for a few months. Upper GI endoscopy was normal and an initial colonoscopy revealed ulcers in the ascending colon which failed to respond to medical therapy. She eventually underwent right hemicolectomy for nonresolution of symptoms and developed the same complaints after 3 months. (A) Axial CTA image and (B) MIP image in arterial phase demonstrate a focal area of mural enhancement at posterior wall of the collapsed transverse colon (arrows, A and B). (C) Coronal and (D) sagittal MIP images show multiple prominent and tortuous feeding vessels (yellow arrows, C and D) reaching up to the lesion (white arrows, C and D).

(CTA: computed tomography angiography; GI: gastrointestinal; MIP: maximum intensity projection)

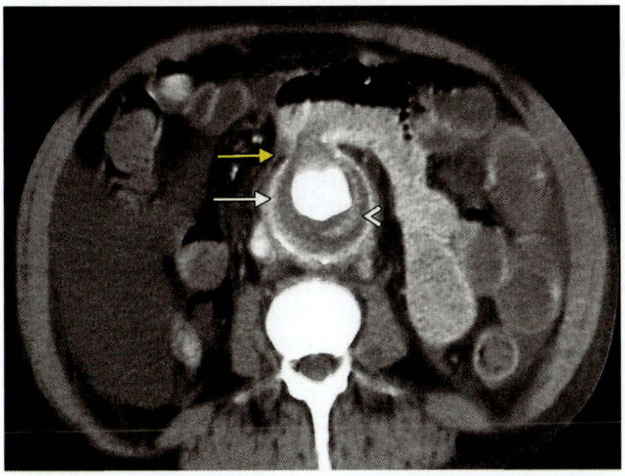

FIG. 4: Aortic aneurysm with an aortoenteric fistula in a 68-year-old male with a history of melena—axial computed tomography angiography (CTA) image in arterial phase shows a dilated abdominal aorta (white arrow) with an eccentric thrombus and intramural hematoma (arrowhead). A defect within the anterior aortic wall with subsequent communication with duodenum is also appreciated (yellow arrow).

TABLE 3: Summary of indications and imaging features of gastrointestinal hemorrhage on CT and catheter angiography.

Points under consideration	CT angiography	Catheter angiography DSA
Role/indication as per ACG/SAR consensus guidelines[2]	• Should be performed as the first diagnostic study in hemodynamically unstable patients • First-line study in hemodynamically stable patients where the suspicion of active bleeding is high • Not indicated as a first-line test in hemodynamically stable patients in whom bleeding has subsided	• Active contrast extravasation on CTA • In LGIH, if CTA is negative for GI bleeding, CA is not indicated • For UGIH, prophylactic embolization of the suspected vessel should be considered in absence of findings of CTA • In case of recurrent intermittent GIH and all other modalities have failed to identify the source of bleeding, provocative CA can be performed to identify and treat the culprit lesion
Imaging features	• Presence of intraluminal bleed—contents with attenuation ≥60 HU is a sign of recent hemorrhage • Sentinel clot sign—presence of hyperdense clotted blood, is typically located closest to the bleeding site • Contrast extravasation **(Figs. 1A to D)**—accumulation of extravasated contrast material in bowel lumen; typically changes in size, attenuation, shape, and location on venous/delayed phases • *Pseudoaneurysm* **(Figs. 1A to D)**—a well-defined lobular focus or an outpouching along an arterial branch; follows the attenuation of the arterial blood pool during later phases but remains unchanged in size and shape • Specific cause—e.g., bowel abnormalities	• Extravasation of contrast **(Fig. 5)**—contrast puddling or staining that persists beyond the capillary and venous phases • *Pseudoaneurysm* • Opacification of intestinal folds on delayed phases due to luminal extravasation of contrast medium **(Fig. 5)** • Pseudo vein appearance **(Fig. 5)**—due to extravasated contrast flowing to the most dependent part in the GIT filled with clotted blood, mimicking the appearance of a vein. However, unlike the venous phase, it persists for a much longer time • Other findings—arteriovenous fistula, abnormal blush, neovascularity, or hyperemia • Hemobilia and hemosuccus pancreaticus—opacification of common bile and pancreatic ducts, respectively

(ACG/SAR: American College of Gastroenterology/Society of Abdominal Radiology; CA: conventional angiography; CT: computed tomography; CTA: CT angiography; DSA: digital subtraction angiography; GI: gastrointestinal; GIH: GI hemorrhage; GIT: GI tract; LGIH: lower GIH; UGIH: upper GIH)

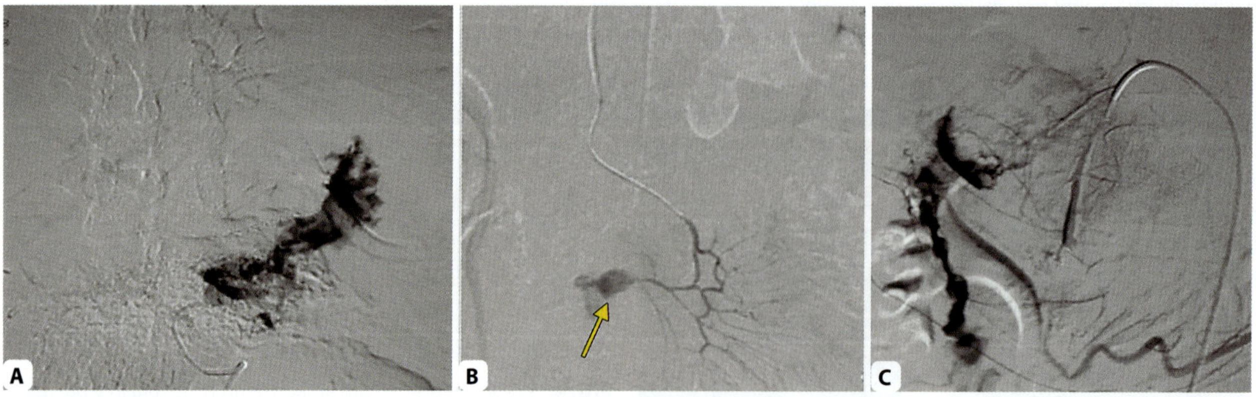

FIGS. 5A TO F: *Continued*

Continued

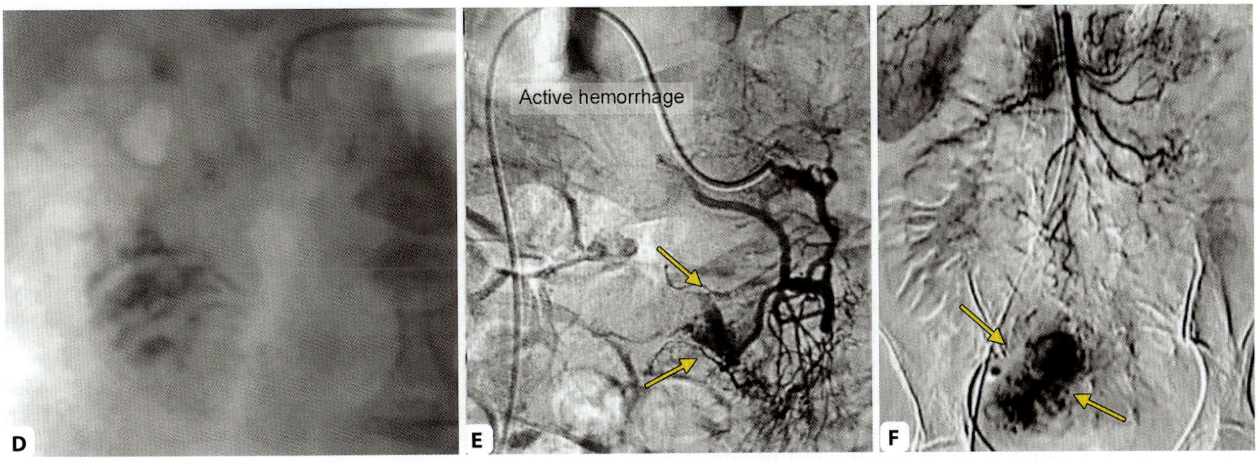

FIGS. 5A TO F: Signs of GIH on DSA: (A) Active contrast extravasation from left gastric artery as evident by irregular contrast puddling beyond the confines of arterial anatomy; (B) Pseudoaneurysm (arrow) from the jejunal branch of SMA; (C) Overt opacification of the second part of duodenum on obtaining SMA run; (D) Opacification of intestinal folds; (E) Pseudovein sign as evident by contrast pooling within the dependent bowel (arrows), simulating venous appearance; and (F) Tumor blush (arrows) on SMA angiogram in a patient with ileal GIST.

(DSA: digital subtraction angiography; GIH: gastrointestinal hemorrhage; GIST: gastrointestinal stromal tumor; SMA: superior mesenteric arteries)

Conventional Angiography

Conventional angiography (CA) with the intention to treat with embolization is most commonly performed for patients with active GIH, including unstable patients who are not appropriate candidates for or have failed endoscopic management.[17] Angiography is also utilized in postoperative and postinterventional GIH. In acute GIH, angiography has an approximate detection rate of 0.5 mL/min.[18]

The patient should undergo CTA ideally before performing angiography. There are several advantages of performing a CTA before which include the following:

- CT assists in planning the DSA by identifying the source artery, including information about variant anatomy
- Allows procedure to be completed faster (e.g., faster catheterization)
- Reduced number of DSA exposures, thereby reducing radiation exposure

Hence, a CTA is routinely advocated in GIH even when eventual DSA is planned already.

Conventional angiography additionally remains a valuable diagnostic tool in patients with recurrent or continued obscure GIH in whom other investigations have failed to detect a source. Provocative angiography with heparin or tissue plasminogen activator (tPA) and carbon dioxide (CO_2) angiography can be performed to evaluate and treat patients with obscure and recurrent GI bleeding if all other methods have failed to diagnose the source of bleeding.[2]

Technical Details

Preprocedural considerations include optimizing the patient's renal and coagulation status. The procedure typically begins through a common femoral artery access. A flush aortogram is practically obsolete due to the advent of CTA. Selective angiograms of celiac and superior mesenteric arteries (SMA) are performed in UGIH to image the site of bleeding suspected based on prior imaging studies. Similarly, in LGIH, the SMA and inferior mesenteric arteries (IMA) should be interrogated to evaluate all potential bleeding sources and collateral vessels. Rosch celiac 1 (RC1) catheter, cobra, and SIM1 catheters are routinely utilized for this purpose.[19] Selective cannulation of the arteries is followed by superselective studies of the major branches using various visceral angiographic catheters. A coaxial microcatheter system (2.5–2.8 F) through diagnostic catheter should be used to reach the site of bleeding.

For diagnostic angiograms, flow rates for contrast injection should be kept high (approximately, 20 mL volume, 5–6 mL/s for celiac and SMA, and 2–3 mL/s for IMA) with a rapid frame rate in arterial phase (~3 frames/s) which can be reduced (1 frame/2–5 seconds) for the capillary and venous phases. The imaging time should be long enough (~30–40 seconds, until opacification of the portal system) to identify slow extravasation, suspected venous occlusion, and vascular malformations. If CTA is not available, sequential angiograms of all major branches of celiac (gastroduodenal, hepatic, and left gastric), superior (middle colic, right colic, ileocolic, major jejunal/ileal branches), and inferior mesenteric arteries (left colic and superior rectal) are obtained. This is essential to increase the detection rate (~0.5 mL/min with selective angiography).

Bowel gas and peristalsis may interfere with the acquisition of mesenteric artery angiograms and can be reduced with antispasmodic drugs such as buscopan and glucagon.[20] The sensitivity of DSA approaches 63–90% and

40–86% for UGIH and LGIH, respectively, and specificity is 100%.[20,21] Various positive angiographic findings, which are seen in about 24–78% patients of GIH, are described in **Table 3** and **Figure 5**.

Provocative Angiography

Provocative angiography may be done in patients of GIH when no cause is found on routine imaging.[22,23] The procedure involves injection of heparin, tPA, and vasodilator (tolazoline) into the artery through the catheter, which is followed by DSA to demonstrate any bleeding source.[23] The instillation increases blood flow into the vessel, relieves vasospasm, and lyses any small clot, thereby improving detection rates. Provocative angiography has identified a cause in up to 33% patients of GIH with normal routine DSA.[22] However, one has to be careful and be prepared to handle acute crises while performing this technique; sometimes, it may lead to life-threatening hemorrhage due to relief of vessel spasm.

Carbon Dioxide Angiography

Carbon dioxide angiography is useful in patients of renal failure and those who are allergic to iodinated contrast agents. CO_2 is an inert, highly soluble gas which is excreted by lungs. It is utilized as a negative contrast agent, displacing the blood volume in lumen of the vessel, with resultant decreased attenuation of X-ray beam. The injections are performed by hand with careful handling to prevent contamination by room air. The low viscosity of CO_2 allows demonstration of subtle bleeding and therefore has been suggested in the evaluation of obscure GIH.[24]

Radionuclide Studies

Radionuclide studies play a vital role in the evaluation of obscure GIH when endoscopy and CTA fail to detect a source.[2,25] These procedures are utilized in cases where bleeding is slow or intermittent as scanning can be done for longer periods. Additionally, they can detect minimal bleeding with detection at rates as low as 0.04 mL/min. However, they suffer from the drawback of limited spatial resolution. In addition, there can be movement of radionuclide between imaging sessions which impairs the precise localization of the actual bleeding site.

^{99m}Tc sulfur colloid: This tracer is cleared from the blood pool by the reticuloendothelial system and has an approximate half-life of 2.5–3 minutes. If active bleeding occurs during this short time, the tracer extravasates into the bowel which is identified on subsequent imaging. Another drawback is that bleeding into the hepatic or splenic flexures of the colon and UGIH will be obscured due to overlap by normal accumulation of the tracer in liver and spleen. It is therefore no longer advocated routinely due to these disadvantages.[25]

^{99m}Tc-labeled RBC: This consists of labeled RBCs which can extravasate during bleeding with consequent detection. They are the preferred radiopharmaceutical for GIH owing to a long intravascular half-life that allows continuous imaging of the GIT and has therefore replaced ^{99m}Tc-sulfur colloid for evaluation of GIH.[2] As imaging is typically performed for at least 1 hour, intermittent bleeding can also be detected. It is also possible to reimage for up to 24 hours.[26] Another advantage of ^{99m}Tc-RBC scanning is its high sensitivity because it can detect GI bleeding at a rate of as low as 0.04 mL/min in experimental animal models and 0.1 mL/min in clinical studies.[26] The sensitivity and specificity approaches 93% and 95%, respectively, for bleeding rates > 0.04 mL/min. The radiation dose to the patient is lower with ^{99m}Tc RBC scanning compared with CTA.[25,27] However, it can only be performed on hemodynamically stable patients. Additionally, activity seen in the lower GIT may have originated from proximal bowel segments and exact source of bleeding may be missed if frequent views are not obtained.

^{99m}Tc pertechnetate: It is used in cases where bleeding from Meckel's diverticulum is suspected. This tracer accumulates in ectopic gastric mucosa present in the diverticulum and helps in identifying the source of GIH.

Ultrasonography and Magnetic Resonance Imaging

Ultrasonography (USG) has a limited role in the evaluation of patients with GIH. It has a therapeutic role in specific situations such as large superficial aneurysm/pseudoaneurysm, where Doppler USG helps in detection and allows percutaneous intervention.

Similarly, magnetic resonance angiography (MRA) has currently no role in the evaluation of acute GIH. Longer scan times, lower spatial resolution, and need for breath hold limits its use in acute situations. MR enterography (MRE) may find use in patients with chronic or recurrent GIH for evaluation of small bowel abnormalities such as inflammatory bowel disease, tumors, mesenteric ischemia, and vasculitis.

INTERVENTIONAL RADIOLOGY IN GASTROINTESTINAL HEMORRHAGE

Once the bleeding site has been localized on endoscopy or on imaging, attempts are made to control or stop the bleeding. There are three options available for management, which is based on multidisciplinary discussion—endoscopic, radiological, and surgical methods. In general, endoscopy and medical treatments are utilized for initial management whenever feasible **(Table 4)**.

Image-guided interventions, specifically transarterial embolization (TAE) are employed in failure of endoscopic treatment, when the bleeding source is not amenable to endoscopic treatment and in situations where the patient is unstable. In addition to providing definite treatment for bleeding in GIH, TAE assumes an adjunctive role in certain

TABLE 4: Management of gastrointestinal hemorrhage (GIH).

Comment under consideration	Endoscopic	Radiological	Surgical
Indication	Usually first-line management, especially in UGIH	• Failure/unable to perform endoscopic treatment • Massive GIH/GIH in unstable patient • Bridge therapy for acute control in surgical candidates	Tumors, vascular malformations, angioectasias
Agents	• Clips and bands • Thermal ablative procedures such as electrocoagulation and laser ablations • Mucosal sclerosant injection • EUS-guided thrombin/glue injection	Endovascular approach—TAE • *Permanent agents:* - Coils—ideal agents; least risk of complications - PVA—for angioectasias, malformations, and tumors; high risk of bowel infarction - Glue—in patients with coagulopathy or unable to reach target; high risk of bowel infarction • *Temporary agents:* - Gelfoam—preoperative or empirical embolization; risk of bowel infarction - Percutaneous approach—rarely used; thrombin or glue	–

(EUS: endoscopic ultrasound; PVA: polyvinyl alcohol; UGIH: upper GIH; TAE: transarterial embolization)

scenarios. Lesions such as bowel tumors and angioectasias, which ultimately require surgical resection, can be managed with TAE during acute situations, thereby acting as a bridge for future surgery **(Table 4)**.[20]

Radiological approaches used in the treatment of GIH include endovascular and percutaneous techniques.[20,28] TAE as an endovascular approach is used in most cases of GIH due to feasibility, better control, and few rates of complications.[29]

TRANSARTERIAL EMBOLIZATION

Principles of TAE in GIH includes superselective catheterization of the target artery using microcatheter coaxial system followed by instillation of embolic agents into the lesion or feeding artery so as to reduce the arterial perfusion pressure, which facilitates clot formation and ultimately controls the hemorrhage.[28,30] On the other hand, the procedure should also ensure that adequate collateral blood flow to the bowel is maintained so that the risk of bowel infarction is minimized. The latter parameter assumes great importance in LGIH due to lack of a dual blood supply in the bowel distal to ligament of Treitz.[28] The various technical differences to be considered during TAE in UGIH and LGIH are enumerated in **Table 5**.

Managing Upper Gastrointestinal Hemorrhage versus Lower Gastrointestinal Hemorrhage

Few points merit consideration before proceeding with TAE in GIH. Bowel proximal to ligament of Treitz has a dual vascular supply with formation of arcades for perfusion. Consequently, embolization in UGIH involves blocking of both proximal and distal vasculature in relation to the area of interest, also referred to as the "front" and "back" door, respectively **(Figs. 6A to F)**. The procedure is also known as the "sandwich technique" and is performed in a distal-to-proximal fashion, which reduces the risk of "back door" failure **(Figs. 7A to D)**.[2] Embolization in this region carries low chances of ischemia at the expense of higher chances of clinical failure **(Table 5)**.

In contrast, the lower GIT has a terminal vascular supply with few collaterals and hence carries a greater risk of bowel ischemia. This anatomical fact gives the benefit of lesser chances of persistent bleeding. The embolization is done from a single side only and it is absolutely essential to be as selective as possible **(Table 5)**.[28]

Success Rates and Outcomes

When considering nonvariceal UGIH, the clinical success of TAE rates varies widely, ranging between 44% and 100%.[31] Previously conducted studies have reported a 33% rebleeding rate on the first attempt.[32,33] The success rate of embolization for LGIH is above 95%.[34,35]

The reported complication rates are up to 10% and include access site problems, nontarget embolization, bowel ischemia, and infarction. These are highly variable due to the differences in technique, embolization material, and reported complications.[31,36] Bowel ischemia may occur in rare cases and is more commonly seen with glue embolization; this occurs in about 10% of patients and is usually treated conservatively.[37,38] It is due to this reason that only those patients of LGIH who demonstrate active extravasation at the time of the angiography should be treated with targeted embolization.[2]

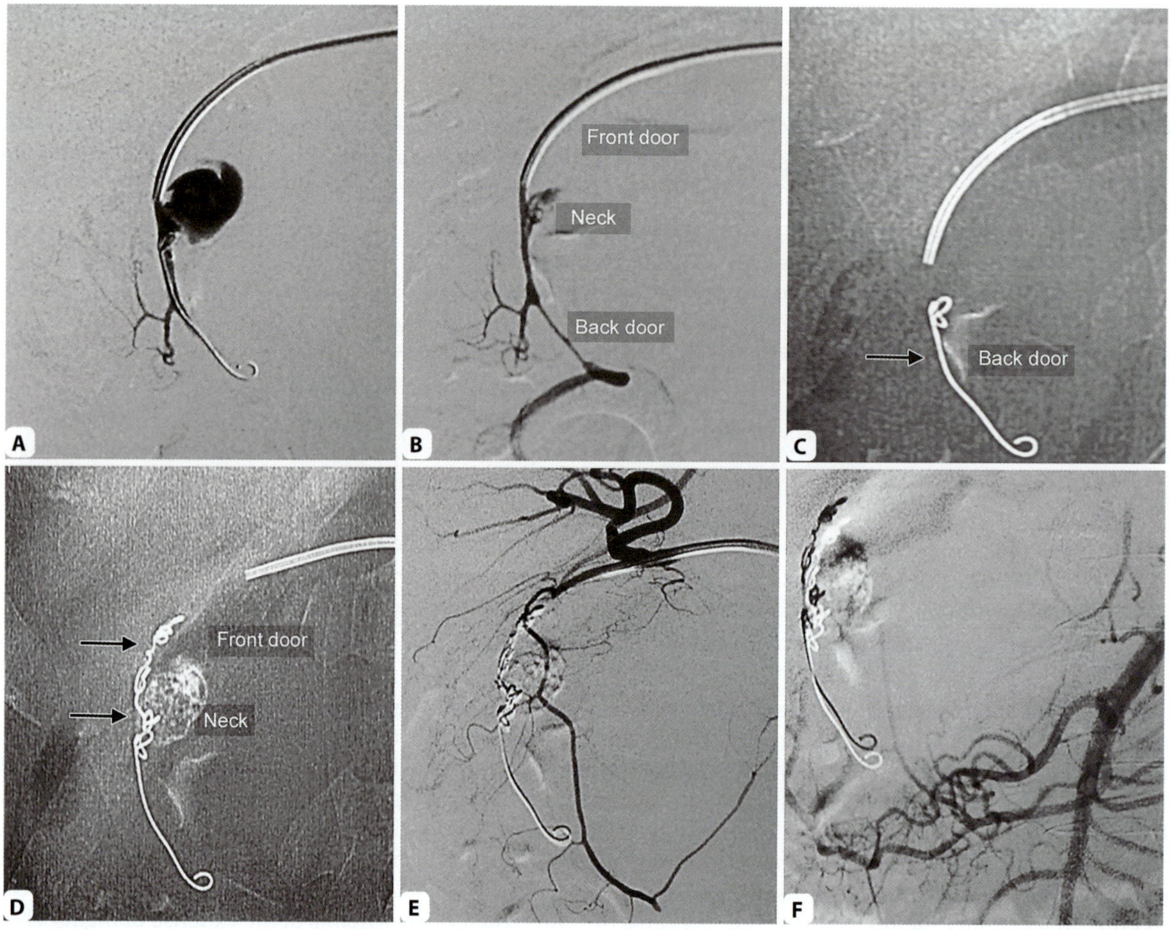

FIGS. 6A TO F: Angiographic embolization technique in UGIH. Spot GDA angiogram images [(A) nonannotated and (B) annotated] shows a large pseudoaneurysm which underwent microcoil embolization. The procedure begins with blocking the distal vasculature in relation to the area of interest or the "back" door with coil (arrow, B and C). This is followed by deployment of another coil for the neck and front door (B and D). Postdeployment angiograms from celiac (E) and SMA (F) ends reveal no residual fill-in of the aneurysm.
(GDA: gastroduodenal artery; SMA: superior mesenteric arteries; UGIH: upper gastrointestinal hemorrhage)

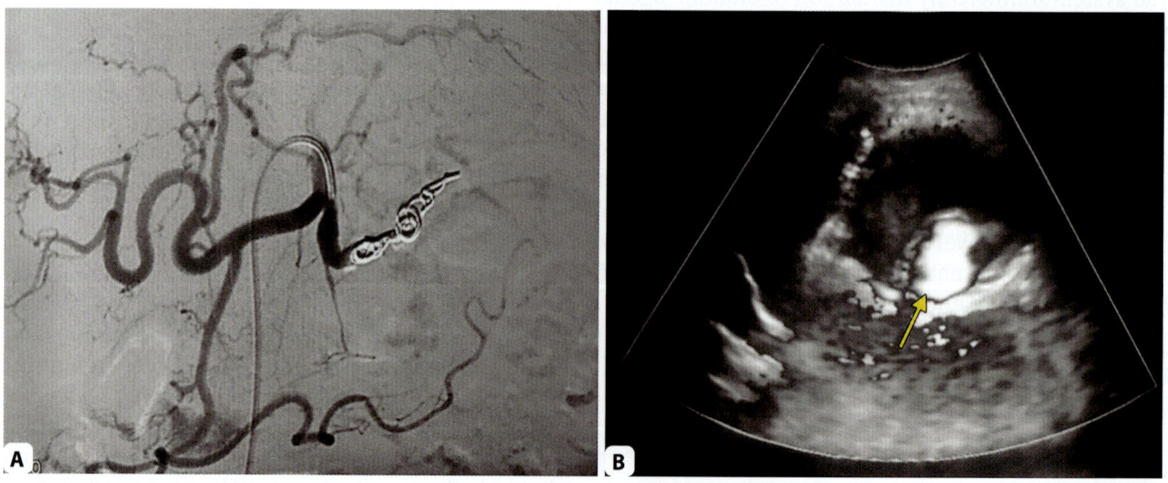

FIGS. 7A TO D: *Continued*

Continued

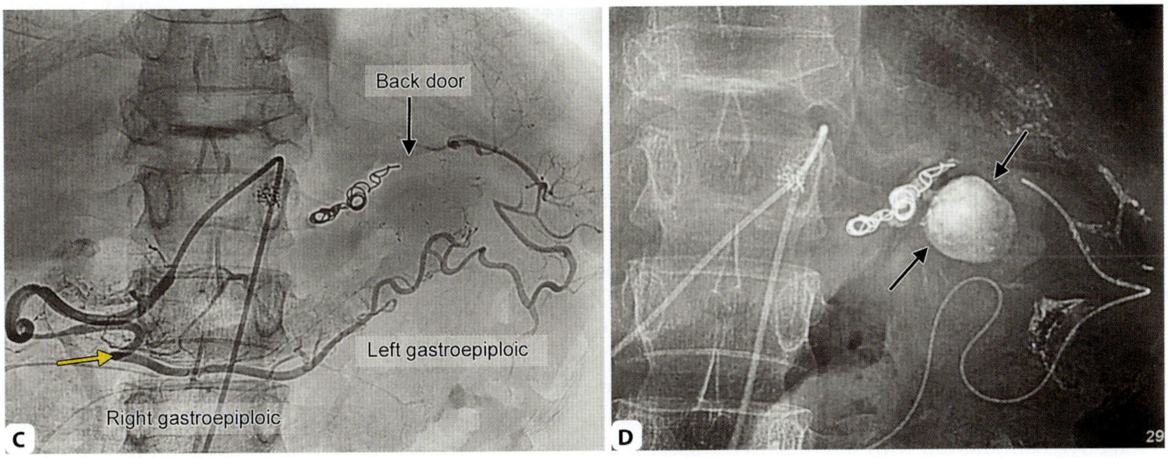

FIGS. 7A TO D: Technical failure of angioembolization due to inadequate blockade of the "back door"—Celiac angiogram image (A) in a 56-year-old male with splenic artery pseudoaneurysm shows coils within the proximal splenic artery without any appreciable pseudoaneurysm. Doppler ultrasonography (USG) image (B) however, shows significant residual flow within the pseudoaneurysm (arrow, B). The residual flow was consequent to extensive collateral network in between gastroepiploic arteries (i.e., GDA and splenic arteries) which resulted in aneurysmal opacification from the distal splenic artery (black arrow, C). The distal arcade was then traversed via a microcatheter followed by glue embolization and subsequent cast formation (arrows, D).

TABLE 5: Technical principles considered during transarterial embolization in UGIH and LGIH.

Upper GI tract	Lower GI tract
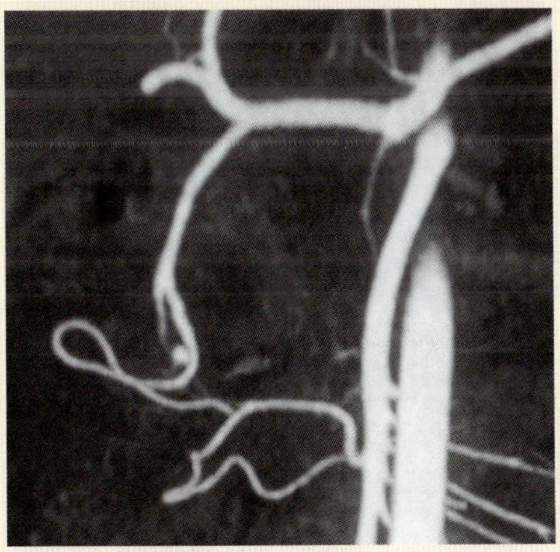	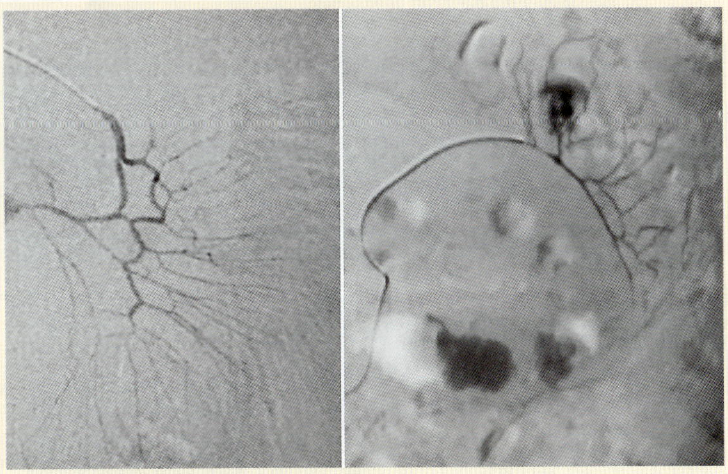
"Multiple arcades" with dual vascularization"	"Terminal branches" and "few collaterals"
Less chance of ischemia	More chance of ischemia
More chance of persistent bleeding from other branches	Less chance of persistent bleeding from other branches
Embolize from "two" sides of arcade	Embolize from "one" side only
As selective as you can but not always crucial	Be *very* selective or do not embolize at all
Note: Do not embolize >4 or more vasa recta in SMA and >5 or more in IMA, if using liquid agents such as glue.	
(GI: gastrointestinal; IMA: inferior mesenteric arteries; LGIH: lower GI hemorrhage; SMA: superior mesenteric arteries; UGIH: upper GI hemorrhage)	

HARDWARE USED IN TRANSARTERIAL EMBOLIZATION

Catheters: Diagnostic Catheters and Microcatheter Coaxial Systems

As described earlier, RC1, cobra, and SIM1 catheters are routinely utilized catheters for cannulating the major arteries and obtaining angiograms.[19] They admit 0.032/0.035 inch guidewires. RC1 catheter is a C-shaped, double-curve catheter having both primary and secondary curves in the same direction **(Figs. 8A to C)**. Sidewinder or SIM1 catheter on the other hand is a reverse-curve catheter utilized in difficult vascular anatomy like acute angulation of the celiac axis or a long celiac axis and provides more stability during superselective cannulation with microcatheter assembly **(Figs. 8A to C)**.

Microcatheters are used for superselective cannulation of the distal branch using a coaxial system with a diagnostic catheter. They are available in various sizes (2.5–2.8 F). Various microcatheter systems are available in market—Progreat (Terumo interventional systems, Tokyo, Japan), Microferret (Cook Medical, Bloomington, USA), FasTracker (Boston Scientific, Massachusetts, USA), and Renegade (Boston Scientific, Massachusetts, USA), one should be familiar with at least one of the microcatheter systems **(Figs. 8A to C)**. Attempts should be made to reach as close as possible to the bleeding site by advancing the microguidewire (0.014–0.018 inches) and microcatheter carefully and steadily while avoiding vessel spasm, dissection, and perforation.

Embolic Materials

Various embolic materials which are used in the management of GIH include permanent occluding agents such as coils or microcoils, particulate agents [polyvinyl alcohol (PVA)], n-butyl cyanoacrylate (nBCA or glue), and vascular plugs **(Table 4 and Figs. 9A to F)**.[28,29] Temporary

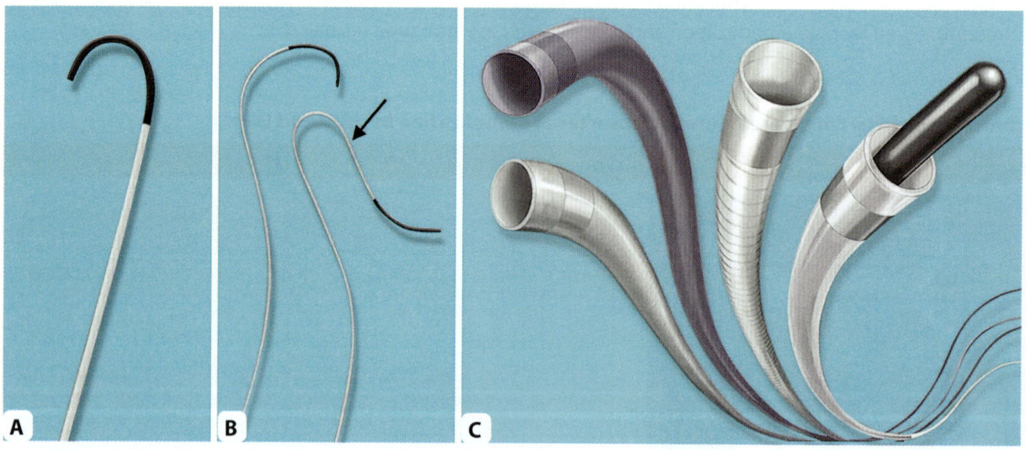

FIGS. 8A TO C: Common catheters utilized in GIH: (A) Rosch celiac 1 (RC1) catheter; (B) Sidewinder/SIM1 (arrow) and cobra catheter; and (C) Microcatheter portfolio.

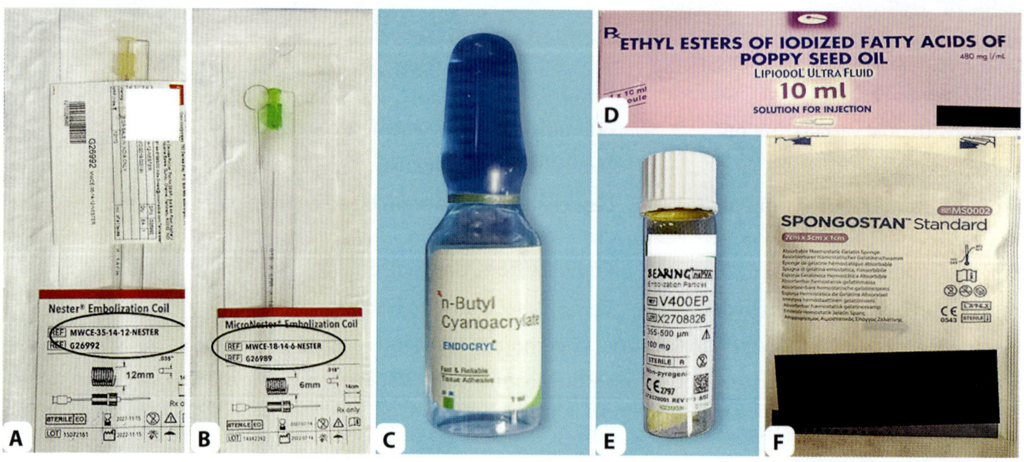

FIGS. 9A TO F: Embolization agents utilized in GIH: (A) Coil and (B) microcoils. Every coil is identified with a 3-digit number (ovals, A and B), with the first digit representing the admitting catheter (i.e., 0.035 or 0.018 inches), the second digit representing the total length of uncoiled form in cm, and the third digit representing the diameter in coiled form. (C) n-Butyl-cyanoacrylate or glue; (D) lipiodol; (E) Polyvinyl alcohol (PVA) particles; and (F) Gelfoam sponge.

embolizing agents include gelatin sponge and autologous blood clot. Wherever a lesion is identified, a permanent embolic agent should be used to avoid recurrence. Temporary agents are used for peroperative and empirical (when bleeding source is not identified) embolization **(Table 4 and Figs. 9A to F)**.

Permanent Agents

Coils

Coils or microcoils are the agents of choice, owing to the high efficacy and least risk of complications. These consist of a metallic component which causes physical occlusion. This is fibered with materials such as nylon, Dacron, or polyester so as to stimulate the thrombogenic process **(Figs. 9A to F)**. Hence, coils rely on the patient's coagulation mechanism for action.[29] A good control of deployment as compared to liquid agents minimizes the risk of nontarget embolization. In addition, detachable-type coils which can be removed after initial deployment if unsatisfactory are also now widely available. As stressed earlier, care should be taken to close both "front and back doors'" when dealing with UGIH **(Figs. 10 and 11)**.

Sizing of coils: It is recommended that the size of the coil/microcoil to be deployed is about 15–20% more than vessel diameter on predeployment angiogram. This roughly translates to one size greater than the vessel diameter.

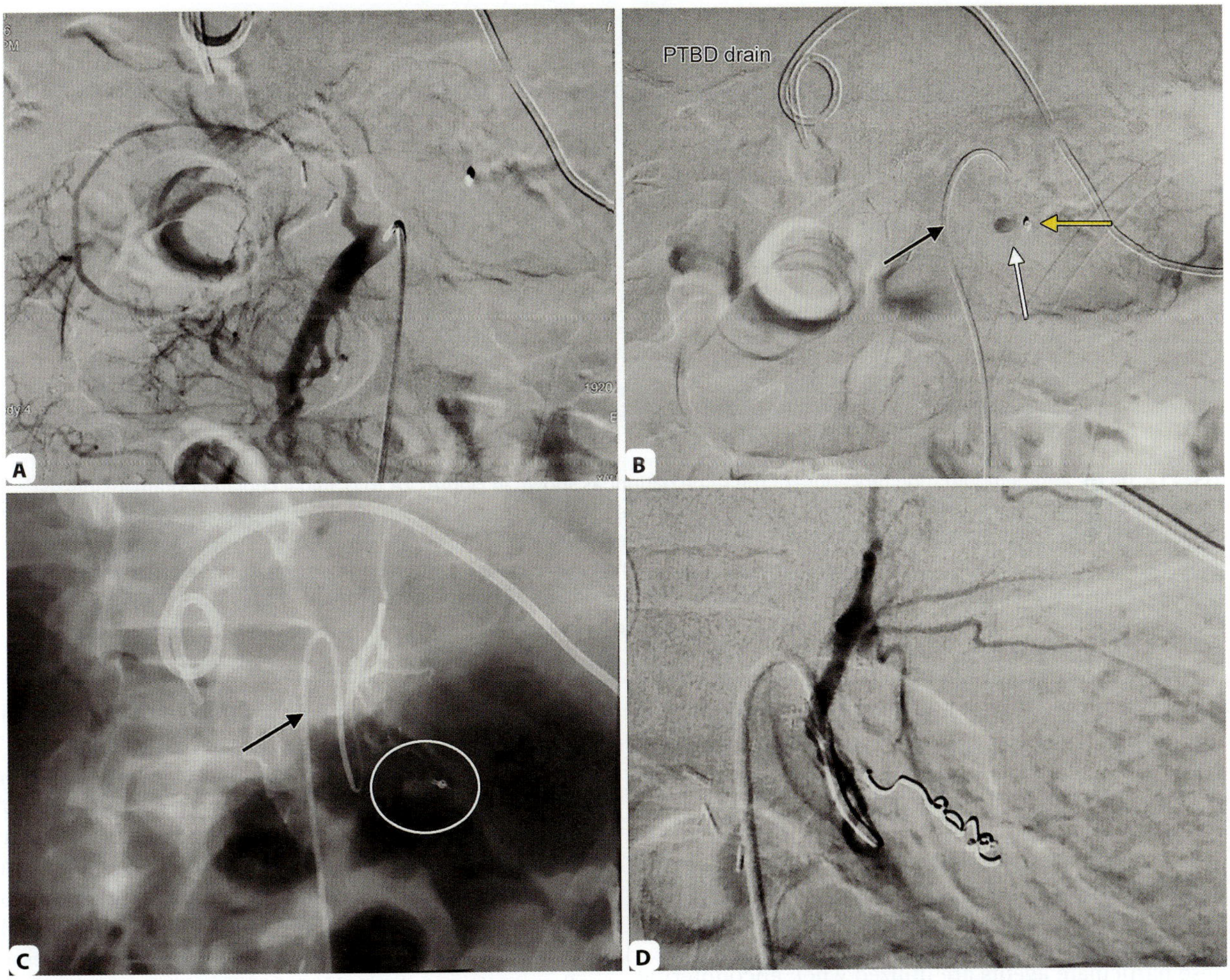

FIGS. 10A TO D: Transarterial embolization in a 65-year-old male who underwent Whipple's operation for periampullary carcinoma and later underwent PTBD in view of bile leak. He developed hematemesis and tachycardia 2 weeks after biliary diversion. The bleed failed to cease on endoscopy with further deterioration of the vitals; hence, an IR opinion was obtained and the patient was taken for DSA directly. An initial SMA angiogram (A) was normal; however, celiac artery angiogram (B) through RC1 catheter (black arrow) revealed a small pseudoaneurysm in the course of gastroduodenal artery (white arrow, B) close to the clip placed by the gastroenterologist (yellow arrow). The culprit branch (oval) was eventually catheterized using a coaxial system with SIM1 catheter (exchanged instead of RC1 catheter in order to provide more stability) and microcatheter system (C, black arrow) followed by deployment of a microcoil. Postdeployment angiogram (D) revealed absence of filling of the pseudoaneurysm.

(DSA: digital subtraction angiography; IR: interventional radiology; PTBD: percutaneous transhepatic biliary drainage; RC1: Rosch celiac 1; SMA: superior mesenteric arteries)

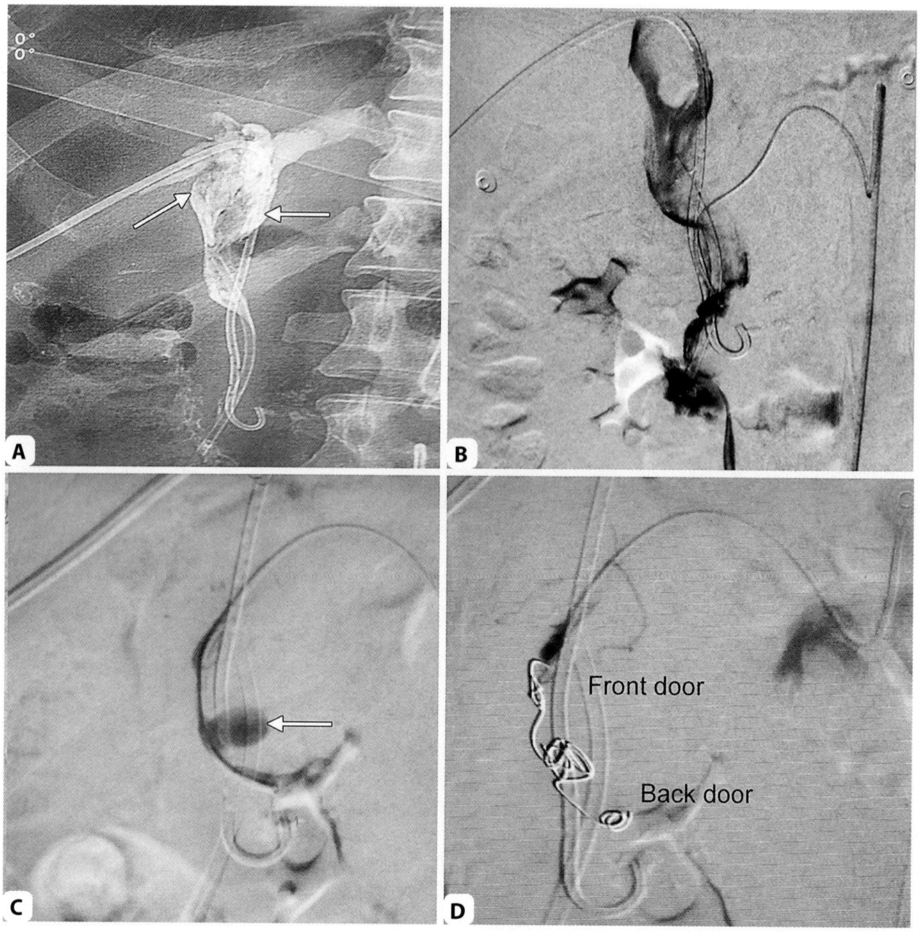

FIGS. 11A TO D: Angioembolization procedure of the same patient as shown in Figures 2A to D. Initial cholangiogram image (A) through the ring biliary catheter shows the presence of multiple filling defects within the opacified CBD (arrows, A), signifying clots and hemobilia. Diagnostic angiogram images (B and C) confirm the pseudoaneurysm in the GDA course (arrows), as observed on CTA (Figs. 2A to D). This was coiled using the "sandwich technique," taking care to include both back and front doors as observed on the postdeployment image (D), resulting in complete blockade and no residual fill-in of the aneurysm.

(CBD: common bile duct; CTA: computed tomography angiography; GDA: gastroduodenal artery)

Deployment of coils: Certain differences exist with regards to the ideal site of coil deployment. When considering SMA territory, they should be deployed as close to the bleeding site **(Figs. 12A to F)** within the vasa recta, while in IMA, deployment at the marginal artery suffices **(Fig. 13A to C)**.

Rebleeding rates with coils vary from 10–30% within the 1st month of intervention.[31]

PVA Particles

These particulate agents are utilized when encountering bleed due to multiple feeders, e.g., in GI tumors **(Figs. 14A to C)**, malformations, and angioectasias **(Figs. 15A to D)**. They can also be used as an alternative to Gelfoam, when the bleeding source is difficult to reach. However, they carry a high risk of bowel infarction.[28]

Glue

NBCA, also known as glue, is another liquid embolic agent, which rapidly polymerizes in contact with ionic surface (blood). It is used along with lipiodol as dilution agent and also to make glue radiopaque while injecting **(Figs. 7 and 9)**. It can be used in situations such as when unable to reach the source and in patients with coagulopathy. A high risk of bowel infarction, however, limits its usage as a standalone agent.[37,38] The use of glue needs technical expertise and should be used with caution in the setting of GIH, otherwise it may lead to serious complications such as bowel infarction and sticking of the catheter to the vessel wall under inexperienced hands.

Temporary Agents

Gelfoam

Gelatin sponge or Gelfoam is a temporary embolizing agent utilized in empirical embolization, situations with difficulty to reach the bleeding, or in combination with coils. It is mixed with iodinated contrast medium to form slurry which helps in visualization during delivery **(Figs. 9A to F)**.

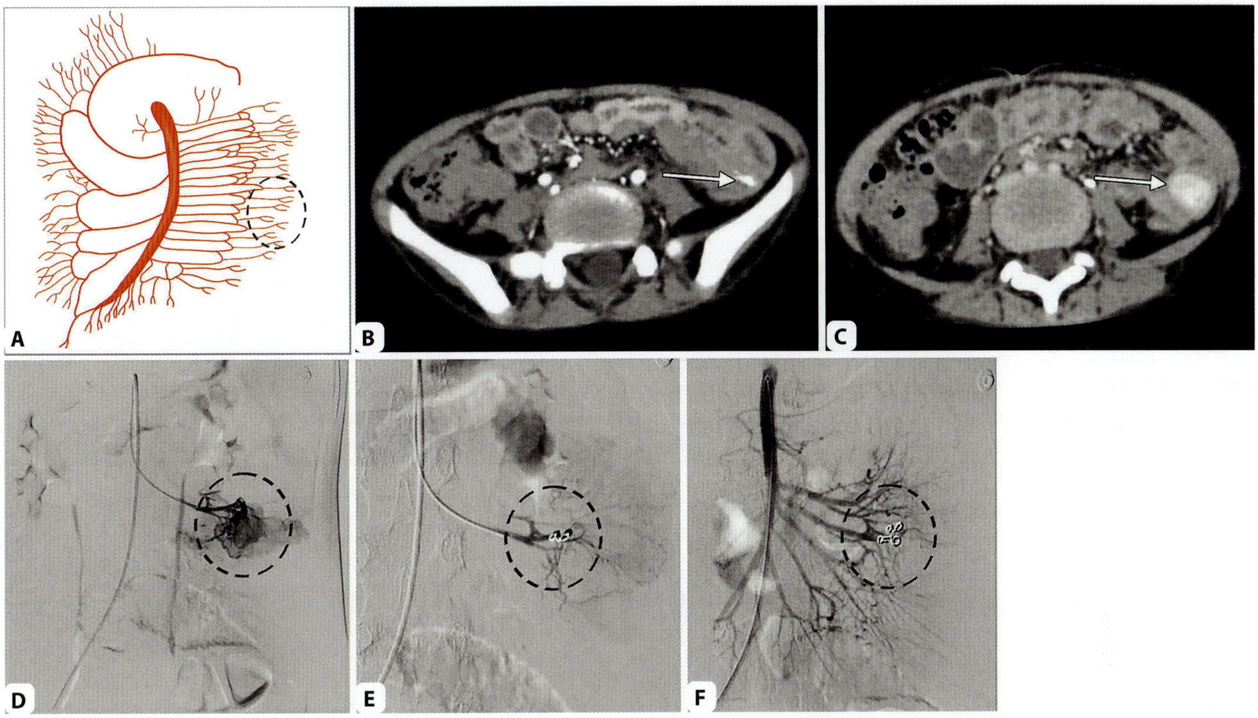

FIGS. 12A TO F: Coil deployment in SMA territory: (A) Schematic representation of the location of deployment at vasa recta (black oval, A). CTA images in (B) arterial and (C) venous phases in a patient with melena show active contrast extravasation within the jejunum (arrows). (D) Spot DSA image shows extravasation from one of the jejunal branches in the arcade (oval, D). Two coils were selectively deployed at the vasa recta as shown on the postembolization images (oval, E and F).

(CTA: computed tomography angiography; DSA: digital subtraction angiography; SMA: superior mesenteric arteries)

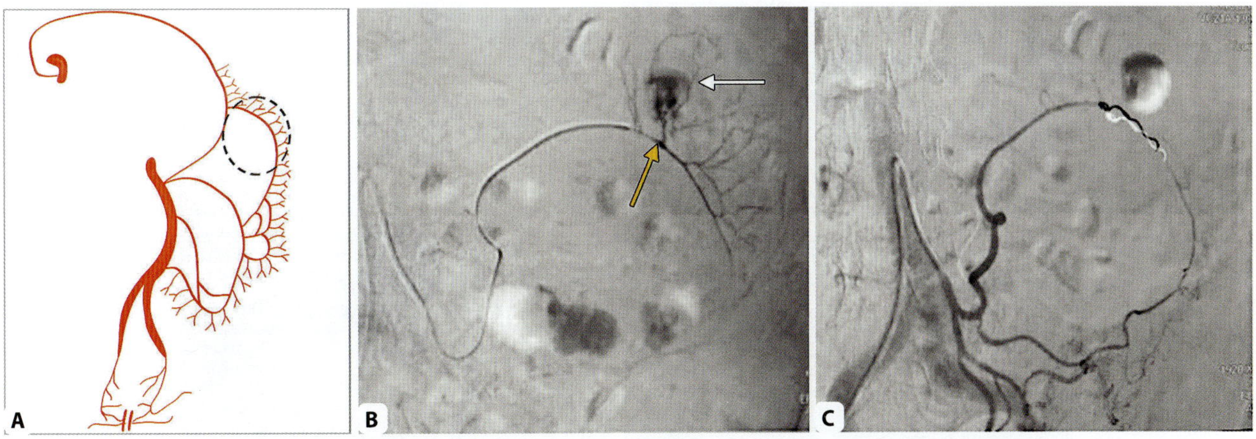

FIGS. 13A TO C: Coil deployment in IMA territory: (A) Schematic representation of the location of deployment at marginal artery (black oval, A). Spot DSA image (B) shows extravasation (white arrow, B) at one of the vasa recta emerging from the marginal artery (yellow arrow, B). The coil was deployed within the marginal artery with the absence of any residual fill-in of the pseudoaneurysm, as seen on postdeployment image (C).

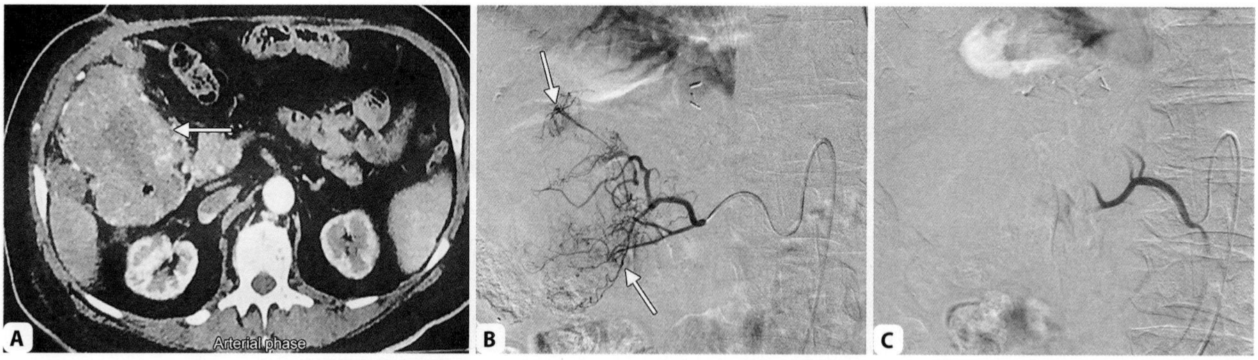

FIGS. 14A TO C: PVA embolization in a patient with colonic malignancy and melena. Axial CECT image demonstrates a large irregular mass within the hepatic flexure with extramural extension (arrow, A). Diagnostic angiogram image of the right branch of SMA (B) shows significant tumor blush which was embolized using PVA particles. Postembolization image (C) showed near complete obliteration of the tumor blush.

(CECT: contrast-enhanced computed tomography; PVA: polyvinyl alcohol; SMA: superior mesenteric arteries)

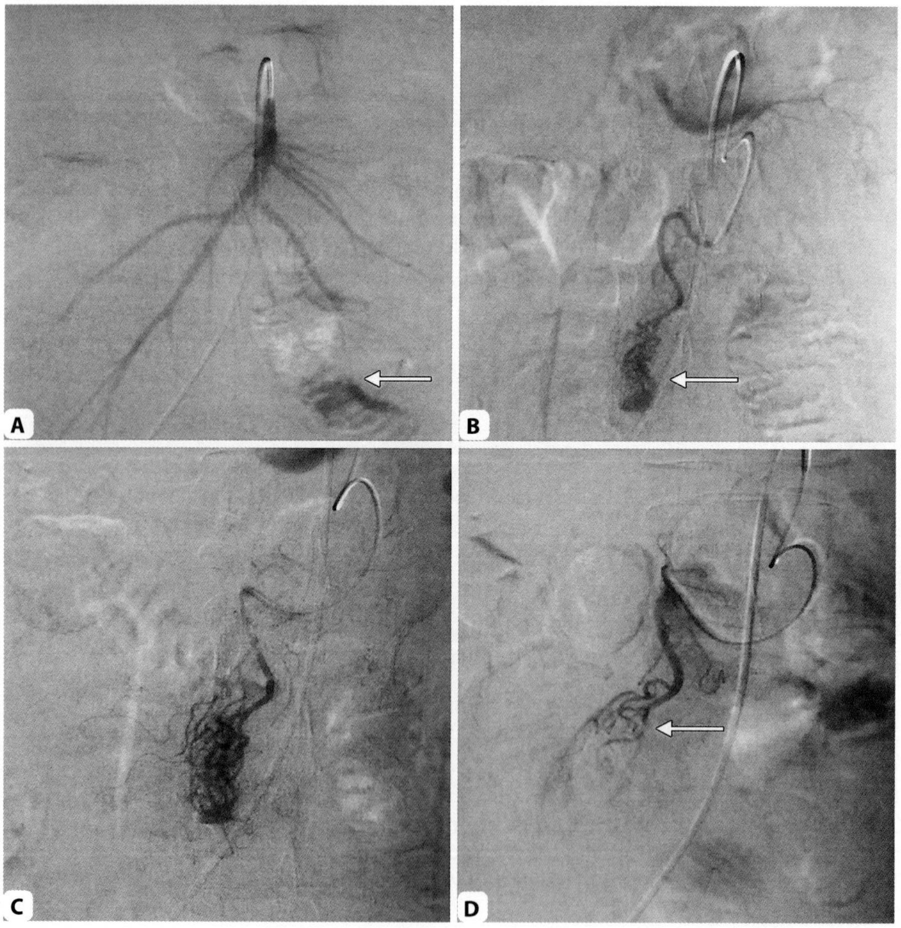

FIGS. 15A TO D: TAE of the patient with angioectasia shown in Figures 3A to D. A repeat surgery was deferred in view of multiple comorbidities and the patient was offered TAE. SMA angiogram (A) and selective angiogram of middle colic artery (B) images show a leash of vessels (arrow, A and B) clustered in the transverse colon. This was selectively catheterized with a microcatheter (C) followed by installation of 300–500 µg PVA particles. Postembolization angiogram shows marked reduction in the abnormal vascularity (arrow, D).

(PVA: polyvinyl alcohol; SMA: superior mesenteric artery; TAE: transarterial embolization)

Availability of future access to the embolized vessel and cost-effectiveness are advantages; however, these need to be weighed against unpredictability and high risk of bowel ischemia especially in lower GI bleeding (LGIB).[29]

Combination of Agents

Combining two agents in areas with rich collateral circulation can minimize rebleeding events, e.g., in UGIH around gastroduodenal artery (GDA) circulation. Popular combinations include coils and Gelfoam, coils and PVA particles, and coils with glue.[29]

PERCUTANEOUS APPROACH

This technique is rarely utilized in GIH when the endovascular approach fails, is not possible, or in cases where the lesion is superficial (e.g., intrahepatic pseudoaneurysm) and is performed by direct puncture of the pseudoaneurysm by a thin needle (22G) under USG guidance followed by injection of embolic agent.[29] Thrombin or glue are most commonly utilized for this purpose. The risks include rupture and nontarget embolization.

Specific Situations

Hemobilia

Hemobilia refers to hemorrhage within the biliary system and most cases result from iatrogenic injury after hepatobiliary interventions **(Figs. 16A to D)**. These include common radiological interventions such as percutaneous transhepatic biliary drainage (PTBD), liver biopsy, and transjugular intrahepatic portosystemic shunt (TIPS), endoscopic procedures such as endoscopic retrograde cholangiopancreatography (ERCP) and biliary stent placement; and hepatobiliary surgical procedures. Infection, inflammatory processes, neoplasms, and trauma are other causes.[39] Hemobilia in these settings may be

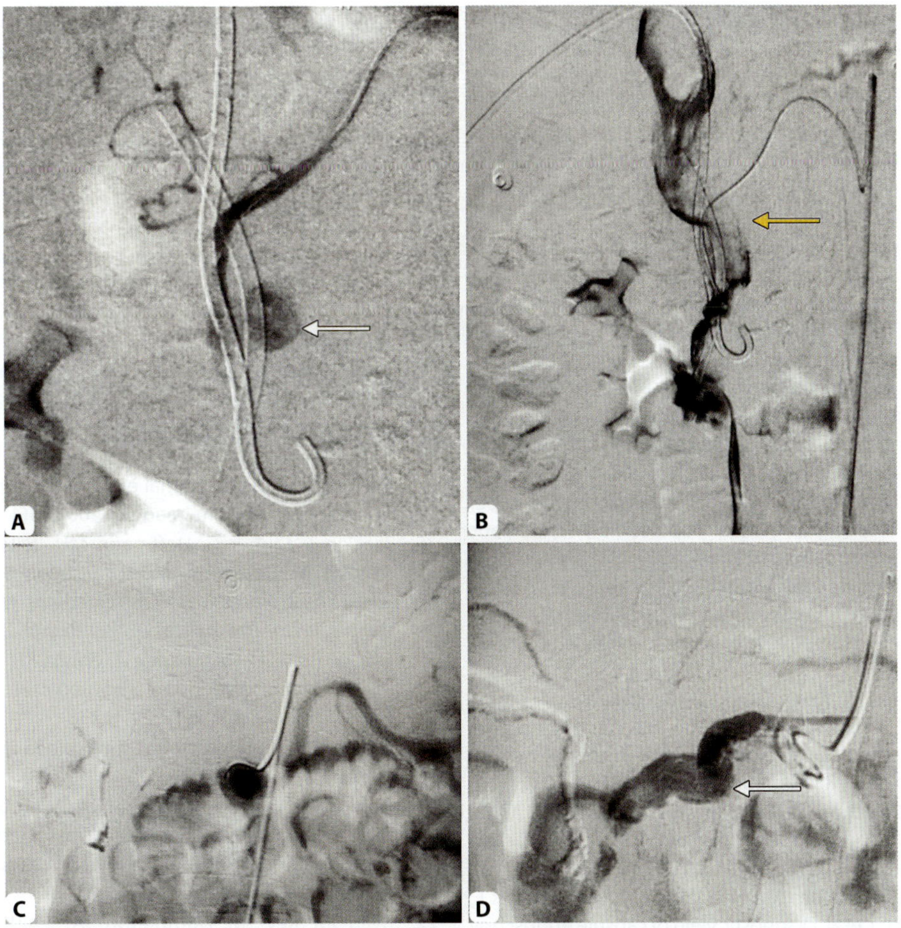

FIGS. 16A TO D: Hemobilia (A and B): Spot images of gastroduodenal artery (GDA) angiogram (A and B) show a pseudoaneurysm along GDA course (white arrow) with subsequent opacification of the common bile duct (CBD) consequent to rupture of pseudoaneurysm into CBD (yellow arrow). Hemosuccus pancreaticus (C and D): Spot images of splenic artery angiogram in another patient (C and D) showing pseudoaneurysm arising from proximal part of splenic artery with opacification of the pancreatic duct due to rupture of pseudoaneurysm into main pancreatic duct (arrow, D).

consequent to arterial or venous injury, direct vascular-biliary fistula creation, or pseudoaneurysm formation.

The classic triad of presentation, i.e., biliary colic, obstructive jaundice, and UGIH may not be observed in all cases, thereby delaying the diagnosis. In the emergent setting, CTA remains the investigation of choice with endoscopy and DSA playing complementary roles in diagnosis and treatment.[39] Typical endoscopic appearance is a demonstration of blood from the ampulla of Vater. The various arterial injuries can be treated by TAE or surgical ligation.

Hemosuccus Pancreaticus

Hemosuccus pancreaticus, also known as pseudohemobilia, refers to upper GIT hemorrhage from the pancreatic duct into the duodenum through ampulla of Vater or major pancreatic papilla.[39,40] The most common cause is pancreatitis with splenic, gastroduodenal, and pancreaticoduodenal arterial injury **(Figs. 16A to D)**. Since both hemobilia and hemosuccus pancreaticus have similar manifestations on endoscopy (i.e., blood at ampulla), imaging can assist in accurate localization and further management.[39,40]

CONCLUSION

Imaging plays a key role in the diagnosis and treatment of GIH and is complementary to endoscopy. An interdisciplinary approach is essential for management. Endoscopy remains the first line of investigation and CTA is the investigation of choice when endoscopy fails to identify the source. CA or DSA is mainly reserved for treatment with coils being the embolic agents of choice in general. Particulate agents and glue are reserved for special situations.

REFERENCES

1. Guglielmo FF, Wells ML, Bruining DH, Strate LL, Huete Á, Gupta A, et al. Gastrointestinal bleeding at CT angiography and CT enterography: imaging atlas and glossary of terms. Radiographics. 2021;41(6):1632-56.
2. Sengupta N, Kastenberg DM, Bruining DH, Latorre M, Leighton JA, Brook OR, et al. The Role of Imaging for GI Bleeding: ACG and SAR Consensus Recommendations. Radiology. 2024;310(3):e232298.
3. Fidler JL, Guglielmo FF, Brook OR, Strate LL, Bruining DH, Gupta A, et al. Management of gastrointestinal bleeding: Society of Abdominal Radiology (SAR) Institutional Survey. Abdom Radiol (NY). 2022;47(1):2-12.
4. Wells ML, Hansel SL, Bruining DH, Fletcher JG, Froemming AT, Barlow JM, et al. CT for evaluation of acute gastrointestinal bleeding. Radiographics. 2018;38(4):1089-107.
5. Gralnek IM, Neeman Z, Strate LL. Acute lower gastrointestinal bleeding. N Engl J Med. 2017;376(11):1054-63.
6. Saydam ŞS, Molnar M, Vora P. Global epidemiology of upper and lower GI bleeding in general population: A systematic review. World J Gastr Surg. 2023;15(4):723.
7. Huprich JE, Alexander JA, Mullan BP, Stanson AW. Gastrointestinal haemorrhage. In: Gore RM, Levine MS (Eds). Gastrointestinal Radiology, 4th edition. Philadelphia: WB Saunders; 2015. pp. 2271-81.
8. Laing CJ, Tobias T, Rosenblum DI, Banker WL, Tseng L, Tamarkin SW. Acute gastrointestinal bleeding: Emerging role of multidetector CT angiography and review of current imaging techniques. Radiographics. 2007;27:1055-70.
9. Jaskolka JD, Binkhamis S, Prabhudesai V, Chawla TP. Acute gastrointestinal haemorrhage: radiologic diagnosis and management. Can Assoc Radiol J. 2013;64:90-100.
10. Van Turenhout ST, Jacobs MA, van Weyenberg SJ, Herdes E, Stam F, Mulder CJ, et al. Diagnostic yield of capsule endoscopy in a tertiary hospital in patients with obscure gastrointestinal bleeding. J Gastrointestin Liver Dis. 2010;19(2):141-5.
11. Strate LL. Lower GI bleeding: epidemiology and diagnosis. Gastroenterol Clin North Am. 2005;34:643-64.
12. Mellinger JD, Bittner JG, Edwards MA, Bates W, Williams HT. Imaging of gastrointestinal bleeding. Surg Clin North Am. 2011;91:93-108.
13. Kim J, Kim YH, Lee KH, Lee YJ, Park JH. Diagnostic performance of CT angiography in patients visiting emergency department with overt gastrointestinal bleeding. Korean J Radiol. 2015;16:541-9.
14. Dane B, Gupta A, Wells ML, Anderson MA, Fidler JL, Naringrekar HV, et al. Dual-Energy CT Evaluation of Gastrointestinal Bleeding. Radiographics. 2023;43(6):e220192.
15. Tse JR, Shen J, Shah R, Fleischmann D, Kamaya A. Extravasation volume at computed tomography angiography correlates with bleeding rate and prognosis in patients with overt gastrointestinal bleeding. Invest Radiol. 2021;56(6):394-400.
16. Yoon W, Jeong YY, Shin SS, Lim HS, Song SG, Jang NG, et al. Acute massive gastrointestinal bleeding: detection and localization with arterial phase multidetector row helical CT. Radiology. 2006;239(1):160-7.
17. Srivastava DN, Sharma S, Pal S, Thulkar S, Seith A, Bandhu S, et al. Transcatheter arterial embolisation in the management of hemobilia. Abdom Imaging. 2006;31(4):439-48.
18. Jaeckle T, Stuber G, Hoffmann MH, Jeltsch M, Schmitz BL, Aschoff AJ. Detection and localization of acute upper and lower gastrointestinal (GI) bleeding with arterial phase multidetector row helical CT. Eur Radiol. 2008;18:1406-13.
19. Ojha V, Raju SN, Deshpande A, Ganga KP, Kumar S. Catheters in vascular interventional radiology: an illustrated review. Diagn Interv Radiol. 2023;29(1):138.
20. Zuckier LS. Acute gastrointestinal bleeding. Semin Nucl Med. 2003;33(4):297-311.
21. Abbas SM, Bissett IP, Holden A, Woodfield JC, Parry BR, Duncan D. Clinical variables associated with positive angiographic localisation of lower gastrointestinal bleeding. ANZ J Surg. 2005;75:953-7.
22. Ryan JM, Key SM, Dumbleton SA, Smith TP. Non localized lower gastrointestinal bleeding: provocative bleeding studies with intraarterial tPA, heparin, and tolazoline. J Vasc Interv Radiol. 2001;12(11):1273-7.
23. Kim CY, Suhocki PV, Miller MJ Jr, Khan M, Janus G, Smith TP. Provocative mesenteric angiography for lower gastrointestinal haemorrhage: results from a single-institution study. J Vasc Interv Radiol. 2010;21(4):477-83.

24. Cho KJ. Carbon dioxide angiography: Scientific principles and practice. Vasc Specialist Int. 2015;31(3):67-80.
25. Grady E. Gastrointestinal bleeding scintigraphy in the early 21st century. J Nucl Med. 2016;57(2):252-9.
26. Dam HQ, Brandon DC, Grantham VV, Hilson AJ, Howarth DM, Maurer AH, et al. The SNMMI procedure standard/EANM practice guideline for gastrointestinal bleeding scintigraphy 2.0. J Nucl Med Technol. 2014;42(4):308-17.
27. RADAR – the RAdiation Dose Assessment Resource. (2015). RADAR Medical Procedure Radiation Dose Calculator and Consent Language Generator. [online] Available from https://www.doseinfo-radar.com/RADARDoseRiskCalc.html [Last accessed June, 2024].
28. Madhusudhan KS, Gamanagatti S, Garg P, Shalimar, Dash NR, Pal S, et al. Endovascular embolisation of visceral artery pseudoaneurysms using modified injection technique with N-butyl cyanoacrylate glue. J Vasc Interv Radiol. 2015;26(11):1718-25.
29. Madhusudhan KS, Venkatesh HA, Gamanagatti S, Garg P, Srivastava DN. Interventional radiology in the management of visceral artery pseudoaneurysms: A Review of Techniques and Embolic Materials. Korean J Radiol. 2016;17(3):351-63.
30. Srivastava DN, Gandhi D, Julka PK, Tandon RK. Gastrointestinal haemorrhage in hepatocellular carcinoma: management with transhepatic arterial embolisation. Abdom Radiol. 2000;25:380-4.
31. Mirsadraee S, Tirukonda P, Nicholson A, Everett SM, McPherson SJ. Embolisation for non-variceal upper gastrointestinal tract haemorrhage: a systematic review. Clin Radiol. 2011;66(6):500-9.
32. Defreyne L, Vanlangenhove P, De Vos M, Pattyn P, Van Maele G, Decruyenaere J, et al. Embolisation as a first approach with endoscopically unmanageable acute nonvariceal gastrointestinal haemorrhage. Radiology. 2001;218(3):739-48.
33. Loffroy R, Rao P, Ota S, De Lin M, Kwak BK, Geschwind JF. Embolisation of acute nonvariceal upper gastrointestinal haemorrhage resistant to endoscopic treatment: results and predictors of recurrent bleeding. Cardiovasc Intervent Radiol. 2010;33(6):1088-100.
34. Hur S, Jae HJ, Lee M, Kim HC, Chung JW. Safety and efficacy of transcatheter arterial embolisation for lower gastrointestinal bleeding: a single-center experience with 112 patients. J Vasc Interv Radiol. 2014;25(1):10-9.
35. Kwon JH, Kim MD, Han K, Choi W, Kim YS, Lee J, et al. Transcatheter arterial embolisation for acute lower gastrointestinal haemorrhage: a single-centre study. Eur Radiol. 2019;29(1):57-67.
36. Ripoll C, Bañares R, Beceiro I, Menchén P, Catalina MV, Echenagusia A, et al. Comparison of transcatheter arterial embolisation and surgery for treatment of bleeding peptic ulcer after endoscopic treatment failure. J Vasc Interv Radiol. 2004;15(5):447-50.
37. Koo HJ, Shin JH, Kim HJ, Kim J, Yoon HK, Ko GY, et al. Clinical outcome of transcatheter arterial embolisation with N-butyl-2-cyanoacrylate for control of acute gastrointestinal tract bleeding. AJR Am J Roentgenol. 2015;204(3):662-6.
38. Yata S, Ihaya T, Kaminou T, Hashimoto M, Ohuchi Y, Umekita Y, et al. Transcatheter arterial embolisation of acute arterial bleeding in the upper and lower gastrointestinal tract with N-butyl-2-cyanoacrylate. J Vasc Interv Radiol. 2013;24(3):422-31.
39. Parvinian A, Fletcher JG, Storm AC, Venkatesh SK, Fidler JL, Khandelwal AR. Challenges in diagnosis and management of hemobilia. Radiographics. 2021;41(3):802-13.
40. Liu B, Contreras FJ, Ward TJ. Hemosuccus pancreaticus. J Vasc Interv Radiol. 2017;8(28):1194.

SECTION

2

Liver

CHAPTER 8

Surabhi Vyas, Ashu Seith Bhalla, Stanzin Spalkit, Smriti Hari

Diffuse Liver Diseases

INTRODUCTION

Diffuse liver diseases encompass a wide spectrum of entities of diverse etiology. Imaging aids in diagnosis, severity assessment/quantification, and complication surveillance. The following conditions are included under the term diffuse liver diseases:

- Steatotic liver disease (SLD)
- Hepatitis
  - Viral
  - Alcoholic
  - Radiation
- Iron overload
- Storage disorder
  - Wilson
- Miscellaneous
  - Granulomatous
  - Amyloidosis
  - Malignant
- Cirrhosis

STEATOTIC LIVER DISEASE

Hepatic steatosis or fatty liver is a benign condition resulting from an excessive accumulation of triglycerides in the form of small or large vacuoles (micro/macrovesicular types) within the hepatocytes. Excess fat deposition in the liver may result from excess synthesis, decreased utilization, impaired release of hepatic lipoproteins, and excess mobilization from fatty tissue.

Hepatic steatosis is associated with hepatocyte injury, liver inflammation, and fibrosis. This was formally recognized by the term "nonalcoholic steatohepatitis" (NASH) in 1980 by Jurgen Ludwig.[1] Subsequently, the term nonalcoholic fatty liver disease (NAFLD) was used to describe the histological spectrum of steatosis to steatohepatitis with its subtypes nonalcoholic fatty liver (NAFL) and NASH.[2]

In 2021, the Delphi consensus statement introduced the new term "steatotic liver disease," which encompasses all underlying causes of hepatic steatosis **(Flowchart 1)**.[3] The previous terminology was deemed inadequate as it relied on exclusionary terms like "nonalcoholic" and carried stigmatizing connotations with phrases such as "alcoholic" and "fatty." To address these shortcomings, the Delphi process led to several key changes: NAFLD was replaced with "metabolic dysfunction-associated steatotic liver disease" (MASLD), which accurately reflects the underlying etiology using nonstigmatizing language. Similarly, NASH was replaced by "metabolic dysfunction-associated steatohepatitis" (MASH). Additionally, a new category, "metabolic dysfunction and alcohol-associated steatotic liver disease" (MetALD), was introduced. This category accounts for patients with metabolic dysfunction who consume alcohol above the MASLD threshold but below that of alcohol-related liver disease (ALD).[4] Finally, "cryptogenic SLD" was introduced to classify cases of steatosis without identifiable metabolic risk factors or other known causes. One crucial aspect of developing this new nomenclature was to ensure seamless integration with existing NAFLD data, allowing for continued research and drug development efforts. By demonstrating a 98% overlap between traditional NAFLD and the newly proposed MASLD, the transition preserves vital datasets.[3]

With the increasing prevalence of obesity, hepatic steatosis has become a major source of liver dysfunction even though in most cases fatty liver is asymptomatic with normal liver function tests. Radiologists are frequently the first to suggest the diagnosis of steatosis. Mild hepatomegaly

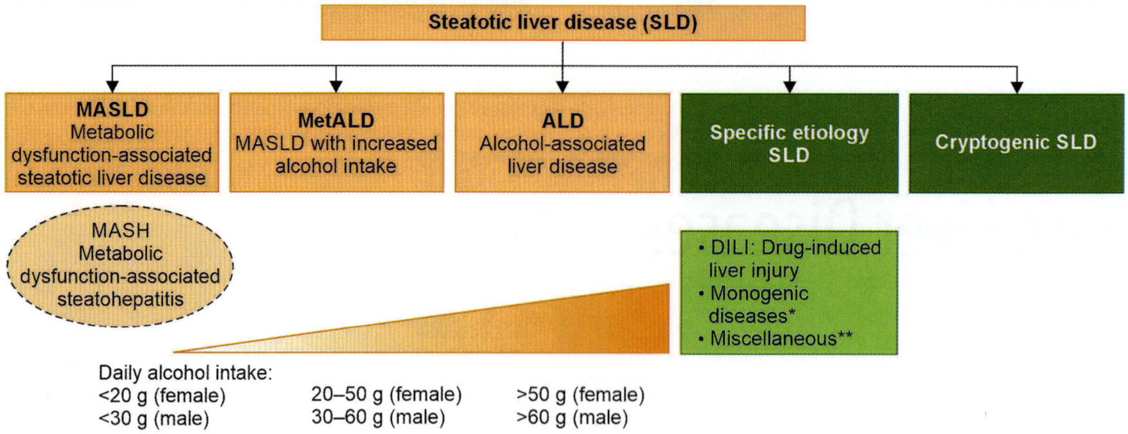

*For example, LALD: Lysosomal acid lipase deficiency, Wilson's disease, hypobetalipoproteinemia, inborn errors of metabolism.
**Hepatitis C virus, malnutrition, celiac disease, human immunodeficiency virus.

FLOWCHART 1: Steatotic liver disease spectrum.[3]

TABLE 1: Steatotic liver disease terminologies.

SLD: Hepatic steatosis of >5% identified by imaging or biopsy					
	Full form	**Metabolic risk factors**	**Alcohol intake**	**Can other causes of steatosis coexist?**	**Disease spectrum**
NAFLD	Nonalcoholic fatty liver disease	Not included	None or minimal	No	Includes steatohepatitis (NASH)
MASLD	Metabolic dysfunction-associated SLD	+/>1 of the 5 CMRF*	Daily intake: • <20 g (females) • <30 g (males)	Yes	Includes steatohepatitis (MASH)
MetALD	Metabolic dysfunction and alcohol-associated steatotic liver disease	+/>1 of the 5 CMRF	Daily intake: • 20–50 g (females) • 30–60 g (males)	Yes (combination etiology)	Can be MASLD/ ALD predominant depending on the extent of alcohol intake
ALD	Alcohol-related liver disease	May be present	Daily intake: • >20 g (females) • >30 g (males)	Yes	Per disease definition
Cryptogenic SLD		Absent	Daily intake: • <20 g (females) • <30 g (males)	No	–
Specific-etiology SLD		Absent	Daily intake: • <20 g (females) • <30 g (males)	Yes (combination etiology)	DILI, monogenic diseases, HCV, HIV, celiac, and malnutrition

*CMRF—based on BMI, fasting serum glucose, blood pressure, plasma triglycerides, and plasma HDL-cholesterol.[3]

(BMI: body mass index; CMRF: cardiometabolic risk factor; DILI: drug-induced liver injury; HCV: hepatitis C virus; HDL: high-density lipoprotein; HIV: human immunodeficiency virus; MASH: metabolic dysfunction-associated steatohepatitis; NASH: nonalcoholic steatohepatitis; SLD: steatotic liver disease)

with or without vague right upper abdominal pain can be present in symptomatic patients. In acute fatty liver associated with pregnancy or alcoholic binge, patients may present with jaundice, acute hepatic failure, or even encephalopathy. **Table 1** outlines the new terminologies.[3]

Ultrasonography

Ultrasonography (USG) findings include hepatomegaly and increased parenchymal echogenicity with impaired visualization of the normally echogenic walls of intrahepatic portal venous branches. There is increased attenuation and poor penetration of the sound beam, resulting in poor visualization of the deeper portion of the liver, diaphragm, hepatic veins, and portal vein radicles **(Fig. 1)**. Echogenicity of the liver can be compared with that of the adjacent kidney as reference. The degree of echogenicity is roughly proportional to the degree of steatosis and tends to parallel biochemical and clinical dysfunction. Focal fat infiltration may produce single or multiple hyperechoic lesions, while areas of focal fat sparing appear hypoechoic in an otherwise hyperechoic liver. In the presence of fatty liver, hepatic hemangiomas may appear hypoechoic, necessitating magnetic resonance (MR) or computed tomography (CT) for their differentiation **(Figs. 2A to C)**. Hepatic steatosis and fibrosis often coexist and produce similar ultrasound (US) findings. Hepatic steatosis can be assessed qualitatively, semiquantitatively, and quantitatively on US.

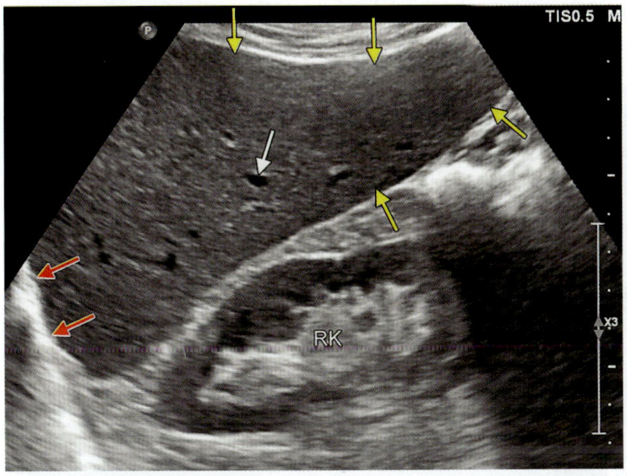

FIG. 1: Normal liver: Parasagittal scan plane shows liver and the right kidney (RK) in the same section. Normal liver has an echogenicity similar to or slightly higher than the adjacent RK, well-demarcated intrahepatic portal vein wall (white arrow), a smooth contour (yellow arrows), and a conspicuous diaphragmatic lining (red arrows).

Qualitative Assessment

On the basis of US findings, fatty liver may be graded qualitatively as **(Figs. 3A to C)**:

- *Mild*: Increased echogenicity with maintained differentiation of intrahepatic vessels, portal vein branches, and diaphragm
- *Moderate*: Partially impaired demarcation of the portal vein and branches and diaphragm
- *Severe*: Markedly impaired demarcation of the portal vein branches and diaphragmatic contour[5]

Semiquantitative Assessment

Semiquantitative assessment can be done by sonographic hepatorenal index (SHRI). In this method, a parasagittal image of the right lobe segment VI of liver and the right kidney is acquired. Region of interest (ROI) is placed on the liver parenchyma and renal cortex, avoiding the vessels, renal pyramid, and renal medulla. A numerical value based on the brightness/echogenicity in the selected pixel is assigned and the ratio between the values of hepatic ROI to renal ROI is calculated to provide the SHRI (cutoff for labeling steatosis is 1.24).[5,6]

Quantitative Assessment of Steatosis

Controlled Attenuation Parameter

Ultrasound elastography (USE) is a noninvasive technique that assesses the hardness of the target organ **(Figs. 4A and B)**. The controlled attenuation parameter (CAP) enables noninvasive evaluation of steatosis by utilizing the characteristics of ultrasonic signals obtained through a transient elastography probe.[7] It operates on the principle that fat alters US propagation, measuring the attenuation

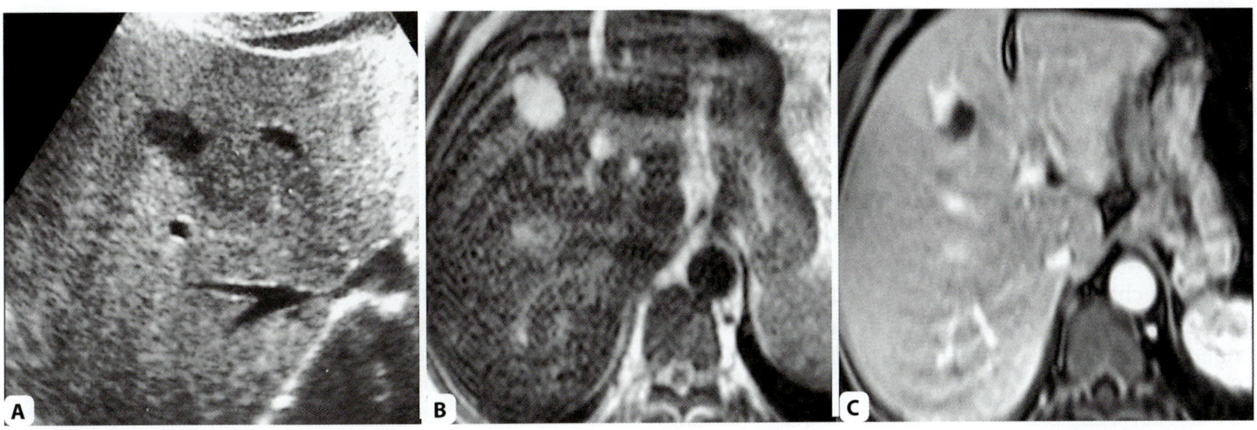

FIGS. 2A TO C: Fatty liver with hypoechoic hemangioma: (A) Transverse ultrasound (US) of the liver shows a small hypoechoic focal lesion against a background of diffusely increased echogenicity of fatty liver. (B) The lesion is hyperintense on T2-weighted (T2W) image, with (C) typical peripheral nodular enhancement, suggestive of hemangioma.

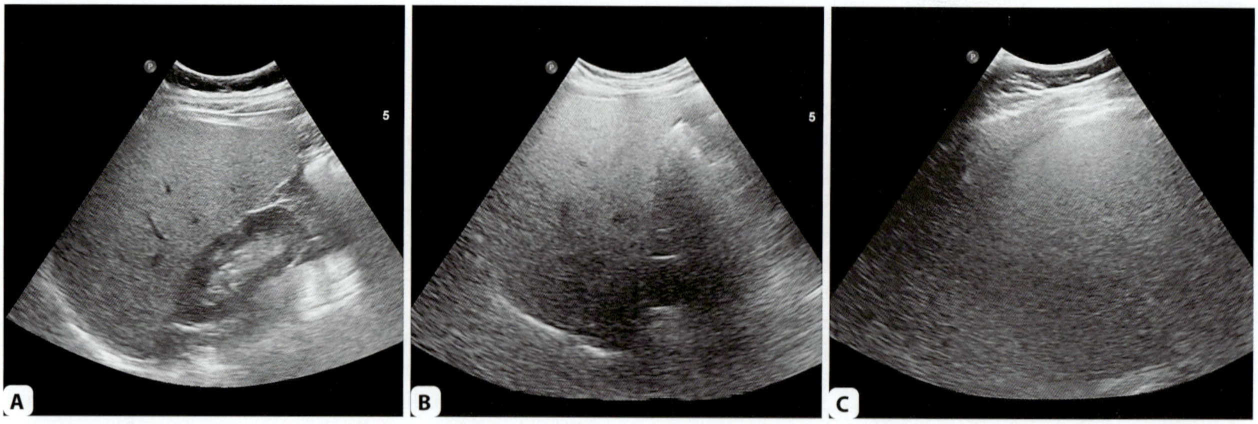

FIGS. 3A TO C: Grades of fatty liver on ultrasound: (A) Mild—echogenicity slightly higher than the adjacent right kidney, well-demarcated intrahepatic portal vein wall and diaphragm. (B) Moderate—partially impaired demarcation of the portal vein branches and diaphragm. (C) Severe—markedly impaired demarcation of the portal vein branches and diaphragmatic contour.

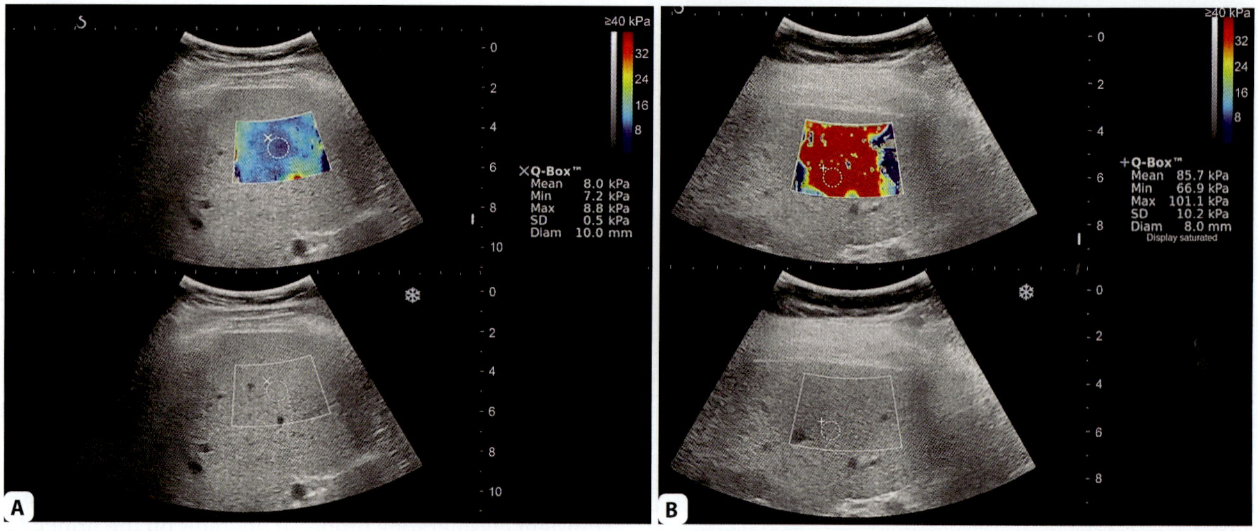

FIGS. 4A AND B: Shear wave elastography of liver showing a mean stiffness of 8 kPa, in case of mild fatty change (A), a higher value of 85.7 kPa in case of chronic liver disease (B). Also noted is irregularity of the hepatic surface in (B).

of US beams across the liver in decibels per meter (dB/m). The optimal CAP cutoff reported for the detection of steatosis was 268 dB/m in a metanalysis by Karlas et al.[8] CAP has been endorsed for rapid point-of-care assessment, exhibiting high accuracy in quantifying liver steatosis, particularly surpassing traditional US methods in detecting mild steatosis and steatosis combined with advanced fibrosis. However, it is important to note that CAP is not an imaging technique; it necessitates a dedicated probe and its effectiveness can be influenced by factors such as the underlying cause of liver disease and metabolic conditions[9] **(Fig. 5)**.

Ultrasound-guided Attenuation Parameter

Ultrasound-guided attenuation parameter (UGAP) utilizes CAP as a reference standard and quantifies the attenuation coefficient (AC) in units of dB/cm/MHz.[10] It integrates US image guidance with AC measurement to identify hepatic steatosis, demonstrating favorable diagnostic accuracy for grading steatosis. AC is determined based on a reference phantom with a known AC. Unlike CAP, liver stiffness does not impact UGAP measurements in assessing hepatic steatosis.[11] UGAP offers advantages such as real-time measurements and consistent sample volumes. Compared to transient and shear wave elastography, which assess tissue stiffness rather than fat content, UGAP offers greater sensitivity in screening for hepatic steatosis, especially in the early stages of MASLD.[12] Studies have shown that the best cutoff values for predicting different grades of liver steatosis with UGAP using CAP as the reference were: S1—192.5 dB/m, S2—231 dB/m, and S3—248 dB/m.[13]

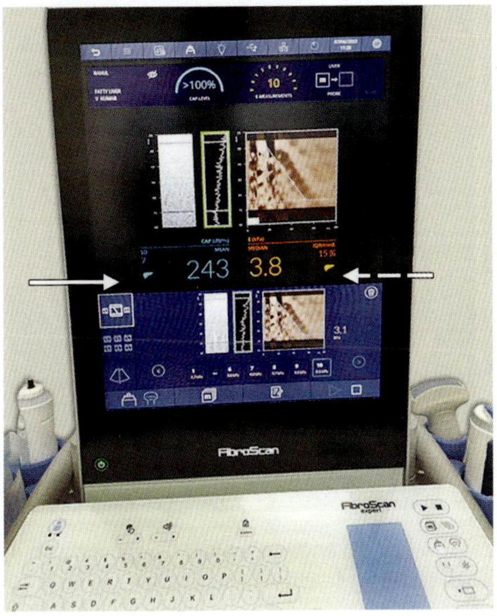

FIG. 5: Vibration-controlled transient elastography: It shows the interface of transient elastography (FibroScan; Echosens, Paris, France). It calculates liver stiffness measurement (LSM) (dashed arrow) and controlled attenuation parameter (CAP) (solid arrow) of 10 consecutive readings and displays the median LSM and CAP values, respectively. The test is considered valid if the ratio of interquartile range (IQR) to median LSM/CAP is <0.3. The median LSM and CAP values in this case were 3.8 kPa (dashed arrow) and 243 dB/m (solid arrow), respectively, with a median LSM/IQR ratio of 0.15, thus suggesting a valid result.

Computed Tomography

There exists an excellent correlation between the CT attenuation of liver and the amount of fat deposition as determined on liver biopsy specimens. Fatty liver is seen as reduced attenuation of the liver parenchyma **(Fig. 6)**. Normal liver attenuation on unenhanced scans is 8–10 Hounsfield units (HU) more than the spleen due to its glycogen content.[14] This relationship is reversed in fatty liver. A threshold CT attenuation value of 45 HU has been shown to be highly specific for moderate-to-severe steatosis.[15] The attenuation is often reduced below that of the normal portal vein and inferior vena cava (IVC) so that these structures stand out, prominently simulating contrast-enhanced image of the liver.[16] Unlike unenhanced scans, contrast-enhanced CT (CECT) is less reliable in the diagnosis of fatty liver. CT has an important role in the detection of incidentally detected steatosis and its initial grading.[17]

Semiquantitative Steatosis Assessment

Liver attenuation index (LAI) can also be calculated as mean liver attenuation–mean splenic attenuation to provide a numeric value. CT-LAI of >5 implies low probability of hepatic steatosis, whereas a value between minus 10 and 5 signifies moderate-to-severe fatty change. A value ≤0 correlates well with significant hepatic steatosis.[17]

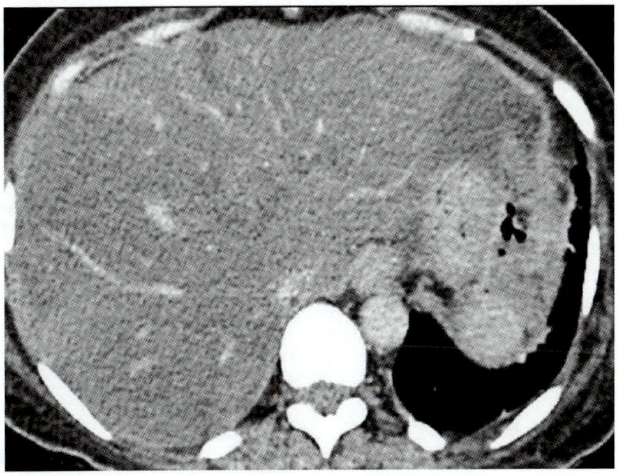

FIG. 6: Fatty liver: Axial computed tomography (CT) image in a case of pancreatitis, showing diffuse decrease in liver attenuation suggestive of fatty infiltration.

Hepatic-to-splenic attenuation ratio: If <0.8 or 1 is highly specific (specificity 100%) for the diagnosis of moderate-to-severe (>30%) macrovesicular steatosis.[18]

Quantitative Steatosis Assessment

Attenuation values at unenhanced CT are linear, correlate strongly with proton density fat fraction (PDFF) and offer an alternative means to quantify liver fat content.

CT-derived equivalent of PDFF (%) = −0.58 × [CT HU] + 38.2 HU[19]

Interpretation: A PDFF of 0% will correspond to approximately 67 HU at unenhanced CT and 0 HU would correspond to 38.2% CT-derived PDFF equivalent.[19]

Decreased attenuation in fatty liver can hamper the detection of hypodense liver lesions such as abscesses or neoplasms. A confident CT diagnosis of focal fat infiltration can be made when it is lobar, segmental, or wedge shaped. In such cases, the area of decreased attenuation typically extends to the liver capsule, without causing a contour bulge and typically has a straight margin. However, MRI may be required for confident differentiation of nodular areas of fat deposition or fat sparing from focal mass lesions.

Dual-energy CT (DECT) has a role in calculation of the hepatic fat [hepatic fat fraction (HFF)], where various material decomposition algorithms allow creation of fat-specific and virtual noncontrast images from the images acquired at tube potentials of 80 and 140 kVP. The liver attenuation is reduced at low energy level and increases at higher energy levels in hepatosteatosis. It has been reported that an increase in attenuation by >10 HU on higher kVP suggests fatty infiltration >25% **(Figs. 7A to C)**.[20] At this time, DECT has no clear advantage over simple attenuation (HU) measurements in noncontrast CT (NCCT). The most likely role of DECT is to separate superimposed iodine or iron overload, which can mask the presence of steatosis at single-energy CT.[19]

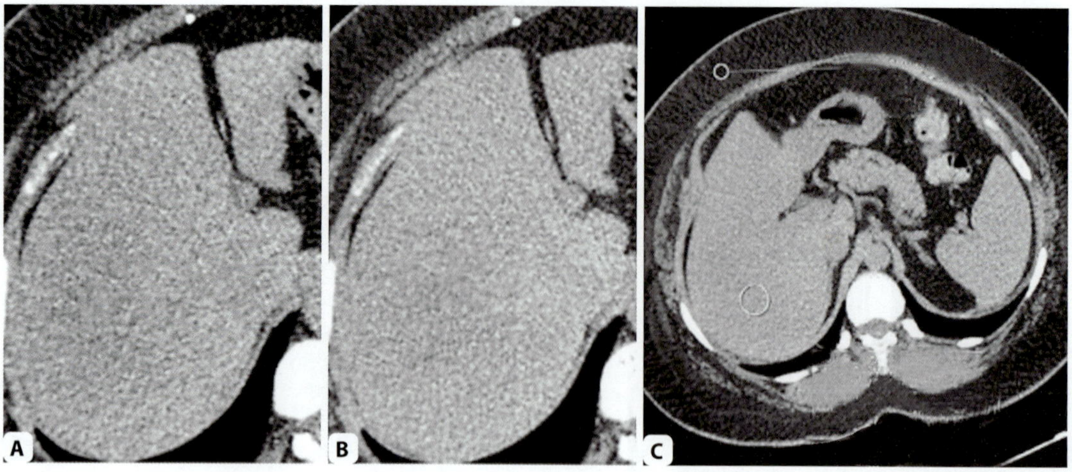

FIGS. 7A TO C: Dual-energy computed tomography (DECT) hepatic steatosis at low keV (A) and higher keV (B) showing an increase in attenuation by >10 HU; (C) liver fat fraction of 14% suggestive of steatosis. Note that the fat fraction of subcutaneous fat is 100%.

Magnetic Resonance Imaging

Magnetic resonance imaging- (MRI)-based techniques for qualitative signal fat fraction estimation include frequency-selective fat suppression and chemical shift-based imaging. In the former, two sets of images are acquired, with and without fat suppression. However, the problem of inadequate fat suppression may preclude adequate signal suppression and thus, the latter is preferred. Although fatty infiltration may demonstrate increased signal intensity of liver on T1- and T2-weighted spin echo images, this increase in signal may not be apparent even with massive fat deposition in liver.[21] Chemical shift imaging is based on acquiring images at two echo times (TEs). Here, fat suppression pulse is not employed. Loss of signal on the opposed phase image when compared with the in-phase image readily identifies excess fat-containing areas in the liver **(Figs. 8A to C)**. On a 1.5T scanner, signals from fat and water are in phase every 4.6 ms, out of phase at 2.3 ms and at their multiples. At 3T, the signals are in phase at 2.3 ms and out of phase at 1.15 ms and at their multiples thereafter. Chemical shift MRI is the investigation of choice in cases with focal nodular or multifocal fat deposition/sparing that may be confused with liver metastases on US or CT. In short, frequency-selective fat suppression leads to bulk fat suppression, whereas chemical shift-based imaging is used to detect intravoxel fat.

Quantitative Steatosis Assessment

There are two MR techniques used for quantitative hepatic fat estimation—chemical shift-encoded MRI (CSE MRI) and MR spectroscopy (MRS). Both make use of the difference in the water and fat proton resonance frequencies to measure signal due to fat fraction [signal fat fraction (SFF) or PDFF].

Magnetic resonance spectroscopy is a direct method of estimating signal fat fraction and since the resonance frequencies of both protons are different, so are their peaks on the spectral tracing. Usually, a single-voxel technique is employed. Multivoxel MR technique is limited by shimming and the inability to acquire a relatively longer sequence in a single breath hold, leading to breathing artifacts. Once the peaks of water and fat are identified, the areas under the peak can be quantified.

Proton Density Fat Fraction

Proton density fat fraction is an advanced MRI technique based on three-dimensional (3D) gradient echo (GRE) imaging that allows quantitative evaluation of liver fat without the inherent limitations of the conventional chemical shift imaging which affects image quality such as choice of imaging parameters, field strength, and coexisting biological factors such as fibrosis, cirrhosis, and iron overload.[22,23]

Proton density fat fraction serves as a quantitative biomarker reflecting the concentration of mobile triglycerides within tissue. It is defined as the ratio of mobile proton density from triglycerides to the total proton density from both mobile triglycerides and water.

PDFF = F/(W + F), where F and W represent signals from protons within mobile triglycerides and mobile water.

This ratio, expressed as a percentage ranging from 0% to 100%, closely corresponds to the fat percentage estimated through histological examination. MRI-PDFF value of ≥5.56% is commonly used to define steatosis and it has been shown to have an excellent sensitivity and specificity to detect and grade steatosis **(Figs. 9A and B)**.[24]

Accurate assessment of PDFF can be achieved through either CSE-MRI or MRS. Both techniques leverage the "chemical shift" phenomenon to distinguish between water and fat proton signals.

While MRS provides high-resolution spectra depicting separate water and fat peaks from a single voxel acquired in a brief breath hold. It suffers from limitations such as limited

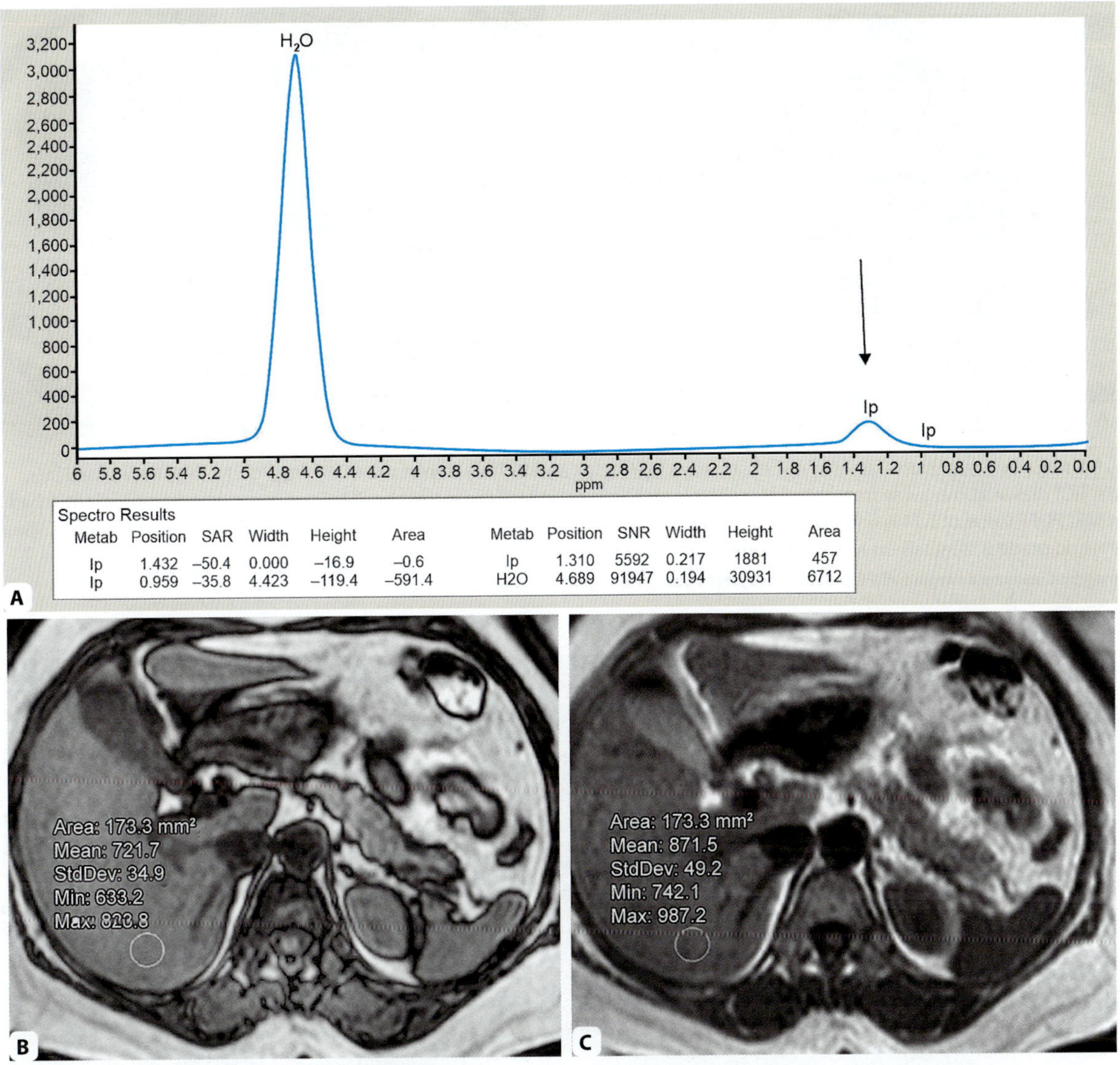

FIGS. 8A TO C: Magnetic resonance spectroscopy (MRS) spectrum in a case of fatty liver (A) showing a lipid peak at 1.3 ppm. Chemical shift magnetic resonance imaging (MRI) of fatty liver shows signal drop of liver parenchyma in the opposed-phase image (B) from in-phase image (C) due to steatosis.

sampling due to small voxel size (using multivoxel MRS increases sample size but also proportionately increases scan time) and requires specialized data processing.

Chemical shift-encoded MRI, on the other hand, utilizes phase and magnitude of MRI signals to fully segregate water and fat proton signals. PDFF is then measured using fat fraction maps, enabling precise, repeatable, and reproducible assessment of liver fat across the entire liver in a short breath hold, typically around 20 seconds. Importantly, this method bypasses the sampling constraints of biopsy and MRS; it is Food and Drug Administration (FDA) approved and commercially available.[25]

However, it is worth noting that while PDFF serves as a reliable biomarker for steatosis, it does not provide insight into steatohepatitis, fibrosis, inflammation, or other endpoints relevant to MASH.[22]

T1 mapping is a novel noncontrast MRI technique that measures the spin lattice relaxation time of a tissue in milliseconds. The T1 value is a direct indicator of the tissue water and the volume of the extracellular space; they are increased in liver fibrosis.[26] Inflammation and iron deposition have opposite effects on T1 such that inflammation increases the T1 values, whereas iron reduces it. It is important to account for elevated hepatic iron as it is a confounding factor in many patients. Therefore, an iron-corrected T1 value (cT1) is used. Multiple studies have found significantly lower T1 values in healthy subjects and patients without fibrosis as compared to patients with significant fibrosis or cirrhosis or those with steatohepatitis.[26-28] Since both active inflammation and fibrosis increase the T1 relaxation time in the liver, it is difficult to determine them in isolation **(Figs. 10A and B)**.[27]

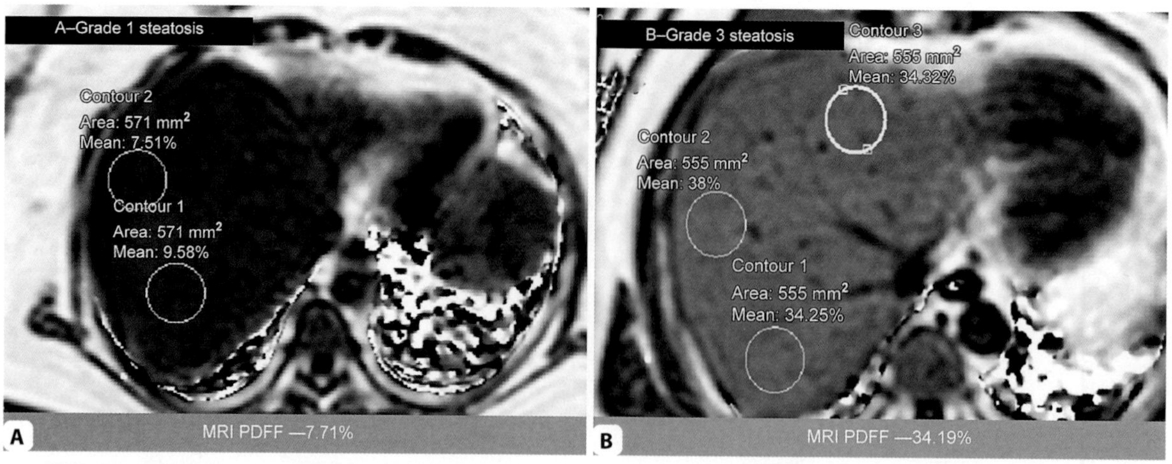

FIGS. 9A AND B: Quantitative assessment of steatosis by MRI: (A and B) They depict the PDFF map of the liver in two patients. Circular ROI drawn above away from the major vessels and liver boundary measures the PDFF value in percentage. Patient A had a mean MRI PDFF value of 7.71% and grade 1 steatosis on histopathology. On the other hand, patient B had a mean MRI PDFF value of 34.19% and grade 3 steatosis on histopathology.

(MRI: magnetic resonance imaging; PDFF: proton density fat fraction; ROI: region of interest)

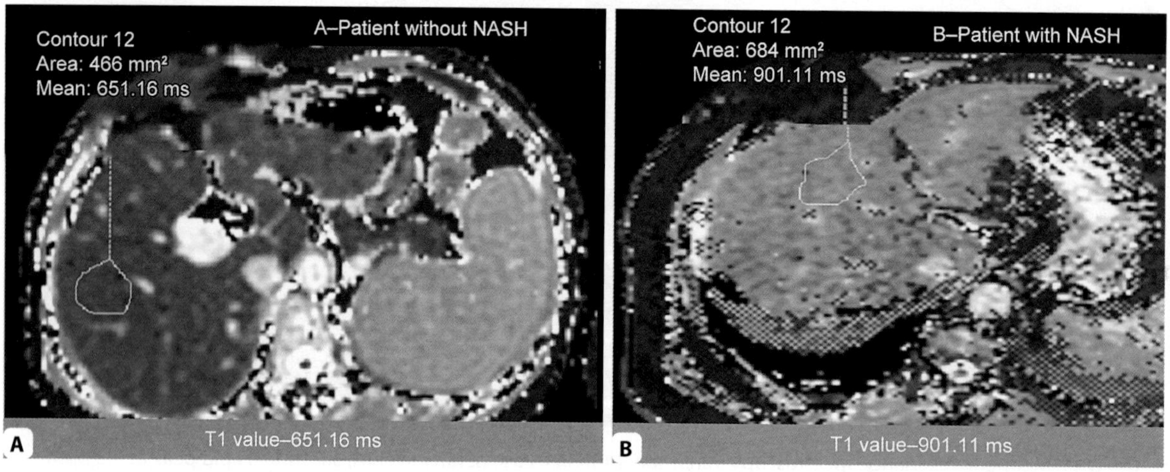

FIGS. 10A AND B: T1 mapping: They illustrate significantly increased liver T1 values in the patient with nonalcoholic steatohepatitis (NASH) (A) on histopathology as compared to the patient who did not have NASH (B). Liver T1 values have been shown to increase in patients who have NASH and those who have fibrosis and can have a potential application to detect NASH noninvasively.

Contrast-enhanced MRI (CEMRI) using gadoxetic acid has been shown to have potential in differentiating simple steatosis from NASH, as the mean liver enhancement is found to be lower in NASH compared with simple steatosis likely due to increased hepatocyte volume reducing the sinusoidal space, and thereby the contrast uptake.[29] Similar observations have been seen using ultrasmall superparamagnetic iron oxide (USPIO), where poor hepatic uptake of USPIO has been seen in patients with NASH than in simple steatosis.[30]

On cross-sectional imaging, fat deposition is most often diffuse. Focal fat deposition and focal fat sparing are less common patterns that typically occur adjacent to the falciform ligament, fissure for ligamentum venosum, porta hepatis, gallbladder fossa, and in the subcapsular portions of the liver. Their characteristic locations, geographic/wedge-shaped configuration with angulated margins, lack of mass effect, presence of normal blood vessels coursing through them, and enhancement similar to normal liver help differentiate these from true lesions. When multifocal or nodular, these may, however, simulate true masses and may require chemical shift MRI for their confirmation **(Figs. 11A to E and Table 2)**.[31]

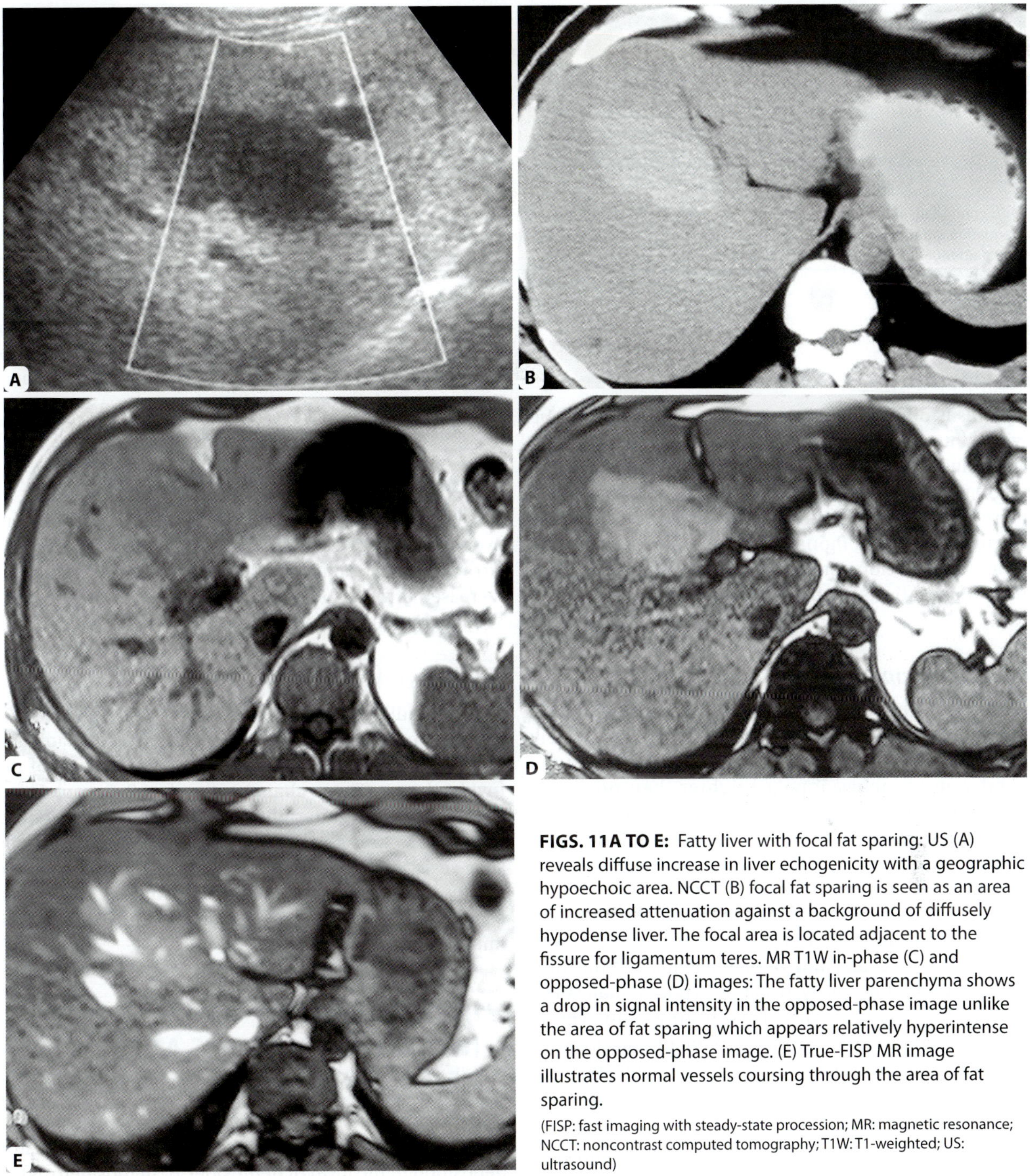

FIGS. 11A TO E: Fatty liver with focal fat sparing: US (A) reveals diffuse increase in liver echogenicity with a geographic hypoechoic area. NCCT (B) focal fat sparing is seen as an area of increased attenuation against a background of diffusely hypodense liver. The focal area is located adjacent to the fissure for ligamentum teres. MR T1W in-phase (C) and opposed-phase (D) images: The fatty liver parenchyma shows a drop in signal intensity in the opposed-phase image unlike the area of fat sparing which appears relatively hyperintense on the opposed-phase image. (E) True-FISP MR image illustrates normal vessels coursing through the area of fat sparing.

(FISP: fast imaging with steady-state procession; MR: magnetic resonance; NCCT: noncontrast computed tomography; T1W: T1-weighted; US: ultrasound)

TABLE 2: Liver steatosis assessment.

Modality	Qualitative	Semiquantitative	Quantitative
USG	• Increased liver echogenicity compared to kidney and spleen • Impaired demarcation of portal vein branches	SHRI	• CAP • UGAP
CT	Reduced attenuation of the liver parenchyma	• LAI • Hepatic-to-splenic attenuation ratio	• Absolute attenuation values • CT-derived PDFF

Continued

Continued

Modality	Qualitative	Semiquantitative	Quantitative
MRI	• Increased signal on fat-only sequences • Drop in signal from in-phase to opposed-phase chemical shift imaging • Decreased signal with fat-suppressed sequences	Signal drop ratio in-phase to opposed-phase	• PDFF: - MRS - CSE-MRI

(CAP: controlled attenuation parameter; CSE-MRI: chemical shift-encoded magnetic resonance imaging; CT: computed tomography; LAI: liver attenuation index; MRS: magnetic resonance spectroscopy; PDFF: proton density fat fraction; SHRI: sonographic hepatorenal index; UGAP: ultrasound-guided attenuation parameter; USG: ultrasonography)

HEPATITIS

Viral Hepatitis

Hepatitis is diffuse inflammation of the liver that can be divided into acute and chronic forms. The latter is in turn, subdivided into persistent and chronic active categories. Imaging is relatively nonspecific but can help to exclude biliary obstruction in acute hepatitis. In chronic hepatitis, imaging is useful in monitoring the progression of the disease, the development of portal venous hypertension, and complications such as hepatocellular carcinoma (HCC).

Ultrasonography

In acute viral hepatitis, liver and spleen are frequently enlarged. Severe acute hepatitis may result in diffusely decreased parenchymal echogenicity against which the portal vein branches appear brighter than normal.[32] This starry-sky pattern is seen in up to 60% of patients with acute viral hepatitis and is best appreciated in thin patients.[33] Gallbladder wall thickening or contraction or both are other nonspecific findings seen in patients with hepatitis. Paradoxical response of gallbladder to fatty food may be seen as dilatation of gallbladder. Severe chronic hepatitis causes coarsening of parenchymal echotexture and increased echogenicity, resulting in poor visualization of portal venous branches. This finding, however, is nonspecific and is also seen in fatty infiltration and cirrhosis. Periportal lymphadenopathy may be seen in hepatitis.

Computed Tomography

Computed tomography attenuation of liver is generally not altered in hepatitis unless fatty infiltration is present. Hepatomegaly, gallbladder wall thickening, and periportal hypodensity can be seen in acute hepatitis and periportal lymphadenopathy is commonly seen in chronic active hepatitis.

Magnetic Resonance Imaging

On MRI, the edematous liver in acute hepatitis may appear heterogeneous, especially on T2-weighted images and early-postcontrast images. Periportal T2-hyperintense signal can also be seen. Likewise, heterogeneous contrast enhancement and T2 hyperintensity signify severe ongoing inflammation in chronic hepatitis, while the absence of patchy enhancement suggests low inflammatory reaction.[34] Progressive enhancement in the delayed phase suggests the presence of liver fibrosis in patients with chronic hepatitis.[35]

Alcoholic Hepatitis

Alcoholic liver disease manifests as three distinct but overlapping entities: Fatty liver, alcoholic hepatitis, and cirrhosis. Unlike acute viral hepatitis, liver echogenicity is increased in acute alcoholic hepatitis due to the presence of concomitant fatty infiltration.

Radiation Hepatitis

In acute radiation hepatitis, CT shows a sharply defined, hypodense area in the liver corresponding to the radiation ports. This represents edema or fatty infiltration of the involved area. These changes manifest 2–6 weeks after therapy and are generally seen in patients receiving a dose of >35 gray to the liver. The CT changes may be seen several weeks after the initiation of the therapy and resolve by 3–5 months. Radiation hepatitis on MRI is seen as geographic areas of edema on T1- and T2-weighted images.[36]

IRON OVERLOAD (HEMOCHROMATOSIS AND HEMOSIDEROSIS)

Hepatic iron overload can be divided into parenchymal iron deposition (hemochromatosis) and reticuloendothelial iron deposition in the form of hemosiderin (hemosiderosis).

In hemosiderosis, the deposition of excess iron is derived from destruction of red blood cells typically due to repeated blood transfusions, chronic hemodialysis, or hemolytic anemia. Because such iron is deposited primarily in the reticuloendothelial system (liver, spleen, lymph nodes, and bone marrow), organ function is generally preserved.

Hemochromatosis on the other hand is a more severe form of iron accumulation (body iron stores up to 50–60 g) that adversely affects organ function. Hemochromatosis may be primary or secondary. Primary hemochromatosis is an autosomal recessive metabolic disorder of excessive iron absorption in duodenum/jejunum. The causes of secondary hemochromatosis include excess iron intake, anemia due to ineffective erythropoiesis requiring multiple blood transfusions, congenital transferrin deficiency, portocaval shunts, and alcoholic cirrhosis.

The excess iron in hemochromatosis is stored as ferritin and hemosiderin in various organs including liver, pancreas, myocardium, joints, and endocrine glands such as pituitary and skin, in decreasing order of severity. Sometimes, iron is deposited in the spleen and kidneys. Brain and nervous tissues are spared. A fibrous tissue reaction is found wherever iron is deposited. Iron deposits are greatest in the liver and pancreas where they can contain 50–100 times the normal amount of iron.

The liver is the first organ to be damaged in hemochromatosis, resulting in hepatomegaly in 95% symptomatic patients. Fibrosis is maximal in periportal areas, resulting in micronodular pigment cirrhosis. Fatty change is unusual. Iron-induced interstitial fibrosis in the pancreas affects endocrine functions to a greater extent than exocrine functions. Skin hyperpigmentation and diabetes mellitus result in so-called bronze diabetes in these patients. Splenomegaly is present in approximately 50% cases; arthropathy of small joints of the hand with or without evidence of chondrocalcinosis on radiographs occurs in 20–50% and cardiac involvement is the presenting complaint in 15% of cases. Diminished sexual activity, loss of body hair, and testicular atrophy can be seen due to decreased production of gonadotropins.

Primary hemochromatosis usually presents in the fourth to sixth decade of life. It is 10 times more frequent in males. Women are generally spared due to iron loss with menstruation and pregnancy. The disease responds favorably to treatment that includes venesection/removal of blood and iron chelators. However, once cirrhosis sets in, it is irreversible and is complicated by the development of HCC in about one third of patients despite adequate therapy.[37] Early diagnosis and treatment of hemochromatosis are therefore of vital importance.

As liver iron is directly related to the body iron, it serves as an accurate estimate of the iron load in the body. Conventionally and historically, estimation of liver iron was performed on the liver biopsy specimen, wherein values of <1.8 mg/g of liver tissue are considered normal[38] and values >15 mg/g are indicative of severe iron overload and risk of early death.[39,40] However, due to the invasive nature of liver biopsy, associated risk of bleeding owing to concomitant thrombocytopenia, and sampling variability, noninvasive iron testing is preferred.

Ultrasonography

Ultrasonography only depicts nonspecific changes of cirrhosis in patients with hemochromatosis and therefore has no role in the diagnosis.

Computed Tomography

Unenhanced CT shows an overall homogeneous increase in density of hepatic parenchyma. While normal liver attenuation is between 45 and 65 HU, in hemochromatosis, this ranges from 70 to 135 HU. The intrahepatic vessels stand out against the background of hyperdense liver. A CT value of 70 HU or more on an unenhanced scan is a sensitive and fairly specific indicator of severe iron overload, although amiodarone treatment and glycogen storage diseases can result in similar increased attenuation **(Fig. 12)**.[21]

Computed tomography also demonstrates increased density in spleen, pancreas, and adrenal and lymph nodes. The increased background liver attenuation in hemochromatosis may hamper detection of HCC in the postcontrast images but facilitates tumor detection in unenhanced scans.

Dual-energy CT has a proven role in the estimation of liver iron concentration (LIC). Iron-specific 3-material decomposition algorithms are used to create virtual iron content (VIC) images which have been used in both in vivo and in vitro studies with good correlation with serum ferritin levels and MR LIC using R2* imaging.[41] The VIC, however, is affected by the iodine-related enhancement.[42]

Magnetic Resonance Imaging

Magnetic resonance imaging is the most sensitive and specific imaging modality for demonstration of hepatic iron overload and also for follow-up of patients under treatment.[34] MRI utilizes the effect of iron present in the liver tissue on the rate of decay of the proton signal. MRI techniques for iron quantification may be performed at both 1.5 or 3T magnets. Higher magnetic strength is preferable at the low iron concentration as the sensitivity of

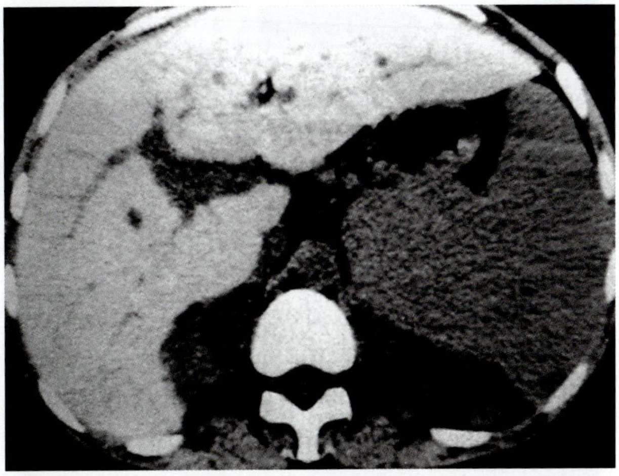

FIG. 12: Primary hemochromatosis: Unenhanced computed tomography (CT) shows markedly increased attenuation of the liver parenchyma.

detection of iron is higher; however, in severe iron overload, 1.5T is preferable due to the limited dynamic range. GRE sequences are more sensitive than spin echo sequences. On MRI, hemochromatosis is characterized by dramatic loss of T1 and T2 signals of the liver (90%) and pancreas (20%) **(Fig. 13)**. A liver/paraspinal muscle (L/M) signal ratio below 0.6 on spin echo T2-weighted images is suggestive of severe iron overload. It correlates well with the amount of iron present in the liver.[21] Iron estimation can also be done by in- and opposed-phase imaging, where contrary to what is seen in fatty infiltration, iron deposition results in loss of signal in the in-phase image which conventionally is acquired at a longer TE than the opposed-phase image **(Figs. 14A to C)**.

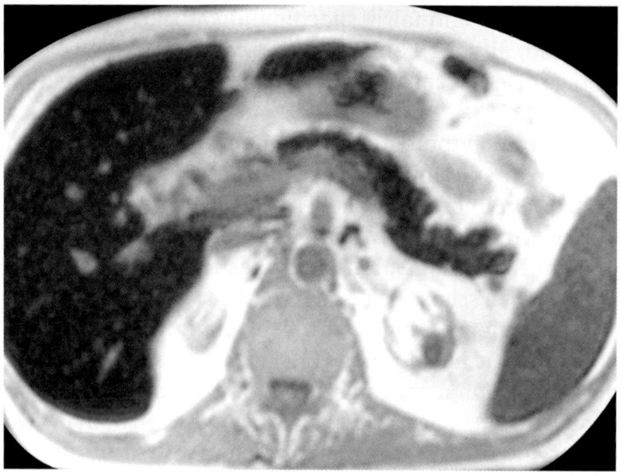

FIG. 13: Primary hemochromatosis: Fast spin echo T2-weighted (FSE T2W) image reveals markedly hypointense signal of the liver and pancreas, while the spleen shows normal signal intensity.

Another method of iron estimation is based on T2 relaxometry. This technique is based on spin echo and gradient echo sequences. MR images are acquired at progressively longer TEs and the rate of signal decay is mathematically estimated. This generates a cross-sectional map of T2 (in spin echo) or T2* (in GRE) relaxation rates. Once the T2 or T2* value is calculated, the LIC in mg of elemental iron/g of liver tissue by dry weight can be estimated by validated calibration curves.[43] LIC can also be calculated by signal intensity ratio (SIR) between the liver and the paraspinal muscles from a set of multiple GRE sequences with fixed repetition time (TR), different TE, and flip angles for 1.5T scanners using an online calculator developed by University of Rennes **(Fig. 15)**.[43]

The MRI techniques of liver iron estimation with relative advantages and disadvantages are summarized in **Table 3**.

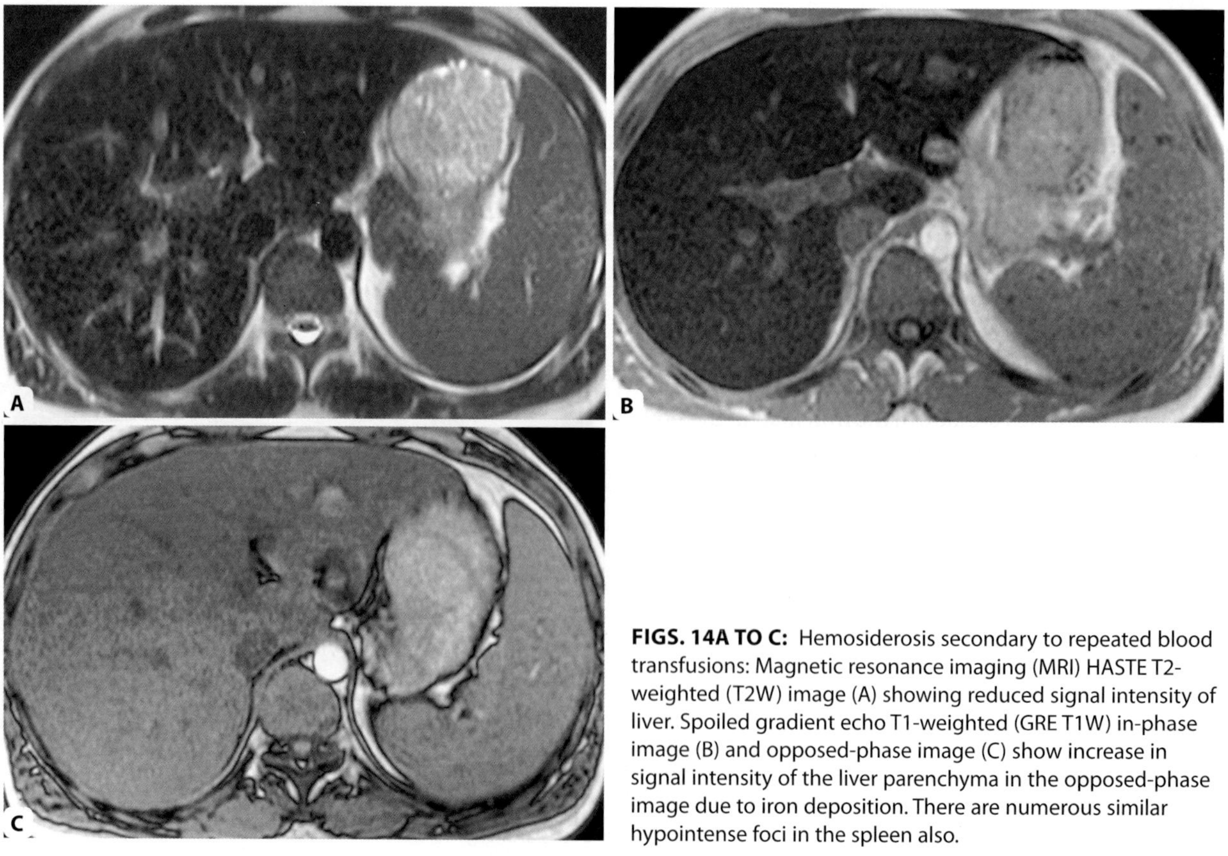

FIGS. 14A TO C: Hemosiderosis secondary to repeated blood transfusions: Magnetic resonance imaging (MRI) HASTE T2-weighted (T2W) image (A) showing reduced signal intensity of liver. Spoiled gradient echo T1-weighted (GRE T1W) in-phase image (B) and opposed-phase image (C) show increase in signal intensity of the liver parenchyma in the opposed-phase image due to iron deposition. There are numerous similar hypointense foci in the spleen also.

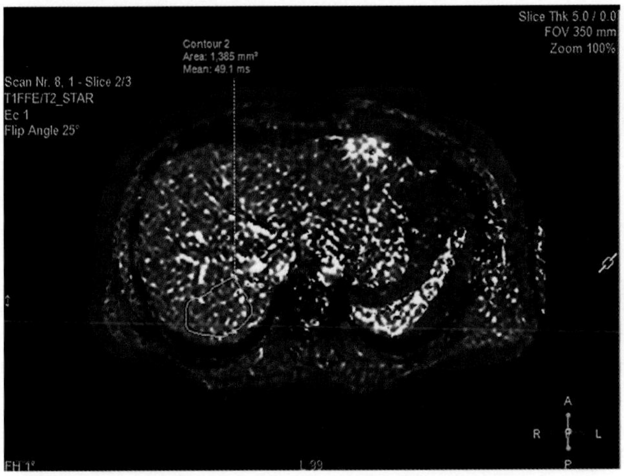

FIG. 15: T2* map is derived by multi-echo gradient echo acquisition and is used to measure the concentration of iron, T2* values reduce with increasing iron accumulation. The T2* value in the above case is 49.1 ms (normal).

Confounders of MRI liver iron estimation:[25]

- The presence of fat and water affects the iron estimation by constructive and destructive interference during gradient echo acquisition using the R2* or SIR. Spin echo acquisition may be affected as fat has a slower relaxation decay than nonfat tissue.
- Fibrosis also decreases R2 and R2* relaxation rates; however, the magnitude of change is insignificant compared to the presence of iron.
- Magnetic field inhomogeneity especially with metallic implants leads to additional signal dephasing and causes overestimation of LICs. The effect is more pronounced with gradient echo sequences.
- Higher field strength, i.e., 3T may show R2 relaxometry confounding in the presence of inhomogeneous radiofrequency deposition.
- Random noise, especially in the presence of high iron concentration, can affect the estimate of iron concentration especially at longer TE.

TABLE 3: MRI techniques of liver iron estimation.

MRI technique	Magnet strength	Principle	Advantages	Limitations
Signal entity ratio method	1.5/3T	Relative signal of the liver and paravertebral muscles using multiple GRE acquisitions. As the liver iron concentration increases, the signal decreases compared to the muscles. The liver-to-muscle signal ratio is then calculated and compared to various calculators to obtain the liver iron concentration	Simple to acquire across various vendors	• Variable result at 3T • Sarcopenia and myosteatosis can confound the results • At mild-to-moderate iron overload, overestimation of liver iron estimation seen
R2-based relaxometry	1.5T	• Spin echo acquisitions at multiple TE using a reference object as a bag of saline • Commercially available single-spin echo acquisition (FerriScan) may also be used • Pixel by pixel R2 map of liver is generated with corresponding liver iron concentration in mg/g or millimol/g	• Reproducible results • R2 mapping can be used at wide range of low-to-moderate iron concentrations at 1.5T	• Long acquisition time, sensitivity to motion • Higher cost • Need for anesthesia in children • Not validated at 3T • Unsuitable for LIC >40 mg/g
R2*-based relaxometry	1.5/3T	2D/3D gradient echo acquisitions at multiple TEs (usually 6–12) in a single breath hold. For high LIC and fatty liver, short TE is used	• Low cost • Well suited for both 1.5/3T • Reproducible results • Wide availability • Rapid acquisition time • Linear relation between iron concentration and R2* • Simultaneous acquisition of liver fat is also done	Very high iron concentration (>40 mg/g at 1.5T and 26 mg/g at 3T) may have limitation of dynamic range

(2D/3D: two dimensional/three dimensional; GRE: gradient echo; LIC: liver iron concentration; MRI: magnetic resonance imaging; TE: echo time)

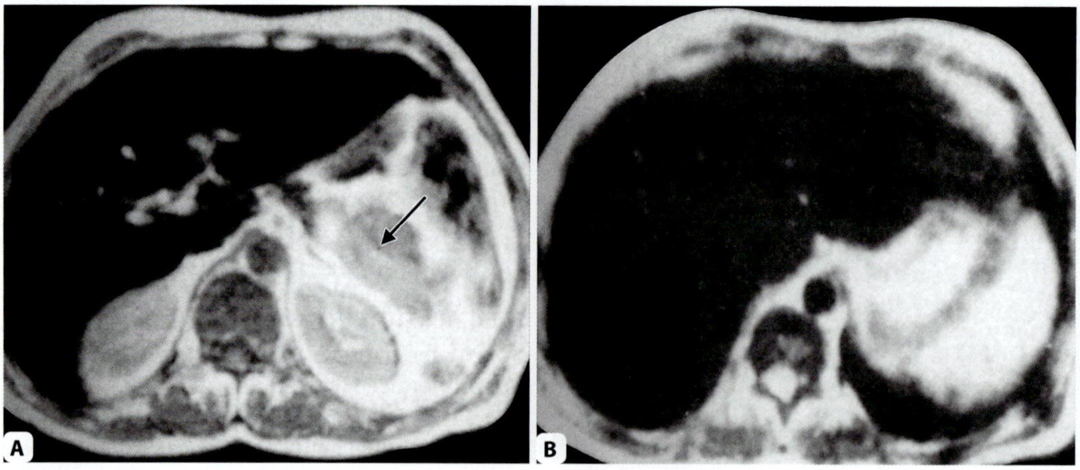

FIGS. 16A AND B: Hemosiderosis: Almost no signal intensity is seen on T1-weighted (A) and T2-weighted axial magnetic resonance (MR) images (B). Normal signal intensity of the pancreas (arrow) helps in differentiation from hemochromatosis. Spleen is not seen because of previous splenectomy in this patient.

Decreased signal intensity in hemochromatosis is also demonstrated in pancreas and myocardium and only occasionally in spleen. In transfusional siderosis, the signal intensity of both spleen and liver is diminished, while the signal of pancreas remains unchanged as it is devoid of reticuloendothelial cells; this feature helps to differentiate transfusional siderosis from hemochromatosis **(Figs. 16A and B)**.

STORAGE DISORDERS

Hepatic storage diseases include conditions which result in accumulation of toxic substances in either the hepatocytes or extracellular tissues and gradually lead to tissue dysfunction and damage and can eventually to cirrhotic changes. Storage disorders include copper accumulation in Wilson's disease, glycogen storage disorders, lysosomal storage disorders, and misfolded insoluble globular protein deposition in alpha-1 antitrypsin deficiency.

Wilson's Disease

Wilson's disease or hepatolenticular degeneration is a rare, inherited autosomal recessive disorder of copper metabolism characterized by impaired biliary excretion of copper. Initially, the excess copper accumulates in the liver. Subsequently, copper deposition occurs in the basal ganglia, renal tubules, cornea, bones, joints, and parathyroid glands. The spectrum of liver injury in Wilson's disease is nonspecific and includes fatty infiltration, acute hepatitis, chronic active hepatitis, cirrhosis, or massive liver necrosis. Development of HCC is extremely rare.

Most patients present in childhood or adolescence with liver disease before the onset of neurologic manifestations. They may have progressive jaundice, ascites, or even fulminant hepatitis. Patients presenting after the age of 20 years can present with a clinical picture simulating chronic active hepatitis or with neurological symptoms such as Parkinson's-like movement disorder and psychiatric disturbance. The Kayser–Fleischer ring is a characteristic corneal pigment that is invariably present. Skeletal changes are seen in over 85% patients with Wilson's disease.[44] These include osteomalacia, chondrocalcinosis, premature osteoarthritis, anterior wedging of dorsal vertebrae, Schmorl's nodes, osteochondritis dissecans, and a periosteal reaction at the trochanters.

Early recognition is important as treatment with penicillamine and zinc can prevent toxic deposition of copper in the liver and brain. Imaging findings of cirrhosis and fatty liver are nonspecific **(Figs. 17A and B)**. Fatty infiltration and excess copper can cancel each other out in advanced Wilson's disease so that a high CT density is usually not seen. Hyperdense nodules may be seen with a hypodense honeycomb pattern on NCCT. On MRI, copper deposition has no ferromagnetic effect on the liver signal intensity as it exists intracellularly in bound form. The changes on MRI are similar to those of cirrhotic liver disease with contour abnormalities and regenerative nodules. A honeycomb pattern consisting of multiple low-intensity nodules surrounded by hyperintense septa on T2-weighted images may be seen. However, this finding is not specific to Wilson's disease.[45] Due to copper deposition, T1 hyperintense and T2 hypointense nodules may be seen on MRI which may show resolution with chelation therapy.[46]

MISCELLANEOUS

Granulomatous Diseases

Granulomatous diseases denote the presence of a focal inflammatory process with the histological features of granuloma. The causes include various viral, bacterial, fungal, and parasitic infections, sarcoidosis, granulomatosis

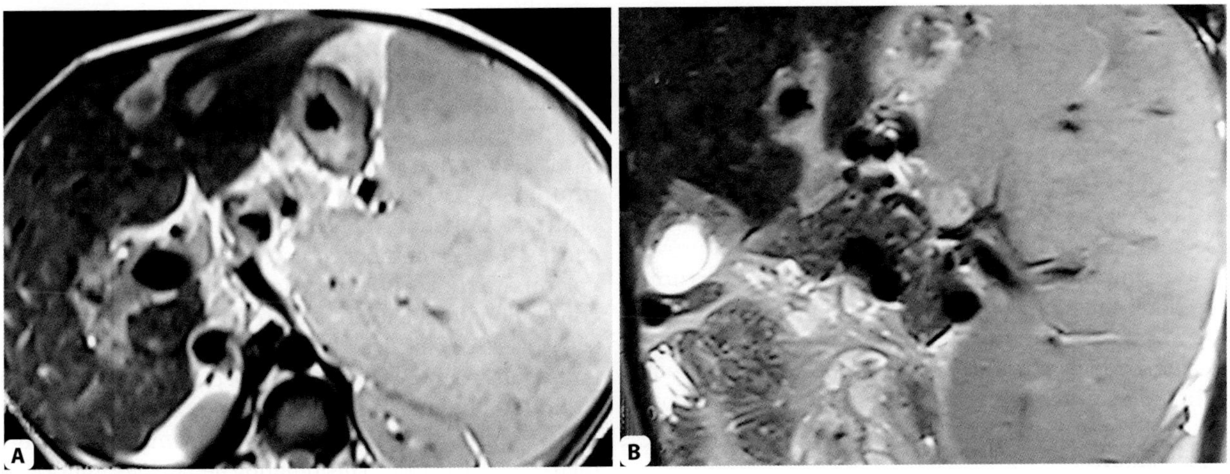

FIGS. 17A AND B: Wilson's disease: (A) Axial and (B) coronal turbo spin echo T2-weighted (TSE T2W) image of a 15-year-old boy showing nonspecific changes of liver cirrhosis with a shrunken liver and massive splenomegaly.

with polyangiitis (Wegener's), and toxic reaction to drugs and chemicals. Biochemical abnormalities in the form of elevated alkaline phosphatase (ALP) and gamma-glutamyl transpeptidase (GGT) is frequently seen in various diffuse infiltrative diseases and alcoholic/viral chronic liver diseases.

Tuberculosis: Miliary tuberculosis is the most common form of hepatic tuberculosis. Usually, it is not accompanied by radiological abnormalities because of its diffuse micronodular nature. Macronodular tuberculomas are uncommon and may be solitary or multiple. These are hypoechoic on US. CT scan shows hypodense masses with or without rim enhancement **(Fig. 18)**. Tubercular cholangitis and tubercular pylephlebitis result from rupture of tubercular nodes/abscess and spread of caseous material into bile ducts and portal vein, respectively. Both these conditions are rare. Multiple small intrahepatic calcifications with no associated masses seen on US and CT represent old healed granulomas.[21]

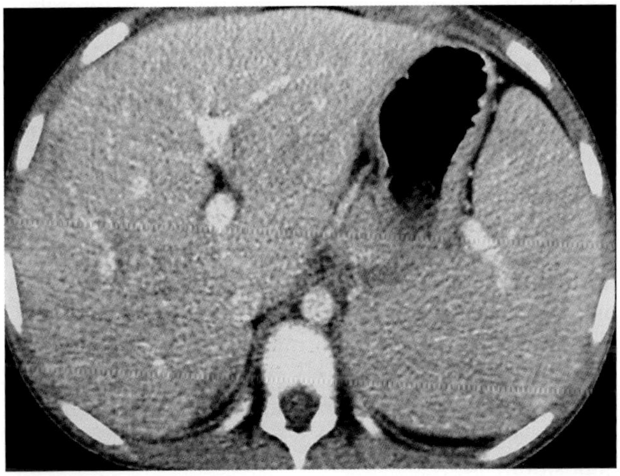

FIG. 18: Granulomatous disease: Contrast-enhanced computed tomography (CECT) of a young adult with disseminated tuberculosis reveals hepatosplenomegaly and ill-defined hypodense lesions in the right lobe of liver.

Sarcoidosis: Liver involvement occurs in 24–79% of patients of sarcoidosis and small (<2 mm) noncaseating granulomas are seen diffusely in the liver.[47] Clinically apparent liver disease is however rare. Cross-sectional imaging most frequently reveals hepatomegaly, often with associated splenomegaly. Less commonly, granulomas are seen as nodular lesions 0.5–2 cm in size in the liver and spleen. These nodular lesions appear hypoechoic on US, hypodense on CT, and hypointense on both T1- and T2-weighted MR images.

Upper abdominal adenopathy is frequently associated with these patients. Occasionally, these nodes enlarge sufficiently to cause biliary obstruction at porta hepatis.

Schistosomiasis: It is a common parasitic infestation with high prevalence in endemic areas such as Africa, South America, Middle East, China, and Japan. The adult worms release ova in portal and mesenteric veins, which embolize to the liver. The host reacts to the ova with a granulomatous inflammation, which is then replaced by fibrous tissue, leading to periportal fibrosis and portal hypertension. On US, periportal fibrosis is seen in the form of thick, echogenic bands replacing the normal portal venous walls, which radiate from porta hepatis to the periphery of the liver. These bands are seen as tubular, round, or oval structures depending on the plane of the section. There may be evidence of portal hypertension. On unenhanced CT, the bands of periportal fibrosis are hypodense and they enhance markedly after contrast administration. They produce round, linear, or branching patterns depending on the plane in which they are sectioned. The portal vein may not enhance if it is thrombosed. Hepatic calcification, if seen, is fairly characteristic and has been termed as "turtle back."[48] It occurs within the capsule and hepatic parenchyma, perpendicular to the capsule looking like a septum. Sometimes, the calcifications may be dense enough to be seen on the plain films.

Liver fluke or Fasciola hepatica: It is a trematode that infests cattle. Humans are accidental hosts. There is an acute phase of hepatic invasion that lasts for 1–3 months and a chronic phase of persistent adult flukes in the biliary tree. In hepatic fascioliasis, CT shows peripheral small, hypodense, serpentine, or nodular lesions whose visibility is improved on dynamic or delayed enhanced CT. The tortuous peripheral channels correspond to the migratory tracts.[49]

There are many other causes of granulomatous infections, which include brucellosis, leptospirosis, syphilis, leishmaniasis, actinomycosis, aspergillosis, and cryptococcosis. These are not associated with any specific radiological features.

Amyloidosis

Amyloidosis is a rare condition characterized by the deposition of an extracellular fibrillar protein in the organs. It may be primary or secondary. Primary amyloidosis is due to the deposition of amyloid light-chain protein (AL). It may occur without preexisting disease or may be seen as a complication of multiple myeloma. Secondary amyloidosis is due to the deposition of amyloid A protein (AA) and is seen with chronic infections, rheumatoid arthritis, ulcerative colitis, Crohn's disease, malignant tumors, and Hodgkin's lymphoma. Clinically, there is smooth, nontender hepatomegaly. Hepatic function is usually preserved despite massive amyloid deposition.

Ultrasound is usually normal except for the presence of hepatomegaly. Rarely, US reveals a heterogeneous echotexture due to nonuniform deposition. Increased liver stiffness is seen on USE which may be due to the protein deposition.[50]

On unenhanced CT scans, amyloid deposition results in hepatomegaly and generalized decreased attenuation. On contrast-enhanced scans, focal areas of decreased enhancement corresponding to nonuniform involvement may be seen. The involved areas may show contrast enhancement in the delayed phase. Concomitant decrease in splenic enhancement may help differentiate amyloid deposition from the fatty liver in appropriate settings. MRI has little role in the assessment of hepatic amyloidosis as there is no significant change in the T2 signal of involved liver.[51] MRI elastography also reveals increased tissue stiffness.

Malignant Liver Disease

Occasionally, a malignant process may diffusely involve the liver. Metastases, particularly from breast cancer, may give rise to diffusely increased heterogeneous echotexture on US. HCC, lymphoma, and leukemia can also be seen as diffusely altered echotexture of the liver. Diagnosis is difficult in such situations and may require biopsy in the appropriate clinical context.[14]

CIRRHOSIS

Cirrhosis is a chronic disease of the liver, which is characterized by fibrosis and nodular regeneration of the liver in response to hepatocellular necrosis. The etiology is diverse which includes viral hepatitis, alcoholism, prolonged cholestasis, hepatic venous outflow tract obstruction, malnutrition, cryptogenic cirrhosis, metabolic causes such as hemochromatosis and Wilson's disease, various toxins, and therapeutic agents. Cirrhosis is conventionally considered as an irreversibly scarred, end-stage disease of the liver. Although the causes are many, the end result is same.[52] The response of the liver to the necrosis is limited, the most important being collapse of hepatic lobules, formation of diffuse fibrous septa, and nodular regrowth of liver cells. The initiating hepatocyte injury leads to inflammation, structural collapse, and fibrogenesis. The resulting fibrosis causes circulatory disturbances, portal hypertension, and intrahepatic cholestasis. A vicious cycle is set up, whereby further hepatocyte injury occurs leading to progression of the disease. Morphologically, cirrhosis is classified into micronodular and macronodular varieties. Micronodular disease is characterized by thick, regular septa, small regenerating nodules of uniform size, and involvement of every lobule. It may represent impaired capacity of regrowth as in alcoholism or malnutrition. Macronodular variety is characterized by septa and nodules of various sizes and the presence of normal liver in between larger nodules.[52]

METAVIR (Meta-analysis of Histological Data in Viral Hepatitis) scoring ***(Flowchart 2)***: This scoring system is used to assess histological samples from liver biopsies, particularly for patients with chronic hepatitis C virus infection. However, it can also be applied to biopsy samples from any type of chronic liver disease. It assesses severity of fibrosis and histological activity reflecting disease stage and grade, respectively.[53]

METAVIR scoring

Grade

Histological activity	
A0	None
A1	Mild
A2	Moderate
A3	Severe

Stage

Fibrosis level		
	Fibrosis in portal tract	Number of septae
F0	–	None
F1	+	None
F2	+	Few
F3	+	Numerous
F4	Cirrhosis	

FLOWCHART 2: METAVIR (Meta-analysis of Histological Data in Viral Hepatitis) scoring.

Significance: METAVIR scoring aids in disease staging, helps in disease prognostication, predicts treatment response, identifies those susceptible to hepatitis C-related HCC, and evaluates the risk of HCC recurrence following treatment.[19]

For MASLD patients, a different histological scoring system is used, known as the NASH Clinical Research Network (NASH CRN): Since there is a large overlap between patients with conventional NAFLD/NASH and those with the newly suggested MASLD/MASH, the NAFLD data and the histological scoring can be generalized to MASLD in order to reduce confusion in clinical practice and drug trials.[3] The clinical research network (CRN) scoring system comprises NAFLD activity score (NAS) and fibrosis scoring.[54]

A regenerative nodule is defined as a hepatocellular nodule containing one or more portal tracts located in a liver that is otherwise abnormal due to either cirrhosis or other severe disease. These nodules are present in all cirrhotic livers and cirrhosis is classified on the basis of size of these on pathologic specimens as micronodular (≤3 mm), macronodular (>3 mm), or mixed. A dysplastic nodule is defined as a nodule of hepatocytes of at least 1 mm in diameter, with dysplasia of low or high grade but no histological criteria for malignancy. Dysplastic nodules are found in 15–25% of cirrhotic livers. Steatosis (fatty infiltration) can occur in either form and either form may result in an enlarged or shrunken liver. Focal confluent fibrosis (or confluent hepatic fibrosis) refers to mass-like fibrosis in advanced cirrhosis, associated with volume loss seen as retraction of overlying hepatic capsule or total shrinkage of segment or lobe.

Clinically, Child's classification is used to determine short-term prognosis. It takes into account jaundice, ascites, encephalopathy, serum albumin, and nutrition status. In the Child–Pugh modification, prothrombin time is used instead of nutritional status as a parameter. The total score classifies patients into grades A, B, or C with increasing severity of disease.[52] Complications of cirrhosis include portal hypertension, variceal bleeding, spontaneous bacterial peritonitis, coagulopathies, hepatic encephalopathy, hepatorenal syndrome, and HCC. Risk of development of HCC in the cirrhotic liver is approximately 3% per year. Although cirrhosis of any etiology may lead to HCC, the risk is particularly high in cirrhosis which occurs secondary to viral hepatitis. Imaging studies play an important role in screening for HCC in cirrhotic patients.

Ultrasonography

Liver is either enlarged or normal in size in the early stage of cirrhosis. A small shrunken liver is seen in advanced cases. Criteria for sonographic diagnosis include heterogeneously increased and coarse parenchymal echotexture, decreased beam penetration through liver, and poor depiction of diaphragm and intrahepatic portal venous walls. These features are common to both fatty infiltration and fibrosis and there is poor interobserver agreement on interpreting these findings. Echogenicity largely depends on gain settings; however, it can be compared with that of adjacent organs in cases of doubt. Normally, the echogenicity of liver and renal cortex is almost equal or that of kidney is slightly lower than liver. In case the kidneys are diseased, comparison may be made with that of splenic echogenicity as spleen has higher echogenicity than normal liver.

Morphological changes in cirrhosis include relative hypertrophy of the caudate lobe and segments 2 and 3 of the left lobe and atrophy of the right hepatic lobe and segment 4 of the left lobe. Sonographically, a right/left lobe ratio of sagittal diameters in midclavicular line and midline, respectively, of 1.3 or less can differentiate cirrhosis from normal liver with 93% accuracy, while a ratio of 1.4 or more excludes cirrhosis.[55] In advanced case of cirrhosis, accentuation of fissures, contour indentations, nodularity, and regenerating nodules are seen. Regenerating nodules vary in size from 2 mm to 2 cm. These may be visible on US as hypoechoic nodules with echogenic border and are difficult to differentiate from small HCC on US. US scanning with a high-frequency probe can depict a nodular liver contour even in early cirrhosis.[56] Atrophy of the liver, along with heterogeneous echotexture and poor beam penetration, however, limits the sonographic detection of small focal lesions in advanced cirrhotic liver. Sonography has poor sensitivity in detection of HCC; it detects only 14% of lesions smaller than 2 cm and its sensitivity for detecting HCC during screening of cirrhotic patients is only 50%.[32,57]

Doppler evaluation is valuable as it provides hemodynamic information. Portal hypertension can be seen in the form of enlarged portal vein, diminution or reversal of portal venous flow, and presence of portosystemic collaterals. Hepatic venous evaluation by Doppler is also helpful. Normal hepatic venous waveform is triphasic with a short phase of reversed flow. The fibrosis and decreased compliance of liver parenchyma leads to decreased amplitude of the phasic variations with loss of reversed flow. Alternatively, there may be a completely flat waveform. These features may be seen even in the early stages of cirrhosis.[33] As the liver atrophies in end-stage cirrhosis, hepatic veins may become attenuated and difficult to visualize. This can cause difficulties when the diagnosis of hepatic venous occlusion is being considered.[55]

The cirrhotic liver can be assessed noninvasively by three USE techniques, transient elastography (fibroscan), acoustic radiation force impulse (ARFI), and shear wave elastography. The hepatic fibrosis correlates with the stiffness values generated on elastography such that value less than 6–7 kPa indicate no or mild fibrosis (F0–F1 METAVIR) and a value >12 kPa suggests cirrhosis (F3–F4 METAVIR).[58]

Contrast-enhanced ultrasound (CEUS) using microbubble contrast agent has a role in characterizing focal liver lesions in cirrhotic liver and in screening of cirrhosis patients for HCCs. It is a useful adjunct to CECT or CEMRI with the benefit of a real-time contrast visualization without renal excretion of the contrast. Both dysplastic nodules and HCCs show arterial phase hyperenhancement on CEUS, similar to CT and MRI.[59]

Computed Tomography

Fatty liver is the most common CT feature of early cirrhosis. Morphological changes in advanced cirrhosis include an overall decrease in liver volume accompanied by atrophy of the right lobe and hypertrophy of left and caudate lobes. The dual arterial supply and shorter intrahepatic course of vessels supplying the caudate lobe along with the fact that caudate vein drains directly into the IVC permits better oxygenation and relative preservation of its function, resulting in compensatory hypertrophy.[60] On the other hand, it is postulated that alcohol and other toxins in the portal vein stream preferentially to the right hepatic lobe. Caudate lobe to right lobe size ratio has been proposed as an objective means of diagnosing cirrhosis. Three lines are drawn: Line 1 is parasagittal through the right lateral wall of main portal vein just caudal to its bifurcation, line 2 is parallel to line 1 through the medial margin of caudate lobe, and line 3 is perpendicular to these lines drawn midway between portal vein and IVC. The distances are measured on line 3. The distance between right abdominal wall and line 1 is right lobe size and distance between line 1 and line 2 is caudate lobe size **(Fig. 19)**. If the caudate lobe to right lobe ratio exceeds 0.65, cirrhosis is likely and it is definitive if it exceeds 0.73.[60] The hepatic fissure, gallbladder fossa, and hilar periportal space are widened due to parenchymal atrophy **(Fig. 20)**. The thickness of the hilar periportal space can be measured on an axial plane where the right portal vein is visible. It is the distance between the anterior wall of the right portal vein and the posterior margin of the medial segment of the left hepatic lobe, ensuring the line is perpendicular to the long axis of the right portal vein. A cutoff value of 10 mm for the anterior hilar periportal space has a sensitivity of 93% and specificity of 92% for diagnosing early cirrhosis on MRI.[60]

These morphological changes are by and large similar irrespective of the underlying etiology of cirrhosis. However, patients with biliary cirrhosis and sclerosing cholangitis tend to have marked caudate lobe hypertrophy and often have atrophy of lateral segments of the left hepatic lobe in addition to atrophy of right lobe.

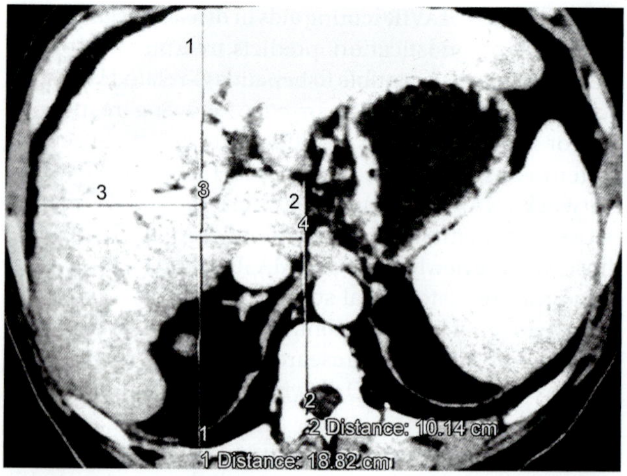

FIG. 19: Computed tomography (CT) scan shows method of measurements of right and caudate lobes. The diameters of right and caudate lobes are measured on line 3 as shown.

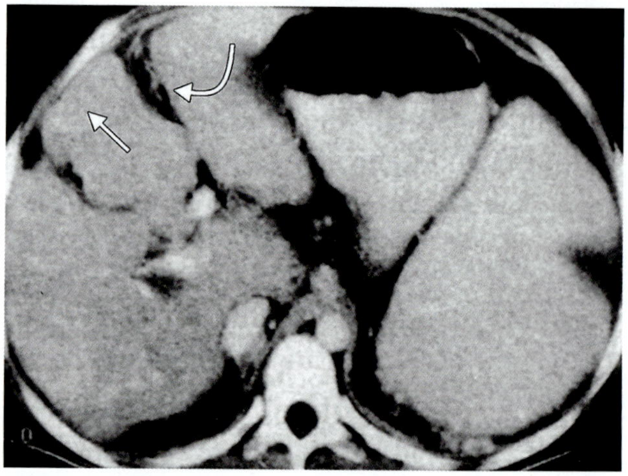

FIG. 20: Cirrhosis: Atrophy of the right lobe and hypertrophy of the caudate lobe with splenomegaly are seen on computed tomography (CT). Widened hepatic fissure (curved arrow), porta, and nodularity of the contour of the liver (straight arrow) are also seen.

Cirrhotic liver often appears heterogeneous on both unenhanced- and enhanced-CT scans due to underlying fibrosis, iron accumulation, regeneration, and altered portal venous flow. Regenerating nodules and atrophy cause nodularity of liver contour. Ancillary CT features in cirrhosis include ascites, splenomegaly, enlargement of the hepatic artery, evidence of portosystemic collaterals, and pericaval fat collection that may appear intraluminal on axial CT scans and increased attenuation of the mesenteric/retroperitoneal fat.[61]

Regenerating nodules are usually <5 mm and are infrequently demonstrated on NCCT, however, may appear hyperdense if they contain iron (siderotic nodules). These do not show arterial phase enhancement and remain isodense to minimally hypodense to the remaining parenchyma on portal venous phase.

Dysplastic nodules, on the other hand, measure 5–10 mm in size and show arterial phase enhancement due to progressive recruitment of hepatic arterial supply. The high-grade dysplastic nodules may even show portal venous washout similar to that of HCCs.

Focal confluent fibrosis that is seen in 30% of patients with advanced cirrhosis can also simulate tumor appearing hypodense on unenhanced CT and isodense to slightly hypodense in CECT. However, typical associated features including wedge-shaped lesions radiating from the porta hepatis, characteristic location in the anterior segments of right lobe and segment 4, delayed enhancement and focal retraction of the overlying liver capsule can help differentiate these from tumor.[62] Similar to hepatitis, patients with cirrhosis can have enlarged upper abdominal lymph nodes and this finding is particularly common in patients with biliary cirrhosis and sclerosing cholangitis. Pseudocirrhosis results from distortion of the hepatic parenchyma due to treated multiple metastatic lesions, usually from breast carcinoma, and can simulate changes in cirrhosis. Similar appearance may also result from pseudomyxoma peritonei or ovarian metastasis due to surface scalloping.

Magnetic Resonance Imaging

Magnetic resonance imaging can often detect cirrhosis at an earlier stage than US or CT.[32] In early cirrhosis, MRI demonstrates fine strands of fibrosis, which are seen as lace-like hypointense fine networks on heavily T2-weighted images. Out-of-phase spoiled GRE images are very sensitive in this regard. These fine fibrotic strands show progressive enhancement following intravenous gadolinium. Enlargement of hilar periportal space, which is a space anterior to right branch of portal vein, is considered as an early manifestation of cirrhosis. It is caused by atrophy of segment 4. Early detection of cirrhosis by MRI is of clinical importance as these patients may benefit from newer treatment options now available.[43] As cirrhosis progresses, MRI demonstrates all features that are seen on CT, including contour nodularity, relative right lobe atrophy and left/caudate lobe hypertrophy, splanchnic vessels enlargement, hepatic arterial enlargement, collaterals, splenomegaly, and ascites. Expansion and widening of interlobar fissures are also seen.

Abnormal hepatic periportal intensity, which is seen as hyperintense rings or track marks surrounding the portal vein branches on T2-weighted images, can be seen in cirrhosis. It is a nonspecific finding and is also seen in many biliary or hepatocellular diseases. Gamna–Gandy bodies in the spleen are seen as multiple, small, low-intensity spots on GRE images. These represent hemosiderin deposits in collagen bundles and may be the result of small hemorrhages and can be seen in portal hypertension due to other causes as well like extrahepatic portal vein obstruction (EHPVO).

Magnetic resonance imaging is the modality of choice for characterizing nodules in cirrhotic liver and can demonstrate regenerating nodules with greater sensitivity than any other modality. While only approximately 25% of regenerating nodules are seen on CT mainly due to their iron content, MR can demonstrate 50% regenerative nodules **(Figs. 21A and B)**. Dysplastic nodules (previously called adenomatous hyperplastic nodules) represent premalignant intermediary phase in the pathway of hepatocellular carcinogenesis **(Figs. 22A to D)**.[32] The MRI appearance of regenerative and dysplastic nodules on various MRI sequences and enhancement phases is summarized in **Table 4**.

Focal confluent fibrosis has T1 and T2 signal similar to HCC, i.e., hypointense on T1 and hyperintense on T2-weighted images. It may show arterial phase enhancement, however, persistent enhancement in delayed phase helps in differentiation from HCC. Moreover, as with CT, characteristic location and associated capsular retraction also helps in differentiation. MRI is useful in differentiating viral from alcoholic cirrhosis. Larger caudate lobe volume, presence of a notch in the outline of right posterior segment of liver, and smaller size of regenerating nodules favors the diagnosis of alcoholic cirrhosis over virus-induced cirrhosis.[63]

MR elastography (MRE) has a role in noninvasive evaluation, staging, and follow-up of hepatic fibrosis. It is based on modified phase contrast sequence, where a mechanical propagation wave is produced in soft tissues usually of frequency 60 MHz. The propagation of the wave in the tissue creates an elastogram using complex algorithms. In various studies, MRE has shown good

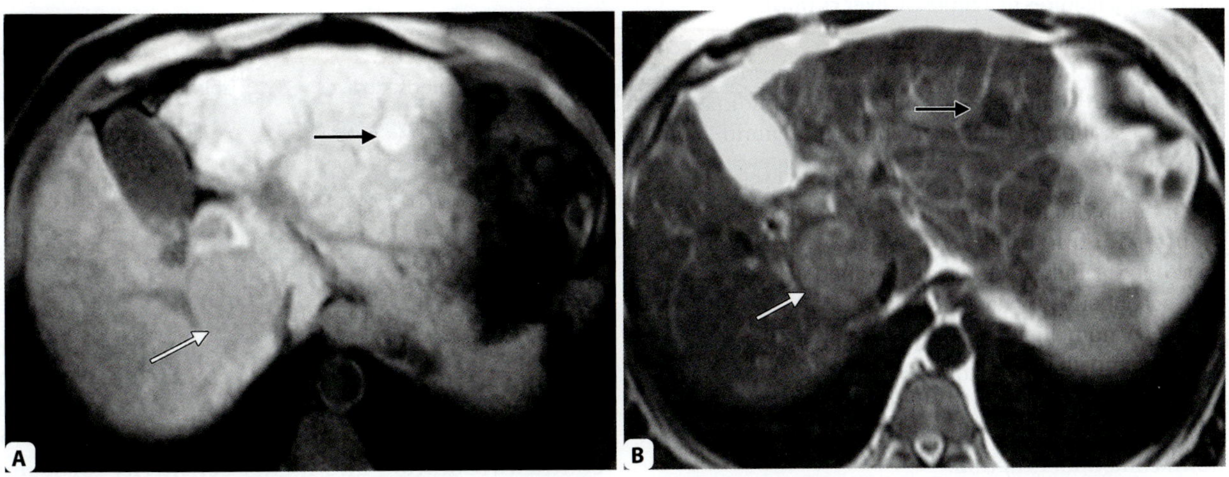

FIGS. 21A AND B: Cirrhosis with regenerative nodule and HCC: Axial T1W (A) and T2W (B) MR images show a well-defined focal lesion in segment VIII of liver (white arrow) which is hypointense on T1 and hyperintense on T2W images suggestive of HCC. A regenerative nodule is also seen in segment II (black arrow) which appears hyperintense on T1 and hypointense on T2W images.

(HCC: hepatocellular carcinoma; MR: magnetic resonance; T1W: T1-weighted; T2W: T2-weighted)

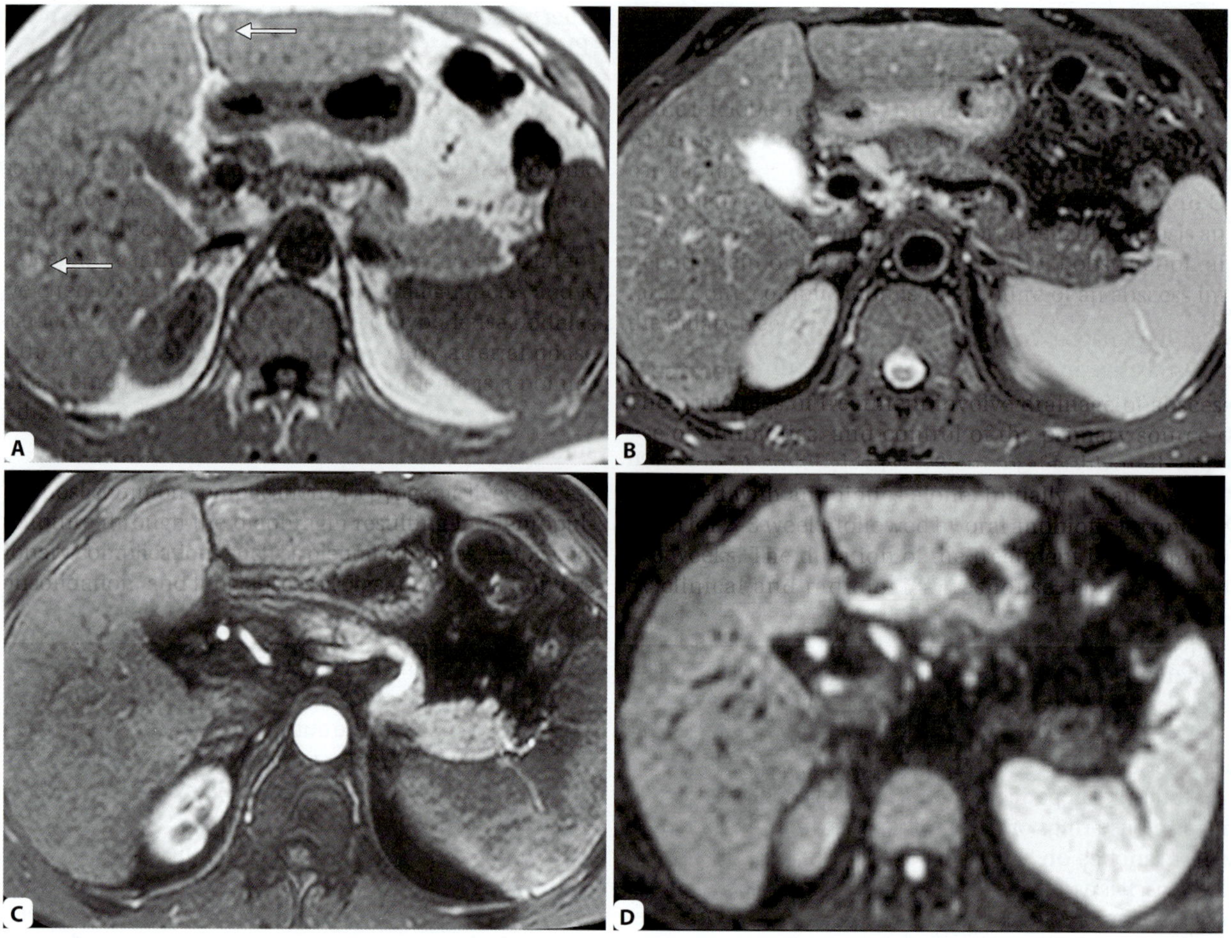

FIGS. 22A TO D: MRI findings of dysplastic nodules: In a patient of viral hepatitis-related chronic liver disease showing irregular liver surface with multiple nodules (arrows) appearing (A) hyperintense on T1W, (B) isointense on T2W, (C) with no arterial phase enhancement. (D) Diffusion-weighted image shows no areas of restricted diffusion.

(MRI: magnetic resonance imaging; T1W: T1-weighted; T2W: T2-weighted)

TABLE 4: MRI features of nodules in liver cirrhosis.

	T1W	T2W	Arterial phase	Venous/delayed phase
Regenerating nodule	Hyperintense	Iso- to hypointense	Isointense to liver	Isointense
Siderotic nodule	Hypointense	Hypointense	Iso- to hypointense	Iso- to hypointense
Low-grade dysplastic nodule	Iso- to hyperintense	Isohypointense	Isointense to liver	No washout
High-grade dysplastic nodule	Iso- to hyperintense	Isohypointense	Hyperenhancing	No washout

(MRI: magnetic resonance imaging; T1W: T1-weighted; T2W: T2-weighted)

agreement with USE, liver biopsy, and other biochemical markers of hepatic fibrosis.[64] The advantages of MRE over USE include the ability to evaluate the entire liver and eliminating the sampling error of USE. Moreover, MRE is unaffected by obesity and presence of ascites, which are known confounders in USE.[65]

CONCLUSION

Diffuse liver diseases may result from a variety of causes, the most important among which are alcoholic liver disease and viral hepatitis due to their wide prevalence and complications such as cirrhosis and HCC. Imaging plays an important role in diagnosis as well as management of diffuse liver diseases. Multiphase CECT remains the workhorse modality; however, MRI with its superior contrast resolution and higher sensitivity for lesion detection and characterization is the modality of choice in indeterminate lesions on CT. New modalities such as USE and various quantitative MR techniques including MRI elastography have further enhanced the imaging evaluation of diffuse liver diseases.

REFERENCES

1. Ludwig J, Viggiano TR, McGill DB, Oh BJ. Nonalcoholic steatohepatitis: Mayo Clinic experiences with a hitherto unnamed disease. Mayo Clin Proc. 1980;55(7):434-8.
2. Schaffner F, Thaler H. Nonalcoholic fatty liver disease. Prog Liver Dis. 1986;8:283-98.
3. Rinella ME, Lazarus JV, Ratziu V, Francque SM, Sanyal AJ, Kanwal F, et al. A multisociety Delphi consensus statement on new fatty liver disease nomenclature. J Hepatol. 2023;79(6):1542-56.
4. Carr RM. Embracing the principles of practice transfer to get the word out on the new metabolic dysfunction-associated steatotic liver disease nomenclature. Hepatol Commun. 2023;7(10):e0275.
5. Skoczylas K, Pawełas A. Ultrasound imaging of the liver and bile ducts - expectations of a clinician. J Ultrason. 2015;15(62):292-306.
6. Borges VF de AE, Diniz ALD, Cotrim HP, Rocha HLOG, Andrade NB. Sonographic hepatorenal ratio: a noninvasive method to diagnose nonalcoholic steatosis. J Clin Ultrasound. 2013;41(1):18-25.
7. De Lédinghen V, Vergniol J, Capdepont M, Chermak F, Hiriart JB, Cassinotto C, et al. Controlled attenuation parameter (CAP) for the diagnosis of steatosis: A prospective study of 5323 examinations. J Hepatol. 2014;60(5):1026-31.
8. Karlas T, Petroff D, Sasso M, Fan JG, Mi YQ, Lédinghen V, et al. Individual patient data meta-analysis of controlled attenuation parameter (CAP) technology for assessing steatosis. J Hepatol. 2017;66(5):1022-30.
9. Sirli R, Sporea I. Controlled Attenuation Parameter for Quantification of Steatosis: Which Cut-Offs to Use? Can J Gastroenterol Hepatol. 2021;2021:6662760.
10. Ogino Y, Wakui N, Nagai H, Igarashi Y. (2021). The ultrasound guided attenuation parameter is useful in quantification of hepatic steatosis in non-alcoholic fatty liver disease. [online] Available from https://onlinelibrary.wiley.com/doi/full/10.1002/jgh3.12615 [Last accessed June, 2024].
11. Imajo K, Toyoda H, Yasuda S, Suzuki Y, Sugimoto K, Kuroda H, et al. Utility of Ultrasound-Guided Attenuation Parameter for Grading Steatosis With Reference to MRI-PDFF in a Large Cohort. Clin Gastroenterol Hepatol. 2022;20(11):2533-41.e7.
12. Zhao Y, Jia M, Zhang C, Feng X, Chen J, Li Q, et al. Reproducibility of ultrasound-guided attenuation parameter (UGAP) to the noninvasive evaluation of hepatic steatosis. Sci Rep. 2022;12(1):2876.
13. Bende F, Sporea I, Şirli R, Bâldea V, Lazăr A, Lupuşoru R, et al. Ultrasound-Guided Attenuation Parameter (UGAP) for the quantification of liver steatosis using the Controlled Attenuation Parameter (CAP) as the reference method. Med Ultrason. 2021;23(1):7-14.
14. Park SH, Kim PN, Kim KW, Lee SW, Yoon SE, Park SW, et al. Macrovesicular hepatic steatosis in living liver donors: use of CT for quantitative and qualitative assessment. Radiology. 2006;239(1):105-12.
15. Pickhardt PJ, Park SH, Hahn L, Lee SG, Bae KT, Yu ES. Specificity of unenhanced CT for non-invasive diagnosis of hepatic steatosis: implications for the investigation of the natural history of incidental steatosis. Eur Radiol. 2012;22(5):1075-82.
16. Hamer OW, Aguirre DA, Casola G, Lavine JE, Woenckhaus M, Sirlin CB. Fatty Liver: Imaging Patterns and Pitfalls. Radiographics. 2006;26(6):1637-53.
17. Lee SW, Park SH, Kim KW, Choi EK, Shin YM, Kim PN, et al. Unenhanced CT for assessment of macrovesicular hepatic steatosis in living liver donors: comparison of visual grading with liver attenuation index. Radiology. 2007;244(2):479-85.
18. Boyce CJ, Pickhardt PJ, Kim DH, Taylor AJ, Winter TC, Bruce RJ, et al. Hepatic steatosis (fatty liver disease) in asymptomatic adults identified by unenhanced low-dose CT. AJR Am J Roentgenol. 2010;194(3):623-8.
19. Starekova J, Hernando D, Pickhardt PJ, Reeder SB. Quantification of Liver Fat Content with CT and MRI: State of the Art. Radiology. 2021;301(2):250-62.
20. Singh D, Das CJ, Baruah MP. Imaging of non alcoholic fatty liver disease: A road less travelled. Indian J Endocrinol Metab. 2013;17(6):990-5.
21. Venbrux AC, Freidman AC. Diffuse hepatocellular diseases. In: Friedman AC, Aachman AH (Eds). Radiology of the Liver, Biliary Tract and Pancreas. St Louis: Mosby Year Book; 1994. pp. 49-167.
22. Caussy C, Reeder SB, Sirlin CB, Loomba R. Non-invasive, quantitative assessment of liver fat by MRI-PDFF as an endpoint in NASH trials. Hepatology. 2018;68(2):763-72.
23. Reeder SB, Hu HH, Sirlin CB. Proton Density Fat-Fraction: A Standardized MR-Based Biomarker of Tissue Fat Concentration. J Magn Reson Imaging. 2012;36(5):1011-4.
24. Idilman IS, Aniktar H, Idilman R, Kabacam G, Savas B, Elhan A, et al. Hepatic Steatosis: Quantification by Proton Density Fat Fraction with MR Imaging versus Liver Biopsy. Radiology. 2013;267(3):767-75.
25. Reeder SB, Cruite I, Hamilton G, Sirlin CB. Quantitative Assessment of Liver Fat with Magnetic Resonance Imaging and Spectroscopy. J Magn Reson Imaging. 2011;34(4):729-49.
26. Hoad CL, Palaniyappan N, Kaye P, Chernova Y, James MW, Costigan C, et al. A study of T_1 relaxation time as a measure of liver fibrosis and the influence of confounding histological factors. NMR Biomed. 2015;28(6):706-14.
27. Breit HC, Block KT, Winkel DJ, Gehweiler JE, Henkel MJ, Weikert T, et al. Evaluation of liver fibrosis and cirrhosis on the basis of quantitative T1 mapping: Are acute inflammation, age and liver volume confounding factors? Eur J Radiol. 2021;141:109789.
28. Eddowes PJ, McDonald N, Davies N, Semple SIK, Kendall TJ, Hodson J, et al. Utility and cost evaluation of multiparametric magnetic resonance imaging for the assessment of non-alcoholic fatty liver disease. Aliment Pharmacol Ther. 2018;47(5):631-44.
29. Bastati N, Feier D, Wibmer A, Traussnigg S, Balassy C, Tamandl D, et al. Noninvasive differentiation of simple steatosis and steatohepatitis by using gadoxetic acid-enhanced MR imaging in patients with nonalcoholic fatty liver disease: a proof-of-concept study. Radiology. 2014;271(3):739-47.
30. Smits LP, Coolen BF, Panno MD, Runge JH, Nijhof WH, Verheij J, et al. Noninvasive Differentiation between Hepatic Steatosis and Steatohepatitis with MR Imaging Enhanced with USPIOs in Patients with Nonalcoholic Fatty Liver Disease: A Proof-of-Concept Study. Radiology. 2016;278(3):782-91.

31. Jang JK, Jang HJ, Kim J, Kim TK. Focal fat deposition in the liver: diagnostic challenges on imaging. Abdom Radiol (NY). 2017;42(6):1667-78.
32. Gore RM. Diffuse Liver disease. In: Gore RM, Levine MS (Eds). Textbook of Gastrointestinal Radiology, 3rd edition. Philadelphia: Saunders Elsevier; 2008. pp. 1685-729.
33. Tchelepi H, Ralls PW, Radin R, Grant E. Sonography of diffuse liver disease. J Ultrasound Med. 2002;21(9):1023-32; quiz 1033-4.
34. Danet IM, Semelka RC, Braga L. MR imaging of diffuse liver disease. Radiol Clin North Am. 2003;41(1):67-87.
35. Martin DR, Semelka RC. Magnetic resonance imaging of the liver: review of techniques and approach to common diseases. Semin Ultrasound CT MR. 2005;26(3):116-31.
36. Semelka RC, Braga L, Armao D. Liver. In: Semelka RC (Ed). Abdominal Pelvic MRI. New York, Wiley-Liss; 2002. pp. 33-318.
37. Kauffman JM, Grace ND. Hemochromatosis. In: Weinstein WM, Hawkey CJ, Bosch J (Eds). Clinical Gastroenterology and Hepatology. Philadelphia: Elsevier–Mosby; 2005. pp. 659-64.
38. Bassett ML, Halliday JW, Powell LW. Value of hepatic iron measurements in early hemochromatosis and determination of the critical iron level associated with fibrosis. Hepatology. 1986;6(1):24-9.
39. Engle MA, Erlandson M, Smith CH. Late Cardiac Complications Of Chronic, Severe, Refractory Anemia With Hemochromatosis. Circulation. 1964;30:698-705.
40. Olivieri NF, Brittenham GM, Matsui D, Berkovitch M, Blendis LM, Cameron RG, et al. Iron-chelation therapy with oral deferiprone in patients with thalassemia major. N Engl J Med. 1995;332(14):918-22.
41. Werner S, Krauss B, Haberland U, Bongers M, Starke U, Bakchoul T, et al. Dual-energy CT for liver iron quantification in patients with haematological disorders. Eur Radiol. 2019;29(6):2868-77.
42. Luo XF, Xie XQ, Cheng S, Yang Y, Yan J, Zhang H, et al. Dual-Energy CT for Patients Suspected of Having Liver Iron Overload: Can Virtual Iron Content Imaging Accurately Quantify Liver Iron Content? Radiology. 2015;277(1):95-103.
43. Gandon Y, Olivié D, Guyader D, Aubé C, Oberti F, Sebille V, et al. Non-invasive assessment of hepatic iron stores by MRI. Lancet Lond Engl. 2004;363(9406):357-62.
44. Gitlin JD. Wilson's disease. In: Zakim D, Boyer TD (Eds). Hepatology: A Textbook of Liver Disease. Philadelphia: Saunders; 2003. pp. 1273-88.
45. Vargas O, Faraoun SA, Dautry R, Guerrache Y, Woimant F, Hamzi L, et al. MR imaging features of liver involvement by Wilson disease in adult patients. Radiol Med (Torino). 2016;121(7):546-56.
46. Hope TA, Ohliger MA, Qayyum A. MR imaging of diffuse liver disease: from technique to diagnosis. Radiol Clin North Am. 2014;52(4):709-24.
47. Karagiannidis A, Karavalaki M, Koulaouzidis A. Hepatic sarcoidosis. Ann Hepatol. 2006;5(4):251-6.
48. Lee D, Shaffer K. Concentric Rings: Updated CT Appearance of Hepatic Schistosomiasis Mansoni. Radiol Case Rep. 2015;1(4):134-9.
49. Pagola Serrano MA, Vega A, Ortega E, González A. Computed tomography of hepatic fascioliasis. J Comput Assist Tomogr. 1987;11(2):269-72.
50. Lanzi A, Gianstefani A, Mirarchi MG, Pini P, Conti F, Bolondi L. Liver AL amyloidosis as a possible cause of high liver stiffness values. Eur J Gastroenterol Hepatol. 2010;22(7):895-7.
51. Srinivasan S, Tan YQ, Teh HS, Lee PJ, Khoo RN. Primary hepatic amyloidosis presenting as nodular masses on the background of diffuse infiltration and extreme liver stiffness on MR elastography. J Gastrointest Liver Dis JGLD. 2014;23(4):437-40.
52. Sherlock S, Dooley J. Hepatic cirrhosis. In: Sherlock S, Dooley J (Eds). Diseases of the Liver and Biliary System, 11th edition. Oxford: Blackwell Science; 2002. pp. 365-8.
53. Bedossa P, Poynard T. An algorithm for the grading of activity in chronic hepatitis C. The METAVIR Cooperative Study Group. Hepatology. 1996;24(2):289-93.
54. Kleiner DE, Brunt EM, Van Natta M, Behling C, Contos MJ, Cummings OW, et al. Design and validation of a histological scoring system for nonalcoholic fatty liver disease. Hepatology. 2005;41(6):1313-21.
55. Goyal AK, Pokharna DS, Sharma SK. Ultrasonic diagnosis of cirrhosis: reference to quantitative measurements of hepatic dimensions. Gastrointest Radiol. 1990;15(1):324.
56. Di Lelio A, Cestari C, Lomazzi A, Beretta L. Cirrhosis: diagnosis with sonographic study of the liver surface. Radiology. 1989;172(2):389-92.
57. Ravindran N, Agarwal A, Li F, Thuluvath PJ. Liver ultrasound in cirrhosis is inadequate for hepatocellular carcinoma surveillance compared to magnetic resonance imaging. [online] Available from https://onlinelibrary.wiley.com/doi/full/10.1002/lci2.57 [Last accessed June, 2024].
58. Ziol M, Handra-Luca A, Kettaneh A, Christidis C, Mal F, Kazemi F, et al. Noninvasive assessment of liver fibrosis by measurement of stiffness in patients with chronic hepatitis C. Hepatology. 2005;41(1):48-54.
59. Giorgio A, Montesarchio L, Gatti P, Amendola F, Matteucci P, Santoro B, et al. Contrast-Enhanced Ultrasound: a Simple and Effective Tool in Defining a Rapid Diagnostic Work-up for Small Nodules Detected in Cirrhotic Patients during Surveillance. J Gastrointest Liver Dis. 2016;25(2):205-11.
60. Giorgio A, Amoroso P, Lettieri G, Fico P, de Stefano G, Finelli L, et al. Cirrhosis: value of caudate to right lobe ratio in diagnosis with US. Radiology. 1986;161(2):443-5.
61. Sangster GP, Previgliano CH, Nader M, Chwoschtschinsky E, Heldmann MG. MDCT Imaging Findings of Liver Cirrhosis: Spectrum of Hepatic and Extrahepatic Abdominal Complications. HPB Surg. 2013;2013:129396.
62. Brancatelli G, Baron RL, Federle MP, Sparacia G, Pealer K. Focal Confluent Fibrosis in Cirrhotic Liver: Natural History Studied with Serial CT. Am J Roentgenol. 2009;192(5):1341-7.
63. Okazaki H, Ito K, Fujita T, Koike S, Takano K, Matsunaga N. Discrimination of alcoholic from virus-induced cirrhosis on MR imaging. AJR Am J Roentgenol. 2000;175(6):1677-81.
64. Kim D, Kim WR, Talwalkar JA, Kim HJ, Ehman RL. Advanced fibrosis in nonalcoholic fatty liver disease: noninvasive assessment with MR elastography. Radiology. 2013;268(2):411-9.
65. Singh S, Venkatesh SK, Wang Z, Miller FH, Motosugi U, Low RN, et al. Diagnostic performance of magnetic resonance elastography in staging liver fibrosis: a systematic review and meta-analysis of individual participant data. Clin Gastroenterol Hepatol. 2015;13(3):440-51.e6.

CHAPTER

9

Sapna Singh, Anjali Prakash, Satyam

Nonneoplastic Focal Lesions of Liver

INTRODUCTION

A focal liver lesion, defined as a distinct abnormality within the liver, is often detected incidentally and can be neoplastic or nonneoplastic.[1] Advances in imaging technologies, particularly multidetector computed tomography (MDCT) and 3T magnetic resonance imaging (MRI), have significantly enhanced the detection and characterization of these lesions, aiding in distinguishing various nonneoplastic focal lesions which vary from developmental to inflammatory.[2,3] The radiologist's acumen in interpreting both typical and atypical imaging attributes is essential for accurate diagnosis, guiding appropriate patient management and mitigating unnecessary anxiety.[4]

DEVELOPMENTAL LESIONS

Hepatic Cyst

Hepatic cysts are benign developmental lesions that do not communicate with the biliary tree. These are observed in 5–18% of the general population with a notable female preponderance (female:male ratio of 5:2).[5] They represent the most common liver lesions. Differentiating primary hepatic cysts from other cystic liver masses is essential for accurate diagnosis and management.

Pathology

Hepatic cyst is also called bile duct cyst and is believed to originate from hamartomatous tissue.[6] Hepatic cyst is a solitary unilocular cyst with a lining composed of a single primary layer of cuboidal bile duct epithelium. Its wall is usually <1 mm thick and is composed of fibrous tissue.

Clinical Features

These are usually asymptomatic and discovered incidentally at routine imaging. Large hepatic cysts can cause compression of adjacent intrahepatic ducts and may rarely be symptomatic.[6]

Imaging Features

Ultrasonography (USG): On USG, a simple hepatic cyst is seen as a well-defined, anechoic, round lesion with smooth, imperceptible walls and posterior acoustic enhancement **(Figs. 1 and 2)**. While thin septations might be observed, features like thick septations, calcifications, nodules, and debris suggest a more complex cyst. US is nearly 100% accurate in diagnosing simple hepatic cysts.[7]

Computed tomography (CT): On CT, a simple hepatic cyst presents as a well-defined, round-to-oval intrahepatic lesion with water-like attenuation (10–15 HU).[8] A homogeneous appearance, sharp margins, and a thin wall without internal septa, nodules, or contrast enhancement are the characteristic imaging findings of a simple hepatic

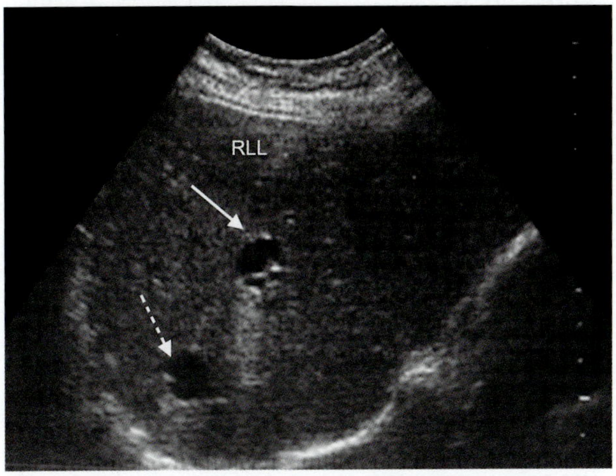

FIG. 1: Conventional ultrasound (US) showing hypoechoic lesions in the right lobe of liver (RLL) with posterior acoustic enhancement and enhanced through transmission—simple liver cysts.

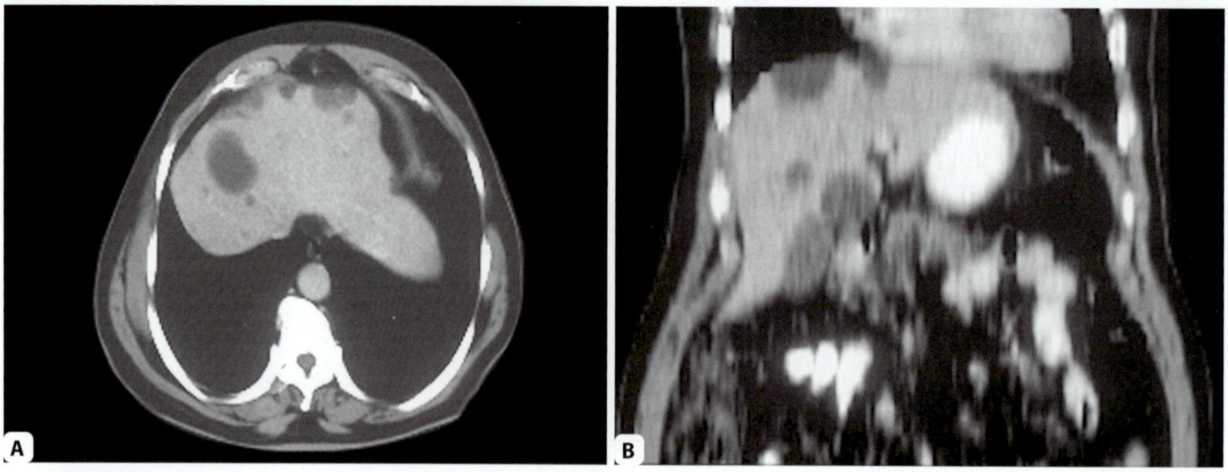

FIGS. 2A AND B: Computed tomography (CT) image revealing multiple hypodense cysts in the liver—simple liver cysts.

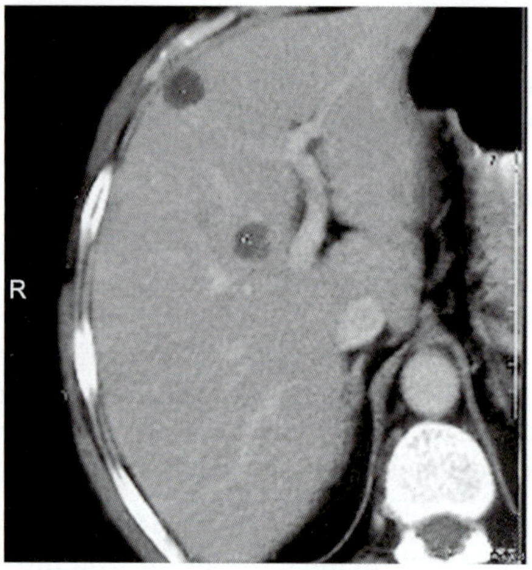

FIG. 3: Computed tomography (CT) image revealing small hypodense lesions in the liver having water attenuation—multiple simple liver cysts.

cyst **(Fig. 3)**. In contrast, a complicated cyst may exhibit internal debris or enhancement, indicative of hemorrhage or infection.

MRI: On MRI, simple hepatic cysts are characterized by well-defined, homogeneous fluid signal intensities, appearing hypointense on T1-weighted (T1W) and markedly hyperintense on T2-weighted (T2W) images **(Figs. 4A and B)**.[9] The increase in signal intensity on higher T2W aids in distinguishing these cysts from metastatic diseases. There is usually no restriction of diffusion signal on diffusion-weighted imaging (DWI), with simple cysts demonstrating decreasing signal intensity with increasing *b* values and appearing strongly hyperintense on the apparent diffusion coefficient (ADC) sequences. The simple cysts may show variations in T1 signal intensity with the presence of proteins or hemorrhage within the cyst, potentially causing a hyperintense appearance on T1W images.

Polycystic Liver Disease

When >10 cysts are present in the liver parenchyma, a polycystic disease should be considered. About 70% of patients with polycystic liver disease have autosomal-dominant polycystic kidney disease, while liver involvement occurs in 30–40% of patients with polycystic kidney disease.[10] Von Meyenburg's complexes and increased fibrous tissue are increasingly seen in the liver which surrounds the cysts in polycystic liver and autosomal-dominant polycystic kidney disease.

Ciliated Hepatic Foregut Cyst

These congenital cysts are histologically similar to bronchogenic and esophageal duplication cysts.[11] They are typically rare and solitary, predominantly located in the medial segment of the left lobe's anterosuperior margin or intersegmentally, often causing a bulge on the liver's outer contour, with a characteristic subcapsular placement. Mostly asymptomatic, they are usually discovered incidentally, though in rare cases, they may cause obstructive jaundice or portal hypertension due to their mass effect on the biliary system or portal vein. Typically, these are unilocular and under 3 cm in size. The diagnosis via CT can be challenging due to fluid attenuation. MRI provides more variable signal intensity on T1W images based on their serous or mucinous content. They appear homogeneously hyperintense on T2W images, with no restricted diffusion or contrast enhancement.[10] Although malignancy is rare, any irregular wall thickness or solid components should raise concerns. Due to this slight risk of malignant transformation, surgical excision is often recommended.

Peribiliary Cyst

The peribiliary cysts represent cystic dilatation of the glands in the bile duct walls. These are associated with cirrhosis, specifically with portal hypertension. On imaging, these

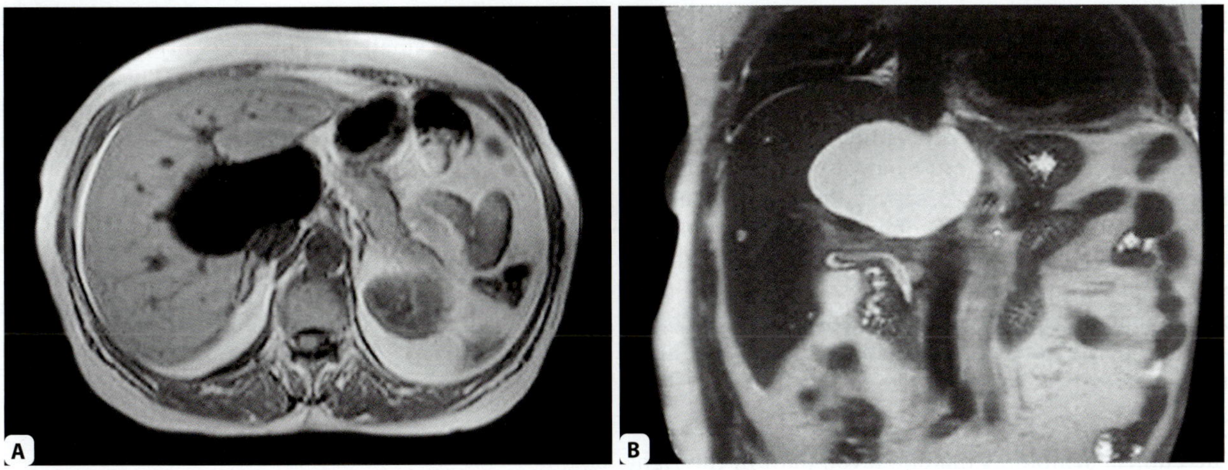

FIGS. 4A AND B: (A) T1-weighted magnetic resonance (T1W MR) image showing a hepatic cyst as a homogeneous sharply marginated hypointense lesion. (B) T2-weighted (T2W) image reveals the cysts to be markedly hyperintense. Few smaller cysts are also seen in the periphery of the right lobe.

cysts are seen as anechoic structures along the portal tracts and may be mistaken for a dilated bile duct. Presence of thin septa within the cysts helps to differentiate these cysts from dilated bile duct.[11] CT shows hypoattenuating structures and MR reveals the cystic nature of the lesions on T2W images.

Bile Duct Hamartoma

Bile duct hamartoma is also called Von Meyenburg's complexes. They are cystic lesions (CL) typically <1.5 cm in diameter diffusely scattered throughout the liver parenchyma.[12]

Pathology

They do not communicate with the biliary tree and are believed to originate from the embryonic bile ducts that fail to involute. They are considered a part of the spectrum of fibropolycystic liver disease that also includes congenital hepatic fibrosis, autosomal-dominant polycystic liver disease, and Caroli disease. Histologically, they consist of focally disordered collections of bile ducts surrounded by abundant fibrous stroma.

Clinical Features

These are usually asymptomatic and are discovered incidentally at imaging.

Imaging Features

On USG, they appear as multiple tiny hyperechoic lesions with comet tail echoes resulting in heterogenous echo pattern of hepatic parenchyma. The CT and MR demonstrate the cystic nature of the lesions, hypointense on T1 and markedly hyperintense on T2W images. They are seen as multiple cysts diffusely scattered in both lobes of the liver and typically measuring 0.5–1.5 cm in diameter and usually showing no enhancement. Very rarely, thin rim enhancement corresponding to the compressed liver parenchyma is seen. At MR cholangiography, no communication with the biliary tree is seen. No enhancement is seen even with the hepato-specific contrast agents as they lack communication with the biliary tree.

On DWI, biliary hamartomas show no evidence of restricted diffusion and behave as simple hepatic cysts, showing no increased signal with increasing "*b*" values and appearing hyperintense on ADC sequences.

Differential Diagnosis

Bile duct hamartomas need to be differentiated from multiple simple cysts. Simple hepatic cysts have a regular outline, while bile duct hamartomas exhibit irregular outline. Hamartomas are typically <1.5 cm in diameter and occur without any renal involvement.

INFECTIVE LESIONS

Bacterial Infections

The bacterial infections in liver are further classified as pyogenic abscess and bacterial granulomatous disease. The pyogenic abscesses are usually polymicrobial. *Escherichia coli* and *Klebsiella pneumoniae* are the most common isolated pathogens. Other organisms seen are *Streptococcus*, *Staphylococcus*, and anaerobes. Bacterial granulomatous diseases are commonly caused by *Mycobacterium tuberculosis* and rarely caused by Brucellosis and *Bartonella* species.

Pyogenic Liver Abscess

A liver abscess can arise through multiple pathways, with the biliary route being the most prevalent due to cholangitis from obstructive biliopathy. Other routes include phlebitis of the portal or superior mesenteric vein secondary to appendicitis, diverticulitis, pancreatitis, and other gastrointestinal (GI) infections. A direct extension from contiguous organs, arterial septicemia secondary to osteomyelitis, endocarditis, pneumonitis, or a post-traumatic or an iatrogenic cause may also be the source of a liver abscess. Cryptogenic abscesses, often seen in diabetic patients, lack a clear source of infection. Biliary-origin abscesses are typically multiple and affect both liver lobes, whereas portal vein-related abscesses are usually solitary, predominantly in the right lobe. Pyogenic abscesses do not show gender preference and mainly affect middle-aged individuals.

Clinical Feature

The clinical symptoms include fever, pain in the right upper quadrant, nausea, vomiting, and malaise. A tender hepatomegaly is seen with leukocytosis being the most common laboratory abnormality.

Imaging Features

Plain film: Elevation of the right hemidiaphragm, hepatomegaly, right pleural effusion, and atelectasis may be seen in case of a large abscess.

USG: Ultrasound (US) can detect hepatic abscesses as small as 1.5 cm with a sensitivity of about 90%. They appear as well-defined lesions with thick, irregular walls **(Fig. 5)**. They are variable in echogenicity and are seen as anechoic in 50%, hyperechoic in 25%, or hypoechoic in 25% cases.[13] Early lesions are hyperechoic and have well-defined margins. Debris, septations, fluid–fluid level, and an air–fluid level may also be seen. Echogenic foci with posterior reverberation artifacts are seen with gas-producing organisms.

CT: On CT scans, abscesses are seen as low-attenuation lesions with a characteristic peripheral rim enhancement **(Figs. 6A and B)**.[14] On administration of intravenous (IV) contrast, a "double target sign" corresponding to perilesional edema[9] and a "cluster sign" representing coalescence of smaller lesions (<2 cm) to form a large abscess are the characteristic features **(Figs. 7 and 8)**.[15] An air–fluid level which is a specific sign of an abscess is seen in <20% of cases and may indicate an enteric communication.

MRI: These are seen as well-defined, rounded lesions hypointense on T1W images and hyperintense on T2W images with intense peripheral rim enhancement on administration of contrast **(Figs. 9A and B)**. Peripheral edema seen as a high signal on T2W images is seen in only one third of the cases.[16] DWI of pyogenic abscesses shows a restricted pattern owing to the high cellularity and viscosity of pus.

Other Features

Liver abscesses can cause transient hepatic attenuation or signal intensity difference **(Fig. 10)**.[17] Gas formation is

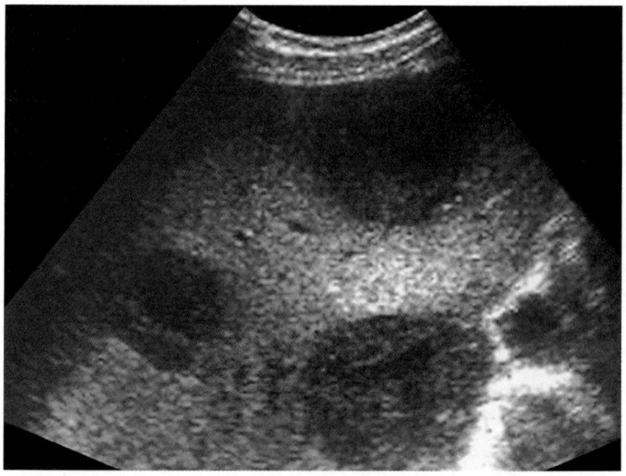

FIG. 5: Ultrasound (US) scan showing three lesions in the liver with well-defined walls and echoes within giving a solid appearance—pyogenic liver abscesses.

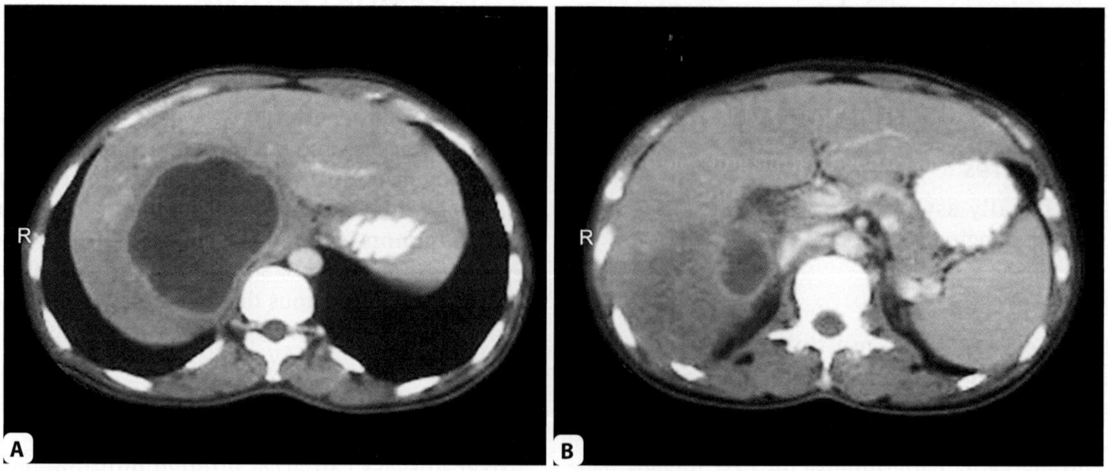

FIGS. 6A AND B: Contrast-enhanced computed tomography (CT) showing irregular hypodense lesions in the liver with enhancing rim—pyogenic liver abscesses.

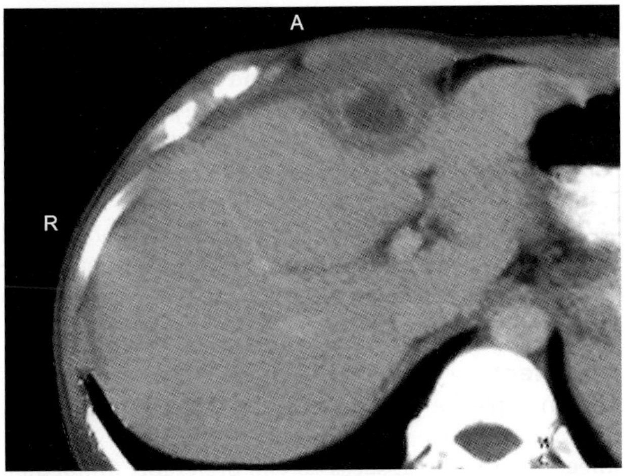

FIG. 7: Contrast-enhanced computed tomography (CT) showing a hypodense lesion with perilesional edema giving a "double-target sign"—pyogenic liver abscess.

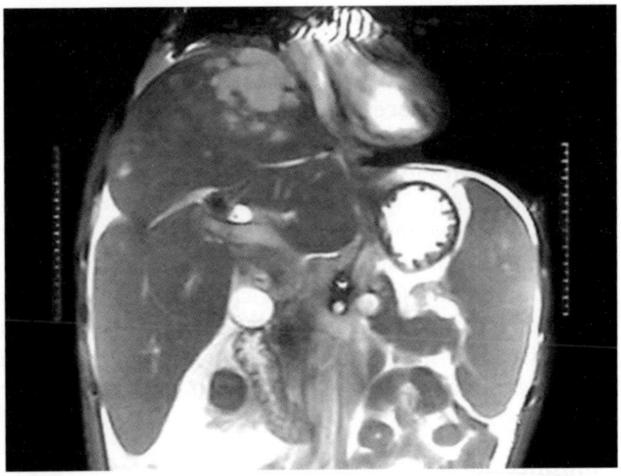

FIG. 8: Magnetic resonance (MR) image showing multiple small abscesses coalescing into a single cavity—"the cluster sign"—pyogenic liver abscesses.

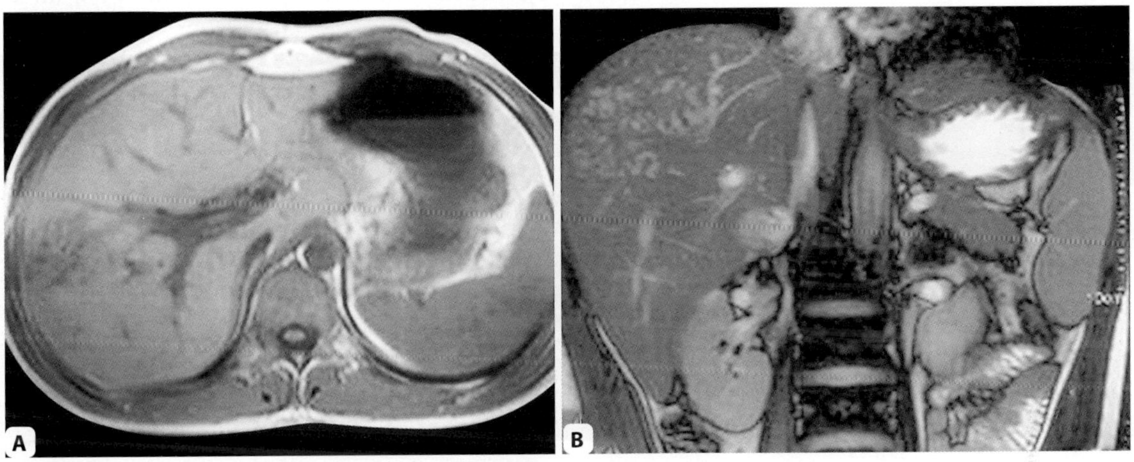

FIGS. 9A AND B: (A) T1-weighted magnetic resonance (MR) image showing an ill-defined area hypointense in signal in the right lobe of liver. (B) T2-weighted image showing the area to have a high signal with multiple small lesions clustering together—liver abscess.

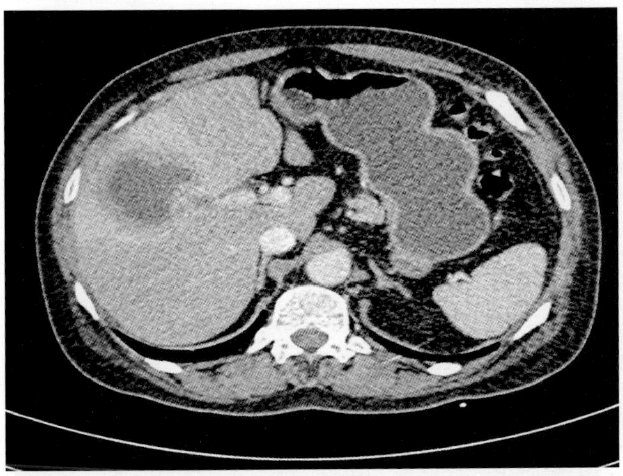

FIG. 10: Contrast-enhanced computed tomography (CT) shows an abscess in the right lobe of liver. There is a geographic area of hyperenhancement peripheral to the abscess compared to the other segments, suggesting transient hepatic attenuation difference (THAD).

seen in an abscess caused by *Klebsiella* infections, giving bubbles or air-fluid levels. *Klebsiella pneumoniae* infections exhibit a distinct "turquoise sign," characterized by slender, branching bands resembling turquoise.[18]

Differential Diagnosis

Pyogenic liver abscesses need to be primarily differentiated from primary or secondary hepatic tumors, amebic abscesses, and hepatic candidiasis. The clinical context and patient history are crucial for an accurate diagnosis.

A transient perilesional enhancement, more commonly seen with pyogenic abscesses, can help distinguish these from hepatic tumors. The presence of an inflammatory capsule with a double-target appearance and progressive outer layer uptake on imaging usually favors an abscess over a neoplasm. Absence of perilesional edema, focal calcification, and nodularity of the lesion wall favors a necrotic tumor over an abscess. When imaging alone cannot differentiate, aspiration or biopsy is required.

A necrotic hepatocellular carcinoma (HCC) with venous invasion can mimic a hepatic abscess complicated by cruoric venous thrombosis. Features such as luminal expansion, arterial phase intraluminal enhancement, and restricted diffusion suggest a tumoral thrombosis.

Amebic liver abscesses (ALAs) are usually unilocular and solitary, involving right lobe of liver with associated ascending colon and caecal wall thickening, while pyogenic liver abscesses are multiple and may not be associated with bowel thickening.

Hepatic candidiasis is seen in patients receiving intensive chemotherapy for hematological malignancies and is characterized by multiple hypoechoic/hypodense nodules in the liver and spleen and showing early arterial phase enhancement on CT. Associated neutropenia is a pointer in the diagnosis.

Complications

The most common complication of a pyogenic liver abscess is rupture through the diaphragm resulting in pleuropulmonary complications such as pleural effusions, empyema, consolidation, and lung abscess **(Figs. 11A to C)**. Rupture into the peritoneal cavity is another serious complication which can be recognized as loculated perihepatic abscess and diffuse peritonitis **(Figs. 12A and B)**. Abscesses located in the left lobe may rarely rupture into the pericardial cavity which is a serious life-threatening complication leading to cardiac tamponade or shock **(Figs. 13A to D)**. Rarely, there is formation of a hepatobronchial fistula **(Figs. 14A to C)**. Vascular complications such as portal vein thrombosis and hepatic vein or inferior vena cava (IVC) obstruction are rare. A rare complication is the rupture of an abscess into the biliary tree.

Treatment

The principles of treatment involve drainage of abscess, use of antibiotics, and control of the primary source of infection. A small abscess <3 cm, preferably unilocular, is treated with antibiotics alone. Initially, IV antibiotic is given for 2–3 weeks followed by oral antibiotic for another 4–8 weeks. The duration of the treatment is determined by clinical and radiological response. For an abscess

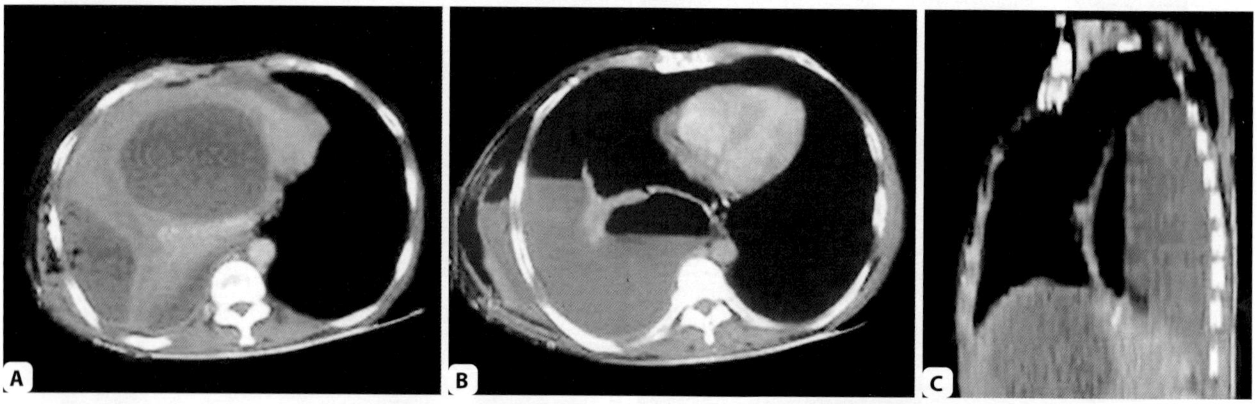

FIGS. 11A TO C: (A) Contrast-enhanced computed tomography (CT) showing two abscesses in the liver with one of lesions showing air loculi and indistinct margins. (B) A large hydropneumothorax is seen in the right pleural cavity. (C) Multiplanar reconstruction showing the communication between the abscess and the right hydropneumothorax—ruptured liver abscess.

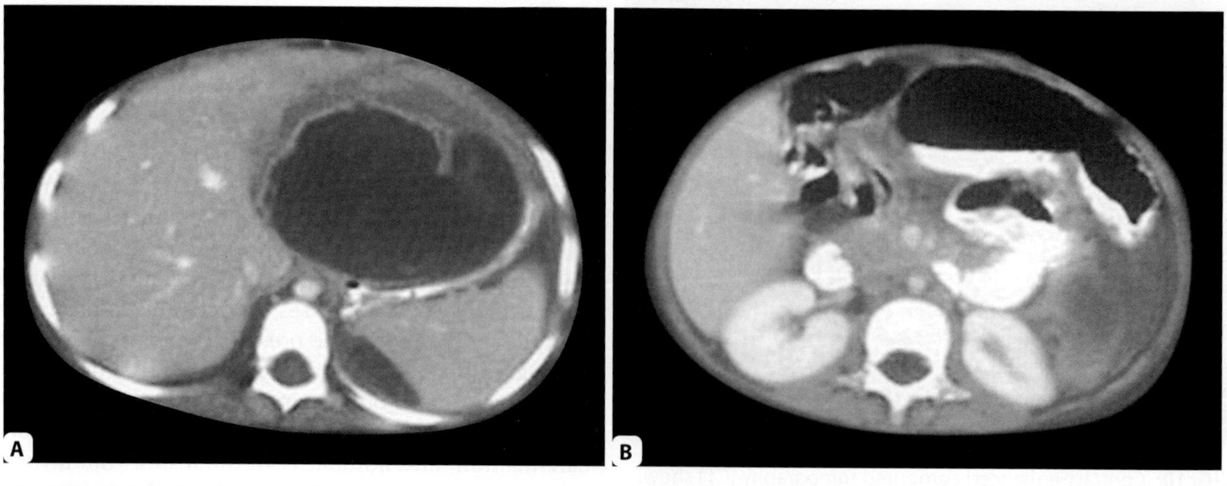

FIGS. 12A AND B: (A) Contrast-enhanced computed tomography (CT) showing a large hypodense lesion with enhancing rim in the left lobe of liver. Perilesional edema is noted. Fluid is seen in the perihepatic and perisplenic region. (B) Fluid is seen in the peritoneal cavity—intraperitoneal rupture of abscess.

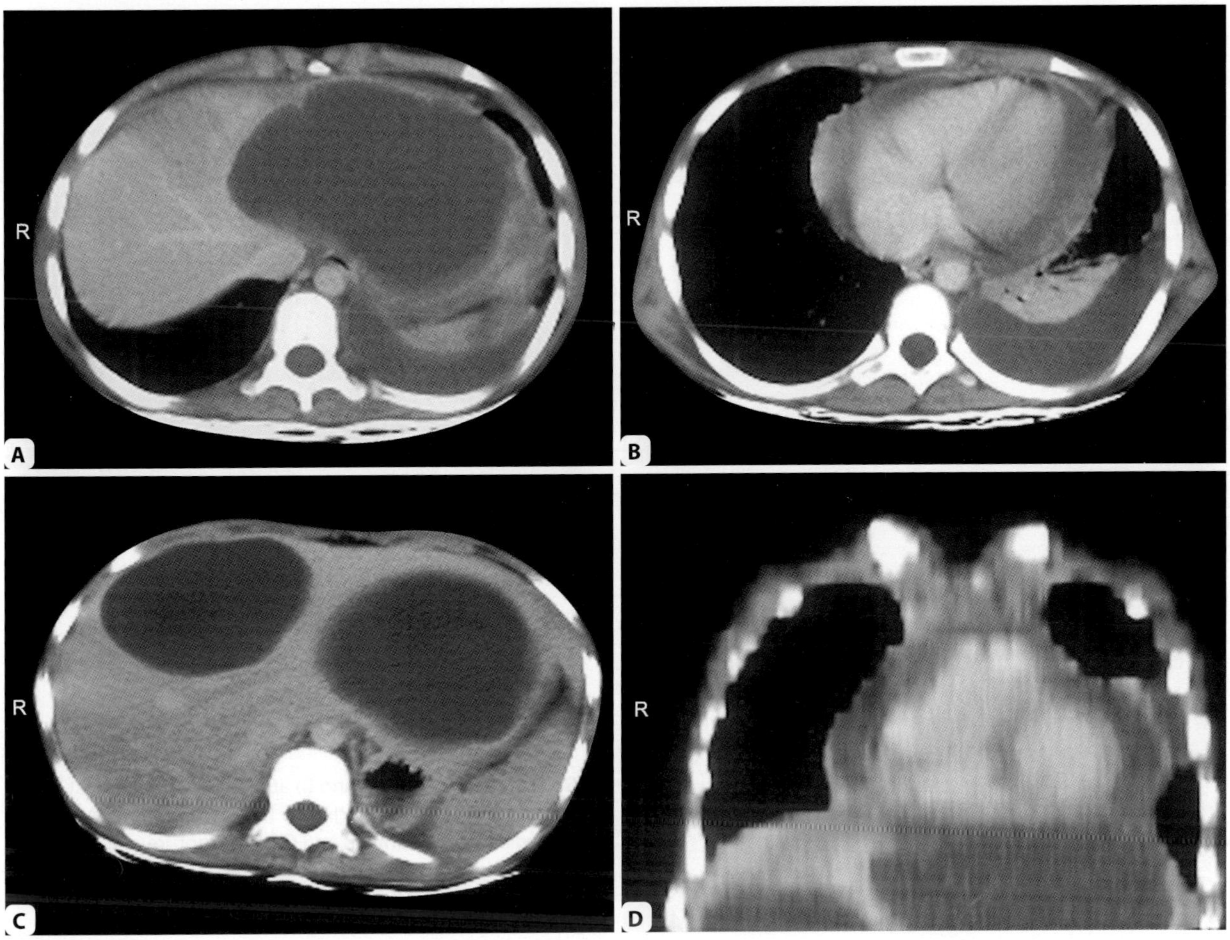

FIGS. 13A TO D: Contrast-enhanced computed tomography (CT) sections reveal large abscesses in the liver with rupture of the left lobe abscess into the pericardium with pericardial and left pleural effusion—pericardial rupture of liver abscess.

< 5 cm and a small abscess < 3 cm not resolving to medical treatment, image-guided percutaneous aspiration can be performed, both for diagnostic and management purposes. This helps in obtaining material for culture and analysis, determining the causative agent and guiding appropriate antibiotic therapy. For all accessible abscesses > 5 cm and unilocular, image-guided percutaneous drainage with catheter placement is done. Surgical drainage is recommended for cases involving peritonitis, abscess rupture, large abscesses in challenging anatomical locations, or when surgery is needed for other reasons.

Hepatic Tuberculosis

Tuberculosis (TB) is a major cause of mortality and morbidity in the tropical countries and its incidence is increasing with the emergence of human immunodeficiency virus (HIV) and acquired immunodeficiency syndrome (AIDS). Hepatic TB accounts for <1% of all tubercular infections,[19] being uncommon due to the low oxygen tension in the liver. The most common route of spread to the liver is hematogenous secondary to a tubercular focus elsewhere in the body, resulting in a miliary pattern. Spread can also occur via the portal vein in cases of involvement of the GI tract or via the lymphatic route in case of rupture of tuberculous lymph node along the portal tract.

Pathology

The histological hallmark of the disease is granuloma formation. Both caseating and noncaseating granulomas are seen. Presence of caseating epithelioid granuloma on histopathology is diagnostic of the disease.

Clinical Features

It most commonly affects people in their second decade of life with a 2:1 male preponderance. The disease is often discovered incidentally, while the patient is being evaluated for nonspecific symptoms. Patients may sometimes present with fever, weight loss, anorexia, and upper abdominal pain. Rarely, patients may present with jaundice due to biliary obstruction caused by periportal adenopathy. Laboratory investigations may reveal elevated hepatic enzymes, though an isolated elevation of alkaline phosphatase rules out the possibility of hepatic parenchymal involvement in TB.

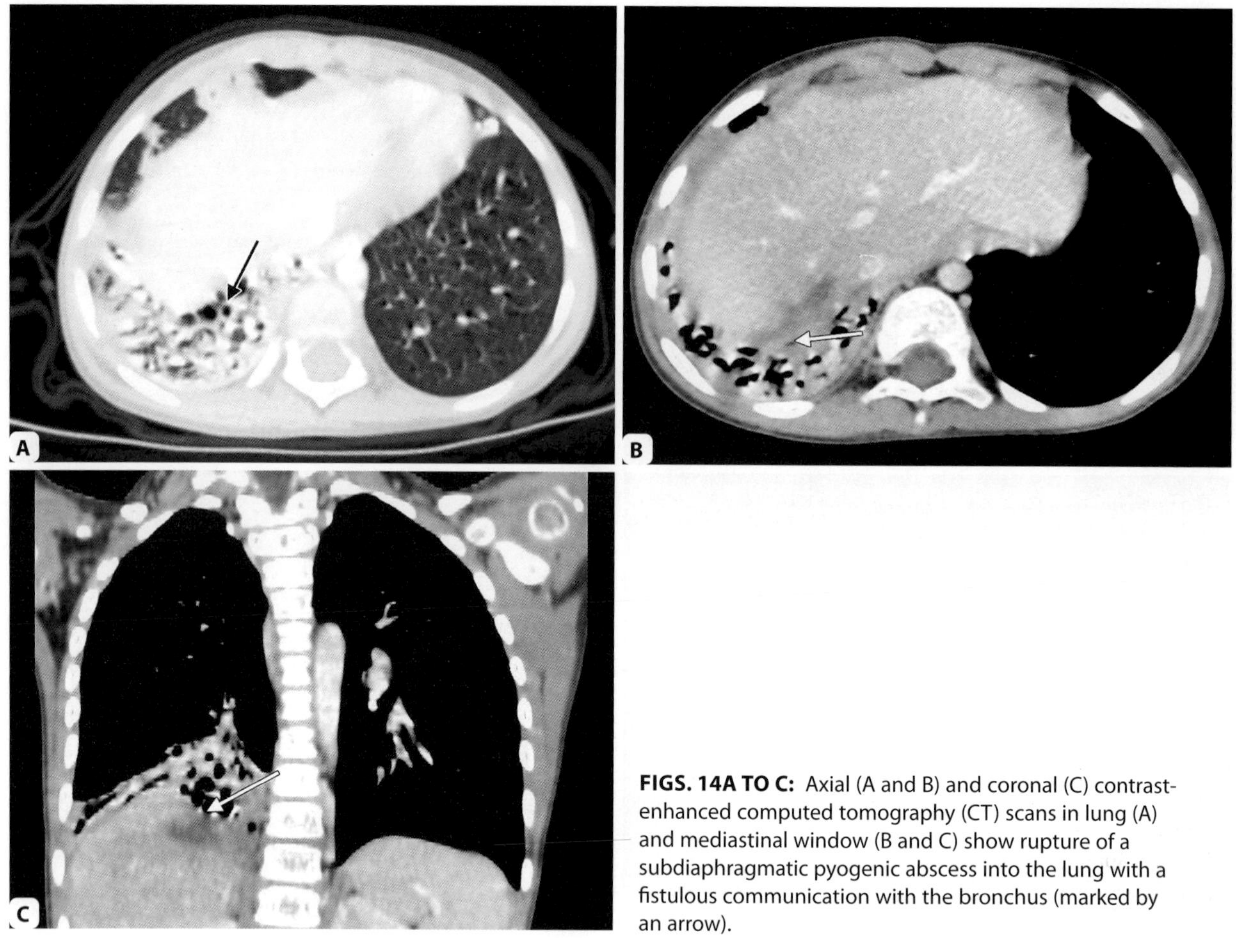

FIGS. 14A TO C: Axial (A and B) and coronal (C) contrast-enhanced computed tomography (CT) scans in lung (A) and mediastinal window (B and C) show rupture of a subdiaphragmatic pyogenic abscess into the lung with a fistulous communication with the bronchus (marked by an arrow).

Imaging Features

The disease can be classified into three forms—parenchymal, serohepatic, and tubercular cholangitis. The parenchymal form can be further subdivided as the micronodular and the macronodular pattern.[20]

Micronodular form/Miliary form Micronodular form is the most common form of hepatic TB and usually occurs secondary to a hematogenous dissemination.[21] A concomitant involvement of the lung may or may not be seen.

The miliary hepatic lesions are multiple in number and are randomly distributed throughout the hepatic parenchyma. They are usually too small (<2 cm) to be resolved by sonography and hepatomegaly may be the only imaging finding observed on US. A diffuse hypoechoic pattern of the liver parenchyma may be seen on sonography as the lesions are hypoechoic compared to the adjacent parenchyma.

On CT, the micronodular pattern is seen as microabscesses with a central hypodensity with peripheral rim enhancement upon administration of contrast **(Figs. 15A and B)**. Chronic lesions may calcify and the lesions may appear as multiple echogenic foci with distal acoustic shadowing on sonography or as multiple calcific foci on CT. This imaging appearance may mimic metastases, leukemic infiltration, or lymphoma or fungal infections.

Magnetic resonance imaging is more sensitive in detecting these diffuse miliary granulomas which appear hypointense on T1W and hyperintense on T2W images.

18-fluorodeoxyglucose positron emission tomography (FDG-PET) may at times provide the only clue to the diagnosis of hepatic TB. There may be a diffuse intense uptake of 18F-FDG. This is known as hepatic super scan appearance and may be the only clue for the diagnosis of miliary hepatic TB as other imaging findings may not reveal any abnormality.

The differential diagnosis includes various other infections such as fungal, brucellosis, *Pneumocystis* jirovecii, sarcoidosis, and Hodgkin's disease, as all of them cause granuloma formation in liver.

Macronodular form The macronodular form is less common than the micronodular variety.[22] Tubercular macronodules are also called pseudotumoral TB, tuberculomas, or tubercular abscesses. These macronodules form as a result of conglomeration of miliary granulomas and may be seen as solitary or multiple complex hepatic masses. The size of the lesion is usually >2 cm. When solitary, the macronodular form may mimic a primary neoplastic lesion or other infective lesions.

On US, there are usually four patterns: (1) Heterogeneously hypoechoic, (2) heterogeneously hyperechoic

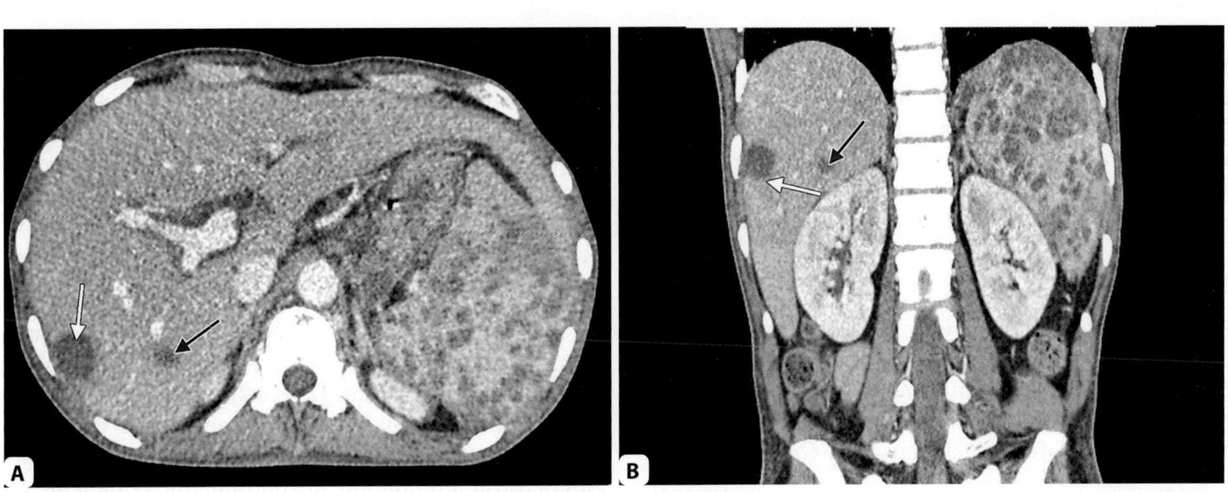

FIGS. 15A AND B: (A) Axial and (B) Coronal contrast computed tomography (CT) show multiple hypodense lesions in the liver and spleen. The lesions are variable varying in size from <2 cm to a large lesion (>2 cm) in the right lobe of liver—micronodular and macronodular hepatic tuberculosis (TB) with multiple splenic tuberculomas.

with anechoic center, (3) predominantly hyperechoic, and (4) hypoechoic with hyperechoic center showing target sign. Sometimes, multiple micronodular lesions coalesce to form a macronodular lesion seen as a multiloculated cystic mass giving a "cluster sign."[23]

On CT, the imaging appearance of the lesion depends on the stage of a hepatic granuloma. The noncaseating granulomas appear as hypodense lesions with surrounding perilesional edema with minimal peripheral contrast enhancement **(Figs. 15A and B)**. The appearance of caseating granuloma depends on the degree and location of internal liquefaction. A tubercular abscess may have a "honeycomb appearance" due to multiple enhancing septae or "cluster sign" due conglomeration of cysts mimicking a pyogenic abscess. Rarely, it may mimic a simple cyst due to extensive necrosis.

On MRI, macronodules have a varying appearance depending on the stage of disease. On T2W image, the tubercular lesions may appear as hypointense, isointense, or hyperintense lesions with a peripheral hypointense rim. These show peripheral or rim enhancement on postcontrast scans known as a "ringed appearance." The peripheral/rim or ring enhancement pattern is helpful in differentiating macronodular form from a neoplastic lesion such as a HCC and hypervascular metastasis. The perilesional edema seen around the tuberculomas is a helpful differentiating feature from cystic metastasis.

Complications such as perihepatic abscess or infective peritonitis may be seen when the macronodular hepatic abscess ruptures. Portal vein thrombosis and consequent portal hypertension are also rare complications of tubercular hepatic abscess.

Serohepatic TB: This rare variety gives rise to a "frosted liver" appearance, owing to a predominant involvement of the subserosal plane of the liver, often inseparable from the fibrous Glisson's capsule. Imaging reveals multiple peripherally located, conglomerated hypodense lesions with an overlying thickened enhancing capsule simulating "sugar coating."[20] There may be associated bulky necrotic gastrohepatic and retroperitoneal adenopathy.

Tubercular cholangitis: This can occur due to a primary involvement of the biliary tree or secondary to an extrinsic compression by enlarged periportal lymph nodes. Imaging findings can vary from bile duct thickening to biliary dilatation and strictures with resultant obstructive biliopathy.[24] Other associated findings include calcification along biliary duct wall and hepatic parenchyma, a characteristic imaging feature of tubercular cholangitis seen on US and CT, which helps to differentiate it from cholangiocarcinoma or sclerosing cholangitis.

As the clinical features of hepatic TB are nonspecific, various imaging findings and concomitant involvement of lymph nodes, spleen, or lung parenchyma by TB may help to narrow the list of differentials. At times, percutaneous aspiration or tissue sampling is necessitated when a noninvasive definitive diagnosis cannot be achieved by imaging alone. Hepatic tuberculomas commonly appear as large epithelioid tumors with conglomerate tubercles and central caseation. Langerhans-type giant cells surrounded by lymphohistiocytic cells, plasma cells, and eosinophils may also be seen. It is important to target the central necrotic center of the TB abscess, as one is more likely to aspirate tubercle bacilli from it. A polymerase chain reaction (PCR) assay in the liver biopsy specimen also helps in establishing the diagnosis. The diagnosis of hepatic TB can be done with laparoscopic biopsy in superficially located lesions.

Treatment

The treatment of choice is antitubercular medication for 1 year. Sometimes, percutaneous drainage of tubercular abscess is also performed, accompanied by local infusion of antitubercular drug into the abscess.

Mustard et al.[25] have proposed several criteria for a successful drainage of a tubercular abscess cavity. These criteria include: (1) A unilocular appearance, (2) accessibility that allows placement of a large-bore catheter, and (3) a sterile compartment. However, in the case of multilocular abscesses where the locules are intercommunicating, a percutaneous drainage can be attempted.

Parasitic Infections

The parasitic infections of liver are further subclassified into: (1) Infection of hepatic parenchyma caused by *Entamoeba histolytica* and *Echinococcus* species; (2) infection of hepatic vessels caused by *Schistosoma* species; and (3) infection of bile ducts caused by *Fasciola* species.

Amebic Abscess

Caused by the protozoan *Entamoeba histolytica*, an ALA is the most common extraintestinal manifestation of amebiasis. The organism may reach the liver from the colon, through the portal vein, via lymphatics, or by direct extension.[26]

Pathology

The cavitary amebic abscess occurs as the liver parenchyma is destroyed. Initially, the lesion contains necrotic tissue including the viable organism. As the lesion becomes larger, central cavitation is apparent with the active organism present in the necrotic tissue lining the cavity. Surrounding this layer is an inflammatory zone of hepatic parenchyma invaded by the organisms. Centrally, the cavity is often filled with a thick fluid resembling "anchovy paste." Frequently solitary, the abscess is most commonly located in the right lobe due to the venous drainage from the typically infected right colon, via the superior mesenteric vein to the portal vein, which preferentially flows into the right lobe of liver **(Figs. 16A and B)**.

Imaging Feature

US: Amebic abscess is seen as a round to oval, solitary lesion in the right lobe of liver, exhibiting fine low-level echoes and usually in continuity with the diaphragm **(Figs. 17A and B)**. A round or oval shape and a hypoechoic appearance with fine echoes are sonographic findings that favor an amebic over a pyogenic liver abscess.[27] **Table 1** shows the differentiating features of amebic and pyogenic liver abscesses.

CT scan: An amebic abscess appears as a low-attenuation lesion and shows evidence of rim enhancement upon contrast administration **(Fig. 18)**. Lesions in the early stage of development have a solid appearance, while older lesions appear cystic.[28] A target appearance due to an outer rim of lower attenuation surrounding the enhancing rim may be seen.

Based on the CT morphology, all amebic abscesses are categorized into three types: Types I, II, and III.[29,30]

Type I abscesses are identified by an absent or incomplete wall, ragged edges, multiple septa, and little or no enhancement. These findings typically indicate an early abscess stage, often seen in severe cases with poor response to medical therapy, necessitating percutaneous drainage. Clinically, these abscesses are associated with severe symptoms, abnormal laboratory results, and a higher risk of complications.

Type II abscesses are characterized by a complete wall with rim enhancement and a relatively smooth outline, indicating a healing phase responsive to drug treatment. Often, a double-target sign is visible, consisting of an inner ring of enhancement due to inflammatory hyperemia and an outer hypodense ring due to localized edema. This stage contrasts with type I, where edema tends to be more widespread. The type II pattern, however, is nonspecific and shares features with pyogenic abscesses.

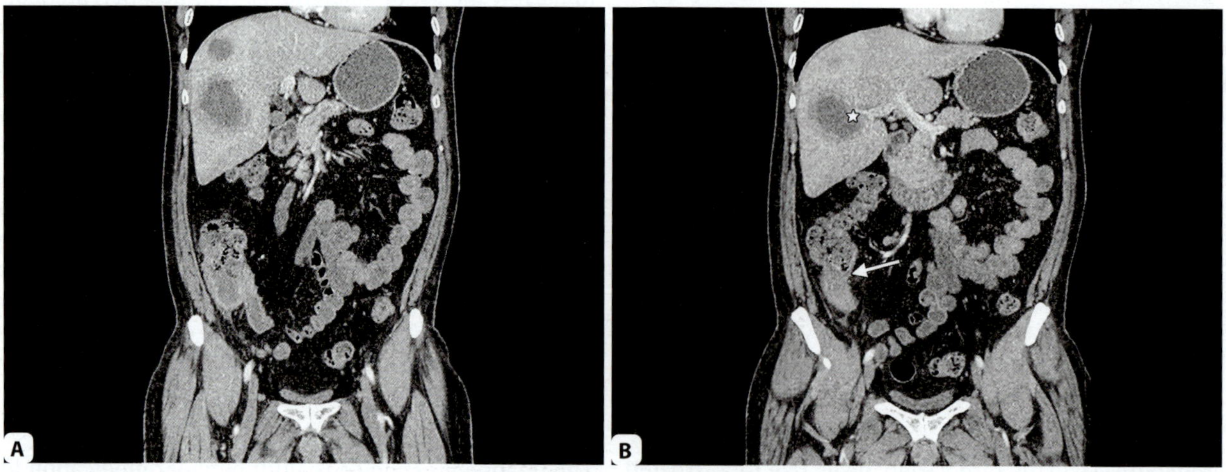

FIGS. 16A AND B: Contrast-enhanced computed tomography (CT) of the abdomen shows two well-defined, peripherally enhancing lesions in the right lobe of liver and circumferential mural thickening of the caecum suggestive of amebic liver abscesses with amebic colitis.

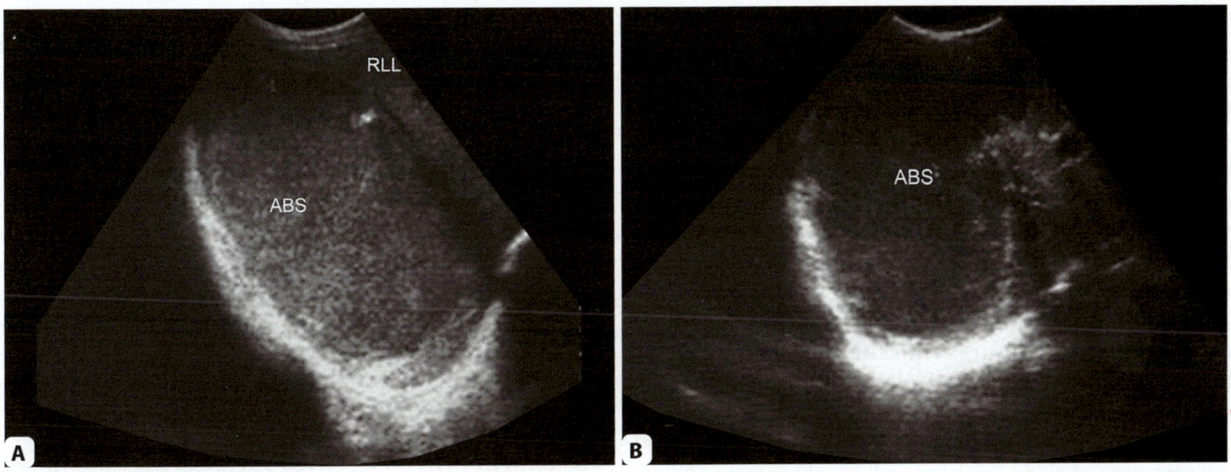

FIGS. 17A AND B: US showing a round hypoechoic lesion with low internal echoes within, with absence of a well-defined abscess wall—amebic liver abscess.
(RLL: right lobe of liver; US: ultrasound)

TABLE 1: Differentiating features of amebic and pyogenic liver abscess.

Variables	ALA	PLA
Causative agent	*E. histolytica*	Polymicrobial, *K. pneumoniae*, *E. coli*, etc.
Ultrasound appearance	Solitary, usually in right lobe, round-to-oval in shape, hypoechoic with low-level internal echoes	Usually, multiple, variable-size hypoechoic lesions, thick walled with internal echo
CT scan appearance	Hypodense round lesion with peripheral enhancement and associated caecal wall thickening	Hypodense lesion with peripheral enhancing wall with perilesional edema showing "double target sign" or "cluster sign." Usually, no associated bowel thickening is seen
MRI appearance	It is hyperintense on T2W with central diffusion restriction	It is hyperintense on T2W with diffusion restriction

(ALA: amebic liver abscess; CT: computed tomography; *E. coli*: *Escherichia coli*; *E. histolytica*: *Entamoeba histolytica*; *K. pneumoniae*: *Klebsiella pneumoniae*; MRI: magnetic resonance imaging; PLA: pyogenic liver abscess; T2W: T2-weighted)

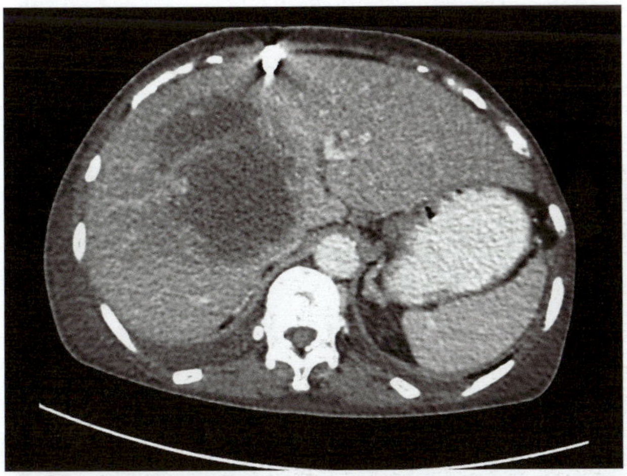

FIG. 18: Contrast-enhanced computed tomography (CECT) axial section shows a large, solitary, well-defined, peripherally enhancing lesion in the right lobe of liver—amebic liver abscess.

Type III abscesses also show a complete wall but are distinguished by a smoother wall that does not enhance with contrast. These abscesses usually develop in cases where the abscess content does not fully resorb after treatment, often appearing as round, thick-walled CL with homogenous content on sonographic studies. This can lead to confusion with benign hepatic cysts. Clinically and biochemically inactive, type III abscesses typically do not require treatment unless they are large enough to cause pain by stretching the liver capsule, in which case percutaneous drainage may be necessary.

MRI: The abscess cavity is seen to have a low signal on T1W and a high signal on T2W images. The central cavity is often surrounded by a rim of high signal intensity, corresponding to hyperemic reactive zone. On contrast administration, this reactive zone shows evidence of enhancement.

Complications

Rupture The most serious complication of an ALA is rupture with incidences reported between 6 and 40%. ALA most commonly ruptures into the thoracic cavity or intraperitoneal space. Less frequently, the abscess may rupture into hollow viscera such as the stomach, duodenum, or colon. Among all types of ruptures, the most severe but fortunately rare is rupture into the pericardium.

Intrathoracic rupture: Pleural empyema, lung abscess, and hepatobronchial fistula

Pleuropulmonary rupture occurs in 7–20% of patients with ALA.[31-33] Abscesses below the diaphragm may rupture in the pleural space, causing amebic empyema **(Figs. 19A and B)**. It is the most frequent intrathoracic complication. Loculations and septations on US indicate amebic empyema. It is important to differentiate amebic empyema from pleural effusions, which are reactionary and resolve without intervention.

Another complication is lung consolidation or abscess when an abscess ruptures into the lung parenchyma, through the diaphragm and pleura. The lung abscess may communicate with bronchi or pleura leading to the formation of a hepatobronchial or bronchopleural fistula.[34] The presence of air in the lung or liver abscess or pleural collections confirms these fistulas.

Intraperitoneal rupture: This occurs in about 7% of cases according to some sources.[31-33] Intraperitoneal ruptures can be classified into two types based on imaging: Contained and free ruptures.[33] A contained rupture typically results in a localized fluid collection near the liver, often in the subphrenic or subhepatic space. This type generally has a favorable prognosis and is more common than free rupture. In contrast, a free rupture leads to fluid spreading throughout the peritoneal cavity, potentially causing generalized peritonitis and having a poorer prognosis. Differentiating between these types is crucial because free ruptures require more intensive and prolonged treatment.

Biliary complications Biliary complications are a common reason for treatment failure, occurring in up to 27% of refractory cases.[28,29] These complications arise from either ductal communication with the abscess or external compression by a large abscess which can be detected by US or CT. The size and location of an abscess can offer clues about potential biliary complications; large (>5–10 cm) and centrally located abscesses near the porta hepatis are more prone to these complications than smaller, subcapsular ones. Aggressive abscesses can destroy liver parenchyma and damage bile ducts, leading to ductal communications. These communications are often subtle and ductal dilatation may not be visible on imaging. The diagnosis frequently comes during percutaneous drainage when bilious fluid is initially aspirated or bile appears persistently thereafter. In rare cases, especially with large and aggressive abscesses, the abscess may rupture into the central bile ducts, leading to duct dilation. Such instances may be confirmed through endoscopic retrograde cholangiopancreatography (ERCP) or magnetic resonance cholangiopancreatography (MRCP).

Secondary bacterial infection Although ALA are typically sterile, secondary bacterial infections complicate 10–20% of cases and recent findings suggest that this incidence might be higher.[34] This complication should be considered in cases that do not respond to treatment, especially when accompanied by persistent high fever and significant leukocytosis (>20,000/μL). The pathway for secondary infection is either from intestinal flora through portal vein or bacterial superinfection, often following unsuccessful needle aspiration or inadequate catheter drainage, which typically occurs when the abscesses are already walled off, presenting symptoms of chronic, indolent disease.

Vascular complications Vascular complications include venous thrombosis, venous compression, and arterial aneurysm.

Venous thrombosis is a complication in this condition and may affect both the portal and hepatic veins, often occurring in the smaller segmental or subsegmental branches. Hepatic vein thrombosis can extend into the IVC **(Figs. 20A and B)** and even reach the right atrium.[35] Although rare, it can lead to a Budd–Chiari-like syndrome. The presence of thrombi in large veins on CT scans can

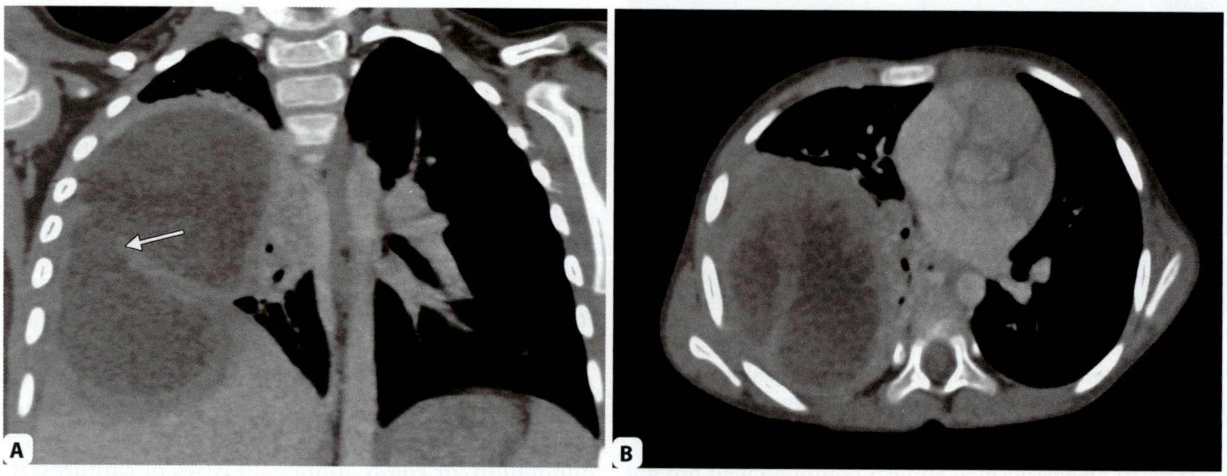

FIGS. 19A AND B: Contrast-enhanced computed tomography (CT) scans showing rupture of a subdiaphragmatic amebic liver abscess through diaphragm into the pleural cavity with adjacent basal atelectasis.

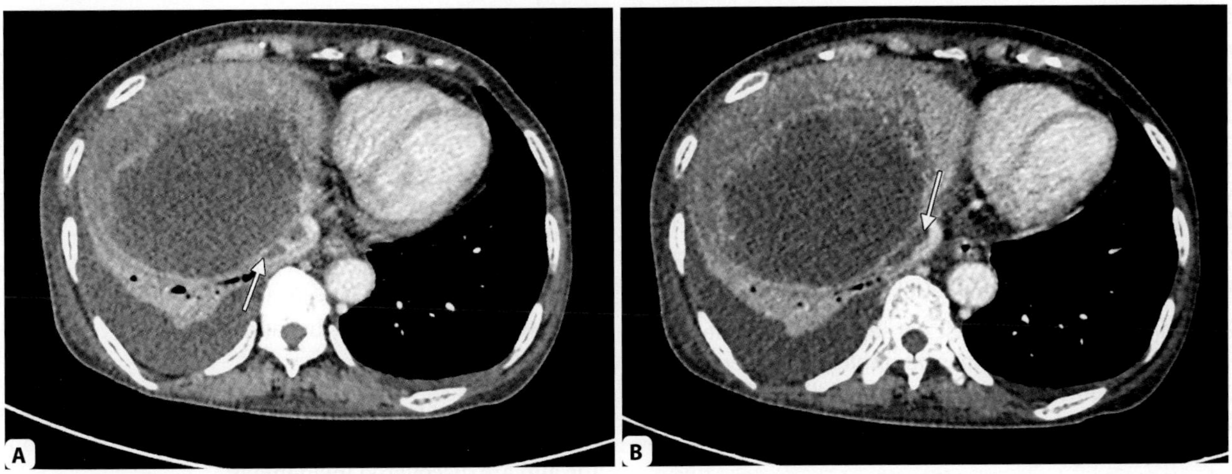

FIGS. 20A AND B: Contrast-enhanced computed tomography (CECT) scans show a large amebic abscess in the right lobe of liver causing compression of the inferior vena cava (IVC) with nonenhancing thrombus within—vascular complication of amebic abscess.

suggest severe ALA and might be indicated by a wedge-shaped hypoattenuating area around the abscess due to thrombosis-led hypoperfusion.

Venous compression is another vascular complication. Compression of the IVC by a large abscess in the caudate lobe can cause leg edema, while portal vein compression near the porta hepatis may lead to splenomegaly and portal hypertension.

Additionally, hepatic artery pseudoaneurysm is a rare complication which requires prompt identification and management to prevent potentially life-threatening outcomes.

Concurrent colitis and perforations Some patients with ALA experience diarrhea and a concurrent colonic involvement is detected in ALA patients undergoing colonoscopy.[36,37] These colonic lesions typically appear as small, discrete ulcers primarily in the cecum or ascending colon, with most of the ulcers localized to the caecum. Contiguous involvement of the appendix (amebic typhloappendicitis) is common. When these ulcers are small and localized, symptoms related to colitis tend to be mild. However, in severe cases, involvement may extend to other segments or lead to caecal perforations. On CT, colitis typically presents as a nonspecific bowel wall thickening **(Figs. 16A and B)**.

Treatment

A definitive diagnosis is generally achieved through a combination of imaging techniques, serological testing, microbial cultures, and percutaneous aspiration findings.

Medical treatment: Unruptured ALA are managed by medical treatment. The drug of choice for the treatment is metronidazole, a nitroimidazole. It is usually followed by luminal amebicide agent such as diloxanide furoate or paromomycin to eradicate the luminal ameba. Aspiration or percutaneous drainage is employed for larger abscesses at risk of rupture or when there is an inadequate response to pharmacological therapy.

Drainage of abscess: The drainage of an abscess is done percutaneously under US or CT guidance either by needle aspiration or by catheter placement depending on the size and number of abscesses.[33]

Indications[33,34]

- Abscess > 5 cm with thin rim of hepatic parenchyma around it
- Impending rupture (thinned parenchyma, i.e., <1 cm) recognized on imaging
- Nonresponse to medical therapy after 3–5 days
- Left lobe liver abscess
- Multiple liver abscesses (to identify the organism)

Percutaneous needle aspiration: It is defined as evacuation or diagnostic sampling of fluid collection with the use of needle (16- or 18-gauge needle) under image guidance, during a single session and removing the needle immediately after aspiration. This helps in obtaining material for culture and analysis, determining the causative agent, and guiding appropriate antibiotic therapy. It is done in abscesses <5 cm with completely liquified content.

Percutaneous drainage with catheter placement: It is defined as catheter placement under image guidance which facilitates the continuous drainage of fluid collections. This procedure aids in locating the fluid collection and ensures the proper placement and maintenance of the drainage system. It can be performed either as a single-stage or as a staged procedure during several sessions. It is the primary intervention for accessible abscesses which are unilocular and >5 cm in size. Under US or CT guidance, a pigtail catheter ranging from 8 to 14 French is placed directly into the abscess cavity to drain the pus under local anesthesia, allowing the contents to drain over several days aided by gravity.[34] Imaging is used to confirm the catheter placement and monitor the drainage process. A pigtail should remain in situ until drainage is minimal. Percutaneous catheter drainage is a more effective technique with a higher success rate than percutaneous aspiration.

Complications

Minor hemorrhage just after intervention, hemorrhage within cavity, or a perihepatic hematoma are few immediate complications. Prolonged catheter drainage can lead to formation of a fistula with the biliary tract. Some cases may develop secondary bacterial infections.

Vascular intervention: In cases of septic thrombophlebitis, endovascular techniques may be employed. Under imaging guidance, thrombolytic agents can be delivered directly to the site of thrombosis or stents may be placed to ensure vascular patency.

Surgical intervention: Surgical drainage is recommended for cases involving peritonitis, abscess rupture, large abscesses in challenging anatomical locations, or when surgery is needed for other reasons. Laparoscopic surgery offers a safe and effective option for patients needing surgical drainage after unsuccessful medical or percutaneous treatments. Preoperative imaging with CT or MRI is critical in planning surgical approach, defining the extent of the disease, and the involvement of other organs.

Hydatid Disease

Echinococcus granulosus (*E. granulosus*) and *Echinococcus multilocularis* (*E. multilocularis*) are responsible for cystic echinococcosis (CE) and alveolar echinococcosis (AE), respectively. *E. granulosus* is more prevalent, but *E. multilocularis* is considered more invasive. **Table 2** elucidates the differentiating features between CE and AE.

Cystic Echinococcosis

Hydatid disease, caused by *E. granulosus,* is also known as cystic echinococcosis. The liver is involved in approximately 75% of cases of echinococcosis, with the right lobe more frequently affected.

TABLE 2: Differentiating features of cystic echinococcosis (CE) and alveolar echinococcosis (AE).

Variables	CE	AE
Elementary lesion	Daughter cyst, internal detached membranes	Microcysts, calcification
Type of growth	Concentric expansion	Vesicle to vesicle, infiltrative spread
Outline of cysts	Well defined	Irregular
Macrocalcification	Peripheral	Internal
Microcalcification	Absent	Present
Biliary dilatation	May be seen	Usually present

Structure of Hydatid Cyst

The hydatid cyst is a trilaminated structure consisting of pericyst, ectocyst, and endocyst. The pericyst is the outermost protective layer made of modified host cells. The ectocyst allows the passage of nutrients, while the endocyst forms the true layer of the cyst, also known as the inner germinal layer. Daughter vesicles (brood capsules), resembling a bunch of grapes, arise from the inner germinal layer. Since the vesicles contain scolices, when they rupture, the scolices pass into the cyst fluid, forming a white sediment known as hydatid sand.[4,38,39]

Clinical Features

Classical symptoms of hydatid disease include abdominal pain and hepatomegaly. The majority may be asymptomatic and are discovered incidentally.

Imaging Features

Plain film: Calcification is seen in 20–30% of hepatic hydatids, usually seen in a curvilinear or a ring-like pattern where the pericyst calcifies. However, calcification of the pericyst does not signify the death of the parasite, which is usually represented by a dense, complete calcification of the cyst.

Ultrasound: USG is crucial for evaluating CE and is classified by the World Health Organization Informal Working Group on Echinococcosis (WHO-IWGE) into six stages, each with distinct imaging characteristics:[40]

1. *CL (Cystic Lesions)*: These are unilocular, anechoic lesions with a barely visible wall **(Fig. 21)**.
2. *CE1*: It features an anechoic lesion with a discernible double-layer wall and contains hydatid sand which moves creating a "snowstorm" sign when the patient repositions.[41,42]
3. *CE2*: It contains multiple septa or cysts so close together that they create a "rosette" appearance within the cyst cavity **(Fig. 22)**.

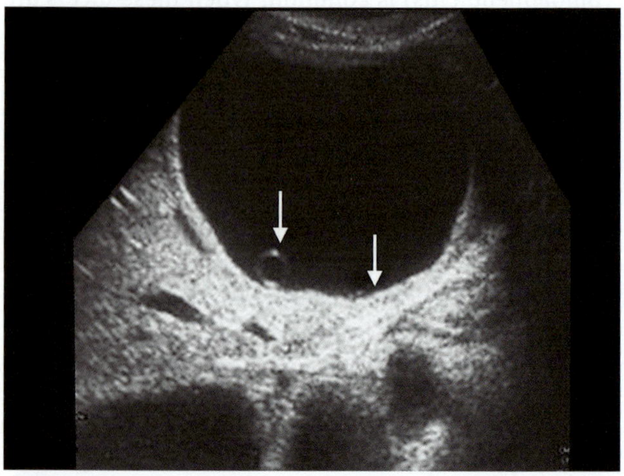

FIG. 21: Ultrasound (US) scan showing a well-defined anechoic cyst with a small cyst within—hydatid cyst.

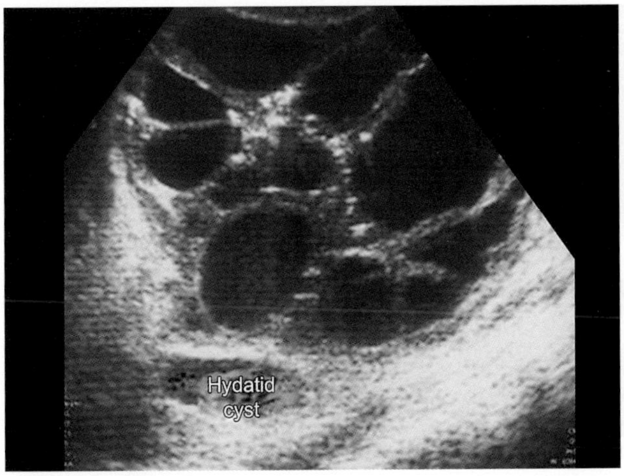

FIG. 22: Ultrasound (US) scan showing a characteristic appearance of cysts enclosed within a cyst giving rise to a honeycomb pattern seen in a hydatid cyst.

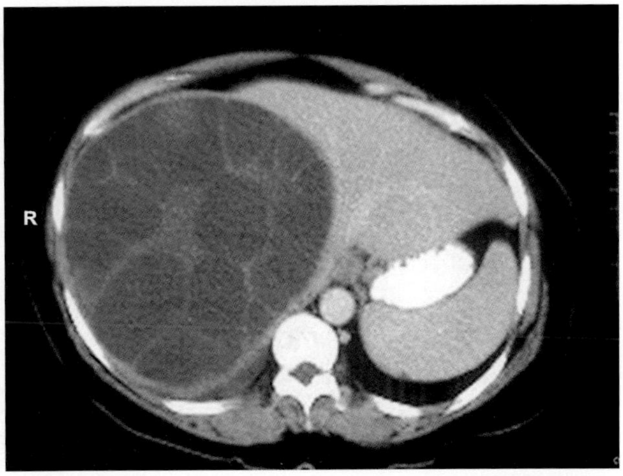

FIG. 24: Computed tomography (CT) scan showing the honeycomb pattern in a hydatid cyst with the multiple septae representing the walls of daughter cysts.

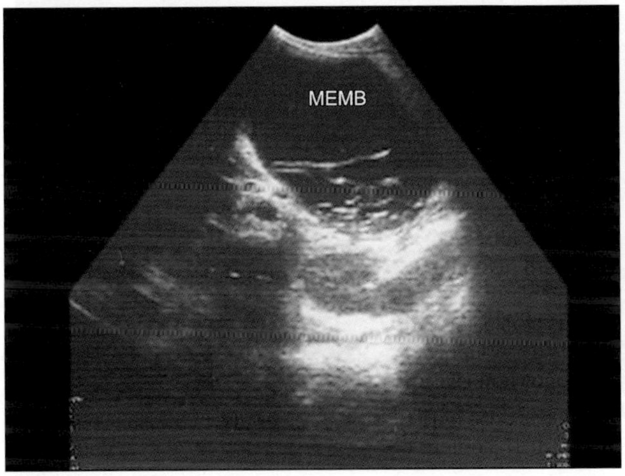

FIG. 23: US scan showing membranes as serpentine linear structures floating within a hydatid cyst.

(MEMB: membrane; US: ultrasound)

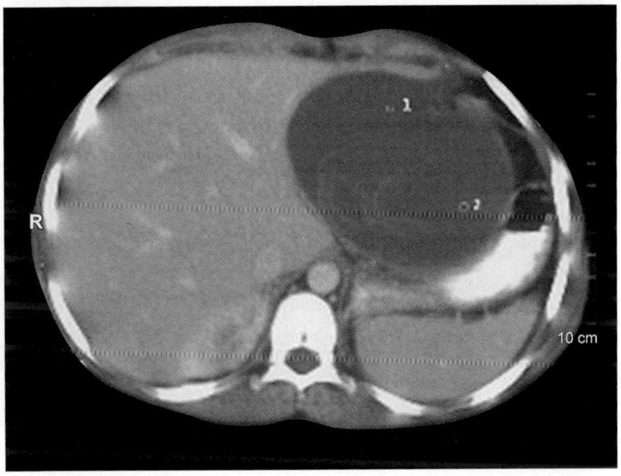

FIG. 25: Contrast-enhanced computed tomography (CECT) scan showing detachment of the laminated membranes from the pericyst seen as linear areas of increased attenuation within the hydatid cyst.

4. *CE3a*: It is characterized by a detached germinal layer floating in the cyst fluid, known as the "water lily" sign **(Fig. 23)**.[38,39]
   CE3b: It contains multiple daughter cysts arranged peripherally in a solid-looking matrix, contrasting with the fluid in CE2.
5. *CE4*: It appears as a heterogeneous mass ranging from hypoechoic to hyperechoic without visible daughter cysts, resembling a "pseudotumor."
6. *CE5*: It shows partial or complete calcification, with a calcified wall appearing as a hyperechoic rim with shadowing.

These US features guide the staging of hydatid cysts and appropriate management strategies. CE1/CE2 represent active stage of disease, CE4/CE5 corresponds to degenerating stages and are nonviable. CE3 denotes transition stage.[43,44]

CT: CT imaging is less sensitive than US in identifying the features of hydatid cysts, with the imaging manifestations varying across different stages. A CL is depicted as a well-defined, unilocular, hypoattenuating lesion with a thin wall. On precontrast CT, the cyst wall appears as a hyperattenuating rim which becomes isoattenuating to the surrounding liver tissue on postcontrast scans.[45] Visible debris within the cyst does not enhance noticeably with contrast. Detached germinal layers are seen as curvilinear hyperattenuating structures, while daughter cysts are identified as hypoattenuating compared to the cyst's matrix **(Figs. 24 and 25)**. Calcifications in the cyst wall are distinctly visible on CT scans **(Figs. 26A and B)**. CT is important for the evaluation of complications of hydatid disease.

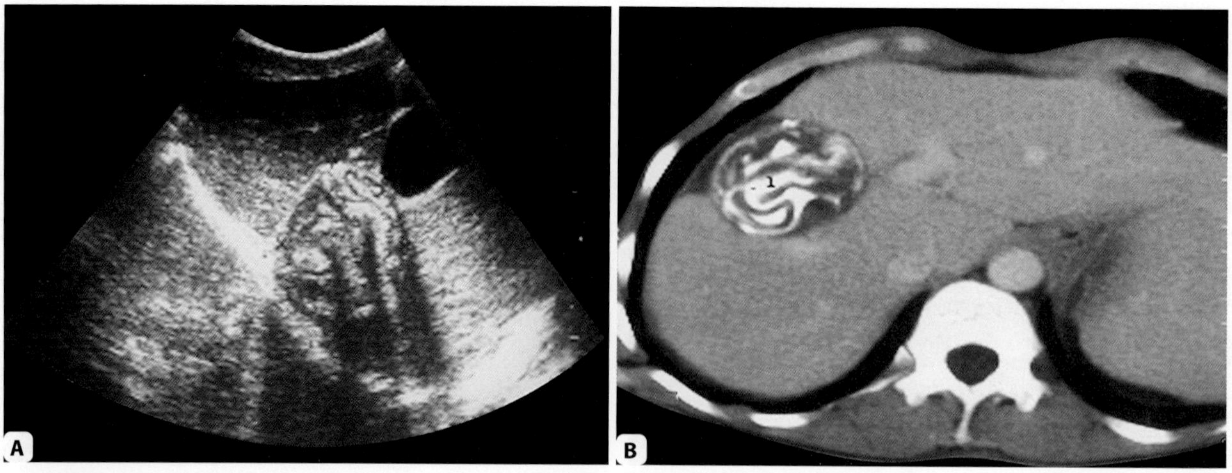

FIGS. 26A AND B: (A) Ultrasound (US) showing dense acoustic shadowing representing calcification in a hydatid cyst. (B) Computed tomography (CT) showing lamellar calcification in the membranes of the hydatid—calcified hydatid.

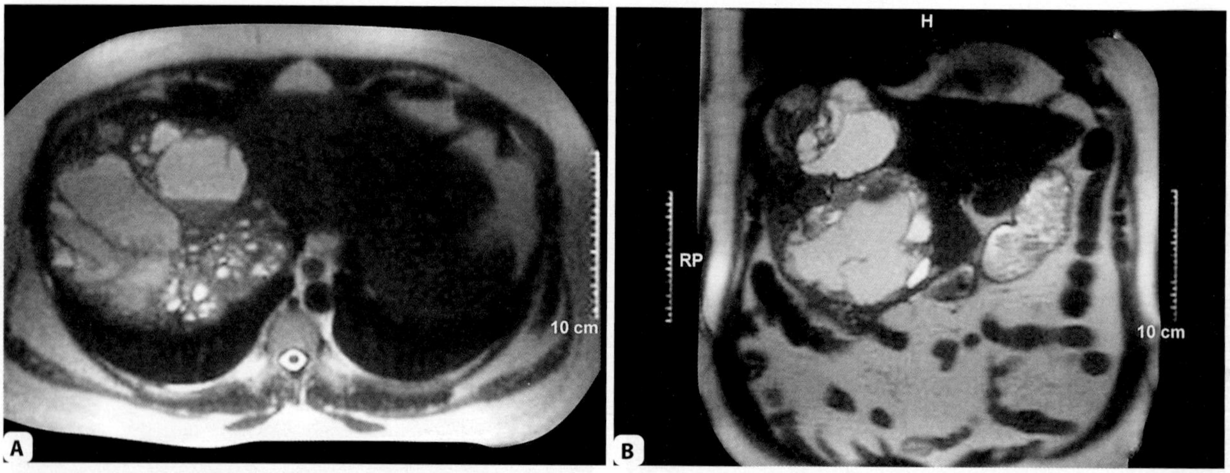

FIGS. 27A AND B: (A) Axial and (B) Coronal magnetic resonance (MR) images showing hepatic hydatids with multiple daughter cysts within appearing hyperintense on the T2-weighted images.

MRI: It is the best modality for imaging a large cyst as it characterizes all components of the cyst separately and helps in staging of disease. The pericyst of a hydatid cyst is clearly visible as a hypointense rim on both T1W and T2W images, and the central cavity appears markedly hyperintense on T2W images and hypointense on T1W images.[39,46,47] Daughter cysts exhibit greater T2 hyperintensity compared to the main cyst **(Figs. 27A and B)**. A collapsed membrane appears T2 hypointense across sequences, creating the "serpent" sign.[48] While there is no postcontrast enhancement in the cyst itself, the fibrous pericyst may demonstrate delayed enhancement. The "ball of wool" sign, indicative of stage CE4, results from the inner layer detaching and folding, making the lesion appear solid. Calcifications within the cyst are identifiable as focal hypointense areas on T2W images. MRI, combined with magnetic resonance cholangiography, enhances the visualization of cystobiliary communications.

Complications

Rupture of hydatid cyst: Usually occurs due to degeneration of the hydatid membranes. This may be a direct or a contained rupture. In direct cyst rupture, there is free spillage of the hydatid material into the peritoneal, pleural, or visceral cavity. A direct cyst rupture can occur when both the pericyst and endocyst rupture, in contrast to a contained rupture where only the endocyst ruptures and the pericyst remains intact. Free-floating membrane seen within cyst known as "water lily sign," curvilinear structures seen within a complex cyst known as "snake/serpent sign," and movement of hydatid sand within the cyst known as "snowstorm pattern" are all indicative of a contained rupture.

Communicating rupture of hepatic hydatids with biliary tree: A passage of cyst contents into the biliary tree constitutes a communicating rupture.[45,48] The direct sign of rupture into the biliary tree is the visualization of the communication between the cyst wall and biliary radicles or the passage of hydatid cyst material into the biliary tree **(Figs. 28A to D)**. US can demonstrate echogenic linear filling structures without posterior acoustic shadow, whereas CT can demonstrate high-attenuation material in the biliary radicles or common bile duct. A loss of continuity of cyst wall in contact with the adjacent bile duct is a pathognomonic sign of bile communication, which is seen infrequently. An air–fluid level or fat–fluid level is the indirect sign of a biliary communication. MR may show the direct fistulous communication between the cyst and biliary tree or may show excretion of hepatobiliary contrast from biliary tree into hepatic hydatid cyst. ERCP has a high sensitivity in the diagnosis of a biliary rupture as it shows the contents as filling defects within biliary tree. However, MRI is preferred over ERCP, owing to the risk of development of biliary fistula in ERCP.

Peritoneal seeding/peritoneal hydatidosis: Peritoneal seeding usually occurs secondary to hepatic hydatid disease, though isolated cases of primary peritoneal echinococcosis can occur. The peritoneal cavity may be involved in 13% of the cases. Cysts are usually multiple, of varying sizes, and may be located anywhere in the peritoneal cavity **(Figs. 29A to C)**[49] known as peritoneal hydatidosis/metastatic hydatidosis. The presentation may be with acute abdomen or with anaphylactic shock as chemical peritonitis may ensue. Peripheral calcifications, daughter cysts, and presence of floating membranes help in differentiating the pelvic seedlings/pelvic hydatids from cystic adnexal masses. An encapsulated multiloculated mass may at times be seen when the peritoneal hydatid disease grows and occupies the entire peritoneal cavity **(Figs. 30A to C)**.

Infection in the Hydatid Cyst

Infection in the hydatid cyst can occur only when both the pericyst and endocyst rupture. Findings suggestive of an infection include a solid appearance, mixed pattern consisting of solid and fluid contents, or air or air–fluid levels within.

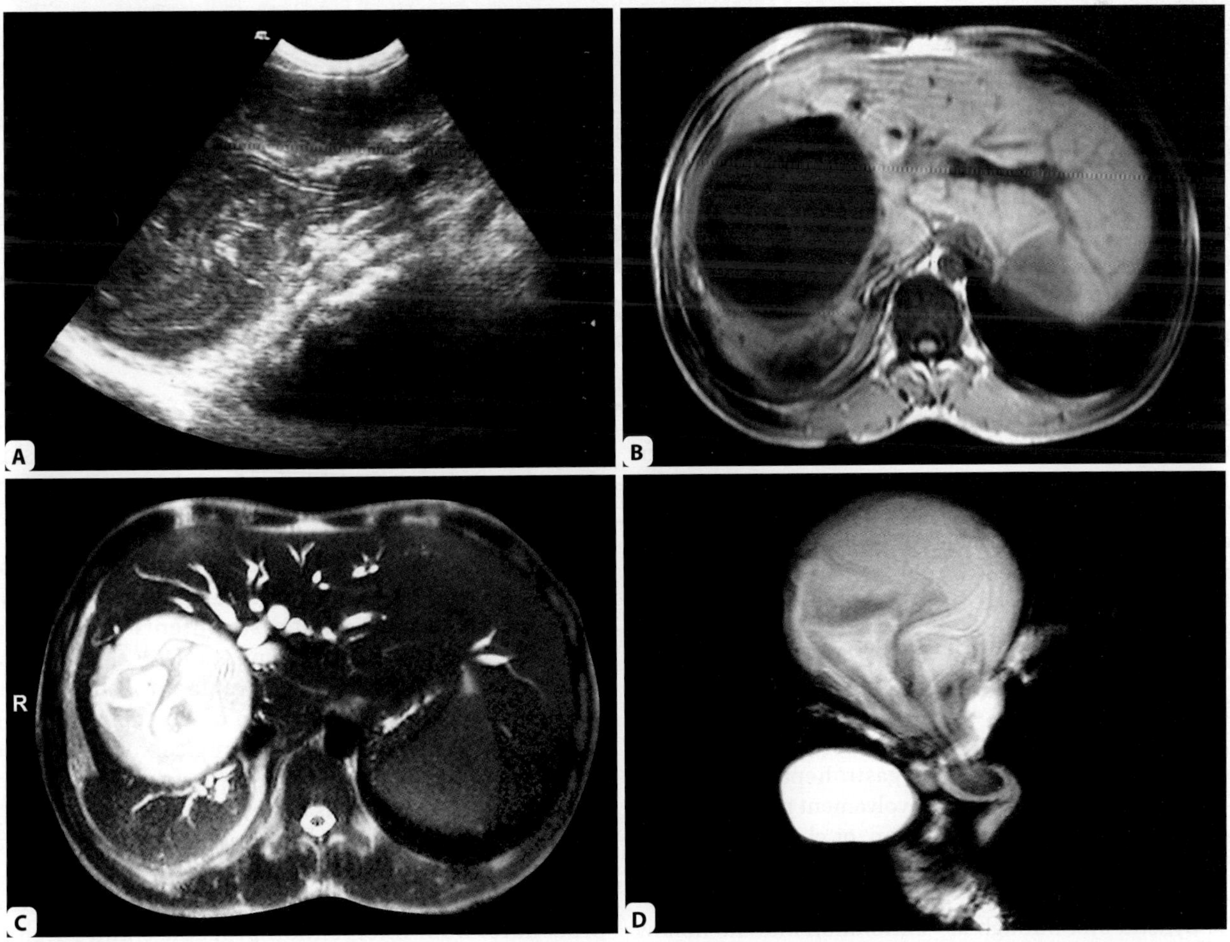

FIGS. 28A TO D: (A) US showing echogenic linear structures within the common bile duct. (B) T1W MR image showing the hydatid cyst as hypointense and T2W image (C) showing it as a hyperintense lesion with multiple linear low-signal structures within s/o membranes. Passage of the cyst contents into the bile duct well depicted on the MRCP image—hydatid cyst with rupture into common bile duct.

(MR: magnetic resonance; MRCP: MR cholangiopancreatography; T1W: T1-weighted; T2W: T2-weighted; US: ultrasound)

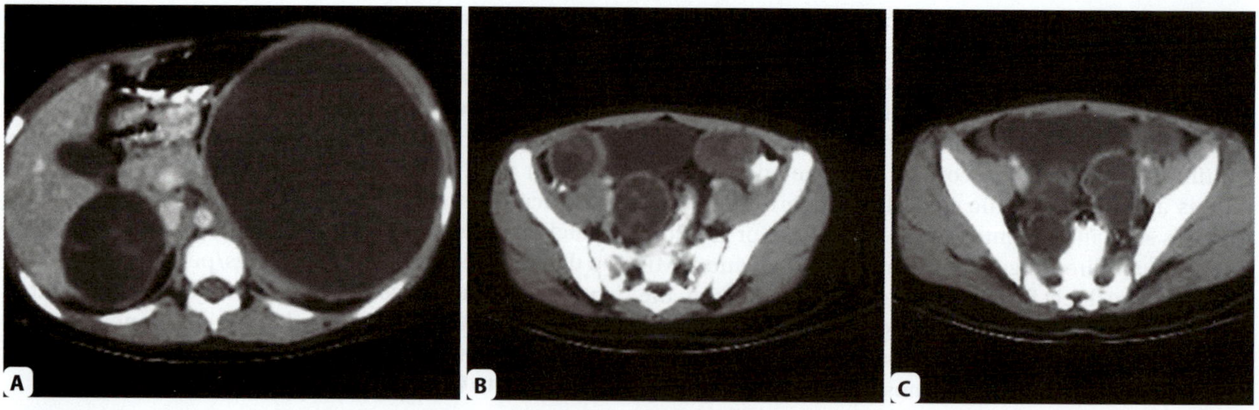

FIGS. 29A TO C: (A) Computed tomography (CT) scan showing hydatid cysts in the liver and spleen. (B and C) Multiple cysts of varying sizes are seen in the peritoneal cavity—peritoneal seeding of hydatid cysts.

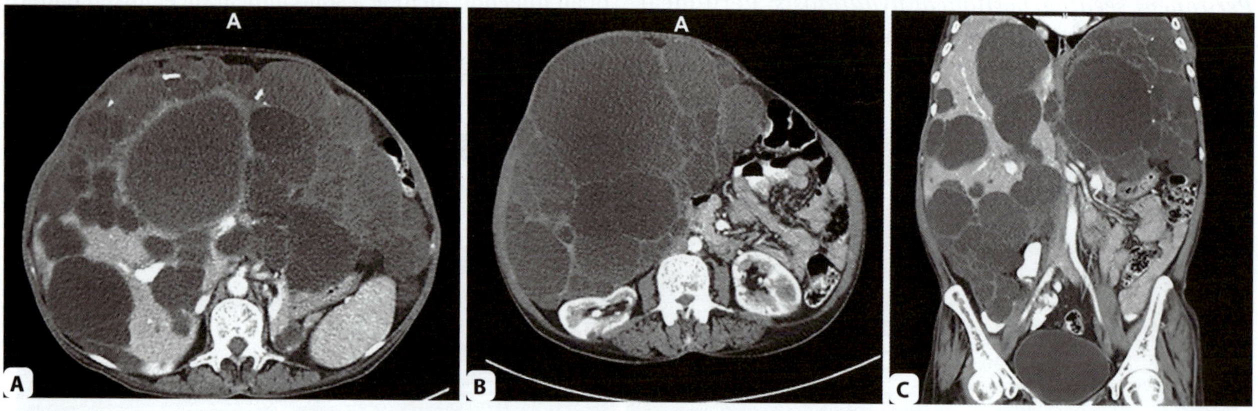

FIGS. 30A TO C: Contrast-enhanced computed tomography (CT) scans revealing a multiloculated mass occupying the entire peritoneal cavity in addition to hydatid cysts within the liver—peritoneal hydatidosis.

Complication due to Mass Effect

A portal cavernoma formation due to compression of the portal vein with secondary thrombosis is a rare complication. It is usually caused by the hydatid cysts located in the caudate lobe.[50] A Budd-Chiari syndrome may develop consequent to compression on hepatic vein/IVC by the hydatid cysts. Large hydatids may cause mass effect on the adjacent structures such as stomach, kidney, or diaphragm.

Other Complications

Hydatid cysts may grow exophytically to involve the bare area of the liver and the gastrohepatic ligament. Transdiaphragmatic thoracic involvement may be seen as pleural effusion, pulmonary lesion, or chronic bronchial fistulas. Sagittal and coronal MRI is best to demonstrate the diaphragmatic defect and the migration of the hydatid cyst through it.[51] Perforation into the hollow viscera is an extremely rare complication seen in only 0.5% of cases. Patients may present with hydatidemesia or hydatidorrhea. Imaging may reveal an air-fluid level or orally administered contrast material inside the hollow viscus.[52,53] Involvement of the abdominal wall may occur due to a direct communication between the cyst and the abdominal wall, sometimes seen due to the cysts passing through a small orifice creating an hourglass configuration.

Treatment

The management of CE varies based on the stage of cyst and includes options such as medical therapy, the puncture-aspiration of cyst contents-installation of proctoscolicidal agent-reaspiration (PAIR), surgical intervention, and a watch-and-wait approach. Medical treatment includes administration of albendazole (ABZ), sometimes for lifetime. However, surgical removal of the cyst or total cystectomy is often the treatment of choice. Percutaneous treatment is done by PAIR.[54] The recently modified catheterization technique (MoCAT) is used for a large cyst; it involves aspiration of cyst content including parasitic membrane and placing a catheter after the procedure. Both intervention procedure and surgical procedure should be followed by ABZ therapy.

Medical treatments, PAIR, and catheterization are generally utilized for CE1 and CE3a stages. ABZ alone is sufficient for small cysts, i.e., <5 cm. In contrast, modified catheterization and surgical procedures are typically favored for managing CE2 and CE3b stages. For CE4 and CE5 stages, which are deemed inactive; a watch-and-wait strategy is often adopted, monitoring the condition without immediate intervention.[44,55]

Puncture-Aspiration of cyst contents-Installation of Protoscolicidal agent-Reaspiration[56,57] The PAIR technique is widely used for the treatment of hepatic hydatid cysts in endemic countries.

Indications: Cysts favorable for PAIR are usually large univesicular cysts (>5 cm in size) which have significant fluid content with intact endocyst and no biliary communication, located in liver, pancreas, spleen, kidney, and bones. It is utilized for CE1 and CE3a stages.

Technique: During and after the procedure, strict monitoring should be done due to the potential for anaphylaxis. This includes obtaining informed consent, ensuring large IV access, administering steroid and antihistamine premedication, and having an adrenaline autoinjector and intubation equipment readily available at the procedure site. Real-time grayscale US is used to continuously visualize the cyst throughout the procedure. A 5 F 40 cm cholangiography needle can be used to drain large univesicular cysts; for smaller or multivesicular cysts, a 22-gauge 20 cm Cook needle can be employed.

The percutaneous drainage of hepatic hydatid cysts is conducted in four sequential steps outlined by the acronym PAIR, which stands for puncture (P), aspiration (A), installation (I), and reaspiration (R).

Step 1—puncture (P): US examination is crucial to determine the cyst's puncture site and to guide the needle through the biopsy port of the probe under real-time imaging. Puncture is ideally performed through the intercostal space into thick liver tissue.

Step 2—aspiration (A): Rapid aspiration of the cyst is performed to decompress its contents and facilitate the detachment of the endocyst (laminated membrane/germinal layer) from the cyst wall. The aspirated fluid is examined for its physical appearance, bilirubin content (using a bilirubin dipstick test), and scolex viability (assessed by motility and a dye test) and is sent for culture and, if possible, for animal inoculation. The presence of yellow fluid or a positive bilirubin test suggests cyst-biliary communication and leads to the termination of the procedure.

Step 3—installation (I): A scolicidal agent, typically hypertonic (20%) saline, is introduced into the cyst cavity, filling about three fourths of its volume and is left in place for 20 minutes. This installation produces a snowflake appearance on the US. Other scolicidal agents used are alcohol 95%, cetrimide in 0.05%, 0.1%, and 0.5%, and povidone-iodine (1%, 5%, and 10%).

Step 4—reaspiration (R): After the installation period, the cyst fluid is reaspirated. US is used to confirm complete detachment of the laminated membrane from the cyst wall. Before removing the needle, normal saline is introduced into the cyst cavity. The reaspirated fluid is again assessed for physical appearance, bilirubin, and scolex viability (via motility and dye test) and is sent for culture and potential animal inoculation. Successful procedure outcomes are defined by the complete detachment of the laminated membranes and nonmotile scolices that absorb the vital dye in the viability tests. If viability tests on reaspirated fluid are positive, the PAIR procedure may be repeated either immediately or within 48 hours.

A routine abdominal US is performed within 24 hours postprocedure to check for cyst appearance and to rule out any leaks. If everything is uneventful, the patient is discharged from the hospital. Follow-up visits occur monthly through clinical, biochemical, and US examinations until the cyst disappears, with 3-monthly follow-ups recommended thereafter.

Modified PAIR technique: It allows for the safe percutaneous drainage of cysts that have multiple septal divisions and large vesicles and it is effective in most cases. This procedure involves puncturing one large vesicle and treating it with hypertonic saline. After puncturing and treating several vesicles, the cyst transforms into a single large cavity with ruptured vesicles, which can then be managed as a unilocular cyst. However, multivesicular cysts with a honeycomb structure are typically not suitable for percutaneous drainage due to technical challenges in the procedure.[56,57]

PAIR in extrahepatic hydatid cysts: PAIR is primarily used for hepatic hydatid cysts but has also been successfully applied to isolated cases involving the pancreas, spleen, kidney, and bone. However, PAIR is contraindicated for lung and brain cysts because these locations lack surrounding host tissue to contain the cyst. Puncturing these cysts can lead to fluid leakage and potential dissemination of the contents.[56,57]

Alveolar Echinococcosis

The causative organism is *E. multilocularis.* It has a tendency to produce multilocular cysts anywhere in the organ or tissue, with the liver being the most common site. Histologically, these cysts resemble alveoli rather than true cysts, unlike hydatid cysts. They range in size from 1–10 mm in diameter but can grow as large as 15–20 cm. The large lesions are not only infiltrative but also voluminous with no clear margin between the lesion and the healthy parenchyma.[57] Some of the lesions are solid infiltrative, heterogeneous with irregular margins, nodular, and dystrophic calcification. These may be difficult to differentiate from malignant lesion of liver.

Imaging Features

Ultrasonography reveals a heterogenous echogenic mass with irregular margins. The mass is composed of cystic vesicles, calcifications, and necrosis and is surrounded by an area of hyperechogenicity due to fibrosis. A "hailstorm pattern" resembling a hemangioma may be observed. Contrast-enhanced US (CEUS) aids in the diagnosis, as AE is characterized by the absence of enhancement or limited peripheral enhancement.[57,58]

Computed tomography shows an infiltrative mass with calcification and absence of contrast enhancement.

Magnetic resonance imaging also reveals a heterogeneous infiltrating hypovascular mass. In AE, the mass is composed of a mix of solid and cystic tissue. On T2W MR image, "a bunch of grapes" or "honeycomb appearance" is seen due to multivesicular lesions.[57,58] The vesicle/microcyst and areas of liquefaction necrosis show high signal on T2W images, while granuloma, coagulative necrosis, and calcification show low signal on T2W images. Microcyst is the key imaging feature for diagnosis of AE. In case of uncertainty between an infiltrative lesion and an AE lesion, the radiologist should look for microcysts on T2W imaging. The microcyst is the pathognomonic elementary lesion of AE. Additionally, diffusion-weighted MRI may aid in the differentiation; increased ADC value will be found in AE lesions but not in infiltrative neoplastic lesions such as cholangiocarcinoma.

The echinococcal cysts involve large regions of the hepatic parenchyma with an affinity for the porta hepatis, with resultant portal hypertension and bile duct stenosis. Irregular margins, cystic and solid components, and an inhomogeneous enhancement pattern characterize the imaging appearances. Calcification begins in a scattered manner initially, but eventually, these become large calcified masses.

Hepatic Schistosomiasis

Hepatic schistosomiasis is a serious parasitic infection of the humans, typically having a chronic and insidious course. Hepatic involvement can occur due to infection with *Schistosoma japonicum, Schistosoma mansoni,* or *Schistosoma haematobium.* Schistosomes penetrate the skin, reaching the bowel lumen where they lodge and release eggs into the mesenteric vein, gaining access to the portal system. Schistosoma eggs cause a chronic inflammatory granulomatous reaction in the portal system, causing periportal fibrosis. Patients may present with hematemesis due to portal hypertension or hematuria due to involvement of the urinary tract.

Imaging Feature

In acute phase, imaging features are nonspecific. Plain X-ray of the abdomen may show hepatosplenomegaly. In the chronic phase, sonography may show periportal echogenicity due to fibrosis around anechoic portal vein, giving a "bull's eye sign."[13] Features of portal hypertension may include splenomegaly, collaterals and free fluid, cirrhosis-like appearance of liver with heterogeneous parenchyma, and irregular contours. On CT, a capsular or peripheral hepatic calcification, considered a hallmark of *Schistosoma japonicum* infection, may be seen. Periportal areas of fibrosis may be appear as low-density band within the porta that show delayed contrast enhancement. Other characteristic findings include pseudoseptations within the liver, bands of calcification, and liver notching. MRI may demonstrate features of portal hypertension and low-signal area within the porta due to fibrosis. Patients with schistosomiasis may develop HCC.

Differential Diagnosis

The cirrhotic appearance of the liver seen in chronic schistosomiasis needs to be differentiated from liver cirrhosis due to other causes. Periportal fibrosis and calcification are the hallmark findings seen in schistosomiasis.

Visceral Larva Migrans

Toxocara canis infection may manifest as nonspecific abdominal symptoms or be discovered during evaluations for peripheral eosinophilia. Imaging reveals variable-sized hypoechoic or isoechoic lesions on US, while CT shows multiple oval or elongated hypoattenuating areas. MRI demonstrates T1W hypointensity and T2W heterogeneous hyperintensity, with lesion locations potentially changing due to larval movement.[59] Visceral larva migrans (VLM) is distinguished from metastases by the absence of peripheral enhancement on venous phase, ill-defined margins, and subtle hypodensity on imaging.

Eosinophilic Liver Abscess

An eosinophilic liver abscess (ELA) is characterized by liver tissue necrosis associated with eosinophil infiltration. This condition, also known as hepatic eosinophilia or eosinophilic granuloma of the liver, is often discovered incidentally in asymptomatic patients who typically exhibit peripheral eosinophilia. The condition generally follows a benign progression. While the migration of parasitic larvae to the liver is a common cause, other factors such as medications, allergies, and cancers are also considered potential contributors to its development. ELAs are rare and can resemble liver metastases on imaging scans. On CT scans, they usually appear as multiple small, hypodense, oval lesions, usually <2 cm.[60] The presence of multiple lesions and a history of parasitic infection can aid in the differential diagnosis, with lesion regression on subsequent imaging also providing diagnostic clues. Nevertheless, a histopathological examination is essential for a definitive diagnosis.

Fascioliasis

Fascioliasis, a foodborne disease caused by *Fasciola hepatica*, affects humans who ingest metacercaria cysts found on freshwater plants. Originating from cercariae released by intermediate host water snails, these cysts penetrate the human duodenum, migrate through the peritoneal cavity to the liver, and mature in the biliary ducts to lay eggs. These eggs are expelled in the stool, continuing the lifecycle. Predominantly found in developing countries, symptoms of fascioliasis include pain in the right hypochondrium, fever, vomiting, and early-stage urticaria. Diagnosis may involve immunological tests and stool parasitology, though stool tests may not always detect the disease early on. Radiology plays a crucial role in early diagnosis and differentiating fascioliasis from other liver conditions.[61,62]

Imaging Features

In the early parenchymal phase, US reveals hypoechoic and hyperechoic liver lesions. CT scan shows subcapsular hypodense clusters that mildly enhance peripherally, indicative of the parasite's entry. MRI displays T2W hyperintense, enhancing subcapsular lesions, with linear lines indicating migration paths.[63,64]

During the late ductal phase, US may show biliary duct dilatation with echogenic walls and periportal hypoechoic lines, in addition to previous liver lesions. CT reveals ductal dilatation with mural thickening and MRI can show linear filling defects in the gallbladder or ducts, representing adult flukes.[64]

Other associated findings may include lymphadenopathy, subcapsular hemorrhage, and hepatic necrosis or worm itself.

Treatment

Treatment includes medical therapy.

Fungal Hepatic Infections

Fungal hepatic infections are uncommon and are usually seen in immunocompromised high-risk patients. Predisposing conditions include hematological malignancies, stem cell or solid organ transplantations, prolonged neutropenia, HIV, and those receiving chemotherapy, etc. Liver is involved secondary to hematogenous spread of mycotic infection from other organs, most commonly from the lungs. Candida is the most common causative organism. Other common fungi are Aspergillosis, Histoplasmosis, *Cryptococcus neoformans*, and mucormycosis. Early diagnosis is important to avoid complications and initiate appropriate treatment.

Hepatic Candidiasis

Imaging Features

USG: Sonographically, four major patterns are seen:[65]

1. "Wheel within a wheel" in which the central hypoechoic region of necrotic tissue and fungal debris is seen surrounded by hyperechoic zone of inflammatory cells, which is further surrounded by a hypoechoic peripheral rim representing fibrosis.
2. "Bull's eye" or "target lesion" in which a hypoechoic rim surrounds a hyperechoic center. This signifies active fungal infection.
3. A "uniformly hypoechoic" appearance which represents fibrosis. It is a nonspecific but the most common sign.
4. "Uniformly echogenic" develops in later stage of infection.

CT scan: The arterial phase of contrast-enhanced CT (CECT) is the most sensitive phase for the diagnosis of candidiasis. The most common pattern is multiple small, rounded hypoattenuating areas surrounded by hyperattenuating rim giving "bull's eye" appearance on the arterial phase.[48,66] Other patterns include hyperattenuating lesions, hypoattenuating lesions, and lesions causing transient hepatic enhancement. Multiple punctate foci of increased attenuation due to calcification can be seen on NCCT.[67]

MRI: It is superior to other modalities in detecting fungal lesions and their appearance varies according to the phase of lesion. In the acute phase, the nodular lesions appear hypointense on the T1W image and hyperintense on the T2W image with no perilesional edema. Absence of perilesional edema differentiates fungal infection from other infections The lesion is hyperintense on both sequences in the subacute phase; however, it shows subtle hypointensity on T1W image and iso- to mildly hyperintense on T2W imaging with no postcontrast enhancement in chronic phase.

Differential Diagnosis

Differential diagnosis of hepatic candidiasis includes TB, sarcoidosis, metastases, leukemia, lymphoma, and sometimes even focal fatty infiltration. Chest X-ray is important to rule out TB and sarcoidosis and history of malignancy points toward metastasis. Fungal microabscesses involve the spleen very commonly and hence, a concomitant involvement of spleen aids in making the diagnosis. Associated neutropenia helps in diagnosis of fungal infection and tissue sampling helps in confirmation.

Hepatic Histoplasmosis

Histoplasmosis, caused by inhaling *Histoplasma capsulatum* spores, typically affects immunocompromised individuals like those who are HIV positive or transplant recipients.[67] While the liver is rarely the initial infection site, it often becomes involved in progressive disseminated disease that originates in the lungs or upper respiratory tract. Imaging of liver for histoplasmosis is neither very specific nor sensitive. Typically, there are multiple small nodules in the liver parenchyma, which may appear similar to those seen in TB, candidiasis, or other disseminated fungal diseases.

Viral Infections

Viral Hepatitis

Acute viral hepatic infections are primarily caused by hepatitis A, B, C, D, and E viruses. Imaging features of acute hepatitis are nonspecific; they are mainly used to exclude other conditions with similar clinical signs, such as biliary obstruction or diffuse liver metastases. Typically, acute hepatitis on US presents with hepatomegaly, reduced liver echogenicity, and increased echogenicity of the portal vein wall, known as the "starry sky" sign.[48] On CT, common findings include hepatomegaly, heterogeneous hepatic enhancement during the arterial phase, low-attenuation zones in the parenchyma, periportal hypoattenuation, and possibly enlarged hepatic hilum lymph nodes. MRI findings are consistent with those on CT, featuring a hyperintense periportal halo on T2W images and a hypointense image on T1W images.

Human Immunodeficiency Virus

Liver involvement is common in patients with HIV, who often also suffer from chronic viral infections such as hepatitis B and C. Common findings seen on US include thickening of the gallbladder and biliary duct walls, along with duct dilatation. On CT, nonspecific findings are seen such as hepatomegaly and periportal lymphadenopathy. Due to frequent associations with biliary and pancreatic disorders in HIV patients, contrast-enhanced MRI along with MRCP are recommended in a single session. This approach helps evaluate biliary tract lesions and anomalies in liver and pancreatic parenchyma. Imaging findings often include long-segment biliary stenosis, papillary stenosis, and acalculous cholecystitis. Primary sclerosing cholangitis is a key differential diagnosis for HIV cholangiopathy.[48]

Rare Infections

Brucellosis

Brucellosis presents with hepatomegaly and can manifest as solitary or miliary hepatic abscesses. On US, the solitary lesions appear as a well-delineated heteroechoic lesion, while miliary abscesses present as multiple hypoechoic subcentimetric lesions. On CECT, lesions appear as hypoattenuating with thick peripheral enhancement and perilesional transient perfusion disorder. On MRI, they appear as hyperintense lesion on T2W images (size up to 15 mm) with thick peripheral enhancement seen on postcontrast images.

Bartonellosis

Bartonellosis typically presents with painful lymphadenopathy near the cat bite or scratch site.[68] If there is hepatic involvement, multiple necrotizing granulomas, measuring up to 3 cm, may be seen throughout the hepatic parenchyma. On US, these granulomas are seen as nonspecific hypoechoic nodules throughout the liver parenchyma. On noncontrast CT (NCCT), these nodules appear hypodense and may remain unchanged, become isodense, or show rim enhancement on contrast administration.[69] On MRI, they are hypointense on T1W images and hyperintense on T2W images with the peripheral enhancement. A history of contact with cats in an immunocompetent child or young adult can be helpful in differentiating Bartonellosis from other similar appearing lesions seen in TB, sarcoidosis, lymphoma, and fungal infection.

Spirochetal Infections

Liver infections caused by spirochetes have become rare since the advent of antibiotics. Spirochetal hepatitis can progress to cirrhosis and is characterized histologically by the presence of gummas, both caseating and noncaseating granulomas, and focal necrosis near the hepatic veins.[69] Liver involvement typically occurs during the secondary and tertiary stages of syphilis, with focal gummas developing 1–10 years postinfection. Due to the infrequency of hepatic involvement, imaging findings are limited. However, potential imaging findings on CT include low-attenuation lesions with peripheral enhancement. Calcifications, though rare, may also be observed.

Fransicella Turarensis

Francisella tularensis, a gram-negative coccobacillus endemic to many parts of North America, most commonly presents as ulceroglandular tularemia. If left untreated, the disease can spread to multiple organs, with liver involvement in 75% of cases affecting extralymphatic organs.[69] This infection frequently leads to granulomatous hepatitis and can result in hepatic abscesses that often appear solid on CT scans.

Actinomycosis of the Liver

Actinomycosis of the liver, caused by the slow-growing, gram-positive *Actinomyces*, is rare, primarily affecting the cervicofacial and ileocecal regions. In the abdomen, the liver is involved in 15% of cases, representing 5% of all actinomycosis cases.[69] Imaging may show either single or multiple lesions and it typically presents as a single hypoattenuating mass. On MRI, these lesions often appear hypointense on T1W images and hyperintense on T2W images, with variable contrast enhancement.

Pneumocystis Jirovecii Infection of Liver

Pneumocystis jirovecii causes commonly an opportunistic infection in immunocompromised and HIV-infected individuals, primarily affecting the lungs. Liver involvement is uncommon. But when it is involved, CT scans may show multiple hypodense lesions in the liver and spleen.[69] Differentiating these infections from neoplastic processes can be particularly challenging if the infection first presents in patients with previously unrecognized retroviral infections. An accurate diagnosis relies significantly on the patient's clinical and medication history, immune status, and any associated lung findings.

Hepatic Sarcoidosis

Sarcoidosis is a systemic disease characterized by the formation of granulomas. While its precise cause remains unclear, the presence of noncaseating granulomas in tissue samples is a hallmark feature. Although the lungs are the most frequently affected organ, sarcoidosis can impact almost any body part. The liver is the third most commonly involved organ following the lungs and lymph nodes, typically as part of the systemic manifestation of the disease.[69] Liver involvement may be seen in 40–70% of patients.[19] Hepatic involvement of sarcoidosis usually coexists with pulmonary sarcoidosis; however, isolated involvement of liver may develop in 13% of cases. The lesions are usually too small to be resolved by sonography and sarcoidosis may be seen as nonspecific diffuse parenchymal heterogeneity, an increased parenchymal echogenicity or coarsening of the liver echotexture. CT and MRI typically show the lesions as having a low attenuation/low signal with no enhancement seen on the postcontrast images.[69] The definitive diagnosis can be made with a biopsy.

MISCELLANEOUS LESIONS

Fatty Infiltration

Fatty infiltration of the liver is a common occurrence resulting from increased deposition of triglyceride in hepatocytes. This condition arises from a variety of nutritional disturbances or toxic insults to the liver, including obesity, nutritional deficiencies, diabetes mellitus, pregnancy, steroids, hepatotoxic drugs, and alcoholism. The development of fatty infiltration is a dynamic process and changes may be seen in a few weeks of an insult and may regress within days. Most characteristically, the fatty involvement is uniform or geographic in distribution. However, occasionally, it may be nodular or multifocal when it is indistinguishable from other focal hepatic lesions. Features suggesting the true nature of the process are sharp angular boundaries to the lesions and no evidence of displacement or effacement of venous structures. Chemical shift imaging on MRI will show focal fatty infiltration as an area of signal drop on the opposed-phase images as compared to the in-phase images.

Another well-recognized variant is focal sparing of small areas of normal liver in a more generalized fatty infiltration. The spared area appears as an echo-poor focal mass. A characteristic location for the spared area is the quadrate lobe anterior to the portal vein bifurcation or related to the gallbladder bed. The shape of the spared area or pseudomass is typically ovoid. Its location has led to the suggestion that the sparing relates to alteration of blood flow in this area.

Hematoma

The most common causes of hematoma are surgery and trauma. Hepatic lacerations, rib fractures, and free fluid favor the diagnosis of a post-traumatic hematoma, while iatrogenic hematoma usually occurs along a surgical plane. An intra- or perihepatic hematoma can also occur due to bleeding in a hepatocellular adenoma. The CT appearance of a hematoma depends on the age of the blood products. While acute and subacute hematomas have a higher-attenuation value due to aggregated fibrin components; a chronic hematoma has a fluid attenuation. On MRI, subacute hematomas show a hyperintense signal on both T1W and T2W images. Gradient echo images are very sensitive for the detection of blood products.

Biloma

A rupture of the biliary system can produce bilomas. These may occur spontaneously, owing to trauma or following surgery. They can occur in an intrahepatic or perihepatic location. Pseudocapsule formation occurs due to the intense inflammatory reaction induced due to bile extravasation. On imaging, bilomas appear as well-defined cystic lesion within the porta. No septations or calcification are usually seen **(Figs. 31A to C)**. Clinical history, location, and imaging appearance help in establishing the diagnosis.

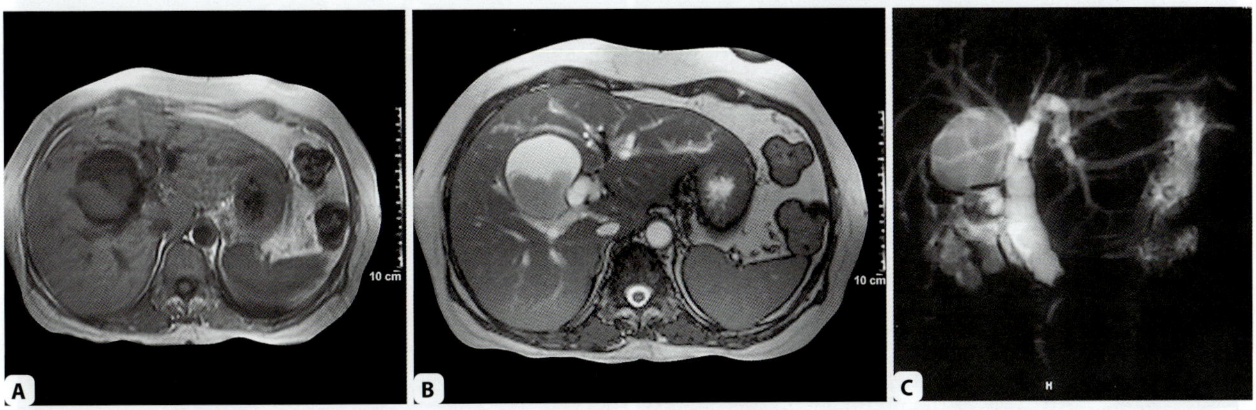

FIGS. 31A TO C: (A) MR image in a postcholecystectomy patient showing a well-defined hypointense lesion in the gallbladder fossa s/o biloma. (B) T2-weighted MR images show a hyperintense signal in the cyst with a fluid–fluid level (due to inspissated bile/sludge). (C) MRCP image depicting the biloma.

(MR: magnetic resonance; MRCP: MR cholangiopancreatography)

Peliosis Hepatis

Peliosis hepatis is a benign vascular lesion characterized by sinusoidal dilatation and blood-filled hepatic spaces. In 50% of cases, no cause can be found. In the remaining, the causative factors range from toxins [arsenic, polyvinyl chloride (PVC)], drugs (steroids and oral contraceptives) to infections (*Bartonella* and tuberculous bacillus) and malignancies (HCC), renal and cardiac transplantation, and diabetes. A variable echogenicity with internal vascularity is seen on US. On NCCT scans, a hypoattenuating area with an early brisk enhancement is noted on the postcontrast scans. Peliosis hepatis on MR is seen to be typically hypointense on T1W and hyperintense on T2W images.

Hereditary Hemorrhagic Telangiectasia of Liver

Hereditary hemorrhagic telangiectasia (HHT) is an autosomal-dominant disorder where vascular malformation may be seen on nose, GI tract, skin, liver, lung, and brain. Here, there is a direct communication between arterioles and venules without any intervening capillaries. Caraco criteria[70] of diagnosis of HHT include: (1) Epistaxis, (2) presence of visceral telangiectasias, (3) cutaneous mucosal vascular malformation, and (4) positive family history. Three of the four criteria should be present to make the diagnosis of HHT. The liver is involved in about 75% of people. In a known case of HHT, involvement of liver is suspected when there is GI bleed, presence of ascites, and abdominal pain. Doppler study can show abnormal tortuous vessel in the liver. Multiple liver arteriovenous malformation (AVM) can be seen on CECT and MRI. An enlarged hepatic artery (>7 mm) and heterogenous liver enhancement in the arterial phase with a homogeneity seen in portal venous phase are the characteristic imaging findings.

Inflammatory Pseudotumor

Hepatic inflammatory pseudotumor (IPT) is a benign lesion consisting of inflammatory cells and fibrosis.[71] They are of two types—fibrohistiocytic and lymphoplasmacytic type. These may occur at any age; they are more common in the young.

Although the exact etiopathogenesis is unknown, it is postulated that they may occur secondary to an inciting hepatic infection. There is also an association between immunoglobulin G4 (IgG4)-related disease and IPT, which are also known as IgG4-related hepatopathy. It develops in close association with sclerosing cholangitis and the most common site is the hepatic hilum. Its imaging features closely resemble cholangiocarcinoma and histopathological confirmation is a must for planning treatment.[69]

On US, IPT may appear as heterogeneous hyperechoic lesions with increased transmission. These are seen as large hypoattenuating lesions on NCCT. CECT reveals central hypodensity with thick peripheral hyperdensity which may mimic a necrotic malignant mass **(Figs. 32A and B)**. The hypodense center corresponds to inflammatory infiltrates, while the hyperdense periphery corresponds to fibroblastic proliferation. On MRI, the lesions are typically hypointense on T1W and hyperintense on T2W images. Contrast-enhanced MRI reveals intense enhancement of the lesions with rapid washout and periportal involvement. It is difficult to differentiate this condition from a primary or metastatic neoplasm and biopsy may be required.[71]

CONCLUSION

There are myriad nonneoplastic focal liver lesions, with some of these having fairly specific imaging characteristics allowing for a confident diagnosis. An accurate patient history and relevant clinical data combined with imaging findings allow for an improved lesion diagnosis.

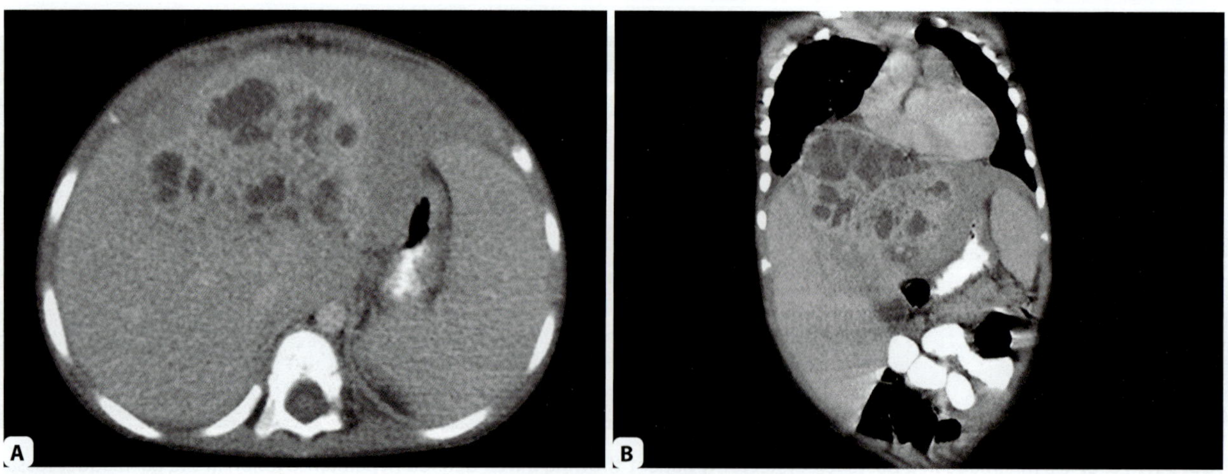

FIGS. 32A AND B: Contrast computed tomography (CT) reveals a mass with central hypodensity and thick peripheral hyperdensity in a child—inflammatory pseudotumor.

REFERENCES

1. Semaan A, Branchi V, Marowsky AL, Von Websky M, Kupczyk P, Enkirch SJ, et al. Incidentally detected focal liver lesions – a common clinical management dilemma revisited. Anticancer Res. 2016;36(6):2923-32.
2. Ata Soy C, Akyar S. Multidetector CT contributions in liver imaging. Eur Radiol. 2004;52:2-17.
3. Winterer JT, Kotter E, Ghanem M. Detection and characterization of benign focal liver lesions with multislice CT. Eur Radiol. 2006;16:2427-43.
4. Bächler P, Baladron MJ, Menias C, Beddings I, Loch R, Zalaquett E, et al. Multimodality imaging of liver infections: differential diagnosis and potential pitfalls. Radiographics. 2016;36(04):1001-23.
5. Tran Cao HS, Marcal LP, Mason MC, Yedururi S, Joechle K, Wei SH, et al. Benign hepatic incidentalomas. Curr Probl Surg. 2019;56(9):100642.
6. Van Sonnenberg E, Wroblicka JT, D'Agostino HB, Mathieson JR, Casola G, O'Laoide R, et al. Symptomatic hepatic cysts: Percutaneous drainage and sclerosis. Radiology. 1994;190: 387-92.
7. Dewbury KC. Benign focal liver lesions. In: Meire H, Cosgrove D, Dewbery K (Eds). Abdominal and General Ultrasound, 2nd edition. London: Churchill Livingstone; 2001.
8. Blumke DA, Fishman EK. Spiral CT of liver tumors. In: Fishman EK, Jeffrey RB (Eds). Spiral CT Principles, Techniques and Clinical Application, 2nd edition. Philadelphia: Lippincott Raven; 1998.
9. Mathieu D, Vilgrain V, Mahfouz A, Anglade MC, Vullierme MP, Denys A. Benign liver tumors. Magn Reson Imaging Clin N Am. 1997;5:255-88.
10. Vachha B, Sun MR, Siewert B, Eisenberg RL. Cystic lesions of the liver. AJR. 2011;196(4):W355-66.
11. Borhani AA, Wiant A, Heller MT. Cystic Hepatic Lesions: A review and an algorithmic approach. AJR. 2014;203: 1192-204.
12. Oto A, Tamm EP, Szklaruk J. Multidetector Row CT of the Liver. Radiol Clin N Am. 2005;43:827-48.
13. Mortele KJ, Segatto E, Ros PR. The infected liver: radiologic–pathologic correlation. Radiographics. 2004;24(4):937-55.
14. Halvovsen RA, Korobkin M, Foster WL, Silverman PM, Thompson WM. The variable CT appearance of hepatic abscesses. AJR. 1984;141:941-6.
15. Jeffrey RB, Tolentino CS, Chang FC, Federle MP. CT of small pyogenic hepatic abscesses: The cluster sign. AJR. 1988;151: 487-9.
16. Balci NC, Semelhar RC, Noone TC, Siegelman ES, de Beeck BO, Brown JJ, et al. Pyogenic hepatic abscesses: MRI findings on T1 and T2 weighted and serial Gadolinium Enhanced Gradient Echo Images. J Magn Reson Imaging. 1999;9:285-90.
17. Gabata T, Kadoya M, Matsui O, Kobayashi T, Kawamori Y, Sanada J, et al. Dynamic CT of hepatic abscesses: significance of transient segmental enhancement. AJR Am J Roentgenol. 2001;176(3):675-79.
18. Kim SB, Je BK, Lee KY, Lee SH, Chung HH, Cha SH. Computed tomographic differences of pyogenic liver abscesses caused by Klebsiella pneumoniae and non-Klebsiella pneumoniae. J Comput Assist Tomogr. 2007;31(01):59-65.
19. Chong V. Hepatobiliary tuberculosis: a review of presentations and outcomes. South Med J. 2008;101:356-61.
20. Yu RS, Zhang SZ, Wu JJ, Li RF. Imaging diagnosis of 12 patients with hepatic tuberculosis. World J Gastroenterol. 2004;10(11): 1639-42.
21. Tatco VR, Margarita AM, Santos M, Austine JU. The many faces of hepatic tuberculosis. WFPITB Corner. 2015;2:1-6.
22. Kakkar C, Polnaya AM, Koteshwara P, Smiti S, Rajagopal KV, Arora A. Hepatic tuberculosis: a multimodality imaging review. Insights Imaging. 2015;6:647-58.
23. Burrill J, William CJ, Bain G, Conder G, Hine AL, Misra RR. Tuberculosis: A Radiologic Review. Radiographics. 2007;27: 1255-73.
24. Chong VH, Lim KS. Hepatobiliary tuberculosis. Singap Med J. 2010;51:744-51.
25. Mustard RA, Mackenzie RL, Gray RG. Percutaneous drainage of a tuberculous liver abscess. Can J Surg. 1986;29:449-50.
26. Gupta RK. Amoebic liver abscess. a report of 1000 cases. Int Surg. 1984;69:261-4.
27. Philips RL. Computed tomography and ultrasound in the diagnosis and treatment of liver abscesses. Australas Radiol. 1994;38:165-69.
28. Radin DR, Ralls PW, Colletti PM, Halls JM. CT of amoebic liver abscess. AJR. 1988;150:1297-301.
29. Priyadarshi RN, Sherin L, Kumar R, Anand U, Kumar P. CT of amebic liver abscess: different morphological types with different clinical features. Abdom Radiol (NY). 2021;46: 4148-58.
30. Priyadarshi RN, Kumar R, Anand U. Amebic liver abscess: Clinico-radiological findings and interventional management. World J Radiol. 2022;14(8):272-85.
31. Peters RS, Gitlin N, Libke RD. Amoebic liver abscess. Ann Rev Med. 1981;32:161-74.
32. Reed SL. Amoebiasis: an update. Clin Infect Dis. 1992;14: 385-93.
33. Priyadarshi RN, Prakash V, Anand U, Kumar P, Jha AK, Kumar R. Ultrasound-guided percutaneous catheter drainage of various types of ruptured amebic liver abscess: a report of 117 cases from a highly endemic zone of India. Abdom Radiol. 2019;44:877-85.
34. Singh S, Chaudhary P, Saxena N, Khandelwal S, Poddar DD, Biswal UC. Treatment of liver abscess: prospective randomized comparison of catheter drainage and needle aspiration. Ann Gastroenterol. 2013;26:332-9.
35. Priyadarshi RN, Kumar P, Kumar R, Anand U, Shyama. Venous thrombosis and segmental hypoperfusion in amebic liver abscess: MDCT demonstration and its implications. Abdom Radiol (NY). 2020;45:652-60.
36. Sachdev GK, Dhol P. Colonic involvement in patients with amoebic liver abscess: endoscopic findings. Gastrointest Endosc. 1997;46:37-9.
37. Premkumar M, Devurgowda D, Dudha S, Kulkarni A, Joshi YK. Clinical and Endoscopic Management of Synchronous Amoebic Liver Abscess and Bleeding Colonic Ulcers. J Assoc Physicians India. 2019;67:14-8.
38. Beggs I. The radiology of hydatid disease. AJR. 1985;145: 639-48.

39. Doyle DJ, Hanbidge AE, O'Malley ME. Imaging of hepatic infections. Clin Radiol. 2006;61(9):737-48.
40. Agudelo Higuita NI, Brunetti E, McCloskey C. Cystic Echinococcosis. J Clin Microbiol. 2016;54(3):518-23.
41. Lewall DB. Hydatid disease: biology, pathology, imaging and classification. Clin Radiol. 1998;53(12):863-74.
42. Polat P, Kantarci M, Alper F, Suma S, Koruyucu MB, Okur A. Hydatid disease from head to toe. Radiographics. 2003;23(2): 475-94.
43. Czermak BV, Akhan O, Hiemetzberger R, Zelger B, Vogel W, Jaschke W, et al. Echinococcosis of the liver. Abdom Imaging. 2008;33(2):133-43.
44. Kern P, Menezes da Silva A, Akhan O, Mullhaupt B, Vizcaychipi KA, Budke C, et al. The Echinococcoses: Diagnosis, Clinical Management and Burden of Disease. Adv Parasitol. 2017;96:259-369.
45. Pedrosa I, Saiz A, Arrazola J, Ferreirós J, Pedrosa CS. Hydatid disease; Radiologic and pathologic features and complications. Radiographics. 2000;20:795-817.
46. Katranci N, Elmas N, Yilmaz F, Mentes A. Correlative CT, MRI and histological findings of hepatic Echinococcus alveolaris: a case report. Comput Med Imaging Graph. 1999;23(3):155-9.
47. Vilgrain V. Cystic lesions of the liver. Gastroenterol Clin Biol. 2001;25(4 Suppl):B167-77.
48. Kumar A, Garg D, Gupta P. Radiological approach to liver infection. J Gastrointest Abdom Radiol ISGAR. 2023;6:101-8.
49. Karavias DD, Vagianos CE, Kakkos SK, Panagopoulos CM, Androulakis JA. Peritoneal echinococcosis. World J Surg. 1996;20:337-40.
50. Gil–Egea MJ, Alameda F, Girvent M, Riera R, Sitges-Serra A. Hydatid cyst in the hepatic hilum causing a cavernous transformation in the portal vein. Gastroenterol Hepatol. 1998;21:227-9.
51. Gomez R, Moreno E, Loinaz C, De la Calle A, Castellon C, Manzanera M, et al. Diaphragmatic or transdiaphragmatic thoracic involvement in hepatic hydatid disease surgical trends and classification. World J Surg. 1995;19:714-9.
52. Mendez JV, Arrazola J, Lopez J, Antela Lopez J, Mendez Fernandez R, Saiz Ayala A. Fat-fluid level in hepatic hydatid cyst: A new sign of rupture into the biliary tree? AJR. 1996; 167:91-4.
53. Jain R, Sawhney S, Berry M. Hydatid disease: CT demonstration and follow-up of a cystogastric fistula. AJR. 1992;158:212.
54. Balli O, Balli G, Cakir V, Gur S, Pekcevik R, Tavusbay C, et al. Percutaneous Treatment of Giant Cystic Echinococcosis in Liver: Catheterization Technique in Patients with CE1 and CE3a. Cardiovasc Intervent Radiol. 2019;42(8):1153-9.
55. Brunetti E, Tamarozzi F, Macpherson C, Filice C, Piontek MS, Kabaalioglu A, et al. Ultrasound and Cystic Echinococcosis. Ultrasound Int Open. 2018;4(3):E70-8.
56. Khuroo MS. Percutaneous Drainage in Hepatic Hydatidosis-The PAIR Technique: Concept, Technique, and Results. J Clin Exp Hepatol. 2021;11(5):592-602.
57. Calame P, Weck M, Cote A, Brumpt E, Richou C, Turco C, et al. Role of radiologist in the diagnosis and management of the two forms of hepatic echinococcosis. Insight Imaging. 2022;13(1):68.
58. Liu W, Delabrousse É, Blagosklonov O, Wang J, Zeng H, Jiang Y, et al. Innovation in hepatic alveolar echinococcosis imaging: best use of old tools, and necessary evaluation of new ones. Parasite. 2014;21:74.
59. Gupta P, Sinha SK, Malik S, Dhaka N, Srinivasan R, Kochhar R. Hepatic visceral larva migrans: a diagnostic enigma. Trop Doct. 2018;48(04):345-7.
60. Kwon JW, Kim TW, Kim KM, Lee SH, Cho SH, Min KU, et al. Clinical features of clinically diagnosed eosinophilic liver abscesses. Hepatol Int. 2011;5(4):949-54.
61. Dusak A, Onur MR, Cicek M, Firat U, Ren T, Dogra VS. Radiological imaging features of Fasciola hepatica infection - a pictorial review. J Clin Imaging Sci. 2012;2:2.
62. Gonzalo-Orden M, Millán L, Alvarez M, Sánchez-Campos S, Jiménez R, González-Gallego J, et al. Diagnostic imaging in sheep hepatic fascioliasis: ultrasound, computed tomography and magnetic resonance findings. Parasitol Res. 2003; 90(05):359-64.
63. Koç Z, Ulusan S, Tokmak N. Hepatobiliary fascioliasis: imaging characteristics with a new finding. Diagn Interv Radiol. 2009; 15(04):247-51.
64. Ramanan RV, Dhus U, Ramamurthy A, Parameswaran SA, Piramanayagam P, Gopalakrishnan R. Human fascioliasis: diagnosis by typical computed tomography features and response to nitazoxanide in 16 patients from India. Trop Gastroenterol. 2019;39(03):149-54.
65. Shirkhoda A. CT findings in hepatosplenic and renal candidiasis. J Comput Assist Tomogr. 1987;11:795-8.
66. Pastakia B, Shawker TH, Thaler M, O'Leary T, Pizzo PA. Hepatosplenic candidiasis: wheels within wheels. Radiology. 1988;166(2):417-21.
67. Metser U, Haider MA, Dill-Macky M, Atri M, Lockwood G, Minden M. Fungal liver infection in immunocompromised patients: depiction with multiphasic contrast-enhanced helical CT. Radiology. 2005;235(01):97-105.
68. Malekzadeh S, Widmer L, Salahshour F, Egger B, Ronot M, Thoeny HC. Typical imaging finding of hepatic infections: a pictorial essay. Abdom Radiol. 2021;46:544-61.
69. Karaosmanoglu D, Uysal A, Karcaaltincaba M, Akata D, Ozmen MN, Kraeft J, et al. Non neoplastic hepatopancreatobiliary lesions simulating malignancy: can we differentiate. Insights Imaging. 2020;11:21.
70. Shovlin CL, Guttmacher AE, Buscarini AE, Buscarini E, Faughnan ME, Hyland RH, et al. Diagnostic criteria for hereditary haemorrhagic telangiectasia (Rendu-Osler-Weber syndrome). Am J Med Genet. 2000;91:66-7.
71. Alobaidi M, Shirkhoda A. Benign Focal Liver Lesions: Discrimination from malignant mimickers. Curr Probl Diagn Radiol. 2004;33:239-53.

CHAPTER **10**

Ankur Goyal, Shrea Gulati, Sanjay Kumar Meena, Raju Sharma

Neoplastic Focal Lesions in Noncirrhotic Liver

INTRODUCTION

Focal liver lesions in noncirrhotic liver present a diverse array of diagnostic and therapeutic challenges, necessitating a nuanced understanding of their etiology, classification, diagnostic modalities, and management strategies. They may be symptomatic or incidentally detected. The gamut of radiological investigations such as ultrasonography (US), contrast-enhanced ultrasound (CEUS), computed tomography (CT), and magnetic resonance imaging (MRI) play a crucial role in the characterization of these lesions. While hepatocellular cancer (HCC) is the most feared focal lesion in patients with underlying liver cirrhosis, a variety of neoplastic lesions may be seen in the noncirrhotic liver. The management necessitates a multidisciplinary approach, encompassing radiologists, hepatologists, surgeons, and oncologists. This chapter outlines the approach toward a focal neoplastic lesion in the noncirrhotic liver. The lesions will be divided into benign, malignant, and rare neoplastic lesions **(Box 1)** followed by a brief overview of pediatric neoplastic liver lesions.

BOX 1 Classification of neoplastic lesions in noncirrhotic liver.

- *Benign lesions*:
  - Hepatic hemangioma
  - Focal nodular hyperplasia
  - Hepatocellular adenoma
  - Mucinous cystic neoplasm
- *Malignant lesions*:
  - Hepatocellular cancer
  - Fibrolamellar hepatocellular cancer
  - Mass-forming intrahepatic cholangiocarcinoma
  - Epithelioid hemangioendothelioma
  - Angiosarcoma
  - Metastasis
  - Hepatic lymphoma
- *Rare neoplastic lesions*:
  - Perivascular epithelioid cell tumor
  - Lipoma
  - Teratoma
  - Neurofibroma
  - Inflammatory pseudotumor
  - Primary hepatic neuroendocrine tumor
- *Pediatric neoplastic liver lesions*:
  - Hepatoblastoma
  - Mesenchymal hamartoma
  - Infantile hepatic hemangioma

BENIGN NEOPLASTIC LIVER LESIONS

Hepatic Hemangioma

Hemangioma is the most common solid-appearing lesion of the liver with an incidence of 20%.[1] It is often incidentally found on imaging, being two to five times more common in females, often attributed to the hormonal characteristics.[2] Though traditionally considered to be the most common benign neoplasm, currently, it is no longer considered neoplastic, rather it belongs to the category of low-flow venous malformations according to the International Society for the Study of Vascular Anomalies 2018 (ISSVA 2018). These lesions are often asymptomatic and associated with low risk of complications usually not requiring surgical resection. The typical forms are usually well-defined round lesions seen in the peripheral parenchyma or along the hepatic veins and include cavernous/typical hemangiomas and flash-filling hemangiomas (FFH).[3]

Cavernous (Typical) Hemangioma

Cavernous (typical) hemangioma is the most common subtype of hemangioma named after the cavernous vascular spaces seen on histopathological examination. Smaller lesions show typical findings on US in the form of a homogeneously hyperechoic lesion with posterior acoustic enhancement; however, larger lesions may appear heterogeneous due to thrombosis or fibrosis. US has a sensitivity of 96% and a specificity of 60% and is diagnostic in case of small lesions (<3 cm) showing typical features.[4] However, hypervascular metastasis and even HCC may appear similar and thus, diagnosis of hemangioma cannot be made on US alone in the presence of a primary malignancy or chronic liver disease (CLD).[5] CEUS shows a characteristic peripheral nodular enhancement in the early phase followed by centripetal filling-in and is thus never hypoenhancing in any phase (compared to the rest of the liver). This feature is especially useful in the diagnosis of hypoechoic hepatic hemangioma (HH) as well as in distinguishing hemangiomas from echogenic metastases which may occur in gastrointestinal and hypervascular primary malignancies **(Figs. 1A and B)**.[6] The findings on multiphasic cross-sectional modalities follow the blood pool in each phase. On unenhanced CT, hemangiomas are hypodense; on the arterial phase, the typical pattern is a peripheral discontinuous nodular enhancement followed by progressive slow centripetal filling **(Figs. 2A to D)**. In the late phases, the lesion gets completely filled and appears isodense/hyperdense to the background liver. Atypical forms, however, can show areas of thrombosis, hemorrhage, fibrosis, cystic degeneration, and calcification.[3] MRI is the best imaging modality in the diagnosis of HH with a sensitivity of 90–100% and a specificity of 91–99%.[7] MRI reveals a well-defined, lobulated, smooth homogenous lesion, brightly hyperintense on T2-weighted images (similar to fluid) described as the classical "light bulb sign."[8] This is considered as one of the hallmark MR features for diagnosing a hemangioma. The high T2 signal of these lesions causes them to appear bright on diffusion-weighted images (DWI) as well as the apparent diffusion coefficient maps—"T2 shine-through effect."[3] The absence of hepatocytes in these lesions makes them appear hypointense in the hepatobiliary phase. Since malignant lesions can also appear hyperintense on T2-weighted images, increasing the echo time causes the signal from malignant lesions to decrease and HH to increase, helping in differentiation.[5] While HH shows peripheral nodular enhancement in the arterial phase and retention in the delayed phase, hypervascular neoplastic lesions show arterial enhancement and washout in the delayed phase, allowing differentiation.

Flash-filling Hemangiomas

Flash-filling hemangiomas are also referred to as rapidly filling or (relatively) high-flow hemangiomas and previously termed capillary hemangiomas. Lesions are usually smaller (<1 cm) and have smaller vascular spaces. On CT and MRI, these show intense homogenous enhancement in the arterial phase, with attenuation matching the aorta in each phase **(Figs. 3A to C)**. FFH may be associated with arterioportal shunting with surrounding perilesional enhancement corresponding to transient hepatic attenuation differences (THAD).[9]

Hepatic hemangioma can show atypical findings on imaging **(Table 1 and Figs. 4A to H)**, in which case differentiation from close mimickers may be difficult. Multiple hemangiomas may be seen in 10–50% of the cases. Diffuse HH, characterized by multiple hemangiomas is a rare condition, characterized by entire liver studded with innumerable HH, which is seen more frequently in newborns, where the entire liver involvement results in arteriovenous shunting and high-output cardiac failure. Two morphological patterns are described, a multinodular form characterized by multiple small discrete and coalescent

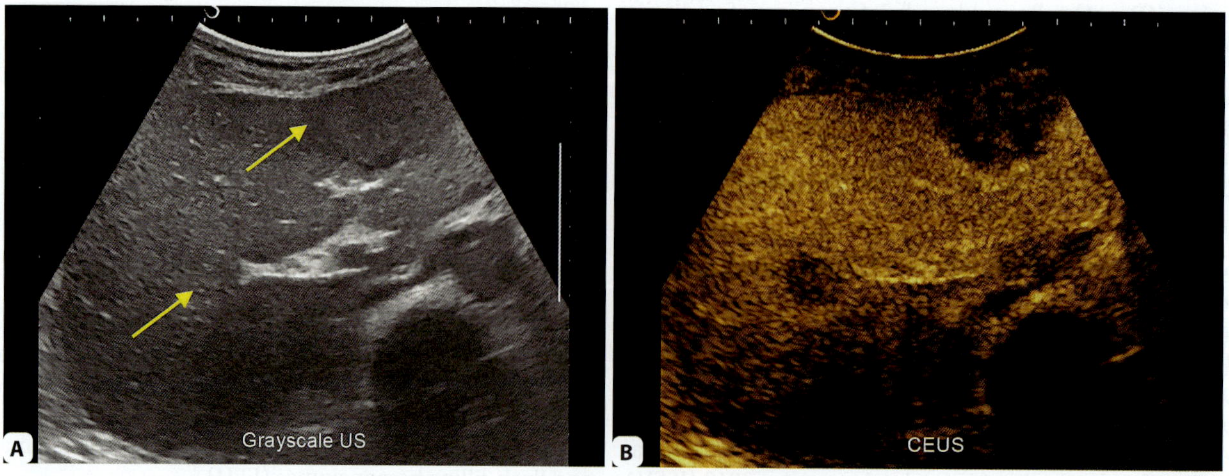

FIGS. 1A AND B: Metastases from colon cancer on contrast-enhanced ultrasound (CEUS): (A) Grayscale ultrasound (US) shows multiple ill-defined lesions which are isoechoic-to-mildly hyperechoic (arrows). The larger lesion shows a hypoechoic halo. (B) CEUS depicts these lesions to be hypoenhancing as compared to surrounding liver parenchyma, helping in differentiation from hemangioma.

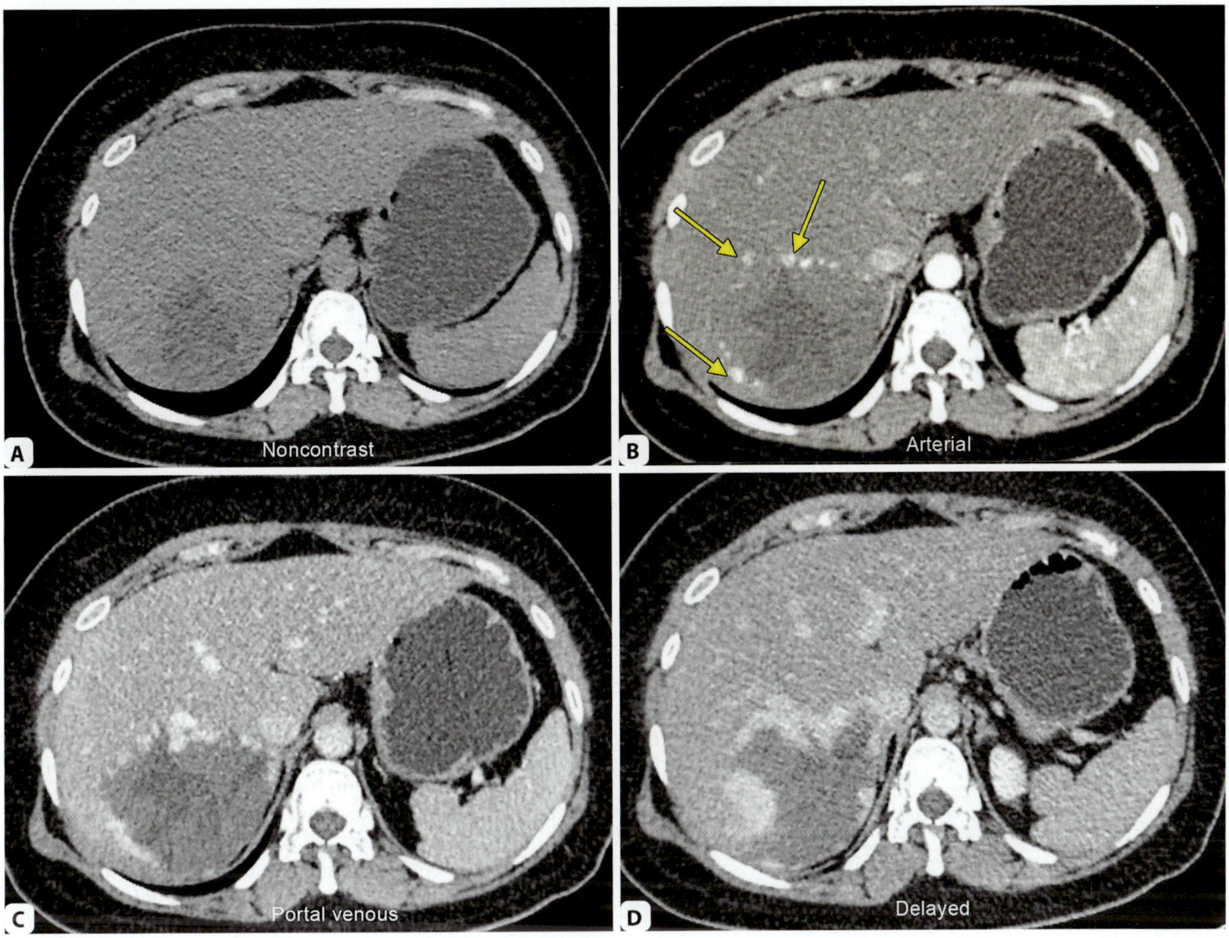

FIGS. 2A TO D: Hemangioma: Axial computed tomography (CT) (A) unenhanced image shows a hypodense lesion in segment VII of the liver. (B) Arterial phase shows peripheral discontinuous nodular enhancement; (C) venous and (D) delayed phase images show progressive centripetal filling in with the enhancement matching that of the blood pool in each phase.

nodules and a diffuse pattern consisting innumerable poorly defined lesions replacing the entire liver.[10] Coexistent hemangioma and focal nodular hyperplasia (FNH) can be seen in 20% of the cases with the association being stronger in patients with multiple FNH.[11] The proposed mechanism is that FNH develops as a hyperplastic response to altered blood supply which occurs in case of hemangiomas. The association also tends to be common in women who are taking oral contraceptive pills (OCPs).

Focal Nodular Hyperplasia

Focal nodular hyperplasia is a benign lesion characterized by hepatocyte hyperplasia without normal development of portal tracts, occurring in the background of a normal liver. It is the second most common incidental liver lesion after hemangioma. The lesion is almost eight times more common in women and commonly occurs between the third and fifth decades.[12] While the exact pathogenesis in not well understood, it is believed to be a hyperplastic response to abnormal blood flow.[13] Most lesions are asymptomatic and they have no malignant potential. There is very low risk of complications such as rupture or hemorrhage.[14] Therefore, asymptomatic FNH does not require any treatment or imaging follow-up in patients without any underlying liver disease or known malignancy.[15] US reveals a solitary well-circumscribed, unencapsulated lobulated lesion, usually isoechoic to the background liver parenchyma. Color and power Doppler may demonstrate a central feeding artery with "spoke wheel pattern" of branching vessels in the radiating septae.[16] CEUS has a good diagnostic accuracy of 87% for FNH and may show a typical centrifugal pattern of enhancement with spoke wheel pattern or an eccentric feeding vessel in the arterial phase.[17] They are often termed "stealth lesions" as they are isodense-to-mildly hypodense on unenhanced CT and isointense on T1 and iso-to-mildly hyperintense on T2-weighted images, thus making detection difficult.[18,19] Owing to the prominent arterial supply, these lesions show marked homogenous enhancement on the arterial phase and become isodense or isointense on the venous phase images with a central scar **(Figs. 5A to F)**. The central scar is composed of fibrous and myxoid tissue and shows T2 hyperintensity and delayed enhancement at 2–5 minutes (detectable in

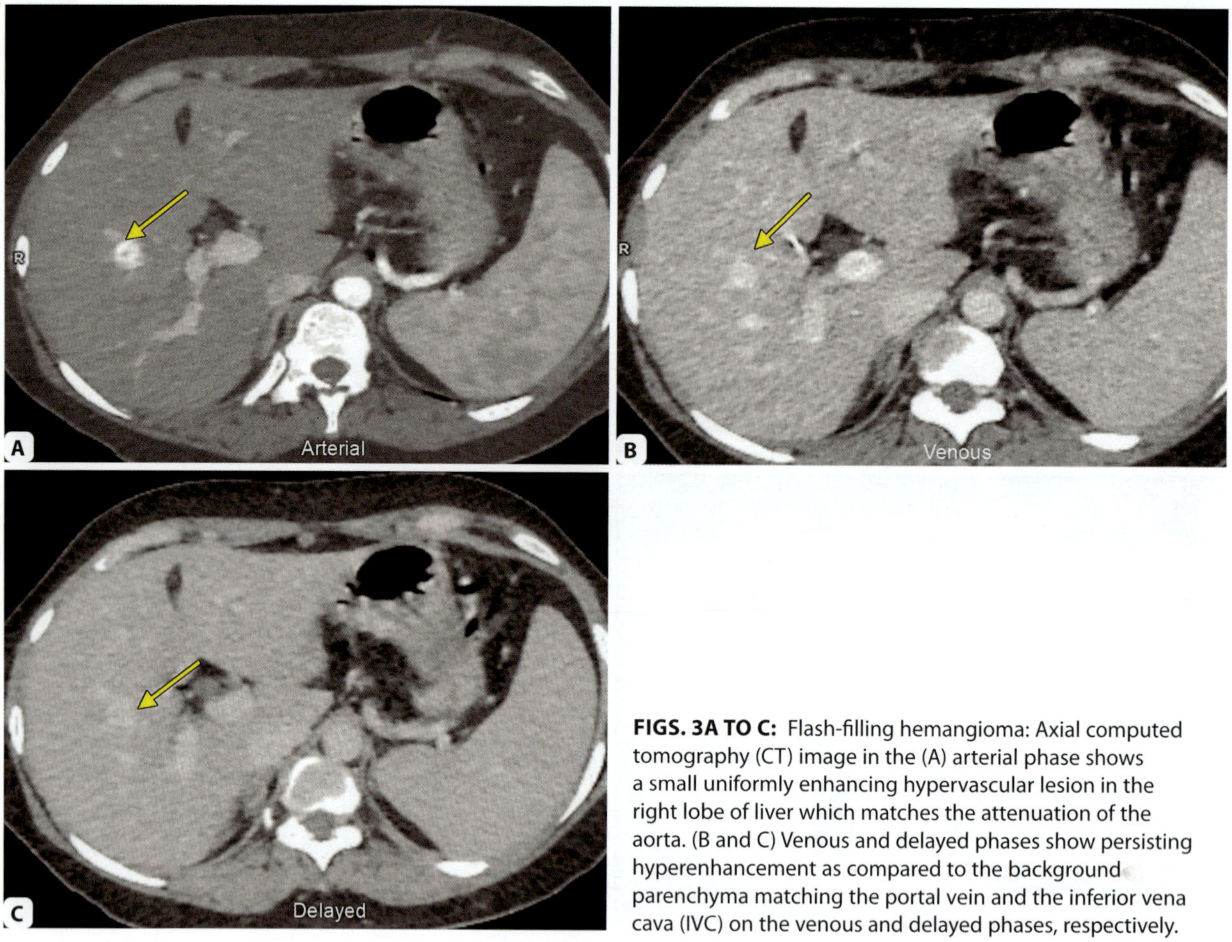

FIGS. 3A TO C: Flash-filling hemangioma: Axial computed tomography (CT) image in the (A) arterial phase shows a small uniformly enhancing hypervascular lesion in the right lobe of liver which matches the attenuation of the aorta. (B and C) Venous and delayed phases show persisting hyperenhancement as compared to the background parenchyma matching the portal vein and the inferior vena cava (IVC) on the venous and delayed phases, respectively.

TABLE 1: Variant/Atypical findings in liver hemangiomas.

Atypical findings in liver hemangiomas	Comments
Echogenic rim on ultrasound	Most common atypical finding
Centrifugal progression of enhancement (inside-out enhancement)	Explained by central vascular spaces and peripheral fibrosis
Sclerosing/Hyalinized hemangioma	• Show central areas of sclerosis • Irregular shaped, associated capsular retraction, wedge-shaped surrounding THED • *Differentials*: Metastasis, cholangiocarcinoma
Giant hemangioma	• Size > 5 cm, may be symptomatic • US—heterogenous, CT—central areas hypodense on CT • Progressive enhancement seen on multiphasic imaging, but complete filling in is not seen due to cystic degeneration/liquefaction, central septae T1/T2 hypointense • *Complications*: Intralesional hemorrhage, intraperitoneal rupture, Kasabach–Merritt syndrome
Calcifications	• Calcified HH show poor enhancement • *Differentials*: Granulomatous infections, parasitic infections, benign and malignant neoplasms (metastasis, adenoma, mucinous cystic neoplasm, fibrolamellar carcinoma, and cholangiocarcinoma)
Fluid–fluid levels	Can mimic complicated cysts, mucinous cystic neoplasm, and necrotic metastasis
Multicystic hemangioma	Often misdiagnosed as mucinous cystic neoplasm
Exophytic pedunculated hemangiomas	• May be misdiagnosed as tumors from other organs • *Complication*: Lesion may twist around the pedicle causing infarction/hemorrhage

Continued

Continued

Atypical findings in liver hemangiomas	Comments
Hemangiomas with capsular retraction	• Described in sclerosed hemangiomas (70% cases) • *Differentials*: Metastasis, cholangiocarcinoma, epithelioid hemangioendothelioma
Hemangioma with biliary dilatation	Centrally located hemangiomas can have ductal dilatation caused by the mass effect exerted by the lesion
Hemangiomas with arterio-portal/arteriovenous shunts	• Associated with flash-filling hemangiomas • Surrounding areas of THED

(CT: computed tomography; HH: hepatic hemangioma; THED: transient hepatic enhancement difference; US: ultrasound)

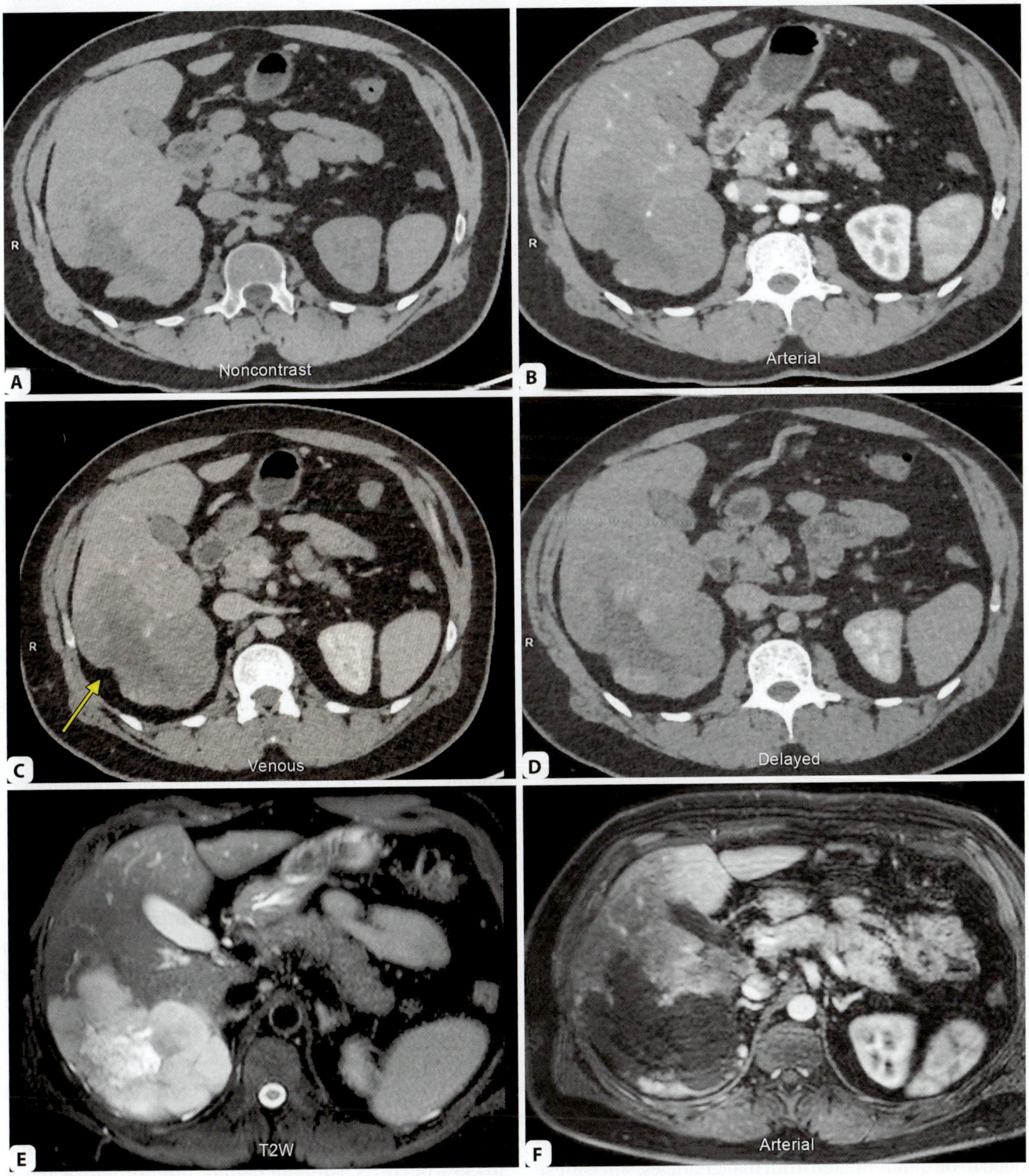

FIGS. 4A TO H: *Continued*

Continued

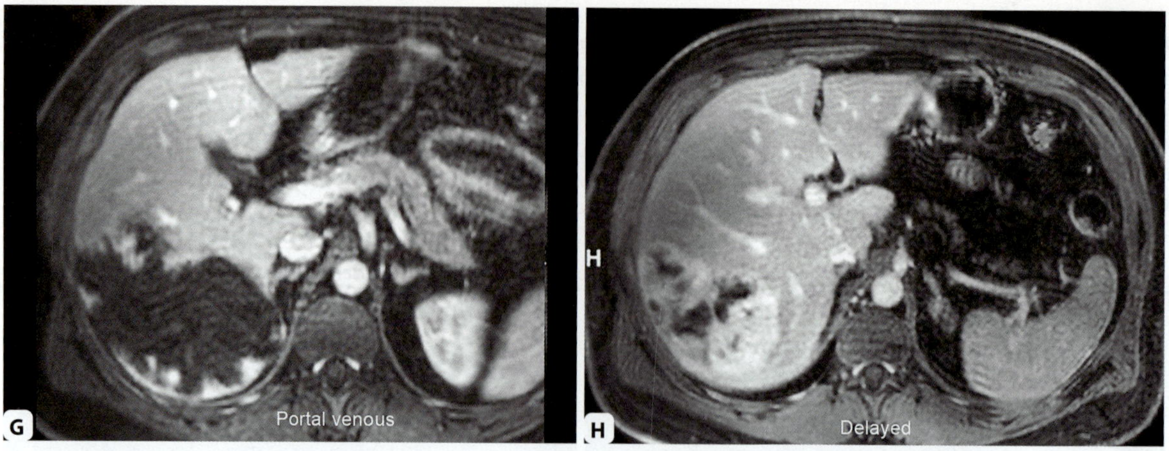

FIGS. 4A TO H: Sclerosing hemangioma: (A) Axial CT images in the (B) arterial phase show a large well-defined lesion with lobulated margins in segments VI and VII of the liver showing peripheral discontinuous nodular enhancement and (C) venous and (D) delayed phases show progressive filling in. There is overlying capsular retraction seen (arrow in C). Axial MR images of the same patient (E) T2W image shows the lesion to be hyperintense with central area of greater hyperintensity. (F) Arterial phase shows peripheral discontinuous nodular enhancement. (G) Venous and (H) Delayed phases show progressive filling in. The contrast enhancement matches that of blood pool in each phase. The lesion shows less enhancement and less hyperintensity of T2W images compared to a typical hemangioma.

(CT: computed tomography; MRI: magnetic resonance imaging; T2W: T2 weighted)

60% of the lesions on CT and 80% of the lesion on MRI).[18] Since a central scar can be seen in fibrolamellar carcinoma (FLC), differentiating the two entities is important **(Table 2)**. The hepatobiliary-specific MR contrast agents such as gadobenate dimeglumine and gadoxetic acid are useful in the diagnosis of FNH. These lesions show retention of contrast and T1 hyperintensity in the hepatobiliary phase due to the presence of functioning hepatocytes with the expression of organic anionic transporter peptide (OATP) receptors and abnormal biliary channels which do not communicate with the normal surrounding biliary system. This helps in the differentiation from hypervascular metastasis, hepatic adenomas (HCAs), and HCC.[20] The caveat here is that some HCAs (inflammatory type and beta-catenin activated) and some well-differentiated HCCs can appear isointense or hyperintense in the delayed phase after hepatobiliary contrast administration.[21]

Focal nodular hyperplasia-like lesions may be seen in patients with underlying vascular disturbances—Budd-Chiari syndrome, cardiogenic congestive hepatopathy, congenital absence of the portal vein, Fontan-associated liver disease, cavernous transformation of portal vein, hereditary hemorrhagic telangiectasia, nodular regenerative hyperplasia, and in patients on certain chemotherapeutic drugs such as oxaliplatin **(Figs. 6A to C)**.[12] These lesions are radiologically, microscopically, and immunohistochemically identical to FNH, except that they occur in a background of an abnormal liver caused by abnormalities in hepatic inflow, outflow, and microvascular disturbances. These may be a source of diagnostic confusion and need to be differentiated from malignancies, since these are benign, silent lesions and are managed conservatively.

Hepatocellular Adenoma

Hepatocellular/liver cell adenoma comprises a group of varied hepatic neoplasms characterized by proliferation of mature hepatocytes occurring in a background of a noncirrhotic liver. This entity is categorized into specific subtypes based on novel molecular signatures and histopathological findings. The updated classification described eight subtypes of HCA: Inflammatory, hepatocyte nuclear factor 1α (HNF-1α) inactivated, β-catenin mutated exon 3, β-catenin mutated exon 7/8, mixed inflammatory and β-catenin mutated exon 3, mixed inflammatory and β-catenin mutated exon7/8, sonic hedgehog (SHH), and unclassified **(Table 3)**.[22,23] The risk factors include obesity, alcohol consumption, anabolic steroid use, OCP, glycogen storage diseases, and McCune-Albright syndrome. The highest incidence is seen in women of reproductive age group. Hepatic adenomatosis requires the presence of more than 10 adenomas **(Figs. 7A to F)**.[24] While most HCAs are asymptomatic and incidentally detected, they are prone to complications such as hemorrhage and malignant transformation which vary depending on the size and the molecular subtype.[25] The risk factors for malignant transformation include male sex, size > 5 cm, β-catenin mutations, and telomerase reverse transcriptase (TERT) promoter mutations.

Hepatocyte Nuclear Factor 1α Inactivated Hepatocellular Adenoma

This group of tumors is usually sporadic and comprises 30–35% of HCAs. Familial hepatic adenomatosis has been related to germline mutations of HNF-1α and maturity-onset

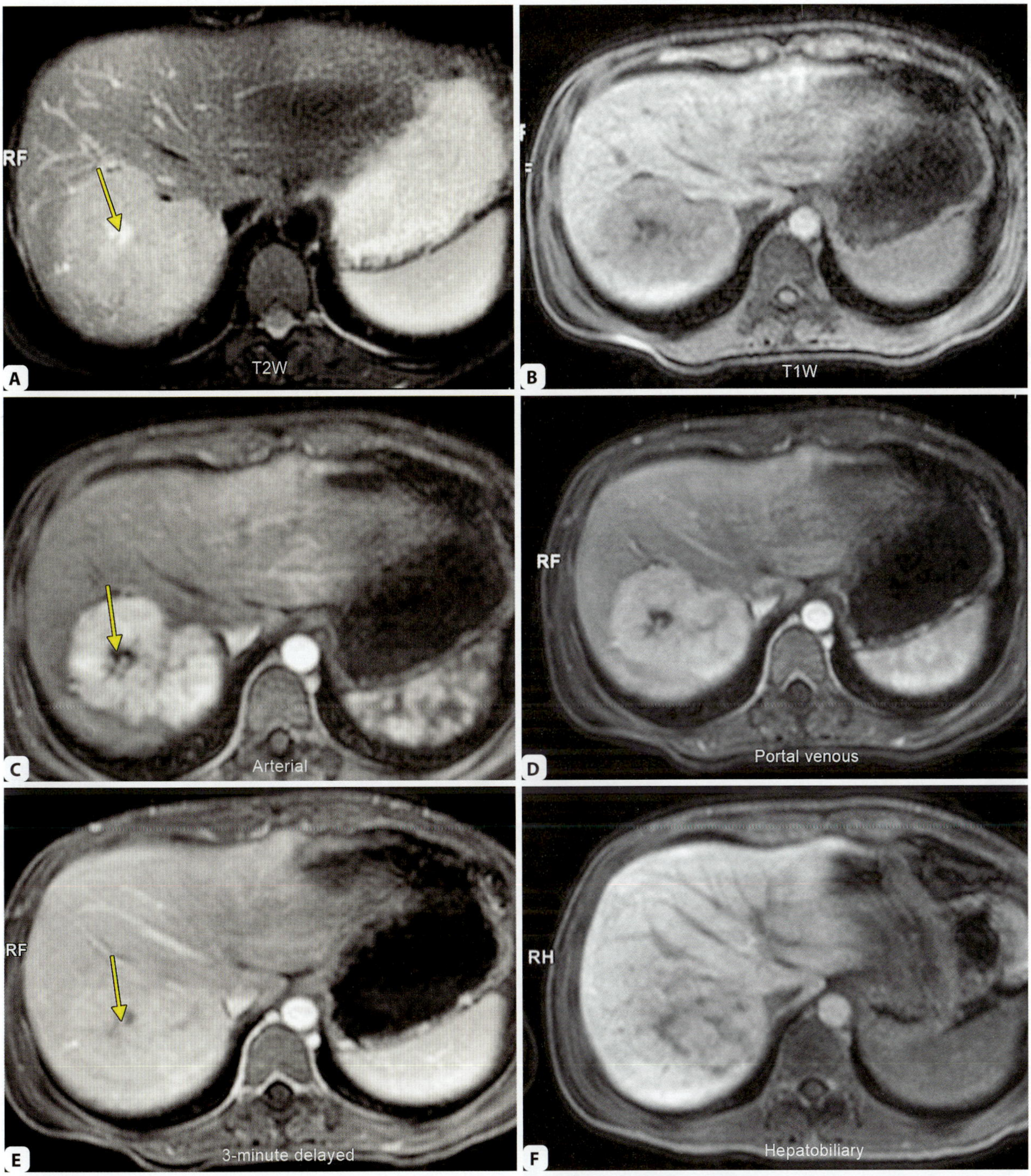

FIGS. 5A TO F: Focal nodular hyperplasia: Axial MRI shows a well-circumscribed lesion in segment VII of the liver appearing (A) T2 mildly hyperintense with central hyperintense scar (arrows in A, C and E) and (B) T1 hypointense. Late arterial phase MRI (C) shows intense nonrim APHE with central nonenhancing scar; (D) portal venous phase showing persistent enhancement of the lesion; (E) 3-minute delayed phase showing persistent enhancement in the lesion with filling into the scar; and (F) hepatobiliary phase showing retention of contrast at 1 hour.

(APHE: arterial phase hyperenhancement; MRI: magnetic resonance imaging; T1W: T1 weighted; T2W: T2 weighted)

TABLE 2: Comparison of FNH and FLC.

	FNH	FLC
Entity	Benign—hyperplasia of hepatocytes	Malignant
Arterial phase	Hyperenhancing	Hyperenhancing
Venous phase	Isodense to liver	Washout may be seen
T1-weighted MRI	Isointense	Hypointense
T2-weighted MRI	Iso- to mildly hyperintense	Hyperintense
Hepatobiliary phase	Retention of contrast	No retention of contrast
Diffusion restriction	Usually absent	Present
Uptake on Tc-m99 labeled colloid scan	Present	Absent
Central scar	Present	Present
T2 signal of scar	Hyperintense	Hypointense
Scar size	<2 cm	>2 cm
Scar calcification	Absent	Present in 35–70%
Scar enhancement	Delayed enhancement	May be seen

(FLC: fibrolamellar carcinoma; FNH: focal nodular hyperplasia; MRI: magnetic resonance imaging)

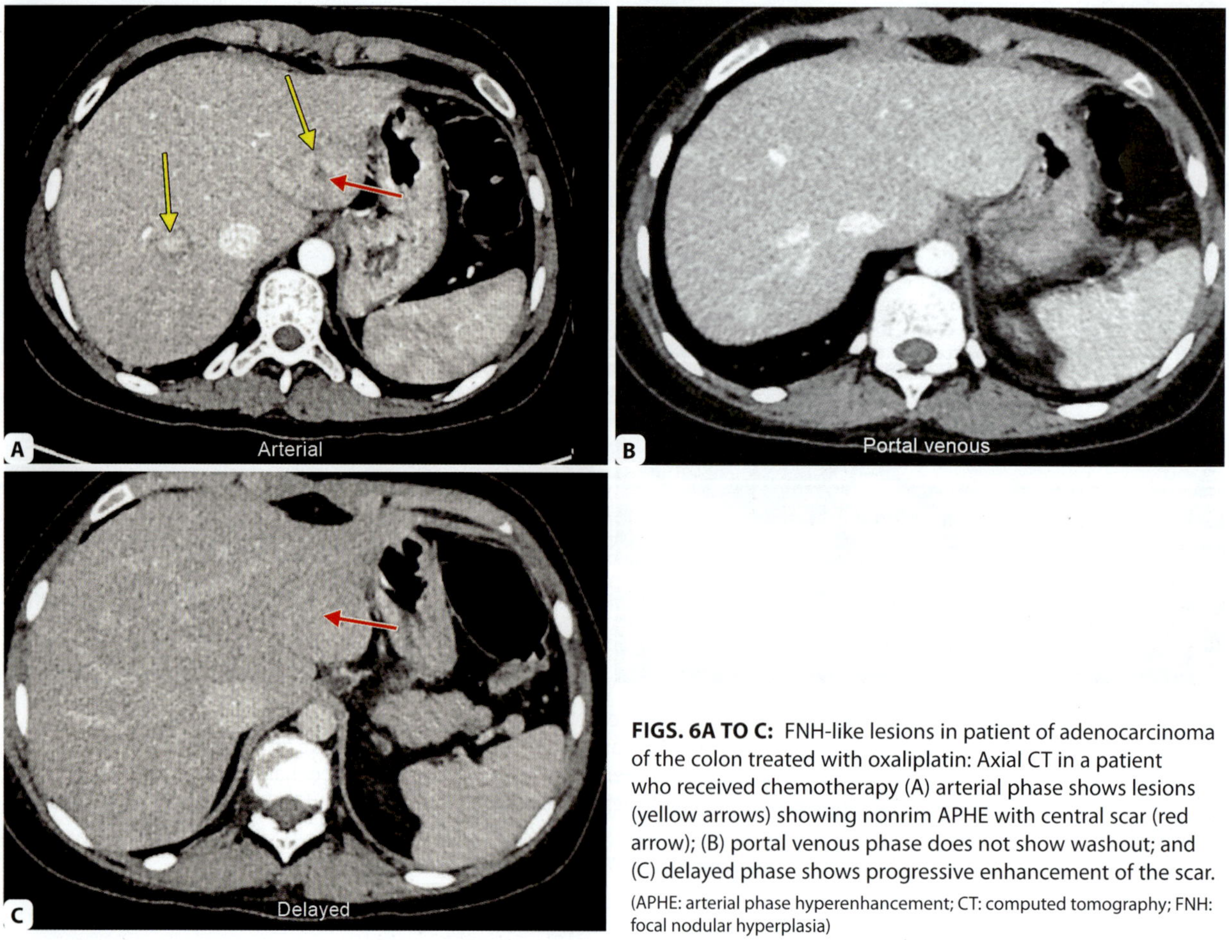

FIGS. 6A TO C: FNH-like lesions in patient of adenocarcinoma of the colon treated with oxaliplatin: Axial CT in a patient who received chemotherapy (A) arterial phase shows lesions (yellow arrows) showing nonrim APHE with central scar (red arrow); (B) portal venous phase does not show washout; and (C) delayed phase shows progressive enhancement of the scar.

(APHE: arterial phase hyperenhancement; CT: computed tomography; FNH: focal nodular hyperplasia)

TABLE 3: Summary of subtypes of HCA.

Subtype of HCA	Epidemiology and risk factors	Imaging features	Risk of malignancy	Risk of bleeding
Inflammatory	• *Most common* • *Risk factors*: Obesity, OCP, fatty liver, alcohol, and glycogen storage disorder	• Atoll sign • Crescent sign • Can show contrast retention in hepatobiliary phase	Low	High
HNF-1α inactivated	• OCP use • More common in females	• Uniform signal loss on opposed-phase imaging • Hypointense in hepatobiliary phase	Low	Low
β-catenin mutated exon 3	Males, androgen use	• Hyperintense signal on T1 and T2—hemorrhage • May show washout in portal venous, delayed enhancing capsule • Contrast retention in the hepatobiliary phase	Highest	Low
β-catenin mutated exon 7/8	• OCP use • More common in females	No specific imaging features, hypointense on hepatobiliary phase	Low	High
Mixed inflammatory and β-catenin mutated exon 3	• OCP use • More common in females	Features of both β-catenin and inflammatory	High	Low
Mixed inflammatory and β-catenin mutated exon 7/8	• OCP use • More common in females • Obesity alcohol use	Features of both β-catenin and inflammatory	Low	Low
SHH	• OCP use • Obesity	• Hyperintense signal on T1 and T2—hemorrhage • Hypointense on hepatobiliary phase	Low	Highest
Unclassified	OCP use	No specific imaging features	Medium	Medium

(HCA: hepatocellular adenoma; HNF-1α: hepatocyte nuclear factor 1 alpha; OCP: oral contraceptive pill; SHH: sonic hedgehog)

diabetes of the young 3 (MODY-3). The molecular hallmark of these lesions is biallelic inactivation of HNF 1α and loss of liver fatty acid-binding protein (LFABP) expression and macrovesicular fat at immunohistochemistry and histopathology. The nonfunctioning HNF-1α protein results in lipogenesis, causing deposition of intracellular fat which manifests on MRI as loss of signal on the opposed-phase T1-weighted MR images **(Figs. 8A to F)**.[26] They show isointense-to-mildly hyperintense signal on T2-weighted images and nonretention of contrast in the hepatobiliary phase attributed to the decreased OATP1B1/3 expression. Postcontrast studies show arterial phase hyperenhancement (APHE) which persists in the portal venous and the delayed phase images.[27] The incidence of complications such as hemorrhage and malignant transformation is low. US displays these lesions to be hyperechoic, owing to the presence of intracellular fat, thereby closely mimicking hemangiomas. On CEUS, they show peak enhancement in the arterial phase and appear isoechoic to the background liver during portal venous and delayed phases.[28] This subtype is intensely avid on fluorodeoxyglucose positron emission tomography (FDG-PET) with maximal standardized uptake values (SUV_{max}) being as high as 12.5, attributed to the overexpression of glucose transporters.[29]

Inflammatory Hepatocellular Adenoma

This variety of HCA is the most common subtype (5–40%) with the risk factors being high body mass index (BMI), OCP usage, fatty liver, alcohol use, and glycogen storage disorder. These tumors have sustained activation of the interleukin 6/Janus kinase/signal transduced and activation and hence, patients may have inflammatory symptoms such as fever, elevated total leukocyte count, elevated fibrinogen level, and C-reactive protein.[30] On histology, the patchy inflammatory infiltrate stains are positive for serum amyloid A and C-reactive protein. On MRI, the "atoll sign"—hyperintense signal along the periphery of the lesion on T2-weighted image is characteristic of inflammatory HCAs.[31,32] The peripheral rim represents the atoll, the lesion represents the lagoon, and the background liver represents the ocean. This sign has an excellent specificity of 97% for the inflammatory subtype.[33] Another sign described is the "crescent sign"—partial rim which appears hyperintense on T2-weighted image and shows APHE and persistence on the portal venous and delayed phases, which represents focal sinusoidal dilatation.[26,32] These lesions have an increased tendency to undergo hemorrhage. Owing to the expression of OATP receptors, inflammatory HCAs may

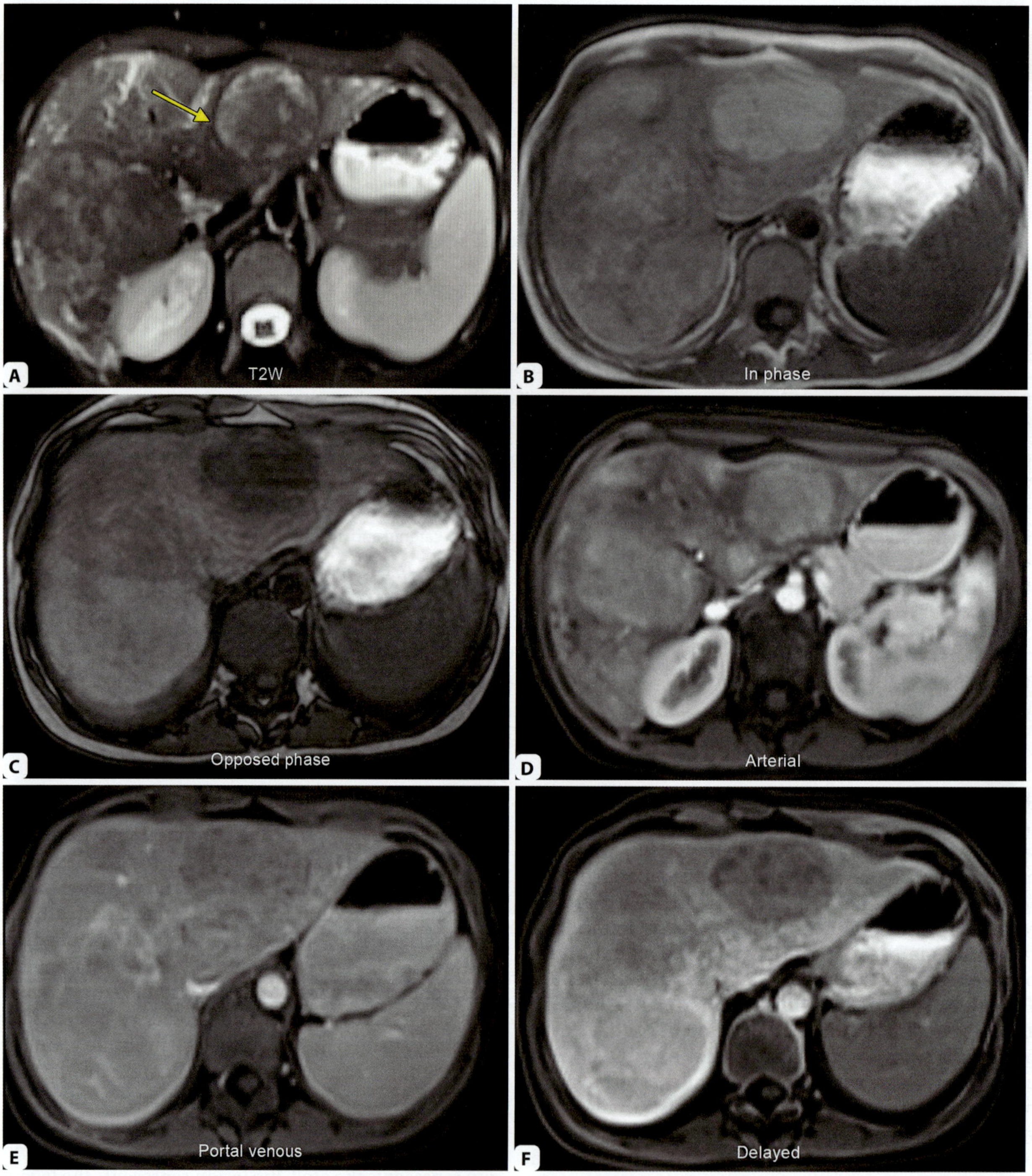

FIGS. 7A TO F: Hepatic adenomatosis: (A) T2-weighted (T2W) image shows a circumscribed mildly hyperintense lesion in the left lobe of the liver (arrow). Multiple similar lesions were seen in both lobes of the liver. (B) In-phase image shows the lesion to be hyperintense with (C) opposed-phase image showing signal drop, suggesting intravoxel fat. (D) Arterial phase demonstrates nonrim arterial phase hyperenhancement (APHE) within the lesion. (E) Portal venous phase shows washout and (F) hepatobiliary phase acquired at 1 hour does not show retention of contrast. These features were suggestive of hepatic adenoma and since the patient had multiple lesions in both lobes (>10), a final diagnosis of adenomatosis was made.

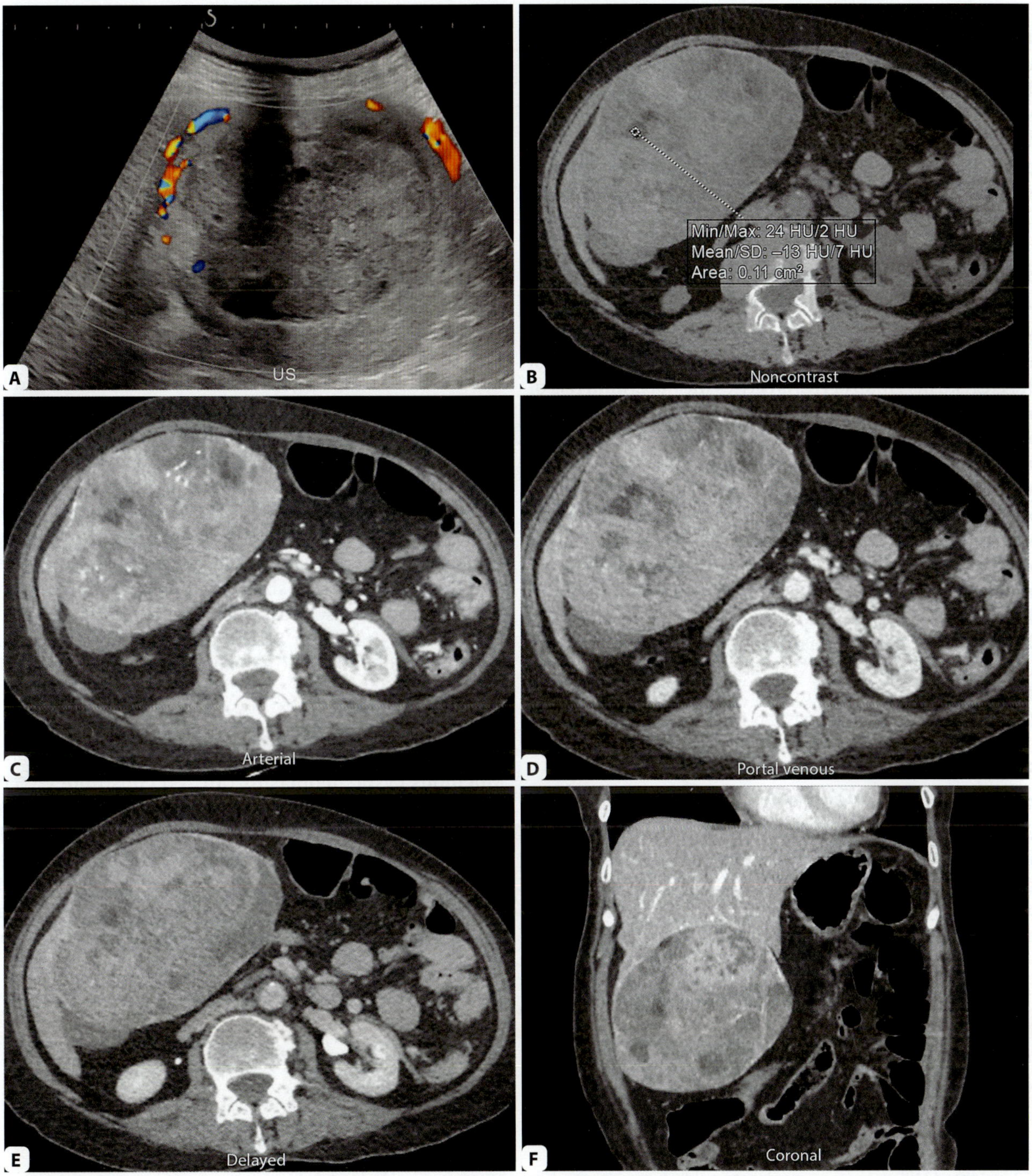

FIGS. 8A TO F: Hepatic adenoma: (A) US image of the liver shows a large heterogeneously hypoechoic mass lesion arising in a noncirrhotic background. Axial CT (B) noncontrast image shows a large circumscribed lesion with exophytic component showing internal areas of fat and hemorrhage within. (C) Arterial phase image shows nonrim APHE. (D) Portal venous phase image shows mild washout and (E) delayed phase image shows washout. (F) Coronal image better depicts the lesion.

(APHE: arterial phase hyperenhancement; CT: computed tomography; US: ultrasound) show contrast retention on the hepatobiliary phase and therefore mimic FNH. Postcontrast imaging demonstrates avid enhancement in the arterial phase which persists during the portal venous phase. An interesting observation on CEUS is that these lesions may show washout on the venous phase. This is explained by the concept that gadolinium and iodine-based contrast agents can diffuse into the interstitial spaces, while contrast agents used in CEUS are purely intravascular.[28]

β-catenin Mutated Hepatocellular Adenoma (Exon 3 and Exon 7/8)

β-catenin mutated HCAs are subcategorized into exon 3 and exon 7/8 mutated HCAs and together they comprise 10% of the HCAs. This group of HCAs carries the maximum risk of malignant transformation, the risk being higher in exon 3 mutations which are more common in men with androgen use.[34] Imaging features are nonspecific with variable hyperintense signals on T1- and T2-weighted images based on the presence of hemorrhage and necrosis. A proportion of these demonstrate heterogeneous enhancement on the arterial phase and washout on the portal venous/delayed images and even the enhancing capsule, making them difficult to differentiate from HCC. 80% of β-catenin HCAs display iso- or hyperintensity on the hepatobiliary phase and therefore can mimic FNH **(Table 4)**. Contrast retention during the hepatobiliary uptake is strongly predictive of β-catenin mutated subtype HCAs and risk of malignancy.[35]

β-catenin-activated Inflammatory Hepatocellular Adenoma

This subtype of HCAs shows features of both the β-catenin-activated HCA and the inflammatory HCAs. Hyperintense signal on T2 along with APHE indicate the inflammatory component, while contrast retention on hepatobiliary phase signifies the β-catenin component and risk for malignancy.

Sonic Hedgehog Hepatocellular Adenoma

Sonic hedgehog HCA is a newer molecular subtype with activation of the SHH pathway due to mutation of the *INHBE* gene, identified in 2017 and constitutes 4% of the HCAs. OCP use and obesity predisposes to these lesions and they have a high risk of bleeding even with lesions < 5 cm in size.[23] Hemorrhage within the lesion gives rise to a T1 hyperintense signal and variable T2 signal.[36] Arterial phase images show hyperenhancement with or without washout on the portal venous and delayed phase.

The management strategy for HCAs depends upon the sex, size of the lesion, molecular subtype, and the presence of or propensity of complications such as hemorrhage and malignant change. In male patients and β-catenin exon 3 mutated lesions, surgical resection is recommended in view of the high risk of malignant transformation.[37,38] The first-line management strategy in women includes OCP discontinuation and weight reduction with 6-monthly monitoring with MRI. Lesions showing reduction in size during monitoring, those <5 cm in size, and HNF-1α-inactivated HCA (on MRI) can be managed conservatively. On the other hand, lesions > 5 cm in size, exophytic lesions, and those not showing size reduction on serial MRI are considered for biopsy and further surgical management.[37,38] HCA with β-catenin or SHH mutations require surgical excision, while other HCAs can be considered for MRI-based follow-up.

Mucinous Cystic Neoplasm

Mucinous cystic neoplasms (MCNs) constitute <5% of cystic lesions in the liver. The mean age of presentation is 45 years for biliary cystadenoma with female predominance, while biliary cystadenocarcinoma occurs a decade later and does not display female predominance.[39] The high incidence among females is explained by the presence of ovarian-type stroma on histopathology in 60–100% cases

TABLE 4: Comparison of FNA with HCA.

	FNH	HCA
Appearance	Homogenous	Heterogenous owing to fat, hemorrhage
Central scar	Present	Absent
T1-weighted MRI	Hypointense	• Signal drop in opposed phase image (HNF-1α) • Hyperintense due to hemorrhage
T2-weighted MRI	Iso- to mildly hyperintense, homogeneous with T2 hyperintense scar	Moderately hyperintense and heterogeneous
Arterial phase	Homogeneous APHE	Heterogeneous APHE
Venous phase	Isodense to liver	Washout may be seen in some subtypes (β-catenin)
Hepatobiliary phase	Retention of contrast	No retention of contrast (except in inflammatory and β-catenin-activated types)
Uptake on Tc-m99 labeled colloid scan	Present	Absent

(APHE: arterial phase hyperenhancement; FNH: focal nodular hyperplasia; HCA: hepatocellular adenoma; HNF-1α: hepatocyte nuclear factor 1 alpha; MRI: magnetic resonance imaging)

that typically express estrogen and progesterone receptors.[40] In the vast majority of patients, it is asymptomatic and therefore picked up incidentally on imaging; however, it may also present with nonspecific symptoms such as abdominal pain and distention.[41] On US, these lesions manifest as anechoic cystic lesions which have thick irregular walls and internal septations. The presence of septal thickening, septal calcification, papillary infolding, and mural nodules within a cystic lesion is characteristic for biliary cystic neoplasms.[42] Mural nodules and papillary projections are more likely to be seen in biliary cystadenocarcinoma. CT is a good modality to evaluate the size and complete extent of the lesion.[43] Most lesions are isodense to fluid on CT and demonstrate contrast enhancement in the mural nodules and the septations. The presence of biliary duct dilatation, single cysts, and lesions in the left lobe of the liver can be predictive of MCN on CT.[44] On MRI, the lesions appear as multiloculated cystic lesions appearing T1 hypointense and T2 hyperintense with irregular thick walls and T2 hypointense septations and mural nodules within **(Figs. 9A to E)**.[45] Magnetic resonance cholangiopancreatography (MRCP) can demonstrate the presence of internal septations

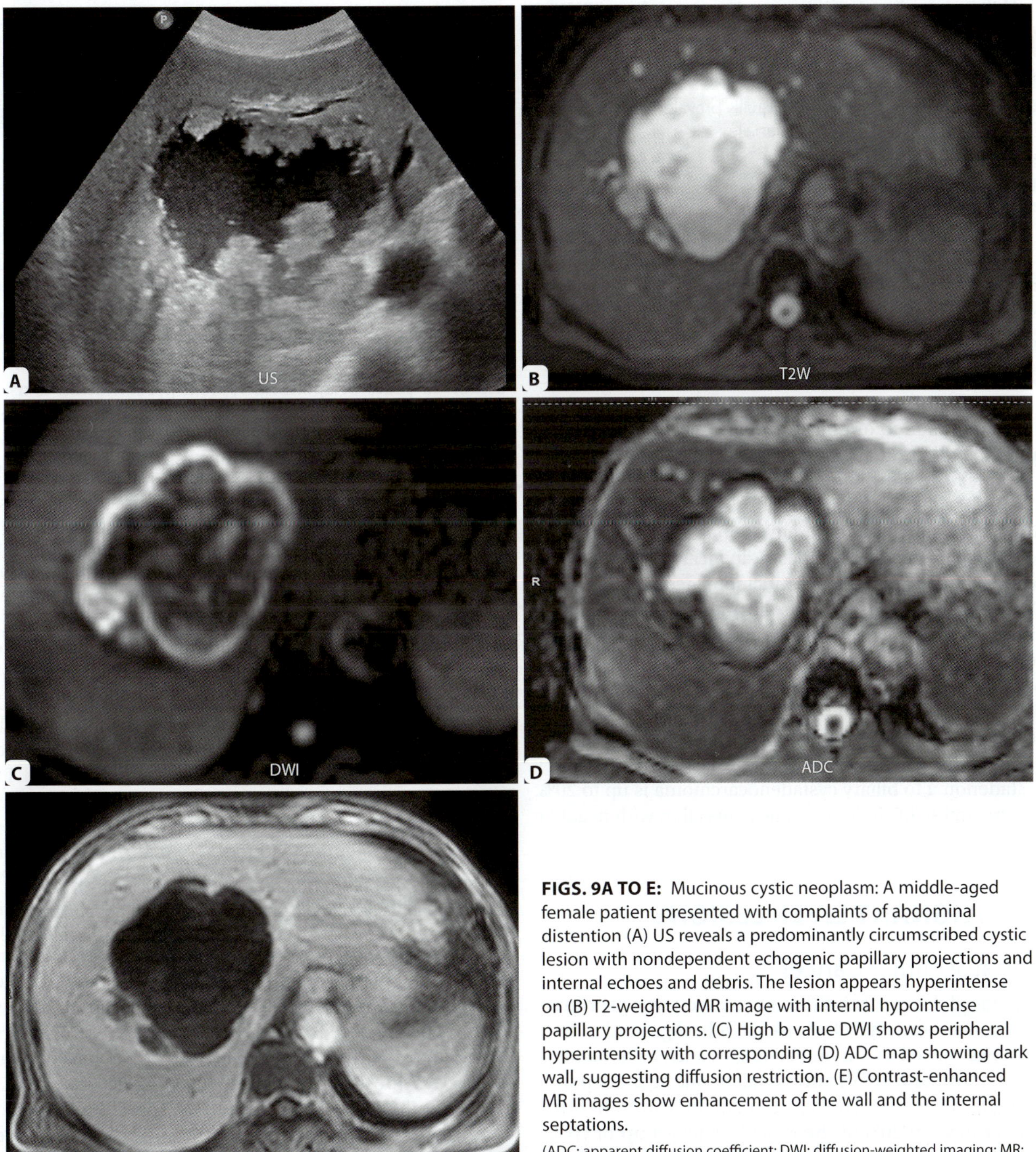

FIGS. 9A TO E: Mucinous cystic neoplasm: A middle-aged female patient presented with complaints of abdominal distention (A) US reveals a predominantly circumscribed cystic lesion with nondependent echogenic papillary projections and internal echoes and debris. The lesion appears hyperintense on (B) T2-weighted MR image with internal hypointense papillary projections. (C) High b value DWI shows peripheral hyperintensity with corresponding (D) ADC map showing dark wall, suggesting diffusion restriction. (E) Contrast-enhanced MR images show enhancement of the wall and the internal septations.

(ADC: apparent diffusion coefficient; DWI: diffusion-weighted imaging; MR: magnetic resonance; T2W: T2 weighted; US: ultrasound)

TABLE 5: Mucinous cystic neoplasm versus liver hydatid.

	Mucinous cystic neoplasm	Hydatid cyst of liver
Lobe of liver usually affected	Left lobe	Right lobe
Cyst wall enhancement	Cyst wall shows enhancement	No cyst wall enhancement
Septae	Septae can show calcification and enhancement	Septae do not show calcification or enhancement
Ultrasonography (USG) appearance	No floating membranes	Floating membranes
Daughter cysts	Never seen	Pathognomonic

TABLE 6: Differentiation between mucinous cystic neoplasm and biliary intraductal papillary mucinous neoplasm (IPMN).

Mucinous cystic neoplasm	Biliary IPMN
Mean age 45 years	Mean age 58 years
Female predominance	Equally prevalent in males and females
Smooth tumor wall with septa inside the tumor resulting in a "cysts-in-cyst" appearance	–
–	Papillary projections
–	Demonstration of cystic tumor and intrahepatic bile duct communication along with the presence of distal mucin is characteristic of biliary IPMN

and the absence of communication with the biliary tree. The differential diagnosis of patients with complex cystic lesions of the liver includes MCN, hydatid cyst **(Table 5)**, post-traumatic cyst, liver abscess, polycystic disease, hemorrhagic cyst, embryonal sarcoma, primary or metastatic necrotic neoplasm, atypical simple cyst, and biliary intraductal papillary mucinous neoplasm (IPMN) **(Table 6)**.[46] The role of cyst fluid carcinoembryonic antigen (CEA), carbohydrate antigen 19-9 (CA 19-9), and serum tumor markers remains controversial. Aspiration of suspected biliary cystic neoplasms should be avoided because of low likelihood of identifying malignant cells and risk of pleural and peritoneal dissemination.[47]

The risk of malignant transformation of biliary cystadenoma to biliary cystadenocarcinoma is up to 20%. The treatment of choice is surgical resection with negative margins.

MALIGNANT LIVER LESIONS

Hepatocellular Cancer

Hepatocellular cancer is the most common type of primary liver cancer and typically arises in a background of liver cirrhosis caused by varying etiologies such as hepatitis B and C (HBV and HCV) and nonalcoholic steatohepatitis (NASH). However, HCC can occur in a noncirrhotic background in 20% of the cases.[48] This group of HCCs usually presents at an advanced stage as they are usually asymptomatic; patients have higher hepatic reserve and there is no periodic surveillance. Moreover, in noncirrhotic HCC, the alpha-fetoprotein (AFP) elevation is less frequent (31–67% vs. 63–84%) as compared to HCC in cirrhotic liver and hence, the sensitivity decreases. Discussion of imaging of HCC is beyond the scope of this chapter and will be dealt with in a separate chapter.

Fibrolamellar Hepatocellular Carcinoma

Fibrolamellar hepatocellular carcinoma (FLC) is a rare hepatic neoplasm predominantly occurring in young individuals in a noncirrhotic background with unique clinicopathological features distinct from conventional HCC **(Table 7)**. The mean age of presentation is 25 years with 65–85% of fibrolamellar HCC occurring in patients under 40 years of age. The typical presentation is as a solitary large circumscribed mass in a noncirrhotic liver with normal AFP levels. US can show a lobulated solid mixed echogenicity liver lesion with a central echogenic scar which may or may not show calcification.[49] CT remains the workhorse for diagnosis with most lesions having lobulated margins, appearing hypodense on the noncontrast images, showing heterogeneous arterial enhancement with variable appearance on the portal venous phase, (48% are isoattenuating to the liver, 36% are hypoattenuating, and 16% are hyperattenuating to the liver on portal venous phase).[50] A central scar **(Figs. 10A to D)** is seen in 20–71% cases and the scar characteristically shows central calcification in up to 68% cases.[51] On MRI, the lesion is hypointense on T1, hyperintense on T2, and may show diffusion restriction along with a central T1 and T2 hypointense central scar, in contrast to the FNH scar which is hyperintense on T2.[52] Delayed phase images show contrast retention within the scar attributable to the vessels and myxomatous tissue within the scar in 25–65% of FLCs.[50] The important differentials based on imaging for FLC are FNH, HCA, hemangioma, and conventional HCC. Its differentiation from other entities is essential in deciding the management and biopsy is needed to make a final diagnosis. Histopathological examination shows plump polygonal cells in a fibrous stroma.[53] FLC displays immunopositivity for Hep Par 1 (positive in conventional HCC), CK7 [positive in intrahepatic cholangiocarcinoma (ICC)], and CD68.[54] In 50% patients, there is associated lymphadenopathy at the hepatic hilum or along the hepatoduodenal ligament which shows similar imaging

TABLE 7: Contrasting features of fibrolamellar HCC versus conventional HCC.

	Fibrolamellar HCC	Conventional HCC
Mean age of occurrence	25 years	65 years
Sex predilection	None	More common in men
Underlying CLD	Absent in 95%	Present
Serum AFP	Normal	Raised
Serum haptocorrin	Raised	–
Serum vitamin B12 binding capacity	Raised	–
Serum neurotensin	Raised	–
Des gamma carboxy prothrombin	Elevated	Elevated
Portal vein thrombosis	Uncommon	Common

(AFP: alpha-fetoprotein; CLD: chronic liver disease; HCC: hepatocellular cancer)

appearance as the index lesion.[55] Metastatic disease can be seen in 20–30% patients with disease spread occurring to the lungs, peritoneum, and the adrenal gland.[56] Surgery is the mainstay of treatment—resection and transplantation along with lymphadenectomy; however, recurrence rates are up to 50%.[57] Chemotherapy is not as effective in management of FLC as it is for conventional HCC; however, platinum-based regimens are used in metastatic disease. The overall prognosis is better than conventional HCC, owing to the absence of underlying CLD and the low risk for portal vein thrombosis.[58]

Mass Forming Intrahepatic Cholangiocarcinoma

Intrahepatic cholangiocarcinoma is the second most common primary hepatic malignancy after HCC. Caroli's disease, primary sclerosing cholangitis, choledochal cyst, familial polyposis, hepatolithiasis, congenital hepatic fibrosis, clonorchiasis, and a history of exposure

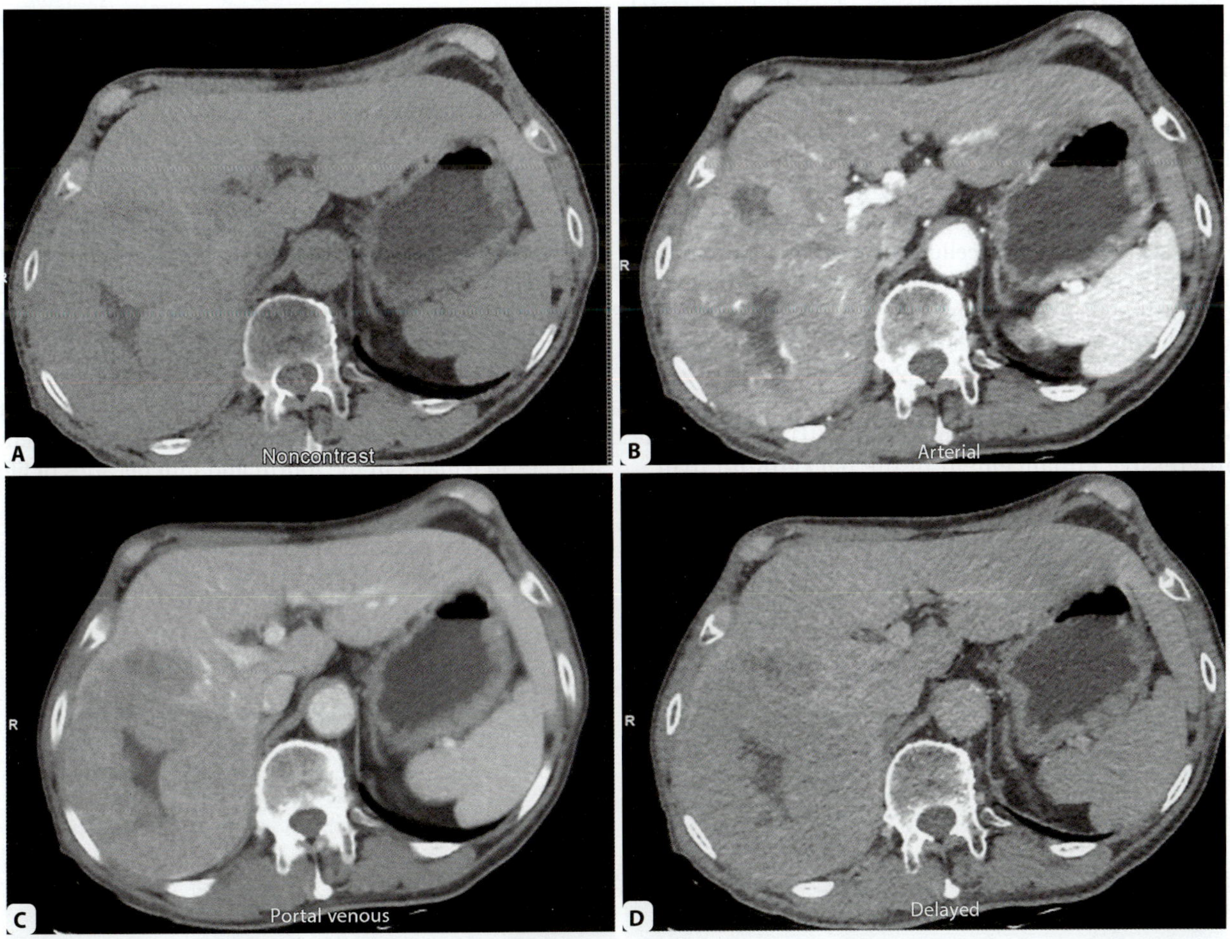

FIGS. 10A TO D: Fibrolamellar HCC: In a background of noncirrhotic liver, (A) noncontrast CT shows a hypodense lesion with (B) arterial phase showing nonrim APHE; (C) venous phase showing washout; and (D) delayed phase showing a central nonenhancing scar. US-guided biopsy confirmed fibrolamellar HCC.

(APHE: arterial phase hyperenhancement; CT: computed tomography; HCC: hepatocellular carcinoma; US: ultrasound)

to thorotrast are risk factors for the development of cholangiocarcinoma (CCA), in addition to background CLD. The clinical presentation is with abdominal pain, anorexia, and weight loss. Jaundice occurs when major ducts are obstructed. CCAs are categorized according to their anatomic location as extrahepatic, peripheral intrahepatic, and hilar intrahepatic and based on their growth pattern or morphologic subtype as mass forming, periductal infiltrating, or intraductal. ICC arise in small intrahepatic bile ducts, accounting for 10% of total cases of CCA. Mass-forming subtype is the most common type of ICC. US appearance may be as a homogeneous mass with intermediate to increased echogenicity and a peripheral hypoechoic halo with tumors > 3 cm in size appearing hyperechoic, while smaller tumors are iso- to hypoechoic.[59] There may be associated upstream biliary dilatation as well as overlying capsular retraction. CEUS can demonstrate early peripheral hyperenhancement followed by fast and marked peripheral washout versus HCC which shows hyperenhancement with slower and less marked washout.[60] The typical CT appearance of a mass-forming ICC is a hypodense mass with irregular peripheral enhancement in the arterial phase and gradual centripetal enhancement on portal venous and delayed phases.[61] Histologically, the peripheral portion of the tumor shows viable tumor cells, while the central portion is composed of coagulative necrosis with fewer tumor cells and varying degree of fibrous stroma.[62] The mass shows heterogeneous high signal intensity on T2-weighted imaging and low signal intensity on T1-weighted imaging. Dynamic contrast-enhanced MRI with extracellular contrast material exhibits prominent peripheral rim enhancement with centripetal or gradual progressive enhancement **(Figs. 11A to H)**. Rarely, mass-forming ICCs can demonstrate a pseudowashout pattern during the transitional phase (late dynamic phase between the portal venous and hepatobiliary phases of gadoxetate disodium-enhanced MRI), owing to the progressive enhancement of the background liver.[63] While it was thought that mass-forming ICCs usually do not show retention of contrast in the hepatobiliary phase attributable to the absence of OATP expression, recent studies have shown that mass-forming ICC can show a targetoid appearance or a heterogeneous hypointensity with intermingled hyperintensity on hepatobiliary phase images due to the fibrous stroma.[63,64] On DWI, 52–75% of mass-forming ICCs exhibit characteristic targetoid diffusion restriction with a central dark area reflecting fibrosis and necrosis of the tumor and a peripheral bright/restricted area representing highly cellular and vascular tumor cells.[65,66] The target sign on DWI which is seen in 50% of ICCs is useful in distinguishing ICC from HCC.[65,66] Additional features of ICC include intrahepatic biliary dilatation, satellite nodules, overlying capsular retraction, and vascular invasion. Involvement of portal vein branch by the mass can result in atrophy of the ipsilateral segment/lobe and hypertrophy of the contralateral lobe. The most important differentials include sclerosing hemangioma and HCC. The presence of upstream biliary dilatation, satellite nodules, diffusion restriction, and portal vein invasion helps in differentiating ICC from hemangioma. The features which help in differentiation from HCC from ICC are summarized in **Table 8**. Distinguishing between the two entities is important because patients with ICC are taken off the transplant list.

Epithelioid Hemangioendothelioma

Epithelioid hemangioendothelioma (EHE) is a rare, low-to-intermediate-grade malignant tumor of endothelial origin with malignant potential being intermediate between that of hemangioma and angiosarcoma.[67] It is composed of epithelioid and histiocyte-like vascular endothelial cells in mucus or fibrotic matrix.[68] The risk factors include vinyl chloride exposure, OCP intake, asbestos, colloidal thorium oxide, trauma repair, and viral hepatitis. These lesions tend to occur in females in the fourth and fifth decades of life.

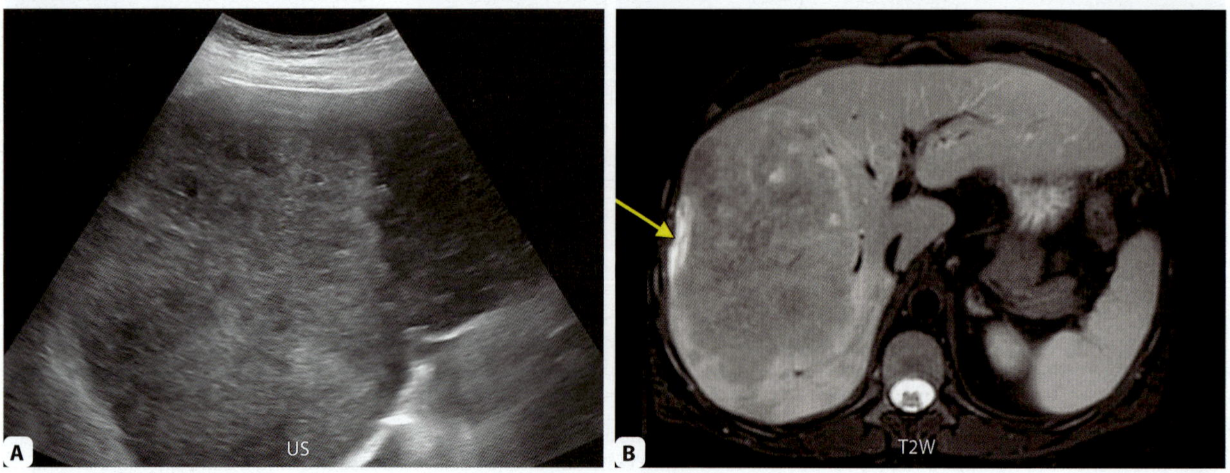

FIGS. 11A TO H: *Continued*

Continued

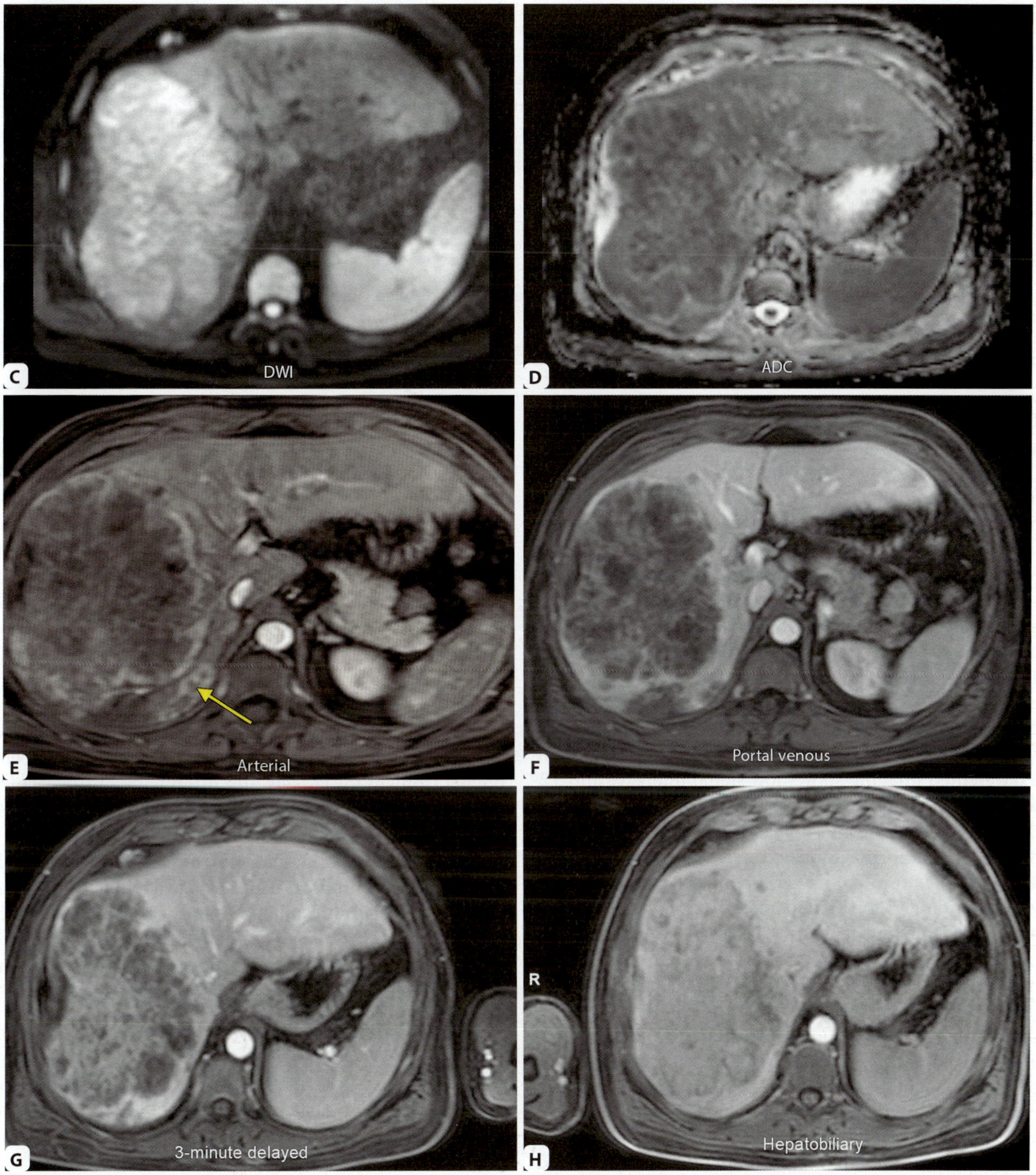

FIGS. 11A TO H: Intrahepatic cholangiocarcinoma: In a 41-year-old male patient, (A) US image shows a large heterogeneously hyperechoic lesion occupying a large part of the right lobe of the liver. No intrahepatic biliary dilatation was seen. (B) Axial T2W MRI shows a large heterogeneous mass occupying segments V, VI, VII, and VIII causing overlying capsular retraction (arrow). Axial (C) DWI and (D) ADC images depict that the lesion appears hyperintense on DWI and hypointense on ADC, indicating diffusion restriction. (E) Arterial phase image shows peripheral rim enhancement with additional satellite lesions in segment VII (arrow). (F) Portal venous phase and (G) 3-minute delayed phase shows progressive enhancement and (H) hepatobiliary phase shows retention of contrast on the 1-hour delayed phase.

(ADC: apparent diffusion coefficient; DWI: diffusion-weighted imaging; MRI: magnetic resonance imaging; T2W: T2 weighted; US: ultrasound)

TABLE 8: Differentiation of ICC from HCC.

	ICC	HCC
Background liver parenchyma	Noncirrhotic	Cirrhotic
Contrast enhancement	Thick peripheral rim enhancement with progressive filling in during portal venous and delayed phases	Arterial nonrim enhancement with washout in portal venous and delayed phase
Vascular involvement	Vascular thrombosis may be seen	Vascular thrombosis is more common
Capsular retraction	Characteristic feature	Less common
Biliary ductal dilatation	May be present	Absent
AFP levels	Usually normal	Elevated
CA 19-9	Elevated	Normal
Contrast-enhanced ultrasound	Early and marked washout on venous and delayed phase	Late and mild washout on delayed phase

(AFP: alpha-fetoprotein; CA 19-9: carbohydrate antigen 19-9; HCC: hepatocellular cancer; ICC: intrahepatic cholangiocarcinoma)

The lung, peritoneum, spleen, lymph nodes, and bone are the most common sites of extrahepatic involvement.[69] In 50% patients, there may be abnormal liver function tests. Morphologically, it can present as single, multiple, or diffuse and the multifocal form is most common. The multifocal variant is more common and lesions often have a peripheral and subcapsular distribution which may become confluent to involve the entire liver. Lesions are usually hypoechoic on US; however, they may show a hyperechoic center giving rise to a "bull's eye" appearance. The appearance on CT is usually as hypodense lesions on unenhanced CT with central foci of calcification seen in 25% cases.[70] There may be surrounding fibrosis and scarring resulting in capsular retraction **(Figs. 12A to G)**.[71] On MRI, T1-weighted imaging shows low signal intensity and T2-weighted imaging shows high signal intensity, owing to the myxomatous stroma.[72] The presence of calcification, necrosis, or hemorrhage makes the T2 signal heterogenous. The enhancement patterns on contrast-enhanced MRI vary according to the blood supply. Multifocal lesions are subdivided into four categories based on the enhancement patterns: (1) Slightly irregular homogeneous enhancement; (2) peripheral enhancement with central low signal intensity in the arterial phase and enhancing lesions surrounded by a thin hypointense ring in the portal venous and delayed phases ("black target-like" sign); (3) nodular enhancement in the central part of the lesion in the arterial phase surrounded by ring-like enhancement in the portal venous and delayed phases ("white target-like" sign); and (4) peripheral nodular enhancement in the arterial phase and centripetal enhancement in the portal venous and delayed phases, an enhancement pattern that is more commonly seen in hemangioma.[72] In the hepatobiliary phase, the peripheral rim of the tumor is hypointense and the central core shows retention of contrast owing to the fibrous stroma.[72] The "lollipop sign" has been described with respect to EHE and is the tapering or an abrupt termination of a portal or a hepatic venous radicle at the margin of the lesion.[73] The "stripe-like'" sign is described as a linear conglomeration of subcapsular lesions.[72] On DWI, the lesion displays a targetoid pattern of diffusion restriction. The differential diagnosis in case of solitary lesions include other lesions which may show capsular retraction such as mass-forming CCA, scirrhous HCC, confluent hepatic fibrosis, and sclerosing hemangioma. The hallmark features pointing toward a diagnosis of EHE include lollipop sign, multilayered target-like appearance, absent CA 19-9 elevation, absent biliary dilatation, and absent background liver cirrhosis and enhancement pattern. The multinodular form needs to be differentiated from multifocal metastasis (such as those originating from breast or colon cancer) and multifocal HCC. On histopathology, EHE shows epithelioid and dendritic cells in a background of myxoid stroma with the development of sclerosis. The tumor cells have a tropism for vessels and often show intravascular extension. The tumor stains are positive for endothelial markers (factor VIII-related antigen, CD31, and CD34). Podoplanin is a specific marker expressed in EHE, which helps in differentiation from other vascular tumors. In localized disease and solitary lesions, surgical resection is the treatment of choice. Patients with multifocal disease require orthotopic transplants. The prognosis is better than angiosarcoma and long-term survival rates are good.

Angiosarcoma

Angiosarcoma is a primary mesenchymal tumor of endothelial cell origin, which can affect the soft tissues of the scalp, head and neck, breast, or liver. While hepatic angiosarcoma is a rare tumor contributing to only 2% of liver malignancies, it remains the third most common primary liver cancer.[74] The tumor is highly aggressive and is metastatic at the time of presentation in 60% of the cases. Exposure to carcinogens such as radiation, thorotrast, vinyl chloride, and arsenic are associated with increased risk.[75] Genetic predisposition is reported in patients with hemochromatosis and neurofibromatosis.[76] The incidence is three times higher in males and the disease usually occurs in 50–79 years age group. The signs and symptoms are usually nonspecific with dull aching pain, abdominal

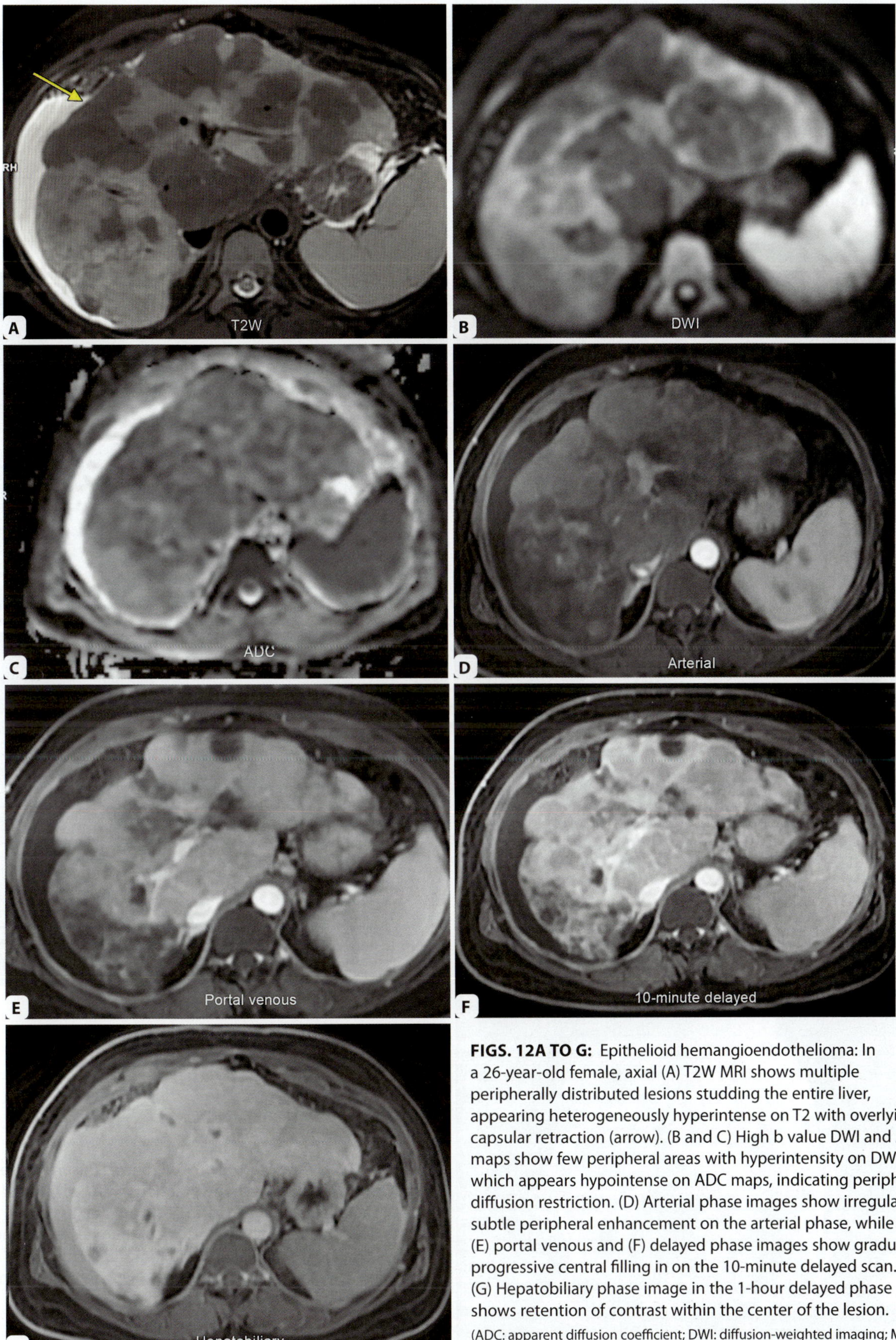

FIGS. 12A TO G: Epithelioid hemangioendothelioma: In a 26-year-old female, axial (A) T2W MRI shows multiple peripherally distributed lesions studding the entire liver, appearing heterogeneously hyperintense on T2 with overlying capsular retraction (arrow). (B and C) High b value DWI and ADC maps show few peripheral areas with hyperintensity on DWI which appears hypointense on ADC maps, indicating peripheral diffusion restriction. (D) Arterial phase images show irregular subtle peripheral enhancement on the arterial phase, while (E) portal venous and (F) delayed phase images show gradual progressive central filling in on the 10-minute delayed scan. (G) Hepatobiliary phase image in the 1-hour delayed phase shows retention of contrast within the center of the lesion.

(ADC: apparent diffusion coefficient; DWI: diffusion-weighted imaging; MRI: magnetic resonance imaging; T2W: T2 weighted) fullness, malaise, and fatigue. In contrast to HCC, AFP elevation is not seen. Advanced/disseminated malignancies show elevated liver enzymes, increased bilirubin levels, and altered albumin-globulin ratio. Lesions may present as a solitary large mass, multiple small lesions, or in a mixed pattern. The multifocal pattern occurs as a dominant mass surrounded by multiple smaller lesions and is the most common imaging appearance. These tumors show necrosis as well as hemorrhagic areas which appear hyperdense on unenhanced CT and hyperintense on T1-weighted images. Blood fluid levels may be seen with varying stages of the hemorrhage. Postcontrast scans show bizarre and nonconforming patterns of hypervascularity within and around the rim of the lesions in the arterial phase **(Figs. 13A to E)**.[77] Venous phase shows progressive enlargement of the areas to form branching or scaffold-like patterns. Lesions can also show centripetal filling in of contrast similar to hemangiomas.[78] The enhancement is less than but parallels

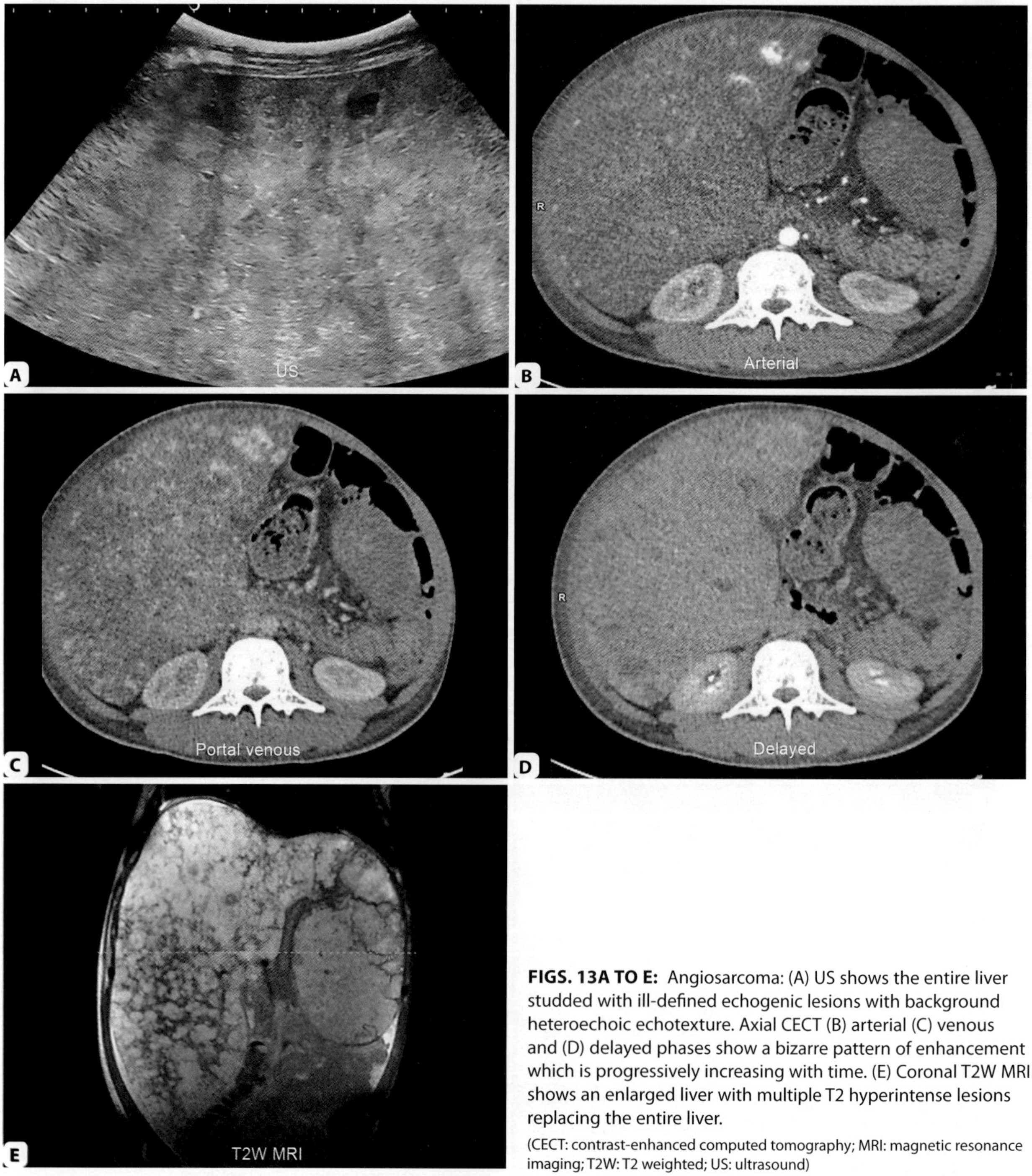

FIGS. 13A TO E: Angiosarcoma: (A) US shows the entire liver studded with ill-defined echogenic lesions with background heteroechoic echotexture. Axial CECT (B) arterial (C) venous and (D) delayed phases show a bizarre pattern of enhancement which is progressively increasing with time. (E) Coronal T2W MRI shows an enlarged liver with multiple T2 hyperintense lesions replacing the entire liver.

(CECT: contrast-enhanced computed tomography; MRI: magnetic resonance imaging; T2W: T2 weighted; US: ultrasound)

TABLE 9: Differentiation of hemangiomatosis from angiosarcoma.

	Hemangiomatosis	Angiosarcoma
T2 appearance	T2 bright light bulb appearance	Heterogenous, internal hypointense areas and disorganized vessels
Vascular invasion	Uncommon	Common
Diffusion restriction	Uncommon	Common
Enhancement characteristics	Peripheral discontinuous nodular enhancement	Irregular bizarre patterns of enhancement on the arterial phase
Enhancement pattern with respect to blood pool	Matches blood pool	Enhancement patterns parallel blood pool but are always lower intensity than blood pool

the blood pool.[77] Small lesions may not depict arterial phase enhancement and even in large lesions, significant parts of the lesion may remain unenhanced even in the equilibrium phase.[79] DWI show a heterogeneous pattern of diffusion restriction, however much less than metastasis and other malignancies. Angiosarcoma is avid on FDG-PET and is a good modality to assess the metastasis and extent of spread of disease. Spontaneous rupture of the tumor and intraperitoneal hemorrhage are the most feared complications which may be seen in up to 27% cases.[80] The differential diagnosis includes hypervascular lesions such as hemangiomatosis, hypervascular metastasis, and multifocal HCC **(Table 9)**. Angiosarcoma may be differentiated from HCC by the absence of underlying CLD, absent AFP elevation, and the presence of thrombocytopenia, bizarre enhancement, and splenic metastasis. Biopsy is required for diagnosis and a plugged biopsy can be done with caution and adequate preparation to handle hemorrhagic complications. On histopathological examination, these lesions show poorly formed vessels and sheets of epithelioid and spindle cells.[81] The sinusoidal type shows blood-filled dilated sinusoids. The atypical cells are positive for endothelial markers such as ERG, factor VIII-related antigen, CD31, and CD34.

Metastasis

Metastasis to the liver is the most common malignant lesion involving the liver, being more common than HCC. A large number of malignancies, including cancers of the gastrointestinal system (e.g., colorectum, stomach, pancreas, and biliary), genitourinary system (e.g., kidney and prostate), gynecologic system (e.g., ovary, endometrium, and cervix), neuroendocrine system, and breast; soft-tissue sarcomas; melanomas; and lymphomas—can show secondaries to the liver. While the presence of metastasis to the liver was previously deemed as an unresectable disease, with progress in treatment options, metastatic lesions are amenable to resection depending upon the size, number, and the location of the lesions. Since the liver function tests are normal in 50% of the patients with metastasis, imaging is essential for detection. US is often the first line of investigation, owing to its easy availability and low cost. The sensitivity is variable 40–77% with poor sensitivity in picking up small-sized lesions. Liver metastases can have a variable appearance on US being hypoechoic, hyperechoic, isoechoic, or even cystic. Hyperechoic metastasis can be seen in primaries from colon, gastrointestinal tumors, islet cell tumors, carcinoids, choriocarcinoma, and renal cell carcinoma (RCC). The typical appearance of metastases is the targetoid or "bull's eye" appearance due to the presence of a hypoechoic rim around the lesion **(Figs. 14A to D)**. Metastasis from mucinous gastrointestinal tract tumors and primary ovarian, breast, lung, renal, and thyroid cancer can show calcification.[82] Metastasis from most primaries is either isodense or hypodense on noncontrast CT. Majority of the metastases are hypovascular in the portal venous phase and may show a complete ring of enhancement in the arterial phase **(Figs. 15A to C)**. Hypervascular metastases arise from primary tumors, such as neuroendocrine tumor (NET), RCC, thyroid carcinoma, choriocarcinoma, pheochromocytoma, malignant melanoma, and sarcomas. These appear hypodense on unenhanced CT images, with moderate hyperintensity on T2-weighted images and cause diffusion restriction. Dynamic contrast-enhanced CT and MRI depict early enhancement on arterial phase images and washout on portal venous phase images which can mimic HCC.[83] MRI has a better diagnostic accuracy than CT in the detection of liver metastasis. A combination of T2-weighted images and DWI is a sensitive technique to pick up metastasis. Liver-specific contrast agents such as gadobenate and gadoxetic acid improve the detection of lesions since metastases appear hypointense on hepatobiliary phase. Cystic appearance of metastasis (very hypodense on CT and high signal intensity on T2-weighted imaging) can be due to (1) necrosis as in metastases from NET, gastrointestinal stromal tumor (GIST), sarcoma, melanoma, angiosarcoma, testicular carcinoma, or squamous cell carcinoma; (2) cystic metastasis from mixed solid-cystic primaries such as intraductal papillary mucinous carcinoma of the pancreas, adenoid cystic carcinoma, or ovarian serous and mucinous carcinoma cystic components of the primary; and (3) hyperintensity due to the primary histological features (mucinous/myxoid component).[84] Rapid growth of hypervascular metastasis beyond their blood supply can result in necrosis and the inner margin of the tumor shows ragged margins in such lesions.[85] Metastasis from NET, melanoma, angiosarcoma, ovarian carcinoma, RCC, leiomyosarcoma, and squamous

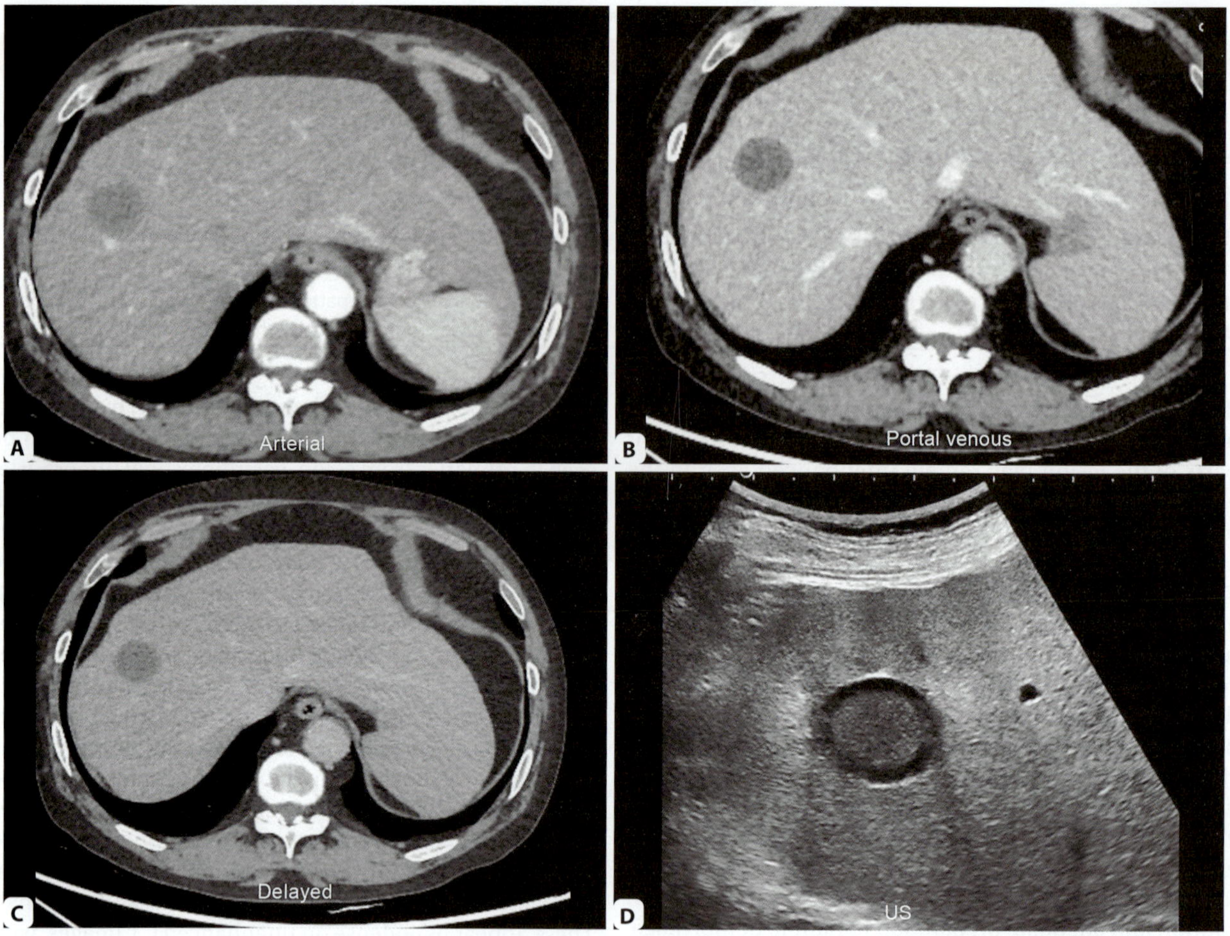

FIGS. 14A TO D: Hypodense solitary liver metastasis in mucinous adenocarcinoma of the colon: In patients with mucinous adenocarcinoma of the colon, axial contrast-enhanced computed tomography (CECT) images in the (A) arterial, (B) venous, and (C) delayed phases show a solitary hypovascular lesion showing minimal peripheral rim enhancement. (D) Ultrasound (US) image shows the lesion to have a classical targetoid appearance indicating metastasis.

cell carcinoma can show intratumoral hemorrhage, causing T1 hyperintensity and fluid–fluid levels on T2-weighted images depending upon the degree and duration of hemorrhage.[86] Marked hyperintensity on fat-suppressed T1-weighted images suggests the presence of paramagnetic substance melanin and is characteristic of malignant melanoma.[87] The important differentials of metastases include hemangiomas, multifocal HCC, and inflammatory granulomas. Inflammatory granulomas (sarcoidosis and tuberculosis) are hypodense/T2 hypointense on imaging and may have lymphadenopathy and additional splenic lesions. US-guided sampling may help establish the final diagnosis. Despite the advances in imaging, subcentimetric and subcapsular lesions may remain underdetected on imaging.

Desmoplastic reaction occurring surrounding the metastasis occurring in subcapsular location can lead to hepatic capsular retraction which is reported with primaries from lung, breast, and colorectal adenocarcinomas.[88] Cirrhosis-like morphology can develop after chemotherapy in the treatment of metastatic breast cancer and gastrointestinal primaries. While the actual metastatic lesions in the liver may regress after chemotherapy, the liver morphology may become nodular and look cirrhotic. This is referred to as pseudocirrhosis, since there is no bridging fibrosis, although there is capsular retraction, atrophy, and volume redistribution.

Hepatic Lymphoma

Hepatic lymphoma can be classified into primary and secondary (metastatic) forms with non-Hodgkin's lymphoma being more common in both the forms.[89] Primary hepatic lymphoma (PHL) is extremely rare, accounting for <1% of all non-Hodgkin's lymphoma.[90] The diagnosis of a primary lymphoma requires the presence of disease only involving the liver and the hilar lymph nodes and concomitant absence of any distant disease in the form of nonregional lymphadenopathy, splenic involvement, or bone marrow disease within 6 months of

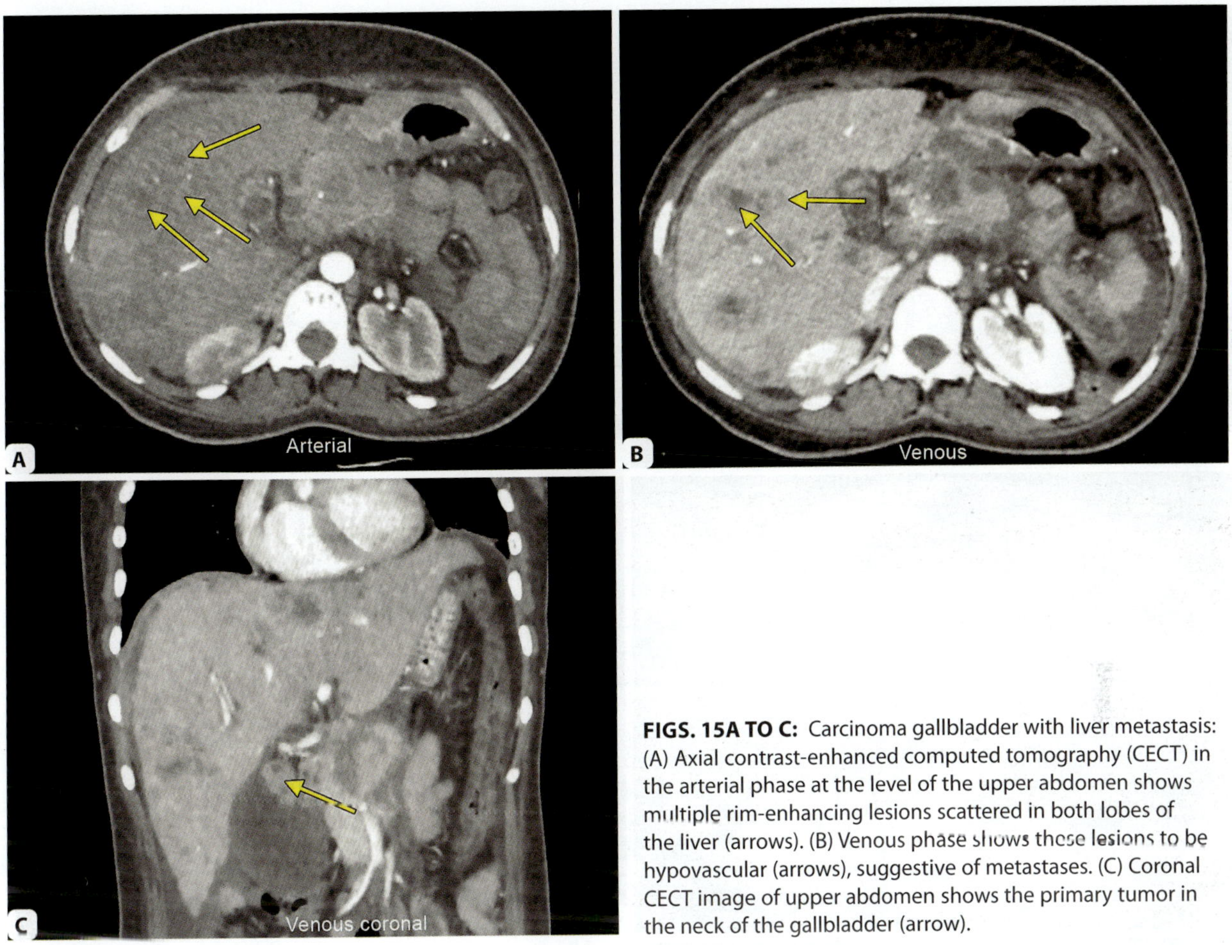

FIGS. 15A TO C: Carcinoma gallbladder with liver metastasis: (A) Axial contrast-enhanced computed tomography (CECT) in the arterial phase at the level of the upper abdomen shows multiple rim-enhancing lesions scattered in both lobes of the liver (arrows). (B) Venous phase shows these lesions to be hypovascular (arrows), suggestive of metastases. (C) Coronal CECT image of upper abdomen shows the primary tumor in the neck of the gallbladder (arrow).

diagnosis.[91] Prolonged immunosuppression and infections with human immunodeficiency virus (HIV), Epstein–Barr virus (EBV), HBV, and HCV have been implicated as risk factors for PHL.[92] The disease tends to occur in males in the fourth and fifth decades.[93] The clinical manifestations include hepatomegaly, right upper quadrant pain, jaundice, and symptoms in the form of fever, weight loss, and night sweats. Elevation of serum lactate dehydrogenase (LDH) and beta-2 microglobulin may be seen.[94] The most common histopathological subtype is diffuse large B-cell lymphoma (DLBCL).[95] Imaging plays an important role in diagnosis, staging, guiding sampling, and in monitoring response to treatment and follow-up.

Imaging Features

Primary hepatic lymphomas occur as solitary masses in 60% of the cases and have a dominant mass among lesions in multifocal PHLs. US usually shows these masses to be solid, rounded, well-defined, lobulated, hypoechoic masses. However, these lesions can appear anechoic (owing to dense cell arrangement) and mimic cysts. On CT, the lesions are usually hypodense without any calcifications **(Figs. 16A to E)**. T2-weighted MR images show the lesion to be only mildly hyperintense with marked diffusion restriction owing to the high cellularity and low or minimal postcontrast enhancement. In the hepatobiliary phase, lymphomas usually do not show contrast retention. A targetoid appearance can be seen in 15% of the PHLs in the form of a peripheral rim which appears hypoechoic on US, mildly T2 hyperintense, shows postcontrast enhancement, and intense diffusion restriction with a more echogenic central scar showing more T2 hyperintensity and progressive centripetal filling of contrast in the delayed and hepatobiliary phases.[96] FDG-PET CT shows uptake and is a good modality to evaluate complete disease extent and response to treatment.

Similar to lymphomas elsewhere, the lesions tend to insinuate around vessels and bile ducts without any significant mass effect or caliber change referred to as the "vessel penetration sign." As compared to PHLs which are more likely to be heterogeneous, secondary lymphomas are usually more homogenous. In secondary forms of lymphoma, diffusely infiltrating lesions and ill-defined periportal infiltrating soft tissue masses can be seen. The diffusely infiltrating form of secondary lymphoma may present only with hepatomegaly and in such circumstances, FDG-PET avidity and diffusion restriction on MRI are excellent in recognition of the involvement.

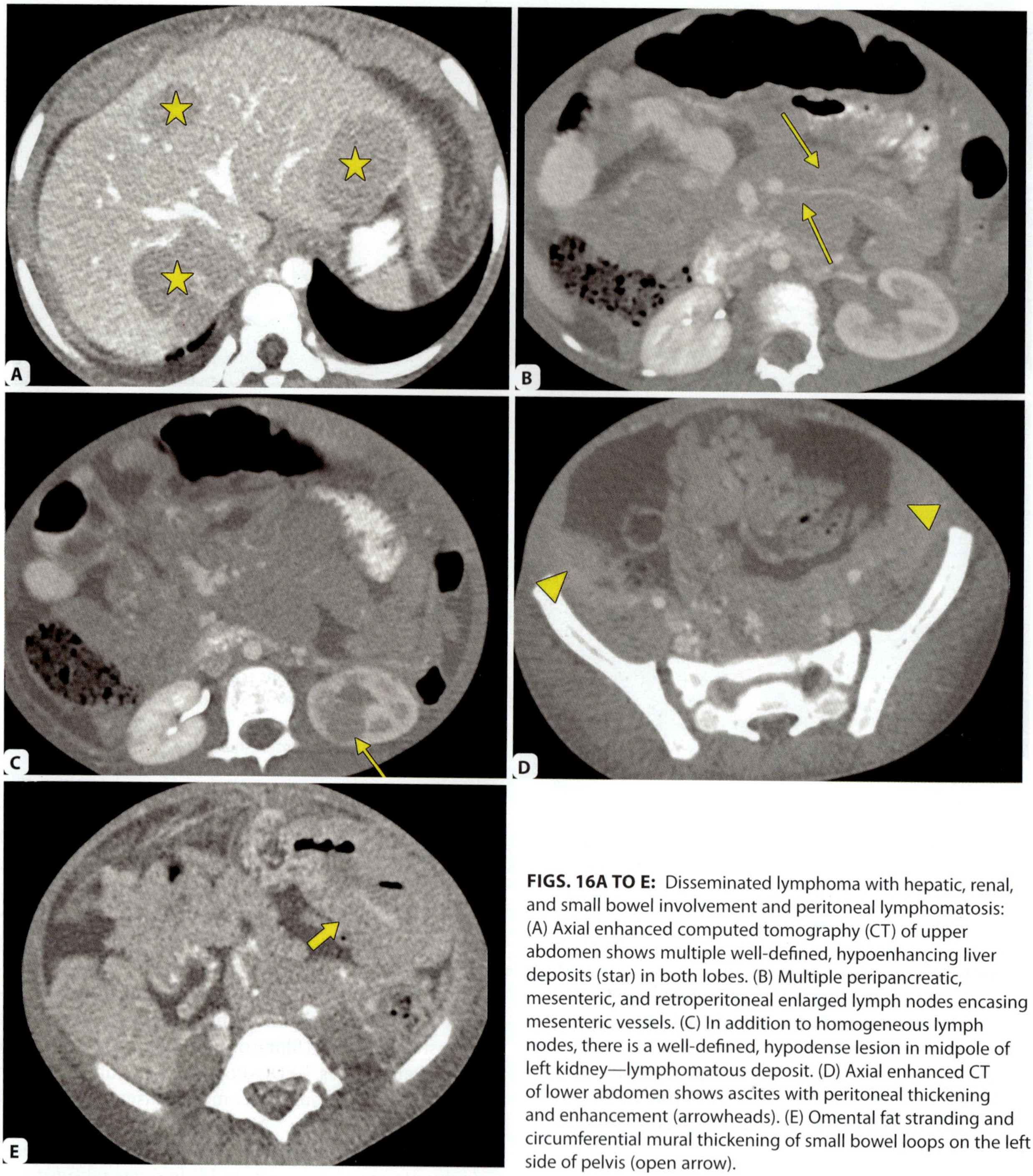

FIGS. 16A TO E: Disseminated lymphoma with hepatic, renal, and small bowel involvement and peritoneal lymphomatosis: (A) Axial enhanced computed tomography (CT) of upper abdomen shows multiple well-defined, hypoenhancing liver deposits (star) in both lobes. (B) Multiple peripancreatic, mesenteric, and retroperitoneal enlarged lymph nodes encasing mesenteric vessels. (C) In addition to homogeneous lymph nodes, there is a well-defined, hypodense lesion in midpole of left kidney—lymphomatous deposit. (D) Axial enhanced CT of lower abdomen shows ascites with peritoneal thickening and enhancement (arrowheads). (E) Omental fat stranding and circumferential mural thickening of small bowel loops on the left side of pelvis (open arrow).

Differential Diagnosis

- PHLs need to be differentiated from secondary forms of lymphoma involving the hepatic parenchyma **(Table 10)**.
- *Cysts and abscesses*: The anechoic appearance of these lesions may mimic benign pathologies; however, the absence of posterior acoustic shadowing and the presence of lateral edge shadowing can indicate the solid nature. The absence of internal moving echoes is also helpful. CT and MRI are diagnostic to identify the solid nature of lymphoma.
- *HCC*: Raised AFP levels, APHE, washout, associated portal vein thrombosis, less intense diffusion restriction, and background liver cirrhosis favor HCC.
- *Metastasis*: The presence of a known primary malignancy can help differentiate it from secondary hepatic lymphoma.

TABLE 10: Differentiation of primary hepatic lymphoma from secondary hepatic lymphoma.

Features	Primary hepatic lymphoma	Secondary hepatic lymphoma
Distribution	• Solitary • Even multifocal lesions show a dominant mass	*Usually multifocal*: Other morphological patterns include diffusely infiltrating and periportal infiltrating types
Morphology	Heterogenous on T1 and T2 and shows heterogeneous enhancement	Homogenous lesions
Enhancement	May show arterial phase hyperenhancement and washout	Hypovascular
Targetoid pattern	Seen in 15% of cases	Absent
Periportal lymphadenopathy	Present	Present
Infrarenal lymphadenopathy	Absent	Present
Splenomegaly	Absent	Present
Bone marrow involvement	Absent	Present

- *CCA*: The presence of hepatic capsular retraction, biliary dilatation, and lobar atrophy favor CCA.
- *Pseudolymphoma*: It is a non-neoplastic-reactive proliferation of lymphoid tissue at extranodal sites. It is a rare incidental lesion that is usually detected on autopsy and may be seen in elderly females with autoimmune hepatitis. Few hallmarks include APHE with washout on the venous/delayed phase, hypointensity on the hepatobiliary phase, and intense avidity on FDG-PET. The confirmation of diagnosis requires a biopsy and treatment options include chemotherapy, radiotherapy, and resection. Adverse prognostic factors include old age, advanced stage, aggressive histological subtypes, bulky disease, immunosuppression, and LDH elevation.

RARE NEOPLASTIC LIVER LESIONS

Perivascular Epithelioid Cell Tumor

Perivascular epithelioid cell tumor (PEComas) are a group of mesenchymal tumors which are histologically characterized by proliferation of both epithelioid cells and spindle cells in variable proportions and are positive for melanocytic (HMB-45 and melan-A) and myoid markers (desmin, smooth muscle actin, and myosin).[97] The most common cytogenetic abnormality is deletion of 16p involving the *TSC2* gene. The PEComa family of tumors includes angiomyolipoma (AML), lymphangioleiomyomatosis, clear-cell sugar tumor, clear-cell myomelanocytic tumor of falciform ligament/ligamentum teres and PEComas—not otherwise specified (NOS).[98] PEComas arising in the right lobe of the liver tend to have AML histology, while those arising along the falciform ligament tend to have PEComa-NOS histology.[97] Out of these, the most common pathological type is AML. These lesions may be incidentally detected in asymptomatic patients or present with nonspecific symptoms such as abdominal pain, distention, and fullness. These lesions tend to be more common in females in the fifth and sixth decades of life. Multiple PEComas may be seen in association with tuberous sclerosis (TSC) in which lesions also present at an earlier age. Liver AMLs may contain macroscopic fat seen as low attenuation on CT or they may be lipid-poor AMLs which are hypervascular. The lipid-poor AMLs get their signal intensity based on the relative proportion of the epithelioid and the myomatous components. The epithelioid components are vascular and are T2 hyperintense and show intense arterial phase enhancement and washout on the venous phase, while the myomatous components show T2 hypointense signal and show hypoenhancement in the arterial phase and progressive enhancement in the venous and delayed phases.[99] Lesions may show diffusion restriction and appear hypointense on the hepatobiliary phase. The presence of abundant distorted vessels in the center of the lesions as well as presence of an early-draining hepatic vein are unique features.[100] While most lesions are benign, few lesions can show features of malignancy with local recurrence and distant metastasis.[101] Folpe et al. have proposed a categorization of PEComas into benign, uncertain malignant potential (UMP), and malignant neoplasms. The features which are suspicious for malignancy include size > 5 cm, infiltrative nature, high nuclear grade and cellularity, mitotic activity > 1/50 high power fields (HPFs), coagulative necrosis, and vascular invasion.[102] The differential diagnosis includes hypervascular lesions such as HCA, FNH, HCC, and hemangioma. The presence of macroscopic fat, relative T2 hypointense signal, tortuous intratumoral vessels, and an early draining vein favor a diagnosis of PEComa. The absence of contrast retention on the hepatobiliary phase in PEComas helps differentiate it from FNH, HCA, and well-differentiated HCC. The absence of a scar differentiates it from FLC and FNH; the absence of necrosis and hemorrhage differentiates it from HCA and HCC; and the lack of matching blood pool enhancement differentiates it from hemangioma. Owing to the potential risk of malignancy, surgical resection is the mainstay of treatment.[100] Mammalian targets of rapamycin (mTOR) inhibitors such as everolimus have been used in the management of metastatic disease.

Soft Tissue (Mesenchymal) Tumors

Lipomas are benign mesenchymal tumors which are rarely encountered in the liver and do not pose a risk of malignant transformation. US appearance is of a homogeneously hyperechoic lesion. On CT, the lesion shows macroscopic fat matching the density of mesenteric or retroperitoneal fat. Lesions appear hyperintense on T1- and T2-weighted images and show loss of signal on T1-weighted fat suppressed sequences. Chemical-shift MRI shows variable loss of signal in these lesions with the presence of hypointense chemical shift artifact around the hepatic lipomas.

Inflammatory pseudotumor also referred to as inflammatory myofibroblastic tumor of the liver is an uncommon, benign tumor histologically composed of inflammatory cells and fibrous stroma. The presence of T2 hypointensity on MRI and mild delayed contrast enhancement may point toward this diagnosis.

Neurofibromas are soft tissue tumors which may rarely be seen in the liver **(Figs. 17A to C)**, especially in association with neurofibromatosis type 1.

Teratoma

The liver is an extremely rare site for teratoma, constituting <1% of all teratomas. They are discovered incidentally and can cause abdominal distension, nausea, and vomiting due to compression of adjacent structures. US shows hypo- or anechoic components representing cystic portion and hyperechoic areas denoting calcifications or macroscopic fat. Fat-fluid levels due to the presence of sebum are considered pathognomonic of teratoma. CT is the diagnostic modality of choice and demonstrates macroscopic fat and areas of calcification within **(Figs. 18A and B)**.

Primary Hepatic Neuroendocrine Tumors

Primary hepatic NETs (PHNETs) are peptide-secreting tumors analogous to NETs at other sites. PHNETs are rare as compared to hepatic metastasis, arising from NET elsewhere in the abdomen. The origin of these tumors is postulated to be from intestinal metaplasia of biliary tract or heterotopic pancreatic/adrenal tissue in the liver.[103] Most cases are reported to be in middle-aged females in fourth and fifth decades. The clinical signs and symptoms are nonspecific such as abdominal pain and fullness and presence of carcinoid syndrome is rare. Elevated serum chromogranin and 24-hour urine 5-hydroxyindoleacetic acid are seen in the majority of the patients. The imaging appearance varies depending on the tumor grade. Grade 1 (G1) and grade 2 (G2) tumors are usually seen as solitary masses in the right lobe, while grade 3 (G3) tumors are seen as multiple masses

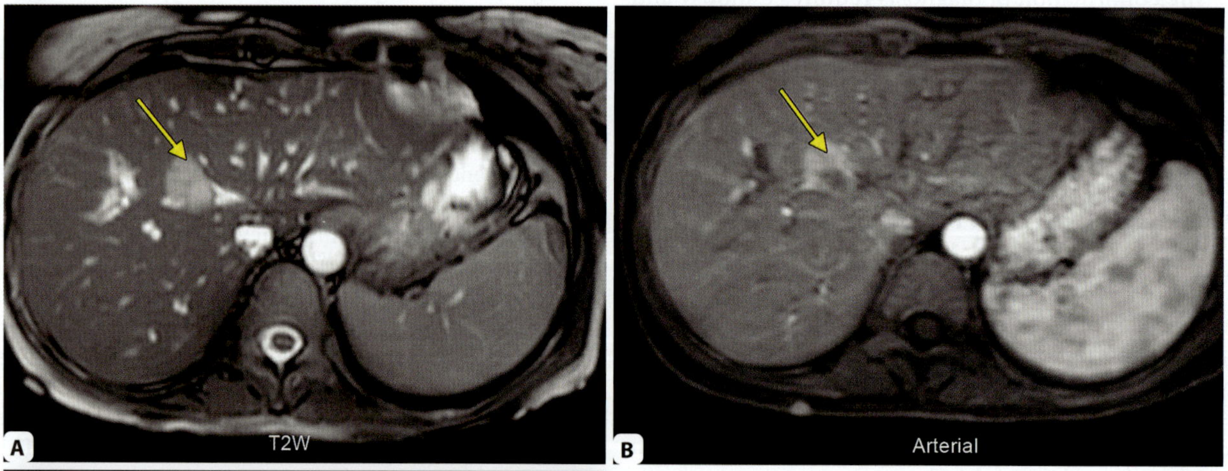

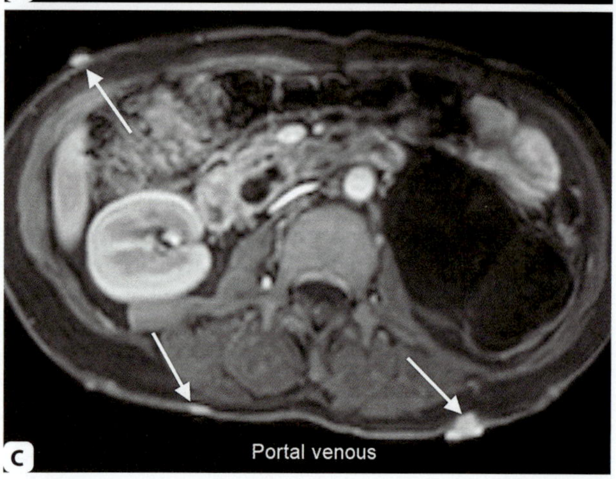

FIGS. 17A TO C: Neurofibroma of the liver: In a patient with neurofibromatosis type 1, axial (A) T2-weighted (T2W) image shows a hyperintense lobulated lesion (arrows) in segment VIII of the liver. (B) Arterial phase shows lesion enhancement (arrows). Lower abdomen in (C) portal–venous phase shows multiple, small, enhancing lesions in the skin (arrows)—cutaneous neurofibromas.

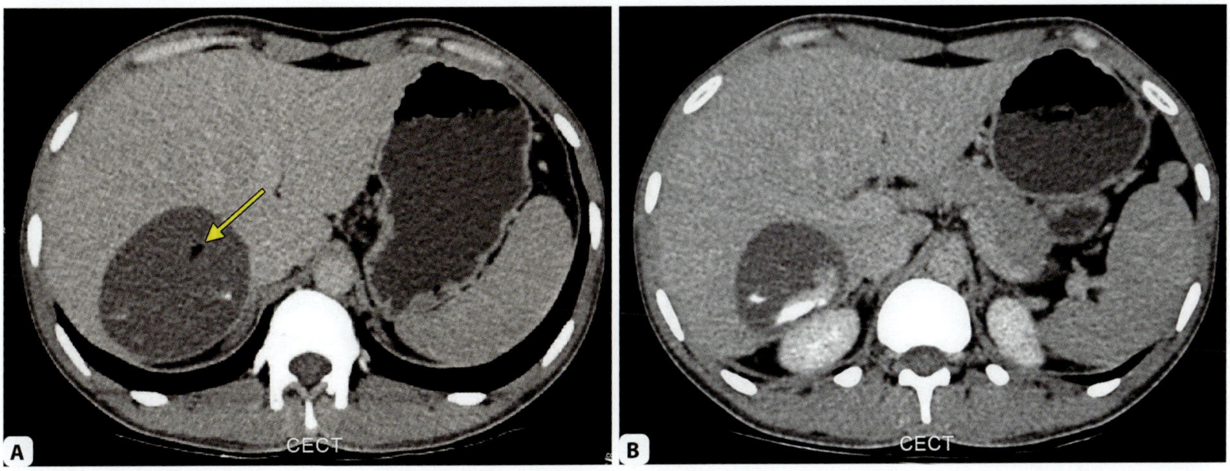

FIGS. 18A AND B: Hepatic teratoma: (A and B) Axial contrast-enhanced computed tomography (CECT) of the upper abdomen shows a well-defined, round, hypodense mass with macroscopic fat (arrow) and coarse calcifications seen in segments VI and VII of liver consistent with hepatic teratoma.

or as a dominant mass with surrounding satellite lesions. These lesions appear hypodense on unenhanced CT, appearing hyperintense on T2-weighted images and show heterogeneous peripheral arterial phase enhancement with hyperenhancement persisting on the venous and delayed phases. DWI show intense restriction. While areas of cystic necrosis, hemorrhage, and blood–fluid levels may be seen, calcification is rare. The incidence of necrosis, hemorrhage, and diffusion restriction is higher in G3 tumors.[104] Akin to NETs elsewhere, uptake is seen on somatostatin receptor scintigraphy (SRS) and Ga-68 DOTANOC PET/CT, which is highly specific. Differentials include hypervascular lesions such as HCC, HCA, PEComa, and hypervascular metastasis. The presence of peripheral APHE, normal AFP level, and absent background CLD helps differentiate it from HCC. Features such as intralesional fat and OCP intake favor HCA. The presence of a known malignancy and multiple lesions favors a diagnosis of metastasis. DOTANOC uptake is highly specific for NET and the presence of additional uptake on DOTANOC elsewhere suggests extrahepatic NET with liver metastasis. However, since bowel NET can be occult on endoscopy and DOTANOC scan, making a final diagnosis of a PHNET requires at least 1-year follow-up after surgery so that an occult extrahepatic primary is ruled out.[105] The treatment of choice for localized disease is surgical resection and the prognosis tends to be better than HCC and intra-HCC (IHCC). Metastatic tumors that are DOTANOC positive can be treated with peptide receptor radionuclide therapy.

NEOPLASTIC LIVER LESIONS IN PEDIATRIC PATIENTS

Most of the abovementioned focal liver lesions discussed occur during adulthood. In the pediatric population, the neoplastic lesions occurring in the liver are distinct entities, including hepatoblastoma, mesenchymal hamartoma, infantile HH (IHH), and congenital HH. Although a detailed discussion of these entities is beyond the scope of this chapter, a brief summary is presented further.

Hepatoblastoma

Hepatoblastoma represents the most common primary malignant lesion of the liver in children with 90% of tumors occurring under the age of 5 years. Markedly elevated serum AFP is a useful marker and increasing levels are of significance in diagnosis, as well as monitoring therapy and detecting recurrence. On imaging, the tumor is a well-circumscribed, homogenous, lobulated mass. US displays most of these lesions to be hyperechoic as compared to the background liver. The mixed variants of the tumor can show areas of necrosis, hemorrhage, and calcification **(Figs. 19A and B)**. CT appearance reveals a circumscribed mass which is hypodense compared to the background liver. CT is an excellent modality in the depiction of portal vein or inferior vena cava invasion. On MR, lesions appear hyperintense on T2 with T2 hypointense fibrotic septa which show postcontrast enhancement. The most common site of metastasis is the lungs and CT chest is mandatory in assessing the extent of disease. The pretreatment extent of disease (PRETEXT) staging system is used for classifying the extent of involvement.

Mesenchymal Hamartoma

Mesenchymal hamartoma is the second most common benign hepatic tumor occurring in the pediatric population. This lesion presents usually in the first 2 years of life with a median age of 10 months.[106] It is twice as common in male children and tends to affect the right lobe of the liver more commonly than the left lobe. AFP levels are normal.[107] Sonography reveals a mixed solid cystic mass with the solid portions appearing echogenic and the cystic portions appearing anechoic with multiple thin septations. On CT, the lesion appears as a complex cystic

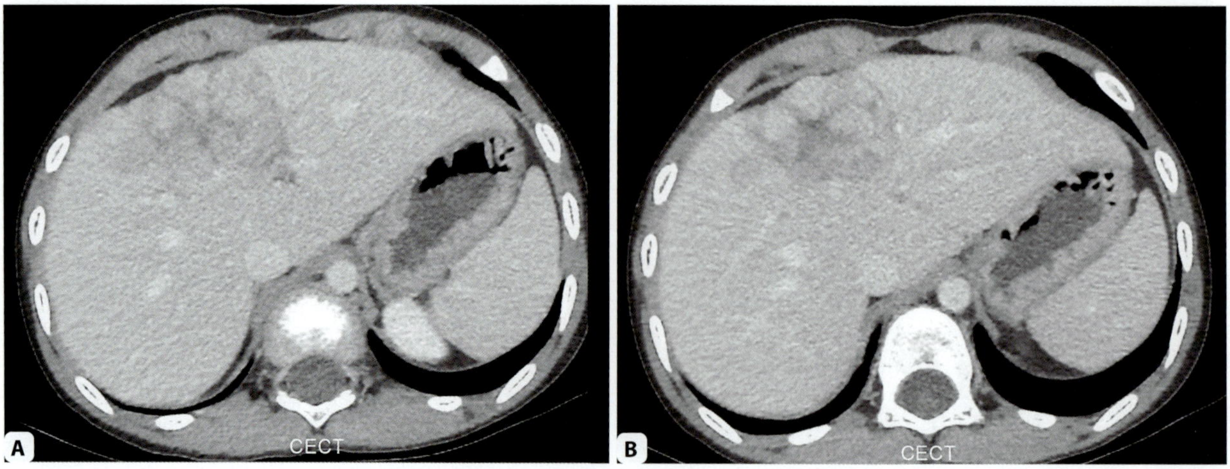

FIGS. 19A AND B: Hepatoblastoma in a 4-year-old male child. Axial (A) contrast-enhanced computed tomography (CECT) of upper abdomen shows a heterogeneously hypoenhancing mass with few nonenhancing areas in segments IVa, IVb, and VIII. (B) CECT shows close abutment with the right and left branches of the portal vein and the mass is reaching up to the capsule.

TABLE 11: Classification of infantile hepatic hemangioma.

	Focal	Multifocal	Diffuse
Onset	Already present at birth	Usually develop after few weeks after birth	Usually develop after few weeks after birth
Development and growth	Form antenatally and fully developed at birth and undergo involution	Growth occurs in the first few weeks to months after birth	Rapid growth occurs after birth
Association with cutaneous hemangiomas	In 15% of cases, cutaneous hemangiomas are associated	Frequent	Frequent
GLUT-1 staining	Negative	Positive	Positive
MRI	Solitary well-defined lesion, hypointense on T1 and hyperintense on T2 with progressive centripetal enhancement	Multiple lesions scattered within the liver with normal intervening hepatic parenchyma	Innumerable lesions studding the entire liver
Symptoms and complications	Often asymptomatic, few cases may have anemia or thrombocytopenia	Few cases asymptomatic, while others can show high output cardiac failure secondary to blood shunting	Usually symptomatic with cardiac failure, hypothyroidism, and abdominal compartment syndrome

(GLUT-1: glucose transporter-1; MRI: magnetic resonance imaging)

mass with cystic components showing fluid attenuation, stromal components appearing hypoattenuating, and the septations showing contrast enhancement.[108] Mesenchymal hamartoma does not demonstrate calcifications or hemorrhage. MR findings depend upon the relative cystic and stromal contents, with the solid portions appearing as both T1 and T2 hypointense and cystic areas appearing as T2 hyperintense and showing variable signals on T1 depending upon the protein content. The differentials include hepatoblastoma, infantile hemangioendothelioma, undifferentiated embryonal sarcoma, and cystic lesions such as simple, hydatid, choledochal, and mesenteric cysts.

Infantile Hepatic Hemangioma

Infantile HH is the most common benign hepatic tumor occurring in infants with females being more commonly affected than males. Three subtypes have been described: Focal, multifocal, and diffuse **(Table 11)**.

Most lesions present during the first 6 months of life. Abdominal examination may reveal palpable abdominal mass and bruit. As a result of the arteriovenous shunting within the lesion, congestive heart failure can occur. Spontaneous rupture can result in hemoperitoneum or Kasabach–Merritt syndrome (thrombocytopenia as a

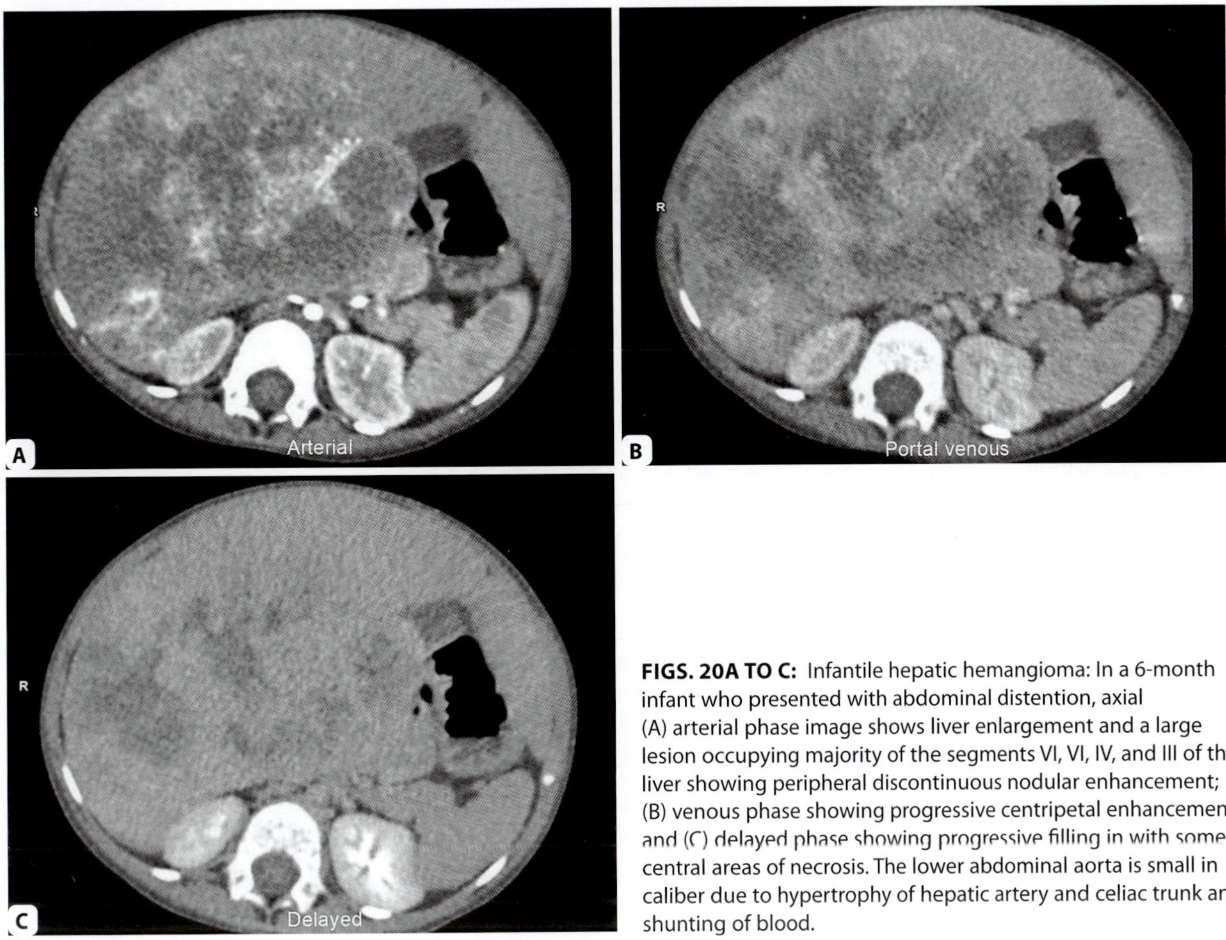

FIGS. 20A TO C: Infantile hepatic hemangioma: In a 6-month infant who presented with abdominal distention, axial (A) arterial phase image shows liver enlargement and a large lesion occupying majority of the segments VI, VI, IV, and III of the liver showing peripheral discontinuous nodular enhancement; (B) venous phase showing progressive centripetal enhancement; and (C) delayed phase showing progressive filling in with some central areas of necrosis. The lower abdominal aorta is small in caliber due to hypertrophy of hepatic artery and celiac trunk and shunting of blood.

result of platelet sequestration). Ultrasound appearance of these lesions is variable ranging from hyperechoic and hypoechoic to anechoic lesions with echogenic septations. Narrowing of the aorta below the origin of the celiac artery with prominent celiac artery, common hepatic artery, and draining veins is a classical feature and results from hypervascularity of these lesions **(Figs. 20A to C)**. Noncontrast CT shows hepatomegaly with hypodense lesions and peripheral centripetal progressive enhancement on the enhanced phases. IHH stain positive for glucose transporter-1 (GLUT-1) except for the focal type. Thus, the latter type may actually represent a form of congenital hemangioma.

CONCLUSION

The approach for characterizing a focal lesion in the noncirrhotic liver **(Flowchart 1)** is a challenging task and requires ruling out non-neoplastic causes first. Ultrasound helps in differentiating solid from cystic lesions, which is a key step in suggesting the diagnosis. If the lesion appears cystic on ultrasound, the neoplastic possibilities include MCN and cystic metastasis. Solid lesions on US have a much longer list of differentials. In the presence of a known primary malignancy, focal liver lesion should be considered metastatic unless proven otherwise. Lesions showing hypervascularity in the arterial phase include hemangioma, HCA, FNH, FLC, HCC, and metastasis from NET, melanoma, RCC, and breast cancer. FNH is commonly seen in young women and appears isodense/isointense to the background liver with a central T2-hyperintense scar. Thick, irregular peripheral rim enhancement with peripheral washout along with upstream biliary dilatation and capsular retraction are features of ICC. The liver-specific MR contrast agents have helped in the evaluation of FNH, HCA, and HCC. Imaging may not always be able to arrive at a final diagnosis and sampling may be required, especially in the scenario of uncommon and rare liver lesions.

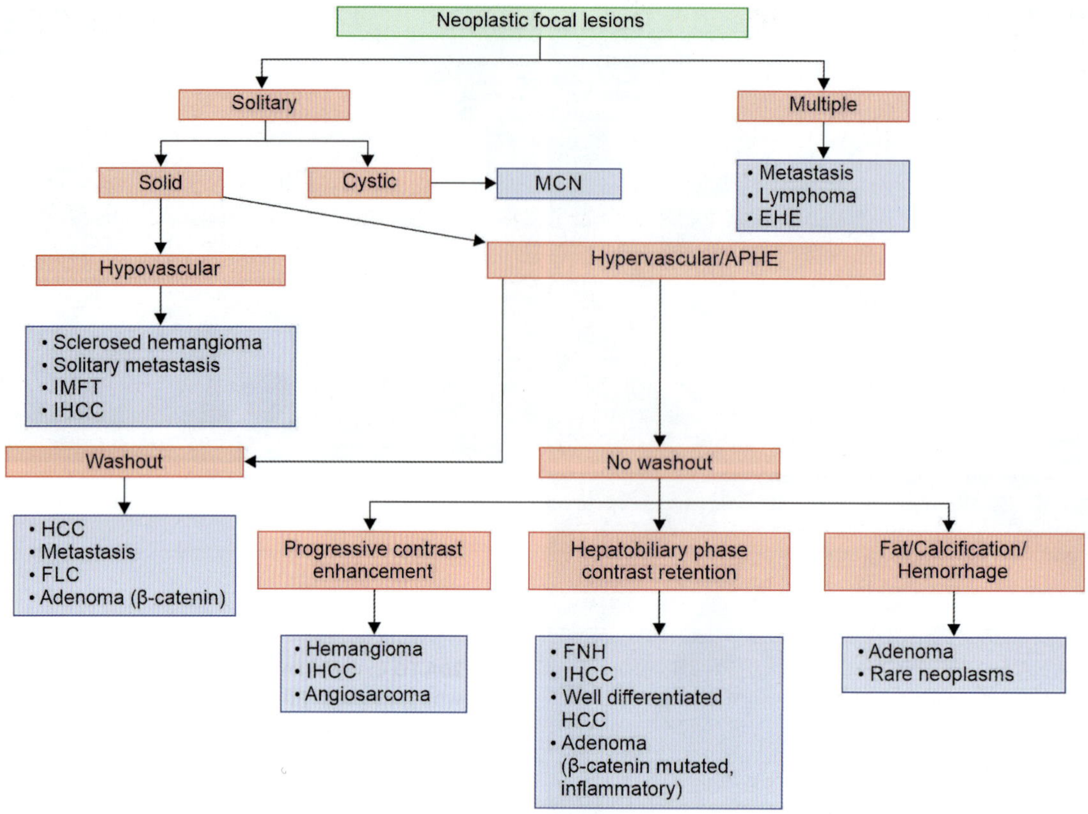

FLOWCHART 1: Imaging approach to neoplastic focal liver lesion.

(APHE: arterial phase hyperenhancement; EHE: epithelioid hemangioendothelioma; FLC: fibrolamellar carcinoma; FNH: focal nodular hyperplasia; HCC: hepato-cellular cancer; IHCC: intra-HCC; IMFT: inflammatory myofibroblastic tumor; MCN: mucinous cystic neoplasms)

REFERENCES

1. Caseiro-Alves F, Brito J, Araujo AE, Belo-Soares P, Rodrigues H, Cipriano A, et al. Liver haemangioma: common and uncommon findings and how to improve the differential diagnosis. Eur Radiol. 2007;17(6):1544-54.
2. Klotz T, Montoriol PF, Da Ines D, Petitcolin V, Joubert-Zakeyh J, Garcier JM. Hepatic haemangioma: common and uncommon imaging features. Diagn Interv Imaging. 2013;94(9):849-59.
3. Mamone G, Di Piazza A, Carollo V, Cannataci C, Cortis K, Bartolotta TV, et al. Imaging of hepatic hemangioma: from A to Z. Abdom Radiol N Y. 2020;45(3):672-91.
4. Toro A, Mahfouz AE, Ardiri A, Malaguarnera M, Malaguarnera G, Loria F, et al. What is changing in indications and treatment of hepatic hemangiomas. A review. Ann Hepatol. 2014;13(4):327-39.
5. Leon M, Chavez L, Surani S. Hepatic hemangioma: What internists need to know. World J Gastroenterol. 2020;26(1): 11-20.
6. Fang L, Huang BJ, Ding H, Mao F, Li CL, Zeng MS, et al. Contrast-enhanced ultrasound (CEUS) for the diagnosis of hypoechoic hepatic hemangioma in clinical practice. Clin Hemorheol Microcirc. 2019;72(4):395-405.
7. McFarland EG, Mayo-Smith WW, Saini S, Hahn PF, Goldberg MA, Lee MJ. Hepatic hemangiomas and malignant tumors: improved differentiation with heavily T2-weighted conventional spin-echo MR imaging. Radiology. 1994;193(1):43-7.
8. Mamone G, Miraglia R. The "light bulb sign" in liver hemangioma. Abdom Radiol N Y. 2019;44(6):2327-8.
9. Kim KW, Kim TK, Han JK, Kim AY, Lee HJ, Choi BI. Hepatic hemangiomas with arterioportal shunt: findings at two-phase CT. Radiology. 2001;219(3):707-11.
10. Guerra A, Infante A, Rinninella E, Spinelli I, Mazziotti MA, De Gaetano AM, et al. A peculiar case of diffuse hemangiomatosis of the left hepatic lobe in an asymptomatic adult patient: case report and literature review. Eur Rev Med Pharmacol Sci. 2017;21(7):1593-7.
11. Vilgrain V, Boulos L, Vullierme MP, Denys A, Terris B, Menu Y. Imaging of atypical hemangiomas of the liver with pathologic correlation. Radiographics. 2000;20(2):379-97.
12. LeGout JD, Bolan CW, Bowman AW, Caserta MP, Chen FK, Cox KL, et al. Focal Nodular Hyperplasia and Focal Nodular Hyperplasia-like Lesions. Radiographics. 2022;42(4):1043-61.
13. Wanless IR. The pathogenesis of focal nodular hyperplasia of the liver. J Gastroenterol Hepatol. 2004;19(s7):S342-3.
14. Kinoshita M, Takemura S, Tanaka S, Hamano G, Ito T, Aota T, et al. Ruptured focal nodular hyperplasia observed during follow-up: a case report. Surg Case Rep. 2017;3:44.
15. Gore RM, Pickhardt PJ, Mortele KJ, Fishman EK, Horowitz JM, Fimmel CJ, et al. Management of Incidental Liver Lesions on CT: A White Paper of the ACR Incidental Findings Committee. J Am Coll Radiol JACR. 2017;14(11):1429-37.

16. Wang LY, Wang JH, Lin ZY, Yu ML, Lu SN, Chuang WL, et al. Hepatic focal nodular hyperplasia: findings on color Doppler ultrasound. Abdom Imaging. 1997;22(2):178-81.
17. Claudon M, Dietrich CF, Choi BI, Cosgrove DO, Kudo M, Nolsøe CP, et al. Guidelines and good clinical practice recommendations for Contrast Enhanced Ultrasound (CEUS) in the liver - update 2012: A WFUMB-EFSUMB initiative in cooperation with representatives of AFSUMB, AIUM, ASUM, FLAUS and ICUS. Ultrasound Med Biol. 2013;39(2):187-210.
18. Mortelé KJ, Praet M, Van Vlierberghe H, Kunnen M, Ros PR. CT and MR imaging findings in focal nodular hyperplasia of the liver: radiologic-pathologic correlation. AJR Am J Roentgenol. 2000;175(3):687-92.
19. Yen YH, Wang JH, Lu SN, Chen TY, Changchien CS, Chen CH, et al. Contrast-enhanced ultrasonographic spoke-wheel sign in hepatic focal nodular hyperplasia. Eur J Radiol. 2006;60(3):439-44.
20. Purysko AS, Remer EM, Coppa CP, Obuchowski NA, Schneider E, Veniero JC. Characteristics and distinguishing features of hepatocellular adenoma and focal nodular hyperplasia on gadoxetate disodium-enhanced MRI. AJR Am J Roentgenol. 2012;198(1):115-23.
21. Schima W, Koh DM, Baron R. Focal Liver Lesions. In: Hodler J, Kubik-Huch RA, von Schulthess GK (Eds). Diseases of the Abdomen and Pelvis 2018-2021: Diagnostic Imaging. Cham (CH): Springer; 2018.
22. Bioulac-Sage P, Sempoux C, Balabaud C. Hepatocellular adenoma. Classification, variants and clinical relevance. Semin Diagn Pathol. 2017;34(2):112-25.
23. Nault JC, Couchy G, Balabaud C, Morcrette G, Caruso S, Blanc JF, et al. Molecular Classification of Hepatocellular Adenoma Associates With Risk Factors, Bleeding, and Malignant Transformation. Gastroenterology. 2017;152(4):880-94.e6.
24. Torbenson M. Hepatic Adenomas: Classification, Controversies, and Consensus. Surg Pathol Clin. 2018;11(2):351-66.
25. Beaufrère A, Paradis V. Hepatocellular adenomas: review of pathological and molecular features. Hum Pathol. 2021;112: 128-37.
26. Bise S, Frulio N, Hocquelet A, Alberti N, Blanc JF, Laurent C, et al. New MRI features improve subtype classification of hepatocellular adenoma. Eur Radiol. 2019;29(5):2436-47.
27. Katabathina VS, Khanna L, Surabhi VR, Minervini M, Shanbhogue K, Dasyam AK, et al. Morphomolecular Classification Update on Hepatocellular Adenoma, Hepatocellular Carcinoma, and Intrahepatic Cholangiocarcinoma. Radiographics. 2022;42(5):1338-57.
28. Laumonier H, Cailliez H, Balabaud C, Possenti L, Zucman-Rossi J, Bioulac-Sage P, et al. Role of contrast-enhanced sonography in differentiation of subtypes of hepatocellular adenoma: correlation with MRI findings. AJR Am J Roentgenol. 2012;199(2):341-8.
29. Lee SY, Kingham TP, LaGratta MD, Jessurun J, Cherqui D, Jarnagin WR, et al. PET-avid hepatocellular adenomas: incidental findings associated with HNF1-α mutated lesions. HPB. 2016;18(1):41-8.
30. Calderaro J, Nault JC, Balabaud C, Couchy G, Saint-Paul MC, Azoulay D, et al. Inflammatory hepatocellular adenomas developed in the setting of chronic liver disease and cirrhosis. Mod Pathol. 2016;29(1):43-50.
31. Guo Y, Li W, Cai W, Zhang Y, Fang Y, Hong G. Diagnostic Value of Gadoxetic Acid-Enhanced MR Imaging to Distinguish HCA and Its Subtype from FNH: A Systematic Review. Int J Med Sci. 2017;14(7):668-74.
32. Zulfiqar M, Sirlin CB, Yoneda N, Ronot M, Hecht EM, Chernyak V, et al. Hepatocellular adenomas: Understanding the pathomolecular lexicon, MRI features, terminology, and pitfalls to inform a standardized approach. J Magn Reson Imaging JMRI. 2020;51(6):1630-40.
33. Auer TA, Fehrenbach U, Grieser C, Penzkofer T, Geisel D, Schmelzle M, et al. Hepatocellular adenomas: is there additional value in using Gd-EOB-enhanced MRI for subtype differentiation? Eur Radiol. 2020;30(6):3497-506.
34. Rebouissou S, Nault JC. Advances in molecular classification and precision oncology in hepatocellular carcinoma. J Hepatol. 2020;72(2):215-29.
35. Reizine E, Ronot M, Ghosn M, Calderaro J, Frulio N, Bioulac-Sage P, et al. Hepatospecific MR contrast agent uptake on hepatobiliary phase can be used as a biomarker of marked β-catenin activation in hepatocellular adenoma. Eur Radiol. 2021;31(5):3417-26.
36. Védie AL, Sutter O, Ziol M, Nault JC. Molecular classification of hepatocellular adenomas: impact on clinical practice. Hepatic Oncol. 2018;5(1):HEP04.
37. Mittal S, Gopal P, Khatri G, Singal AG. Evaluation and Management of Hepatocellular Adenomas. Clin Liver Dis. 2021;17(2):57-60.
38. Aziz S, Sey M, Marotta P, Driman D, Parfitt J, Teriaky A, et al. Recurrent Hepatocellular Carcinoma After Liver Transplantation: Validation of a Pathologic Risk Score on Explanted Livers to Predict Recurrence. Transplant Proc. 2021;53(6):1975-9.
39. Läuffer JM, Baer HU, Maurer CA, Stoupis C, Zimmerman A, Büchler MW. Biliary cystadenocarcinoma of the liver: the need for complete resection. Eur J Cancer. 1998;34(12): 1845-51.
40. Zen Y, Pedica F, Patcha VR, Capelli P, Zamboni G, Casaril A, et al. Mucinous cystic neoplasms of the liver: a clinicopathological study and comparison with intraductal papillary neoplasms of the bile duct. Mod Pathol. 2011;24(8):1079-89.
41. Ahanatha Pillai S, Velayutham V, Perumal S, Ulagendra Perumal S, Lakshmanan A, Ramaswami S, et al. Biliary Cystadenomas: A Case for Complete Resection. HPB Surg. 2012;2012: 501705.
42. Xu HX, Lu MD, Liu LN, Zhang YF, Guo LH, Liu C, et al. Imaging features of intrahepatic biliary cystadenoma and cystadenocarcinoma on B-mode and contrast-enhanced ultrasound. Ultraschall Med. 2012;33(7):E241-9.
43. Korobkin M, Stephens DH, Lee JK, Stanley RJ, Fishman EK, Francis IR, et al. Biliary cystadenoma and cystadenocarcinoma: CT and sonographic findings. AJR Am J Roentgenol. 1989;153(3):507-11.
44. Kim JY, Kim SH, Eun HW, Lee MW, Lee JY, Han JK, et al. Differentiation between biliary cystic neoplasms and simple cysts of the liver: accuracy of CT. AJR Am J Roentgenol. 2010;195(5):1142-8.
45. Alobaidi M, Shirkhoda A. Malignant cystic and necrotic liver lesions: a pattern approach to discrimination. Curr Probl Diagn Radiol. 2004;33(6):254-68.
46. Soochan D, Keough V, Wanless I, Molinari M. Intra and extra-hepatic cystadenoma of the biliary duct. Review of literature and radiological and pathological characteristics of a very rare case. BMJ Case Rep. 2012;2012:bcr0120125497.

47. Teoh AYB, Ng SSM, Lee KF, Lai PBS. Biliary cystadenoma and other complicated cystic lesions of the liver: diagnostic and therapeutic challenges. World J Surg. 2006;30(8):1560-6.
48. Desai A, Sandhu S, Lai JP, Sandhu DS. Hepatocellular carcinoma in non-cirrhotic liver: A comprehensive review. World J Hepatol. 2019;11(1):1-18.
49. Friedman AC, Lichtenstein JE, Goodman Z, Fishman EK, Siegelman SS, Dachman AH. Fibrolamellar hepatocellular carcinoma. Radiology. 1985;157(3):583-7.
50. Ichikawa T, Federle MP, Grazioli L, Madariaga J, Nalesnik M, Marsh W. Fibrolamellar hepatocellular carcinoma: imaging and pathologic findings in 31 recent cases. Radiology. 1999;213(2):352-61.
51. McLarney JK, Rucker PT, Bender GN, Goodman ZD, Kashitani N, Ros PR. Fibrolamellar carcinoma of the liver: radiologic-pathologic correlation. Radiographics. 1999;19(2):453-71.
52. Brandt DJ, Johnson CD, Stephens DH, Weiland LH. Imaging of fibrolamellar hepatocellular carcinoma. AJR Am J Roentgenol. 1988;151(2):295-9.
53. Chagas AL, Kikuchi L, Herman P, Alencar RSSM, Tani CM, Diniz MA, et al. Clinical and pathological evaluation of fibrolamellar hepatocellular carcinoma: a single center study of 21 cases. Clinics. 2015;70(3):207-13.
54. Lin CC, Yang HM. Fibrolamellar Carcinoma: A Concise Review. Arch Pathol Lab Med. 2018;142(9):1141-5.
55. Ganeshan D, Szklaruk J, Kundra V, Kaseb A, Rashid A, Elsayes KM. Imaging features of fibrolamellar hepatocellular carcinoma. AJR Am J Roentgenol. 2014;202(3):544-52.
56. El-Serag HB, Davila JA. Is fibrolamellar carcinoma different from hepatocellular carcinoma? A US population-based study. Hepatology. 2004;39(3):798-803.
57. Chun YS, Zimmitti G. Fibrolamellar variant of hepatocellular carcinoma. Recent Results Cancer Res. 2013;190:101-10.
58. Darcy DG, Malek MM, Kobos R, Klimstra DS, DeMatteo R, La Quaglia MP. Prognostic factors in fibrolamellar hepatocellular carcinoma in young people. J Pediatr Surg. 2015;50(1):153-6.
59. Chung YE, Kim MJ, Park YN, Choi JY, Pyo JY, Kim YC, et al. Varying appearances of cholangiocarcinoma: radiologic-pathologic correlation. Radiographics. 2009;29(3):683-700.
60. Fábrega-Foster K, Ghasabeh MA, Pawlik TM, Kamel IR. Multimodality imaging of intrahepatic cholangiocarcinoma. Hepatobiliary Surg Nutr. 2017;6(2):67-78.
61. Ros PR, Buck JL, Goodman ZD, Ros AM, Olmsted WW. Intrahepatic cholangiocarcinoma: radiologic-pathologic correlation. Radiology. 1988;167(3):689-93.
62. Maetani Y, Itoh K, Watanabe C, Shibata T, Ametani F, Yamabe H, et al. MR imaging of intrahepatic cholangiocarcinoma with pathologic correlation. AJR Am J Roentgenol. 2001;176(6):1499-507.
63. Jeong HT, Kim MJ, Chung YE, Choi JY, Park YN, Kim KW. Gadoxetate disodium-enhanced MRI of mass-forming intrahepatic cholangiocarcinomas: imaging-histologic correlation. AJR Am J Roentgenol. 2013;201(4):W603-11.
64. Kang Y, Lee JM, Kim SH, Han JK, Choi BI. Intrahepatic mass-forming cholangiocarcinoma: enhancement patterns on gadoxetic acid-enhanced MR images. Radiology. 2012;264(3):751-60.
65. Park HJ, Kim YK, Park MJ, Lee WJ. Small intrahepatic mass-forming cholangiocarcinoma: target sign on diffusion-weighted imaging for differentiation from hepatocellular carcinoma. Abdom Imaging. 2013;38(4):793-801.
66. Kim R, Lee JM, Shin CI, Lee ES, Yoon JH, Joo I, et al. Differentiation of intrahepatic mass-forming cholangiocarcinoma from hepatocellular carcinoma on gadoxetic acid-enhanced liver MR imaging. Eur Radiol. 2016;26(6):1808-17.
67. Antonescu C. Malignant vascular tumors—an update. Mod Pathol. 2014;27 Suppl 1:S30-8.
68. Kou K, Chen YG, Zhou JP, Sun XD, Sun DW, Li SX, et al. Hepatic epithelioid hemangioendothelioma: Update on diagnosis and therapy. World J Clin Cases. 2020;8(18):3978-87.
69. Gurung S, Fu H, Zhang WW, Gu YH. Hepatic epithelioid hemangioendothelioma metastasized to the peritoneum, omentum and mesentery: a case report. Int J Clin Exp Pathol. 2015;8(5):5883-9.
70. Mamone G, Miraglia R. The "Target sign" and the "Lollipop sign" in hepatic epithelioid hemangioendothelioma. Abdom Radiol N Y. 2019;44(4):1617-20.
71. Miller WJ, Dodd GD, Federle MP, Baron RL. Epithelioid hemangioendothelioma of the liver: imaging findings with pathologic correlation. AJR Am J Roentgenol. 1992;159(1):53-7.
72. Gan L, Chang R, Jin H, Yang L. Typical CT and MRI signs of hepatic epithelioid hemangioendothelioma. Oncol Lett. 2016;11(3):1699-706.
73. Alomari AI. The lollipop sign: a new cross-sectional sign of hepatic epithelioid hemangioendothelioma. Eur J Radiol. 2006;59(3):460-4.
74. Molina E, Hernandez A. Clinical manifestations of primary hepatic angiosarcoma. Dig Dis Sci. 2003;48(4):677-82.
75. Mani H, Van Thiel DH. Mesenchymal tumors of the liver. Clin Liver Dis. 2001;5(1):219-57, viii.
76. Huerta-Orozco LD, Leonher-Ruezga KL, Ramírez-González LR, Hermosillo-Sandoval JM, Sandoval-Alvarado J de J, Morán-Galaviz RE. Hepatic angiosarcoma and liver transplantation: case report and literature review. Cir Cir. 2015;83(6):510-5. [Spanish].
77. Kim B, Byun JH, Lee JH, Park BJ, Kwon HJ, Lee JH, et al. Imaging findings of primary hepatic angiosarcoma on gadoxetate disodium-enhanced liver MRI: comparison with hepatic haemangiomas of similar size. Clin Radiol. 2018;73(3):244-53.
78. Thapar S, Rastogi A, Ahuja A, Sarin S. Angiosarcoma of the Liver: Imaging of a rare salient entity. J Radiol Case Rep. 2014;8(8):24-32.
79. Bruegel M, Muenzel D, Waldt S, Specht K, Rummeny EJ. Hepatic angiosarcoma: cross-sectional imaging findings in seven patients with emphasis on dynamic contrast-enhanced and diffusion-weighted MRI. Abdom Imaging. 2013;38(4):745-54.
80. Locker GY, Doroshow JH, Zwelling LA, Chabner BA. The clinical features of hepatic angiosarcoma: a report of four cases and a review of the English literature. Medicine (Baltimore). 1979;58(1):48-64.
81. Yasir S, Torbenson MS. Angiosarcoma of the Liver: Clinicopathologic Features and Morphologic Patterns. Am J Surg Pathol. 2019;43(5):581-90.
82. Sica GT, Ji H, Ros PR. CT and MR Imaging of Hepatic Metastases. Am J Roentgenol. 2000;174(3):691-8.
83. Lincke T, Zech CJ. Liver metastases: Detection and staging. Eur J Radiol. 2017;97:76-82.
84. Silva AC, Evans JM, McCullough AE, Jatoi MA, Vargas HE, Hara AK. MR Imaging of Hypervascular Liver Masses: A Review of Current Techniques. Radiographics. 2009;29(2):385-402.

85. Matsushita N, Douhara A, Ueno H, Asada S, Murata K, Yanase K, et al. Intraductal papillary-mucinous carcinoma with portal vein tumor thrombus and multifocal liver metastasis: An autopsy case. Mol Clin Oncol. 2021;14(5):101.
86. Sommer WH, Zech CJ, Bamberg F, Auernhammer CJ, Helck A, Paprottka PM, et al. Fluid-fluid level in hepatic metastases: a characteristic sign of metastases of neuroendocrine origin. Eur J Radiol. 2012;81(9):2127-32.
87. Kelekis NL, Semelka RC, Woosley JT. Malignant lesions of the liver with high signal intensity on T1-Weighted MR images. J Magn Reson Imaging. 1996;6(2):291-4.
88. Blachar A, Federle MP, Sosna J. Liver Lesions With Hepatic Capsular Retraction. Semin Ultrasound CT MRI. 2009;30(5):426-35.
89. Rajesh S, Bansal K, Sureka B, Patidar Y, Bihari C, Arora A. The imaging conundrum of hepatic lymphoma revisited. Insights Imaging. 2015;6(6):679-92.
90. Howell JM, Auer-Grzesiak I, Zhang J, Andrews CN, Stewart D, Urbanski SJ. Increasing incidence rates, distribution and histological characteristics of primary gastrointestinal non-Hodgkin lymphoma in a North American population. Can J Gastroenterol. 2012;26(7):452-6.
91. Anthony PP, Sarsfield P, Clarke T. Primary lymphoma of the liver: clinical and pathological features of 10 patients. J Clin Pathol. 1990;43(12):1007-13.
92. Alves AMA, Torres US, Velloni FG, Ribeiro BJ, Tiferes DA, D'Ippolito G. The many faces of primary and secondary hepatic lymphoma: imaging manifestations and diagnostic approach. Radiol Bras. 2019;52(5):325-30.
93. Razik A, Malla S, Goyal A, Gamanagatti S, Kandasamy D, Das CJ, et al. Unusual Primary Neoplasms of the Adult Liver: Review of Imaging Appearances and Differential Diagnosis. Curr Probl Diagn Radiol. 2022;51(1):73-85.
94. Padhan RK, Das P, Shalimar. Primary hepatic lymphoma. Trop Gastroenterol. 2015;36(1):14-20.
95. Chim CS, Choy C, Ooi GC, Liang R. Primary hepatic lymphoma. Leuk Lymphoma. 2001;40(5-6):667-70.
96. Tomasian A, Sandrasegaran K, Elsayes KM, Shanbhogue A, Shaaban A, Menias CO. Hematologic malignancies of the liver: spectrum of disease. Radiographics. 2015;35(1):71-86.
97. Armah HB, Parwani AV. Perivascular epithelioid cell tumor. Arch Pathol Lab Med. 2009;133(4):648-54.
98. Handa A, Fujita K, Kono T, Komori K, Hirobe S, Fukuzawa R. Radiological findings of perivascular epithelioid cell tumour (PEComa) of the falciform ligament. J Med Imaging Radiat Oncol. 2016;60(6):741-3.
99. Tan Y, Xiao EH. Hepatic perivascular epithelioid cell tumor (PEComa): dynamic CT, MRI, ultrasonography, and pathologic features—analysis of 7 cases and review of the literature. Abdom Imaging. 2012;37(5):781-7.
100. Maebayashi T, Abe K, Aizawa T, Sakaguchi M, Ishibashi N, Abe O, et al. Improving recognition of hepatic perivascular epithelioid cell tumor: Case report and literature review. World J Gastroenterol. 2015;21(17):5432-41.
101. Tirumani SH, Shinagare AB, Hargreaves J, Jagannathan JP, Hornick JL, Wagner AJ, et al. Imaging Features of Primary and Metastatic Malignant Perivascular Epithelioid Cell Tumors. Am J Roentgenol. 2014;202(2):252-8.
102. Folpe AL, Kwiatkowski DJ. Perivascular epithelioid cell neoplasms: pathology and pathogenesis. Hum Pathol. 2010;41(1):1-15.
103. Kellock T, Tuong B, Harris AC, Yoshida E. Diagnostic Imaging of Primary Hepatic Neuroendocrine Tumors: A Case and Discussion of the Literature. Case Rep Radiol. 2014;2014:e156491.
104. Wang LX, Liu K, Lin GW, Jiang T. Primary hepatic neuroendocrine tumors: comparing CT and MRI features with pathology. Cancer Imaging. 2015;15(1):13.
105. Song JE, Kim BS, Lee CH. Primary hepatic neuroendocrine tumor: A case report and literature review. World J Clin Cases. 2016;4(8):243-7.
106. Gupta R, Parelkar SV, Sanghvi B. Mesenchymal hamartoma of the liver. Indian J Med Paediatr Oncol. 2009;30(4):141-3.
107. Chung EM, Cube R, Lewis RB, Conran RM. Pediatric Liver Masses: Radiologic-Pathologic Correlation Part 1. Benign Tumors. Radiographics. 2010;30(3):801-26.
108. Gray SC, Pienaar JA, Sofianos Z, Varghese J, Warnich I. Hepatic mesenchymal hamartoma: An uncommon but important paediatric diagnosis. SA J Radiol. 2020;24(1):1891.

CHAPTER 11

Raju Sharma, Shivanand Gamanagatti, Anjali Sah, Anuradha Sharma

Focal Lesions in Cirrhotic Liver: LI-RADS

INTRODUCTION

Liver cirrhosis represents the end stage of chronic liver disease, characterized by regenerative nodules and bridging fibrosis on histopathology. Common causes of cirrhosis are chronic viral hepatitis (hepatitis B or C), alcohol-associated liver disease (ALD), and metabolic dysfunction-associated steatotic liver disease (MASLD). With the widespread availability of hepatitis B vaccine and directly acting antivirals, infectious causes of cirrhosis are expected to decline. On the other hand, the prevalence of MASLD-related cirrhosis is on the rise, especially in developed nations.

A variety of focal lesions are encountered on radiological evaluation in cirrhotic livers. These include benign hepatocellular nodules (regenerative nodules and low-grade and high-grade dysplastic nodules), hepatocellular carcinoma (HCC), non-HCC malignancies [intrahepatic cholangiocarcinoma (iCCA), combined hepatocellular cholangiocarcinoma (cHCC-CCA), metastases], nonhepatocellular benign lesions (cysts and hemangiomas), and confluent hepatic fibrosis, as well as pseudolesions (perfusion anomalies). Radiologists need to be aware of the imaging features of these focal lesions to reach an accurate diagnosis and guide appropriate management. Focal hepatic neoplastic lesions may also be seen on imaging following some form of locoregional treatment; these are outside the purview of this chapter and will be covered elsewhere.

LIVER IMAGING REPORTING AND DATA SYSTEM

The Liver Imaging Reporting and Data System (LI-RADS) is a comprehensive system for standardizing liver imaging technique, interpretation, reporting, and data collection in patients at risk for or with HCC. It is endorsed by the American College of Radiology (ACR) and is consistent with the American Association for the Study of Liver Diseases (AASLD) and National Comprehensive Cancer Network (NCCN) guidelines.[1] It covers both surveillance by ultrasound (US) as well as diagnosis by contrast-enhanced US (CEUS), multiphase computed tomography (CT), or magnetic resonance imaging (MRI). It also allows for assessment of treatment response on CT or MRI following locoregional therapies for HCC. The first version of LI-RADS was proposed in 2011 and has undergone several major refinements and updates since then. By delineating standardized criteria and terminology, LI-RADS facilitates clearer communication among radiologists, oncologists, and other healthcare providers, ultimately improving patient care and outcomes in the realm of HCC management.

IMAGING MODALITIES

Ultrasound

Ultrasound plays an important role in the screening and surveillance of patients at high risk of developing HCC. US at 6-month intervals is recommended for the surveillance of patients at high risk for HCC. Longitudinal and transverse images of the right and left lobes of the liver should be obtained, as well as color Doppler images of the main portal vein and its right and left branches. The advantages of US are lack of exposure to ionizing radiation, widespread availability, and low cost, whereas its drawbacks include operator dependence, poor performance in patients with large body habitus, hepatic steatosis, or markedly heterogeneous liver parenchyma.

Contrast-enhanced Ultrasound

Contrast-enhanced US is performed after injection of microbubble contrast agents which comprise an inert gaseous core (sulfur hexafluoride in SonoVue®, octafluoropropane in Definity®) surrounded by a stabilizing phospholipid shell. On precontrast scan, the target nodule and optimal patient position, scan plane, and breathing technique for its visualization are determined. Contrast bolus is administered through a peripheral intravenous line (0.2 mL Definity or 1.5–2.4 mL SonoVue®). Timer is started following the end of contrast injection when commencing saline flush (5–10 mL at 2 mL/s). Continuous scanning is done till 1 minute from the start of contrast injection covering the entire arterial phase (10–20 seconds till 30–45 seconds after contrast injection), followed by intermittent scanning every 30 seconds to minimize microbubble injection covering portal venous (30–45 seconds till 120 seconds after contrast injection) and late phases (120 seconds till 4–6 minutes after contrast injection). Low mechanical index (< 0.3) is required to reduce microbubble destruction.

Due to its capacity for real-time imaging with high temporal resolution, CEUS can detect early arterial phase enhancement which may be missed on multiphase CT or MRI. This enables the detection of HCCs that appear hypovascular on CT or MRI and the depiction of peripheral discontinuous nodular enhancement in flash-filling hemangiomas which would appear as homogeneously enhancing hypervascular nodules on CT or MRI. As these contrast agents are purely intravascular or blood pool agents, they directly reflect perfusion and are more sensitive for the detection of washout in comparison to CT or MRI. They are also able to differentiate the washout pattern of HCC which has late onset after 60 seconds and is mild as compared to non-HCC malignancies which show early-onset washout before 60 seconds that is marked. Another advantage of CEUS is the non-nephrotoxic nature of the microbubble contrast agents, which enables them to be safely used in patients with renal dysfunction.[2] Drawbacks of CEUS include those of grayscale US, as well as the inability to perform CEUS assessment of observations that are not well visualized on US and the inability to assess multiple observations with a single injection.

The present version of CEUS LI-RADS is primarily applicable to pure blood pool agents, such as SonoVue® but not to combined blood pool/Kupffer cell agents, such as Sonazoid®. This distinction is due to the difference in *mechanism of action* and *imaging properties* of these contrast agents. SonoVue® and other pure blood pool agents enhance the vascular phase of imaging as they remain confined within the circulation. They do not accumulate inside Kupffer cells or hepatocytes. On the other hand, the contrast agent Sonazoid® has the unique ability to aggregate in Kupffer cells found in the sinusoids of the liver. Hence, it prolongs the hepatic enhancement phase for at least an hour.[3] Therefore, an additional postvascular phase, also known as Kupffer phase, is acquired with Sonazoid®, beginning from 10 minutes post injection till 60 minutes. Malignant lesions such as HCC tend to become hypoechoic in this phase due to depletion of Kupffer cells, whereas benign lesions remain isoechoic to hyperechoic. Screening for any hypoechoic lesions is done in the Kupffer phase; any defects seen in this phase are reevaluated after a second injection of Sonazoid® to look for arterial phase enhancement to confirm the diagnosis of HCC. This is known as defect reperfusion imaging.

Computed Tomography

Multiphase CT involves the acquisition of CT images in late arterial, portal venous, and delayed phases after contrast injection **(Table 1)**. LI-RADS requires acquisition on multidetector CT scanners with a minimum of eight detector rows for accurate diagnosis of HCC. Late arterial

TABLE 1: CT protocol for characterization of liver lesions.*

Phases**	Late arterial phase	PVP	Delayed phase
Phase timing	35–45 seconds after starting contrast injection	60–75 seconds after starting contrast injection	2–5 minutes after starting contrast injection
Coverage	Liver	Whole abdomen and pelvis	Liver
Appearance on CT	Portal vein enhanced, hepatic vein not yet enhanced	• Portal veins and hepatic veins enhanced • Enhancement of liver parenchyma at peak	• Enhancement of portal and hepatic veins less than venous phase • Enhancement of liver parenchyma less than in PVP
Significance	Lesions such as HCC, FNH, adenoma, etc., enhance optimally	Hypovascular lesions such as metastases and abscesses are best seen	Fibrotic lesions such as cholangiocarcinoma and scirrhous metastases are best seen

*Contrast—1.5–2 mL/kg body weight of low-osmolar iodinated contrast medium (300 mg/mL or higher) is given at 3–5 mL/s followed by 30–40 mL saline chaser at the same rate.

**An additional noncontrast scan is recommended after locoregional treatment such as TACE.

(CT: computed tomography; FNH: focal nodular hyperplasia; HCC: hepatocellular carcinoma; PVP: portal venous phase; TACE: transarterial chemo-embolization)

phase is preferred in the imaging protocol because HCC enhances more strongly in the late arterial phase than in the early arterial phase. Advantages of CT include high spatial resolution and widespread availability. It enables assessment of observations where US is limited such as in patients with large body habitus, fatty liver, or deep-seated focal lesions. Due to fast acquisition, there is less chance of image quality degradation by motion artifacts or in patients with gross ascites. Disadvantages of CT include exposure to ionizing radiation and inferior contrast resolution compared to MRI.

Magnetic Resonance Imaging

Magnetic resonance imaging for assessment of focal lesions in cirrhosis requires acquisition of multiple sequences which are summarized in **Table 2**. LI-RADS requires MRI to be performed on scanners of field strength >1.5 Tesla with multichannel-phased array coils. Similar to CT, multiphase postcontrast imaging is done after injection of extracellular or hepatobiliary contrast agents. Precontrast as well as postcontrast three-dimensional T1-weighted (3D T1W) sequences are acquired. Bolus tracking is recommended for arterial phase; portal venous and delayed phases are acquired at 60–80 seconds and 2–5 minutes after the start of contrast injection. If using hepatobiliary contrast agents, an additional hepatobiliary phase (HBP) is acquired at 20 minutes with gadoxetate or at 1 hour with gadobenate (MultiHance®). With gadoxetate, the 2–5 minute-postcontrast phase is termed transitional phase instead of delayed phase; at this time, the hepatic parenchyma and vessels are of similar signal intensity. Evaluation of subtracted images is essential for determining enhancement in focal lesions which are intrinsically hyperintense on T1W sequences.

The advantages of MRI are its superior soft tissue contrast resolution and acquisition of multiple sequences which enable assessment of ancillary features (AFs) suggestive of HCC and increase the diagnostic confidence. The disadvantages of MRI include lack of easy availability, longer examination times, and occurrence of dielectric artifact in patients with ascites. To overcome the disadvantage of long examination times, recently, abbreviated MRI protocols have been proposed for HCC surveillance in which the entire examination can be completed within 15 minutes. There are three strategies for abbreviated MRI, including nonenhanced imaging, dynamic contrast-enhanced imaging, and HBP imaging.[4] Nonenhanced abbreviated MRI comprises T1W (in-phase and opposed-phase), T2-weighted (T2W), and diffusion-weighted images (DWI). Dynamic contrast-enhanced abbreviated MRI implies acquisition of nonenhanced, arterial, portal venous, and delayed images after administration of an extracellular contrast agent. HBP abbreviated MRI requires administration of hepatobiliary contrast agent gadoxetate disodium 15 minutes prior to scan, followed by acquisition of T2W, diffusion-weighted, and HBP T1W sequences. However, a positive result on an abbreviated MRI study may require recalling the patient for a complete MRI study.[4]

LI-RADS SURVEILLANCE ULTRASOUND (V2024)

The LI-RADS surveillance US algorithm was first introduced in 2017 and has been updated in 2024 based on recent clinical evidence. The target population for the application of US LI-RADS has been listed in **Box 1**. The US LI-RADS algorithm incorporates two key components: *US category* and *US visualization score*. In addition, *alpha-fetoprotein (AFP) levels* also affect the management algorithm.

BOX 1 Target population for USG LI-RADS surveillance.

- *Cirrhosis of any etiology with*:
  - Child–Pugh A and Child–Pugh B
  - Child–Pugh C if candidate is on the transplant list
- *Noncirrhotic with chronic HBV infection with*:
  - Family history of HCC
  - Males >40 years or females >50 years from an endemic country
  - Those from Africa at an earlier age
  - Those with a PAGE-B scored ≥ 10 in Western populations on antiviral therapy

(HBV: hepatitis B virus; HCC: hepatocellular carcinoma; LI-RADS: Liver Imaging Reporting and Data System; USG: ultrasonography)

TABLE 2: Multiparametric MRI protocol for characterization of liver lesions.

Sequences	Plane of acquisition	Fat suppression	Slice thickness
T2W (SSFSE/HASTE)	Axial, coronal	Optional	<8 mm
T1W dual-echo gradient (in and opposed phase)	Axial	None	<8 mm
Diffusion-weighted imaging (>2 b values including b 0–50 and b 400–1,000 s/mm^2)	Axial	Not applicable	<8 mm
3D T1W precontrast and postcontrast sequences*	Axial, coronal	Strongly recommended	<5 mm

*Contrast—injected at 1–2 mL/s followed by 30–40 mL saline chaser at the same rate.

(3D: three dimensional; HASTE: half-Fourier acquisition single- shot turbo spin-echo; SSFSE: single-shot fast spin echo; T1W: T1 weighted; T2W: T2 weighted)

Ultrasound Category

The US category summarizes the primary findings of the examination and decides on further management. There are three distinct categories:

1. *US-1 (negative)*: If there is no focal lesion or only the presence of definitively benign findings, such as focal fatty sparing, simple cysts, or previously confirmed hemangiomas, then US-1 category is assigned. The recommended management strategy in this setting is to continue routine surveillance every 6 months.[5,6]
2. *US-2 (subthreshold)*: This category denotes the presence of one or more focal lesions, each measuring < 10 mm, that may not be definitively benign. Such patients require close follow-up with short-interval US examinations every 3–6 months.[5,6] If the lesion remains stable in size for 2 years or more, the patient can be recategorized at US-1.
3. *US-3 (positive)*: This category signifies the presence of > 1 observation measuring 10 mm or larger and not definitively benign. Such observations necessitate further evaluation by triple-phase CT/MRI or CEUS.[5,6] Examples include solid nodules measuring ≥ 10 mm in any echogenicity, newly identified thrombi in portal or hepatic veins, or focal parenchymal distortion measuring ≥ 10 mm in size.

   (*Tie-breaking rules*: As surveillance tests aim to have high sensitivity, if unsure between any two US categories, one should select the one reflecting higher degree of suspicion, i.e., one should assign US-2 category if unsure between US-1 and US-2 and assign US-3 category if unsure between US-2 and US-3.)

Ultrasound Visualization Score

The US Visualization Score is for evaluating the adequacy and quality of the scan, thereby giving information about the expected sensitivity of the US examination in detecting HCC. There are three possible scores:

1. *VIS-A (no or minimal limitations)*: The liver appears homogeneous or mildly heterogeneous and is visualized in near entirety.
2. *VIS-B (moderate limitations)*: The liver shows heterogeneous echotexture and some portions of liver and diaphragm are not visualized. Thus, there is decreased sensitivity for detection of nodules < 10 mm.
3. *VIS-C (severe limitations)*: Severe heterogeneity of liver parenchyma, > 50% of right/left lobe not visualized, > 50% of diaphragm not seen. In all VIS-C categories, ultrasonography (USG) should be repeated at short intervals or an alternate imaging modality should be performed for surveillance (abbreviated MRI or multiphase CT).

AFP positive: Patients with either no lesion or benign lesions on screening US but with raised AFP levels (> 20 ng/mL), AFP levels showing an increasing trend on two consecutive tests or doubling of AFP levels should be evaluated with triple-phase CT/MRI.

LI-RADS CONTRAST-ENHANCED ULTRASOUND (V2017)

With regard to diagnosis, there are two modules of LI-RADS—one is CEUS LI-RADS (V2017) and the other is CT/MRI LI-RADS (V2018). CEUS is a recently added tool in the LI-RADS framework. While it shares similarities with the CT/MRI LI-RADS, there are certain key differences between these modalities in terms of types of contrast used and imaging method. Visibility of the liver nodule on conventional B-mode US is a prerequisite for the application of CEUS LI-RADS. In addition, while conducting the study, it is essential to use approved contrast agents such as SonoVue®, Luminity®, or Definity®. Use of other newer contrast agents such as Sonazoid® is limited to some countries such as Japan, China, Norway, and South Korea and is not addressed in the current version of CEUS LI-RADS.[5]

The target population for the application of CEUS LI-RADS has been listed in **Box 2**.

Contrast-enhanced US LI-RADS categories: Observations refer to any focal abnormality that is distinct from the background liver parenchyma. This term is preferred over the word "nodule" or "lesion" as many of these focal abnormalities in a cirrhotic liver may not be true lesions but may represent changes of perfusion alteration, hypertrophic pseudomass, or an artifact. The LI-RADS category is a scoring system assigned to observations detected during imaging studies. The observations are classified as ranging from LR-1 to LR-5, representing a gradient from definitely benign to definitely HCC. Observations on CEUS are categorized as:

- *CEUS LR not categorizable (LR-NC)*: Those observations that cannot be assigned to a particular category due to image degradation or omission fall under LR-NC.[7,8] In such cases, alternate imaging modalities such as CT/MRI should be performed.

BOX 2 Target population for CEUS LI-RADS.

- Patients at high risk for HCC, namely those with:
  - Cirrhosis
  - Chronic hepatitis B infection
  - Current or prior HCC
- To avoid misinterpretation and unnecessary testing, it should not be applied to patients:
  - Without the abovementioned risk factors
  - < 18 years of age
  - With cirrhosis due to congenital hepatic fibrosis
  - With cirrhosis due to vascular disorders such as Budd–Chiari syndrome, chronic portal vein occlusion, or cardiac congestion
- In addition, LI-RADS categories should not be assigned to patients with biopsy-proven malignancies or pathologically proven benign lesions of nonhepatocellular origin

(CEUS: contrast-enhanced ultrasound; HCC: hepatocellular carcinoma; LI-RADS: Liver Imaging Reporting and Data System)

- *CEUS LR tumor in vein (LR-TIV)*: Lesions showing the unequivocal presence of enhancing soft tissue within a vein (portal or hepatic vein), regardless of visualization of definitive liver nodules are categorized as LR-TIV. CEUS also plays an important role in differentiating between tumor thrombus and bland thrombus based on the timing of contrast agent arrival to the vein. Early arrival (same time as hepatic artery enhancement) favors TIV. Arrival several seconds (~10 seconds) after hepatic artery enhancement favors bland thrombi.[9]
- *CEUS LR-1*: This category is assigned to definitely benign observations such as simple hepatic cysts (anechoic, posterior acoustic enhancement, and no contrast enhancement in any phase), hemangiomas (variable echogenicity with peripheral discontinuous globular enhancement in arterial phase and progressive centripetal filling-in on portal venous and late phases), focal fatty infiltration/sparing (nonmass-like hypoechoic or hyperechoic parenchyma with isoenhancement in all phases in characteristic sites such as gallbladder fossa or anterior to right portal vein in segment IV).
- *CEUS LR-2*: Observations which are probably benign (regenerative or low-grade dysplastic nodules) are categorized as LR-2. These include distinct isoenhancing nodules < 10 mm, nonmass-like isoenhancing observation in sites which are atypical for focal fatty infiltration/sparing, and CEUS LR-3 nodules with stable size for > 2 years.
- *CEUS LR-M* ***(Figs. 1A to D)***: Nodules that have imaging features suggestive of malignant lesions but not specific to HCC fall under this category. Imaging features include arterial phase rim enhancement, early washout (< 60 seconds), and/or marked washout within 2 minutes of contrast injection.[10]
- *CEUS LR-3 to LR-5* ***(Figs. 2A to D)***: Based on the CEUS LI-RADS major imaging features, the CEUS diagnostic table **(Table 3)** should be applied for nodules not fitting into the above-described categories.

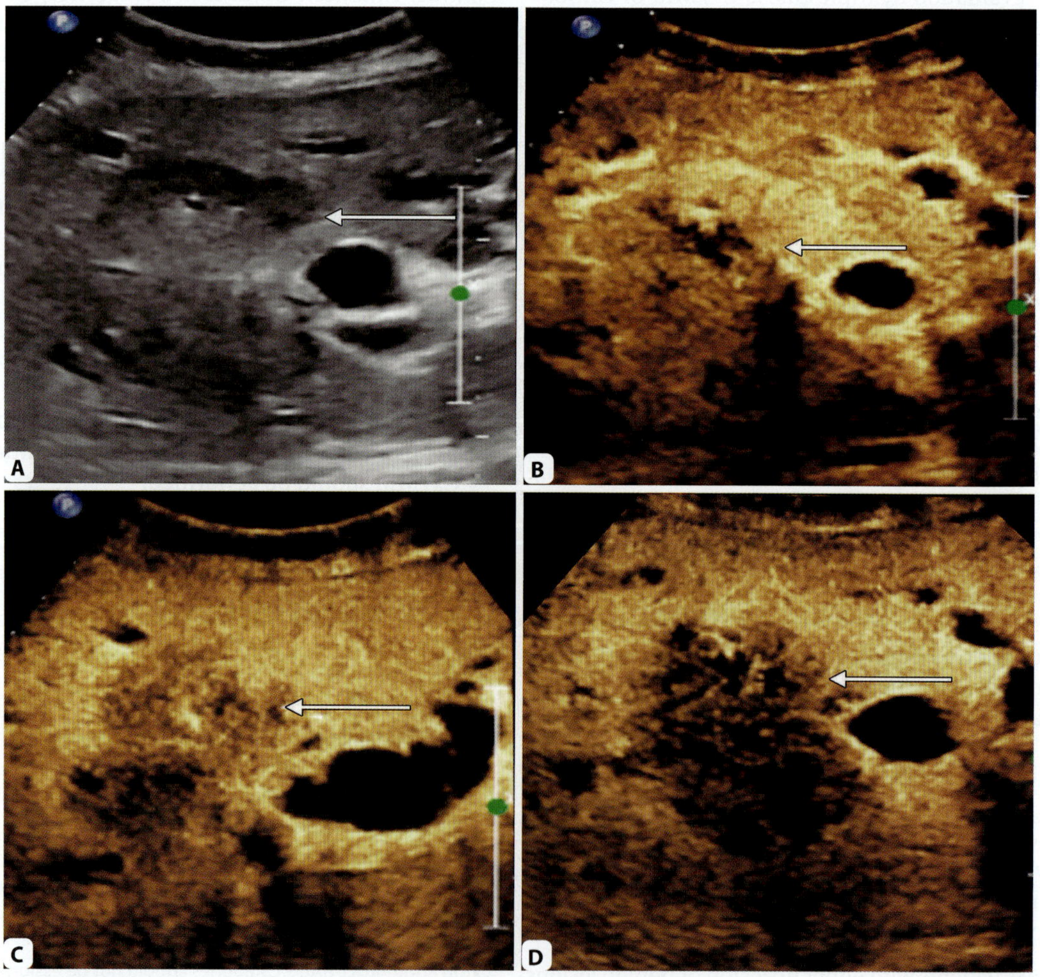

FIGS. 1A TO D: Contrast-enhanced ultrasound (CEUS) LR-M: (A) Grayscale ultrasound shows a hypoechoic mass (arrow) in the right lobe of the liver. (B) On CEUS acquired at 30 seconds after injection of SonoVue®, there is mild arterial phase enhancement; (C) at 70 seconds postinjection, there is early washout and (D) 120 seconds after contrast injection, marked washout is seen.

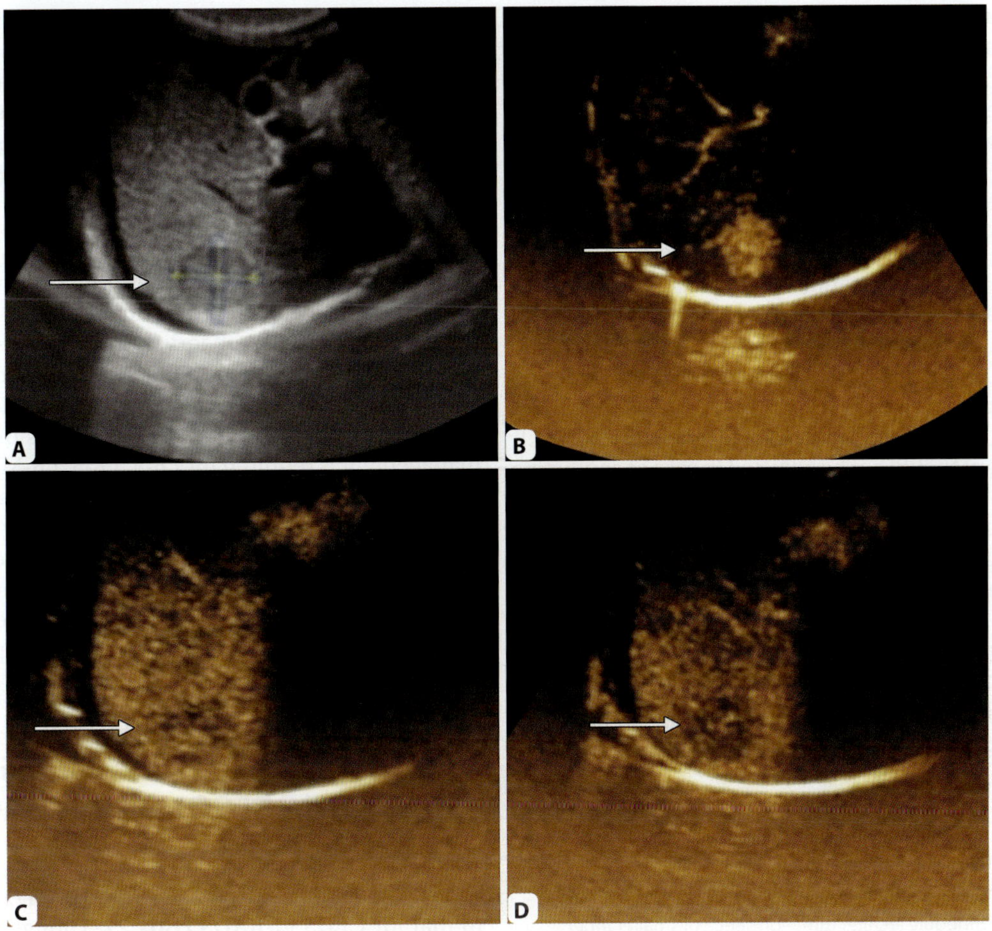

FIGS. 2A TO D: Contrast-enhanced ultrasound (CEUS) LR-5: (A) Grayscale ultrasound shows a 2 cm hypoechoic lesion (arrow) in segment VII of the liver. (B) Entire observation shows arterial phase hyperenhancement (25 seconds). (C and D) Observation shows mild and late washout in portal venous (75 seconds) and late phases (135 seconds).

TABLE 3: CEUS diagnostic table.

APHE	No APHE		APHE (not rim, not peripheral discontinuous globular)	
Nodule size (mm)	< 20	>20	< 10	>10
No washout	CEUS LR-3	CEUS LR-3	CEUS LR-3	CEUS LR-4
Late and mild washout	CEUS LR-3	CEUS LR-4	CEUS LR-4	CEUS LR-5

(APHE: arterial phase hyperenhancement; CEUS: contrast-enhanced ultrasound)

The major features of CEUS LI-RADS are:

- *Arterial phase hyperenhancement (APHE)*:
  - Enhancement of the entire or a portion of the nodule should be greater than that of the adjacent liver in the arterial phase.
  - It should not have rim or peripheral discontinuous globular type of enhancement, as these are features of LR-M observations and hemangiomas, respectively.[10]
- *Washout*:
  - A temporal reduction in enhancement of the whole or part of a nodule resulting in hypoenhancement in comparison to the liver parenchyma at any time, including arterial, portal venous, and late phases.[11]
  - Presence of APHE is not necessary for determining washout.
  - Washout can be classified based on timing (early or late) or degree (mild or marked). If washout is detected earlier than 60 seconds, it is considered early washout and if detected after 60 seconds, it is called late washout.
  - Mild washout occurs when a nodule is hypoenhancing compared to the liver, but it still demonstrates substantial enhancement 2 minutes after contrast injection. On the other hand, marked washout is characterized by a more pronounced hypoenhancing appearance, where the nodule may appear almost black with minimal internal

enhancement or resemble a punched-out defect by 2 minutes of contrast injection.[11]

- HCC and its precursors show mild and late washout, while iCCA and metastases show rapid and marked washout.[11]

Ancillary Features

The CEUS AFs complement the major features and can be used optionally by the examiner for category adjustment and increasing diagnostic confidence. Based on additional imaging features favoring malignancy or benignity, the CEUS LI-RADS category can be upgraded or downgraded by one category, respectively. However, no lesion can be upgraded to LR-5 category based solely on the AFs. The LI-RADS category should not be adjusted in case of conflicting AFs, i.e., the presence of some AFs favoring benignity and others favoring malignancy. The AFs used in CEUS LI-RADS have been summarized in **Box 3**.

(*Tie-breaking rules*: As diagnostic tests aim to have high specificity, if unsure between any two CEUS LI-RADS categories, one should select the one reflecting a lower degree of certainty. For instance, if unsure between LR-1 and LR-2, one should assign the LR-2 category which indicates lower certainty of benignity. Similarly, if unsure between LR-4 and LR-5, one should assign LR-4 indicating lower certainty of malignancy. Also, if unsure between LR-4/LR-5 and LR-M, one should classify observation as LR-M to indicate lower certainty of hepatocellular origin.)

BOX 3 CEUS LI-RADS ancillary features.*

- AFs favoring malignancy in general, not HCC in particular
  - Definite growth—unequivocal spontaneous increase in observation size
- AFs favoring HCC in particular
  - Nodule-in-nodule architecture—presence of smaller inner nodule with imaging features different from larger outer nodule
  - Mosaic architecture—presence of randomly distributed internal compartments, usually with different imaging features
- AFs favoring benignity
  - Size stability > 2 years—no significant change in observation size measured on examinations > 2 years apart in the absence of treatment
  - Size reduction—unequivocal spontaneous decrease in size over time

*If unsure about the presence of any ancillary feature, characterize that feature as absent.

(AFs: ancillary features; CEUS: contrast-enhanced ultrasound; HCC: hepatocellular carcinoma; LI-RADS: Liver Imaging Reporting and Data System)

Management Recommendations

For noncategorizable observations, repeat CEUS or a multiphase CT/MRI should be done within 3 months. For CEUS LR-1 and LR-2 observations, patients can return to 6-monthly routine surveillance US. LR-3 observations require either a repeat CEUS or multiphase CT/MRI within 6 months. Multidisciplinary team discussion for further management is required for LR-4, LR-5, LR-M, and LR-TIV observations. LR-4 observations may be biopsied, treated, or followed up with repeat or alternative imaging in 3 months. LR-5 observations are typically not biopsied, whereas biopsy and/or tumor marker correlation may be needed for LR-M and LR-TIV observations before determining the treatment plan. Important biomarkers for hepatic tumors are summarized in **Table 4**.

LI-RADS COMPUTED TOMOGRAPHY/MAGNETIC RESONANCE IMAGING (V2018)

Target population for diagnostic LI-RADS CT/MRI is similar to that for CEUS LI-RADS (**Box 2**). Though visibility on precontrast imaging is not a prerequisite for application of CT/MRI LI-RADS, the LI-RADS categories cannot be assigned on a noncontrast CT or noncontrast MR. As discussed previously, the LI-RADS category should not be assigned to any pathology-proven benign or malignant lesions.

Computed Tomography/Magnetic Resonance Imaging LI-RADS Categories

The classification of observations from LR-1 to LR-5 using CT/MRI LI-RADS is similar to CEUS LI-RADS. The key difference between them lies in the number of major features and AFs used to assign categories LR-3 to LR-5.

TABLE 4: Tumor markers.

Biomarker	Normal range	Significance (elevated in)
Alpha-fetoprotein (AFP)	0–9 ng/mL	Hepatocellular carcinoma
Protein induced by vitamin K absence-II (PIVKA-II)	< 40 mAU/mL	Hepatocellular carcinoma
Carbohydrate antigen 19-9 (CA 19-9)	< 37 U/mL	• Intrahepatic cholangiocarcinoma • Pancreatic and biliary malignancies
Carcinoembryonic antigen (CEA)	< 5 ng/mL	• Intrahepatic cholangiocarcinoma • Metastases (gastrointestinal, lung, and breast)

- *LR-NC*: Lesions in which the technical quality of the scan does not allow evaluation of the major features.
- *LR-TIV* ***(Figs. 3A to F)***: Observation should be categorized as LR-TIV, if there is unequivocal enhancing soft tissue within the vein, regardless of the presence of discrete liver mass. Indirect signs include occluded vein with ill-defined walls, occluded vein with restricted diffusion, obscured vein in contiguity with parenchymal mass, and heterogeneous vein enhancement not due to artifact. TIVs are most commonly seen in HCC but

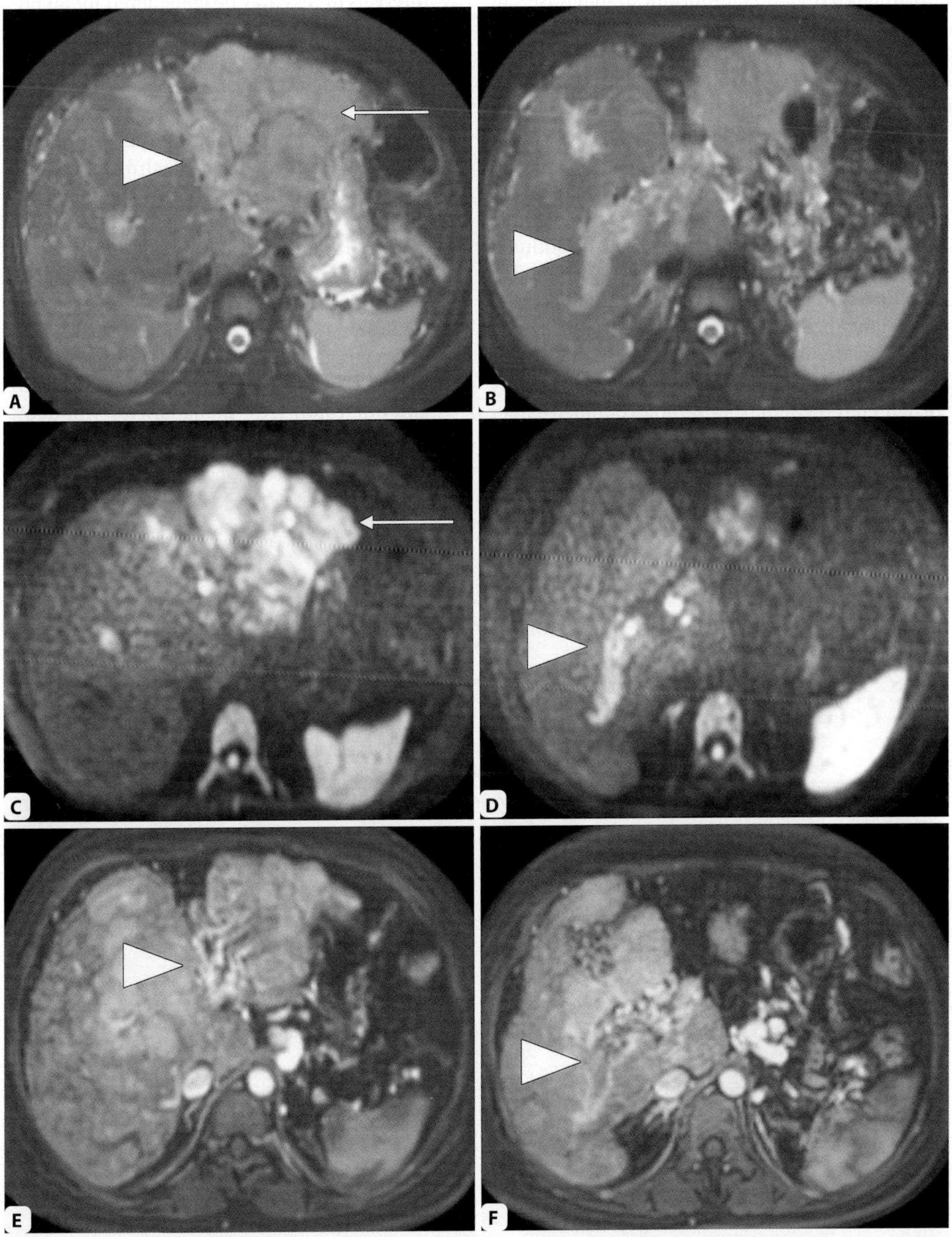

FIGS. 3A TO F: LR-TIV observation: (A and B) Axial T2W images show hyperintense mass (arrow) in segment II of left lobe of liver with similar signal intensity thrombus (arrowheads) in left portal vein, extending to the portal vein bifurcation and right portal vein. (C and D) DWI shows restricted diffusion within the left lobe mass (arrow), as well as in the tumor thrombus. (E and F) Postcontrast T1W FS images show thread-and-streak appearance of tumor thrombus (arrowheads).

(DWI: diffusion-weighted images; T1W: T1 weighted; T2W: T2 weighted) can also be observed in patients with iCCA or cHCC-CCA.[12] If LR-TIV is contiguous with an LR-5 or LR-M observation, it should be reported as LR-TIV definitely due to HCC and LR-TIV may be due to non-HCC malignancy, respectively. For all other categories of associated observations, it should be reported as LR-TIV probably due to HCC. It is important to diagnose LR-TIV, as it is a contraindication for liver transplantation due to the increased risk of tumor recurrence and poor postsurgery outcome. In all LR-TIV categories, a biopsy should be performed if the tumor in the vein is not attributed to HCC and/or if biomarkers suggest a non-HCC malignancy.

- *LR-1*: All definitely benign observations are categorized as LR-1. Examples of LR-1 observations include simple cysts, definitive hemangioma **(Figs. 4A to D)**, confluent fibrosis, focal fatty infiltration or sparing **(Figs. 5A to D)**, perfusion alterations, hypertrophic pseudomass, etc. USG surveillance at 6-month intervals is recommended for LR-1 observations.
- *LR-2* ***(Figs. 6A to D)***: All LR-2 observations are probably (but not definitely) benign. The examples outlined earlier are categorized as LR-2 unless there is definite certainty. Atypical imaging appearance of benign entities may also be categorized as LR-2. Also, a distinctive solid nodule <20 mm with no major feature of HCC, no LR-M and no AF of malignancy can be categorized as LR-2 (e.g., siderotic nodules). Follow-up CT or MRI at 6-month intervals or less may be considered for all LR-2 lesions.
- *LR-M* ***(Figs. 7A to D)***: This category should be assigned to malignant-appearing observations that do not have typical imaging features of HCC. These lesions often exhibit nonspecific or atypical features on imaging such as target-like imaging morphology (including rim APHE, peripheral washout, delayed central enhancement, targetoid appearance on DWI/HBP), infiltrative appearance, marked restricted diffusion, etc. It is important to understand that categorizing an observation as LR-M does not exclude diagnosis of HCC as certain variants of HCC, such as scirrhous HCC or steatohepatitic HCC, may have targetoid appearance on imaging. The common differentials of LR-M include iCCA, cHCC-iCCA, HCC with atypical imaging features, and other non-HCC malignancies. About 5% of LR-M

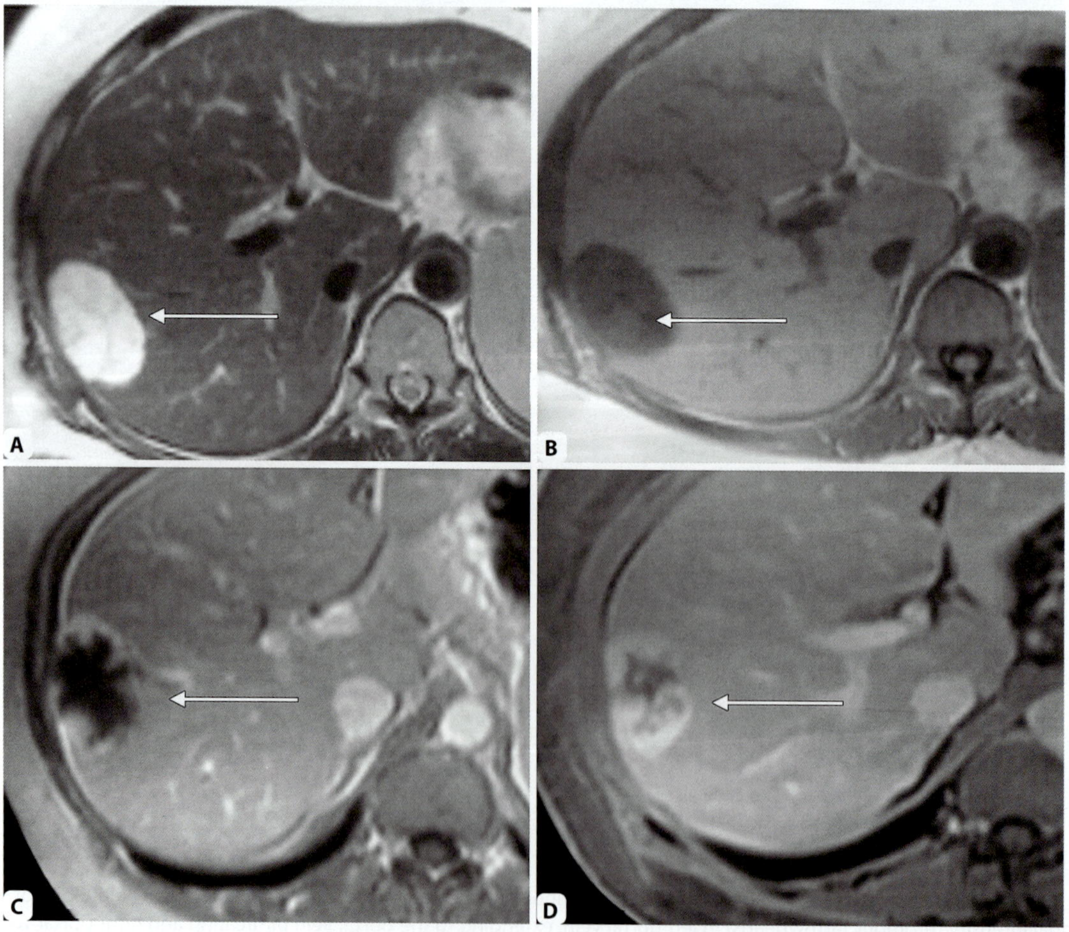

FIGS. 4A TO D: LR-1 (hepatic hemangioma): Axial T2W image (A) shows a markedly hyperintense oval lesion in the right lobe of liver (arrow). The lesion is hypointense on T1-weighted (T1W) image (B) with discontinuous peripheral nodular enhancement in arterial phase (C) and progressive fill-in on venous phase (D).

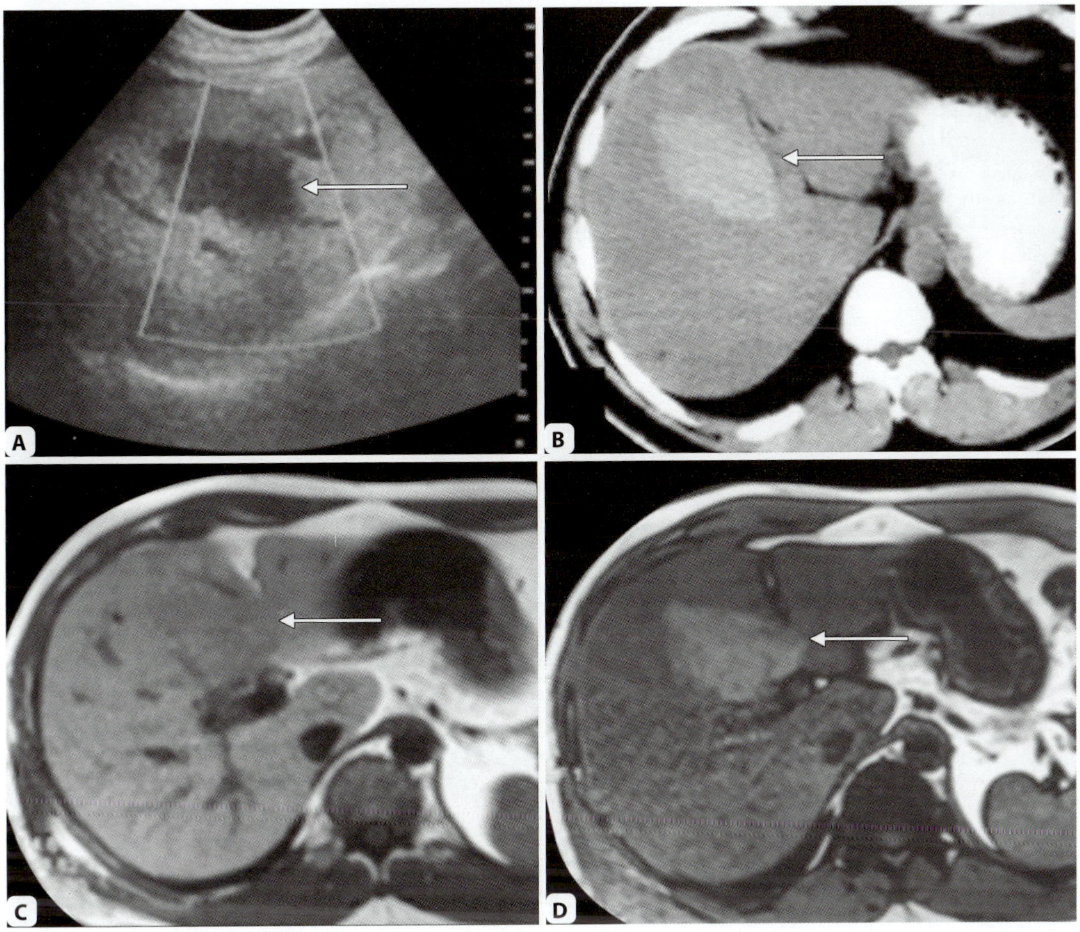

FIGS. 5A TO D: LR-1 (focal fatty sparing): (A) Grayscale ultrasound shows a geographic hypoechoic lesion (arrow) in segment IVb of liver with background hepatic steatosis. (B) noncontrast computed tomography (NCCT) shows the lesion is hyperdense compared to the rest of the hepatic parenchyma. (C) The lesion is hypointense on T1-weighted (T1W) in-phase images. (D) The lesion appears hyperintense as background liver parenchyma shows loss of signal on opposed phase images.

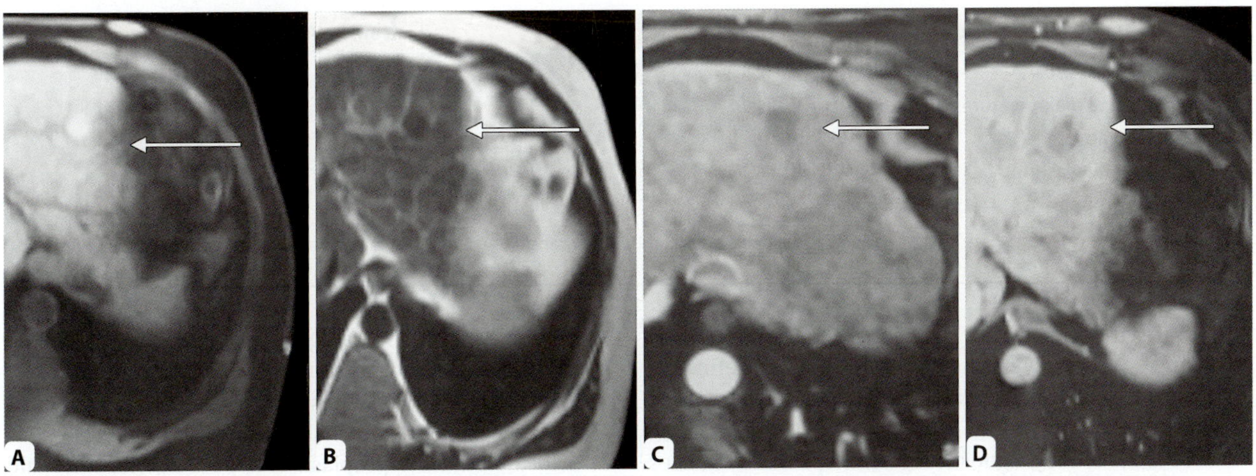

FIGS. 6A TO D: LR-2 observation: (A) T1-weighted (T1W) image showing a small hyperintense lesion in segment II of liver. (B) On T2-weighted (T2W) image, the lesion appears hypointense. (C) No contrast enhancement seen on arterial phase and (D) no washout on venous phase.

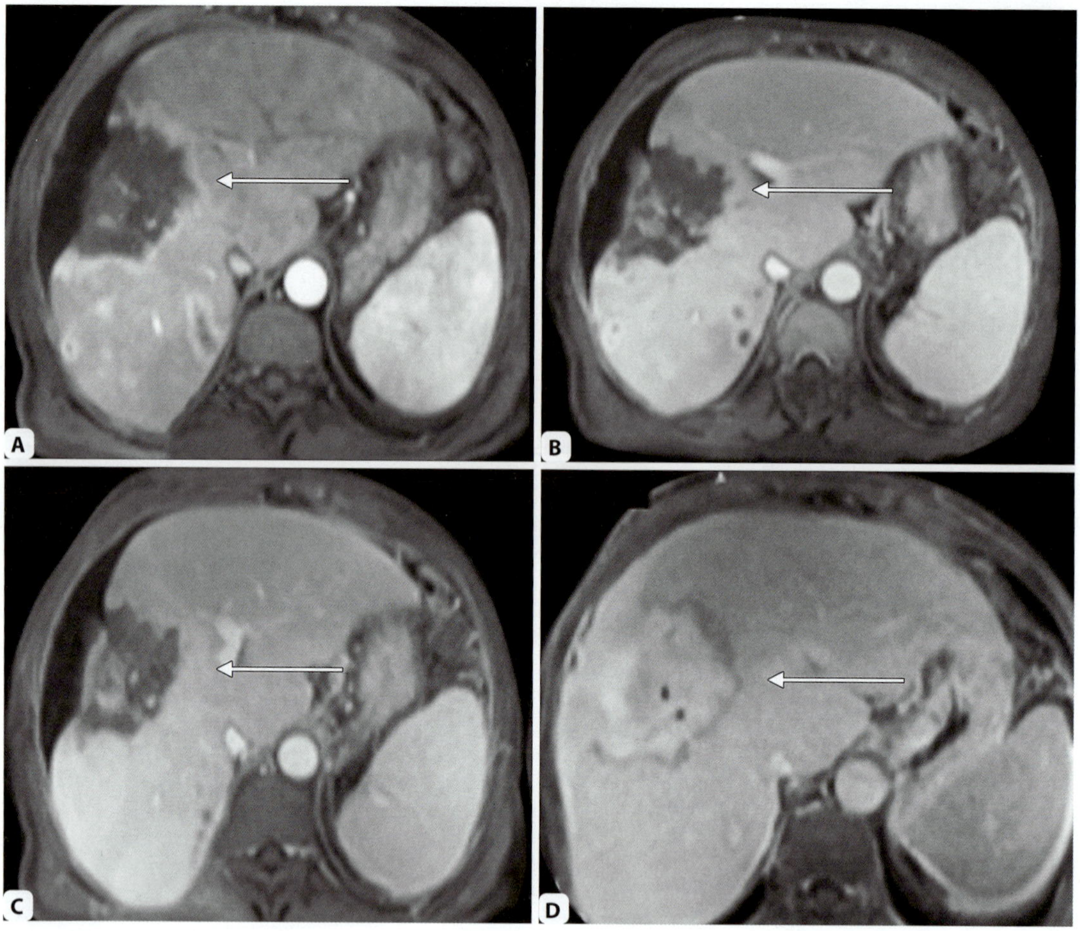

FIGS. 7A TO D: LR-M: (A) Multiphase MR in arterial phase showing a mass in right lobe with rim APHE in the arterial phase, (B and C) with peripheral washout and progressive centripetal enhancement on venous and delayed phase images. (D) Hepatobiliary phase shows retention of contrast within the lesion.

(APHE: arterial phase hyperenhancement; MR: magnetic resonance)

TABLE 5: CT/MRI diagnostic table.

Arterial phase hyperenhancement (APHE)		No APHE		Nonrim APHE		
Observation size (mm)		<20	>20	<10	10–19	>20
Count additional major features:	None	LR-3	LR-3	LR-3	LR-3	LR-4
• Enhancing capsule	1	LR-3	LR-4	LR-4	LR-4/5*	LR-5
• Nonperipheral washout • Threshold growth	>2	LR-4	LR-4	LR-4	LR-5	LR-5

*Observations are categorized as LR-4, if additional major feature is enhancing capsule and as LR-5, if additional major feature is nonperipheral washout or threshold growth.

lesions turn out to be benign. Such lesions often require further evaluation with biopsy for definitive diagnosis and to form individualized management plans accordingly.

- *LR-3 to LR-5*: The diagnostic algorithm primarily utilizes five *major features* to categorize lesions as LR-3, LR-4, or LR-5 **(Table 5)**. Following the initial categorization based on major features, the application of AFs can reclassify the final assessment by upgrading or downgrading the category as discussed in the subsequent section. The higher the LI-RADS category assigned, the greater the likelihood that it represents HCC or malignancy.
- *LR-3* ***(Figs. 8A to C)***: These observations have an intermediate probability of malignancy.[1] Nodules suggestive of focal nodular hyperplasia or hepatic adenoma should also be categorized as LR-3 rather than LR-2, as these are diagnoses of exclusion in high-risk patients. Among LR-3 lesions, approximately 37% turn out to be HCC, with another 39% showing malignant characteristics.[13] Hence, follow-up imaging by the same or alternative

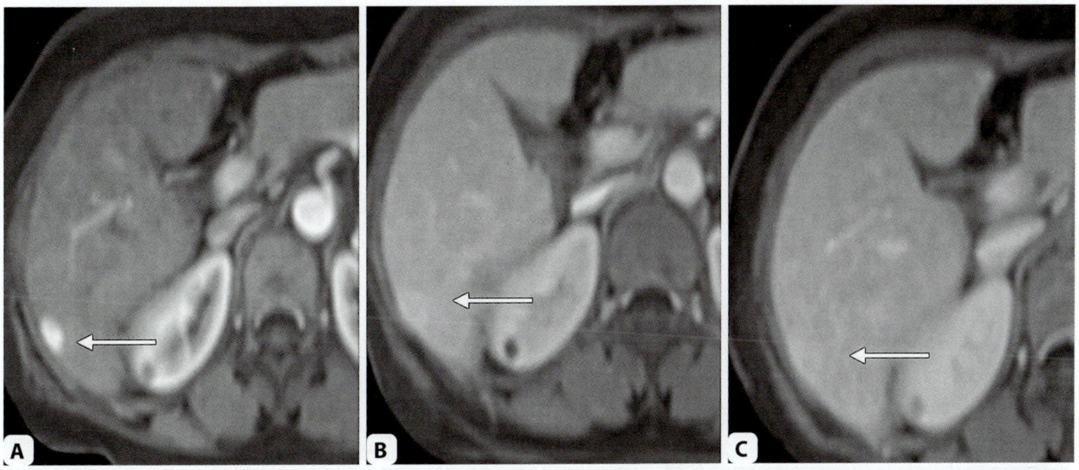

FIGS. 8A TO C: LR-3 observation: Axial T1 PG image (A) shows a small lesion in right lobe showing nonrim arterial phase hyper-enhancement (APHE) in arterial phase (A) and iso+enhancing on venous (B) and delayed phase images (C) with no evidence of washout/enhancing capsule formation.

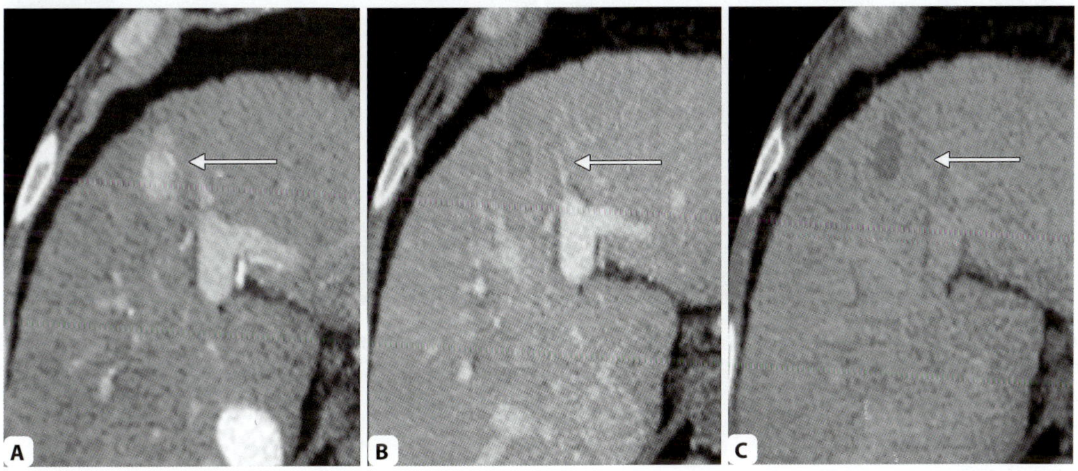

FIGS. 9A TO C: LR-4 observation: A 17 mm lesion in segment V of liver demonstrating (A) nonrim arterial phase, (B) with washout on venous and (C) 3-minute delayed phase.

modality at a 3–6 month interval is advised for all LR-3 lesions.

- *LR-4* ***(Fig. 9A to C)***: Observations characterized by imaging features that are suggestive of HCC but lack definitive diagnostic criteria. About 74% of LR-4 observations are due to HCC and 81% are malignant. Hence, multidisciplinary discussion for the management of such lesions is warranted, which may include repeat imaging within 3 months, biopsy of the lesion, or treatment without histological confirmation.
- *LR-5* ***(Figs. 10A to D)***: These observations show imaging features that are diagnostic for HCC, with a specificity of approximately 95%.[14] Such lesions can be referred for treatment without the need for any tissue diagnosis. Biopsy may be indicated in some scenarios such as if the patient is being recruited for some clinical trials or in cases where molecular characterization is desired. Both APHE and observation size > 10 mm are "required" criteria for diagnosing LR-5 lesions. Additional major features include nonperipheral washout, threshold growth, and enhancing capsule.

The major features ***(Figs. 11A to E)*** *of CT/MRI LI-RADS are*:

- *Nonrim APHE*: This feature is said to be present if there is nonrim type of hyperenhancement in the entire or a portion of observation compared to the liver during the arterial phase. However, it is important to note that its absence does not rule out the possibility of HCC. In some cases, HCC lesions may not demonstrate APHE due to various factors such as some histological subtype or the presence of underlying liver disease.
- *Nonperipheral washout*: Washout is defined as a temporal reduction in the enhancement of the lesion resulting in hypoenhancement compared to the rest of the liver parenchyma in the portal venous or delayed phase. This feature can be applied even in the absence

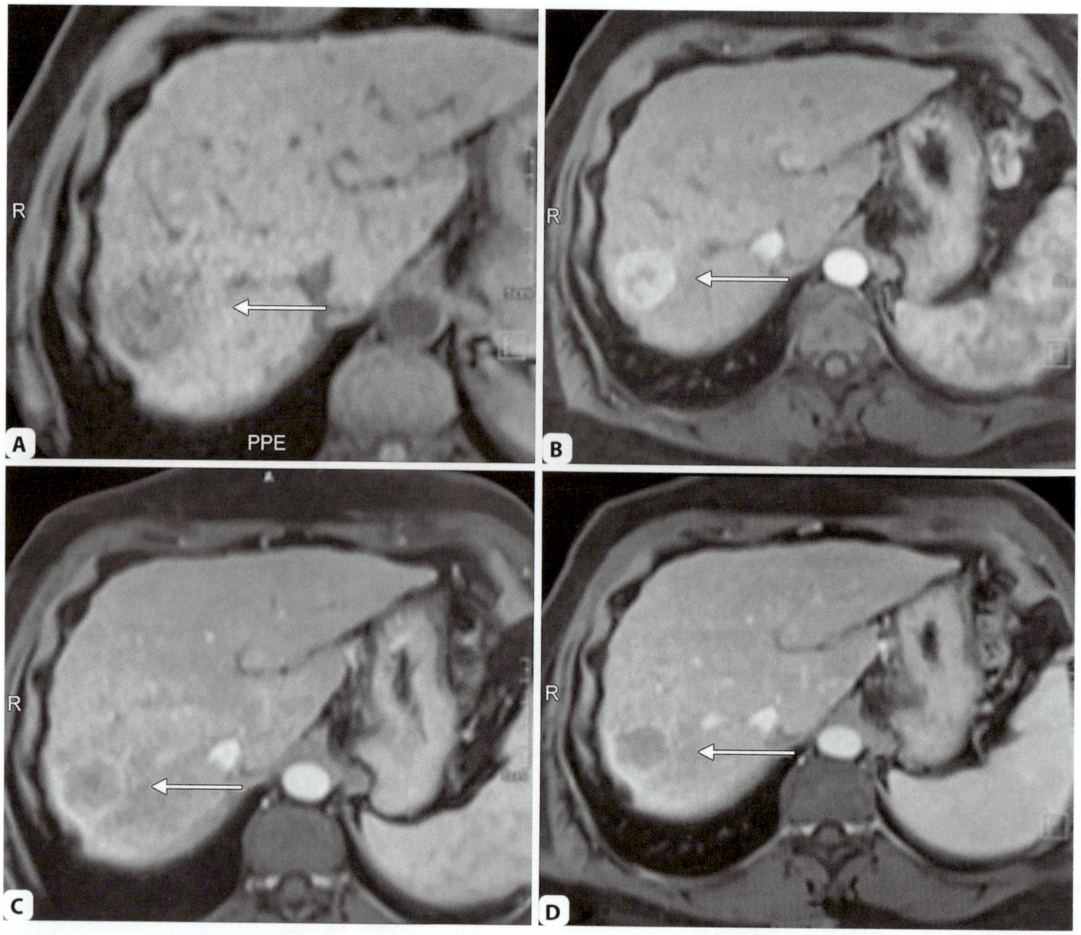

FIGS. 10A TO D: LR-5 observation: Axial T1W noncontrast image (A) shows an oval lesion in the right lobe of liver (arrow). (B) The lesion shows nonrim arterial phase hyperenhancement (APHE) in arterial phase and (C) washout on venous and (D) delayed phases with enhancing capsule formation.

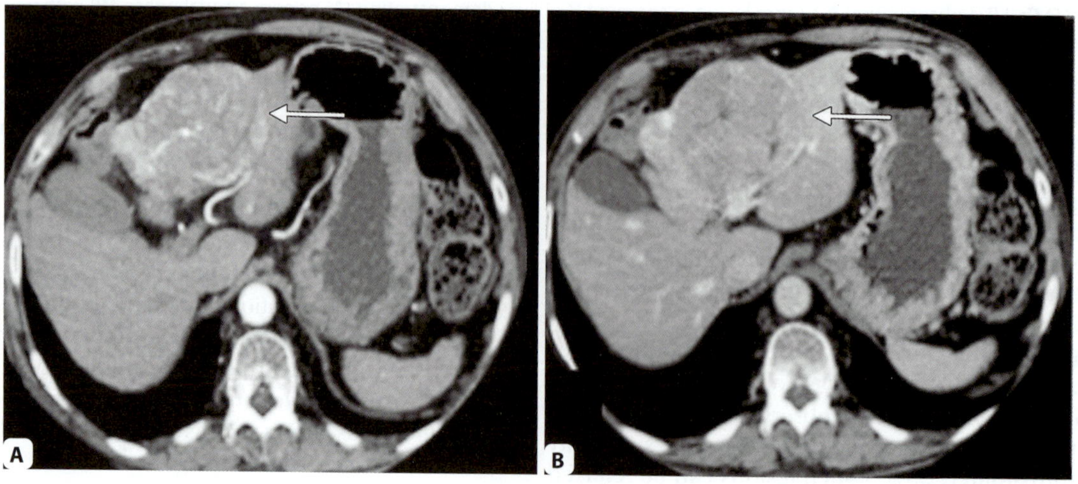

FIGS. 11A TO E: *Continued*

Continued

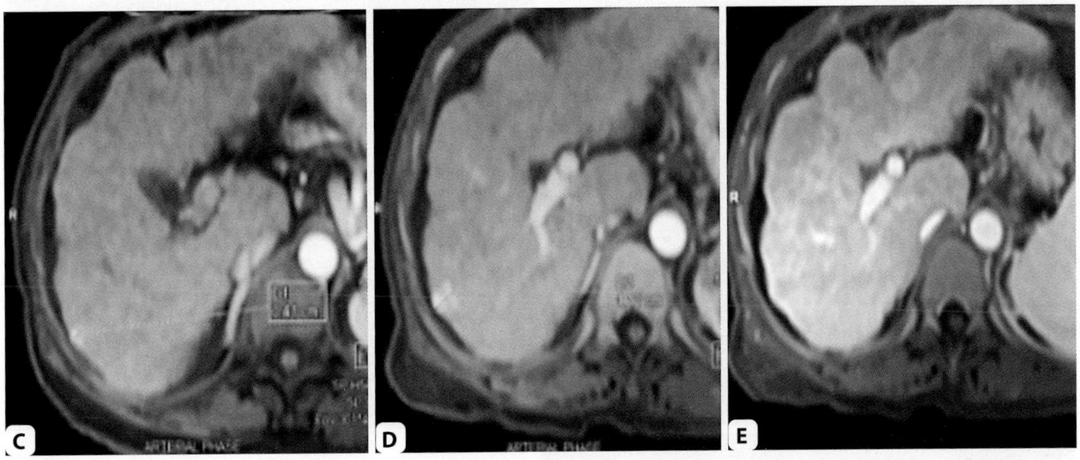

FIGS. 11A TO E: CT/MRI LI-RADS major features: (A) Arterial phase CT shows observation (arrow) with nonrim APHE in segment IVa of liver. (B) The observation shows nonperipheral washout with enhancing capsule on portal venous phase. (C to E) Axial postcontrast T1W images of another patient demonstrating threshold growth of an observation. Initial MRI (C) showing a 4 mm observation with nonrim APHE. Follow-up MRI (D and E) after 6 months shows observation has increased in size to 11 mm with nonrim APHE and nonperipheral washout.

(APHE: arterial phase hyperenhancement; CT: computed tomography; LI-RADS: Liver Imaging Reporting and Data System; MRI: magnetic resonance imaging; T1W: T1 weighted)

of APHE.[13] If temporal reduction in enhancement leads to isoenhancement in all subsequent phases, it is termed *fade* **(Figs. 12A to C)**. Fade is *not* a major feature or AF of CT/MRI LI-RADS. However, if washout is there even in part of the observation while rest of the observation shows fade, washout is considered to be present.

- *Enhancing capsule*: It is a smooth enhancing rim around most or all of an observation, best seen in portal venous/delayed phase.
- *Observation size*: The size of the observation should be measured from one outer edge to another and should include the enhancing capsule, if present. It should be measured in the phase, sequence, or plane in which the margins are best seen. If possible, one should avoid measuring the size in the arterial phase (due to periobservation enhancement) or DWI sequence (due to anatomical distortion).
- *Threshold growth*: It is defined as an increase in size of a mass by ≥50% in ≤6 months. It should be applied only after comparison with previous CT/MR images of good quality, preferably using the same imaging phase, sequence, and plane for measurement. Comparison should not be done with previous US or CEUS studies.

Ancillary Features

The use of AFs, also known as additional features, to further refine the preliminary LI-RADS category is optional. Similar to CEUS LI-RADS, they can be used to either upgrade or downgrade a category after application of the major features. The purpose of including the AFs is to improve the confidence level of the examiner in making a diagnosis. The various AFs favoring malignancy, benignity, or HCC in particular have been listed in **Box 4** and some are illustrated in **Figures 13A to D**. Cases identified to have one or more AF/AFs favoring HCC or malignancy, in addition to the major features, can be upgraded by one level till LR-4, but no lesion can be upgraded to LR-5 category based solely on the AFs. On the other hand, the presence of one or more features suggestive of benignity can result in downgrading of the category by one level. If AFs of both malignancy and benignity are present, then the category should not be changed. It is important to note that the absence of AFs should not be used to downgrade a category. Also, the presence of AFs should not be used to change LR-TIV or LR-M to a different category.

(*Tie-breaking rules*: As for CEUS LI-RADS, if unsure between two categories, the examiner should select the category with a lower level of certainty. For instance, if unsure about the presence of tumor in vein (TIV)—do not categorize it as LR-TIV.)

Management Recommendations

For noncategorizable observations, repeat or alternative diagnostic imaging should be done within 3 months. For negative CT/MRI exams (no observations) and LR-1 and LR-2 observations, patients can return to 6-monthly routine surveillance US. LR-3 observations require either a repeat or alternative diagnostic imaging in 3–6 months **(Figs. 14A to E)**. Multidisciplinary team discussion for further management is required for LR-4, LR-5, LR-M, and LR-TIV observations. Management of LR-4, LR-M, and LR-TIV observations may include biopsies, whereas LR-5 observations having high specificity for HCC are typically not biopsied.

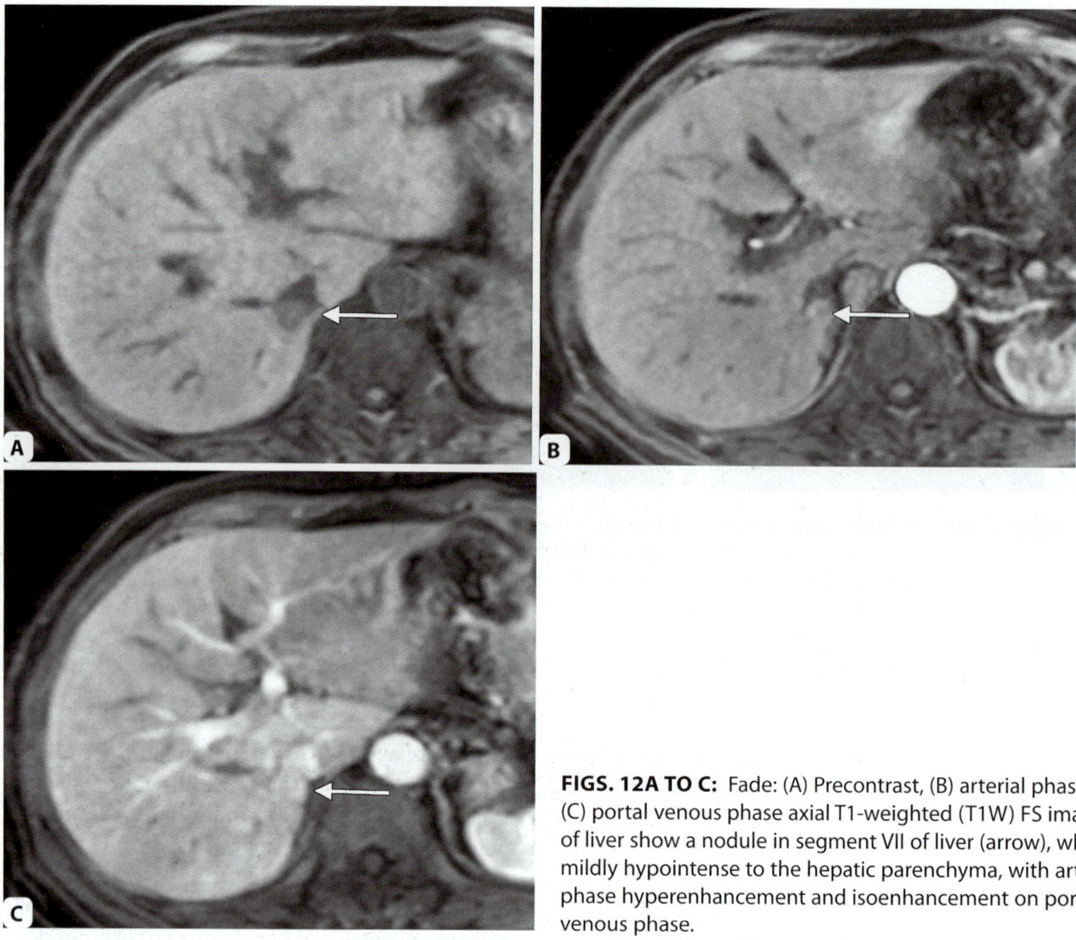

FIGS. 12A TO C: Fade: (A) Precontrast, (B) arterial phase, and (C) portal venous phase axial T1-weighted (T1W) FS images of liver show a nodule in segment VII of liver (arrow), which is mildly hypointense to the hepatic parenchyma, with arterial phase hyperenhancement and isoenhancement on portal venous phase.

BOX 4 Ancillary features for CT/MRI LI-RADS.*

- *Ancillary features favoring malignancy in general*:
  - US visibility as discrete nodule—visibility as discrete nodule on nonenhanced US corresponding to observation detected on CT/MRI
  - Subthreshold growth—unequivocal size increase less than threshold growth
  - Corona enhancement—periobservational enhancement in late arterial/early portovenous phase
  - Fat sparing or iron sparing in solid mass—relative paucity of fat or iron in solid mass with respect to steatotic or iron-overloaded background liver, respectively
  - Restricted diffusion—intensity of DWI unequivocally higher than liver and/or ADC unequivocally lower than liver
  - Mild-to-moderate T2 hyperintensity—hyperintensity on T2W images mildly or moderately higher than liver and similar to or less than that of noniron-overloaded spleen
  - Transitional phase hypointensity—intensity on transitional phase unequivocally less, in whole or in part, than liver
  - HBP hypointensity—intensity on HBP unequivocally less, in whole or in part, than liver
- *Ancillary features favoring HCC in particular*:
  - Nonenhancing "capsule"—capsule appearance not visible as an enhancing rim
  - Mosaic architecture—presence of randomly distributed internal compartments, usually with different imaging features
  - Nodule-in-nodule architecture—presence of smaller inner nodule with imaging features different from larger outer nodule
  - Fat in mass, more than in adjacent liver—excess fat in mass, in whole or in part, relative to adjacent liver
  - Blood products in mass—intralesional or perilesional hemorrhage in absence of trauma or intervention
- *Ancillary features favoring benignity*:
  - Size stability for > 2 years, no significant change in observation size measured on examinations > 2 years apart in the absence of treatment
  - Size reduction—unequivocal spontaneous decrease in size over time
  - Parallels blood pool enhancement—temporal pattern in which enhancement matches that of blood pool
  - Undistorted vessels—vessels traversing an observation without displacement or deformation

Continued

Continued

- Iron in mass, more than in liver—excessive iron in a mass relative to background liver
- Marked T2 hyperintensity—intensity on T2W images markedly higher than liver and similar to fluid-filled structures
- HBP isointensity—intensity on HBP nearly identical to liver

*If unsure about the presence of any ancillary feature, characterize that feature as absent.

(ADC: apparent diffusion coefficient; CT: computed tomography; DWI: diffusion-weighted images; HBP: hepatobiliary phase; HCC: hepatocellular carcinoma; LI-RADS: Liver Imaging Reporting and Data System; MRI: magnetic resonance imaging; T2W: T2 weighted; US: ultrasound)

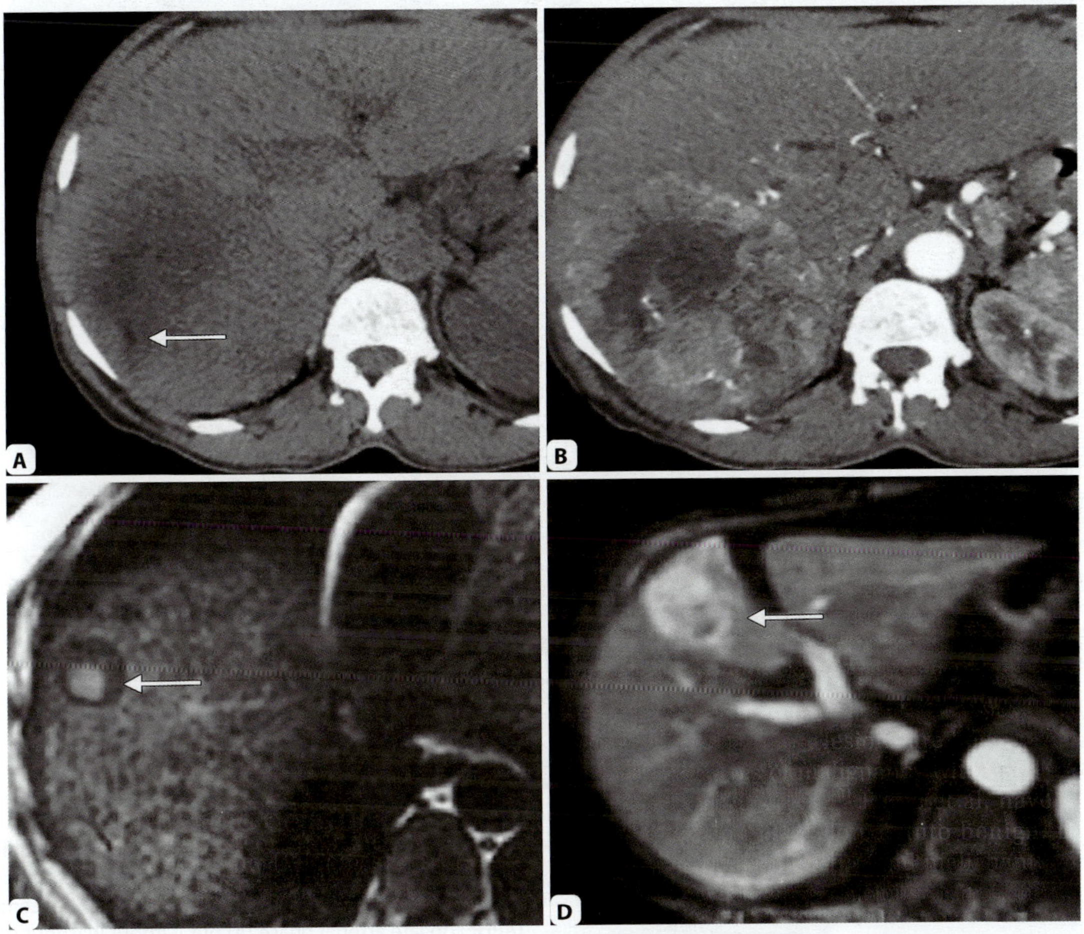

FIGS. 13A TO D: CT/MRI LI-RADS ancillary features favoring HCC in particular: (A) Noncontrast and (B) arterial phase CECT of a patient with HCC in the right lobe of liver with fat in mass (arrow) more than in adjacent liver. (C) Axial T2W MRI shows nodule-in-nodule appearance of HCC (arrow) developing in a dysplastic nodule. (D) Axial postcontrast T1W FS image in late arterial phase shows HCC in segment IV (arrow) with mosaic architecture.

(CECT: contrast-enhanced computed tomography; CT: computed tomography; HCC: hepatocellular carcinoma; LI-RADS: Liver Imaging Reporting and Data System; MRI: magnetic resonance imaging; T1W: T1 weighted; T2W: T2 weighted)

Differences between CEUS LI-RADS and CT/MRI LI-RADS

Both CEUS LI-RADS and CT/MRI LI-RADS are diagnostic algorithms for liver observations in patients at high risk for HCC. However, there are some salient differences between them which are tabulated in **Table 6**.

LIMITATIONS OF LI-RADS

- Differentiation of HCC from non-HCC malignancies is difficult with current major features, with many atypical HCC accounting for LR-M observations, and some non-HCC malignancies are also incorrectly categorized as LR-4 or LR-5.

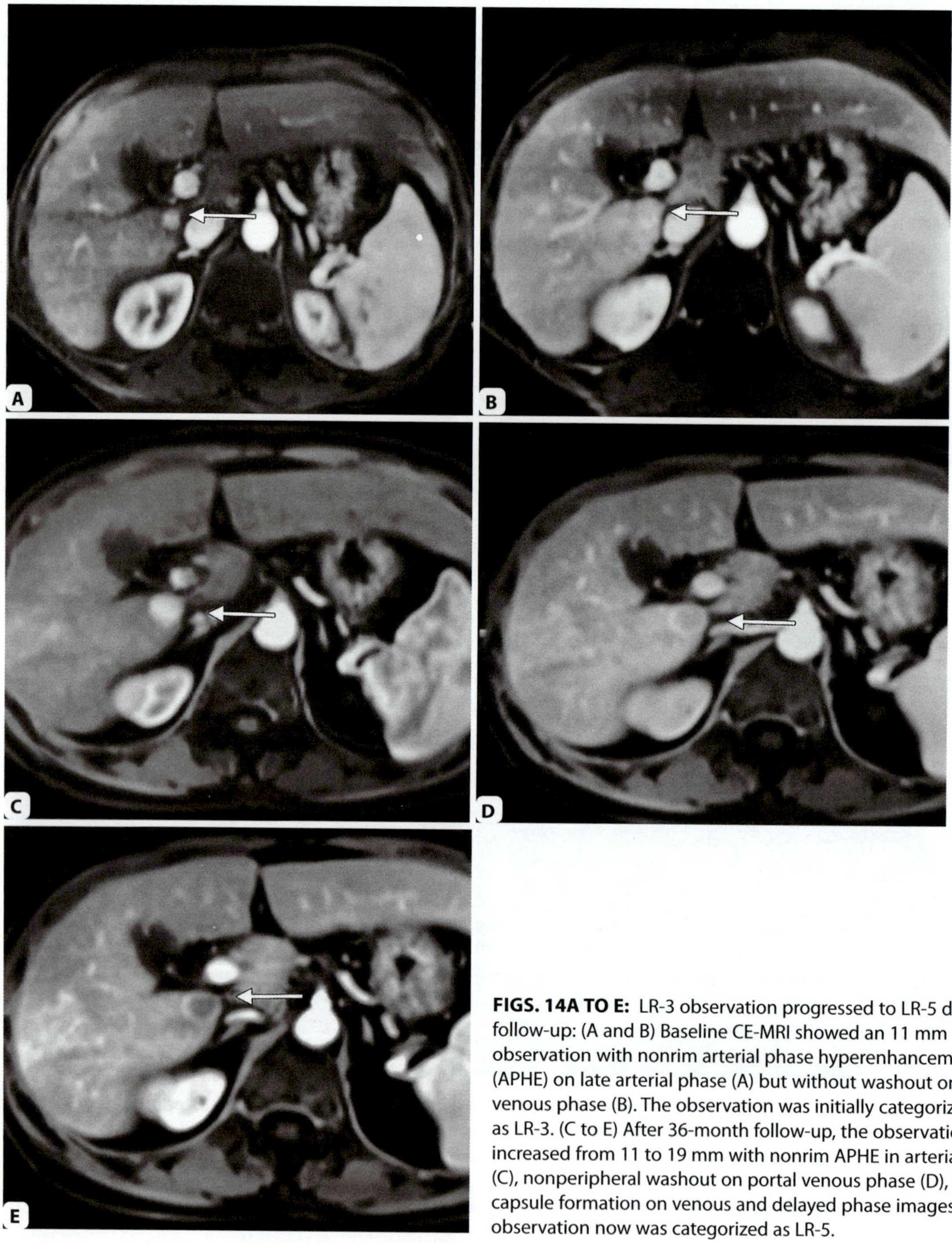

FIGS. 14A TO E: LR-3 observation progressed to LR-5 during follow-up: (A and B) Baseline CE-MRI showed an 11 mm observation with nonrim arterial phase hyperenhancement (APHE) on late arterial phase (A) but without washout on portal venous phase (B). The observation was initially categorized as LR-3. (C to E) After 36-month follow-up, the observation increased from 11 to 19 mm with nonrim APHE in arterial phase (C), nonperipheral washout on portal venous phase (D), and capsule formation on venous and delayed phase images (E). The observation now was categorized as LR-5.

TABLE 6: Differences between CEUS LI-RADS and CT/MRI LI-RADS.

	CEUS LI-RADS	CT/MRI LI-RADS
Latest version	2017	2018
Use	Diagnosis only	Diagnosis, staging, and treatment response
Contrast		
Type of agents	Blood pool	Extracellular or hepatobiliary
Number of injections	One to multiple (if required)	One
Safety profile	Safer	Less safe

Continued

Continued

	CEUS LI-RADS	CT/MRI LI-RADS
Major features		
APHE	Higher sensitivity due to better temporal resolution, size thresholds < 10 and > 10 mm	Lower sensitivity; size thresholds < 10 mm, 10–19 mm, and > 20 mm
Washout	True washout; classified as per timing (early/late) and degree (mild/marked)	True or apparent washout; classified as peripheral or nonperipheral
Capsule	Not a feature	Major feature
Growth	Not a major feature (definite growth is an ancillary feature)	Threshold growth is a major feature
Ancillary features	Few	Many
Observation visibility on precontrast imaging	Necessary	Not necessary
Evaluable number of observations	One to few	One to many
Vascular pseudolesions	Not depicted	Frequently detected
High operator expertise	Required	Not required

(APHE: arterial phase hyperenhancement; CEUS: contrast-enhanced ultrasound; CT: computed tomography; LI-RADS: Liver Imaging Reporting and Data System; MRI: magnetic resonance imaging)

- Use of AFs is optional and all are given equal weightage. However, certain AFs such as HBP hypointensity and restricted diffusion may warrant greater weightage than other AFs on account of their stronger association with malignancy.
- Regional differences in HCC are not addressed in the current version of LI-RADS.[15]
- CT/MRI LI-RADS deals with diagnosis, staging, and treatment response assessment, but prognostic implications of different LI-RADS categories are not clear and require further research.
- Ideally, an observation should be assigned the same LI-RADS category irrespective of the imaging modality used. However, intrinsic differences between CEUS, CT, and MRI lead to different categorization of the same observation on different modalities. Interobserver variability can also cause assignment of different LI-RADS categories to the same observation. Further refinements are necessary to eliminate these variations.
- Current version of CEUS LI-RADS is based on the use of blood pool agents such as SonoVue® and Definity® and does not allow for use of Sonazoid® which is a Kupffer cell agent. A consensus statement by the Asian Federation of Societies for Ultrasound in Medicine and Biology (AFSUMB) recommends the use of US contrast agent Sonazoid® with defect reperfusion imaging in postvascular (Kupffer phase) for surveillance of small HCCs in cirrhotic patients.[16] However, this has not been incorporated in the surveillance module of LI-RADS either.

FOCAL LESIONS IN CIRRHOTIC LIVER

In cirrhosis, there is distortion and replacement of normal liver parenchyma by fibrous and regenerative tissue, which pose significant challenges in detecting and diagnosing liver nodules on imaging.[2] Hence, familiarity with the typical and atypical imaging features of these lesions is necessary for accurate diagnosis. Although HCC is the most common tumor in cirrhotic liver, several other benign and malignant lesions can occur in this setting.[17,18]

Nonhepatocellular Benign Lesions

Cysts (Figs. 15A to C)

Most of the simple hepatic cysts can be categorized as LR-1. Cysts with mild atypical features or hypodense lesions too small to be characterized may be categorized as LR-2. Peribiliary cysts can also be seen in cirrhosis, particularly in patients with fibrocystic liver disease or ALD. These are formed due to obstruction of peribiliary glands. In contrast to dilated intrahepatic biliary radicles which are situated on one side of the portal vein, peribiliary cysts are clustered on both sides of the portal vein. Their imaging features are similar to simple hepatic cysts—thin-walled with fluid density/signal intensity and no internal enhancement. Occasionally, von Meyenburg complexes or biliary hamartomas can be seen in cirrhotic livers. These appear as multiple small cysts, usually up to 15 mm size, scattered in both lobes of the liver with characteristic comet-tail artifact on US.

Hemangiomas (Figs. 16A and B)

Unlike the general population, the prevalence of hemangioma is less common in cirrhotic liver, and also the imaging features may not be classical. HCC often mimics hemangioma on USG because of hyperechogenicity resulting from necrosis, fatty changes, or fibrosis.[19] In patients with early cirrhosis, hemangioma usually shows classical features on CEUS, multiphase CT, or MRI as peripheral nodular enhancement with centripetal progressive fill-in,[20,21] with bright signal on T2, and high signal on

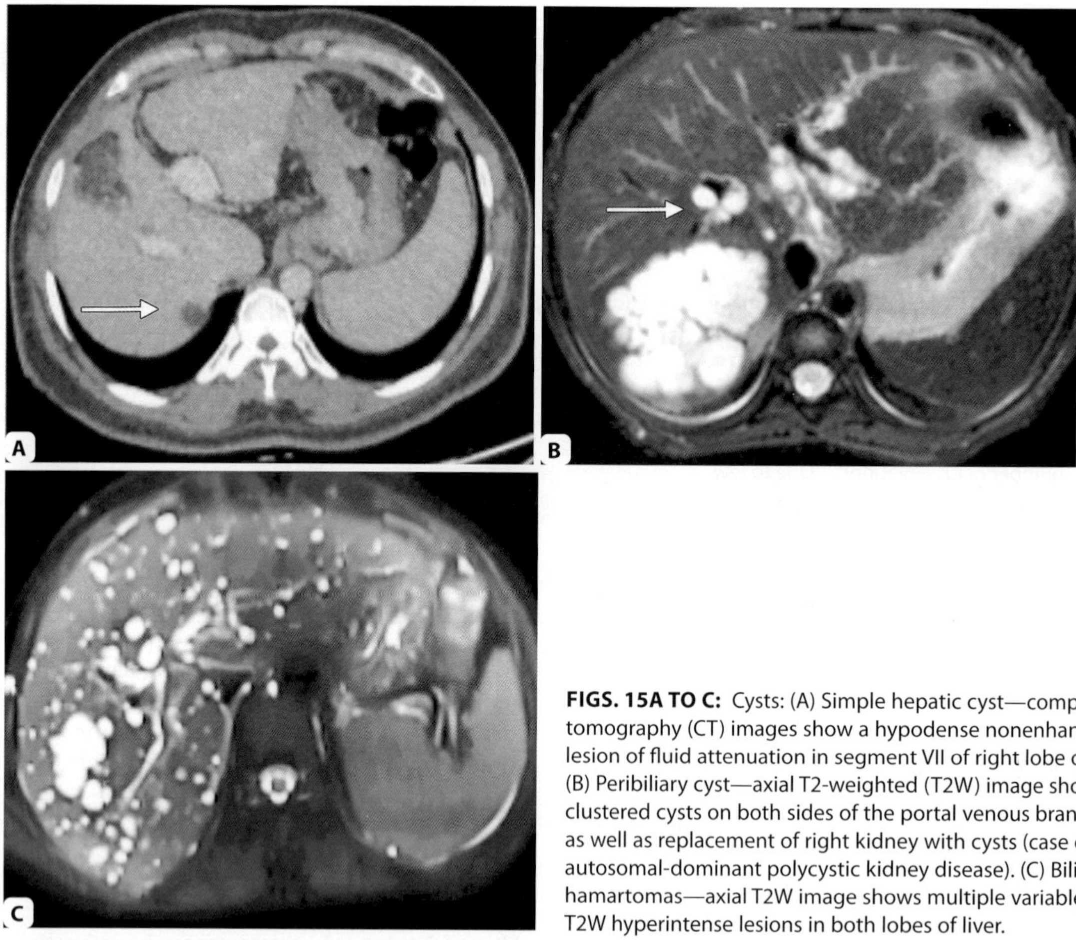

FIGS. 15A TO C: Cysts: (A) Simple hepatic cyst—computed tomography (CT) images show a hypodense nonenhancing lesion of fluid attenuation in segment VII of right lobe of liver. (B) Peribiliary cyst—axial T2-weighted (T2W) image shows clustered cysts on both sides of the portal venous branches as well as replacement of right kidney with cysts (case of autosomal-dominant polycystic kidney disease). (C) Biliary hamartomas—axial T2W image shows multiple variable-sized T2W hyperintense lesions in both lobes of liver.

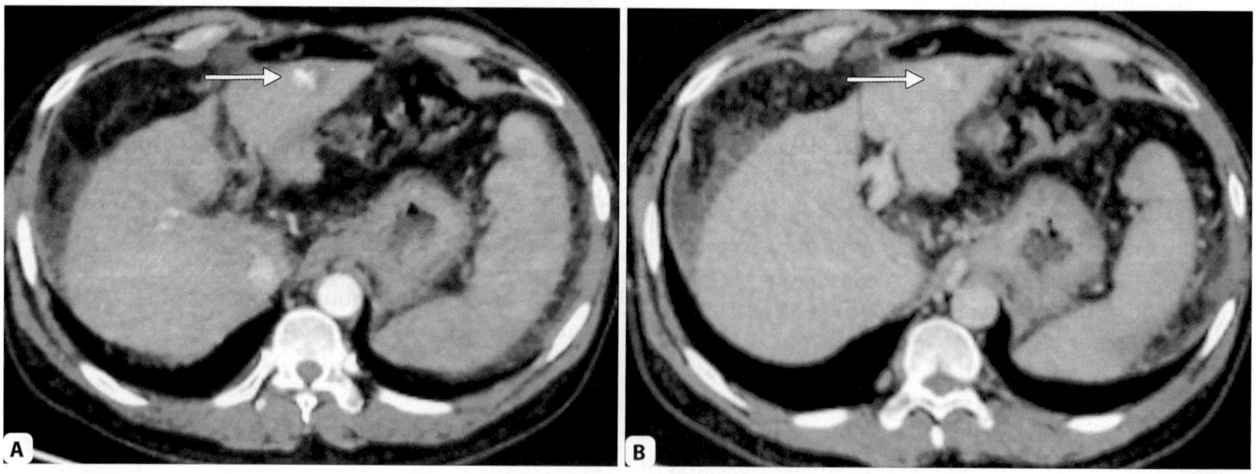

FIGS. 16A AND B: Hemangioma: (A) Arterial phase image shows lesion with peripheral nodular enhancement (arrow). (B) Venous phase image shows progressive fill-in. Enhancing component is isoattenuating to the blood pool on both phases.

DWI. However, with increasing fibrosis, it may become hypovascular with loss of this enhancement pattern, leading to diagnostic confusion.[22,23] These sclerosing hemangiomas are usually irregular in shape unlike hypovascular HCC which are spherical. Comparison with previous imaging can also help identify signs of stability. In cases where previous imaging is not available or if hemangioma demonstrates atypical features, then it can be categorized at LI-RADS 2, 3, or 4, depending upon the level of suspicion and managed accordingly.[24] Diagnosis of flash-filling hemangiomas in cirrhotic livers is also challenging; CEUS can be a useful problem-solving tool in these cases. Due to its superior temporal resolution, it can demonstrate discontinuous peripheral nodular enhancement in these lesions which is not evident on multiphase CT or MRI.

Confluent Hepatic Fibrosis (Figs. 17A to F)

Confluent hepatic fibrosis results from chronic liver injury, the most common etiologies being alcohol-related cirrhosis and primary sclerosing cholangitis.[25] It occurs more commonly in the anterior and medial segments of the liver, involving segments IV, V, and VIII. On noncontrast CT scans, it appears as a single peripheral wedge-shaped hypodense area with apex pointing toward hilum and a broad base toward the capsular surface and associated capsular retraction or flattening. Gradual enhancement with

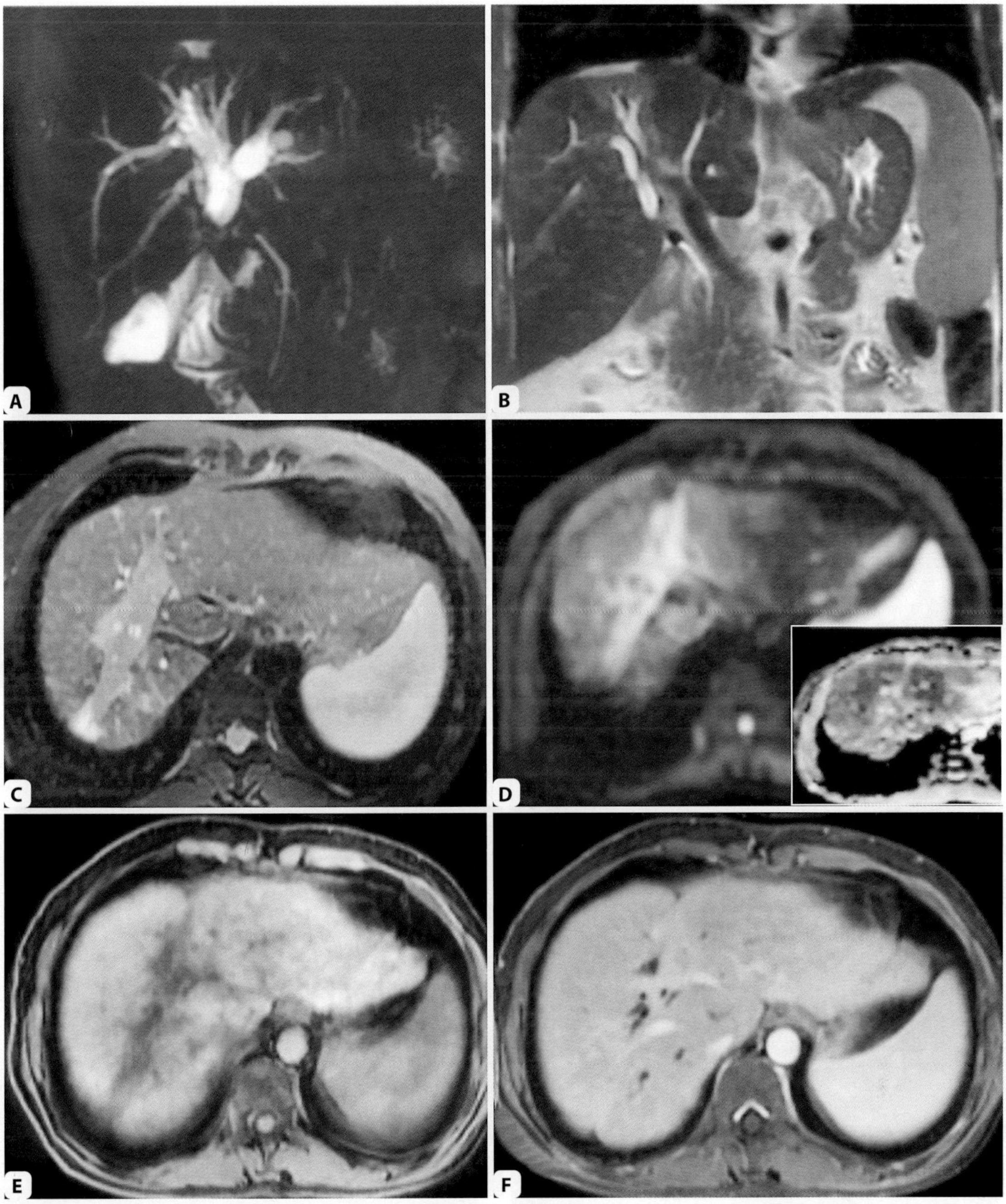

FIGS. 17A TO F: Confluent hepatic fibrosis—patient with secondary biliary cirrhosis: (A) Coronal MRCP image shows intrahepatic biliary ductal dilatation due to hepaticojejunostomy site stricture. (B) Coronal HASTE image shows wedge-shaped confluent hyperintense lesion in segments VIII/IVa with overlying capsular retraction. (C) Axial T2W fat-suppressed image shows band-like T2W hyperintense lesion in segments VIII and IVa. (D) Axial diffusion-weighted image (inset—ADC map)—the lesion does not show restricted diffusion. (E) The lesion is hypointense on axial precontrast T1W fat-suppressed image, (F) with enhancement on delayed phase.

(ADC: apparent diffusion coefficient; MRCP: magnetic resonance cholangiopancreatography; T1W: T1-weighted; T2W: T2-weighted)

retention of contrast on delayed phase images is seen on dynamic contrast scans, reflecting the presence of fibrosis. Trapped and crowded enhancing vessels may be seen traversing through the lesion in 15% of the cases.[26] On MRI, it appears hypointense on T1 and moderately hyperintense on T2 with no diffusion restriction. With the use of liver-specific contrast agents, it does not show any retention of contrast in the HBP due to a lack of normal hepatocytes. The presence of capsular retraction and progressive enhancement are key imaging features for differentiating it from HCC. The presence of characteristic morphologic features, specific location, and absence of suspicious enhancement patterns may lead to confident diagnosis and categorization as LI-RADS 1 or 2, depending on the level of confidence. Rarely, it may show enhancement in the arterial phase due to active ongoing inflammation mimicking HCC on imaging.[27] Biopsy is warranted in such cases.

Pseudolesions (Perfusion Abnormalities)

Several factors can contribute to development of transient hepatic attenuation differences (THAD) **(Figs. 18A and B)** and transient hepatic intensity differences (THID) **(Figs. 19A and B)**, including arterioportal shunting/fistula, various benign and malignant tumors, biliary obstruction, portal vein obstruction, etc. THAD and THID phenomenon is characterized by hyperenhancement in the arterial phase followed by isoenhancement or isointensity in the subsequent phases. They may be occult on all noncontrast sequences. Three morphological patterns have been described: Peripheral wedge shaped, nodular enhancement, and florid type. Although these perfusion abnormalities are benign and usually categorized as LI-RADS 1 or 2, they may be associated with malignancies such as HCC. If present, HCC nodules are generally present at

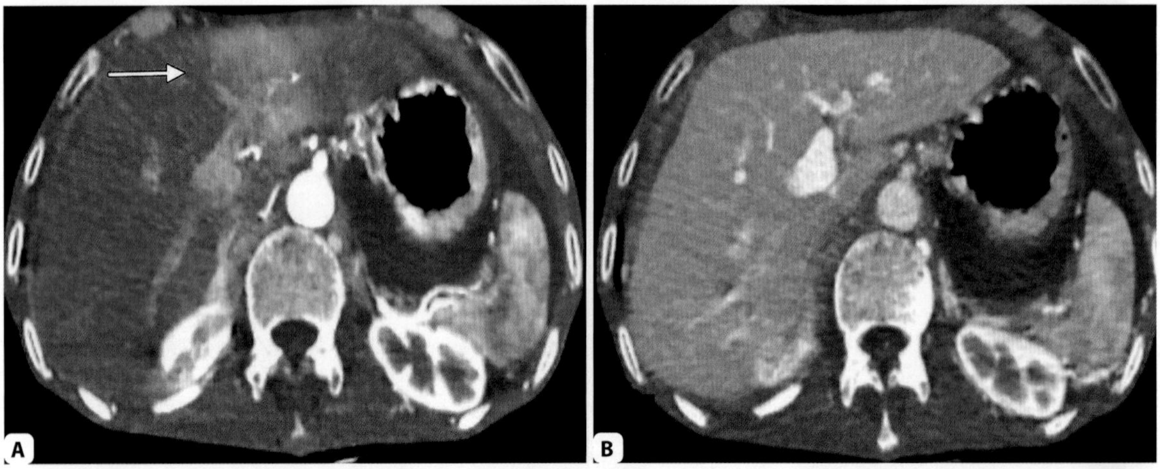

FIGS. 18A AND B: Transient hepatic attenuation difference. (A) Axial contrast-enhanced images in arterial phase, (B) showing wedge-shaped area of hyperenhancement in segment III (arrow) which becomes isodense to liver on venous phase images.

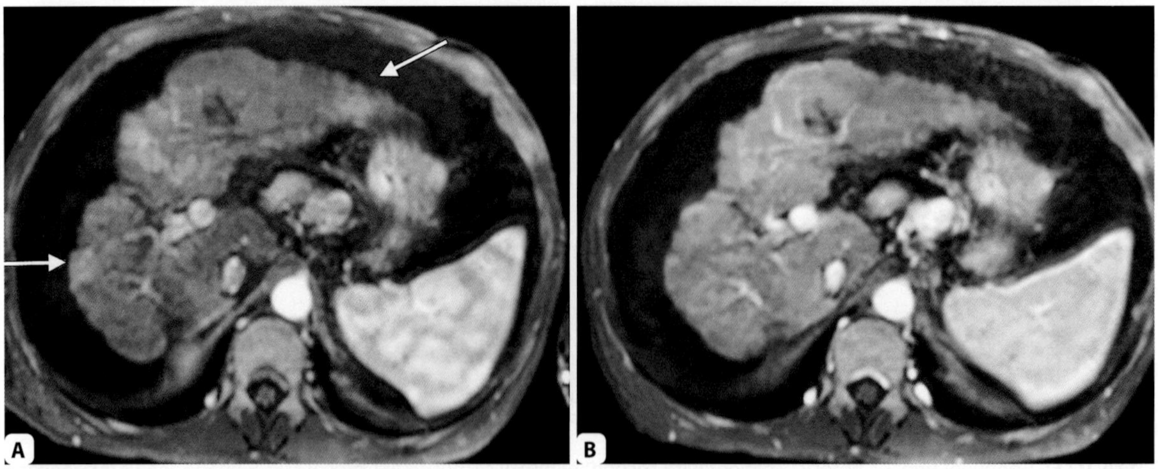

FIGS. 19A AND B: Transient hepatic intensity difference—axial image in the arterial phase shows multiple wedge-shaped enhancing areas in the right lobe of the liver (A, arrows). (B) The lesions are isoenhancing to the background liver parenchyma in the venous phase images.

the apex of the wedge-shaped THID/THAD phenomenon.[24] Hence, the apex of these areas should be examined carefully for the presence of any mass.

Benign Hepatocellular Nodules (Table 7)

Focal Nodular Hyperplasia-like Lesions (FNH-like lesions) (Figs. 20A to C)

These are lesions which are pathologically identical to FNH but occur in a background of abnormal liver. Microvascular disturbances in cirrhosis predispose to the development of FNH-like lesions (previously known as regenerative nodules). These are benign nodules with no malignant potential (do not touch lesions) present in 3–15% cirrhotic livers. Similar to conventional FNH, FNH-like lesions are isointense to liver parenchyma on noncontrast T1W and T2W sequences and may have a T2W hyperintense central scar. They show APHE, but in contrast to HCC, there is no washout in venous or delayed phases. Majority of them are isointense or hyperintense on the HBP. Given the overlap of imaging features with HCC, FNH-like lesions should be classified as LR-3.[28] On CEUS, regenerative nodules show no enhancement during the arterial phase and remain isoechoic in the portal and late phases, reflecting the absence of abnormal arterial supply within the nodule.[29,30]

Dysplastic nodules (Figs. 21 to 23): Premalignant

Dysplastic nodules represent an intermediate step in the progression toward HCC in cirrhotic livers. In the initial phases of hepatocarcinogenesis, there is a decline in the density of portal triads. This accounts for arterial phase isoenhancement or hypoenhancement of dysplastic nodules. Their signal intensity features often overlap with those of early well-differentiated HCCs. Siderotic nodules are usually low-grade or high-grade dysplastic nodules.

Malignancies

Hepatocellular Carcinoma

Hepatocellular carcinoma is the most common primary malignancy of the liver. On noncontrast USG, HCC can have variable appearance depending upon the size, echotexture of background liver, etc. Small lesions appear hypoechoic, while larger lesions can be heterogeneous due to fibrosis, necrosis, fatty changes, etc. Diffuse infiltrative HCC may be difficult to diagnose from background cirrhosis. On CEUS, HCC classically enhances in the arterial phase and shows mild and late washout in the venous/delayed phase.[10] Multiphase CT/MR is the standard imaging modality for the diagnosis of HCC. Increase in density of unpaired

TABLE 7: Cirrhosis-associated hepatocellular nodules.

Nodule	Histology	T1W	T2W	Arterial phase hyperenhance-ment	Venous/ delayed phase washout	Hepatobiliary phase
Regenerative nodules	Benign, resembling other background nodules	Isointense	Isointense	Absent*	Absent	Isointense
Siderotic nodules	Dysplastic nodules with increased iron content	Hypointense	Hypointense	Absent	Absent	Isointense
Low-grade dysplastic nodule	Clonal expansion of cells without atypia	Hyperintense	Iso- to hypo-intense	Absent	Absent	Isointense
High-grade dysplastic nodule	• Clonal expansion of cells with atypia • Lack of stromal invasion	Hyperintense	Iso- to hypo-intense	Present	Absent	Isointense
Early HCC	• Well-differentiated malignancy • Stromal invasion present • Replacing growth	Iso/hypo/ hyperintense	Hyperintense	Present	Present	Hypointense
Progressed HCC	• Moderate-to-poorly differentiated malignancy • Expansile growth • Vascular invasion and metastases	Iso/hypo/ hyperintense	Hyperintense	Present	Present	Hypointense†

* Arterial phase enhancement is present in regenerative nodules associated with Budd–Chiari syndrome.

† 5% of HCC express OATP and appear isointense on hepatobiliary phase.

(HCC: hepatocellular carcinoma; OATP: organic anion transporting polypeptide; T1W: T1 weighted; T2W: T2 weighted)

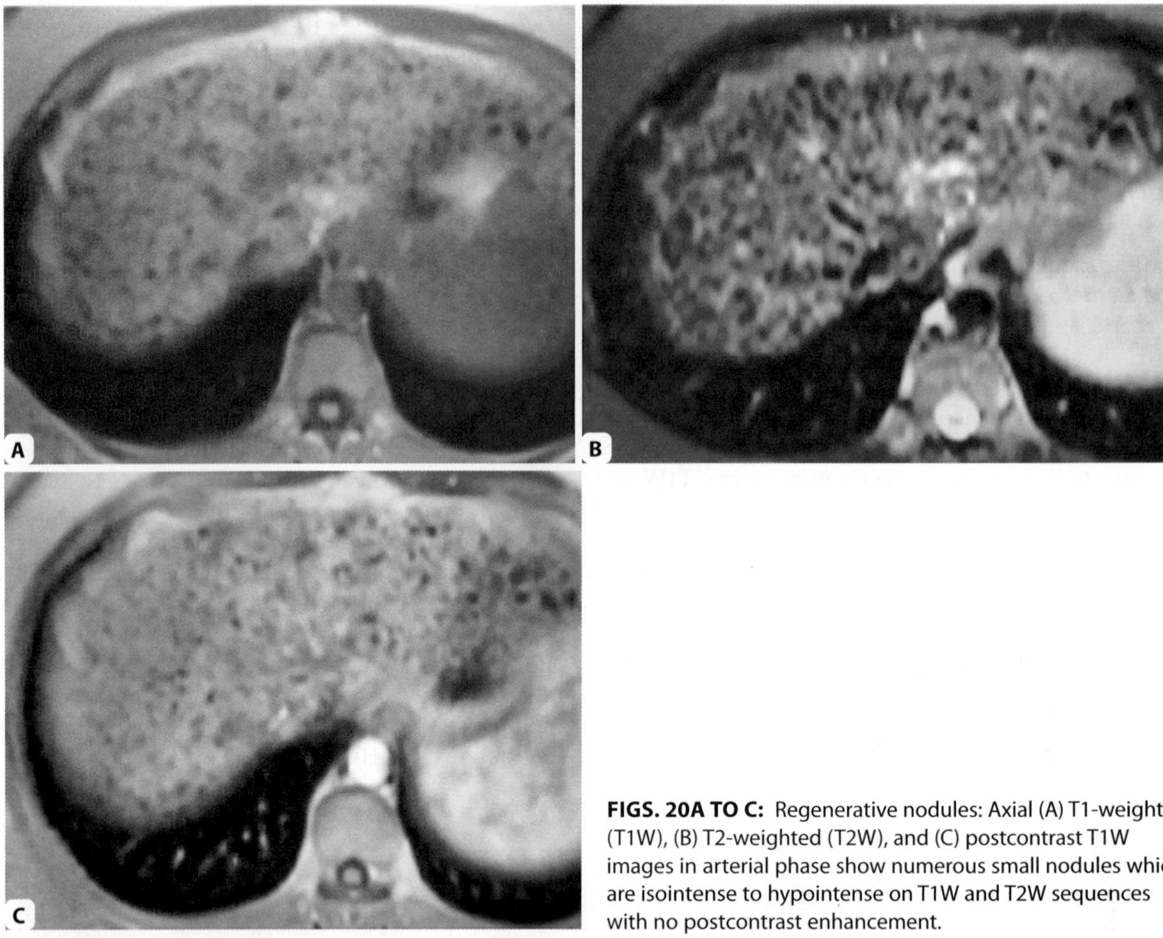

FIGS. 20A TO C: Regenerative nodules: Axial (A) T1-weighted (T1W), (B) T2-weighted (T2W), and (C) postcontrast T1W images in arterial phase show numerous small nodules which are isointense to hypointense on T1W and T2W sequences with no postcontrast enhancement.

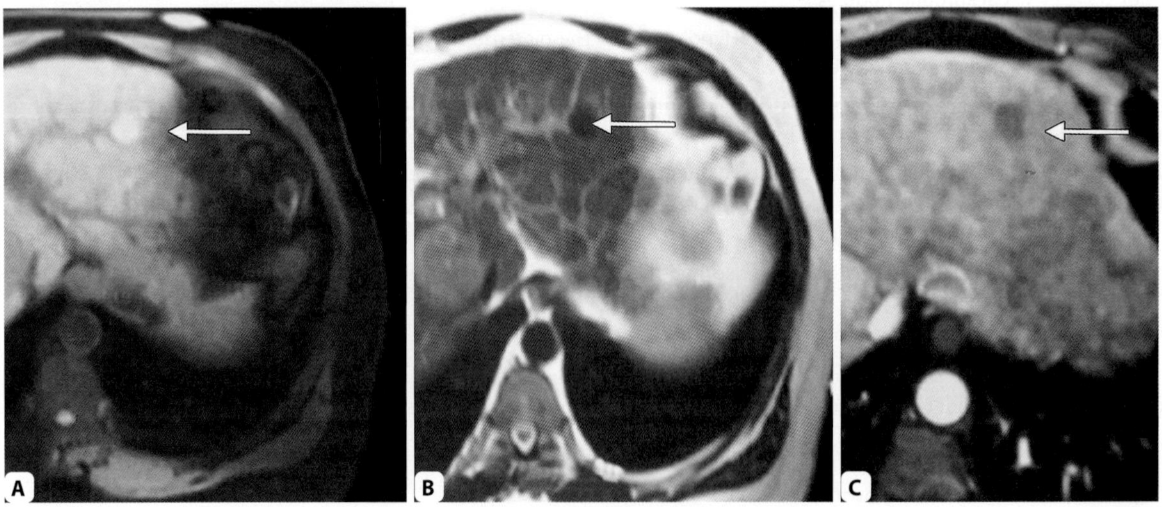

FIGS. 21A TO C: Low-grade dysplastic nodule: Axial (A) T1-weighted (T1W), (B) T2-weighted (T2W), and (C) postcontrast T1W images in arterial phase show a small nodule in left lobe of liver (arrow) which is hyperintense on T1W and hypointense on T2W sequences with no postcontrast enhancement.

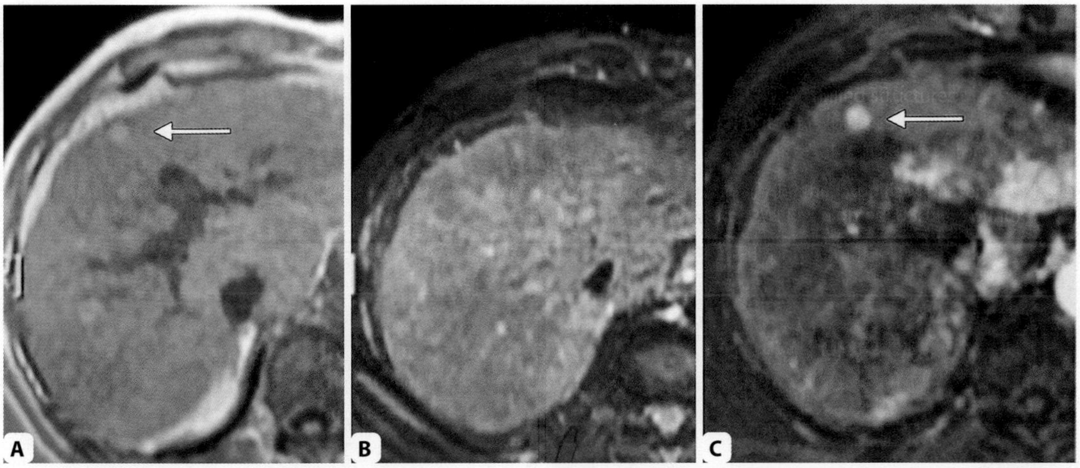

FIGS. 22A TO C: High-grade dysplastic nodule: Axial (A) T1-weighted (T1W), (B) T2-weighted (T2W), and (C) postcontrast T1W images in arterial phase show a small 8 mm nodule in left lobe of liver (arrow) which is hyperintense on T1W and isointense on T2W sequences with arterial phase hyperenhancement.

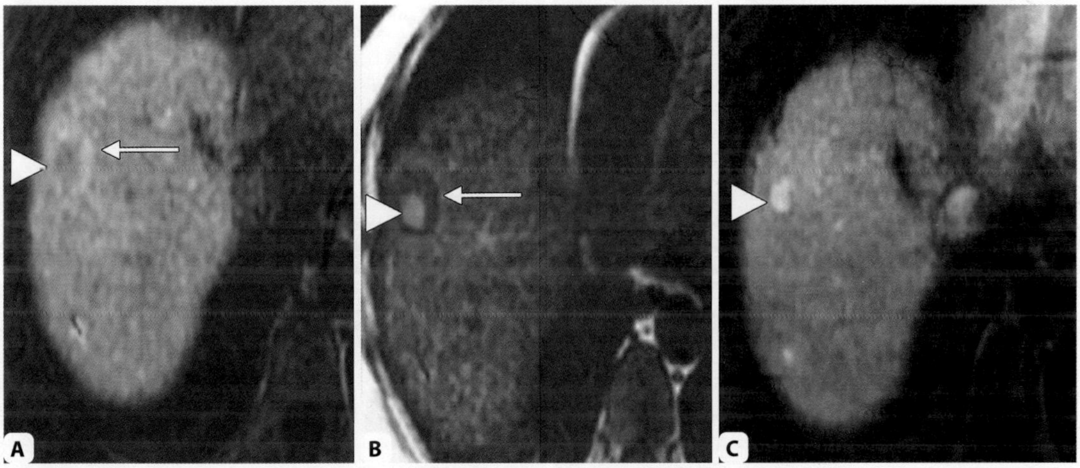

FIGS. 23A TO C: High-grade dysplastic nodule with early hepatocellular carcinoma (HCC) (nodule-in-nodule appearance): Axial (A) T1-weighted (T1W), (B) T2-weighted (T2W), and (C) postcontrast T1W images in arterial phase show a dysplastic nodule (arrowhead) which is predominantly hyperintense on T1W and hypointense on T2W sequences. Within the dysplastic nodule is a smaller nodule (arrow) which is hypointense on T1W and hyperintense on T2W and shows arterial phase hyperenhancement indicative of an early HCC.

arteries and reduction in portal venous inflow leads to the nonrim APHE and nonperipheral washout appearance characteristic of HCC, whereas expansile growth pattern causes the capsule formation **(Figs. 24A to F)**. Organic anion transporting polypeptide (OATP) expression progressively declines in HCC, accounting for their HBP hypointensity. However, 5% of HCCs express OATP and can therefore appear isointense on the HBP.

Morphologically, HCC can be of three patterns on imaging—nodular, multifocal, or diffuse. Nodular HCC appears as a well-circumscribed mass; there may be associated satellite nodules which are smaller nodules located within 2 cm of the dominant nodule **(Figs. 25A to D)**. Multifocal HCC refers to the presence of synchronous or metachronous nodules, either due to intrahepatic metastases from HCC or due to multicentric hepatocarcinogenesis **(Figs. 26A to D)**. Diffuse or infiltrative HCC involves multiple hepatic segments and can even involve an entire lobe or the entire liver. It appears ill-defined with minimal arterial phase enhancement and heterogeneous washout. Tumor thrombus is frequently associated with diffuse HCC and it has the worst prognosis among the three morphological patterns of HCC **(Figs. 27A to D)**.[31]

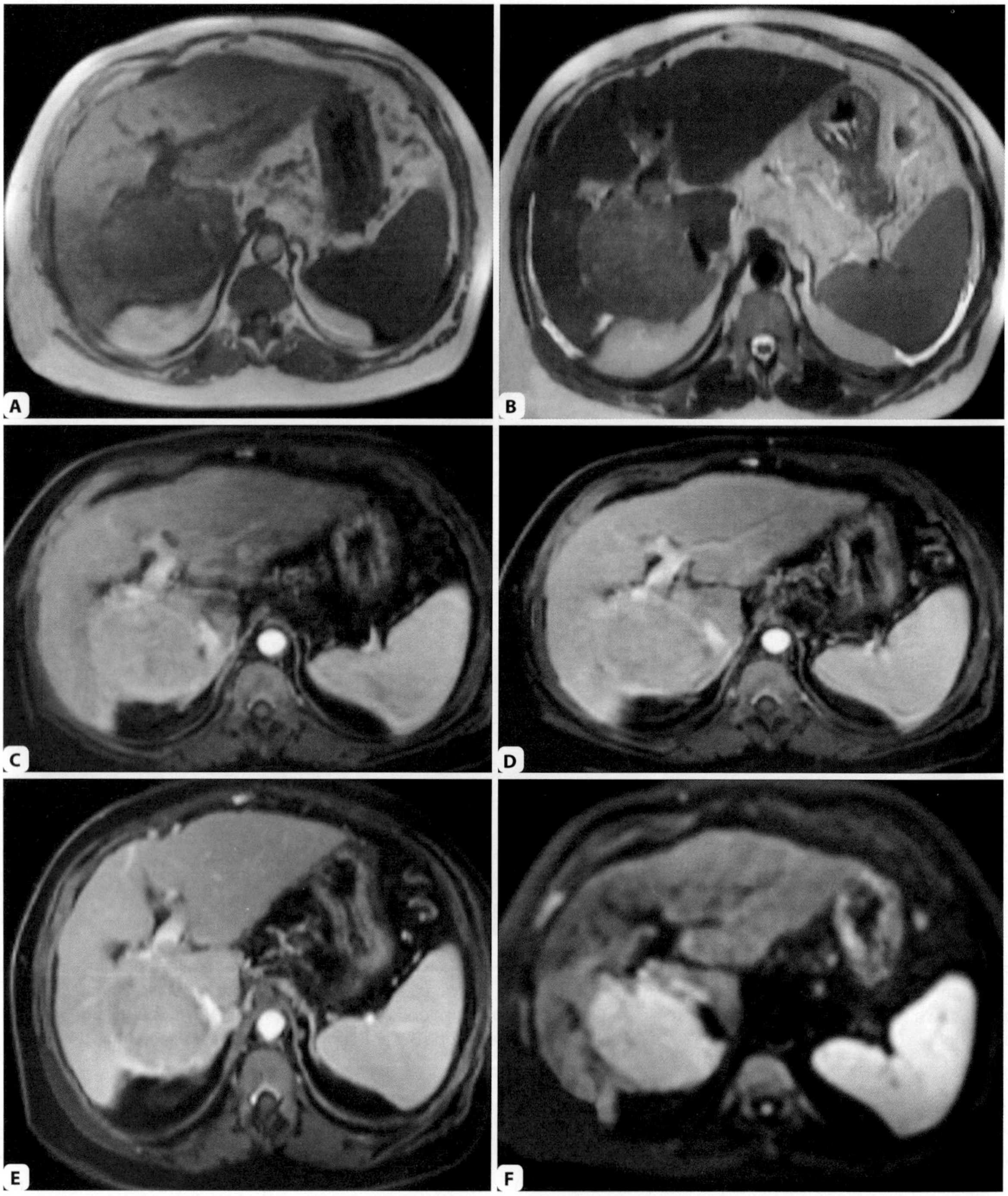

FIGS. 24A TO F: Hepatocellular carcinoma: The axial (A) T1-weighted (T1W) image shows a hypointense mass in segment VI and VII of liver which is (B) hyperintense on T2-weighted (T2W) image. (C) Arterial phase T1W image shows nonrim hyperenhancement in the lesion. (D) Venous and (E) delayed phase images showing contrast washout and enhancing capsule. (F) Diffusion-weighted images at b value 500 shows the lesion is hyperintense, suggesting restricted diffusion.

Though the majority of cases (65%) are not otherwise-specified HCC (NOS-HCC), the remainder are classified into eight histopathological subtypes as per the 5th edition of the World Health Organization (WHO) classification, molecular and imaging features of which are summarized in **Table 8**.[32] More broadly, HCCs can be classified as proliferative or nonproliferative types. Proliferative HCCs are more aggressive with a poorer prognosis compared to the nonproliferative ones. Macrotrabecular massive, scirrhous, clear cell, fibrolamellar, sarcomatoid HCCs are proliferative HCCs, whereas steatohepatitic and β-catenin-mutated HCCs are nonproliferative. Imaging

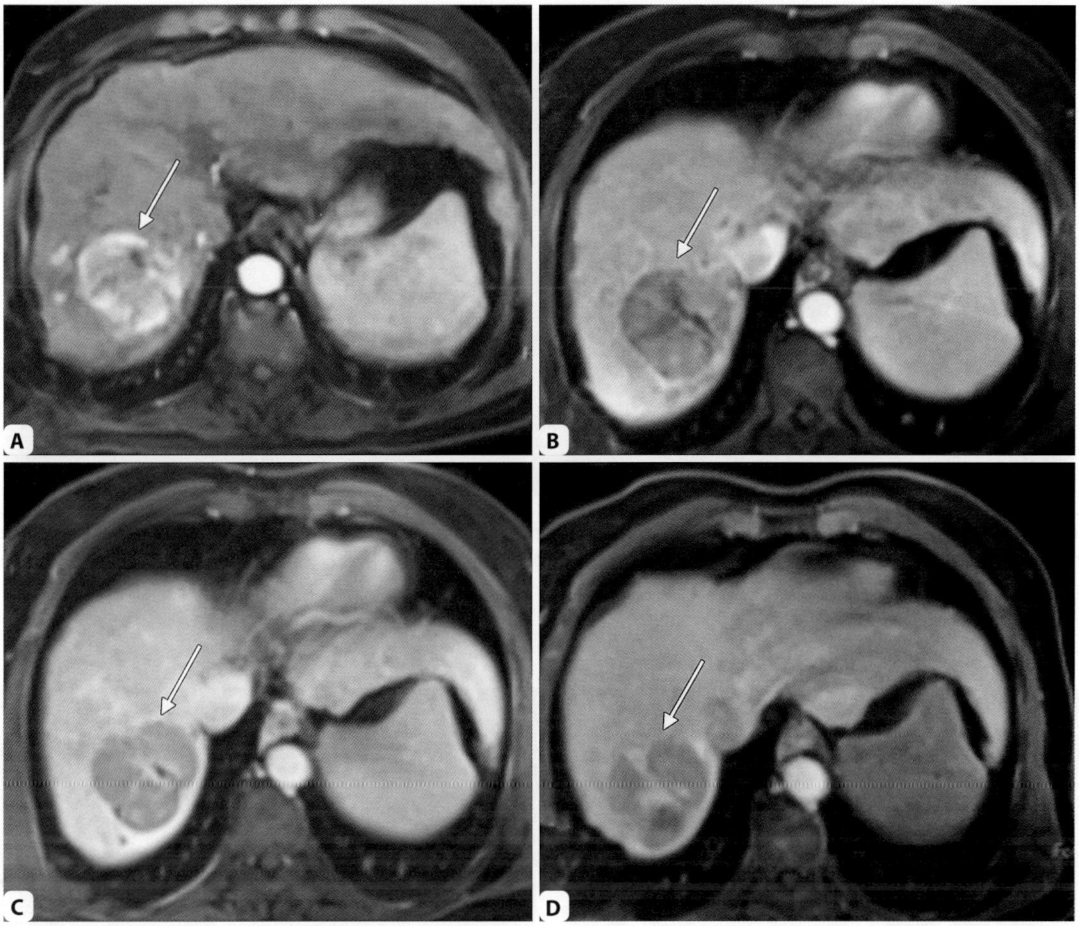

FIGS. 25A TO D: Solitary HCC: The axial (A) T1 PG image shows an observation (arrow) with nonrim APHE lesion in segment VII of liver, (B) showing washout on venous phase and (C) enhancing capsule formation on delayed phase images. (D) HBP shows nonretention of contrast within the lesion.

(APHE: arterial phase hyperenhancement; HBP: hepatobiliary phase; HCC: hepatocellular carcinoma)

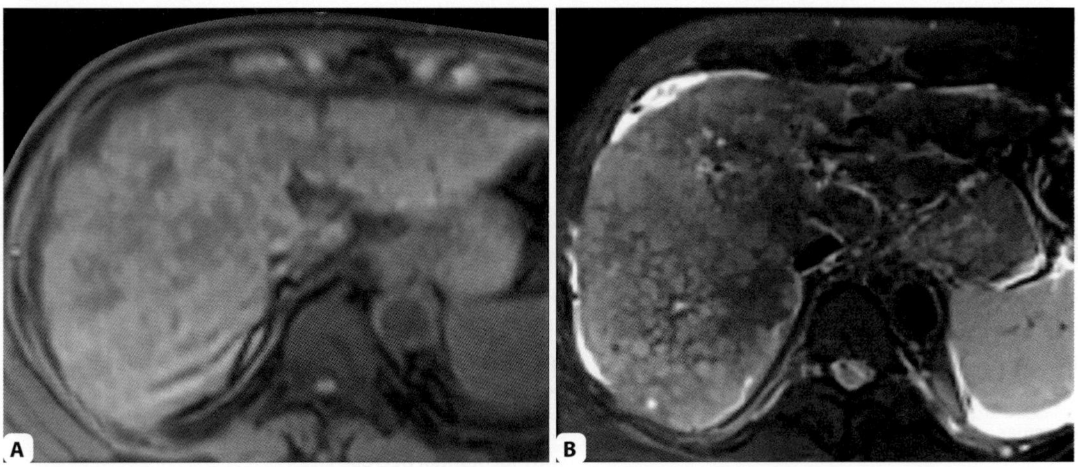

FIGS. 26A TO D: *Continued*

Continued

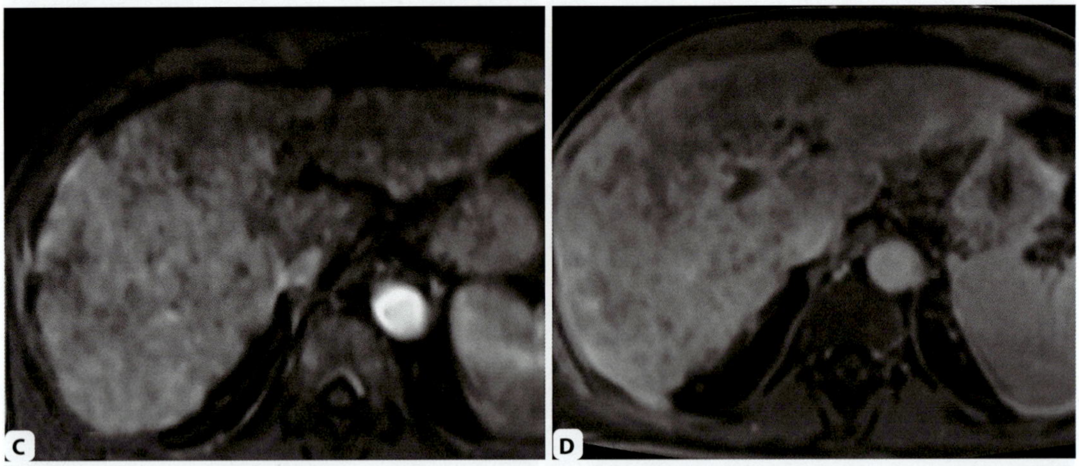

FIGS. 26A TO D: Multifocal HCC: (A) Multiple iso- to hypointense lesions throughout the liver on axial T1 fat-saturated images. (B) The lesions are hyperintense on axial T2W images, (C) show avid enhancement on axial T1 FS arterial phase and (D) washout on venous phase.

(HCC: hepatocellular carcinoma; T1W: T1 weighted; T2W: T2 weighted)

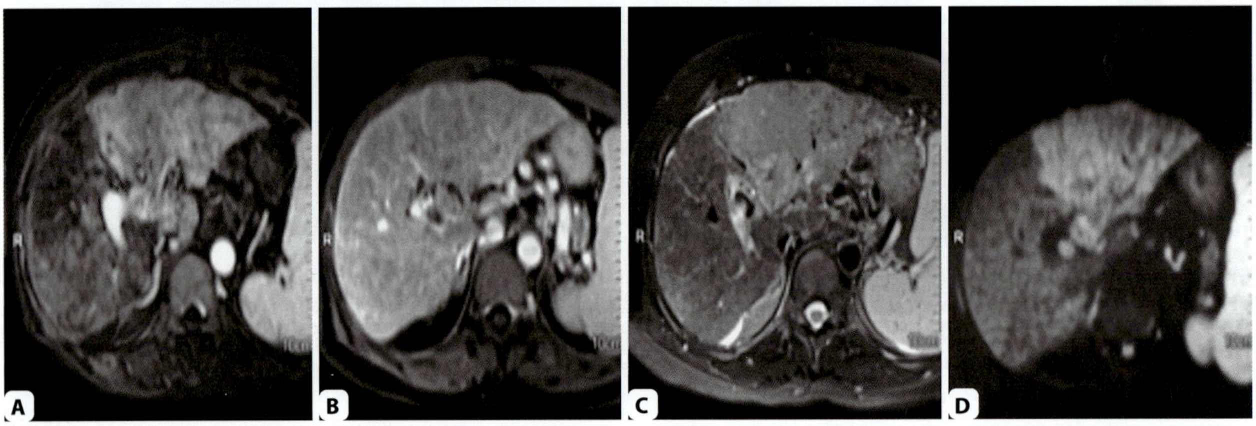

FIGS. 27A TO D: (A) Infiltrative HCC: Geographic area of nonrim APHE, (B) seen in left lobe of liver showing washout on portal venous phase. (C) The lesion appears hyperintense on T2WI and (D) shows restricted diffusion on DWI. Background liver shows cirrhotic changes.

(APHE: arterial phase hyperenhancement; DWI: diffusion-weighted images; T2WI: T2-weighted images)

TABLE 8: Histological variants of HCC.

Subtype	Molecular features	Imaging features	Prognosis (compared to conventional HCC)
Steatohepatitic	Activation of IL-6/JAK/STAT pathway	LR-5 features with intralesional fat and background steatosis	Similar
Clear cell	IDH1	LR-5 features with intralesional fat, pseudocapsule	Better
Macrotrabecular massive	TP53 mutations, FGF19 amplification	Large size (> 5 cm), LR-5 or LR-M features with substantial necrosis	Worse

Continued

Continued

Subtype	Molecular features	Imaging features	Prognosis (compared to conventional HCC)
Scirrhous	TSC1/TSC2 mutations, TGF-β pathway activation	LR-M features	Similar/worse
Fibrolamellar	Microdeletion on chromosome 19 with DNAJB1-PRKACA translocation	Central scar and calcification	Similar
Chromophobe	ALT	Limited data	Similar
Neutrophil rich	G-CSF production	Limited data	Worse
Lymphocyte rich	Not known	Limited data	Better

(ALT: alternative lengthening of telomeres; FGF19: fibroblast growth factor 19; G-CSF: granulocyte colony-stimulating factor; HCC: hepatocellular carcinoma; IDH1: isocitrate dehydrogenase 1; IL-6: interleukin-6; JAK: Janus tyrosine kinase; TGF-β: transforming growth factor-beta; TP53: tumor protein P53; TSC1/TSC2: tuberous sclerosis complex 1/2)

features which serve as surrogate markers of proliferative HCCs are larger size of tumor, multifocal lesions, satellite nodules, infiltrative growth pattern, tumor thrombus, biliary involvement, rim-APHE, peritumoral hypointensity on HBP, and lower apparent diffusion coefficient (ADC) values.[33]

Intrahepatic Cholangiocarcinoma

Intrahepatic cholangiocarcinoma is the second most common primary hepatic malignancy. It typically presents as an irregular lobulated hypoechoic mass with well-defined margins on USG. On CEUS, it shows heterogeneous enhancement in the arterial phase with marked washout on the venous phase within 60 seconds.[34] On multiphase CT and MR, it shows thick irregular rim enhancement in arterial phase with peripheral washout and progressive central enhancement on venous and 15-minute delayed scans **(Figs. 28A to F)**. On T2W images, the lesion appears hyperintense or hypointense depending on the amount of fibrous component. On DWI and in HBP, it shows targetoid appearance. The presence of adjacent biliary radicle dilatation, capsular retraction, and/or atrophy favors the diagnosis of CCA.

Based on their growth patterns, CCAs could be mass forming, periductal infiltrating, intraductal growing, or mixed patterns. iCCA are also classified on the basis of size of bile duct involvement as small duct or large duct type **(Table 9)**; cirrhosis-associated iCCA are mostly mass-forming small duct type.[33,35]

Combined Hepatocellular Cholangiocarcinoma

Combined hepatocellular cholangiocarcinoma is a unique primary liver malignancy displaying features of both hepatocytic and biliary differentiation within the same tumor. This entity has a more aggressive and worse prognosis compared to classical HCC and is similar to iCCA. iCCAs have a propensity to metastasize to extrahepatic sites relatively early in their development. The risk factors for the development of cHCC-CCA are similar to those of classical HCC.[36] An increase in both serum AFP and CA 19-9 levels at the same time may suggest the diagnosis of cHCC-CCA, but such elevations are only observed in a minority of patients.[37] The imaging features of cHCC-CCA are varied with overlapping features of both phenotypes. The imaging appearance varies depending on the proportion of each cell type. The US appearance is nonspecific; it may be heterogeneously hypoechoic or hypoechoic with a central hyperechoic focus.[38] On CT and MRI, tumors with a predominant HCC component may show APHE in an early phase and washout in venous/delayed as seen in classical HCC. In contrast, tumors with predominant biliary differentiation show rim enhancement in the arterial phase with progressive centripetal enhancement in venous/delayed phase images, biliary radicle dilatation, or capsular retraction similar to mass-forming iCCA **(Figs. 29A to F)**. MRI features such as the presence of intralesional fat/hemorrhage, washout, and progressive enhancement in the same tumor favor a diagnosis of cHCC-CCA.

Metastases

Metastases from extrahepatic tumors are far more uncommon in cirrhotic livers compared to noncirrhotic ones. Several reasons have been postulated for this such as hepatic fibrosis, reduced portal venous flow, and hepatofugal flow.[39] A retrospective study by Mahdi et al. found liver metastases constituted only 1.7% of masses in cirrhotic livers.[40] Majority of liver metastases have LR-M features with rim APHE. However, the diagnosis of hypervascular metastases from neuroendocrine tumors, renal cell carcinoma, thyroid carcinoma, etc. in cirrhotic livers is challenging as they may have nonrim APHE with washout appearance similar to HCC **(Figs. 30A to C)**.

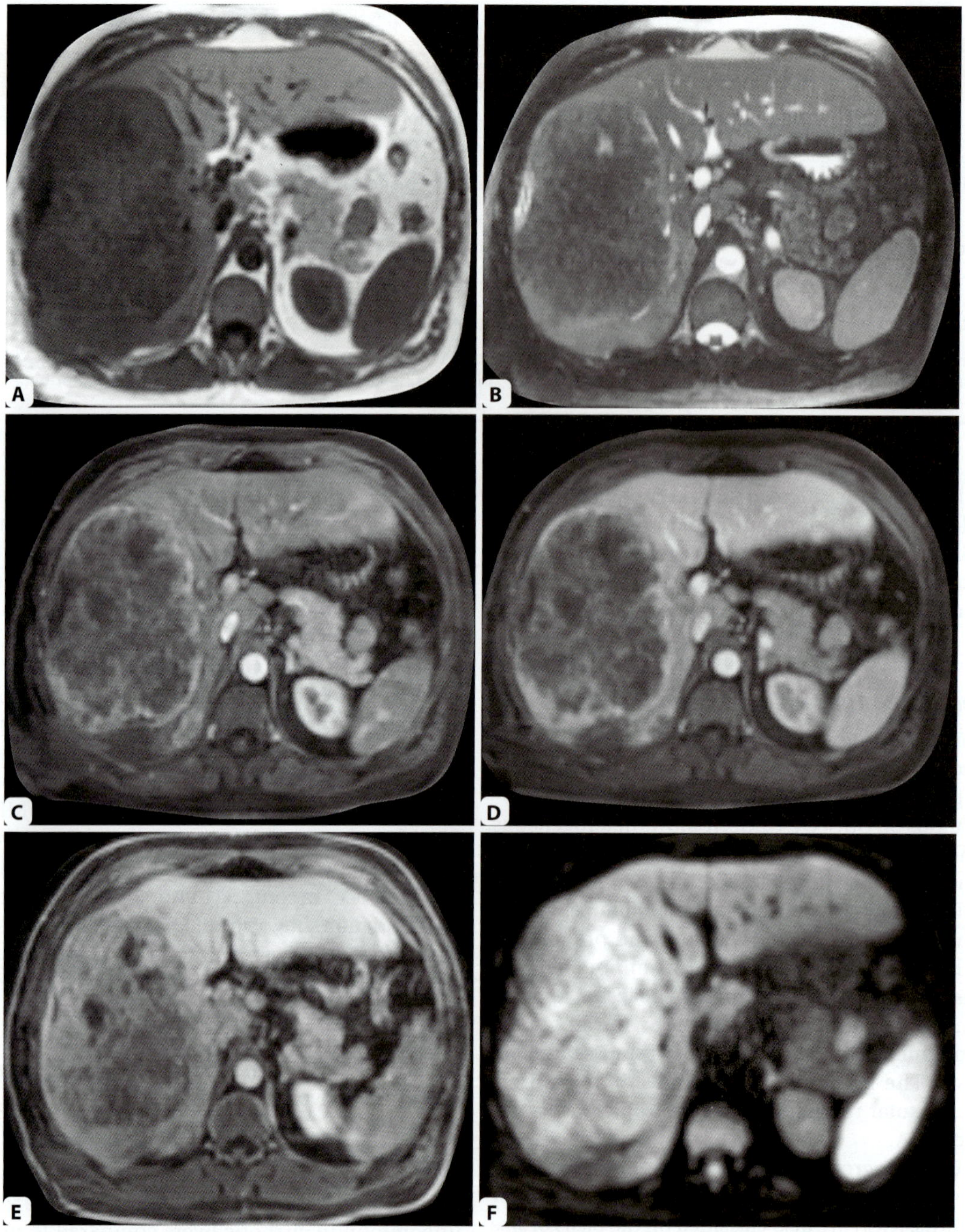

FIGS. 28A TO F: Intrahepatic cholangiocarcinoma: (A) Axial T1W images showing lobulated hypointense mass in the right lobe with capsular retraction. (B) Axial T2W images show heterogeneously hypointense nature of the lesion. (C) On contrast-enhanced images, the lesion shows thick peripheral enhancement in arterial phase, (D and E) with gradual filling in of the lesion in venous and delayed phases. (F) Axial DWI showing restriction of diffusion in the lesion.

(DWI: diffusion-weighted imaging; T1W: T1 weighted; T2W: T2 weighted)

TABLE 9: Small duct versus large duct type of intrahepatic cholangiocarcinoma.

	Small duct type	Large duct type
Level of biliary involvement	Small peripheral bile ducts and ductules	Large central intrahepatic bile ducts
Cells of origin	In the canals of hering from hepatic stem progenitor cells	In the peribiliary glands from biliary tree stem progenitor cells

Continued

Continued

	Small duct type	Large duct type
Molecular alterations	IDH1, IDH2, and FGFR2 mutations	KRAS and TP53 mutations
Risk factors	Nonbiliary cirrhosis and chronic viral hepatitis	Primary sclerosing cholangitis, choledochal cysts, liver fluke infestation
Growth pattern	Mass forming	Mass forming or periductal infiltrating
Histological features	Lymphovascular and perineural invasion less frequent, stromal dysplasia less (nonscirrhous)	Lymphovascular and perineural invasion more frequent, stromal dysplasia more (scirrhous)
Imaging features		
Biliary dilatation	Usually not present	Usually present
Area of arterial phase enhancement	Larger	Smaller
Area of delayed phase enhancement and HBP iso/hyperintensity	Smaller	Larger
Target appearance on HBP	Less common	More common
Area of diffusion restriction	Larger	Smaller
Prognosis	Good	Worse

(FGFR2: fibroblast growth factor receptor 2; HBP: hepatobiliary phase; IDH1: isocitrate dehydrogenase 1; TP53: tumor protein P53)

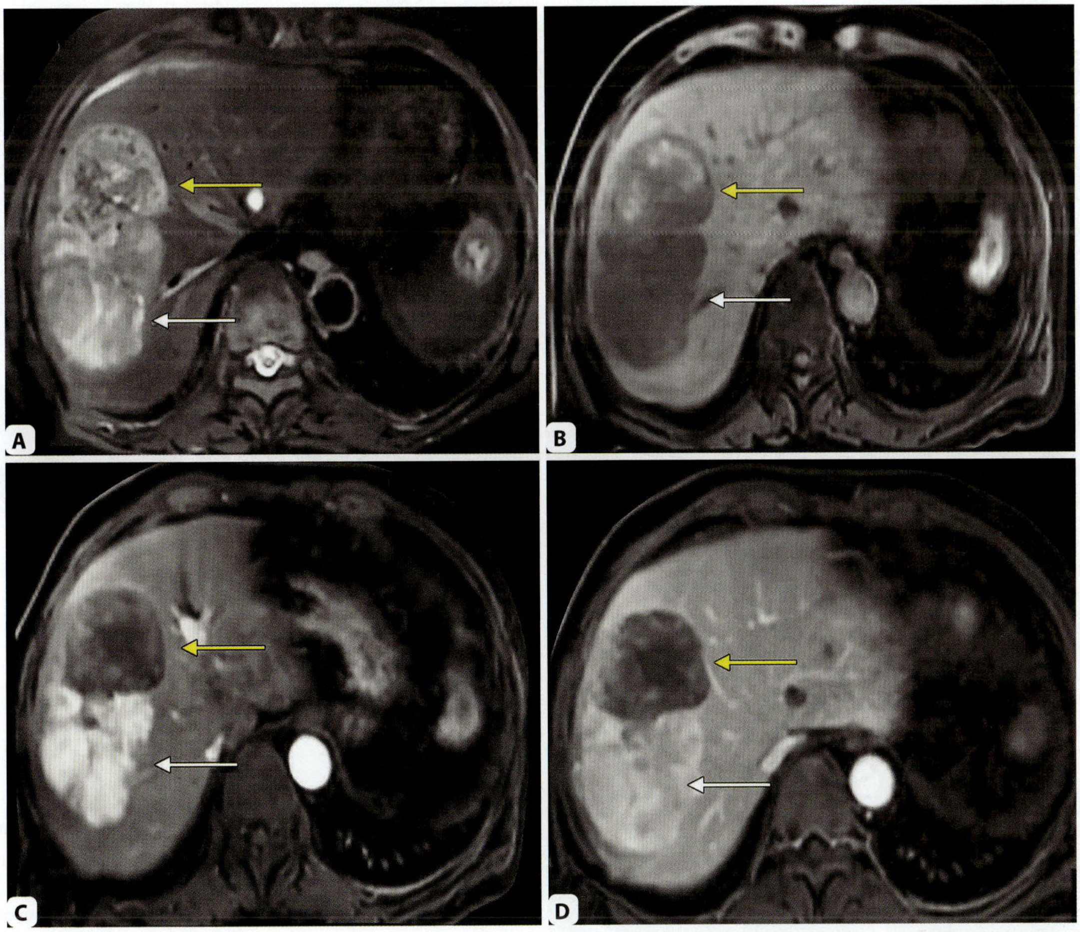

FIGS. 29A TO F: *Continued*

Continued

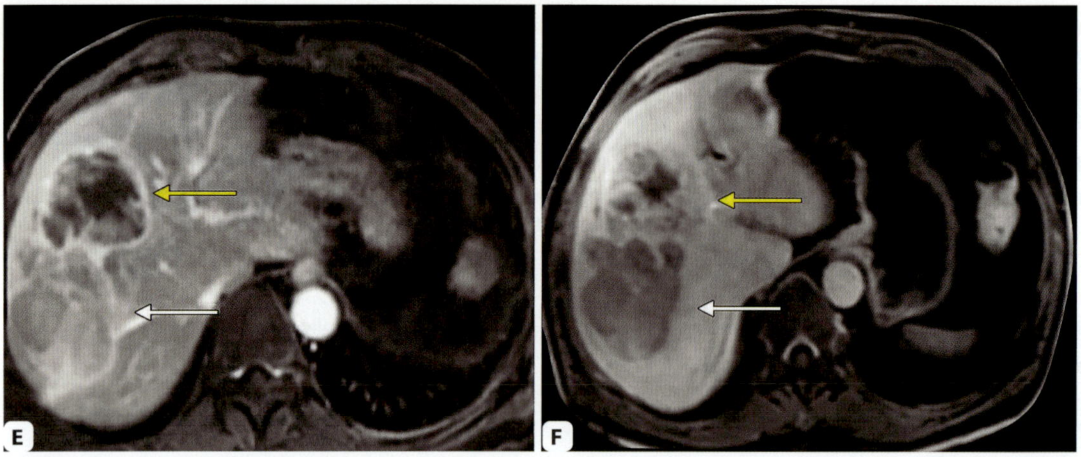

FIGS. 29A TO F: Biphenotypic tumor (combined hepatocellular-cholangiocarcinoma): Hepatocellular carcinoma (HCC) (white arrow) and iCCA (yellow arrow) in the same lesion. (A) The posterior part of tumor is T2 hyperintense and (B) T1 isointense and (C) shows nonrim arterial phase hyperenhancement (APHE) with washout and capsule formation on (D) venous and (E) delayed phases, and (F) hypointensity on hepatobiliary phase. However, the anterior component of tumor shows heterogeneous signal on (A) T2-weighted and (B) T1-weighted images, (C) with rim APHE, progression of centripetal enhancement on (D) venous and (E) delayed phases, and (F) a targetoid appearance on hepatobiliary phase.

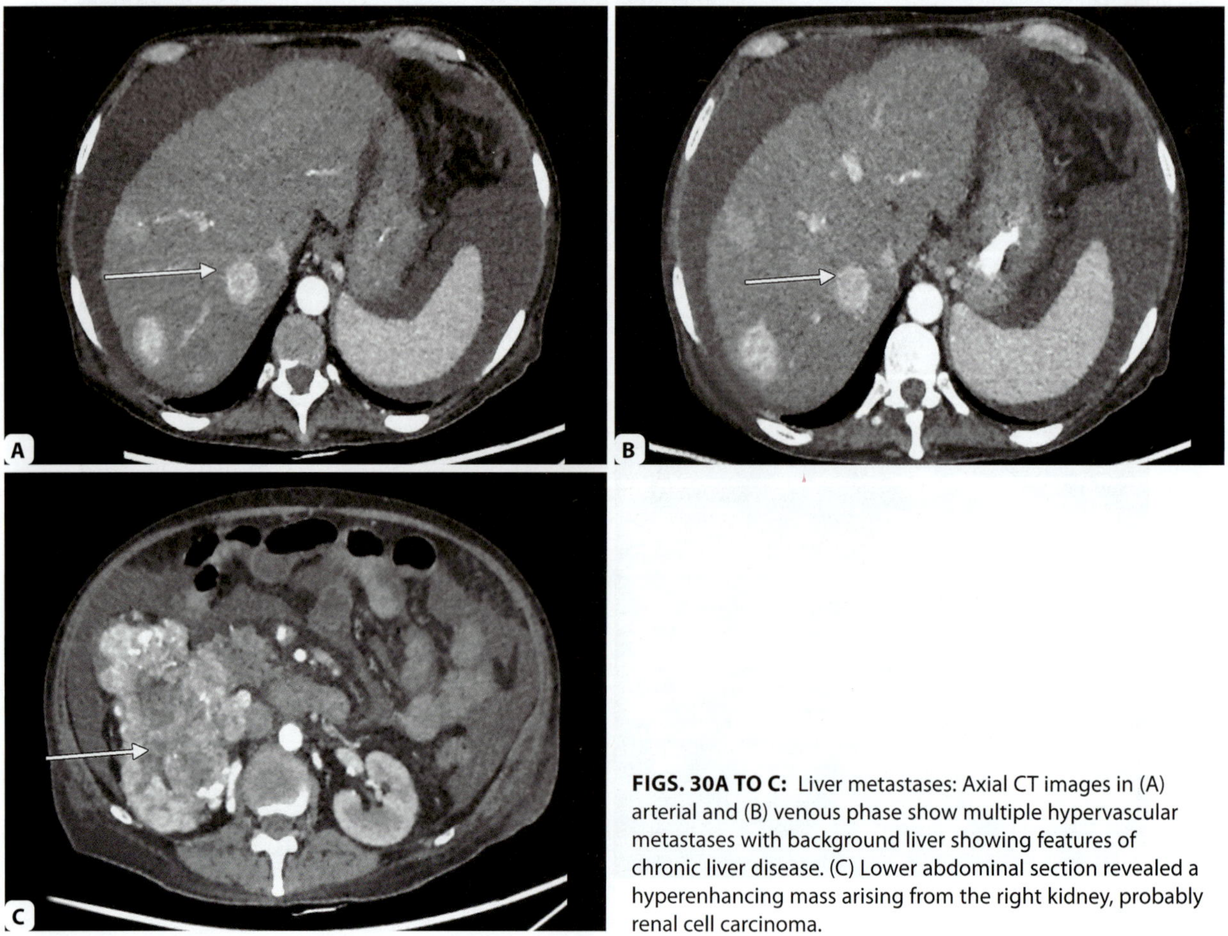

FIGS. 30A TO C: Liver metastases: Axial CT images in (A) arterial and (B) venous phase show multiple hypervascular metastases with background liver showing features of chronic liver disease. (C) Lower abdominal section revealed a hyperenhancing mass arising from the right kidney, probably renal cell carcinoma.

CONCLUSION

While HCC continues to be the most common liver cancer in cirrhotic patients, patients with cirrhosis have a higher risk of developing other malignancies such as iCCA and cHCC-CCA. Benign hepatocellular and nonhepatocellular nodules can also occur in cirrhosis. Due to substantial differences in prognosis and treatment approaches, it is imperative to distinguish between these entities. Therefore, careful assessment and a multimodality diagnostic approach are essential for correctly differentiating between various liver lesions in patients with cirrhosis. By standardizing reporting, LI-RADS is very useful in facilitating collaboration among physicians, radiologists, and pathologists to ensure comprehensive evaluation and optimize patient outcomes.

REFERENCES

1. Santillan C, Chernyak V, Sirlin C. LI-RADS categories: concepts, definitions, and criteria. Abdom Radiol. 2018;43(1):101-10.
2. Liu X, Tan SBM, Awiwi MO, Jang HJ, Chernyak V, Fowler KJ, et al. Imaging Findings in Cirrhotic Liver: Pearls and Pitfalls for Diagnosis of Focal Benign and Malignant Lesions. Radiographics. 2023;43(9):e230043.
3. Kang HJ, Lee JM, Yoon JH, Yoo J, Choi Y, Joo I, et al. SonazoidTM versus SonoVue® for Diagnosing Hepatocellular Carcinoma Using Contrast-Enhanced Ultrasound in At-Risk Individuals: A Prospective, Single-Center, Intraindividual, Noninferiority Study. Korean J Radiol. 2022;23(11):1067.
4. An JY, Peña MA, Cunha GM, Booker MT, Taouli B, Yokoo T, et al. Abbreviated MRI for Hepatocellular Carcinoma Screening and Surveillance. Radiographics. 2020;40(7):1916-31.
5. American College of Radiology. (2024). LI-RADS® Ultrasound Surveillance v2024 Core. [online] Available from https://www.acr.org/-/media/ACR/Files/RADS/LI-RADS/LI-RADS-US-Surveillance-v2024-Core.pdf [Last accessed July, 2024].
6. Morgan TA, Maturen KE, Dahiya N, Sun MRM, Kamaya A; American College of Radiology Ultrasound Liver Imaging and Reporting Data System (US LI-RADS) Working Group. US LI-RADS: ultrasound liver imaging reporting and data system for screening and surveillance of hepatocellular carcinoma. Abdom Radiol. 2018;43(1):41-55.
7. Elsayes KM, Kielar AZ, Chernyak V, Morshid A, Furlan A, Masch WR, et al. LI-RADS: a conceptual and historical review from its beginning to its recent integration into AASLD clinical practice guidance. JHC. 2019;6:49-69.
8. Wilson SR, Lyshchik A, Piscaglia F, Cosgrove D, Jang HJ, Sirlin C, et al. CEUS LI-RADS: algorithm, implementation, and key differences from CT/MRI. Abdom Radiol. 2018;43(1):127-42.
9. American College of Radiology. (2017). CEUS-LI-RADS® v2017 CORE (For CEUS with Pure Blood Pool Agents). [online] Available from https://www.acr.org/-/media/ACR/Files/RADS/LI-RADS/CEUS-LI-RADS-2017-Core.pdf [Last accessed July, 2024].
10. Chammas MC, Bordini AL. Contrast-enhanced ultrasonography for the evaluation of malignant focal liver lesions. Ultrasonography. 2022;41(1):4-24.
11. Yang HK, Burns PN, Jang HJ, Kono Y, Khalili K, Wilson SR, et al. Contrast-enhanced ultrasound approach to the diagnosis of focal liver lesions: the importance of washout. Ultrasonography. 2019;38(4):289-301.
12. Bae JS, Lee JM, Jeon SK, Yoo J, Park SJ, Yoon JH, et al. LI-RADS Tumor in Vein at CT and Hepatobiliary MRI. Radiology. 2022;302(1):107-15.
13. American College of Radiology. (2018). CT/MRI LI-RADS® v2018 CORE. [online] Available from https://www.acr.org/-/media/ACR/Files/RADS/LI-RADS/LI-RADS-2018-Core.pdf [Last accessed July, 2024].
14. Elmohr M, Elsayes KM, Chernyak V. LI-RADS: Review and updates. Clin Liver Dis (Hoboken). 2021;17(3):108-12.
15. Kim YY, Choi JY, Sirlin CB, An C, Kim MJ. Pitfalls and problems to be solved in the diagnostic CT/MRI Liver Imaging Reporting and Data System (LI-RADS). Eur Radiol. 2019;29(3):1124-32.
16. Lee JY, Minami Y, Choi BI, Lee WJ, Chou YH, Jeong WK, et al. The AFSUMB Consensus Statements and Recommendations for the Clinical Practice of Contrast-Enhanced Ultrasound using Sonazoid. Ultrasonography. 2020;39(3):191-220.
17. Brancatelli G, Baron RL, Peterson MS, Marsh W. Helical CT Screening for Hepatocellular Carcinoma in Patients with Cirrhosis: Frequency and Causes of False-Positive Interpretation. Am J Roentgenol. 2003;180(4):1007-14.
18. Choi SH, Lee JM, Yu NC, Suh KS, Jang JJ, Kim SH, et al. Hepatocellular Carcinoma in Liver Transplantation Candidates: Detection with Gadobenate Dimeglumine-Enhanced MRI. Am J Roentgenol. 2008;191(2):529-36.
19. Jang HJ, Kim TK, Lim HK, Park SJ, Sim JS, Kim HY, et al. Hepatic Hemangioma: Atypical Appearances on CT, MR Imaging, and Sonography. Am J Roentgenol. 2003;180(1):135-41.
20. Bajenaru N, Balaban V, Săvulescu F, Campeanu I, Patrascu T. Hepatic hemangioma - review. J Med Life. 2015;8:4-11.
21. KS Dorji, Cheewadhanaraks S. Hepatic hemangioma in cirrhosis: Two case reports. ASEAN J Radiol. 2020;21(1):21-33.
22. Brancatelli G, Federle MP, Blachar A, Grazioli L. Hemangioma in the Cirrhotic Liver: Diagnosis and Natural History. Radiology. 2001;219(1):69-74.
23. Wu XF, Bai XM, Yang W, Sun Y, Wang H, Wu W, et al. Differentiation of atypical hepatic hemangioma from liver metastases: Diagnostic performance of a novel type of color contrast enhanced ultrasound. WJG. 2020;26(9):960-72.
24. Jha RC, Mitchell DG, Weinreb JC, Santillan CS, Yeh BM, Francois R, et al. LI-RADS Categorization of Benign and Likely Benign Findings in Patients at Risk of Hepatocellular Carcinoma: A Pictorial Atlas. Am J Roentgenol. 2014;203(1):W48-69.
25. Park YS, Lee CH, Kim BH, Lee J, Choi JW, Kim KA, et al. Using Gd-EOB-DTPA-enhanced 3-T MRI for the differentiation of infiltrative hepatocellular carcinoma and focal confluent fibrosis in liver cirrhosis. Magn Reson Imaging. 2013;31(7):1137-42.
26. Ramanathan S, Raghu V, Virmani V, Sheikh A, Al Heidous M, Tirumani S. Unveiling the unreal: Comprehensive imaging review of hepatic pseudolesions. Clin Imaging. 2021;80:439-53.
27. Vilgrain V, Lagadec M, Ronot M. Pitfalls in Liver Imaging. Radiology. 2016;278(1):34-51.
28. LeGout JD, Bolan CW, Bowman AW, Caserta MP, Chen FK, Cox KL, et al. Focal Nodular Hyperplasia and Focal Nodular Hyperplasia-like Lesions. Radiographics. 2022;42(4):1043-61.

29. Wu W, Chen M, Yan K, Dai Y, Yin S, Yang W, et al. Evaluation of contrast-enhanced ultrasound for diagnosis of dysplastic nodules with a focus of hepatocellular carcinoma in liver cirrhosis patients. Chin J Cancer Res. 2015;27(1):83-9.
30. Quaia E, Calliada F, Bertolotto M, Rossi S, Garioni L, Rosa L, et al. Characterization of Focal Liver Lesions with Contrast-specific US Modes and a Sulfur Hexafluoride-filled Microbubble Contrast Agent: Diagnostic Performance and Confidence. Radiology. 2004;232(2):420-30.
31. Reynolds AR, Furlan A, Fetzer DT, Sasatomi E, Borhani AA, Heller MT, et al. Infiltrative Hepatocellular Carcinoma: What Radiologists Need to Know. Radiographics. 2015;35(2): 371-86.
32. Fowler KJ, Burgoyne A, Fraum TJ, Hosseini M, Ichikawa S, Kim S, et al. Pathologic, Molecular, and Prognostic Radiologic Features of Hepatocellular Carcinoma. Radiographics. 2021;41(6):1611-31.
33. Katabathina VS, Khanna L, Surabhi VR, Minervini M, Shanbhogue K, Dasyam AK, et al. Morphomolecular Classification Update on Hepatocellular Adenoma, Hepatocellular Carcinoma, and Intrahepatic Cholangiocarcinoma. Radiographics. 2022;42(5):1338-57.
34. Bartolotta TV, Randazzo A, Bruno E, Taibbi A. Focal liver lesions in cirrhosis: Role of contrast-enhanced ultrasonography. WJR. 2022;14(4):70-81.
35. Joo I, Lee JM, Yoon JH. Imaging Diagnosis of Intrahepatic and Perihilar Cholangiocarcinoma: Recent Advances and Challenges. Radiology. 2018;288(1):7-13.
36. Li R, Yang D, Tang CL, Cai P, Ma K sheng, Ding SY, et al. Combined hepatocellular carcinoma and cholangiocarcinoma (biphenotypic) tumors: clinical characteristics, imaging features of contrast-enhanced ultrasound and computed tomography. BMC Cancer. 2016;16(1):158.
37. Beaufrère A, Calderaro J, Paradis V. Combined hepatocellular-cholangiocarcinoma: An update. J Hepatol. 2021;74(5):1212-24.
38. Stavraka C, Rush H, Ross P. Combined hepatocellular cholangiocarcinoma (cHCC-CC): an update of genetics, molecular biology, and therapeutic interventions. JHC. 2018;6:11-21.
39. Möller K, Safai Zadeh E, Görg C, Dong Y, Cui X, Lim A, et al. Focal liver lesions other than hepatocellular carcinoma in cirrhosis: Diagnostic challenges. J Transl Int Med. 2023;10(4):308-27.
40. Mahdi Z, Ettel MG, Gonzalez RS, Hart J, Alpert L, Fang J, et al. Metastases can occur in cirrhotic livers with patent portal veins. Diagn Pathol. 2021;16(1):18.

CHAPTER 12

Shivanand Gamanagatti,
Rajendra Behera, Anuradha Sharma

Interventional Radiology Treatment and Response Assessment of Liver Tumors

INTRODUCTION

Liver is among the most common sites for primary and secondary tumors. Hepatocellular carcinoma (HCC) represents >90% of the primary liver tumors and is the second important cause of cancer related death. Its incidence and mortality is on the rise world over.[1] Metastatic liver tumors are even more common particularly in cases of colorectal carcinoma where about 20% of the cases have metastases at the outset and about half of them are likely to develop during its course.[2] Surgery remains the first line of therapy for these patients and the options of resection or liver transplant provide best outcomes of 5-year survival ranging from 60 to 80%.[3] However, the vast majority of these patients are unsuitable for surgery due to the advanced disease at diagnosis, poor liver reserve, and performance status. Furthermore, limited infrastructure, organ shortage, and long-waiting period deny timely liver transplantation in many.

Over the last two decades, a large number of radiological interventions consisting of either ablative techniques or angiographic procedures have evolved, which are effective in prolonging survival **(Box 1 and Table 1)**. Being widely available, safe and efficacious, these minimally invasive techniques have become widely popular and have emerged as the alternative therapeutic options to surgery for both primary and secondary liver malignancies. This chapter focuses on the armamentarium of the currently available image-guided interventional treatments used in the management of liver tumors.

BOX 1 Radiological interventions for liver tumors.

Percutaneous ablative techniques
- Chemical ablation:
  - Ethanol
  - Acetic acid
- Thermal ablation:
  - Radiofrequency ablation
  - Microwave ablation
  - Laser ablation
  - Cryoablation
  - High-intensity focused ultrasound ablation
- Nonthermal ablation:
  - Irreversible electroporation (IRE) or nano knife

Intra-arterial procedures
- Transarterial embolization
- Transarterial chemoembolization (TACE)
- Transarterial chemotherapy (TAC)
- Transarterial rhenium/Yttrium therapy (TART)

Portal vein embolization

TABLE 1: Survival rate of various interventional techniques, surgical resection and liver transplantation for treatment of HCC.[4]

		Survival (%)					
Procedure	**No. of patients**	**1st year**	**2nd year**	**3rd year**	**5th year**	**7th year**	**10th year**
Surgical resection	25,066	88.2	78.4	69.5	54.2	42.0	29.0
Transplant	183	74.2	69.3	63.4	56.7	NA	NA
Ablation	27,150	92.8	81.4	68.6	45.6	29.8	15.7
TACE	19,569	77.8	59.0	44.2	24.2	14.0	6.5

(HCC: hepatocellular carcinoma; TACE: transarterial chemoembolization)

TREATMENT OF MALIGNANT TUMORS

Hepatocellular Carcinoma

The Barcelona Clinic Liver Cancer (BCLC) staging, which was updated in 2022, is the most validated and widely used staging system for HCC **(Flowchart 1)**.[5] According to this system, HCC is staged based on the tumor burden (single nodule, multinodular, portal venous invasion, and extrahepatic spread), functional status of liver (Child–Pugh score, albumin–bilirubin score, and model for end-stage liver disease score) and the performance status (as per Eastern Cooperative Oncology Group) of the individual. It also recommends the therapeutic options for the different stages of HCC. Amongst the interventional therapies, ablation is indicated for BCLC-0 (very early stage) and BCLC-A (early stage); whereas intra-arterial therapies are indicated for BCLC-B (intermediate stage). Both ablative and intra-arterial therapies are termed *locoregional therapies* as they exclusively target the tumor tissue while sparing the adjoining normal hepatic parenchyma. The BCLC 2022 update also introduces the concept of *treatment stage migration*, which allows for a shift to a treatment option recommended for a more advanced stage in certain patients based on their clinical profile.

Pretreatment Assessment for Locoregional Therapy

The pretreatment evaluation includes laboratory studies namely complete blood count, liver function tests, coagulation profile, and alpha-fetoprotein (AFP) levels. Cross-sectional imaging, either multiphasic computed tomography (CT) or magnetic resonance imaging (MRI) is also essential for staging of the disease. Treatment planning is done by careful appraisal of the imaging for the size, number and location of the tumors, presence of macrovascular (portal vein) invasion, and presence of extrahepatic disease. Holistic multidisciplinary treatment is required, which involves treating the tumor,

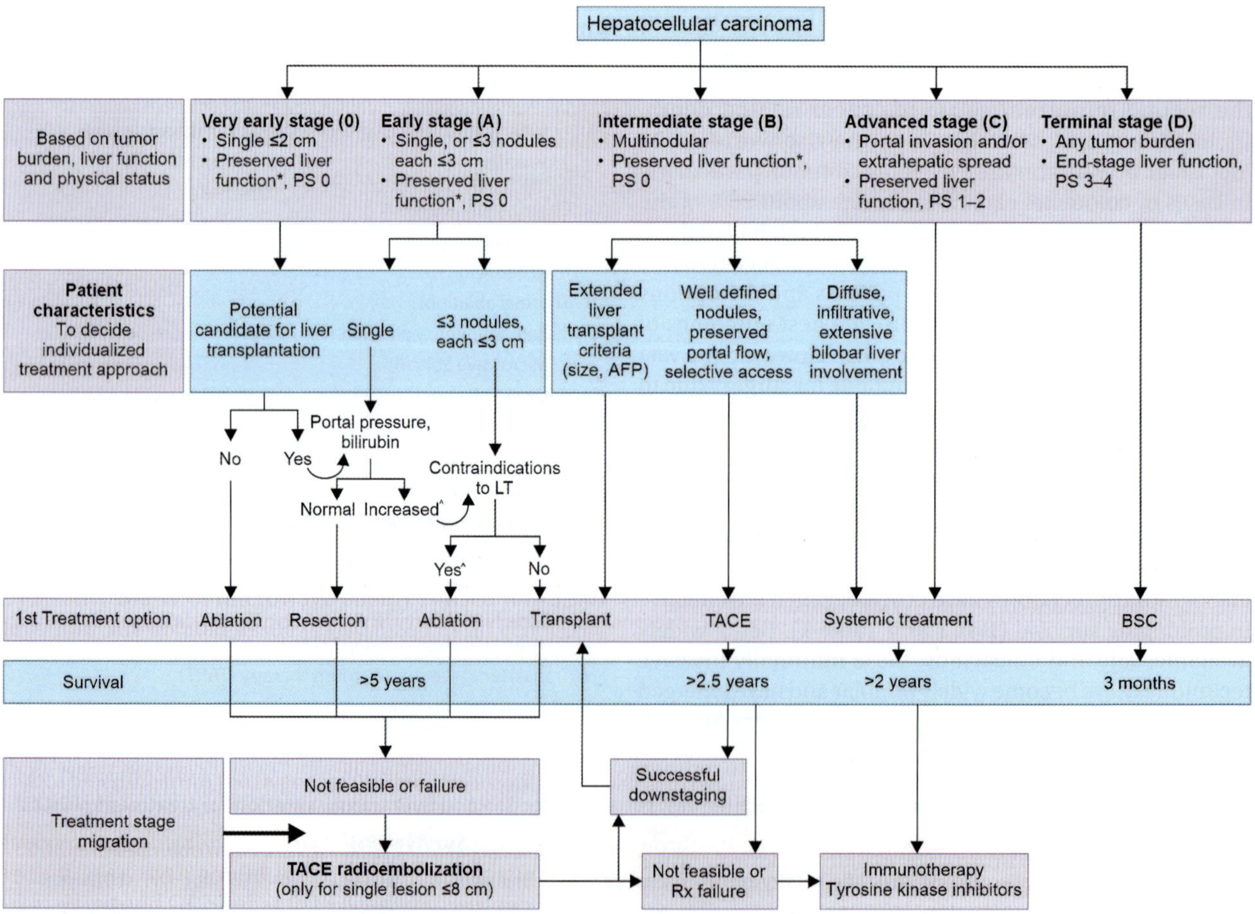

* Except for those with tumor burden acceptable for transplant.

^ Resection may be considered for single peripheral HCC with adequate remnant liver volume.

FLOWCHART 1: BCLC staging 2022.[5]

(AFP: alpha-fetoprotein; BCLC: Barcelona Clinic Liver Cancer; BSC: best supportive care; PS: performance status; LT: liver transplantation; TACE: transarterial chemo-embolization)

Source: Adopted from BCLC staging and treatment strategy in 2022.

the underlying tumor etiology (mostly viral hepatitis) and the associated deranged liver function.

Percutaneous Ablative Therapy

Percutaneous ablative therapy involves the direct application of chemical or energy-based therapy to treat tumors. It is the recommended treatment for unresectable early HCC. It aims at destroying the viable tumor tissue while creating a safety margin of 0.5–1 cm around it. Percutaneous ablation is safe, easy to perform, and well tolerated, with a very low major and minor complication rate. It is most beneficial in treating early small tumors, as best outcome of complete response (CR) following ablation is related to the size of the tumor (90–100% in tumors of 2 cm, 50% in the tumors of 5 cm).[6]

Selection criteria for ablation: Ideal HCC patients for ablation are those who are Child–Pugh class A/B cirrhosis, have a performance status of 0–1, tumor size smaller than 5 cm (ideal <3 cm), well-defined intrahepatic tumor with hepatic parenchyma all around, solitary or multifocal (not >3 in number) with absence of vascular invasion and extrahepatic disease.

Absolute contraindications to ablation are presence of vascular invasion, tumor located <1 cm from the main biliary duct, intrahepatic biliary dilatation, exophytic tumor, or uncorrectable coagulopathy. Relative contraindications are the presence of bilioenteric anastomosis, superficial lesions, lesions close to gallbladder or any part of gastrointestinal tract, ascites, low platelet count (<50,000/mm^3), pacemaker/defibrillator, and hepatic failure.[7]

Chemical Ablation

Chemical ablation involves the use of percutaneous ethanol injection (PEI) or percutaneous acetic acid injection (PAI) into the tumor. PEI is the earliest technique which has been extensively studied and its role in treating small HCCs has been well-established.[8] It is inexpensive and can be readily performed with imaging guidance without the use of any special equipment.

- *Mechanism of ethanol/acetic acid ablation:* Neoplastic and non-neoplastic tissue is made up of cellular, interstitial, and vascular compartments. Chemical agents with relatively low molecular weight, such as ethanol and acetic acid, when injected into the tumor, penetrate the cellular compartment remote from the point of injection, through the tumor interstitium. HCCs have extracellular volumes more than twice that of noncancerous liver which results in a high interstitial fluid pressure and interstitial diffusion coefficient that favors easy diffusion of these low-molecular-weight agents.[9] As ethanol distributes through the tumor interstitium, its cytotoxic mechanisms are exerted through a combination of cytoplasmic dehydration, denaturation of cellular proteins, and small vessel thrombosis. These effects result in coagulative necrosis. The cytotoxic mechanisms of acetic acid are similar to those of ethanol, which include protein denaturation, dissolution of cellular basement membranes, and destruction of interstitial collagen.
- *Technique of chemical ablation:* Percutaneous chemical ablation is usually performed with real-time ultrasound guidance and local anesthesia. A 20–22 gauge end-hole or conical tip multiside-hole needle is used. Infusion is performed slowly in 0.1–0.2 mL aliquots with continuous ultrasound monitoring **(Figs. 1A to F)**. When the tumor becomes echogenic, the needle is withdrawn while injecting a long-acting local anesthetic agent such as Bupivacaine for local pain relief. If performed under CT-guidance, iodinated contrast is mixed with ethanol/acetic acid for visualization of the ablation zone **(Figs. 2A to D)**.
- *Volume of alcohol and acetic acid injection:* Strength of the chemical agents used are 95% absolute alcohol (ethanol) or 50% acetic acid. Volume estimation is based on the volume of the tumor and an "ablation margin" of 1 cm beyond the periphery of the lesion. For PEI, the volume is calculated using the formula: $V = 4/3\pi (r + 0.5)^3$, where V is the target volume of ethanol, r the radius of the lesion (in centimeters), and 0.5 for the correction for the additional "surgical margin". For PAI, the maximum total volume of acetic acid required to ablate the tumor is three times the maximum diameter of the tumor. This total dose is injected over multiple sessions (1–2 mL of acetic acid per tumor per session per week) performed once or twice weekly under ultrasound guidance.
- *Advantage of PAI over PEI:* Both PAI and PEI are effective in treating small HCC < 3 cm. PAI has high diffusion capacity because of which smaller volume of acetic acid and fewer treatment sessions are required to achieve the same degree of cell kill as that with ethanol.[10] PAI has an advantage of infiltrating the tumor septae and capsule of tumors, whereas ethanol is unable to do so. Due to this limitation, PEI is unable to ablate the small satellite nodules and create a safety margin. Local tumor recurrence rate is therefore higher in PEI than PAI [37% and 8%, respectively ($p < 0.001$)].[11]
- *Complications:* Chemical ablation is a safe procedure with low complication rate; major complications are rare. Minor complications in the form of transient pain, fever, and transient renal failure (with acetic acid) may be encountered. Rarely, transient hemoglobinuria may occur immediately following PAI and this clears on its own. Major complications are rare and include hemorrhage, liver necrosis, and abscess formation. Although PEI is performed with a small-caliber needle, substantial hemorrhage has been reported. Therefore, correction of underlying coagulopathy should be performed (target international normalized ratio ≤ 1.4, platelet count ≤ 50,000/mm^3).[1,2]

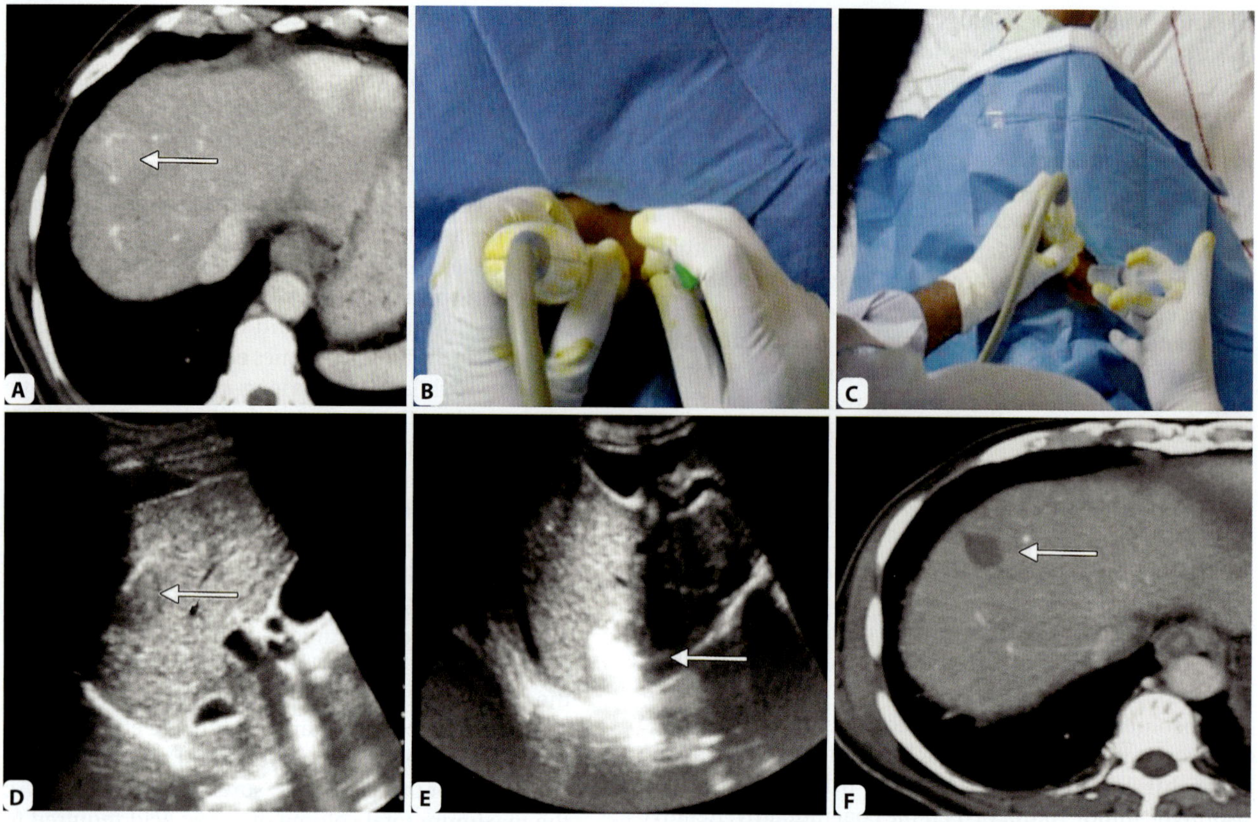

FIGS. 1A TO F: USG-guided percutaneous acetic acid injection (PAI). Contrast-enhanced computed tomography (CECT) abdomen reveals enhancing lesion (arrow) in segment VIII of liver (A). Photographs showing ultrasound-guided placement of 21G lumbar puncture needle in the liver lesion (B) followed by intralesional injection of acetic acid (C). Grayscale ultrasound shows hypoechoic liver lesion (arrow) with needle placement in its center (D). Postablation ultrasound shows good coverage of the lesion which has become completely hyperechoic (E). Follow-up CECT (F) after 1 month shows no residual enhancement within the lesion (LR-TR nonviable).

Thermal Ablation

There are five types of thermal ablative techniques (See **Box 1**):

1. Radiofrequency ablation (RFA)
2. Microwave ablation (MWA)
3. Cryoablation
4. High-intensity focused ultrasound (HIFU)
5. Laser ablation

Radiofrequency Ablation

The first experiments with thermal ablation of living tissue were described by D´Arsonval as early as 1868, while the use of thermal ablation for treatment of malignant hepatic lesions was first shown by McGahan et al. and Rossi et al. in 1990.[12,13] Since then, RFA has evolved as the most popular ablative technique world over.

Principle of RFA

RFA Induces thermal injury to the tumor tissue by electromagnetic energy deposition. The patient is a part of a closed-loop circuit which includes an RF generator, an electrode needle, and a large dispersive electrode (ground pads). RF energy is delivered as an alternating current at a frequency of 375–500 kHz within the tumor. This produces ionic agitation around the needle tip because of the relatively high electrical resistance of the tissue in comparison to the metal electrodes. Ionic agitation causes frictional heat around the electrode with resultant coagulative necrosis. The thermal damage is dependent on the tissue temperature achieved and duration of heating. A temperature of 50–55°C for 4–6 minutes produces irreversible cellular damage.

Types of RFA Electrodes

There are various types of electrodes which have either monopolar or bipolar technology **(Figs. 3A and B)**; difference between the two technologies is elaborated in **Table 2**. Bipolar and multipolar technology is a recent advance in RFA which has eliminated the need of a grounding pad and is also more effective in ablating large areas.[14,15]

The electrodes are broadly divided into the cooled tip or noncooled tip type depending upon the presence of the continuous cooling system. In the cooled tip type, there is

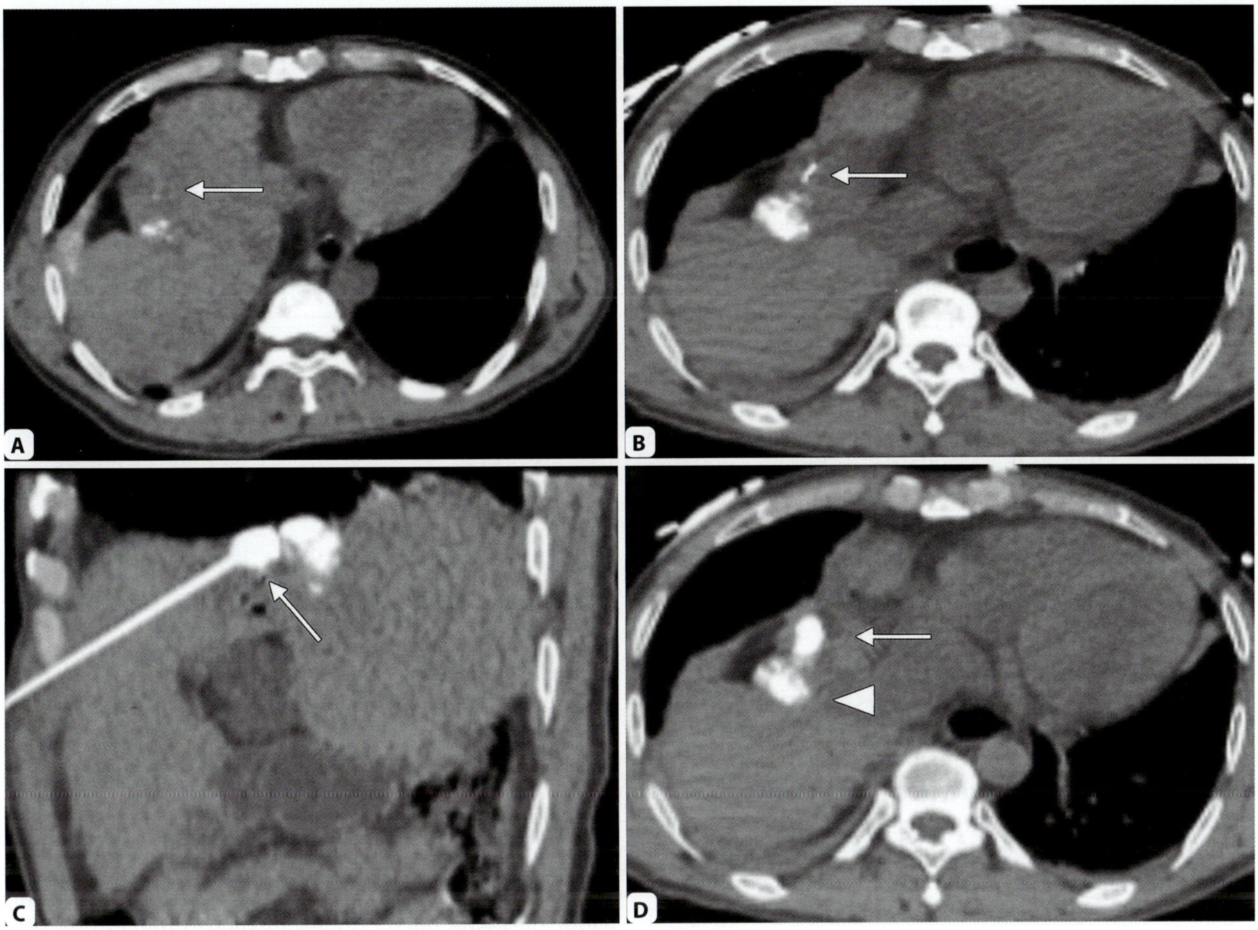

FIGS. 2A TO D: CT-guided percutaneous acetic acid injection (PAI). (A) NCCT abdomen reveals post-TACE lipiodol deposition with overlying capsular retraction in right lobe of liver (arrowhead) with hypodense residual lesion anterior to it (arrow). (B) CT-guided placement of needle in recurrent lesion (arrow). (C) Sagittal reformat showing oblique needle trajectory to residual tumor with intralesional contrast and acetic acid injection(arrow); with post-TACE lipiodol deposition posterior to it (arrowhead). (D) Post-PAI CT shows good coverage of residual lesion by contrast (arrow).

(NCCT: noncontrast computed tomography; TACE: transarterial chemoembolization)

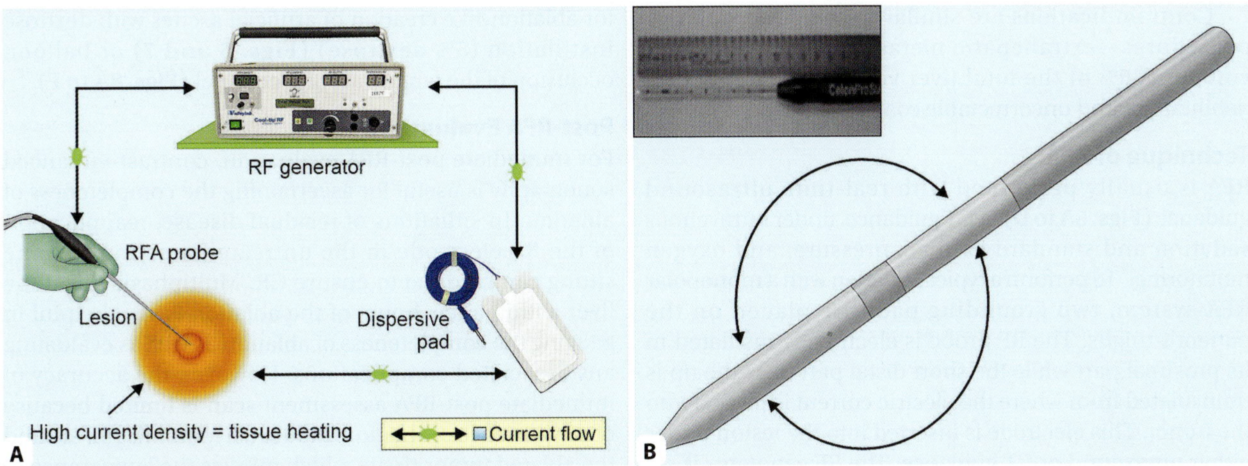

FIGS. 3A AND B: (A) Closed circuit of radiofrequency ablation (RFA) with monopolar electrode. The RFA probe acts as cathode, patient is part of the circuit, while grounding pads act as the anode. (B) With bipolar electrode, anode and cathode are both incorporated in it and grounding pads are not needed to complete the circuit.

TABLE 2: Monopolar versus bipolar radiofrequency ablation (RFA) technology.

Monopolar system	Bipolar system
Circuit is completed inside the patient (patient is part of the complete circuit)	Circuit is completed with the lesion
Grounding pads are required	No grounding pads
Multiple lesions cannot be treated at same time	Multiple lesions can be ablated at same time
Arrhythmias may occur	

continuous saline circulation through the electrode which produces cooling of the needle tip and prevents tissue charring. The heat is generated away from the electrode which results in coagulation necrosis of the tumor tissue. Based upon the array configuration, the electrodes may be single, clustered, multitined, or saline perfused **(Figs. 4A to F)**.

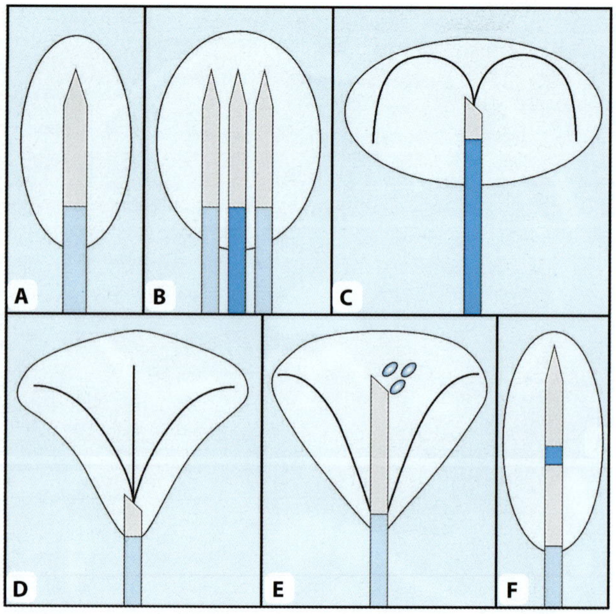

FIGS. 4A TO F: Radiofrequency ablation (RFA) electrode designs: (A) Monopolar single electrode; (B) Clustered electrode; (C) Tined electrode; (D) Multitined; (E) Saline perfused; (F) Bipolar single electrode.

Note: The area marked around each electrode represents the shape of ablating zone.

Patient Selection

RFA ideally suited for smaller lesions < 3 cm size. Although RFA can be done for tumors up to 5 cm diameter, chances of complete ablation diminish with increase in tumor diameter. The technique can also be used to treat multiple lesions; up to three lesions can be safely treated in single or multiple sittings. Lesions close to main branches of portal or hepatic veins are difficult to treat as continuous high blood flow in these vessels will have cooling effect because the thermal energy will be dissipated away, which is known as "heat sink effect". If the lesion is close to the liver capsule or gallbladder, chances of peritonitis or cholecystitis respectively are high. For these reasons, lesions that do not have at least one centimeter of normal liver parenchyma separating it from the liver capsule, gallbladder, porta hepatis, or major vessels are considered a relative contraindication for RFA.

Contraindications are similar to the other ablative procedures—extrahepatic metastatic disease, tumor volume >30% of the total liver volume, sepsis, severe debilitation, and uncorrectable coagulopathies.

Technique of RFA

RFA is usually performed with real-time ultrasound guidance **(Figs. 5A to D)** or CT guidance, under intravenous sedation and standard cardiac, pressure, and oxygen monitoring.[8] To perform a typical ablation with a monopolar RFA system, two grounding pads are placed on the patient's thighs. The RF probe is electrically insulated in its proximal part while the short distal part near the tip is uninsulated from where the electric current is passed into the tumor. This electrode is inserted into the lesion under either ultrasound or CT guidance. The RF generator is set for the wattage, timer, and temperature as per the device instructions (vendor specific). A pulsed RF energy is applied for 15–30 minutes, which causes a rise of the temperature at the target site from 80 to 110°C. Once there is ionic agitation within the tissue, microbubbles are seen forming around the electrode which make the lesion echogenic and obscure the tumor margins. After successful ablation, additional energy is applied during the withdrawal of the electrode under monitoring by real time ultrasound to prevent seeding of tumor cells in the probe track.

Technical Modifications

Tumors close to critical structures require special procedures for ablation-like creation of artificial ascites with dextrose instillation (5% dextrose) **(Figs. 6 and 7)** or balloon occlusion of the larger vascular channel **(Figs. 8A to F)**.[16]

Post-RFA Evaluation

For immediate post-RFA evaluation, contrast-enhanced sonography is useful for ascertaining the completeness of ablation. In situations of residual disease, reapplication of the RF electrode in the untreated area in the same sitting can be done to ensure CR. Multiphasic CT of the liver within a few hours of the ablation is also helpful in gauging the completeness of ablation as well as evaluating any associated complications. However, the accuracy of immediate post-RFA assessment scan is limited because of the presence of ablation-induced hyperemic rim around the ablated tumor tissue which mimics the appearance of residual viable tumor. The reactive hyperemia generally resolves in a months' time, when more accurate assessment of tumor response can be made on imaging.

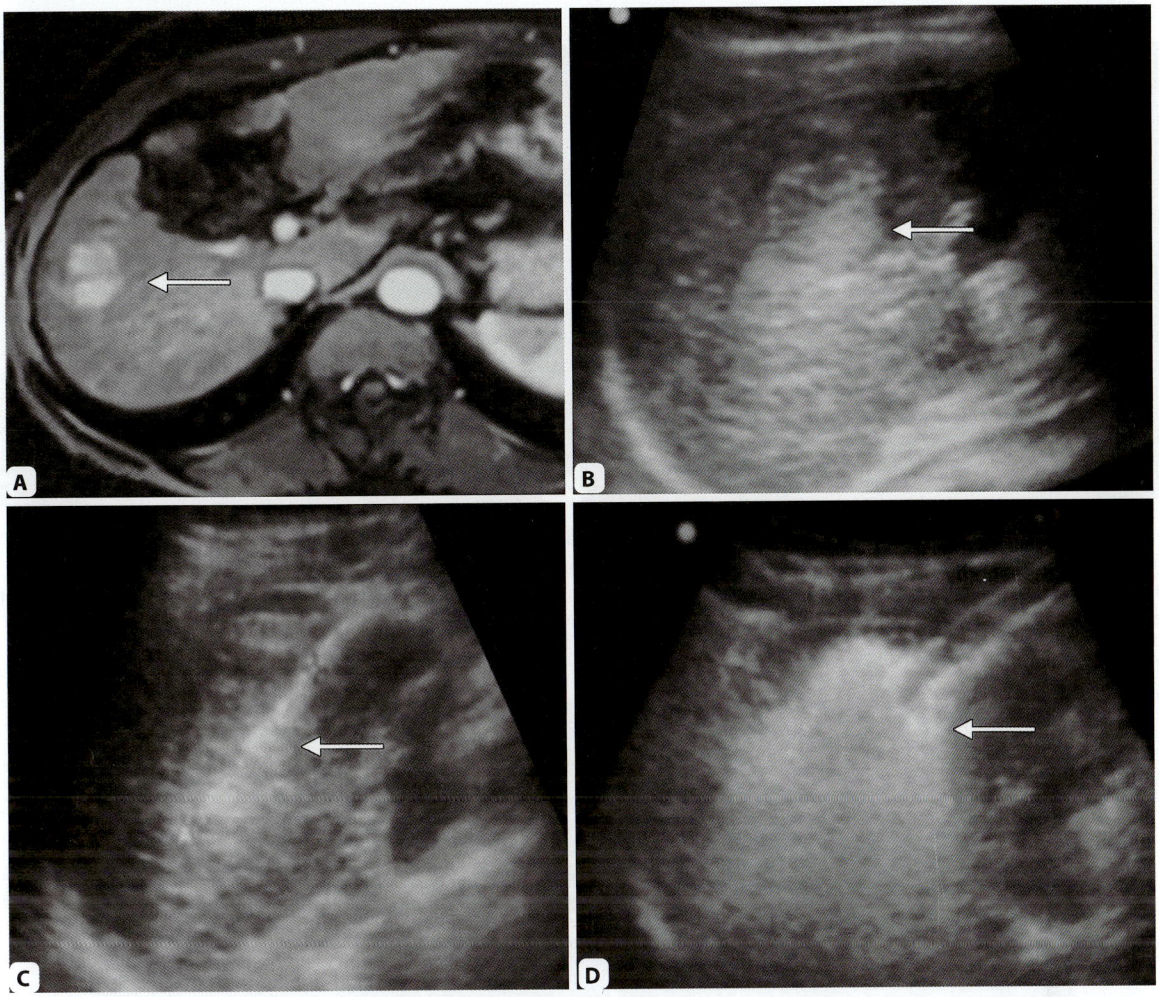

FIGS. 5A TO D: Ultrasound-guided radiofrequency ablation (RFA). (A) MRI shows HCC in segment V of liver (arrow). (B) Ultrasound shows the tumor is hyperechoic (arrow). (C) Ultrasound-guided placement of RFA electrode in the tumor (arrow). (D) Postablation echogenic appearance of the liver lesion (arrow).

(HCC: hepatocellular carcinoma; MRI: magnetic resonance imaging)

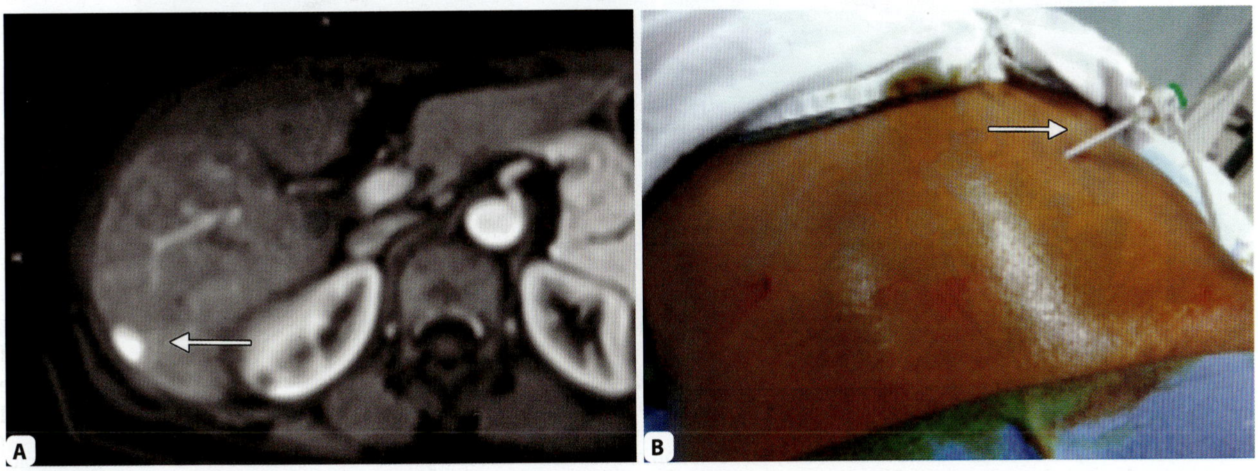

FIGS. 6A TO D: *Continued*

Continued

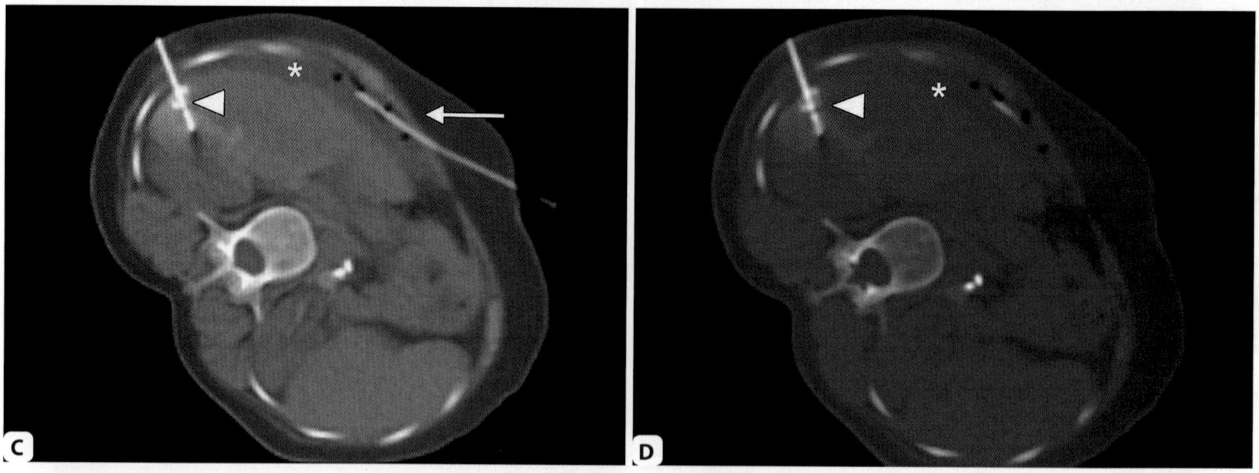

FIGS. 6A TO D: Creation of artificial ascites for radiofrequency ablation (RFA) of surface lesion. (A) Axial postcontrast T1W-fat suppressed image shows hypervascular lesion in subcapsular location in segment VI of liver (arrow). (B) Placement of 6F vascular sheath in perihepatic space for instillation of 5% dextrose for creation of artificial ascites (arrow). (C and D) Subsequent placement of RFA electrode in the liver lesion (arrowhead) with sheath in situ (arrow) and perihepatic fluid (asterisk).

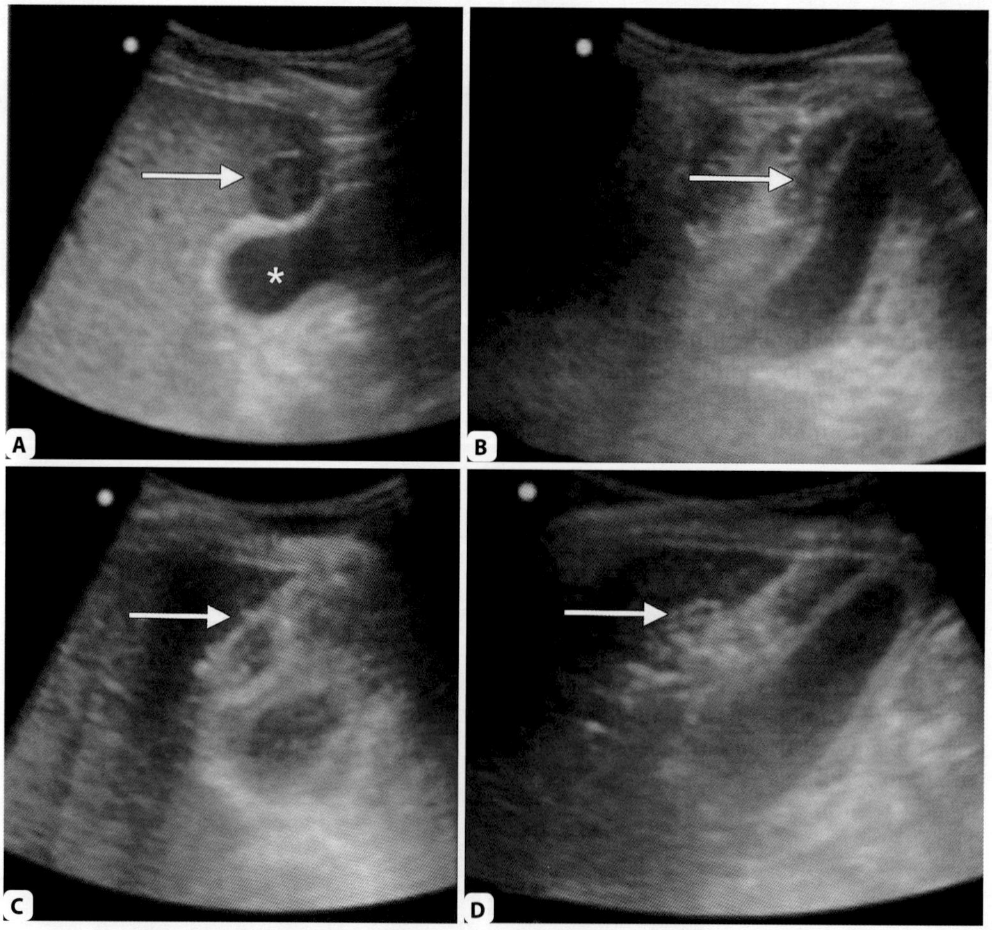

FIGS. 7A TO D: Hydrodissection for radiofrequency (RF) ablation of liver lesion close to gallbladder. (A) Ultrasound shows hypoechoic liver lesion (arrow) abutting the gallbladder (asterisk). (B) Hydrodissection by instillation of 5% dextrose between liver and gallbladder (arrow). (C) Placement of RF electrode in liver lesion (arrow). (D) Echogenic appearance of liver lesion during RF ablation (arrow).

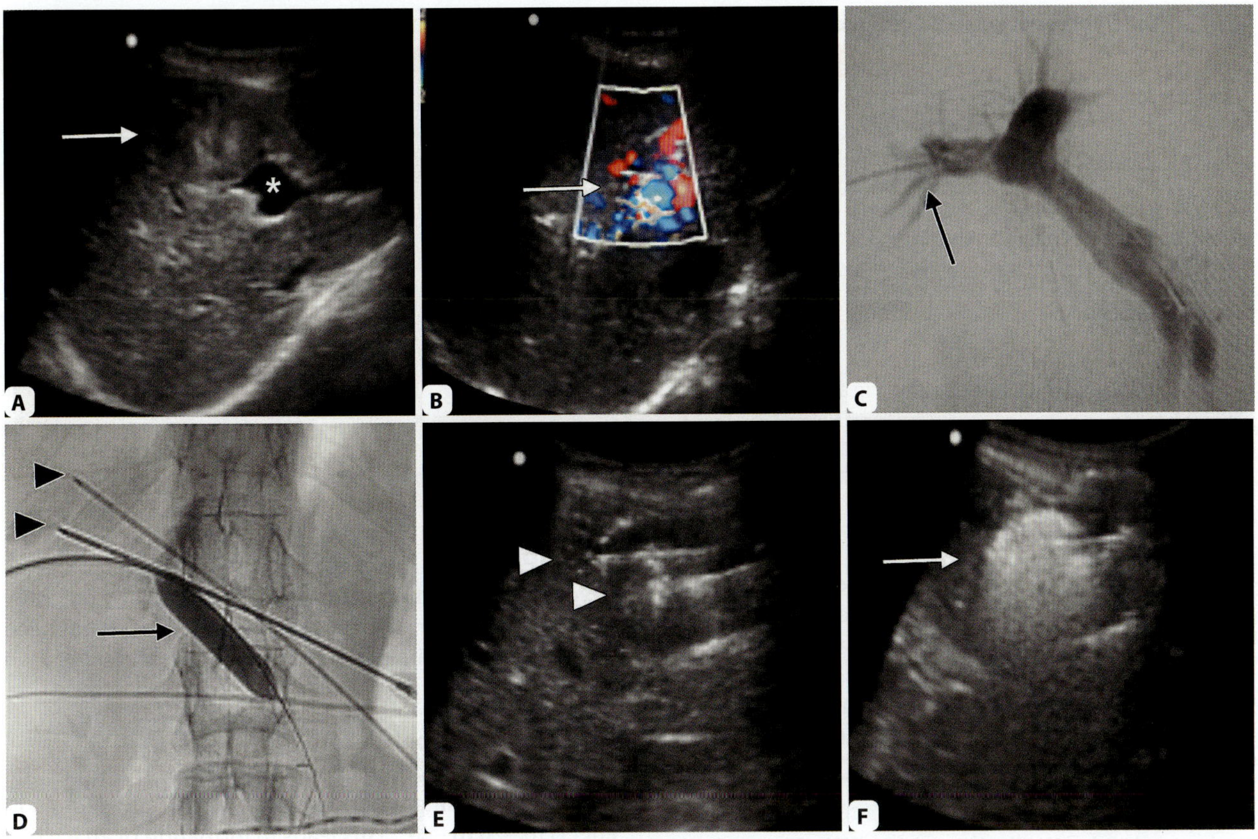

FIGS. 8A TO F: Balloon occlusion of portal vein for central hepatocellular carcinoma (HCC). (A) Grayscale ultrasound shows heteroechoic liver lesion (arrow) abutting the left portal vein (asterisk). (B) Color Doppler image showing the flow in left portal vein (arrow) (C) Portography after percutaneous puncture of right portal vein (arrow). (D) Balloon inflation in the main portal vein (arrow) and placement of radiofrequency (RF) electrodes (arrowheads) in liver lesion. (E) Ultrasound showing the two RF electrodes (arrowheads) in situ in liver lesion. (F) Echogenic appearance of liver lesion due to microbubble formation after RF ablation (arrow).

Complications

RFA is a safe procedure with a mortality rate as low as 0.1–0.3% and major complication rate of 2.2–3.1%. Minor complication rate ranges from 5 to 8.9%. Pain or fever is common and is usually self-limiting. Peritoneal hemorrhage, bile duct injury, hepatic abscess, and intestinal perforation are some of the adverse outcomes rarely encountered.[17,18] Late complication of tumor seeding along the needle track is also known to occur but is highly uncommon (0.5–0.8%).

Limitations of RFA

Complete tumor response is difficult to achieve in larger tumors >5 cm for which newer electrodes are coming into existence. Moreover, combination of RFA with other available treatment modalities is being used for larger tumors with improved results.[19] Tumors adjacent to large blood vessels are difficult to treat due to the "heat-sink effect"—a perfusion-mediated tissue cooling reducing the extent of coagulation necrosis produced by thermal ablation.[20]

Microwave Ablation

The MWA is a more recently developed technique of thermal ablation. It uses electromagnetic waves (900–2,459 MHz frequency) generated from one or more thin microwave antennas that are applied directly to the tumor to create heat and friction that destroys the tumor.[21]

Benefits of MWA

In comparison to RFA, MWA is faster with a more uniform and larger ablation zone due to improved convection profile and higher intratumoral temperature as it is less susceptible to the heat-sink effect and has a higher thermal efficiency. Also, unlike RFA, microwaves are able to penetrate charred tissue that builds up around the antenna.[22] Therefore, the benefit of MWA over RFA is its ability to do multiple ablations at the same time, and the potential to destroy larger-sized tumors faster and with less pain. Grounding pads are also not required in MWA.

Salient differences between RFA and MWA are summarized in **Table 3**.

TABLE 3: Differences between radiofrequency ablation and microwave ablation.

	Radiofrequency ablation	Microwave ablation
Electromagnetic energy used	High-frequency alternating current (375–500 kHz)	Electromagnetic radiation (900–2,459 MHz)
Time for ablation	Longer	Shorter
Heating	Nonuniform	Uniform
Intratumoral temperature attained	Lower	Higher
Ablation zone	Smaller	Larger
Pain during procedure	More	Less
Susceptibility to heat-sink effect	More	Less
Number of lesions which can be treated in a single session	Single	Multiple
Grounding pads	Required with monopolar systems	Not required

Principle of MWA

Oscillating charge of microwaves causes rapid flipping of water molecules which are dipolar. Heat is generated by friction from agitated water molecules; which in turn leads to cell death by coagulative necrosis. A less important mechanism of action is ionic polarization—microwaves cause ionic displacement which results in conversion of kinetic energy to thermal energy.[23]

Patient Selection

Patient selection is similar as for RFA. However, it is preferred over RFA for lesions > 3 cm and up to 5 cm in diameter. MWA is also preferred over RFA for lesions situated in proximity to major blood vessels.

Technique of MWA

Procedure is done under general anesthesia or conscious sedation. Ultrasound **(Figs. 9A to F)** or CT guidance is employed for placement of 14–17-gauge microwave antenna in the lesion. Microwaves are transmitted from the generator via a coaxial cable to the antenna. Duration of ablation depends on tumor volume but is typically < 10 minutes. Aim is to ablate tumor as well as 1 cm of normal parenchyma around the lesion (A0 ablation). Typically, 100 W of microwave energy is used for tumor ablation. The ablated tissue is visualized as an echogenic cloud on ultrasound. Following ablation of the tumor, the tract is also ablated with 75 W pulses of microwave energy while withdrawing the microwave antenna 0.5 cm at a time. This prevents tumor seeding along the tract and also reduces risk of bleeding from the liver capsule. For lesions with poor visibility on ultrasound, TACE or transarterial lipiodol injection may be done before MWA, as lipiodol deposition within the lesion would make it more conspicuous on ultrasound and CT. Similar to RFA, hydrodissection can be done for lesions close to gallbladder, bowel, or diaphragm.[23]

Complications

MWA can cause complications such as hemoperitoneum, pleural effusion, fever, hepatic pseudoaneurysm, biliary dilatation, and liver abscess formation.[24]

Cryoablation

Cryoablation is a unique form of thermal ablative therapy in which the tumor is frozen rather than heated. It has been more widely used in kidney, prostate, lung, and bone than in liver tumors.

Principle of Cryoablation

High-pressure argon gas expands within the tip of the cryoprobe causing a temperature drop (Joule-Thomson effect) to –20 to –40°. This leads to formation of an ice ball that results in cell death due to intracellular ice formation and cellular dehydration; as well as by indirect mechanism of microvascular thrombosis.[25]

Patient Selection

Cryoablation is safer and preferred over other thermal ablative techniques in cases of tumors in critical locations such as in the vicinity of the gallbladder, diaphragm, or bowel.[26]

Technique of Cryoablation

The procedure is done under local anesthesia and conscious sedation, as it causes less pain compared to other thermal ablation techniques.[27] Ultrasound, CT, or MRI guidance can be used. On CT and MRI, the entire ice ball is seen as a hypodense area and signal void respectively, which is useful in monitoring the ablation zone during the procedure. On ultrasound, only the hyperechoic near edge of the ice ball is visualized. 17G cryoprobes are inserted into the tumor; the number of cryoprobes used depends on the size and shape of the tumor. Typically, at least two probes are used for a synergistic effect. As per the "2-to-1 rule", distance between the cryoprobes should be <2 cm and cryoprobes should be within 1 cm of the tumor edge. A dual freeze-thaw-freeze cycle (freeze time 10–20 minutes; thaw time 5–10 minutes) is usually employed. Argon gas is delivered during the freeze phase, whereas helium is circulated for thawing. Ice ball is monitored during the procedure to extend 10 mm beyond the tumor margin; with this, the lethal isotherm will extend 5 mm beyond the tumor margin.[26]

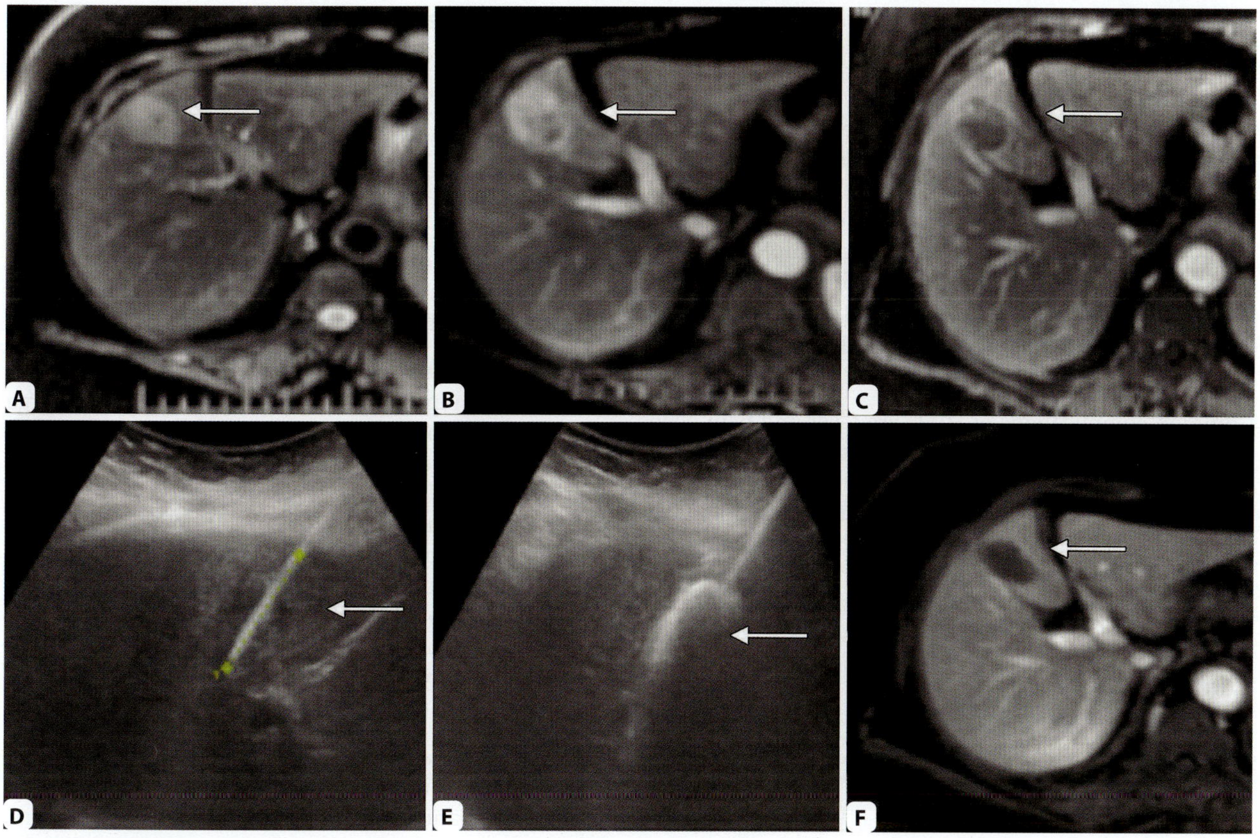

FIGS. 9A TO F: MWA of HCC. (A) Axial T2W fat suppressed image shows a hyperintense mass in segment IVa of liver (arrow). (B) Postcontrast axial T1W arterial phase image shows nonrim APHE in the mass (arrow). (C) The mass shows washout with enhancing capsule in the portovenous phase (arrow). (D) Ultrasound-guided placement of microwave antenna in the mass (arrow). (E) Following microwave ablation, the mass becomes hyperechoic (arrow). (F) Follow-up MRI 1 month after MWA shows no residual enhancement in the lesion (arrow)—LR-TR nonviable.

(HCC: hepatocellular carcinoma; MRI: magnetic resonance imaging; MWA: microwave ablation)

Complications

Cryoshock is a rare complication following large hepatic ablation with multiorgan failure and coagulopathy due to release of cytokines such as interleukin 6 (IL-6) and tumor necrosis factor-α (TNF-α). This has a high mortality of up to 40%.[28] Other reported complications include thrombocytopenia, acute kidney injury due to myoglobinuria, hemoperitoneum, and hemothorax.[29]

Response Assessment

Early postprocedure imaging can be done on the day of procedure to assess technical success and for any complications. Typically, follow-up MRI is performed at 1, 3, 6, 9, and 12 months and then annually. A benign thin periablation enhancement can be seen in initial months following cryoablation; this usually resolves by 4–6 months. Involution of the ablation zone occurs after 2–3 months due to fibrous scarring; overlying capsular retraction may ensue. The involution is more marked in cryoablation compared to heat-based thermal ablative techniques.[30]

High-intensity Focused Ultrasound

The HIFU is a noninvasive transcutaneous technique of thermal ablation. As it does not involve percutaneous puncture, there is reduced risk of hemorrhage and no risk of tumor seeding along the ablation tract.

Principle of HIFU

HIFU involves the focusing of ultrasound beam on target lesion with an acoustic lens. The ultrasound is converted to thermal energy; which causes increase in target tissue temperature to >55° with resultant coagulative necrosis.[31] At higher acoustic energies, inertial cavitation also occurs. Damage to surrounding tissues is minimal.

Indications/Patient Selection

As for other ablative techniques, HIFU is indicated in patients of Child A cirrhosis with single tumor < 5 cm or up to 3 tumors < 3 cm. It is the ablative technique of choice in patients with coagulopathy or ascites where other locoregional therapies are contraindicated. It is also effective in tumors close to major vessels like inferior vena cava, portal, or hepatic veins.

Technique of HIFU

The procedure is done under general or epidural anesthesia. Ultrasound or MRI guidance can be used. Preprocedure rib resection (2 weeks prior to HIFU), creation of artificial ascites, or hydrothorax may be needed for a better acoustic window. 0.8–1.8 MHz ultrasound beam is employed; up to 300 W of acoustic power is delivered to the target lesion. CR can be achieved in 91% of tumors of <3 cm, and the 1 and 3 years survival rates are 87.7% and 62.4%, respectively.[31]

Complications

Common complications of HIFU are fever and pain. Skin burns at application site or osteonecrosis of ribs along the pathway of the ultrasound beam can also occur.[32] Like other thermal ablative techniques, damage to gallbladder, adjacent bowel loops, and secondary infection with liver abscess formation may occur.

Laser Ablation

Principle of Laser Ablation

Optical fibers transmit laser light which is absorbed and distributed within the tumor. Light is converted to heat energy in the target tumor tissues and produces coagulation necrosis of the tumor.

Patient Selection

It is safe and highly effective in HCCs < 4 cm (complete ablation achieved in 82–97% tumors ≤ 5cm).[33] Laser ablation can also be used in patients with liver metastases.[34] As the diameter of needles used is smaller than that of RFA electrodes or MWA antennas, laser ablation is preferable for at-risk or difficult to access locations; or to treat multiple lesions in single session.

Technique of Laser Ablation

Laser ablation is performed under conscious sedation and local anesthesia. Ultrasound, CT, or MRI guidance is employed. Neodymium-doped yttrium aluminum garnet (Nd:YAG, wavelength 1,064 nm) and diode (wavelength 800–980 nm) lasers are the most commonly used, as penetration of light is optimal in the near infrared spectrum.[35] Bare tip quartz fibers (300–600 μm) are inserted through one or multiple 21-gauge needles into the tumor. Single fiber, when illuminated, releases 1,800 J producing an ablation zone of 12–16 mm diameter. For larger lesions, 2–4 fibers can be inserted and a pullback technique can be used.

Complications

Laser ablation is a relatively safe procedure with a major complication rate of 1.5%, minor complication rate of 6.2%, and mortality of 0.8%.[36] Its major complications include liver failure/segmental infarction, hepatic abscess, bile duct injury, and hemorrhage (hepatic, intraperitoneal, and gastrointestinal). Minor complications encountered with laser ablation are pleural effusion, fever, and pain.

Irreversible Electroporation

Irreversible electroporation is a nonthermal energy-based ablation technique.

Principle of Irreversible Electroporation

Applied pulsed electric fields cause formation of nanopores in the lipid bilayer of cell membranes. This disrupts cellular homeostasis and causes apoptotic cell death. Walls of blood vessels and bile ducts are composed of predominantly extracellular connective tissue which is resilient to the effects of irreversible electroporation.[37]

Indications/Selection Criteria

Tumors < 5 cm in size which are in close vicinity of large blood vessels (abutment of single remaining portal vein or hepatic vein, unreconstructable invasion of inferior vena cava), gallbladder, or major bile ducts (within 1 cm of common hepatic duct, right or left hepatic ducts); as thermal ablation procedures would be less effective in these locations on account of heat-sink effect due to vascular proximity; and would be more likely to cause complications such as bile leak, hemobilia, biliary occlusion, or cholangitis due to biliary proximity.[38]

Technique

The procedure is done under general anesthesia with complete neuromuscular blockade to reduce muscle stimulation. Nanoknife device (Angiodynamics, Latham, NY) with monopolar (single pole on one probe) or bipolar (two poles on same probe) probes is used. Probes are inserted percutaneously into the lesion using CT or ultrasound guidance. If monopolar probes are used, at least two probes have to be inserted in a parallel orientation 1.5–2 cm apart. 90 high-voltage direct current electrical pulses (1,500–3,000 V, 25–45 A) are delivered. Electrocardiogram (ECG) synchronization is done with electric pulses delivered during the ventricular refractory period to minimize cardiac arrhythmias.[39]

Complications

Cardiac arrhythmias, brachial plexus injury, portal vein thrombosis, pneumothorax, and pleural effusion have been reported to occur as complications of irreversible electroporation.

Response Assessment

Follow-up is done with contrast-enhanced CT or MRI at 1, 3, 6, and 12 months postprocedure. Irreversibly electroporated tissue is surrounded by a penumbra of reversibly electroporated tissue; the latter appears hyperintense on T2W sequences and shows arterial phase enhancement up to 1 month after the IRE.[40] Ablation zone shrinks over time and may even disappear completely.

Intra-arterial Procedures

Image-guided intra-arterial procedures are the most commonly used palliative treatment options for the patients of HCC as the vast majority have advanced disease at the outset which precludes the use of curative options. Being palliative in nature, the primary goal of the therapy is to improve the quality of life and prolong survival; and the treatment invariably needs to be repeated in situations of disease progression or recurrences.

Transarterial Chemoembolization

Transarterial chemoembolization (TACE) is a combination of intra-arterial injection of chemotherapeutic drugs followed by embolization of the feeding supply to the tumor.

Principle of TACE

Normal liver has a dual blood supply from hepatic artery and portal vein; whereas HCC is supplied by hepatic artery alone. This forms the basis for TACE. In conventional TACE (cTACE), the chemotherapeutic drug emulsion prepared by mixing the chemotherapeutic drugs with lipiodol is delivered intra-arterially, which results in up to 100-fold higher drug dose compared to systemic chemotherapy, and causes extensive tumor necrosis. The effect is further augmented by the additional embolization of the feeding arteries (branches from the hepatic arteries) by either gelfoam pledgets or polyvinyl alcohol (PVA) particles causing ischemic necrosis of the tumor.[41-43] Gelfoam embolization creates a hypoxic environment in the tumor bed and tissue hypoxia inhibits the active efflux of the chemotherapeutic drug by making transmembrane P-glycoprotein, an ATP-dependent pump ineffective.

Agents Used

Doxorubicin (10–100 mg), epirubicin (5–120 mg) alone, or in combination with cisplatin (10–100 mg) is the commonly used chemotherapeutic agents. Lipiodol, which acts as a drug carrier, is mixed with chemotherapeutic drugs to prepare a water-in-oil emulsion, using a three-way stopcock and Luer lock syringes and at least 20 pumping exchanges. This drug emulsion is selectively retained within the tumor cells resulting in increased exposure of the neoplastic cells to the chemotherapeutic agents. Lipiodol also enhances the visibility of the emulsion on fluoroscopy.

For better stability of the emulsion, the lyophilized powder form of epirubicin or doxorubicin should be reconstituted in iodinated contrast media rather than normal saline so that the specific gravity of water and oil become similar. Volume of lipiodol should be two to four times more than that of the reconstituted chemotherapeutic agent (most commonly, 2:1 ratio of lipiodol to chemotherapeutic agent is used). The ratio of lipiodol to maximum tumor diameter is 1:2–1:1; maximum dose of lipiodol should not exceed 15 mL.

Patient Selection

TACE is used for treating patients of unresectable HCC of BCLC B stage,[5] unsuitable candidates for local ablative therapies of BCLC A stage and for downstaging the disease to make patients suitable for resection or transplant. These patients are those who have a preserved liver function (Child–Pugh class A,B), multinodular tumors without vascular invasion or extrahepatic spread. Patients who have reduced liver function or hepatic failure (Child–Pugh C), have to be excluded for this treatment since the liver function may further deteriorate due to ischemic damage of the unaffected liver tissue leading to acute liver failure.

Portal vein tumor thrombus has been classified by Liver Cancer Study Group of Japan as follows:

- Vp0—no tumor thrombus in portal vein
- Vp1—tumor thrombus distal to second-order branches of portal vein
- Vp2—tumor thrombus in second-order branches of portal vein
- Vp3—tumor thrombus in first-order branches of portal vein
- Vp4—tumor thrombus in main portal vein; or a portal vein contralateral to primarily involved lobe; or both[44]

Previously, portal vein tumor thrombus was considered a contraindication for TACE. Though TACE has been performed in studies in patients with all grades of portal vein tumor thrombus, its use should be avoided in Vp3 or Vp4 due to risk of liver failure.

Various prognostic systems have also been developed to predicting outcome of TACE such as Selection for TrAnsarterial chemoembolization TrEatment (STATE) score, Hepatoma-Arterial embolization Prognostic (HAP) score, and six-and-twelve score.[45] Proper patient selection is very important to have long-term survival and reduced postprocedure complications. Patients with lower tumor burden do better than higher tumor burden score **(Table 4).**[46]

Technique (Figs. 10A to F)

TACE is performed in the angiography suite, under aseptic precautions with the patient under conscious sedation and through the percutaneous route. To begin with, diagnostic mesenteric and celiac arteriograms are performed using

TABLE 4: Hepatocellular carcinoma (HCC) tumor burden scoring systems.

Scoring system	Calculation	Risk group		
		Low risk	Medium risk	High risk
Tumor Burden Score (TBS)	Square root [(max tum diameter)^2 + (number of tumor)^2]	<3.36	3.36–13.74	>13.74
Six-and-twelve score (SAT)	Largest diameter(cm) + tumor number	<6	>6 but <12	>12
Seven-eleven criteria (SEC)	Largest diameter(cm) + tumor number	<7	>7 but <11	>11

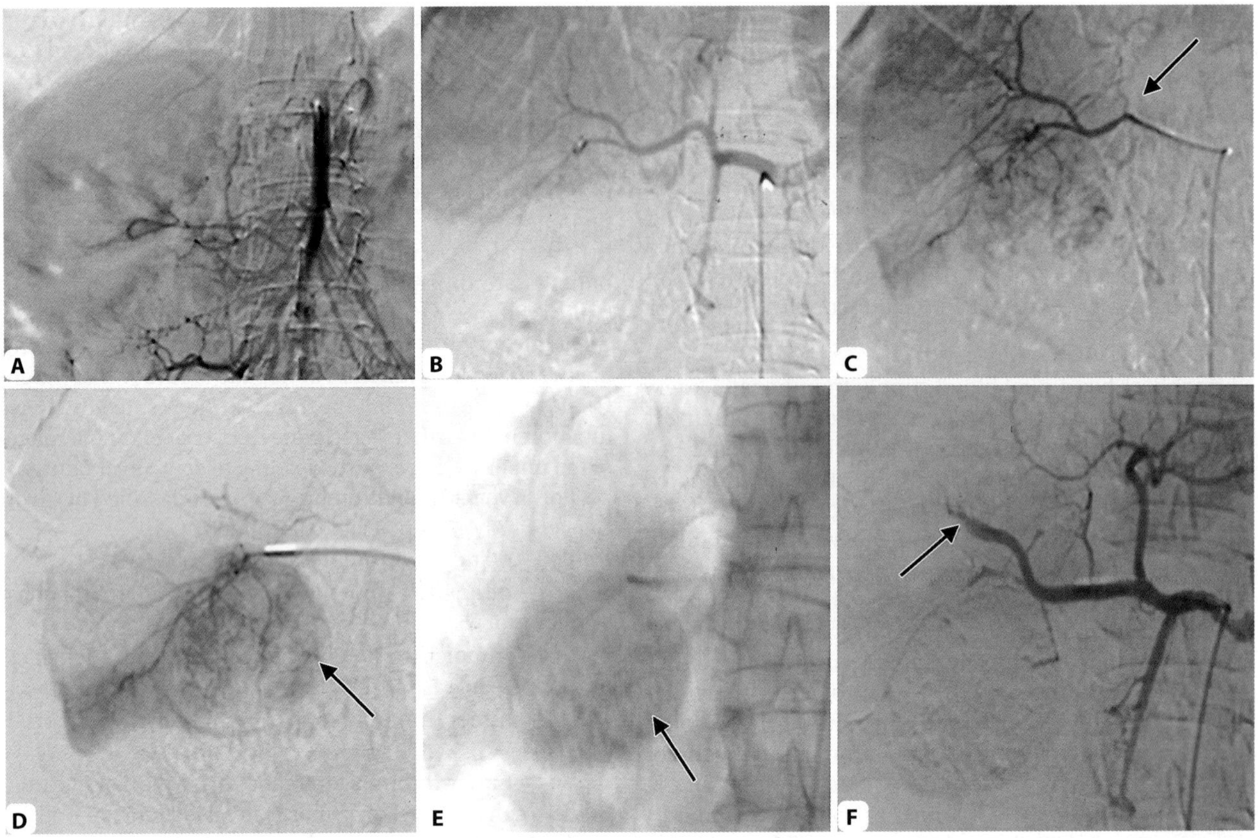

FIGS. 10A TO F: Various steps of angiographic technique of transarterial chemoembolization (TACE): Initial SMA angiogram (A) performed to look for anomalous origin of hepatic artery, followed by celiac axis angiogram. (B) Selective angiogram of the right hepatic artery (arrow) (C) showing abnormal tumor blush (arrow) (D), followed by injection chemotherapeutic emulsion into the tumor bed shows retention of lipiodol (arrow) (E) and stasis of blood flow (F) following gelfoam embolization (arrow).

various preshaped polyurethane catheters (4F or 5F) with the digital subtraction technique to determine the vascular anatomy and feeding tumor supply. Superior mesenteric arteriogram is done for detecting the presence of any accessory or aberrant right hepatic artery arising from the vessel as well as for evaluating the patency of the portal vein. Celiac angiogram should include the left gastric artery to identify any accessory or aberrant left hepatic artery. Cone-beam CT or Dyna-CT, with intra-arterial contrast injection into the hepatic arteries via a pressure injector, is also useful in demonstrating the tumoral feeding vessels.[47]

Depending upon the hepatic arterial anatomy and tumor vascular supply, selective arteriography of the common, left, and right hepatic arteries as per the case is done. Microcatheter, inserted coaxially through the diagnostic catheter, helps to reach the tumor superselectively avoiding vessel spasm and dissection. The placement of the catheter tip in the feeding artery, as close to the tumor as possible, is the most important technical factor undertaken for maximizing the treatment effect on the tumor and minimizing damage to nontumor hepatic tissue. Based on the site of microcatheter position from where infusion of chemotherapeutic emulsion is infused, cTACE can be nonselective (catheter tip in right or left hepatic artery), selective (catheter tip in proximal segmental artery), superselective (catheter tip in distal subsegmental artery), or ultraselective (catheter tip in distal subsubsegmental tumor feeding artery).[48]

After advancement of the microcatheter system to the appropriate segmental or subsegmental vessel supplying the tumor, the chemotherapeutic mixture is injected slowly at the rate of 1 mL/min under continuous fluoroscopic observation avoiding reflux of chemotherapeutic agent into nontarget areas. In case of multiple vascular feeders, the emulsion is injected into all the feeders superselectively in divided doses. Infusion is performed till there is visualization of peritumoral portal venous radicles; though this may be difficult to achieve in cases of large tumor burden. There are three grades of peritumoral portal vein visualization—grade 0 (no visualization), grade 1 (slight visualization), and grade 2 (marked visualization). Better the visualization of portal vein, lower is the rate of local recurrence.[49]

Subsequently, the feeding vessels are embolized by gelfoam pledgets to reduce the blood flow and also the wash out of chemotherapeutic agents into the systemic circulation. Complete stasis should be achieved, i.e., a static contrast column for at least 5 heartbeats. Cone-beam CT is repeated at the end of procedure to assess lipiodol accumulation within the tumor.

The peripheral part of large tumors > 5 cm, exophytic tumors, tumors involving bare area of liver, tumors with extracapsular invasion, previously treated tumors, or patients with stenosis or occlusion of the hepatic artery, may develop supply from extrahepatic collaterals from the inferior phrenic, omental, internal mammary, suprarenal, right renal, intercostal, or lumbar arteries. Parasitic blood supply should be suspected if any of these arteries appear hypertrophied, or if there is a defect in the tumor blush at angiography or in the post-TACE lipiodol retention.[50] Unusual origins of the various arterial supply to the tumor may also be encountered, like the gastroduodenal artery arising close to the origin of the middle or left hepatic artery, the right gastric artery arising from right or proper hepatic artery, or the left hepatic artery arising from the left gastric artery. Use of microcatheter and sometimes coil embolization of these vessels is performed to protect the stomach and duodenum from potential reflux of the chemotherapeutic and embolic agents.

There are no recommendations regarding the volume of emulsion to be injected with reference to the tumor size. In case of significant arterioportal or arteriovenous shunting, a small amount of gelfoam or PVA particles is injected to block the shunt prior to the injection of chemotherapeutic emulsion. If the tumor is very large in size, repeated sessions of TACE may be required to achieve CR; this should be performed on an on-demand basis, i.e., when residual or new tumor is detected on imaging, rather than on a scheduled basis.

Complications of TACE

Postembolization syndrome (noninfectious fever, pain, nausea, and vomiting) is commonly encountered. It is self-limiting and only supportive care is needed. Prophylactic use of steroids has been shown to reduce the occurrence of postembolization syndrome.

Major complications of TACE include hepatic insufficiency, liver abscess (especially in patients with bilioenteric anastomosis or biliary stents), rupture of tumor, and Ischemic complications due to nontarget embolization (cholecystitis, bile duct necrosis, perforation of the alimentary tract, pulmonary lipiodol embolism, diaphragmatic injury, and skin necrosis).[51]

TACE Using Drug-eluting Beads (DEB-TACE) (Figs. 11A to F)

The main target of TACE is to reduce systemic toxicity, increase the therapeutic efficacy, and provide a sustained

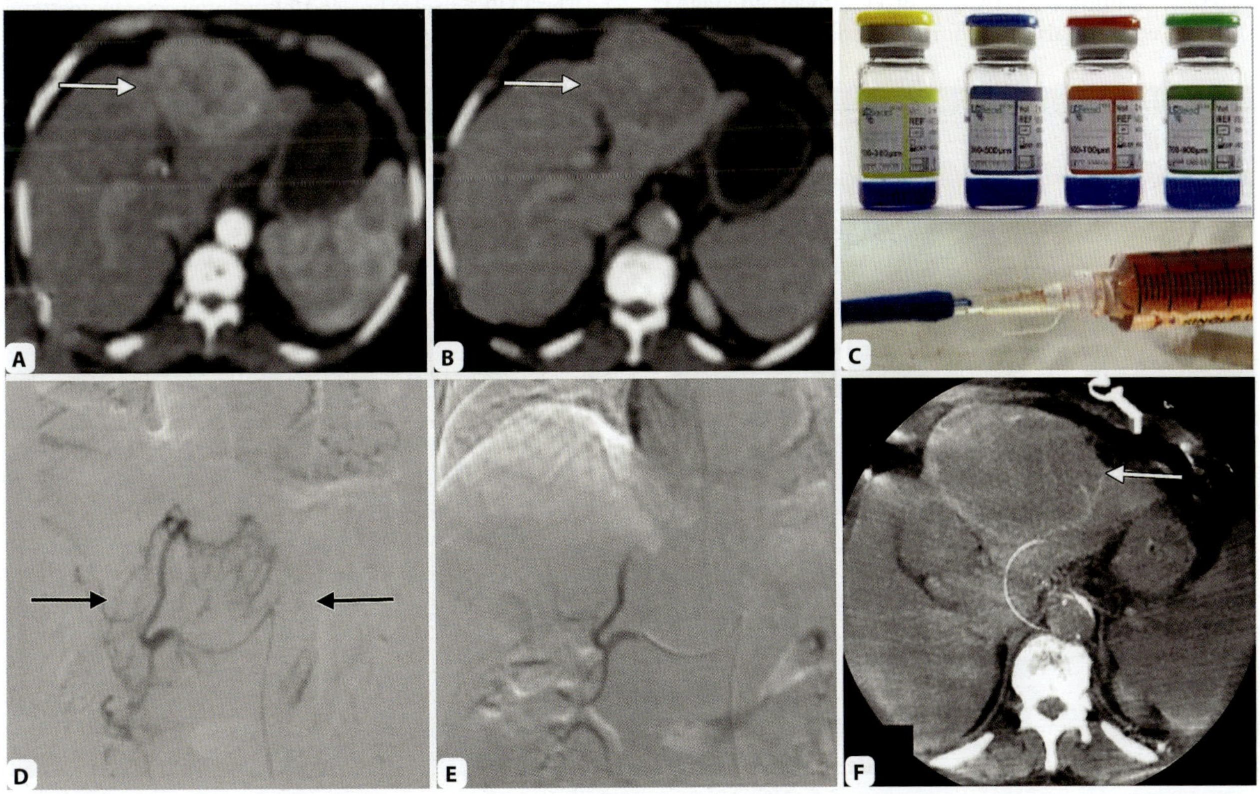

FIGS. 11A TO F: Drug-eluting bead transarterial chemoembolization (DEB-TACE) (A) Postcontrast T1W image in arterial phase shows mass with nonrim arterial phase hyperenhancement in segment III of left lobe (arrow). (B) The mass shows washout with enhancing capsule in portovenous phase (arrow). (C) Drug-eluting beads loaded with doxorubicin in syringe. (D) Tumor blush (arrow) on left hepatic angiogram. (E) Left hepatic artery angiogram following intra-arterial injection of DC beads showing no tumor blush. (F) Cone-beam CT showing coverage of left lobe tumor (arrow).

release of chemotherapy over time without damaging the healthy surrounding hepatic parenchyma. Recently, introduced novel technologies consisting of embolic microspheres (100–300, 300–500, or 500–700 µm size) such as DC-Beads, CalliSphere, or HepaSpheres have the ability to actively sequester doxorubicin hydrochloride from a solution and release it in a controlled and sustained fashion (DEB) over 2 weeks. The mixture of DEB and chemotherapeutic agent is mixed with an equal volume of nonionic contrast medium and injected intra-arterially at 1 mL/min till near-stasis is achieved in the tumor feeding vessel. DEB-TACE has been shown to substantially diminish the amount of chemotherapy that reaches the systemic circulation compared with lipiodol-based conventional TACE, thus significantly increasing the local concentration of the drug and achieving better tumor response rates.[52]

Transarterial Radioembolization (TARE)

Also known as selective internal radiation therapy (SIRT); transarterial radioembolization (TARE) is a safe, effective and promising therapeutic option in patients with inoperable HCC **(Figs. 12A to F)**. Hemodynamic principles and techniques of TARE are similar to TACE. Major limiting factor is the high cost of radioisotope.

Patient Selection

The best candidate for TARE is BCLC-Advanced stage C, i.e., HCC with portal vein tumor thrombosis (PVT), because of the minimal embolic effect of the radioisotope-labeled microspheres.[53] Also used for downstaging prior to resection and bridging to liver transplant in case large tumors without portal vein thrombus.

Agents Used

90Yttrium (90Y)-labeled glass or resin microspheres are most commonly used agents in TARE. 90Y radioembolization can deliver extremely high levels of β radiation (up to 150 Gy) with tolerable exposure to normal parenchyma due to its limited penetration (mean penetration 2.5 mm and maximum penetration 11 mm). Less commonly, TARE is performed by injection of isotopes like ^{131}Iodine + lipiodol, ^{188}Rhenium + lipiodol, and into the hepatic artery.

Technique

A mapping of hepatic tumor and its blood supply is done with technetium-99m-labeled macroaggregated albumin (MAA) followed by single-photon emission CT (SPECT) a few days prior to the TARE procedure to rule out significant hepatopulmonary shunting so as to avoid radiation pneumonitis. Preprocedure mapping also enables tumor volumetry using cone-beam CT for calculation of dose of radioisotope required for the TARE procedure. The rest of the technique of TARE is similar to TACE, except for injection of radioisotope for intra-arterial brachytherapy instead of lipiodol-chemotherapeutic agent emulsion.

The TARE can also be used for radiation segmentectomy or radiation lobectomy. Radiation segmentectomy implies

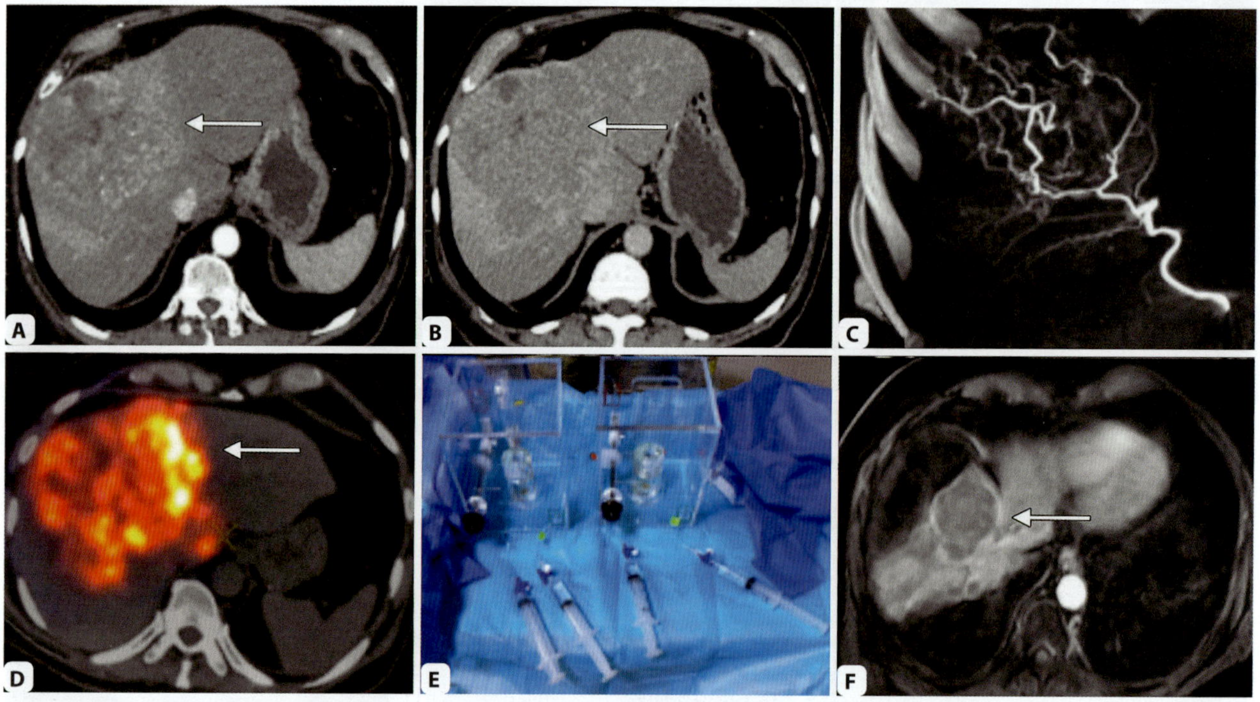

FIGS. 12A TO F: Transarterial radioembolization (TARE) (A) axial CECT (contrast-enhanced computed tomography) (arterial phase) shows hypervascular mass (arrow) in segments VIII and IVa of liver. (B) On axial CECT (portovenous phase), the mass (arrow) shows washout with enhancing capsule. (C) Coronal reformat of cone-beam CT for mapping of hepatic arterial supply for TARE. (D) SPECT-CT (Single-photon emission computed tomography–computed tomography) image demonstrating ^{99m}Tc-MAA uptake by the tumor (arrow). (E) Assembly for administration of 90Yttrium labeled microspheres. (F) Follow-up MRI 6 months after TARE reveals reduction in size of mass (arrow) with capsular retraction and no arterial phase enhancement (LR-TR nonviable).

selective delivery of radioisotope to a maximum of two Couinaud segments; and can be considered an alternative to ablative therapies. In radiation lobectomy, radioisotope is delivered to an entire hepatic lobe to cause its atrophy along with hypertrophy of spared lobe to improve future liver remnant (FLR) volume and facilitate surgical resection.[54]

Complications

Minor complications of TARE are fatigue and transient lymphopenia. Nontarget embolization can occur leading to gastrointestinal ulcers, radiation pneumonitis, radiation-induced cholecystitis, or radiation dermatitis. Other major complications are radioembolization-induced liver disease, biliary necrosis, and liver abscess formation.[51]

Combination Treatment

Currently, in cases with increased tumor burden or larger-sized tumors, multimodality approach is being considered. The regional and local therapies are combined in the same patient either concomitantly or sequentially to produce better results as compared to the use of a single therapy.[55,56] Examples of combination treatment are:

- Ablative therapies of PEI, RFA, or MWA performed after TACE in cases of small residual disease
- In small tumors amenable for ablation but with poor visibility on ultrasound or CT, TACE can be done prior to ablation as lipiodol accumulation will improve tumor visibility **(Figs. 13A to F)**.
- Synergistic effect of TACE which promotes neoangiogenesis due to hypoxia and oral chemotherapy with sorafenib which is antiangiogenic in patients with advanced HCC.
- In patients with postresection recurrence(s), RFA or TACE is undertaken frequently.

Follow-up and Response Assessment after Locoregional Therapies for HCC

Clinical Follow-up

Postprocedure, patients are followed up at 1–2 monthly intervals postprocedure for the assessment of the liver function status and treatment side-effects if any. Various laboratory tests which are done include liver and renal function tests, tumor markers (serum AFP and PIVKA-II if elevated prior to treatment), viral markers (depending upon the etiology of HCC) for monitoring of the hepatitis B or C activity status. If a clinical suspicion of recurrence

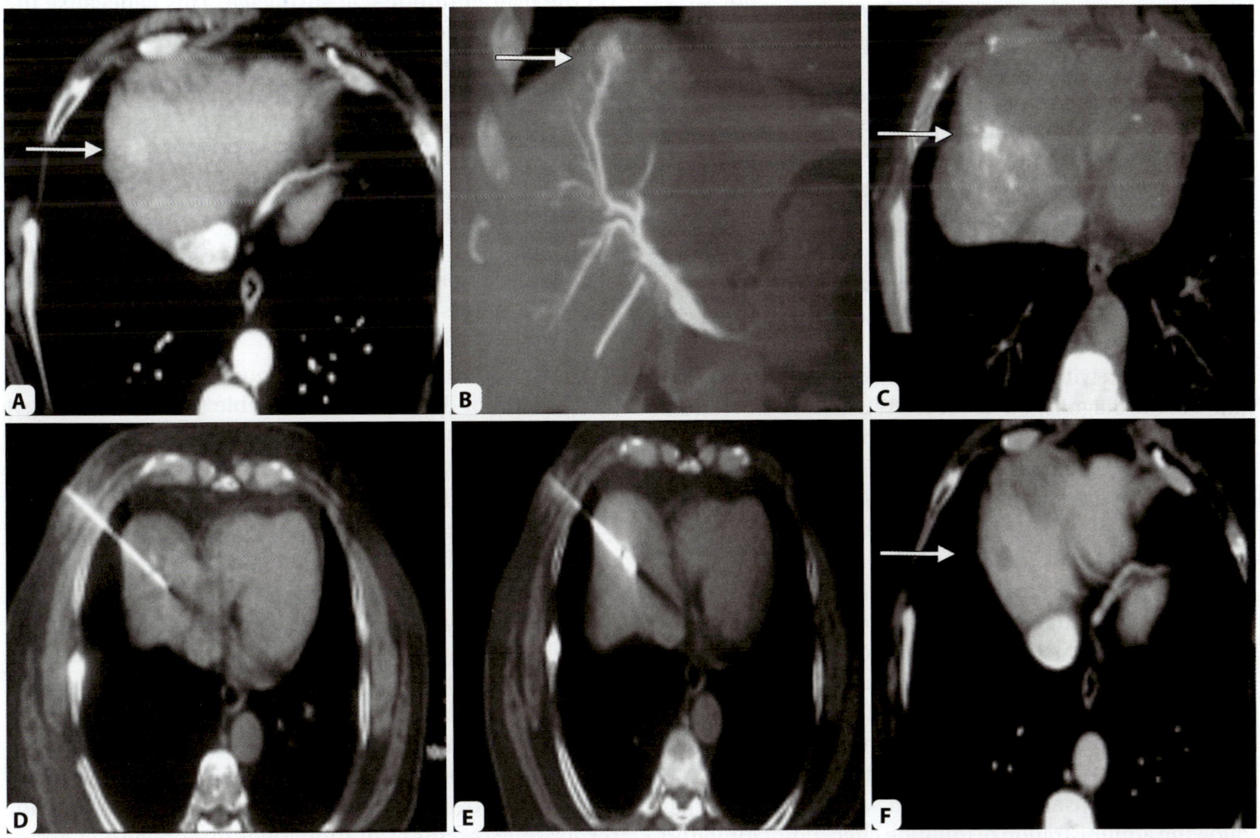

FIGS. 13A TO F: Combination treatment. (A) Axial CECT (contrast-enhanced computed tomography) (arterial phase) shows small hypervascular mass in segment VIII of right lobe of liver (arrow). The mass had poor visibility on ultrasound (not shown). Coronal (B) and axial (C) cone-beam CT after transarterial injection of lipiodol in the tumor to improve its visibility (arrow). (D and E) CT-guided placement of RF electrode in the liver tumor. (F) Follow-up CT shows no residual enhancement in the ablated lesion (arrow)—LR-TR nonviable.

or disease progression arises on follow-up (features of decompensation or rise in AFP), imaging evaluation is asked for and the management done accordingly.

Imaging Follow-up

Accurate assessment of tumor response is extremely important in oncology practice for prolonging survival. Imaging techniques of multiphasic CT and MR are generally recommended and lately, use of contrast-enhanced ultrasound (CEUS) has also been used with promising results.[57,58]

Due to the differences in the principles of imaging techniques and contrast, these modalities have some limitations, advantages, and accuracies in the therapeutic assessment. Response evaluation entails detection of any viable tumor tissue which on contrast imaging techniques [CEUS, multiphase CT (MPCT), and MRI] is seen as an enhancing area at the tumor site, while the nonviable tissue lacks enhancement. On MPCT/MRI, assessment of tumor morphology, resorption of ethiodized oil, overall liver size, and development of new lesions or metastases are looked for. Completely treated tumor invariably shrinks in size over a period of time. One of the major limitations of MPCT is the difficulty in accurate assessment of the residual disease in postlipiodol TACE patients. Lipiodol is radiodense and is seen as a hyperdensity in the tumor site on MPCT, the appearance that is similar to the hyperenhancing viable tumor tissue following contrast injection. This at times leads to masking of the small viable tissue on MPCT resulting in misinterpretation. However, lipiodol retention pattern on CT can act as a surrogate marker for residual disease; incomplete lipiodol deposition is associated with higher rates of recurrent disease in comparison with complete lipiodol deposition.

Magnetic resonance imaging has the highest accuracy in assessment of patients after TACE, as it is not affected by the lipiodol presence.[59] Contrast sequences can be complimented with diffusion-weighted sequences (DWI) to improve the diagnostic accuracy. DWI helps to differentiate inflammatory enhancement (T2-shine through) from the viable tumor (diffusion restriction).[60] Evaluation by CEUS is also not hampered by the lipiodol presence and thus CEUS can diagnose even a small viable tissue with high accuracy.[61]

Initial multiphasic CT or MRI is done at 1, 3, 6, and 12 months postablation, TACE, or systemic chemotherapy with tyrosine kinase inhibitors such as sorafenib or lenvatinib for detection of residual disease on the basis of modified response evaluation criteria in solid tumors (*mRECIST criteria*).[62] However, first imaging should be done at 3 months following radiation-based locoregional therapies such as TARE or stereotactic body radiotherapy (SBRT). Due to pseudoprogression which occurs initially following administration of immune checkpoint inhibitors, the first imaging should be done 8–12 weeks after treatment **(Table 5)**. For the same reason, iRECIST criteria can be applied for response assessment with immune checkpoint inhibitors. Metastatic disease is assessed with RECIST 1.1 irrespective of the treatment given. Subsequent imaging should be done at 3 monthly intervals for intermediate and advanced HCC. However, for very early and early HCC, the interval can be increased to 6 months after the first 2 years.[63]

TABLE 5: Ideal timing of response assessment after locoregional therapy for hepatocellular carcinoma (HCC).

Treatment modality	Time for first imaging study after treatment
Locoregional therapies	
Ablative therapies	1 month
TACE	1 month
TARE	3 months
SBRT	3 months
Systemic therapies	
Tyrosine kinase inhibitors	1 month
Immune checkpoint inhibitors	2–3 months

(SBRT: stereotactic body radiotherapy; TACE: transarterial chemoembolization; TARE: transarterial radioembolization)

Response assessment as per mRECIST criteria is based on the percentage of necrosis, viable tumor tissue, and not on the overall tumor size shrinkage. This is because the locoregional therapies produce tumor destruction and accurate interpretation of the viable and nonviable cells would give the true picture of efficacy of the therapy in the form of complete or partial response (PR). According to the mRECIST criteria, tumor response is categorized as:

- Complete response—disappearance of any intratumoral arterial enhancement in all target lesions **(Figs. 14A to D)**
- Partial response (PR)—more than 30% decrease in sum of diameters of all viable (enhancing) target lesions **(Figs. 15A to D)**
- Progressive disease (PD)—more than 20% increase in the sum of diameters of all viable (enhancing) target lesions **(Figs. 16A to D)**
- Stable disease (SD)—any case that does not qualify for either PR or PD.[62]

If the imaging findings suggest PR or PD, then depending upon the disease stage at that point of time, the decision of further treatment is taken. When CR is achieved, the patient is kept under regular clinical and imaging follow-up.

More recently, Liver Imaging Reporting and Data System (LI-RADS) by American College of Radiology has incorporated the Treatment Response Assessment for nonradiation and radiation-based locoregional therapies **(Figs. 17 to 20)**.[64,65] Whereas mRECIST criteria are used for assessing overall patient response, LI-RADS is used for response assessment of individual tumors and is better suited for routine clinical practice. It is applicable for response assessment of pathologically proven or presumed (LR-4, LR-5, or LR-M) malignancies after locoregional treatment (ablative, transarterial, or external radiation

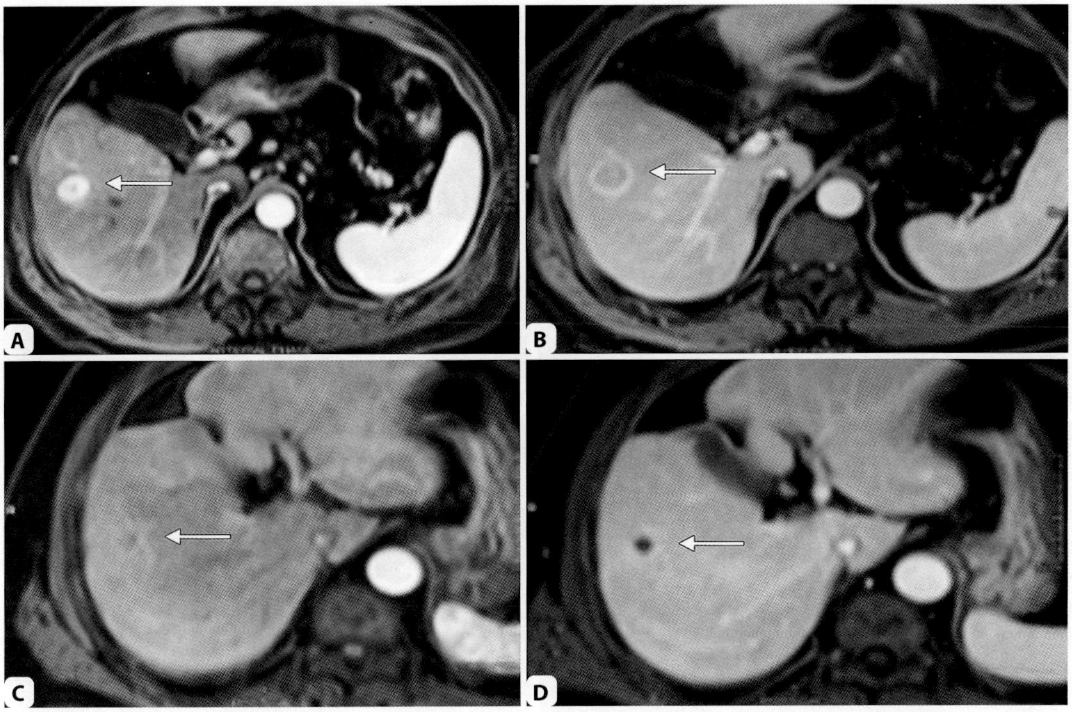

FIGS. 14A TO D: Pretreatment MRI arterial (A) and portovenous phase (B) shows lesion (arrow) with nonrim arterial phase hyperenhancement in segment V of liver with washout and enhancing capsule in the portovenous phase. Follow-up MRI arterial (C) and portovenous phase (D) 1 month after percutaneous acetic acid injection shows faint rim-enhancement in the lesion (arrows) consistent with post-treatment changes—complete response (CR) as per *mRECIST*.

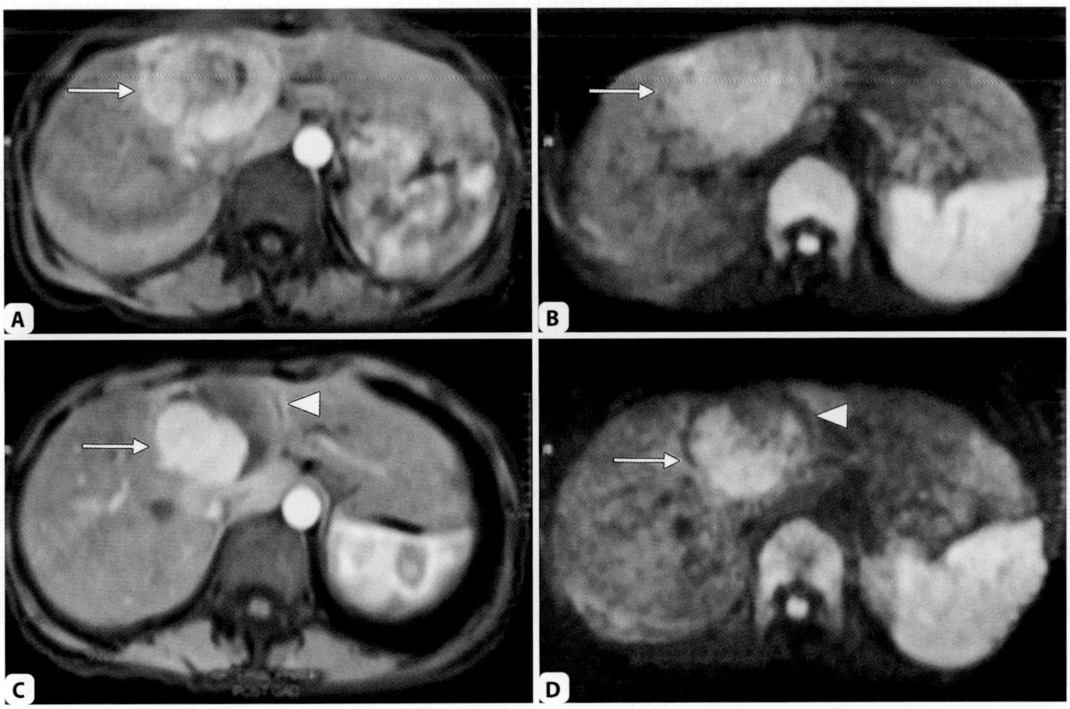

FIGS. 15A TO D: Baseline MRI arterial phase (A) and diffusion-weighted image (B) shows mass (arrow) with nonrim arterial phase hyperenhancement in segment IV of liver with moderate diffusion restriction. Follow-up MRI arterial phase (C) and diffusion-weighted image (D) 1 month after TACE shows residual arterial phase hyperenhancement and diffusion restriction in nearly half of the tumor (arrows)—viable component; rest of the tumor (arrowhead) does not show arterial phase enhancement or diffusion restriction (nonviable)—Partial response (PR) as per *mRECIST*.

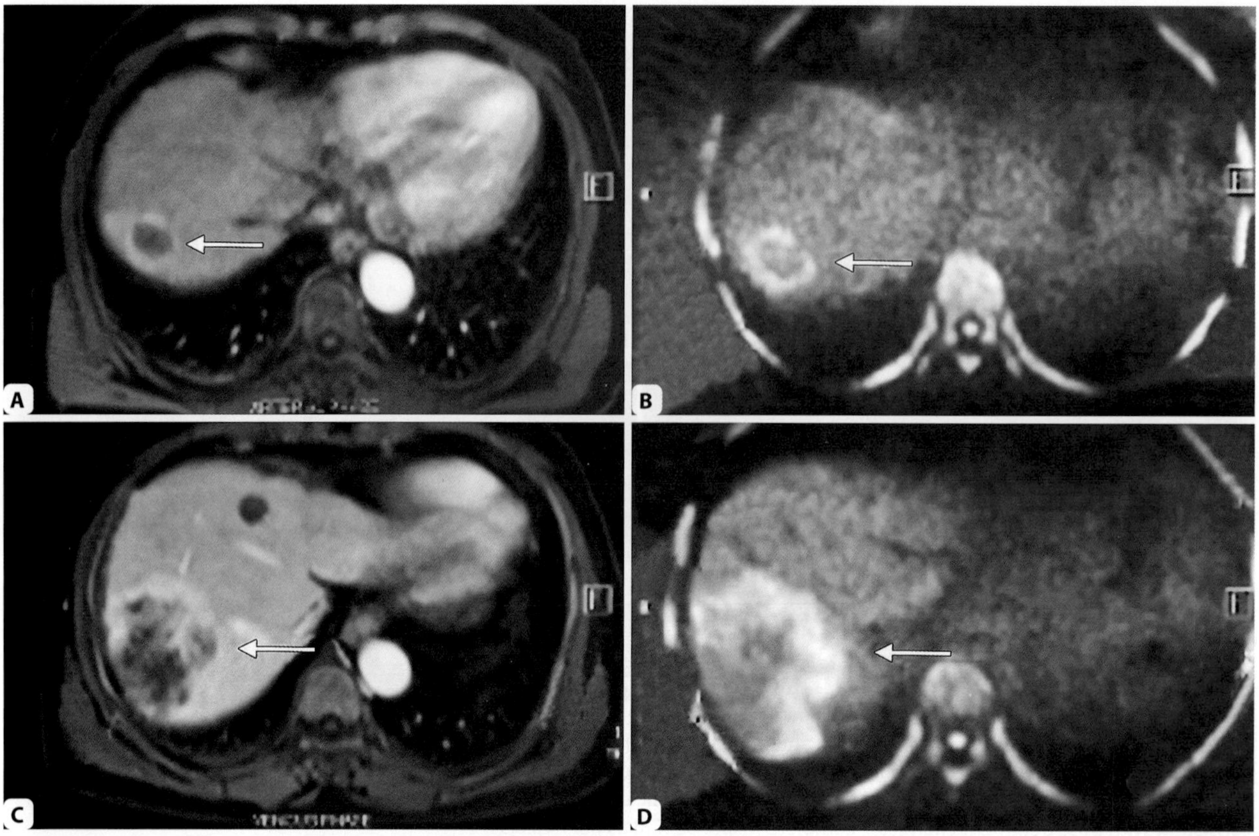

FIGS. 16A TO D: Baseline MRI arterial phase (A) and diffusion-weighted image (B) shows mass (arrow) with nodular peripheral enhancement in arterial phase and peripheral diffusion restriction in segment VII of liver. Follow-up MRI arterial phase (C) and diffusion-weighted image (D) 3 months after TACE shows increase in size of mass (arrows) with arterial phase hyperenhancement and diffusion restriction—Progressive disease (PD) as per *mRECIST*.

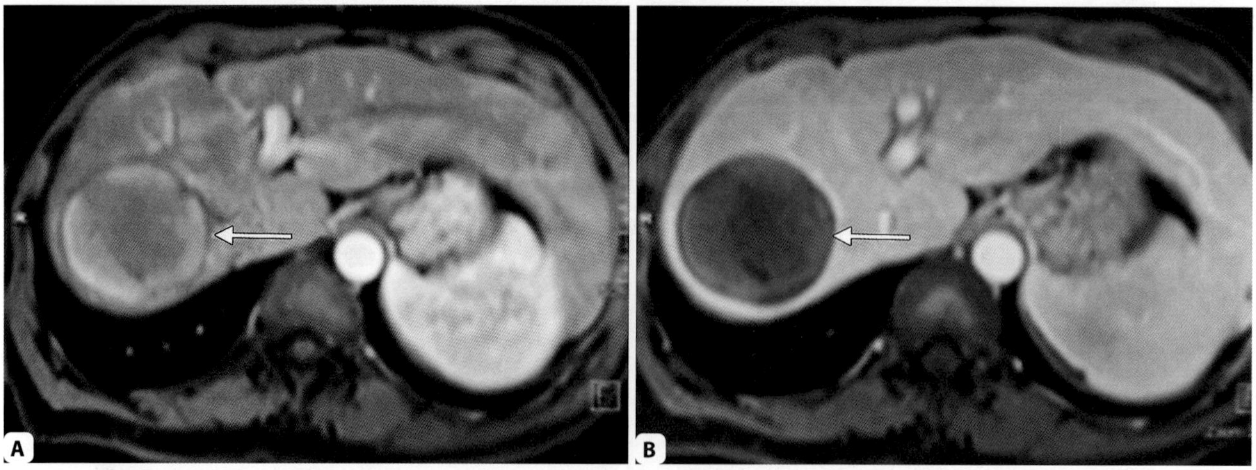

FIGS. 17A TO C: *Continued*

Continued

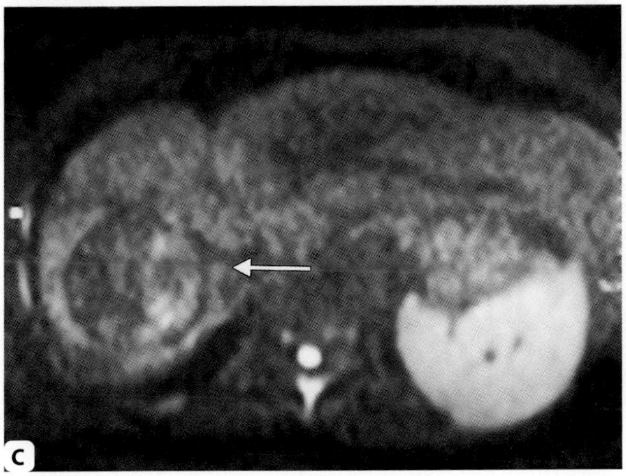

FIGS. 17A TO C: Late arterial (A), portal venous (B), and diffusion-weighted images (C) show HCC postmicrowave ablation (arrow) with thin-rim enhancement and no diffusion restriction—LR-TR nonviable.

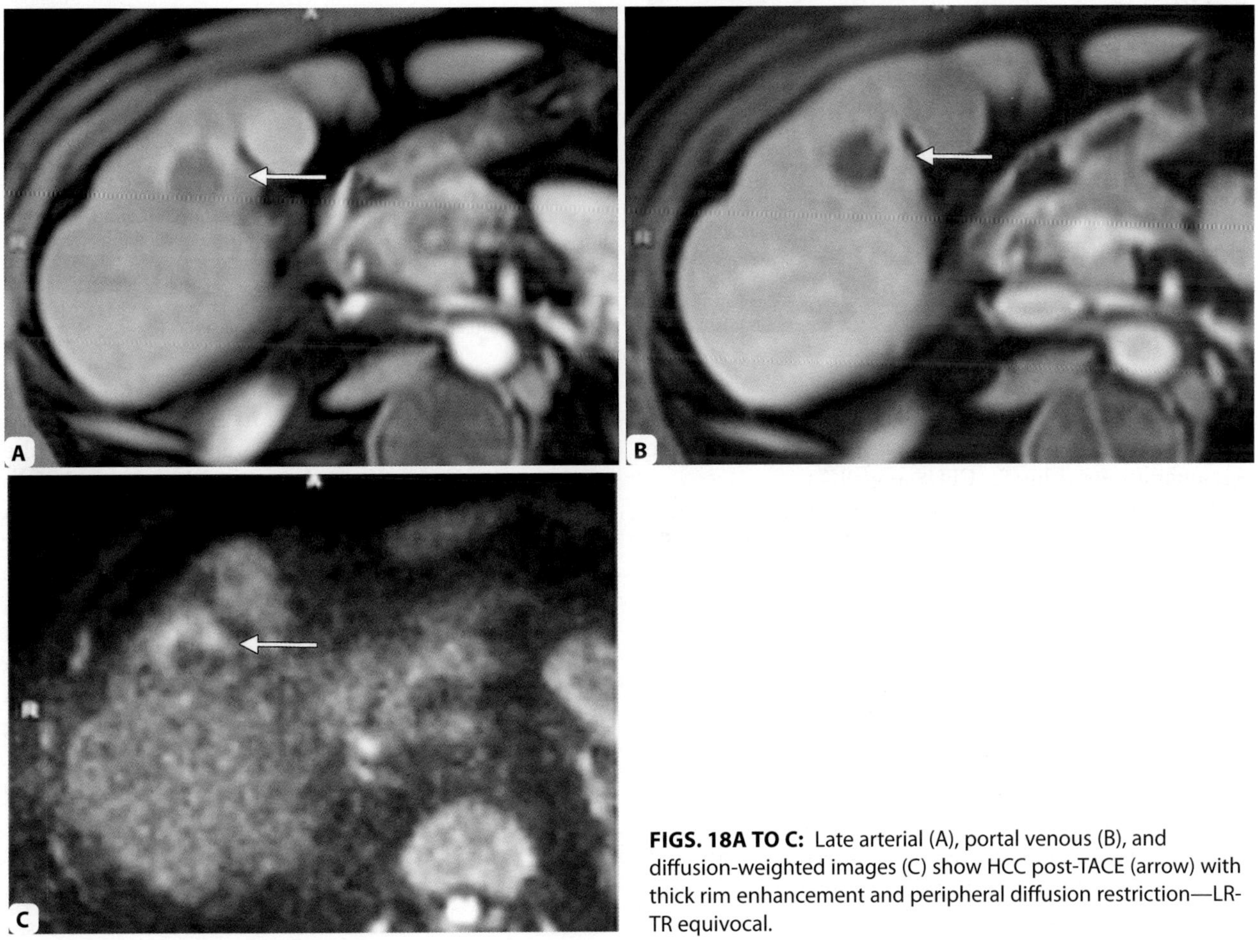

FIGS. 18A TO C: Late arterial (A), portal venous (B), and diffusion-weighted images (C) show HCC post-TACE (arrow) with thick rim enhancement and peripheral diffusion restriction—LR-TR equivocal.

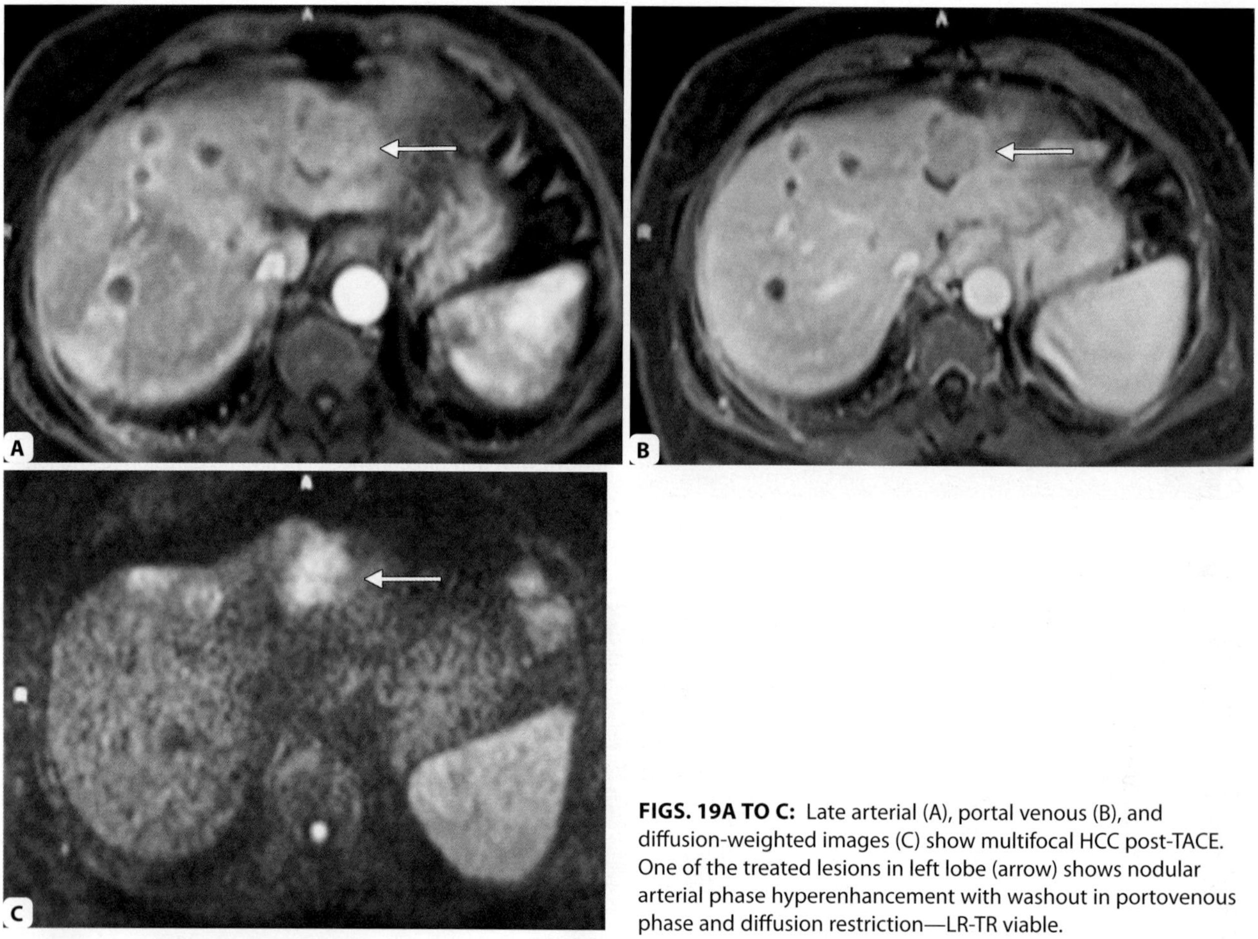

FIGS. 19A TO C: Late arterial (A), portal venous (B), and diffusion-weighted images (C) show multifocal HCC post-TACE. One of the treated lesions in left lobe (arrow) shows nodular arterial phase hyperenhancement with washout in portovenous phase and diffusion restriction—LR-TR viable.

therapy) but not for systemic therapy. It is applicable on MPCT or multiphase MRI; and in the latest update, there is a separate algorithm for CEUS as well.[66]

First step is deciding whether treatment response can be assessed (evaluable) or not (LR-TR nonevaluable in cases of image degradation due to artifacts or omission of requisite images). If evaluable, lesions are categorized as:

- LR-TR nonviable—no mass-like enhancement (complete lesion disappearance, no lesional enhancement, smooth perilesional enhancement, or parenchymal perfusion changes without mass-like enhancement)
- LR-TR equivocal—uncertainty about mass-like enhancement (presence or morphology)
- LR-TR viable—mass-like enhancement (any degree and any phase) which could be nodular, irregular peripheral, or thick rim enhancement

Presence of ancillary features (mild-moderate T2 hyperintensity or diffusion restriction) in areas of uncertain mass-like enhancement can be used to upgrade LR-TR equivocal to LR-TR viable. If unsure whether the tumor is viable or nonviable, it should be categorized as LR-TR equivocal according to the tie-breaking rule.

In contrast to nonradiation-based locoregional therapies, for radiation-based locoregional therapies, the response assessment has to be assessed over time before categorizing an observation as LR-TR viable. Also, the term LR-TR nonprogressing is used instead of LR-TR equivocal for observations with mass-like enhancement which is stable or decreased in size after radiation-based locoregional therapy. For LR-TR viable, LR-TR equivocal or LR-TR nonprogressing observations, measurement is made on any standard orthogonal imaging plane on any phase as a single dimension of enhancing tumor excluding intervening nonenhancing areas.

The LI-RADS treatment response assessment guidelines are summarized in **Flowcharts 2 to 4**.

Outcome of Chemical Ablation

PEI is highly effective in small HCCS of 3 cm size. Complete tumor response is encountered in about 80% of the cases and when the size increases to 5 cm, the CR drops to 50%.[67] In Child's A with early HCC, a 5-year survival rate of 47–53% is seen following PEI.[68] Limited studies on PAI are available. With PAI too, the response rates are better in small masses up to 3 cm. The local tumor recurrence rate is 51% at 1 year and 74% at 3 years. The survival rate at 1 and 3 years is 84%

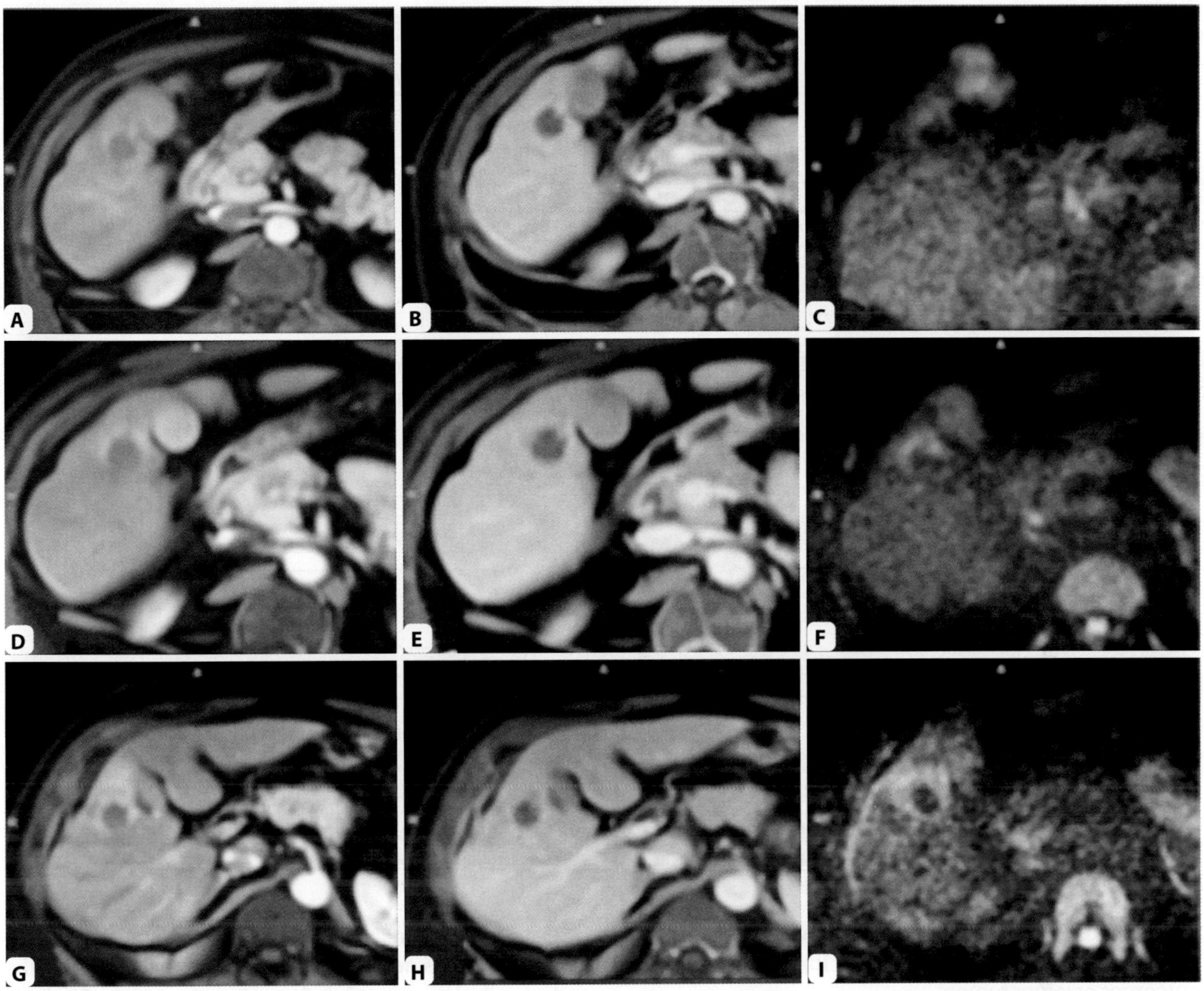

FIGS. 20A TO I: Arterial (A, D, and G), portovenous (B, E, and H), and diffusion-weighted images (C, F, and I) 1, 3, and 6 months after TACE. At 1-month follow-up (A to C), the lesion shows thin peripheral enhancement with no diffusion restriction—LR-TR nonviable. At 3-month follow-up (D to F), the lesion shows thick peripheral enhancement with some peripheral diffusion restriction—LR-TR equivocal. At 6-month follow-up (G to I), the lesion shows nodular enhancement and diffusion restriction—*LR-TR viable.*

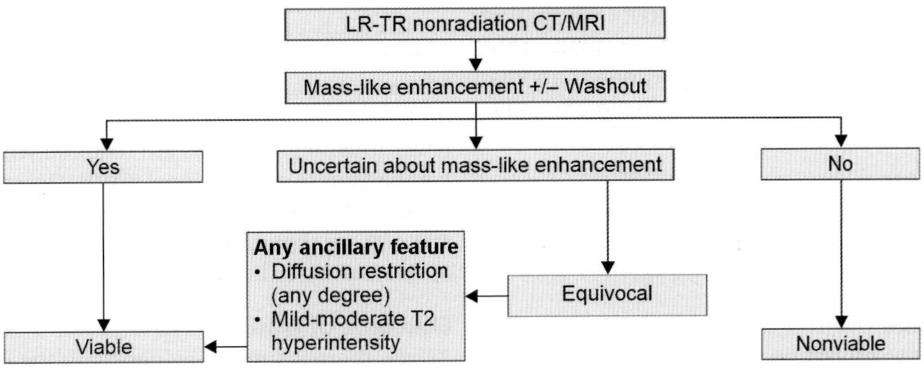

FLOWCHART 2: LI-RADS CT/MRI treatment response assessment for nonradiation-based locoregional therapies.[64]

(CT/MRI: computed tomography/magnetic resonance imaging; LI-RADS: Liver Imaging Reporting and Data System)

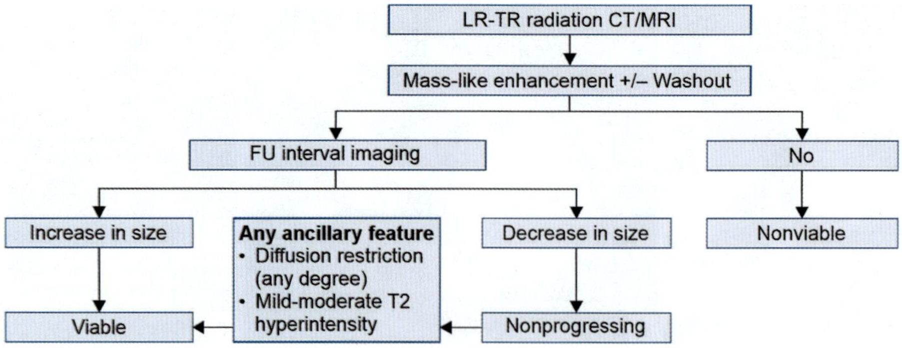

FLOWCHART 3: LI-RADS CT/MRI treatment response assessment for radiation-based locoregional therapies.[65]
(CT/MRI: computed tomography/magnetic resonance imaging; LI-RADS: Liver Imaging Reporting and Data System)

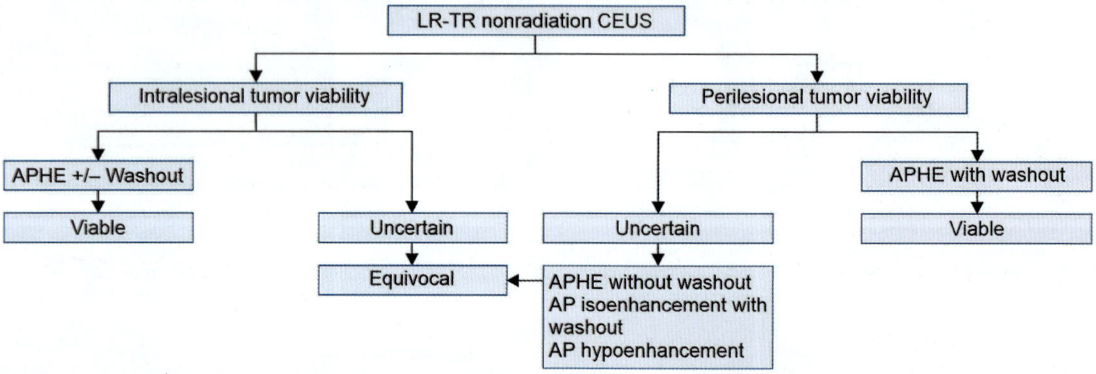

FLOWCHART 4: LI-RADS CEUS treatment response assessment for nonradiation-based locoregional therapies.[66]
(CEUS: contrast-enhanced ultrasound; LI-RADS: Liver Imaging Reporting and Data System)

and 51%, respectively.[11] Combination of PEI or PAI with other treatments is being taken up for improving treatment outcomes of larger tumors.

Outcome of RFA

Like other techniques of ablation, the tumor response depends on the size, number, and location of the tumor as well as the associated liver function. Several studies have reported complete ablation rates of 80–90% in nodules < 3 cm, 50–80% for 3–5 cm, and as low as 25% in nodules > 5 cm.[69] On comparing the outcome of RFA with surgical resection in multinodular HCC, a recent meta-analysis has shown a better survival benefit with resection than RFA; whereas in solitary small HCC of 2 cm, comparable results of RFA and resection have been observed.[70]

Outcome of MWA

MWA is also equivalent to or better than RFA, especially in larger tumors, with complete ablation rates of 98.6% in tumors < 3 cm, and 83.3% for tumors > 3 cm.[71]

Outcome of TACE

TACE is an effective procedure which produces significant tumor response and survival benefit despite tumor size in comparison to supportive care. A survival advantage of 82% and 63% for chemoembolization has been documented in comparison to 63% and 27% for supportive care at 1 and 2 years, respectively.[72,73] The largest Japanese cohort study has depicted a median survival of 34 months and a survival benefit at 1, 3, 5, and 7 years as 82%, 47%, 26%, and 16%, respectively with negligible procedure-related mortality (0.5%).[74] A study from India, TACE performed for relatively larger tumor size [up to16 cm (mean size 6.6–3.92 cm)], the cumulative survival rate at 1, 2, and 3 years was 66%, 47%, and 36.4%, respectively.[75]

Outcome of DEB-TACE

As the DEB produces slow, sustained release of the chemotherapeutic drug, the liver toxicity as well as the systemic toxicity is less. Limited literature is available on long-term follow-up. Improved local response and fewer treatment sessions are required with DEB-TACE in comparison to conventional TACE. Decreased frequency of postembolization syndrome with 100–300 mm versus 400–600 mm beads has also been documented. Less side effects leading to low hospitalization rates are seen.[76,77]

Outcome of TARE

As yet, there is limited evidence on the outcome of 90Y radioembolization in patients with unresectable HCC. The therapeutic efficacy essentially depends upon the radiation effects as opposed to the ischemia associated with chemoembolization or pure embolization. With

90Y, best outcomes occur in patients with preserved liver function (Child's A) regardless of PVT. Those with Child's B liver function and PVT, have poor outcomes.[78,79] The difference in survival between Child's A and B patients has been 17.2 months and 7.7 months; $p = 0.002$, respectively.[80] Rhenium used in one Indian multicentric trial depicted survival rates of 90.5% at 1 year and 30.5% at 3 years.[53] In India, the biggest limitation of TARE usage has been the high cost and limited availability.

Transcatheter Arterial Embolization

In this, the tumor is embolized with intra-arterial temporary or permanent embolizing materials in single or multiple sessions. It has been proved to be a less effective palliative treatment, especially for large and peripherally located HCC due to development of collateral circulation. Transcatheter arterial embolization (TAE) of the tumor may be done as an emergency procedure to reduce gastrointestinal hemorrhage in selected patients. Gastrointestinal hemorrhage from HCC during the natural course of the tumor is unusual. The causes of massive intermittent gastrointestinal bleeding may be either due to varices or due to direct invasion of duodenum **(Figs. 21A to F)**, transverse colon and stomach by the tumor. The variceal bleeding may be consequent to portal hypertension secondary to intratumoral arterioportal shunts. These patients may respond well to TAE.[80] Some studies have shown that TAE is an effective method for palliative treatment in such patients.[80,81]

Portal Vein Embolization

Percutaneous portal vein embolization is an important preoperative treatment in patients who undergo extensive liver resection due to hepatic malignancy. It is performed when FLR volume is <25% in case of normal background liver; or <40% in case of cirrhotic liver. The aim is to occlude the right portal vein either through an ipsilateral or contralateral approach using various embolizing agents such as glue, PVA particles, and coils. This results in compensatory hypertrophy of the FLR, subsequent increase in the functional reserve of the liver, and reduces the risk of postoperative hepatic failure. The procedure is done percutaneously using both ultrasound and angiography guidance. In normal livers, sufficient hypertrophy typically occurs within 2–4 weeks, whereas regeneration in patients with cirrhosis can take ≥4 weeks. This technique is mainly useful in noncirrhotic livers with malignant tumor confined to segments of one lobe **(Figs. 22A to F)**.[82]

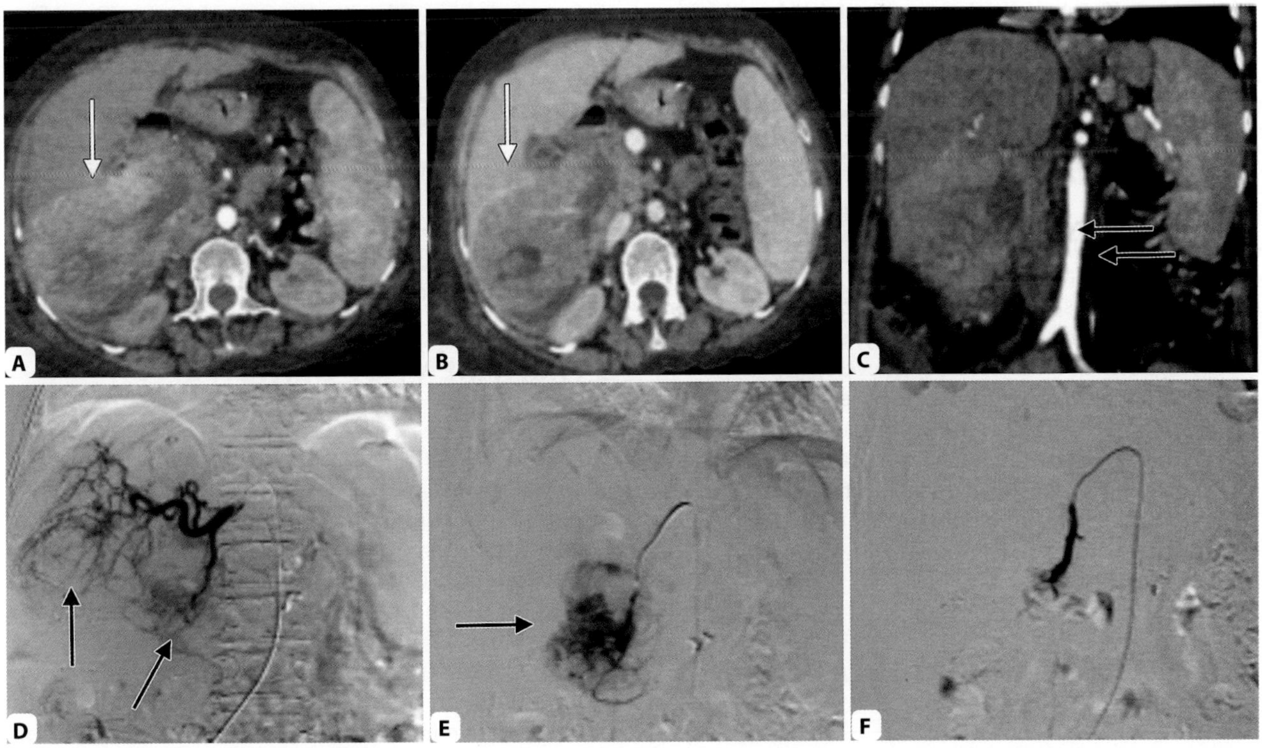

FIGS. 21A TO F: Transarterial embolization for hepatocellular carcinoma (HCC) with duodenal involvement causing melaena. (A and B) Axial CECT (contrast-enhanced computed tomography) (arterial phase A and venous phase B) shows hypervascular mass involving segments V and VI of liver (arrow). (C) Coronal reformat of arterial phase CT shows mass infiltrating second part of duodenum (arrow). (D) Common hepatic angiogram shows tumor blush (arrows) with vascular supply from right hepatic artery and gastroduodenal artery. (E) Selective run of gastroduodenal artery demonstrating tumor blush (arrow). (F) Selective run of gastroduodenal artery after embolization with 100–300 μm polyvinyl alcohol (PVA) particles demonstrating no tumor blush.

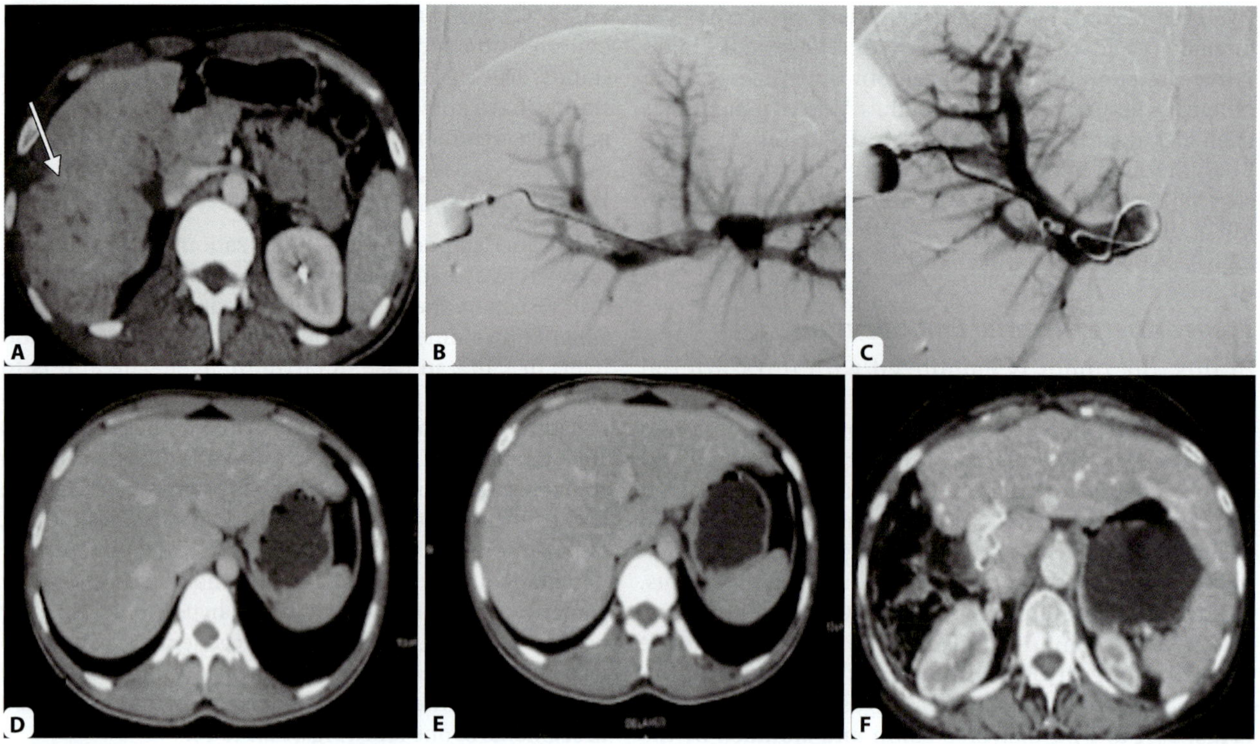

FIGS. 22A TO F: Portal vein embolization. (A) Axial CECT (contrast-enhanced computed tomography) shows large gallbladder mass invading segment V of liver (arrow) with small left lobe of liver. (B) Portography after percutaneous puncture of right branch of portal vein. (C) Selective catheterization of right branch of portal vein for embolization with n-butyl cyanoacrylate glue. (D and E) Postembolization CT after 4 weeks shows improved volume of left lobe of liver. (F) Postright hepatectomy CT shows good volume of residual left lobe of liver.

Hepatic Vein Stenting with Transarterial Chemoembolization

The association of Budd–Chiari syndrome and HCC is favored by two conditions. First, HCC can cause obstruction of the main hepatic veins or inferior vena cava due to endoluminal invasion by the tumor. This produces an acute or fulminant variant of Budd–Chiari syndrome, which has a poor prognosis. Secondly, HCC can develop in patients with chronic Budd–Chiari syndrome; these account for 0.7% of all the cases of HCC. HCC is most common in patients with membranous obstruction of the vena cava. These patients can be managed effectively by combined interventional techniques; hepatic vein stenting or IVC dilatation to relieve the venous obstruction combined with TACE for the HCC **(Figs. 23A to F)**.

TREATMENT OF METASTATIC DISEASES OF LIVER

Short of surgery, such as HCC, interventional techniques of ablation (commonly RFA and MWA) **(Figs. 24A to F)**, and intra-arterial chemotherapy, is the standard treatment recommended for metastases to the liver.[83] Transarterial administration of anticancer drugs (doxorubicin, cisplatin, 5-FU, mitomycin C, and irinotecan), either alone or as hepatic arterial infusion (HAI), or combined with embolization of feeding artery (TACE) **(Figs. 25A to F)** or bland vascular embolization (TAE) is used. TARE with rhenium-188-HDD-lipiodol has also been used in the management of intrahepatic metastases such as from colorectal primaries **(Figs. 26A to F)**.[84-86]

TREATMENT OF BENIGN LIVER TUMORS

Interventional treatment with bland transarterial embolization with particulate embolic agents may be done for benign hepatic tumors such as hemangiomas, focal nodular hyperplasia, or hepatic adenoma. Various studies have shown that TAE of hepatic cavernous hemangioma is a useful procedure in the therapy of symptomatic hemangiomas.[87-89] Indications for embolization of benign hepatic tumors include symptomatic cases (patients with pain, fever, pressure symptoms, breathlessness, and obstructive jaundice), Kasabach–Merritt syndrome (consumptive thrombocytopenia in association with hemangiomas), spontaneous rupture of tumor (hepatic adenomas have highest propensity for hemorrhage and rupture), portal hypertension due to arterioportal fistula or pressure effect on portal vein, and preoperative embolization to reduce intraoperative blood loss **(Figs. 27A to F)**.

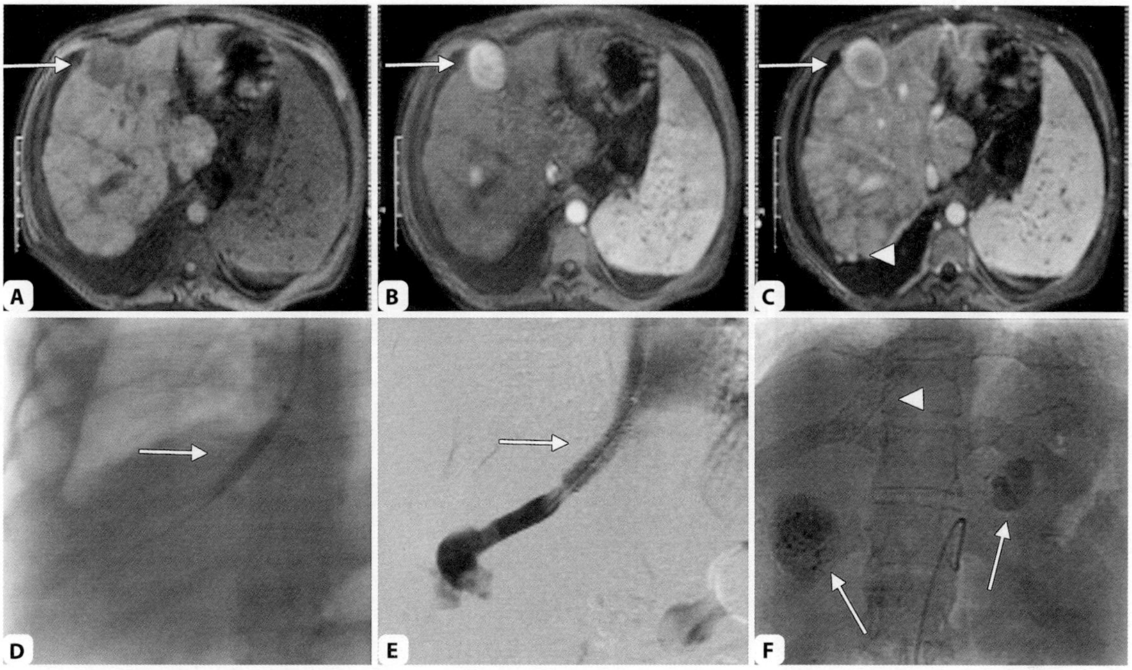

FIGS. 23A TO F: Hepatic vein stenting. (A) Axial precontrast T1W fat-suppressed shows hypointense lesion in liver (arrow). (B) Lesion shows nonrim arterial phase hyperenhancement (arrow). (C) On venous phase, the lesion shows nonperipheral washout (arrow). Background liver shows heterogeneous parenchymal enhancement with nonvisualization of right hepatic venous ostium and surface collaterals over right lobe of liver (arrowhead) indicative of hepatic venous outflow tract obstruction. (D) Initially, balloon angioplasty of right hepatic vein (arrow) was done. (E) Deployment of balloon-mounted stent in right hepatic vein (arrow). (F) Subsequently, TACE was done; fluoroscopic spot image shows lipiodol deposition in HCC in both lobes of liver (arrows) with right hepatic vein stent (arrowhead).

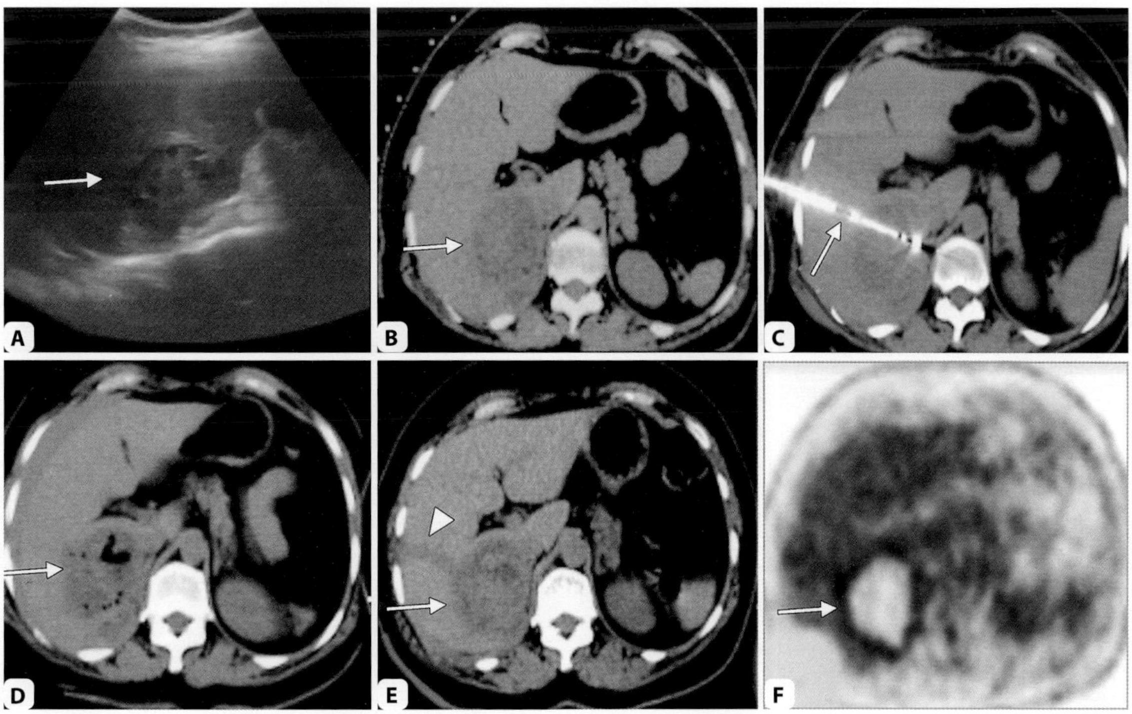

FIGS. 24A TO F: CT-guided microwave ablation (MWA) for hepatic metastasis from neuroendocrine tumor. (A) Ultrasound shows heteroechoic mass in right lobe of liver (arrow). (B) Noncontrast computed tomography (NCCT) showing hypodense mass (arrow) in segment VI of liver. (C) CT-guided placement of microwave antenna (arrow) in the mass. (D) Postablation CT showing air foci within the mass (arrow) and mild hemoperitoneum (asterisk). (E) Follow-up NCCT showing ablation tract (arrowhead) and mass in right lobe (arrow). (F) Follow-up PET-CT shows only peripheral uptake in mass (arrow) consistent with postablation changes.

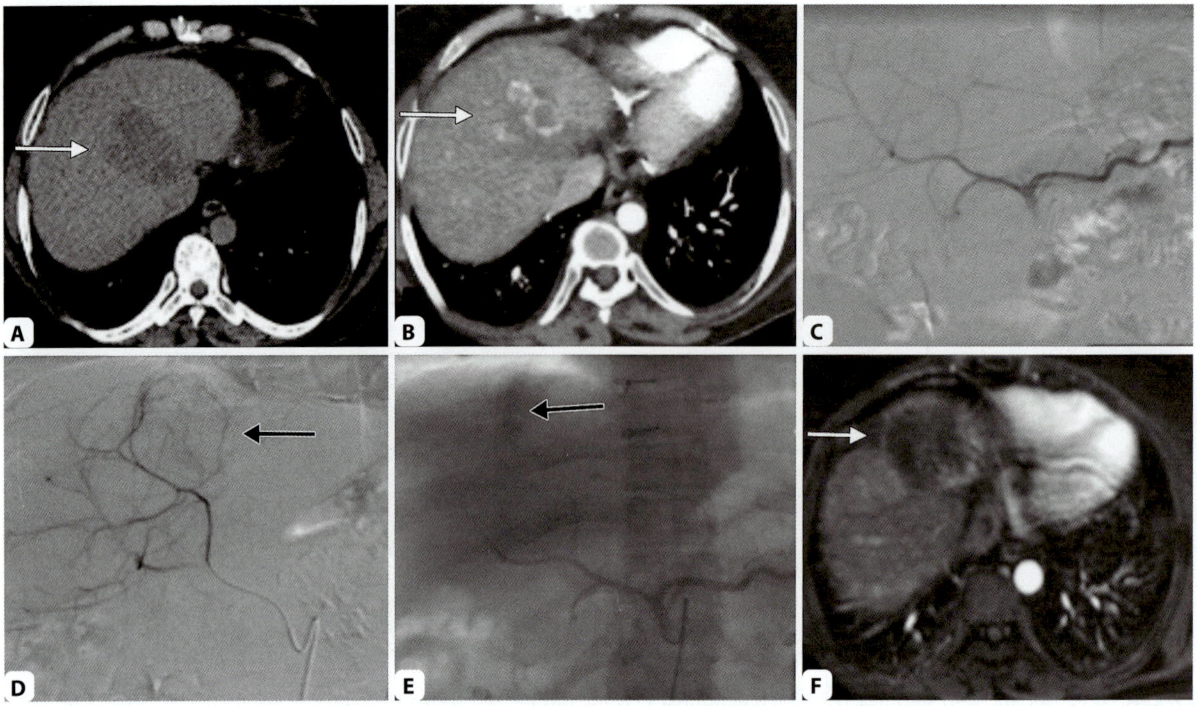

FIGS. 25A TO F: TACE (transarterial chemoembolization) for metastatic germ cell tumor. (A) Axial noncontrast computed tomography (NCCT) showing hypodense lesion in segment IVa of liver (arrow). (B) Arterial phase CT showing rim enhancement in hepatic lesion (arrow). (C) Celiac angiogram (D) hepatic angiogram showing tumor blush (arrow) from left hepatic arterial branches (E) Postembolization run showing lipiodol deposition in the tumor (arrow). (F) Follow-up MRI after 1 month showing no residual enhancement within the tumor (arrow).

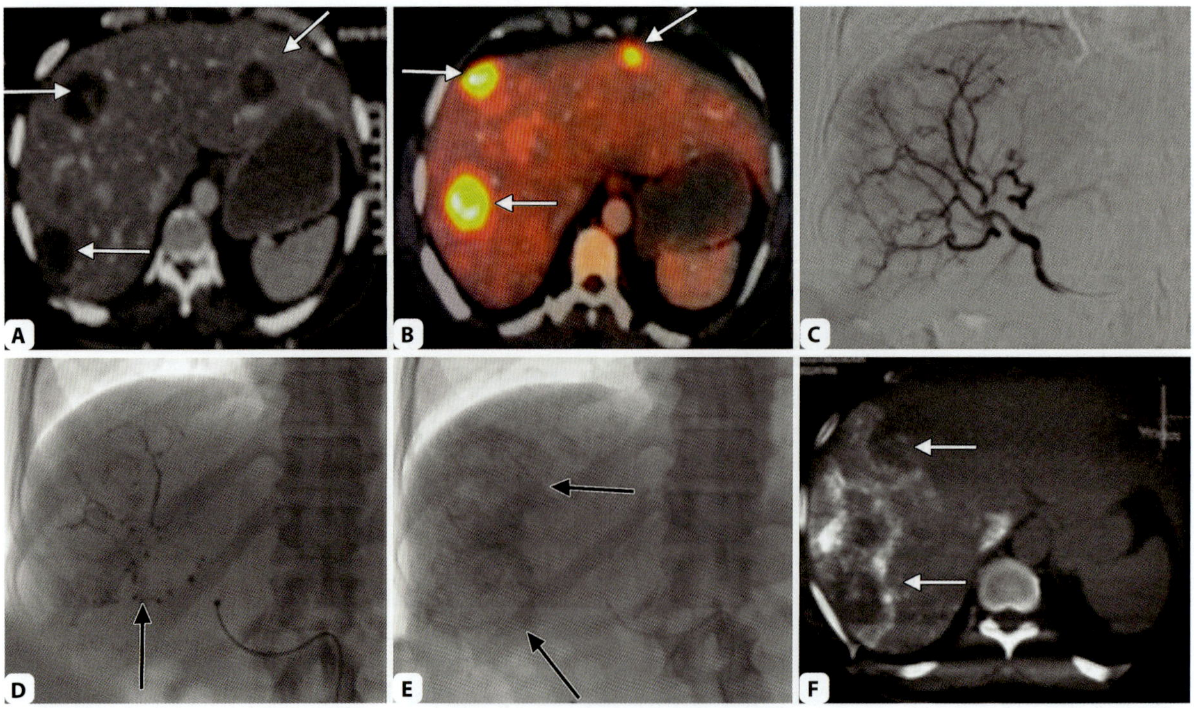

FIGS. 26A TO F: Transarterial radioembolization (TARE) for liver metastases from colorectal carcinoma. (A) Axial CECT (contrast-enhanced computed tomography) shows multiple hypoenhancing liver metastases in both lobes of liver (arrows). (B) PET-CT shows avid FDG uptake by the liver metastases (arrows). (C) Selective catheterization of right hepatic artery. (D) Injection of rhenium-188 microspheres and lipiodol (arrow) into the right hepatic artery. (E) Postembolization deposition of lipiodol in colorectal metastases (arrows). (F) Cone-beam CT showing good lipiodol deposition in the hepatic metastases (arrows).

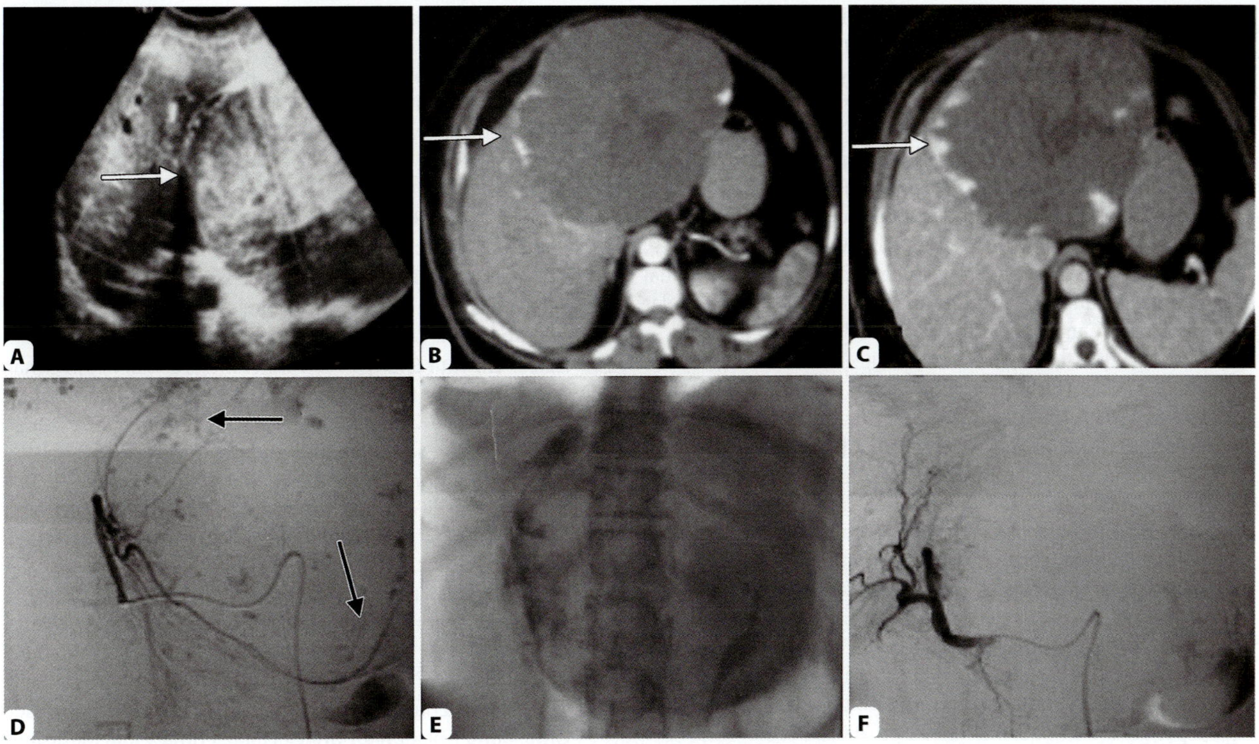

FIGS. 27A TO F: Preoperative embolization of symptomatic giant hemangioma. (A) Ultrasound showing hyperechoic mass in left lobe of liver (arrow). (B) Arterial phase CT showing mass (arrow) with discontinuous peripheral nodular enhancement. (C) Progressive fill-in of mass (arrow) on portal venous phase; enhancing component is isoattenuating to the blood pool. (D) Left hepatic angiogram shows vascular feeders to hemangioma (arrows). (E) Embolization of left hepatic artery branches with 100–300 µm PVA particles. (F) Postembolization run of common hepatic artery shows devascularization of hemangioma.

CONCLUSION

Radiological interventions are established procedures and recommended therapeutic options for liver tumors. A variety of locoregional therapies are available which can be used in isolation or as a part of combination therapy. Treatment is based upon the clinical presentation, stage of the disease, liver function, and the performance status of the patient and varies from case to case. Decision and execution of treatment is a teamwork which aims at providing maximum patient benefit.

REFERENCES

1. International Agency for Research on Cancer: World Health Organization. (2012). GLOBOCAN 2012: Estimated cancer incidence, mortality, and prevalence worldwide in 2012. [online] available from https://www.iarc.who.int/news-events/latest-world-cancer-statistics-globocan-2012-estimated-cancer-incidence-mortality-and-prevalence-worldwide-in-2012/ [Last accessed July, 2024].
2. Lencioni R, Crocetti L, Cioni D, Della Pina C, Bartolozzi C. Percutaneous radiofrequency ablation of hepatic colorectal metastases: Technique, indications, results, and new promises. Invest Radiol. 2004;39:689-97.
3. European Association For The Study Of The Liver; European Organisation For Research And Treatment Of Cancer. EASL-EORTC clinical practice guidelines: management of hepatocellular carcinoma. J Hepatol. 2012;56:908-43.
4. Ikeda M, Mitsunaga S, Shimizu S, Ohno I, Takahashi H, Okuyama H, et al. Current status of hepatocellular carcinoma in Japan. Chin Clin Oncol. 2013;2(4):40.
5. Reig M, Forner A, Rimola J, Ferrer-Fàbrega J, Burrel M, Garcia-Criado Á, et al. BCLC strategy for prognosis prediction and treatment recommendation: The 2022 update. J Hepatol. 2022;76(3):681-93.
6. Livraghi T, Bolondi L, Buscarini L, Cottone M, Mazziotti A, Morabito A, et al. No treatment, resection and ethanol injection in hepatocellular carcinoma: a retrospective analysis of survival in 391 patients with cirrhosis. Italian Cooperative HCC Study Group. J Hepatol. 1995;22:522-6.
7. Foltz G. Image guided percutaneous ablation of hepatic malignancies. Semin Intervent Radiol. 2014;31:180-6.
8. Clark TW, Soulen MC. Chemical ablation of hepatocellular carcinoma. J Vasc Interv Radiol. 2002;13(9 Pt 2):S245-52.
9. Kapoor V, Thaete FL. Percutaneous ethanol and acetic acid ablation of hepatocellular carcinoma. In: Carr BI (Ed). Hepatocellular Cancer. Publisher: United States: Humana Press; 2005. pp. 153-69.

10. Ohnishi K, Nomura F, Ito S, Fujiwara K. Prognosis of small hepatocellular carcinoma (less than 3 cm) after percutaneous acetic acid injection: study of 91 cases. Hepatology. 1996;23: 994-102.
11. Huo TI, Hiang YH, Wu JC, Lee PC, Chang FY, Lee SD. Comparison of percutaneous and acid injection and percutaneous ethanol injection for hepatocellular carcinoma in cirrhotic patients. A prospective study. Scand J Gastroenterol. 2003;7:770-8.
12. Rossi S, Di Stasi M, Buscarini E, Cavanna L, Quaretti P, Squassante E, et al. Percutaneous radiofrequency interstitial thermal ablation in the treatment of small hepatocellular carcinoma. Cancer J Sci Am. 1995;1(1):73-81.
13. McGahan JP, Gu WZ, Brock JM, Tesluk H, Jones CD. Hepatic ablation using bipolar radiofrequency electrocautery. Acad Radiol. 1996;3:418-22.
14. Goldberg SN, Grassi CJ, Cardella JF, Charboneau JW, Dodd GD 3rd, Dupuy DE, et al. Society of Interventional Radiology Technology Assessment Committee and the International Working Group on Image-guided Tumor Ablation. Image-guided tumor ablation: standardization of terminology and reporting criteria. J Vasc Interv Radiol. 2009;20 (Suppl 7):S377-90.
15. Seror O, N'kontchou G, Ibraheem M, Ajayon Y, Barrucand C, Ganne N, et al. Large (> = 5.0 – cm) HCCs: Multipolar RF Ablation with Three Internally Cooled Bipolar Electrodes–Initial experience in 26 patients. Radiology. 2008;248(1):288-96.
16. Yang W, Yan K, Wu GX, Wu W, Fu Y, Lee JC, et al. Radiofrequency ablation of hepatocellular carcinoma in difficult locations: Strategies and long-term outcomes. World J Gastroenterol. 2015;21(5):1554-66.
17. Livraghi T, Solbiati L, Meloni MF, Gazelle GS, Halpern EF, Goldberg SN. Treatment of focal liver tumors with percutaneous radiofrequency ablation: complications encountered in a multicenter study. Radiology. 2003;226:441-51.
18. Lahat E, Eshkenazy R, Zendel A, Zakai BB, Maor M, Dreznik Y, Ariche A. Complications after percutaneous ablation of liver tumors: A systematic review. Hepatobiliary Surg Nutr. 2014;3(5): 317-23.
19. Sheta E, El-Kalla F, El-Gharib M, Kobtan A, Elhendawy M, Abd- Elsalam S, et al. Comparison of single-session transarterial chemoembolization combined with microwave ablation or radiofrequency ablation in the treatment of hepatocellular carcinoma: a randomized-controlled study. Eur J Gastroenterol Hepatol; 2016;28(10):1198-203.
20. Poch FG, Rieder C, Ballhausen H, Knappe V, Ritz JP, Gemeinhardt O, et al. The vascular cooling effect in hepatic multipolar radiofrequency ablation leads to incomplete ablation ex vivo. Int J Hyperthermia. 2016;32(7):749-56.
21. Meloni MF, Chiang J, Laeseke PF, Dietrich CF, Sannino A, Solbiati M, et al. Microwave ablation in primary and secondary liver tumours: Technical and clinical approaches. Int J Hyperthermia. 2016;33(1):15-24.
22. Lubner MG, Brace CL, Ziemlewicz TJ, Hinshaw JL, Lee FT Jr. Microwave ablation of hepatic malignancy. Semin Intervent Radiol. 2013;30(1):56-66.
23. Gala KB, Shetty NS, Patel P, Kulkarni SS. Microwave ablation: How we do it? Indian J Radiol Imaging. 2020;30(2):206-13.
24. Ramalingam R, Mukund A, Anandpara KM, Patidar Y, Sarin SK. Comparative Analysis of Radiofrequency Ablation and Microwave Ablation for Critically Located Hepatocellular Carcinomas Smaller than 5 cm. J Clin Interv Radiol ISVIR. 2021;5(01):22-8.
25. Pusceddu C, Mascia L, Ninniri C, Ballicu N, Zedda S, Melis L, et al. The Increasing Role of CT-Guided Cryoablation for the Treatment of Liver Cancer: A Single-Center Report. Cancers (Basel). 2022;14(12):3018.
26. Aghayev A, Tatli S. The use of cryoablation in treating liver tumors. Expert Rev Med Devices. 2014;11(1):41-52.
27. Song KD. Percutaneous cryoablation for hepatocellular carcinoma. Clin Mol Hepatol. 2016;22(4):509-15.
28. Ní Eochagáin A. Cryoshock following cryoablation for hepatocellular carcinoma. J Clin Anesth. 2022;77:110641.
29. Glazer DI, Tatli S, Shyn PB, Vangel MG, Tuncali K, Silverman SG. Percutaneous Image-Guided Cryoablation of Hepatic Tumors: Single-Center Experience With Intermediate to Long-Term Outcomes. AJR Am J Roentgenol. 2017;209(6):1381-9.
30. Ratanaprasatporn L, Sainani N, Duda JB, Aghayev A, Tatli S, Silverman SG, et al. Imaging findings during and after percutaneous cryoablation of hepatic tumors. Abdom Radiol (NY). 2019;44(7):2602-26.
31. NG KK, Poon RT, Chang SC, Chok KS, Cheung TT, Tung H, et al. High-intensity focused ultrasound for hepatocellular carcinoma: A single center experience. Ann Surg. 2011;253:981-87.
32. Ji Y, Zhu J, Zhu L, Zhu Y, Zhao H. High-Intensity Focused Ultrasound Ablation for Unresectable Primary and Metastatic Liver Cancer: Real-World Research in a Chinese Tertiary Center With 275 Cases. Front Oncol. 2020;10:519164.
33. Pacella CM, Breschi L, Bottacci D, Masotti L. Liver tumors laser ablation. Image-Guid. Laser Ablation. 2020:31-44.
34. Pacella CM, Bizzarri G, Francica G, Bianchini A, De Nuntis S, Pacella S, et al. Percutaneous laser ablation in the treatment of hepatocellular carcinoma with small tumors: analysis of factors affecting the achievement of tumor necrosis. J Vasc Interv Radiol. 2005;16(11):1447-57.
35. Sartori S, Di Vece F, Ermili F, Tombesi P. Laser ablation of liver tumors: An ancillary technique, or an alternative to radiofrequency and microwave? World J Radiol. 2017;9(3):91-6.
36. Gough-Palmer AL, Gedroyc WM. Laser ablation of hepatocellular carcinoma—a review. World J Gastroenterol. 2008;14(47):7170-4.
37. Silk M, Tahour D, Srimathveeravalli G, Solomon SB, Thornton RH. The state of irreversible electroporation in interventional oncology. Semin Intervent Radiol. 2014;31(2):111-7.
38. Meijerink MR, Ruarus AH, Vroomen LGPH, Puijk RS, Geboers B, Nieuwenhuizen S, et al. Irreversible Electroporation to Treat Unresectable Colorectal Liver Metastases (COLDFIRE-2): A Phase II, Two-Center, Single-Arm Clinical Trial. Radiology. 2021;299(2):470-80.
39. Narayanan G, Froud T, Suthar R, Barbery K. Irreversible electroporation of hepatic malignancy. Semin Intervent Radiol. 2013;30(1):67-73.
40. Padia SA, Johnson GE, Yeung RS, Park JO, Hippe DS, Kogut MJ. Irreversible Electroporation in Patients with Hepatocellular Carcinoma: Immediate versus Delayed Findings at MR Imaging. Radiology. 2016;278(1):285-94.
41. Tsochatzis EA, Germani G, Burroughs AK. Transarterial chemoembolization, transarterial chemotherapy, and intra-arterial chemotherapy for hepatocellular carcinoma treatment. Semin Oncol. 2010;37(2):89-93.

42. Davis CR. Interventional radiological treatment of hepatocellular carcinoma. Cancer Control. 2010;17(1):87-99.
43. Ramsey DE, Geschwind JH. New interventions for liver tumors. Semin Roentgenology. 2002;37:303-11.
44. Jiang JF, Lao YC, Yuan BH, Yin J, Liu X, Chen L, et al. Treatment of hepatocellular carcinoma with portal vein tumor thrombus: Advances and challenges. Oncotarget. 2017;8(20):33911-21.
45. Müller L, Stoehr F, Mähringer-Kunz A, Hahn F, Weinmann A, Kloeckner R. Current Strategies to Identify Patients That Will Benefit from TACE Treatment and Future Directions a Practical Step-by-Step Guide. J Hepatocell Carcinoma. 2021;8:403-19.
46. Korean Liver Cancer Association; National Cancer Center. 2018 Korean Liver Cancer Association-National Cancer Center Korea Practice Guidelines for the Management of HCC. Gut Liver. 2019;13(3):227-99.
47. Cho Y, Choi JW, Kwon H, Kim KY, Lee BC, Chu HH, et al. Research Committee of the Korean Liver Cancer Association. Transarterial Chemoembolization for Hepatocellular Carcinoma: 2023 Expert Consensus-Based Practical Recommendations of the Korean Liver Cancer Association. Korean J Radiol. 2023;24(7):606-25.
48. Horikawa M, Miyayama S, Irie T, Kaji T, Arai Y. Development of Conventional Transarterial Chemoembolization for Hepatocellular Carcinomas in Japan: Historical, Strategic, and Technical Review. AJR Am J Roentgenol. 2015;205(4):764-73.
49. Miyayama S, Matsui O, Yamashiro M, Ryu Y, Kaito K, Ozaki K, et al. Ultraselective transcatheter arterial chemoemboliza-tion with a 2-f tip microcatheter for small hepatocellular carcinomas: relationship between local tumor recurrence and visualization of the portal vein with iodized oil. J Vasc Interv Radiol. 2007;18(3):365-76.
50. Moustafa AS, Abdel Aal AK, Ertel N, Saad N, DuBay D, Saddekni S. Chemoembolization of Hepatocellular Carcinoma with Extrahepatic Collateral Blood Supply: Anatomic and Technical Considerations. Radiographics. 2017;37(3):963-77.
51. Lee HN, Hyun D. Complications Related to Transarterial Treatment of Hepatocellular Carcinoma: A Comprehensive Review. Korean J Radiol. 2023;24(3):204-23.
52. Carter S, Martin Ii RC. Drug-eluting bead therapy in primary and metastatic disease of the liver. HPB (Oxford). 2009;11: 541-50.
53. Kumar A, Srivastava DN, Chau TTM, Long HD, Bal C, Chandra P, et al. Inoperable hepatocellular carcinoma: transarterial188 Re HDD-Labeled iodized oil for treatment—Prospective multicenter trial. Radiology. 2007;243:509-19.
54. Miller FH, Lopes Vendrami C, Gabr A, Horowitz JM, Kelahan LC, Riaz A, et al. Evolution of Radioembolization in Treatment of Hepatocellular Carcinoma: A Pictorial Review. Radiographics. 2021;41(6):1802-18.
55. Yamakado K, Nakatsuka A, Ohmori S, Ikoma J, Adachi Y, Takeda K, et al. Radiofrequency ablation combined with chemoembolization in hepatocellular carcinoma treatment response based on tumor size and morphology. J Vasc Interv Radiol. 2002;13:1225-32.
56. Yang M, Yuan JQ, Bai M, Han GH. Transarterial chemoembolization combined with sorafenib for unresectable hepatocellular carcinoma: a systematic review and meta- analysis. Mol Biol Rep. 2014;41:6575-82.
57. Lee JM, Yoon JH, Joo I, Woo HS. Recent advances in CT and MR imaging for evaluation of hepatocellular carcinoma. Liver Cancer. 2012;1:22-40.
58. Minami Y, Kudo M. Therapeutic response assessment of transcatheter arterial chemoembolization for hepatocellular carcinoma: ultrasonography, CT and MR imaging. Oncology. 2013;84(Suppl 1):58-63.
59. Guan YS, Sun L, Zhou X-P, Li X, Zheng XH. Hepatocellular carcinoma treated with interventional procedures: CT and MRI follow-up. World J Gastroenterol. 2004;10:3543-8.
60. Yuan Z, Li WT, Ye XD, Peng WJ, Xiao XS. Utility of diffusion-weighted imaging to assess hepatocellular carcinoma viability following transarterial chemoembolization. Oncol Lett. 2014; 8:831-6.
61. Liu M, Lin MX, Lu MD, Xu ZF, Zheng KG, Wang W, et al. Comparison of contrast-enhanced ultrasound and contrast-enhanced computed tomography in evaluating the treatment response to transcatheter arterial chemoembolization of hepatocellular carcinoma using modified RECIST. Eur Radiol. 2015;25:2502-11.
62. Riccardo Lencioni R, Llovet JM. Modified RECIST (mRECIST) Assessment for Hepatocellular Carcinoma. Semin Liver Dis. 2010;30:52-60.
63. Kumar A, Acharya SK, Singh SP, Duseja A, Madan K, Shukla A, et al. 2023 Update of Indian National Association for Study of the Liver Consensus on Management of Intermediate and Advanced Hepatocellular Carcinoma: The Puri III Recommendations. J Clin Exp Hepatol. 2024;14(1):101269.
64. American College of Radiology. (2024) LI-RADS® CT/MRI Nonradiation TRA v2024 Core. [online] Available from: https://www.acr.org/-/media/ACR/Files/RADS/LI-RADS/LI-RADS-CTMR-Nonradiation-TRA-v2024-Core.pdf [Last accessed July, 2024].
65. American College of Radiology. (2024). LI-RADS® CT/MRI Radiation TRA v2024 Core. [online] Available from: https://www.acr.org/-/media/ACR/Files/RADS/LI-RADS/LI-RADS-CTMR-Radiation-TRA-v2024-Core.pdf [Last accessed July, 2024].
66. American College of Radiology. (2024). LI-RADS® CEUS Nonradiation TRA v2024 Core. [online]. Available from: https://www.acr.org/-/media/ACR/Files/RADS/LI-RADS/LI-RADS-CEUS-Nonradiation-TRA-v2024-Core.pdf [Last accessed July, 2024].
67. Vilana R, Bruix J, Bru C, Ayuso C, Sole M, Rodes J. Tumor size determines the efficacy of percutaneous ethanol injection for the treatment of small hepatocellular carcinoma. Hepatology. 1992;16:353-7.
68. Lencioni R. Locoregional treatment of hepatocellular carcinoma. Hepatology. 2010;52:762-73.
69. Cucchetti A, Piscaglia F, Cescon M, Ercolani G, Pinna AD. Systematic review of surgical resection versus radiofrequency ablation for hepatocellular carcinoma. World J Gastroenterol. 2013;19:4106-18.
70. Duan C, Liu m, Zhang Z, Ma K, Bie P. Radiofrequency ablation versus hepatic resection for the treatment of early stage hepatocellular carcinoma meeting Milan criteria: a systematic review and meta-analysis. World J Surgl Oncol. 2013;11:190.
71. Chung JC, Naik NK, Lewandowski RJ, Deng J, Mulcahy MF, Kulik LM, et al. Diffusion-weighted magnetic resonance imaging to predict response of hepatocellular carcinoma to chemoembolization. World J Gastroenterol. 2010;16(25):3161-7.

72. Llovet JM, Bruix J. Systematic review of randomized trials for unresectable hepatocellular carcinoma: Chemoembolization improves survival. Hepatology. 2003;37:429-42.
73. Yamada R, Sato M, Kawabata M, Nakatsuka H, Nakamura K, Takashima S. Hepatic artery embolization in 120 patients with unresectable hepatoma. Radiology. 1983;148:397-401.
74. Takayasu K, Arii S, Ikai I, et al. Prospective cohort study of trans-arterial chemoembolization for unresectable hepatocellular carcinoma in 8510 patients. Gastroenterology. 2006;131:461-9.
75. Paul SB, Gamanagatti S, Sreenivas V, Chandrashekhara SH, Mukund A, Gulati MS, et al. Trans-arterial chemoembolization in patients with unresectable hepatocellular carcinoma: experience from a tertiary care centre in India. Indian J Radiol Imaging. 2011;21:113-20.
76. Lammer J, Malagari K, Vogl T, Pilleul F, Denys A, Watkinson A, et al. Prospective randomized study of doxorubicin-eluting-bead embolization in the treatment of hepatocellular carcinoma: results of the PRECISION V study. Cardiovasc Interv Radiol. 2010;33:41-52.
77. Prajapati HJ, Dhanasekaran R, El-Rayes BF, Kauh JS, Maithel SK, Chen Z, et al. Safety and efficacy of doxorubicin drug-eluting bead transarterial chemoembolization in patients with advanced hepatocellular carcinoma. J Vasc Interv Radiol. 2013;24:307-15.
78. Geschwind JF, Salem R, Carr BI, Soulen MC, Thurston KG, Goin KA, et al. Yttrium-90 microspheres for the treatment of hepato-cellular carcinoma. Gastroenterology. 2004;127:S194-S205.
79. Salem R, Lewandowski RJ, Mulcahy MF, Riaz A, Ryu RK, Ibrahim S, et al. Radioembolization for hepatocellular carcinoma using Yttrium-90 microspheres: A comprehensive report of long-term outcomes. Gastroenterology. 2010;138:52-64.
80. Srivastava DN, Thulkar S, Sharma S, Pandey GK, Sahni P, Julka PK, et al. Therapeutic radiological interventional procedures in hepatocellular carcinoma. Indian J Gastroenterol. 2002;21:96-8.
81. Srivastava DN, Gandhi D, Julka PK, Tandon RK. Gastrointestinal hemorrhage in hepatocellular carcinoma management with transhepatic arterioembolization. Abdominal Imaging. 2000;25:1-6.
82. Madoff DC, Hicks ME, Vauthey JN, Charnsangavej C, Morello FA Jr, Ahrar K, et al. Transhepatic portal vein embolization: anatomy, indications, and technical considerations. Radiographics. 2002;22(5):1063-76.
83. Gunabushanam G, Sharma S, Thulkar S, Srivastava DN, Rath GK, Julka PK, et al. Radiofrequency ablation of liver metastases from breast cancer: results in 14 patients. J Vasc Interv Radiol. 2007;18(1):67-72.
84. Kumar A, Bal C, Srivastava DN, Thulkar SP, Sharma S, Acharya SK, et al. Management of multiple intrahepatic recurrences after radiofrequency ablation of hepatocellular carcinoma with rhenium-188-HDD lipiodol. Eur J Gastroenterol Hepatol. 2006;18(2):219-23.
85. Kumar A, Srivastava DN, Bal C. Management of postsurgical recurrence of hepatocellular carcinoma with Rhenium 188-HDD labeled iodized oil. J Vasc Interv Radiol. 2006;17(1):157-61.
86. Srivastava DN, Madhusudan KS. Oncologic Imaging. Ind J of Medical and Paediatric Oncology. 2008;29(1): 65-6.
87. Srivastava DN, Sharma S, Yadav S, Nundy S, Berry M. Pedunculated hepatic haemangioma with arteriportal shunt–treated with angioembolization and surgery. Australasian Radiology. 1998;2:151-3.
88. Srivastava DN, Gandhi D, Seith A, Pande GK, Sahni P. Transcatheter arterial embolization in the treatment of symptomatic cavernous haemangioma of the liver: A prospective study. Abdominal Imaging. 2001;26:510-14.
89. Rammohan A, Sathyanesan J, Ramaswami S, Lakshmanan A, Senthil-Kumar P, Srinivasan UP, et al. Embolization of liver tumors: Past, present, and future. World J Radiol. 2012;4(9):405-12.

CHAPTER 13

Chandan Jyoti Das, Sanchita Gupta, Krithika Rangarajan

Imaging in Liver Transplant

INTRODUCTION

Liver transplantation is considered the ideal and accepted treatment for patients with end-stage liver disease (ESLD), with reported 1-year graft and patient survival rates of 80–95% and 5-year rates of 60–85%.[1] Unfortunately, there is inadequate availability of cadaveric liver grafts because of several limitations in organ donation. Hence, transplantation of partial grafts from living and deceased donors has become more popular in the last decade. There has been a paradigm shift in the various imaging techniques concomitant with the technical refinements in partial liver transplantation that allow a precise and better understanding of donor and recipient anatomy before the transplantation.

Pretransplantation evaluation of the extent of liver disease and details of the vascular and biliary anatomy of potential recipients and donors are paramount for successful liver transplantation. In this chapter, we will discuss the indications and contraindications of various liver transplantation techniques, different surgical techniques, and a plethora of imaging modalities used for radiologic evaluation of donors and recipients. We also briefly discuss imaging in various postoperative complications.

INDICATIONS AND CONTRAINDICATIONS FOR LIVER TRANSPLANT

The common indications for liver transplantation include complications of cirrhosis, hepatocellular carcinoma (HCC), autoimmune hepatitis, chronic hepatitis B and C, cholestatic diseases such as primary biliary cirrhosis and primary sclerosing cholangitis, and metabolic diseases such as hemochromatosis and Wilson's disease **(Box 1)**.[2]

BOX 1 Common indications for liver transplantation.

- Cirrhosis with end-stage liver disease and decompensation
  - Hepatocellular carcinoma/hepatoblastoma
- Alcoholic liver disease
- *Hepatitis*: Autoimmune, chronic hepatitis B and C
- *Cholestatic diseases*: Primary biliary cirrhosis and primary sclerosing cholangitis
- *Metabolic diseases*: Hemochromatosis Wilson disease
- *Fulminant hepatic failure*: Viral/toxin/drug-induced

There are few absolute and relative contraindications for transplantation. The absolute contraindications include uncontrolled ongoing sepsis, active abuse of alcohol or other substances, extrahepatic malignancy, severe cardiopulmonary disease, hepatopulmonary syndrome with severe pulmonary hypertension, lack of a psychosocial support system, and some variants of cholangiocarcinoma. The relative contraindications include age > 65 years, human immunodeficiency virus (HIV) infection, HCC (not fitting in established criteria), morbid obesity, and psychological instability.

PATIENT SELECTION

Most patients have ESLD, which is assessed by the model for end-stage liver disease (MELD) scoring system.[2,3] MELD is an objective way to assess patients waiting for liver transplantation and is being used to prioritize the allocation of livers for transplantation.

This scoring system, based on the patient's bilirubin, international normalized ratio (INR), and creatinine, was initially created to predict the 3-month mortality for patients with non-HCC ESLD undergoing a transjugular intrahepatic portosystemic shunt (TIPS) procedure.[2,4] MELD scores range from 6 to 40, with 6 indicating the least sick patients and 40 indicating the sickest patients. It is generally thought that for liver transplantation, waitlisting the patient should have at least 15 MELD points. Conversely, it may be futile to contemplate transplantation for patients with MELD values closer to 40.

HEPATOCELLULAR CARCINOMA

The Milan criteria[5] are accepted by most national deceased donor-based transplant programs worldwide. For patients with HCC to be eligible for transplantation, the tumor must be grade 1 or grade 2, solitary < 5 cm, or may up to 3 nodules with each < 3 cm, with no extrahepatic metastases or evidence of macrovascular invasion.

According to the tumor, node, and metastasis (TNM) staging system, a tumor of any size may be classified as T1 if it does not extend into the blood vessels. Any tumor > 1, T2 tumors may be any size if they extend into the blood vessels; they may also be classified as T2 if they are more than one and smaller than 5 cm. Tumors are characterized as T3 if larger than 5 cm. T4 tumors extend beyond the liver, except for the gallbladder. Transplant priority should be given to stage T2 disease because patients with T1 disease have high survival rates without transplantation, and those with T3 disease have a high rate of recurrence.[5]

Milan criteria are used to assess transplant eligibility for small HCCs. The University of California San Francisco (UCSF) criteria are used for liver transplantation in patients with large tumors, i.e., they have a single tumor that is 6.5 cm or smaller or if three or fewer tumor nodules are present, with the largest being 4.5 cm or smaller. Recently, a cut-off tumor volume of 115 cm^3 has been used to select candidates for transplantation, showing enhanced accuracy of pretransplantation imaging.[6] Factors with high potential for recurrence after living donor liver transplantation (LDLT) include a tumor larger than 6 cm, multiple nodules > 3, a disease that progresses after pretransplantation treatment, gross vascular invasion, and a tumor that is exposed to the liver surface.[7]

Types of Hepatic Transplant

Currently, there are three types of liver transplantations being performed—(1) whole liver cadaveric transplant, (2) split liver cadaveric transplant, and (3) living donor liver transplant **(Table 1)**. Worldwide, cadaveric or deceased donor liver transplantation (DDLT) is the most common type. It is also the most technically straightforward form of liver transplantation and has the advantage of a full-sized donor liver.

Living Donor Liver Transplant

Living donor liver transplantation accounts for approximately 4.0% of the liver transplants performed in the last 10 years but accounts for >85% of the transplants being performed in our country. The advantages of LDLT include the elective nature of the procedure, good quality organs, and the lack of organ injuries due to preservation. The main disadvantage of this technique is the risk related to the healthy donor, with a mortality risk of 0.15–0.20% and a postoperative complication rate of 20–40%. The residual donor liver must be >30% of the total donor hepatic volume to ensure adequate postoperative liver function, and the graft-to-recipient body weight ratio (GRWR) should be >0.8 to minimize the risk of "small-for-size" syndrome in the recipient.[8]

An adult recipient can use either a full-right or full-left hepatic graft (small adults < 50 kg). In the donor right hepatectomy, the liver is split on the right of the middle hepatic vein (MHV), close to Cantlie's line that connects the left border of the suprahepatic inferior vena cava (IVC) to the midpoint of the gallbladder fossa. Generally, the MHV remains with the donor in right hepatectomy, whereas it is harvested when the left donor's hepatectomy is performed.[7]

Hence, variations in the MHV's anatomy are critical to this operation's success and need to be conveyed to the transplant surgeon beforehand. Left donor hepatectomy involves harvesting the MHV en-bloc to obtain an adequate-sized graft with good venous outflow as congestion of the paramedian segment (segment IV) in the recipient is

TABLE 1: Comparison of different hepatic grafts.

	Right hepatectomy	Extended right hepatectomy	Left hepatectomy	Left lateral sectionectomy	Left hepatectomy with segment I
Segments	V, VI, VII, and VIII	V, VI, VII, and VIII + IV	II, III, and IV	II and III	II and III + I
Middle hepatic vein	Excluded	Included	Included	NA	Included
Advantage	Larger than LH	No congestion	Less burden on donor	Less burden on donor	Larger than LH
Disadvantage	Congestion of graft	Increased burden on donor	Twisting of graft	Small graft	Complicated reconstruction of SI anastomosis
Type of recipient	Adult	Adults	Small size adults, bigger children	Small children	Small size adults, bigger children

avoided. As the right hepatic vein (RHV) is dominant in most patients and the caudate lobe usually remains in the donor, congestion of the remnant donor liver after removal of the MHV along with the left hemi liver usually is not clinically significant.

The recipient's left hepatic vein (LHV) and MHV can be enlarged and then anastomosed to the enlarged graft MHV-LHV confluence to provide unimpeded venous outflow to the graft after implantation. Left lateral segmentectomy (segments 2 and 3 with or without the caudate lobe) is suitable for children and smaller recipients (20–30 kg).[7,9]

Split liver cadaveric transplant is the least common type in which a single cadaveric liver is anatomically divided and transplanted into two recipients (usually one adult and one child).[9,10] The right lobe is given to an adult recipient, whereas the left lateral segment is given to a child. Although this helps mitigate the shortage of deceased donor livers available, there are technical difficulties related to the sharing of blood vessels/bile duct and a higher risk of complications in the adult recipient (bile leaks, cut surface bleeding, and segment four necrosis). The most common cadaveric splitting technique involves a transection plane 1 cm to the right of the falciform ligament, resulting in a right extended graft (segments I and IV–VIII) used in adults and a left lateral graft (segments II–III) for a pediatric recipient who is not larger than 30 kg. The common bile duct (CBD), main portal vein, and IVC are included in the right liver graft, and the main arterial trunk is part of the left liver graft. The biliary reconstruction of the left lateral graft usually entails a hepaticojejunostomy in the pediatric recipient.[9,10]

PREOPERATIVE IMAGING MODALITIES

Multidetector computed tomography (MDCT) and magnetic resonance imaging (MRI) are the workhorses of pretransplant imaging and complement each other in evaluating donors and recipients.

Multidetector Computed Tomography

Multidetector computed tomography is frequently used to evaluate the donor and recipient arterial and venous anatomy using intravenous contrast in CT angiography (CTA). Donor liver fat content is also evaluated by an unenhanced scan (by calculating the hepatic attenuation index). Dual-energy CT (DECT) scan has been increasingly used as virtual noncontrast images can be reconstructed from the set of enhanced images, thus obviating the need for a true unenhanced scan that reduces the radiation dose. MDCT/CTA generates a massive amount of data which requires dedicated postprocessing by vendor-specific software for optimal evaluation of the anatomy—the hepatic arteries on three-dimensional (3D) or axial maximum intensity projections (MIPs), the hepatic veins on axial MIPs, portal veins on coronal MIPs, and volume renderings of the hepatic parenchyma. All these can be superimposed on one another for further delineation of the anatomy for the surgeons. MDCT should be judiciously used to reduce the radiation dose as donors are often young and healthy.

Magnetic Resonance Imaging

Magnetic resonance imaging coupled with magnetic resonance cholangiopancreatography (MRCP) is primarily performed to evaluate the biliary system. Hepatobiliary contrast agents such as Gd-BOPTA (Multihance, Bracco Diagnostics, NJ) can be used. The biliary tree is better seen on 3D heavily T2 weighted or 3-D T1 weighted, and postcontrast coronal oblique images. MRI can also evaluate the hepatic parenchyma to characterize incidental focal lesions and the degree of fatty infiltration.

PREOPERATIVE IMAGING EVALUATION

Recipient Evaluation

Imaging of the recipient's liver should be performed as close to the time of transplantation as possible because tumors may grow rapidly, invade local structures, or metastasize, which may affect the stage of disease, management perspective, and surgical technique. *The patient's MELD score determines eligibility* and allows for candidate list prioritization based on medical *needs*. Imaging plays a pivotal role in the care of patients with HCC.[2] Imaging of the recipient consists of a detailed evaluation and description of the arterial, portal venous, and hepatic venous anatomy and the extent of tumor burden in HCC patients awaiting transplant.

For patients with liver lesions, the Organ Procurement and Transplantation Network (OPTN) or Liver Imaging Reporting and Data System (LI-RADS) criteria are used to characterize liver lesions as benign, suspicious for HCC, or definitely HCC.[11,12] The intrinsic signal intensity of the mass, enhancement, washout pattern, capsule appearance, and nodule architecture is frequently used to determine the likelihood that a nodule is HCC. Once the liver nodules are characterized, the Milan/UCSF criteria determine transplant candidacy. Patients with HCC whose tumors are growing at a significant rate or who are expected to wait > 6 months on the transplant list may be offered locoregional therapy, a practice known as "bridging to transplant." Occasionally, some programs use down-staging locoregional therapy for cases where the HCC lesions were beyond the standard listing criteria, provided there is no evidence of extrahepatic disease or macrovascular tumor invasion. In such patients, there is a need for a 3-month waiting period post-downstaging therapy [usually transarterial chemoembolization (TACE)/radiofrequency ablation (RFA)/transarterial radioembolization (TARE)] and reimaging to see whether they fit the listing criteria before being considered for liver transplantation. This is accomplished by alcohol injection, thermal ablation (including radiofrequency and microwave ablation), TARE, and more commonly, TACE.[13] The choice of therapy is based on Barcelona Clinic Liver Cancer Staging (BCLC) criteria, which take into account the number and size of HCC nodules, the patient's Child-Pugh score, and the patient's Eastern Cooperative Oncology Group (ECOG) performance status.[14]

All focal lesions should be described segment-wise along with their relation to major vascular structures, the gallbladder, and central bile ducts because the outcome may be affected. If MDCT is indeterminate for lesion characterization, contrast-enhanced MRI imaging should be performed to characterize the lesion further. It is also critical to perform a CT chest and abdomen to exclude extrahepatic malignancy or spread.

Preoperative Imaging of the Living Donor Liver Transplantation Donor

An accurate preoperative depiction of donor anatomy is essential to determine the suitability of the donor so that hepatectomy may safely be performed without any risk to the donor and, simultaneously, avoid "small-for-size" syndrome in the recipient. This syndrome is characterized by poor bile production, delayed synthetic function, prolonged cholestasis, intractable ascites, and deranged coagulation, which leads to septic complications and high mortality. To avoid small-for-size syndrome, the residual liver volume should exceed 30–35% of the total donor liver volume, and the GRWR should be >0.8 with reference to the recipient.[15] Preoperative imaging of the LDLT donor involves assessment of various features such as vascular and biliary anatomy for relevant variants, MHV anatomy, the hepatic parenchyma for degree of fatty infiltration, iron content, and focal hepatic lesions and last but not the least, calculation of liver volumes. Minor variations of anatomy can be tackled with advanced vascular surgical techniques.

In a study by Tsang et al., the various causes of donor unsuitability were recipient issues such as inadequate remnant volume (57.4%), steatosis (27.7%), a small for size graft (8.9%), and variations of biliary system (5%) hepatic artery (4%), and portal vein (1%) anatomy.[15]

Among the various imaging techniques, MDCT angiography is faster and more cost-effective than MR angiography and is used more often. Two-dimensional or 3D reformations from MDCT in both arterial and portal venous phases provide the best methods of analysis. The MDCT protocol for liver donors varies with institutions. The protocol followed at our institution includes unenhanced CT followed by multiphase contrast-enhanced CT. Four 10 mm sections are obtained first in the unenhanced CT protocol, followed by arterial and portal venous phase contrast-enhanced CT. The details are given in **Table 2**.

TABLE 2: Multidetector computed tomography (MDCT) protocol for living donor liver transplantation (LDLT) donor evaluation.

Phases	Iodinated contrast material	Delay	kVp
Unenhanced CT	—	—	120 kVp
Arterial phase	80–100 mL of with a concentration of 370 mg/mL @ 4–5 mL/sec	30 seconds	100–120 kVp
Portal venous phase	80–100 mL of with a concentration of 370 mg/mL @ 4–5 mL/sec	60–70 seconds	120 kVp

VASCULAR ANATOMY

Preoperative imaging of the hepatic artery, portal, and hepatic veins involves identifying the vessels **(Figs. 1A to C)** and their variations and measuring the diameter at the site of the proposed anastomosis since anastomosis of similar size decreases the risk of thrombosis or stenosis.

Hepatic Arteries

Normal hepatic arterial anatomy (Michel type I) consists of a common hepatic artery arising from celiac axis and dividing into the right and left hepatic arteries, found in only 55% of the population.[16] Replaced right hepatic artery (RHA) from superior mesenteric artery (11%) and replaced left hepatic artery (LHA) from left gastric artery (10%) are other common variations.[16] The term "aberrant" or "replaced" is used when the variant arteries substitute the normal artery, whereas the variant artery that persists in addition to the normal one is termed "accessory". The most common arterial variant is an accessory right or LHA. Since few of these variants are surgically relevant, hence variants should be mentioned in the report. A replaced or accessory RHA will affect right LDLT, whereas a replaced or accessory LHA will affect full left or left lateral segment LDLT. Similarly, the middle hepatic artery (MHA) will affect both right and left LDLT.

The diameter of RHA or LHA is also essential as <2 mm diameter makes future arterial anastomoses prone to thrombosis, and microvascular techniques are often required.

Hepatic Veins

Hepatic venous variants are seen in 16–33% of the population. If not dealt with intraoperatively, these can lead to hepatic insufficiency in the donor or recipient if drainage to a liver segment is compromised.[17] Identification of the exact location and variation of the MHV is paramount for guiding surgical planning because the hepatectomy plane—which, in living donors, is to the right of the MHV along the

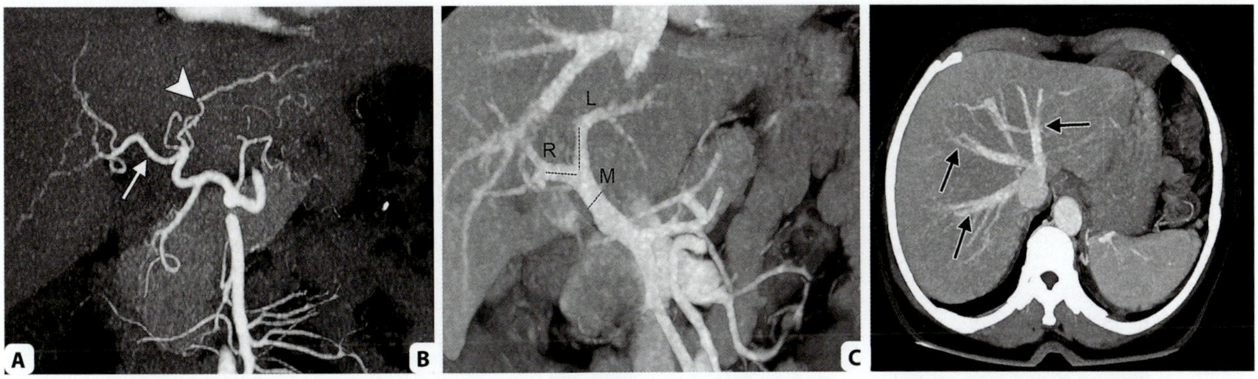

FIGS. 1A TO C: Preoperative work-up of liver donor (A) CT scan in arterial phase showing right hepatic artery (white arrow) and left hepatic artery (arrowhead) from the celiac truck. Caliber and length of the hepatic arteries should be measured. (B) Venous phase images show densely opacified portal vein (M) with measurements of the caliber and length of the main as well as right (R) and left (L) branches. (C) Venous phase showing opacified hepatic veins and their tributaries (black arrows) (segments 5 and 8 being important).

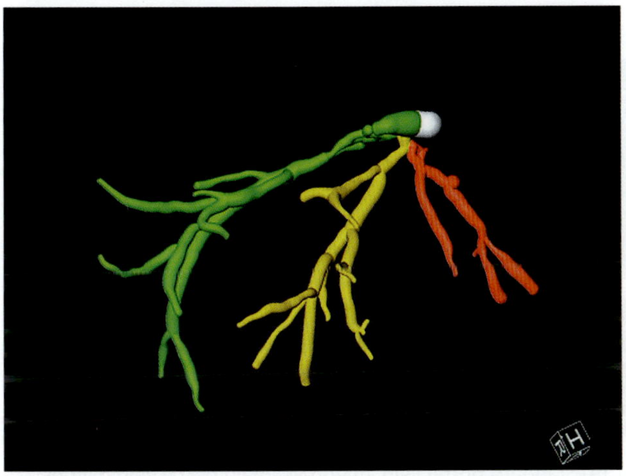

FIG. 2: Three-dimensional model of hepatic venous anatomy.

gallbladder fossa—may be affected.[18] MDCT is frequently used to evaluate hepatic veins **(Fig. 2)**. The usual position of the MHV is between segments VIII and IV. The drainage of segments IVa and IVb should also be mentioned. It is important to determine if an accessory inferior RHV as it is the most common venous variant. If accessory RHV(s) drains VI, VII, and V, a separate anastomosis is needed to preserve drainage of these segments during a right LDLT.

Similarly, the right lobe anterior sector segmental veins (V5 and V8) draining into MHV need to be separately anastomosed to the recipient suprahepatic IVC to preserve drainage of these segments during right LDLT. This is especially needed when the right lobe graft is harvested without the MHV. When the right lobe graft is harvested with the MHV in an MHV-predominant system, care has to be taken to preserve the V4a tributary and terminal part of the MHV in the donor remnant liver.

The most common venous variant is an accessory right inferior hepatic vein. If its caliber is 5 mm or more, a separate anastomosis to the IVC is performed to prevent hepatic congestion. The distance in the coronal plane between the accessory inferior RHV and the RHV is crucial for the surgeon while planning the graft implantation.[19]

Portal Veins

Portal venous anatomic variants are less common, although a few surgically relevant variations exist. 3D CT images can help to find out the variation easily **(Figs. 3 and 4)**.

Few critical findings that can affect the transplant include left branch of portal vein (LPV) from right anterior branch of PV (RAPV) (affects right LDLT, may be a relative contraindication to donation), RAPV from LPV (affects left LDLT, may be a relative contraindication to donation) and trifurcation into right posterior branch of PV (RPPV), RAPV, and LPV (affects both right and left LDLT; right LDLT: must clamp and anastomose these separately; left LDLT: RAPV from graft must be excluded).[20] There has been a described association between portal venous and biliary system variants. Hence, if portal venous variants are identified, these should be examined closely to preclude associated biliary tree variations.[20]

Biliary Anatomy

Biliary anastomosis usually occurs between the donor's CBD and the recipient's common hepatic duct (CHD) in a DDLT. Biliary variations are commonly seen in up to 33% of the population. If not identified preoperatively, this may result in biliary leaks and strictures, leading to substantial morbidity or mortality in the donor and recipient in the postoperative period.[5] Biliary complications are the most common cause of morbidity after split and LDLT, occurring in up to 40% of patients.[20]

Magnetic resonance cholangiopancreatography **(Figs. 5A to C)** and T1 contrast cholangiography **(Fig. 6)** are helpful for a detailed understanding of the biliary anatomy

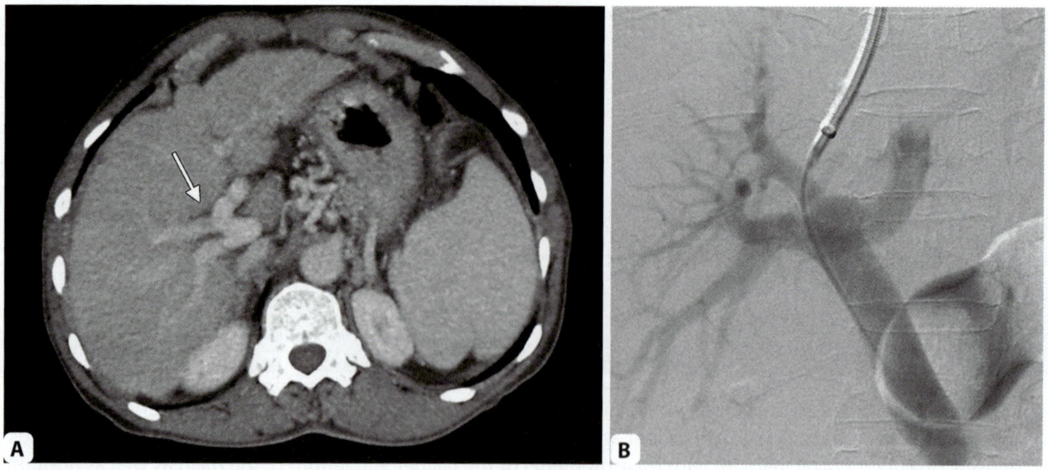

FIGS. 3A AND B: Portal vein trifurcation seen on (A) axial CECT image (marked with arrow) and (B) DSA image after portal venous puncture for TIPS.

(CECT: contrast-enhanced computed tomography; DSA: digital subtraction angiography; TIPS: transjugular intrahepatic portosystemic shunt)

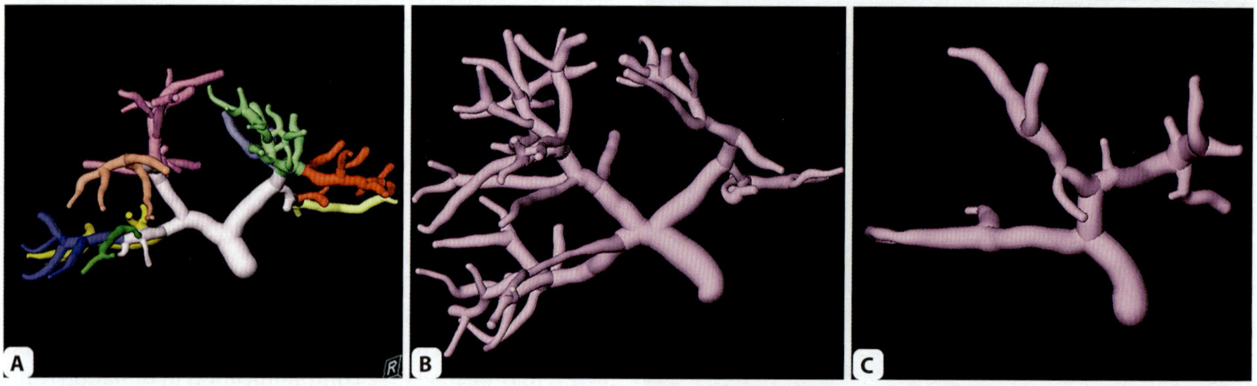

FIGS. 4A TO C: Three-dimensional models of portal venous anatomy. (A) Standard portal vein anatomy—main portal vein divides into the right and left portal veins. (B) Portal vein trifurcation—main portal vein divides into the left portal vein, right anterior portal vein, and right posterior portal vein. (C) Right posterior portal vein arising as the first branch from the main portal vein.

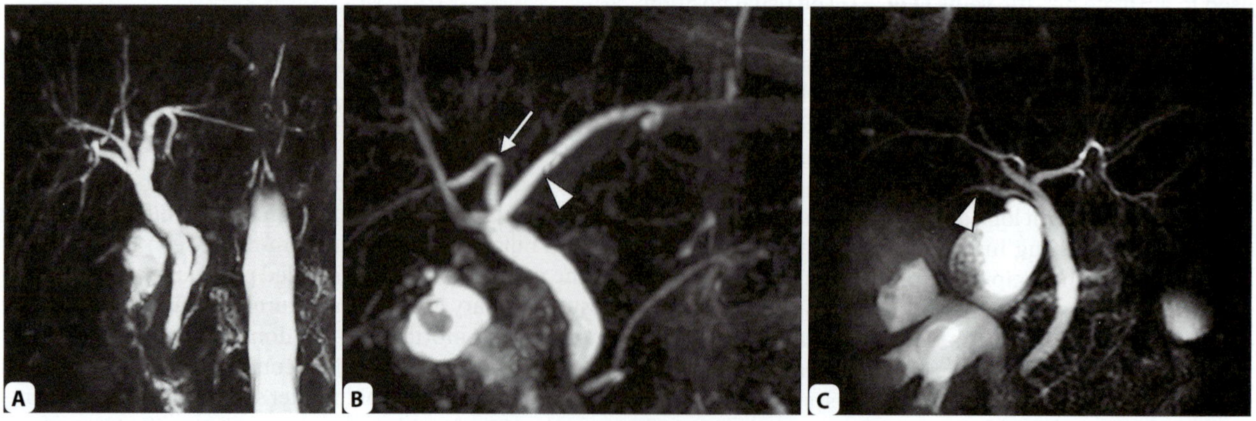

FIGS. 5A TO C: Projective MR cholangiogram images demonstrating common biliary variants. (A) Triple confluence of right anterior, right posterior, and left hepatic duct. (B) Drainage of the right posterior hepatic duct (arrow) into the left hepatic duct (arrowhead). (C) Aberrant drainage of the right posterior duct (arrowhead) into common hepatic duct.

to prevent these types of complications.[21] Variations such as right posterior hepatic duct (RPHD) or right anterior hepatic duct (RAHD) draining into left hepatic duct (LHD) are contraindications to left lobe donation, whereas LHD draining into RAHD or RPHD is contraindications to right lobe donation. To prevent biliary complications and to be sure of the hilar ductal configuration during LDLT, fluoroscopy-based intraoperative cholangiography (IOC) is essential before proceeding with the donor hepatectomy. IOC is repeated after graft removal to ensure there is no biliary leak and to confirm that the caliber of the remnant ductal system is adequate.[21]

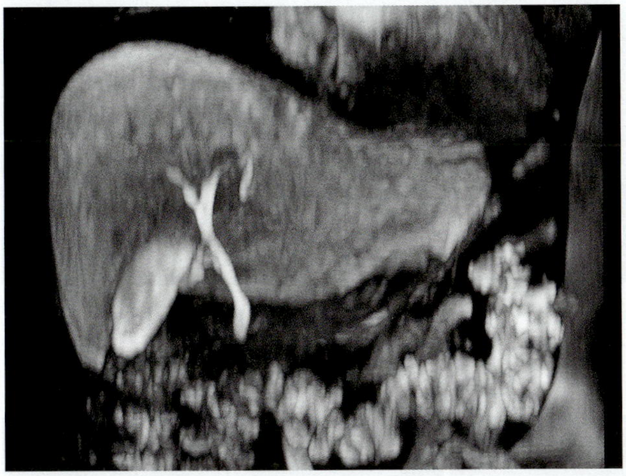

FIG. 6: T1 contrast cholangiography for assessment of pretransplant biliary anatomy.

Liver Parenchyma

The final step of preoperative donor imaging is evaluating the hepatic parenchyma to identify focal or diffuse liver disease (particularly steatosis), any incidental benign or malignant conditions that may preclude segmental donation, and measurement of liver volumes **(Fig. 7)**.

Hepatic steatosis > 30% precludes donation. NCCT findings consistent with this degree of steatosis include hepatic density > 10 HU lower than the spleen, hepatic density < 40 HU, and a hepatic-to-splenic density ratio of <0.8 **(Figs. 8A and B)**.[22]

In MRI, this degree of steatosis corresponds to 30% signal dropout on Dixon-type chemical shift imaging, with liver parenchymal signal dropout normalized to the spleen.

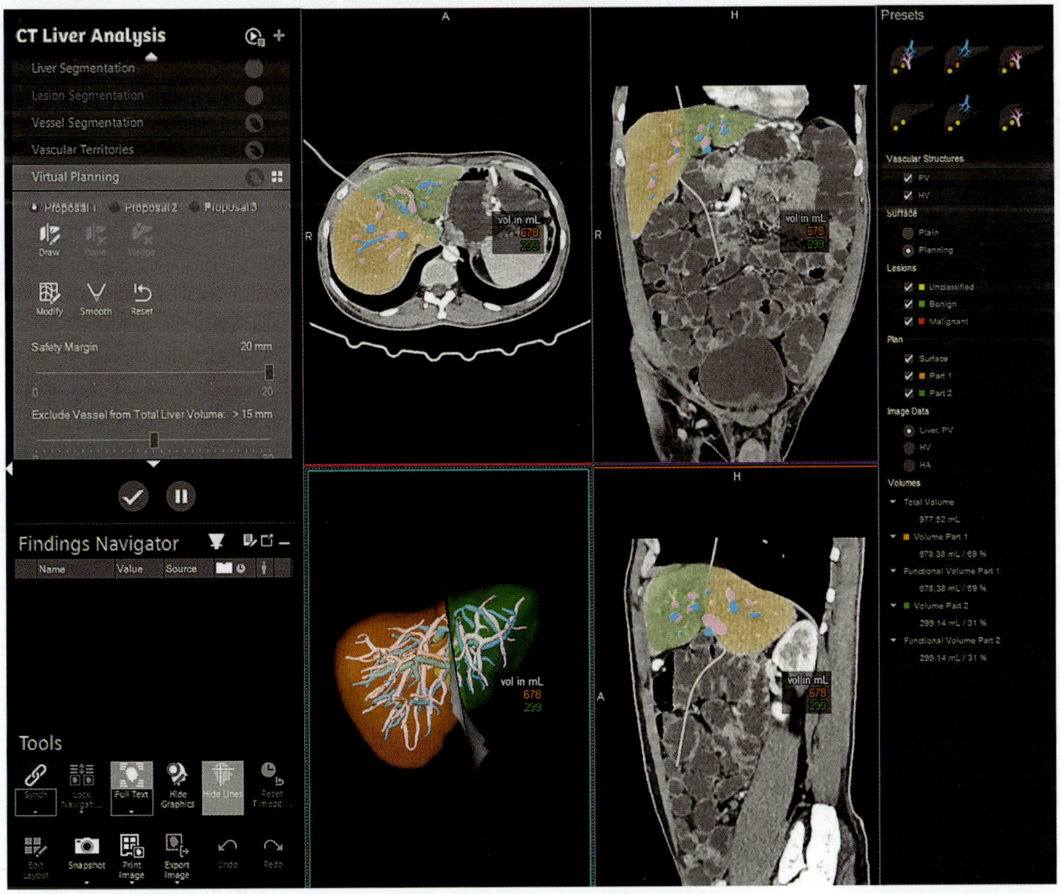

FIG. 7: Liver volumetry showing assessment of total liver volume using vendor-specific software and generation of 3D model of liver. Note the software separately assesses residual and donor liver volume with the line of division along the lateral margin of middle hepatic vein (MHV)

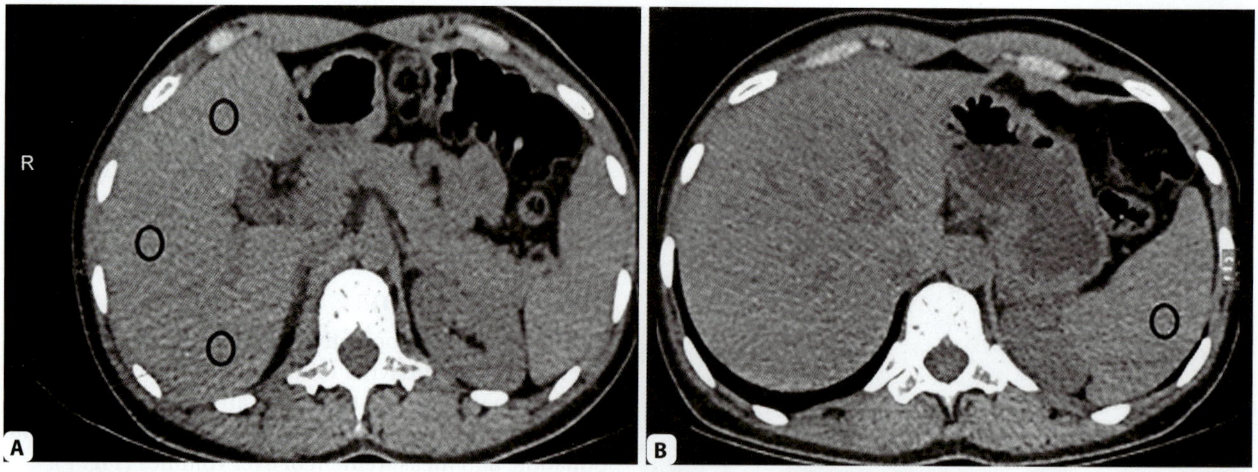

FIGS. 8A AND B: Liver attenuation index (LAI): Regions of interest (ROI) drawn on liver (25 ROI) and splenic (3 ROI) parenchyma avoiding vessels.

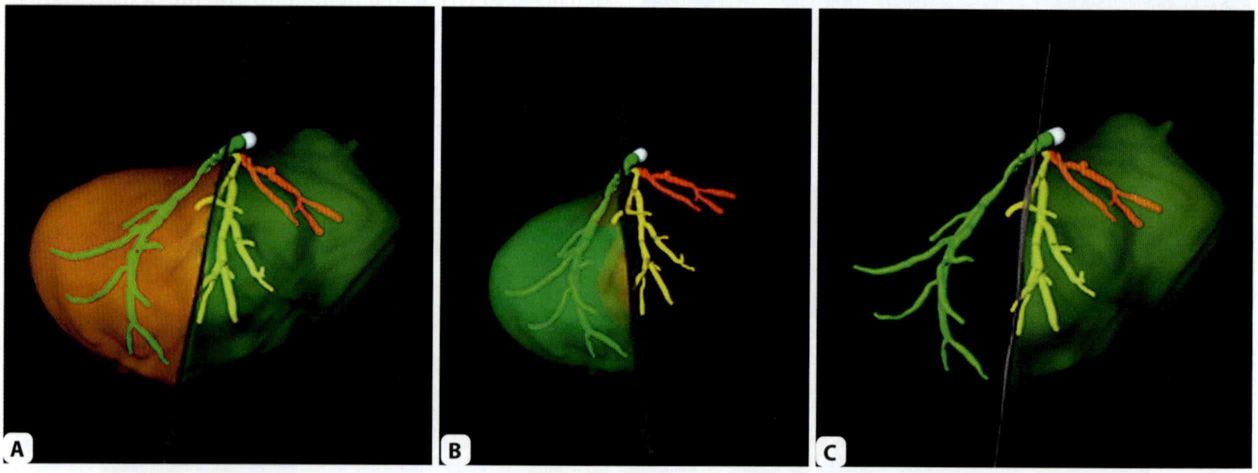

FIGS. 9A TO C: Virtual hepatectomy: Three-dimensional reconstructed CT images of the entire donor liver (A) showing the plane of hepatectomy, which passes to the right of the middle hepatic vein through segment VIII. The potential residual donor liver (B) and the donor segment (C) are also shown.

MR spectroscopy is considered to be better for estimating hepatic steatosis.

Finally, integrated software may be used to calculate the volume of the entire liver, the potential residual volume in the donor, and the potential volume in the recipient by performing a virtual hepatectomy **(Figs. 9A to C)** from the MDCT data set. All the processed images of the vascular tree, biliary system, and liver parenchyma can be superimposed into a single presurgical liver model, which can help as a guide map during surgery.

Safety of Liver Donor

Donor safety is paramount, so the basic idea is to have minimal complications for the living donor. Usually, donor hepatectomy is a safe procedure, although it may be associated with complications such as pleural effusion and infection, which are generally self-limiting. Surgical complications such as biliary leakage and biloma formation may arise, which is seen as persistent biliary output from the surgical drain. MRCP performed with a hepatobiliary contrast agent is very helpful in confirming the leak and localizing the site of the bile duct injury. Postsurgery liver failure is extremely rare as preoperative imaging evaluation of future liver remnant (FLR) is accurate most of the time.

POSTOPERATIVE EVALUATION

Understanding the surgical technique for anastomosis is essential for the evaluation of postoperative complications after orthotopic liver transplant since the majority of complications occur at the site of anastomosis **(Table 3)**. Arterial, portal venous, caval, and biliary anastomosis are required for all liver transplants.

TABLE 3: Surgical technique of DDLT and LDLT.

	DDLT	LDLT
Technical difficulty	Easier compared to LDLT	More challenging (due to complex anastomosis)
	Whole liver/split graft	Right hepatic graft, left hepatic graft, and left lateral sectionectomy graft
Gallbladder	Removed	Removed
PV anastomosis	End-to-end	End-to-end
HA anastomosis	End-to-end	End-to-end
Bile duct anastomosis	End-to-end	End-to-end
IVC/HV anastomosis	End-to-side or side-to-side (piggy-back technique)	End-to-end
Complications	Less	More (due to complex anastomosis, leak from transected hepatic surface)

(DDLT: deceased donor liver transplantation; HA: hepatic arterial; HV: hepatic vein; IVC: inferior vena cava; LDLT: living donor liver transplantation; PV: portal vein)

IMAGING OF POST-TRANSPLANT COMPLICATIONS

The post-transplant period is precarious, with the majority of complications occurring during the first month.[23] These complications may be medical or surgical **(Tables 4 and 5)**. Imaging plays a vital role in the early recognition of surgical complications and excluding them as a cause of graft dysfunction.[24] Knowledge of standard surgical anastomosis techniques and review of the operative notes is essential while reviewing post-transplant imaging.

Doppler US is routinely carried out at the bedside in the postoperative period to detect vascular complications early. Institutional protocols vary regarding the frequency of Doppler after liver transplant, ranging from twice a day in the first postoperative week to every 3–5 days in the first week. Patients at higher risk are imaged more frequently in the postoperative period. This entails a detailed assessment of the hepatic parenchyma, intrahepatic biliary radicals, CBD, hepatic artery, portal vein, hepatic vein/IVC, and intra-abdominal collection. Normal appearance and various Doppler parameters of the hepatic vein **(Figs. 10A to C)**, hepatic artery, IVC, and portal vein **(Figs. 11A and B)** in the postoperative period are described below **(Table 6)**. CT/MR angiography or contrast-enhanced ultrasonography (CEUS) may be used as a problem-solving tool in case of abnormal US findings.

Hepatic Artery Thrombosis

Hepatic artery thrombosis (HAT) is the most common and devastating arterial complication after liver transplant.[25] Early-onset HAT (within the first 30 days after transplant) is a common cause of graft loss with a high mortality rate **(Figs. 12 to 14)**. Incidence is lower in adults compared to pediatric transplants. US Doppler shows a complete absence of flow within the hepatic artery and its branches. The adjacent hepatic parenchyma may also show wedge-shaped areas of heterogenous echotexture on US, representing hepatic infarction. In cases of radioclinical mismatch, CEUS or CTA can help establish the diagnosis. Treatment comprises thrombolysis or thrombectomy by endovascular approach as the first line, followed by urgent retransplant if that fails.[26]

TABLE 4: Common medical complications after liver transplant.

Primary graft dysfunction	• Early allograft dysfunction • Primary nonfunction
Graft rejection	• Hyperacute • Acute • Chronic
Post-transplant infections	• Bacterial • Viral
Others	• Pleural effusion • Hospital-acquired pneumonia • Acute respiratory distress syndrome • Postreperfusion syndrome • Acute kidney injury

TABLE 5: Surgical complications after liver transplant.

Vascular complications	Hepatic artery	Hepatic artery thrombosis
		Hepatic artery stenosis
		Hepatic artery pseudoaneurysm
	Portal vein	Portal vein stenosis
		Portal vein thrombosis
	HV/IVC	HV/IVC stenosis
Biliary complications		Biliary leak
		Extrahepatic biliary stricture
		Intrahepatic biliary stricture

(HV: hepatic vein; IVC: inferior vena cava)

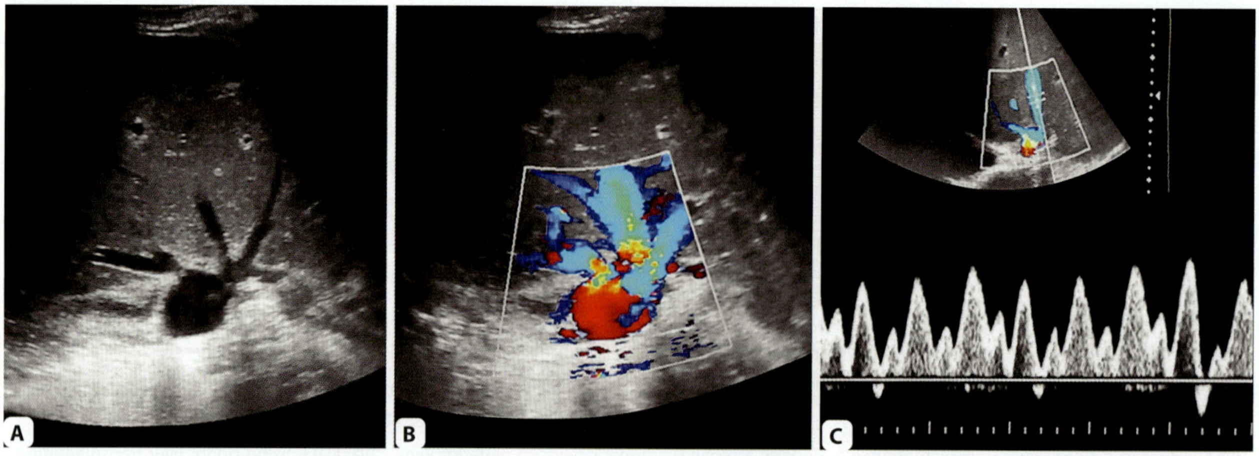

FIGS. 10A TO C: Postoperative ultrasonography: Hepatic veins. Grayscale (A), color flow (B), and Doppler trace (C) images show normal and patent hepatic veins and inferior vena cava.

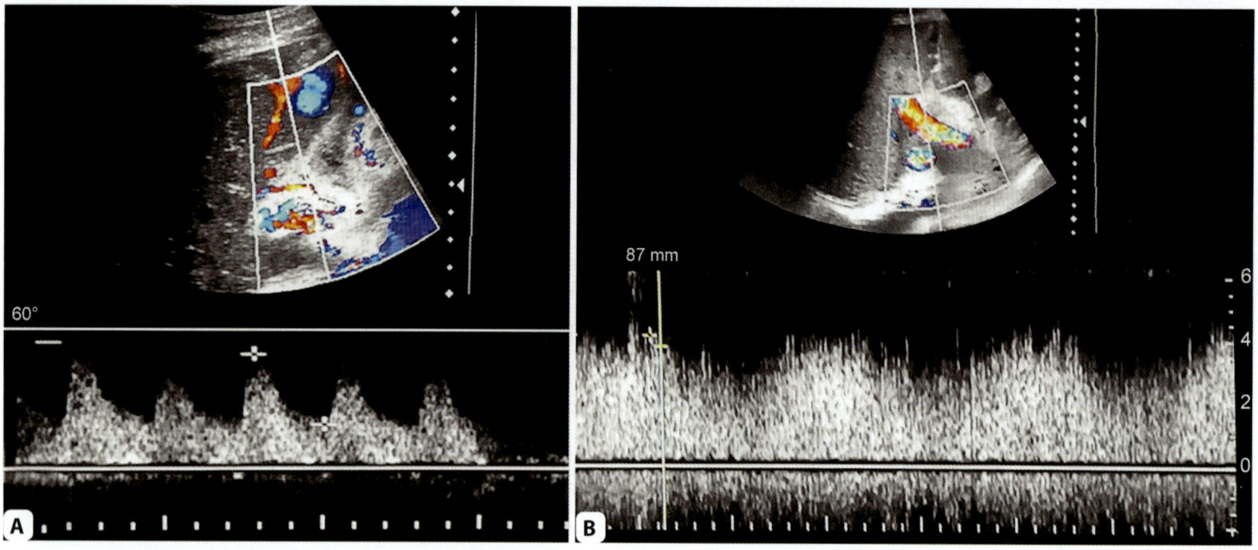

FIGS. 11A AND B: Postoperative ultrasonography: (A) Color Doppler image shows a normal hepatic artery with low resistance flow. (B) Color Doppler image shows a normal portal vein with an undulating spectral waveform.

TABLE 6: Normal flow parameters for hepatic vasculature after transplant.

	Normal Doppler parameters	Postoperative variations
Hepatic artery	Continuous diastolic flow: • PSV: 13–367 cm/s (Variable) • RI: 0.5–0.8 AT < 0.08 seconds	Early postoperative period: • Elevated RI (>0.8)—common • Low RI (<0.6)—increased risk of vascular complications
Hepatic veins	Triphasic flow	Monophasic flow during the early postoperative period due to graft edema
Portal vein	Continuous hepatopetal flow with mild cardiac and respiratory variation	

Delayed Hepatic Artery Thrombosis

It occurs > 30 days after transplant. These patients are frequently asymptomatic due to the development of collateral hepatic circulation from the superior mesenteric artery and diaphragmatic vessels. Since the hepatic artery is the sole supply of the biliary system in the post-transplant period, HAT may lead to ischemia of the biliary tree and resultant strictures. On US, the intrahepatic arteries generally show a low RI (<0.5) and a parvus tardus waveform.

Hepatic Artery Stenosis

Hepatic artery stenosis (HAS) usually affects the anastomotic site with clinical manifestations and Doppler findings similar to delayed HAT. Endovascular stenting of the hepatic artery is the treatment of choice.

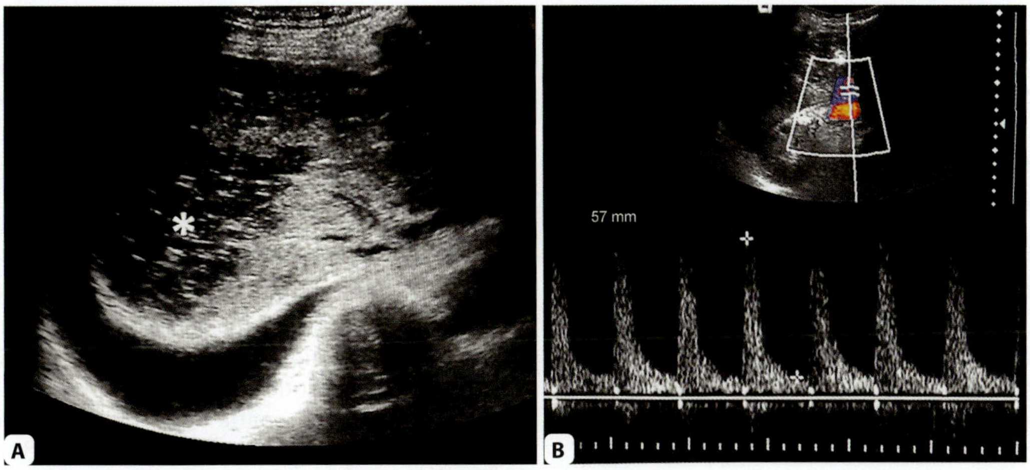

FIGS. 12A AND B: Hepatic artery thrombosis: Postoperative day 2 of a patient after cadaveric liver transplantation. (A) Grayscale ultrasonography shows a wedge-shaped hypoechoic area (asterisk) suggestive of infarct. (B) Color Doppler image at porta shows high resistance flow in hepatic artery proximal to the thrombosis.

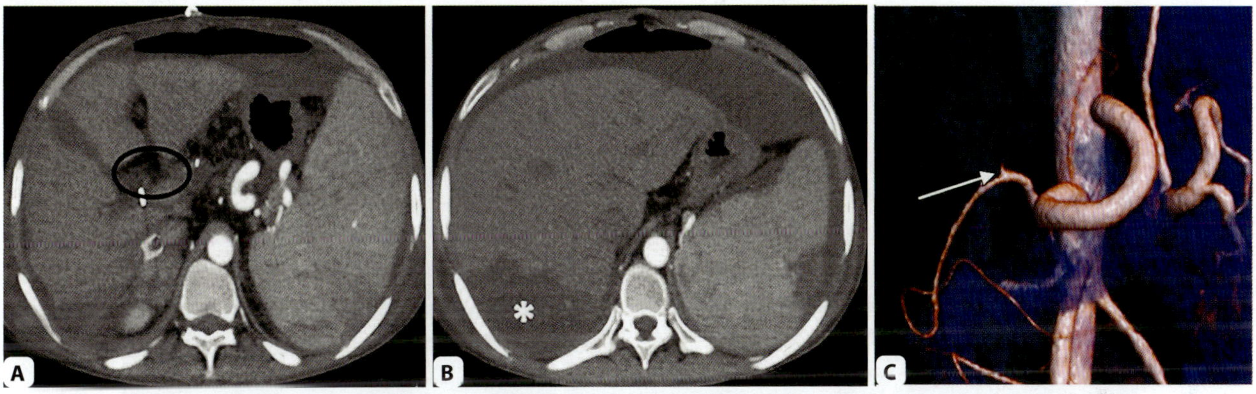

FIGS. 13A TO C: Hepatic artery thrombosis: CT angiography images show nonvisualization of the hepatic artery at porta (ellipse in A) with hypodense area in right posterior segments suggesting infarct (asterisk in B). Volume-rendered image (C) shows an abrupt cut-off of the hepatic artery with a small stump (arrow).

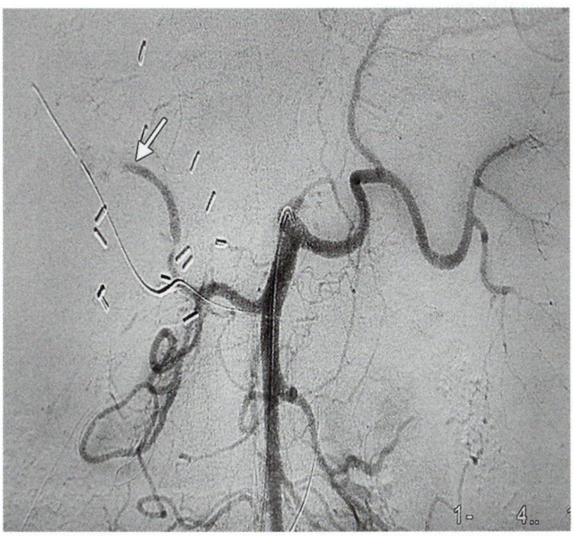

FIG. 14: Postliver transplant hepatic artery thrombosis (HAT): DSA image demonstrates an abrupt cut-off of the hepatic artery (arrow) with nonvisualization of the arterial branches distal to it.

Hepatic Artery Pseudoaneurysms

These are rare; however, they demand immediate management due to the high risk of rupture. These pseudoaneurysms are mycotic and mostly occur at the site of anastomosis **(Fig. 15)**.

Portal Vein

Portal vein thrombosis (PVT) is the most common complication affecting the postoperative portal vein **(Figs. 16 and 17)**.[27] Hypercoagulable states, history of PVT, previous TIPS, and difference in caliber between donor and recipient portal vein are risk factors. PVT appears as a hypoechoic/anechoic filling defect on grayscale US with no or partial color flow within the portal vein on Doppler. Portal vein stenosis is infrequent and usually at the site of the surgical anastomosis. A focal site of narrowing may be seen on grayscale US with increased peak velocity at the site of anastomosis becomes > 125 cm/s (~three times the preanastomotic velocity) and a difference of > 60 cm/s across the anastomosis.

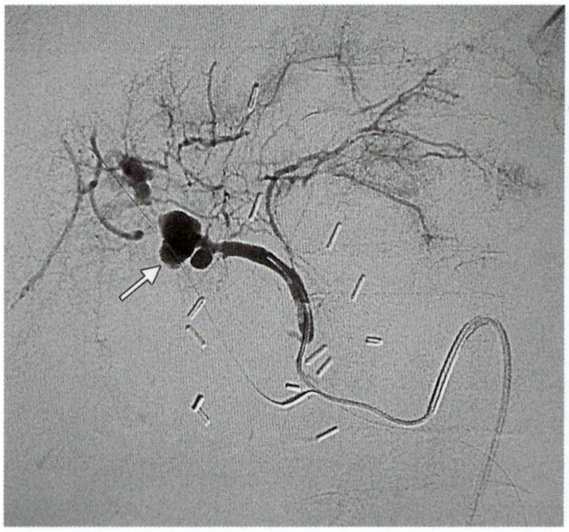

FIG. 15: Postliver transplant hepatic artery pseudoaneurysm (PSA): DSA image demonstrates a large saccular contrast-filled outpouching from the hepatic artery (arrow) at the site of arterial anastomosis.

Hepatic Vein/Inferior Vena Cava

Complications involving the HV/IVC are infrequent (<1%).[28] Stenosis is usually at the site of anastomosis, with increased incidence in LDLT due to complex anastomosis in these cases. Monophasic flow instead of the triphasic pattern is seen in the hepatic vein.

Biliary Complications

Strictures are the most common biliary complication.[29] LDLT is associated with a higher risk of biliary complications due to the complex anastomosis involved during the process. Anastomotic site strictures are more common, occur in the extrahepatic duct, and are not associated with graft dysfunction. Nonanastomotic strictures are less common, involve the intrahepatic duct, and are usually secondary to ischemia. The hepatic artery is the sole supply of the biliary system after transplant **(Figs. 18 and 19)**. MRCP helps delineate the site of biliary obstruction.

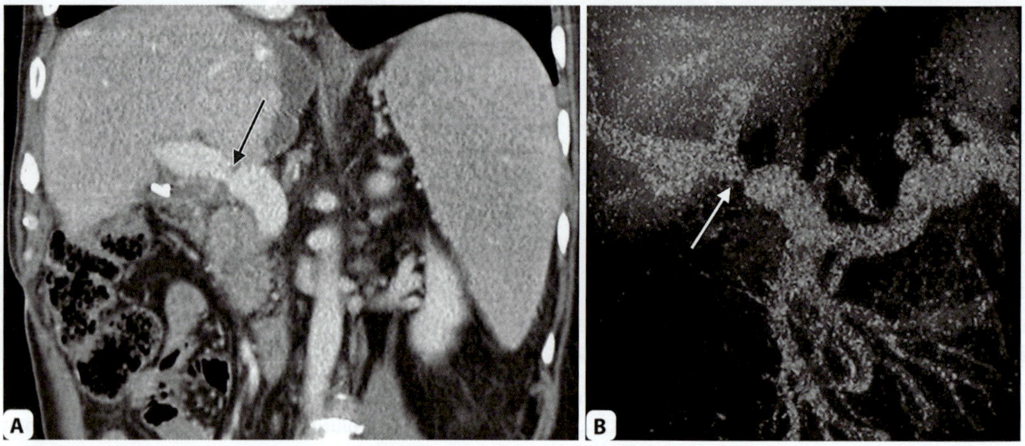

FIGS. 16A AND B: PV narrowing: Coronal (A) and volume rendered (B) contrast-enhanced CT images show short segment portal vein stenosis (arrow) with dilated splenic vein and splenomegaly, suggesting portal hypertension.

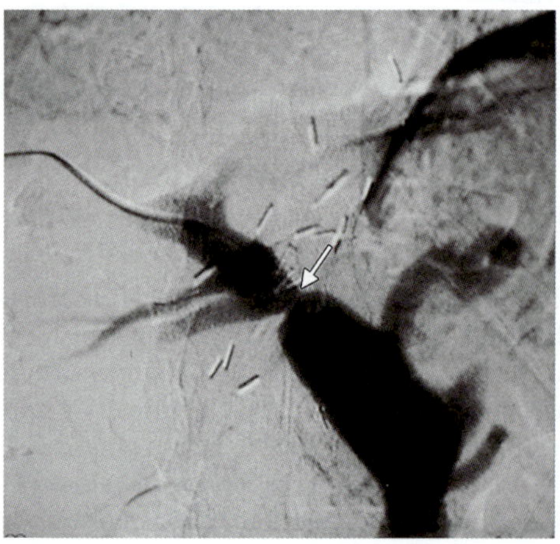

FIG. 17: Postliver transplant portal vein stenosis: The DSA image demonstrates narrowing in the portal vein at the site of portal venous anastomosis (arrow).

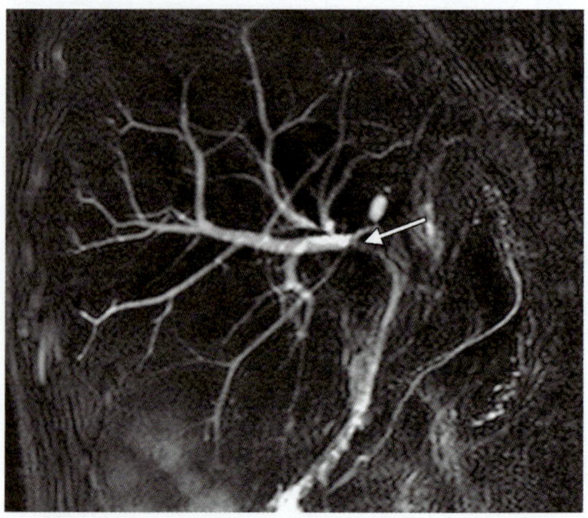

FIG. 18: Biliary stricture: Magnetic resonance cholangiopancreatography (MRCP) in a patient after right lobe liver donor liver transplantation showing short segment narrowing of the bile duct (arrow) at the site of anastomosis with mild intrahepatic biliary radicle dilatation.

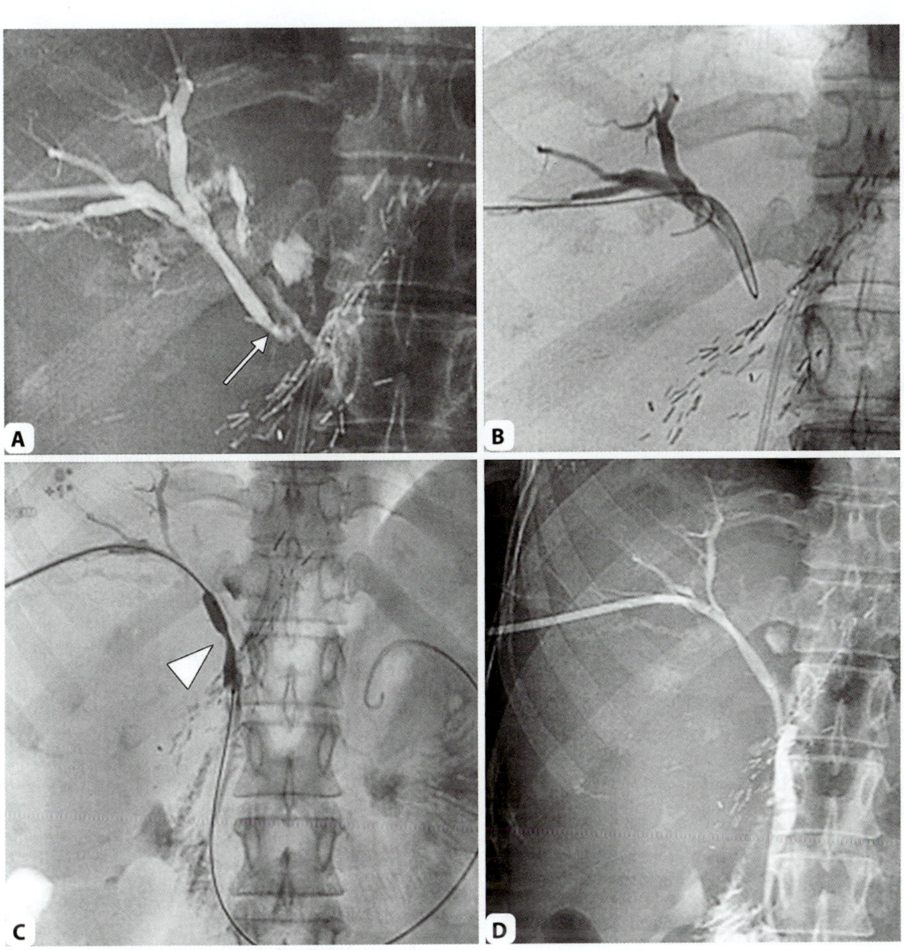

FIGS. 19A TO D: Postliver transplant delayed biliary stricture: (A) Fluoroscopic images demonstrate narrowing of the common bile duct (CBD) at the site of biliary anastomosis (arrow). Percutaneous transhepatic biliary drainage (PTBD) (B) and balloon dilatation (C) were done, resulting in the resolution of the stricture (D).

Bile leak is also a common early postoperative complication and usually occurs at the site of anastomosis **(Fig. 20)**. Hepatobiliary scintigraphy or hepatobiliary-specific contrast agent MRI may be used to detect bile leaks.[30]

In addition to the above-described complications, patients may develop hematomas or infected collections in the abdomen in the postoperative period. They are also at an increased risk of malignancies and post-transplantation lymphoproliferative disorder due to prolonged immunosuppression. Imaging also has a vital role to play in their management.[31]

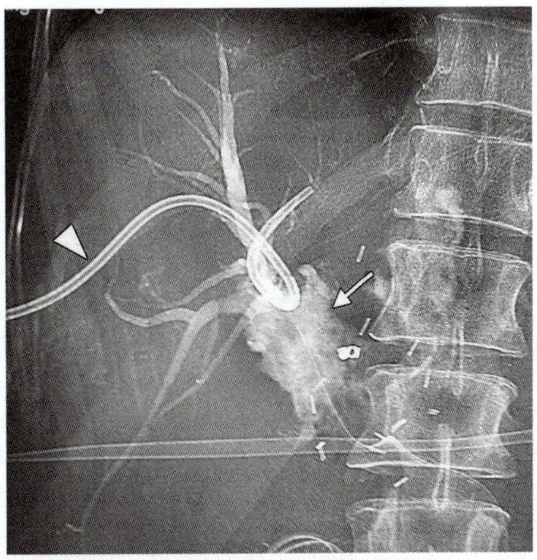

FIG. 20: Postliver transplant biliary leak: Fluoroscopic image shows leakage of contrast from the biliary anastomosis (arrow). A diversion percutaneous transhepatic biliary drainage (PTBD) (arrowhead) was done to allow the anastomotic site to heal.

CONCLUSION

Preoperative imaging in potential liver transplant donors and recipients with CT and MRI is essential for proper candidate selection and preoperative evaluation of the liver parenchyma, vascular, and biliary anatomy in the

BOX 2 Checklist for living donor MDCT reporting.

Liver size (craniocaudal):
- Any evidence of acute or chronic liver disease
- *Any focal lesions*: Yes/No (If yes, describe the number, size, segment, and nature of the lesions)
- Any biliary obstruction or IHBD

Liver fat estimation (on unenhanced or VNC images):
- Mean liver attenuation (in HU)
- Mean splenic attenuation (in HU)
- Liver attenuation Index (in HU)
- Do the intrahepatic vessels appear hypoattenuating compared to the liver parenchyma: Yes/ No

Liver volume analysis:
- Total liver volume (in cc)
- Graft volume (in cc)
- Donor remnant liver volume (in cc)
- Donor remnant liver volume (in percentage of total liver volume)

Hepatic arterial anatomy:
- *Right hepatic artery (RHA)*:
  - Vessel of origin
  - Diameter at origin (in mm)
  - Length before first sectional division (in cm)
  - Any vascular thrombus: Yes/No (If yes, mention the degree of occlusion)
- *Left hepatic artery (LHA)*:
  - Vessel of origin
  - Diameter at origin (in mm)
  - Length before first sectional division (in cm)
  - Any vascular thrombus: Yes/No (If yes, mention the degree of occlusion)
- *Segment IV artery origin*: RHA/LHA/others (mention)
- *Any variant vascular anatomy*: Yes/No (If yes, specify according to Michel classification)
- *Accessory RHA/ LHA/segmental artery (if any)*:
  - Vessel of origin
  - Diameter at origin (in mm)
  - Length before first division (in cm)

Portal venous anatomy:
- *Main portal vein (MPV)*:
  - Length before first division (in cm)
  - Any evidence of portal hypertension: Yes/No
  - Any thrombus: Yes/No. If yes, mention the extent (length and degree of luminal compromise), duration (acute vs. chronic), nature (bland vs. malignant) and the presence of collaterals
- *Right portal vein (RPV)*:
  - Length before first sectional division (in cm)
  - Diameter at origin (in mm)
  - Any thrombus: Yes/No
- *Left portal vein (LPV)*:
  - Length before first sectional division (in cm)
  - Diameter at origin (in mm)
  - Any thrombus: Yes/No
- *Any variant vascular anatomy*: Yes/No. If yes, specify according to Nakamura's classification. If type C, mention the distance between the ostium of the right anterior and posterior sectional portal veins (in cm).
- Accessory RPV/LPV (if any)

Hepatic venous anatomy:
- *Diameters at IVC ostium in milimeter*:
  - Right hepatic vein (RHV)
  - Common middle hepatic vein (MHV) and left hepatic vein (LHV) stump (mention otherwise if separate)
- *Any major (>4 mm) segment V/VIII tributaries into MHV*: Yes/No. If yes, mention the number
- *Any significant segment VI/VII drainage into segment V/VII veins or MHV*: Yes/No. If yes, describe
- *Any accessory inferior RHV*: Yes/No. If yes, specify the number of veins and the vertical distance between these veins and the RHV in centimeter
- Any thrombosis of IVC: Yes/No. If yes, mention the site, extent, and nature

Other abdominal organs: Normal/abnormal. If abnormal, specify

Ascites or lymphadenopathy: Yes/No

Visualized lung bases and bone: Normal/abnormal. If abnormal, specify

(HU: Hounsfield units; IHBD: intrahepatic bile duct; IVC: inferior vena cava; MDCT: multidetector computed tomography)

setting of LDLT. Multiphase liver CT is the modality of choice for pretransplantation assessment of living donors and recipients whereas MRCP is commonly used for evaluating the biliary tree. Understanding the indications for transplantations and the standard surgical techniques is important for a thorough assessment and can help the radiologist craft a clear and meaningful report **(Box 2)**. This reports with the sets of reconstructed images and 3D models, allows the surgeon to safely perform liver transplants thus avoiding post-transplant complications. Imaging is also helpful in detecting various postoperative complications and long-term follow-up for transplant viability.[32]

ACKNOWLEDGMENTS

Authors sincerely acknowledge Dr Sujoy Pal and Dr Nihar Ranjan Dash from the Department of Gastrointestinal Surgery, All India Institute of Medical Sciences, New Delhi, India.

REFERENCES

1. Ioannou GN. Development and validation of a model predicting graft survival after liver transplantation. Liver Transpl. 2006;12(11):1594-606.
2. United Network for Organ Sharing. (2016). National Data Report. [online] Available from http://www.unos.org/ [Last accessed July, 2016].
3. Koffron A, Stein JA. Liver transplantation: indications, pretrans plant evaluation, surgery, and post-transplant complications. Med Clin North Am. 2008;92(4):861-88, ix.
4. Kamath PS, Wiesner RH, Malinchoc M, Kremers W, Therneau TM, Kosberg CL, et al. A model to predict survival in patients with end-stage liver disease. Hepatology. 2001;33(2):464-70.
5. Singh AK, Cronin CG, Verma HA, Boland GW, Saini S, Mueller PR, et al. Imaging of preoperative liver transplantation in adults: what radiologists should know. Radiographics. 2011;31(4):1017-30.
6. Toso C, Trotter J, Wei A, Bigam DL, Shah S, Lancaster J, et al. Total tumor volume predicts risk of recurrence following liver transplantation in patients with hepatocellular carcinoma. Liver Transpl. 2008;14(8):1107-15.
7. Woo HY, Jang JW, Choi JY, You CR, Jeong SW, Bae SH, et al. Living donor liver transplantation in hepatocellular carcinoma beyond the Milan criteria. Liver Int. 2008;28(8):1120-8.
8. Marelli L, Grasso A, Pleguezuelo M, Martines H, Stigliano R, Dhillon AP, et al. Tumour size and differentiation in predicting recurrence of hepatocellular carcinoma after liver transplantation: external validation of a new prognostic score. Ann Surg Oncol. 2008;15(12):3503-11.
9. Tanaka K, Yamada T. Living donor liver transplantation in Japan and Kyoto University: What can we learn? J Hepatol. 2005;42(1):25-8.
10. Foster R, Zimmerman M, Trotter JF. Expanding donor options: marginal, living, and split donors. Clin Liver Dis. 2007;11(2):417-29.
11. Broering DC, Wilms C, Lenk C, Schulte am Esch J 2nd, Schönherr S, Mueller L, et al. Technical refinements and results in full-right full-left splitting of the deceased donor liver. Ann Surg. 2005;242(6):802-12;discussion 812-3.
12. Rosenkrantz AB, Campbell N, Wehrli N, Triolo MJ, Kim S. New OPTN/UNOS classification system for nodules in cirrhotic livers detected with MR Imaging: Effect on hepatocellular carcinoma detection and transplant allocation. Radiology. 2015;274(2):426-33.
13. American College of Radiology. (2016). Liver imaging reporting and data system. [online] Available from http://www.acr.org/quality-safety/resources/LIRADS [Last accessed July, 2016].
14. Prasad MA, Kulik LM. The role of bridge therapy prior to orthotopic liver transplantation. J Natl Compr Canc Netw. 2014;12:1183-91.
15. Forner A, Gilabert M, Gruix J, Raoul JL. Treatment of intermediate-stage hepatocellular carcinoma. Nat Rev Clin Oncol. 2014;11:525-35.
16. Tsang LL, Chen CL, Huang TL, Chen TY, Wang CC, Ou HY, et al. Preoperative imaging evaluation of potential living liver donors: reasons for exclusion from donation in adult living donor liver transplantation. Transplant Proc. 2008;40(8):2460-2.
17. Michels NA. Blood supply and anatomy of upper abdominal organs. Philadelphia, PA: Lippincott; 1955.
18. Fan ST, Lo CM, Liu CL. Technical refinement in adult-to-adult living donor liver transplantation using right lobe graft. Ann Surg. 2000;231:126-31.
19. Sahani D, Mehta A, Blake M, Prasad S, Harris G, Saini S. Preoperative hepatic vascular evaluation with CT and MR angiography: implications for surgery. RadioGraphics. 2004;24(5):1367-80.
20. Erbay N, Raptopoulos V, Pomfret EA, Kamel IR, Kruskal JB. Living donor liver transplantation in adults: vascular variants important in surgical planning for donors and recipients. AJR. 2003;181(1):109-14.
21. Sahani D, D'souza R, Kadavigere R, Hertl M, McGowan J, Saini S, et al. Evaluation of living liver transplant donors: method for precise anatomic definition by using a dedicated contrast enhanced MR imaging protocol. Radiographics. 2004;24:957-67.
22. Itamoto T, Emoto K, Mitsuta H, Fukuda S, Ohdan H, Tashiro H, et al. Safety of donor right hepatectomy for adult-to-adult living donor liver transplantation. Transpl Int. 2006;19(3):177-83.
23. Piekarski J, Goldberg HI, Royal SA, Axel L, Moss AA. Difference between liver and spleen CT numbers in the normal adult: its usefulness in predicting the presence of diffuse liver disease. Radiology. 1980;137:727-9.
24. Sugi MD, Joshi G, Maddu KK, Dahiya N, Menias CO. Imaging of renal transplant complications throughout the life of the allograft: Comprehensive multimodality review. RadioGraphics. 2019;5:1327-55.
25. Agostini C, Buccianti S, Risaliti M, Fortuna L, Tirloni L, Tucci R, et al. Complications in post-liver transplant patients. J Clin Med. 2023;12(19):6173.
26. Orons PD, Sheng R, Zajko AB. Hepatic artery stenosis in liver transplant recipients: prevalence and cholangiographic appearance of associated biliary complications. AJR. 1995;165(5):1145-9.
27. Singh AK, Nachiappan AC, Verma HA, Uppot RN, Blake MA, Saini S, et al. Postoperative imaging in liver transplantation: what radiologists should know. Radiographics. 2010;30(2):339-51.
28. Nghiem HV. Imaging of hepatic transplantation. Radiol Clin North Am. 1998;36(2):429-43.
29. Uzochukwu LN, Bluth EI, Smetherman DH, Troxclair LA, Loss GE Jr, Cohen A, et al. Early postoperative hepatic sonography as a predictor of vascular and biliary complications in adult orthotopic liver transplant patients. AJR. 2005;185(6):1558-70.
30. Fulcher AS, Turner MA. Orthotopic liver transplantation: Evaluation with MR cholangiography. Radiology. 1999;211(3):715-22.
31. Zemel G, Zajko AB, Skolnick ML, Bron KM, Campbell WL. The role of sonography and transhepatic cholangiography in the diagnosis of biliary complications after liver transplantation. AJR. 1988;151(5):943-6.
32. Dupuy DE, Costello P. Cross-sectional imaging of liver transplantation. Semin Ultrasound CT MR. 1992;13(5):399-409.

CHAPTER 14

Naveen Kalra, Sreedhara BC, Ujjwal Gorsi, Mandeep Garg

Imaging and Interventions in Hepatic Venous Outflow Tract Obstruction

INTRODUCTION

Hepatic venous outflow tract obstruction, Budd–Chiari syndrome (BCS), is a rare disorder which can involve the hepatic veins (HVs), inferior vena cava (IVC) or both and is characterized by structural and functional abnormalities of the liver. The term "Budd–Chiari" was coined after George Budd, who reported three cases of HV thrombosis in 1845 and Hans Chiari, who in 1899 described obliterating endophlebitis of the HVs.[1] According to a recent meta-analysis, which included six studies from Asia and Europe, the prevalence and the annual incidence of BCS was 2.40–33.10 per million and 0.168–4.09 per million, respectively.[2] However, taking into consideration the single-center studies from China and India which included hundreds of patients,[3,4] the disease appears to be more common in India, China, South Africa, and Japan as compared to the Western countries.

Based on the level of occlusion, BCS may be classified into three types.[5] In type I, involvement is at the level of IVC alone; in type II, it is at the level of HVs and type III involves both IVC and HVs. It can also be classified based on the underlying cause (primary and secondary) and the duration of symptoms (fulminant, acute, subacute, or chronic BCS).

CLINICAL PRESENTATION

The clinical picture of BCS is dictated by the degree of venous obstruction and the rapidity with which it develops. Usually, the clinical presentation of the syndrome is nonspecific. Sudden and large blockage leads to acute BCS, which presents as abdominal pain (usually severe), ascites, jaundice, tender hepatomegaly, and rapidly developing hepatic failure. The most frequently encountered clinical type is subacute BCS. Having an insidious onset, it may take up to 3 months to become symptomatic. The progress is slow and during the period decompressive collaterals develop. Thus subacute BCS does not present with esophageal bleed. On the other hand, when there is still more insidious gradual venous outflow obstruction it leads to chronic BCS which is characterized by postsinusoidal portal hypertension, prominent abdominal veins, upper GI bleed, pedal edema, ascites, and large nodular liver that develops over many months. Rarely, BCS can present as acute fulminant liver failure when all three HVs are acutely thrombosed.[3] Acute BCS is more frequently reported from the western part of the globe, whereas chronic BCS cases are more often reported from Japan, China, South Africa, and India. Differentiation of acute and chronic forms is vital to determine the prognosis and to plan the treatment. In acute BCS cases, the prognosis is poor with high mortality if not treated, whereas chronic BCS is less ominous and half the patients are alive after 5 years.[6]

ETIOPATHOGENESIS

The BCS is labeled as primary when the outflow obstruction is because of primary venous thrombosis, stenosis, or web. It is classified as secondary when venous outflow is obstructed by extrinsic compression by tumor, cyst, or abscess.[7] These lesions obstruct venous outflow by invasion of the lumen or by extrinsic compression. Most BCS patients have an underlying inherited or acquired hypercoagulable state. Myeloproliferative disease is the most common thrombotic disorder detected. The other associations include JAK2 V617F mutation, factor V Leiden mutation, pregnancy, antiphospholipid antibodies, oral contraceptive pills, paroxysmal nocturnal hemoglobinuria, and protein C and S deficiency. JAK2 V617F mutation may be picked up in 30–50% of BCS cases.[4]

Geographical variation has also been noted in the etiology of BCS.[8] In Asia, the most frequent causes are membranous obstruction of the IVC (MOVC), pregnancy, and infections, while in the West, primary myeloproliferative disorders, hypercoagulable states, steroidal contraceptives, and tumors are responsible in majority of cases. While earlier studies from India found isolated IVC involvement to be the most common disease type, recent studies found the combination of IVC and HV obstruction to be the most frequently reported.[9] Rarely, BCS may occur due to malignant thrombosis of the IVC or main HVs secondary to hepatic, renal, and adrenal neoplasms.[10] Hepatocellular carcinoma (HCC) can produce an acute fulminant variant of BCS by causing obstruction of the HVs or IVC because of endoluminal invasion. However, in up to 20% of patients etiology remains unidentified and classified as idiopathic BCS.[4] Initially when the HVs occlude, the sinusoidal and portal pressures increase and there is hepatic congestion **(Fig. 1A)**. This increase in sinusoidal pressure leads to hypoxic injury to hepatocytes which results in noninflammatory centrilobular cell necrosis especially in perivenular zones. In case the hepatocyte damage is large, patients present with fulminant disease. In case the damage is insidious, the liver slowly develops fibrosis and then cirrhosis **(Fig. 1B)**. The patient will then present with portal hypertension and ascites.

Liver biopsy differentiates BCS from veno-occlusive disease (VOD), an entity that occurs because of nonthrombotic occlusion of HVs by subendothelial swelling on account of sinusoidal wall injury **(Fig. 1C)**. The causes of VOD include ingestion of toxins, drugs (chemotherapeutic agents), and irradiation. The myeloablative regimens in hematopoietic stem cell transplantation combined with high-dose chemotherapeutic agents remain the most common cause of VOD. Cyclophosphamide-containing regimen is the most common causative agent. VOD is also known as sinusoidal obstruction syndrome (SOS). Although VOD mimics BCS and causes hepatic outflow blockade, it has been separately classified from primary BCS and to distinguish from BCS, VOD has been termed as SOS.[11,12]

DIAGNOSTIC TECHNIQUES

Recent developments in imaging modalities and techniques have facilitated delineation of exact vascular abnormalities and their treatment, leading to improvement in survival rates of BCS patients. Most commonly used modalities are ultrasound doppler, magnetic resonance imaging (MRI), and computed tomography (CT). The historical gold

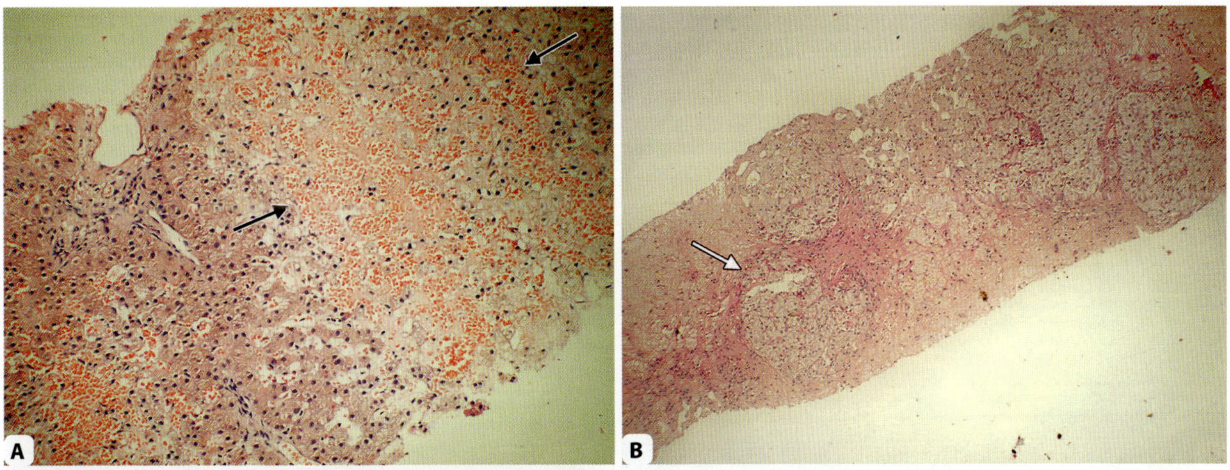

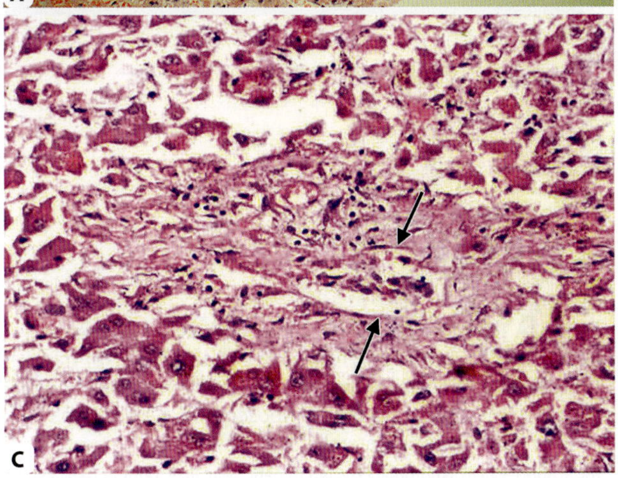

FIGS. 1A TO C: (A) Photomicrograph shows normal portal tract with sinusoidal congestion (arrows) in acute Budd–Chiari syndrome. (B) Photomicrograph shows centrizonal fibrosis (arrow) indicating chronic Budd-Chiari syndrome. (C) Photomicrograph shows occlusion of central vein in acute veno-occlusive disease (arrows).

Courtesy: Professor Ashim Das, Department of Histopathology, PGIMER, Chandigarh, India.

standard, invasive hepatic/IVC venography is currently limited to assessment during therapeutic interventions and/or in rare circumstances for diagnosing when primary noninvasive modalities are inconclusive. Ultrasound Doppler remains the primary investigation of choice for diagnosis due to easy availability and less economical burden, with sensitivity and specificity of >80% in diagnosing BCS. However, the confounding factors such as large body habitus and observer's experience in accurately diagnosing BCS with ultrasound Doppler can be overcome with use of cross-sectional imaging. Both CT and MRI can depict the location and extent of venous thrombosis or stenosis, parenchymal changes and aid in delineating the venous anatomy for therapeutic interventions. MRI is also useful in characterizing the nodules associated with BCS.[13-15]

A recent systematic review and meta-analysis on diagnostic accuracy of noninvasive modalities for diagnosis of BCS documented a pooled sensitivity and specificity of 89% and 68% for Doppler ultrasound, 89% and 72% for CT, and 93% and 55% for MRI, respectively. Overall, MRI showed the highest sensitivity whereas CT showed highest specificity, however, with good diagnostic accuracy all three investigations can be used interchangeably based on the experience and availability.[16]

EVALUATION OF HEPATIC VEINS IN BUDD–CHIARI SYNDROME

Real-time sonography is considered the investigation of choice for initial assessment of BCS. The technique demonstrates the morphological hepatic alterations along with thrombosis/occlusion of HVs or IVC. At the same time, other organs can also be evaluated. The findings picked up on ultrasound include hepatomegaly, heterogeneous liver, and caudate hypertrophy. Additionally, features that suggest HV thrombosis on ultrasonography include nonvisualization of the HV-IVC confluence, distorted or absent HVs, stenosed veins with thick wall echoes **(Fig. 2A)**, hyperechoic HVs **(Fig. 2B)**, portal vein thrombosis, and ascites. Presence of comma-shaped venovenous intrahepatic collaterals is taken as a highly reliable sign **(Fig. 2C)**.[17-21] Subcapsular venous collaterals may also be seen. In case only the HV occlusion is the cause of BCS, at least two of the HVs must be occluded for the disease to be clinically evident.[22]

Liver is usually enlarged but could be normal in size. Advanced chronic BCS may show shrunken liver. Right lobe may be atrophied with associated left lobe hypertrophy. Echotexture is homogenously hypoechoic in acute BCS

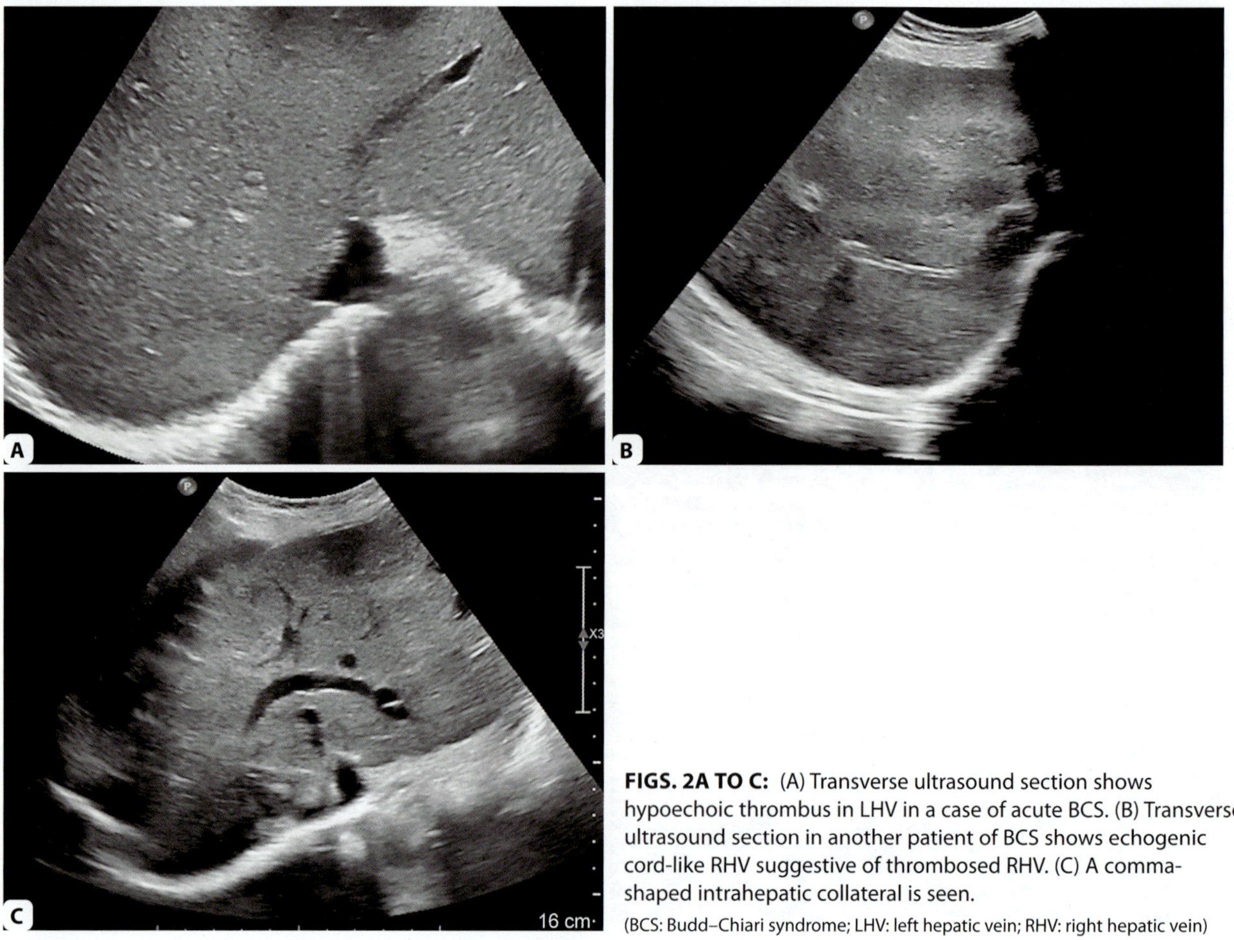

FIGS. 2A TO C: (A) Transverse ultrasound section shows hypoechoic thrombus in LHV in a case of acute BCS. (B) Transverse ultrasound section in another patient of BCS shows echogenic cord-like RHV suggestive of thrombosed RHV. (C) A comma-shaped intrahepatic collateral is seen.

(BCS: Budd–Chiari syndrome; LHV: left hepatic vein; RHV: right hepatic vein)

and nonhomogeneous in chronic BCS. The surface of the liver may be nodular due to changes of cirrhosis. Caudate hypertrophy is seen in 82–91% of the patients and is a useful diagnostic pointer, but is a nonspecific sign and may be seen in cirrhosis secondary to other causes.[23]

Caudate hypertrophy occurs because it has separate venous drainage which is not affected by the thrombotic process and which drains into the IVC directly just distal to the ostia of the HVs. This segment of the liver thus receives uninterrupted supply of hepatotropic agents like insulin. Caudate lobe drainage serves as an outflow for intrahepatic venous collaterals. A caudate vein diameter > 3 mm strongly suggests the diagnosis of BCS in the appropriate clinical background.[24] The accuracy of ultrasound for picking up HV thrombosis has been reported to be 70–87% in the literature.[20,25] The normal diameter of right and middle HVs is <10 mm and that of left HV is <9 mm.[26] The technique has limitations in cases of swollen and nodular, or shrunken and scarred liver in which HVs may be obscured within the hepatic parenchyma. Detection of intraluminal webs and membranes is also limited. Poor visualization of extrahepatic collaterals and possibility of an inadequate scan because of bowel gas are also limiting factors.

Color Doppler combined with grayscale imaging has improved the diagnostic performance as it allows better visualization of HVs by automatically adding flow information. Doppler waveform of HVs in healthy individuals is a triphasic waveform **(Fig. 3A)**.[27] Presence of flat waveform (monophasic flow) or absent or reversed flow in HVs is the most reliable signs of HV thrombosis **(Fig. 3B)**. Veins that are not seen on grayscale imaging because of compression by liver nodules may show flow on color Doppler, thus proving to be normal. The contrast-enhanced ultrasound (CEUS) can also be used for diagnosis and is a useful adjunct to improve the diagnostic accuracy **(Fig. 4)**.[28]

Magnetic resonance imaging can also be utilized for HV evaluation.[29] T2-weighted gradient-echo sequence or multiphase contrast-enhanced images are needed for the evaluation of vessels and collaterals. MR has the distinct advantage of showing HVs in three dimensions but on routine sequences, its ability to ascertain the degree of flow is limited. As reported by multiple authors, Color Doppler is superior to MR for assessing the HVs as the ostial narrowing can be better appreciated on US and additionally, hemodynamic flow across the confluence can be evaluated. The angiographic techniques used for studying the HVs include IVC venography with retrograde HV cannulation, and direct hepatic venography under US guidance following contrast injection into peripheral segment of HV under fluoroscopy to localize the level of obstruction and intrahepatic collaterals. These techniques are the most definitive but are reserved for cases being considered for angioplasty or stent placement where exact delineation of the stenosed segment and its length is necessary for guiding management. In BCS, there is a collateral circulation between the tributaries of the HVs which forms a "spider web". In the initial stage, these collaterals are fine giving rise to a "fine spider web". With long standing BCS, these collaterals form a "coarse spider web".[30] Arteriography in BCS patients would show larger caliber of the hepatic artery as compared to the splenic artery since the blood supply to the liver by the hepatic artery is increased.[31]

Scintigraphy and CT have also been used for the evaluation of BCS. Scintigraphy may show elevated uptake by caudate and left lobe, with patchy uptake of radionuclide in the rest of the liver giving the appearance of hot spots.

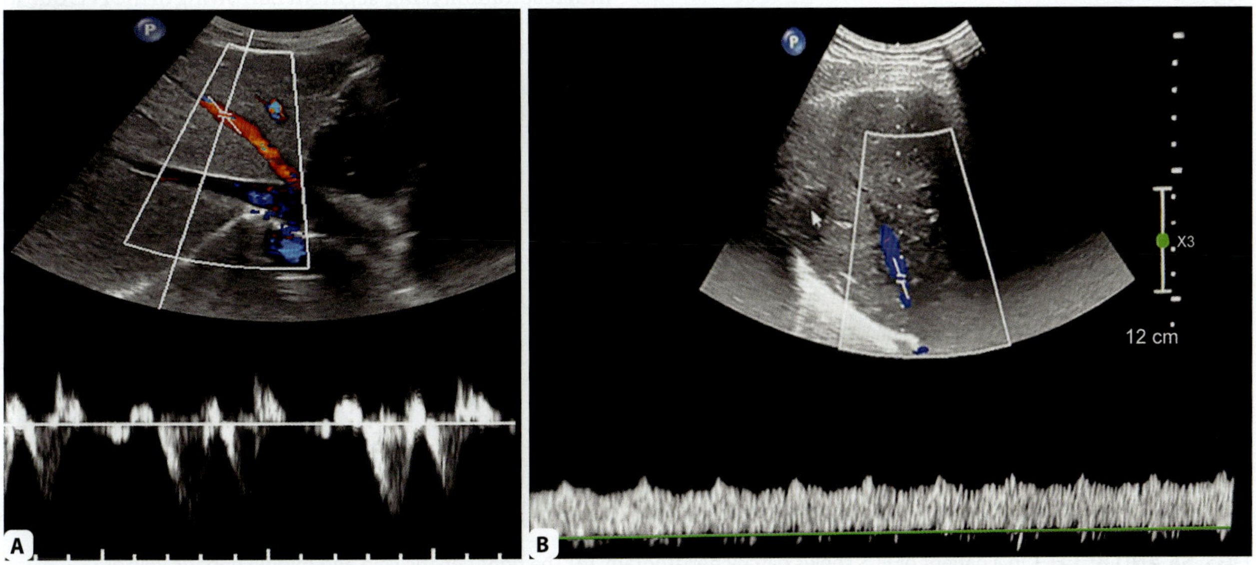

FIGS. 3A AND B: Normal pulsed Doppler tracing in the left hepatic vein (LHV) shows the triphasic waveform. (A) The antegrade flow occurs during the ventricular systole and atrial diastole while retrograde flow occurs during the atrial systole. (B) Color Doppler US with color box placed in the region of RHV in a patient of Budd–Chiari syndrome (BCS) shows uniphasic flow.

On CT, caudate hypertrophy with low attenuation areas elsewhere, right lobe atrophy, nonvisualization of HVs, and nodular liver surface may be seen. On CECT presence of patchy hepatogram, areas of linear, irregular, or wedge-shaped hypoattenuation particularly in the peripheral portions of liver due to fibrosis and parenchymal destruction indicate hepatic venous thrombosis. Dynamic CT may demonstrate thrombus within the HVs and comma-shaped intrahepatic collaterals **(Fig. 5A)**. Presence of areas of hypoattenuation surrounded by areas of increased enhancement can simulate presence of intrahepatic mass lesion. The availability of volume imaging and 3D reconstructions will provide a useful adjunct to axial images for the evaluation of intra- and extrahepatic collaterals **(Fig. 5B)**.[31]

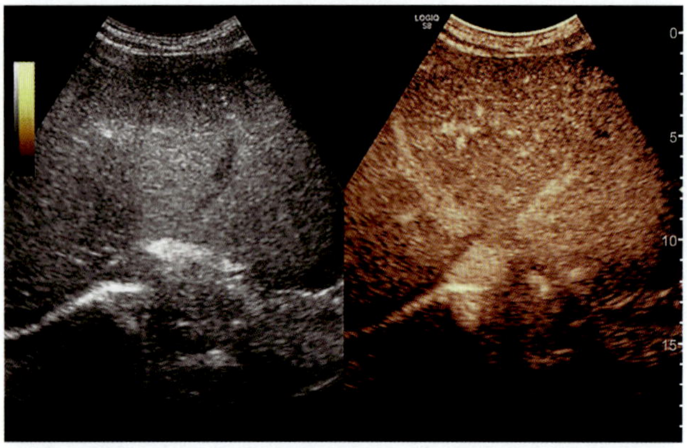

FIG. 4: CEUS in the case of BCS. The hepatic veins are poorly appreciated in the background of heterogenous liver echotexture, with ill-defined hepatic-venous confluence. On CEUS, course of MHV and LHV are well appreciated with stenosis at the level of hepaticovenous confluence.

(BCS: Budd–Chiari syndrome; CEUS: contrast-enhanced ultrasound; LHV: left hepatic vein; RHV: right hepatic vein)

Courtesy: Dr Pankaj Gupta, Department of Radiodiagnosis, PGIMER, Chandigarh, India.

EVALUATION OF INFERIOR VENA CAVA IN BUDD–CHIARI SYNDROME

Inferior vena cava evaluation is an essential component of the imaging in suspected cases of BCS. IVC obstruction alone or in combination with HV obstruction can lead to BCS. Conversely, establishing IVC patency is a must before deciding upon the type of the surgical intervention as mesoatrial shunt is indicated when IVC is obstructed and portocaval/mesocaval shunt in cases of patent IVC.

Incidence of IVC obstruction in BCS varies from 33 to 56%.[32,33] IVC can be obstructed in its intrahepatic portion, suprahepatic portion, or both. The causes of IVC obstruction are membranes, tumor thrombus, and caudate lobe hypertrophy.[20,32,33] Suprahepatic obstruction is generally due to short segment stenosis or IVC webs. Intrahepatic IVC obstruction is most commonly due to compression from the enlarged caudate lobe. Chronic thrombosis of the IVC can evolve into calcification.[31]

Webs are visualized as thin linear filling defects on contrast venography and MR angiography. On ultrasound imaging, webs appear as hyperreflective linear foci, best appreciated in deep inspiration **(Figs. 6A to C)**. Whether these webs represent congenital lesions or they are the result of thrombotic process is an issue which remains disputed.[34] It is quite plausible to assume that both segmental stenosis and IVC web represent the spectrum of same pathological process, i.e., thrombosis.

On real-time ultrasound, short-segment stenosis is seen as an area of narrowing and the caliber of IVC is dilated proximal to the obstruction with loss of phasic variation with respiration. Long-segment narrowing of the IVC due to

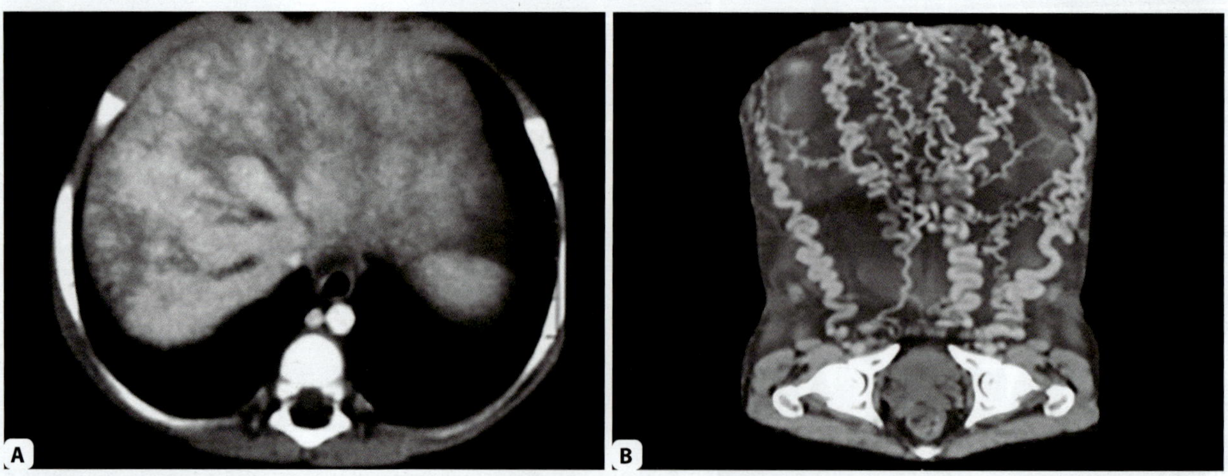

FIGS. 5A AND B: CECT in a patient of BCS shows patchy hepatogram. (A) The right hepatic vein and middle hepatic vein are thrombosed while the left hepatic vein is not visualized. (B) MDCT reconstructed image shows multiple parietal wall collaterals in a patient with type III BCS.

(BCS: Budd–Chiari syndrome; CECT: contrast-enhanced computed tomography; MDCT: multidetector computed tomography)

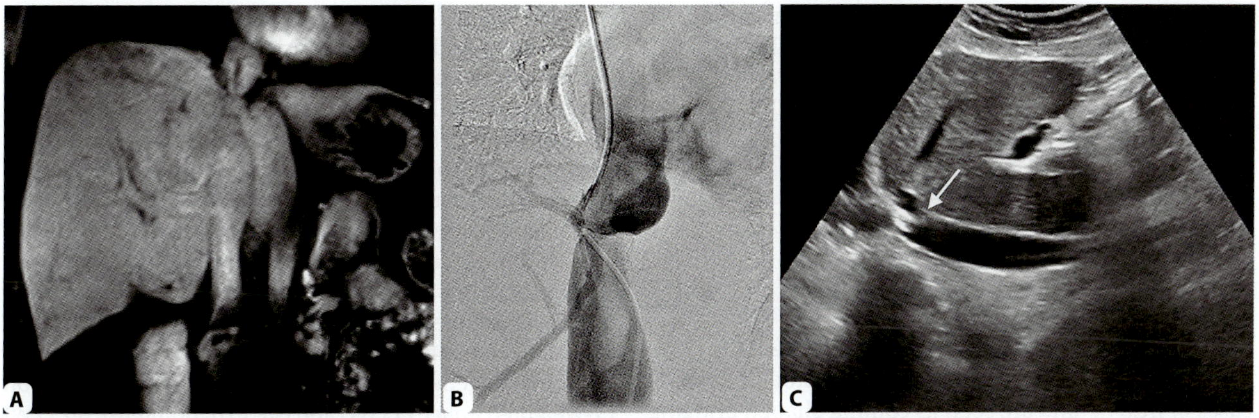

FIGS. 6A TO C: A 45-year-old male presenting with abdominal distention. (A) Coronal T1W VIBE postcontrast image shows a hypointense linear signal in the inferior vena cava (IVC) proximal to cavoatrial junction suggestive of a web. (B) IVC venography with catheters both proximal and distal to the IVC narrowing shows slit-like web. There is filling up of an intrahepatic collateral. (C) Parasagittal gray scale ultrasound in a different patient shows hyperechoic calcified web (arrow).

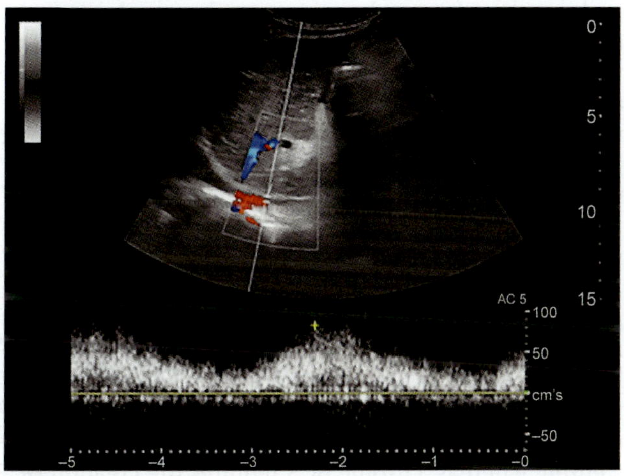

FIG. 7: Color Doppler image shows focal short segment narrowing in the intrahepatic portion of IVC with uniphasic flow pattern and increased flow velocity consistent with stenosis.

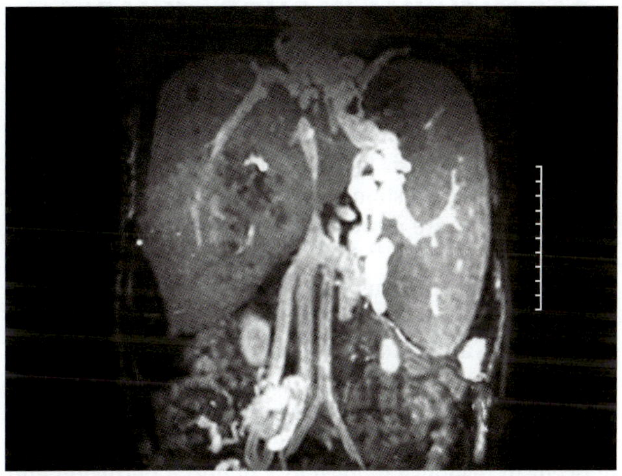

FIG. 8: Coronal contrast-enhanced MR venography shows long segment narrowing of inferior vena cava (IVC) in intrahepatic portion with filling defect proximal to cavoatrial junction. There are multiple collaterals in the retroperitoneum and at the splenic hilum.

caudate lobe enlargement is well depicted. In cases where IVC obstruction is due to tumor thrombi, extension of the tumor into the IVC can be well demonstrated on ultrasound. The limitations of ultrasound are, suboptimal evaluation due to bowel gases, inability to ascertain hemodynamic significance of IVC narrowing and assess exact length of stenosis for treatment planning.

Color Doppler ultrasound combined with real-time 2D imaging is superior to grayscale imaging as it provides better assessment of IVC adding flow information. The normal IVC flow pattern is a triphasic waveform. The flow abnormalities can be either absent flow in cases of IVC occlusion and uniphasic or reversed flow in cases of stenosis.[35] Turbulent flow can be appreciated at the site of short-segment stenosis **(Fig. 7)**.[35,36]

The inferior venocavography is considered the gold standard investigation for evaluation of IVC. However, it has certain limitations particularly for evaluation of HVs. The limitations of IVC venography include nonvisualization of IVC distal to obstruction due to diversion of contrast into the collaterals and suboptimal evaluation of status of HVs either due to stenosis at the confluence or thrombosis leading to difficult cannulation. Thus, in case of suprahepatic obstruction due to web/membrane visualization of IVC above and below the lesion may require double catheter study **(Fig. 6B)**. Lastly, the intrahepatic collaterals which are important parameters for diagnosis of chronic BCS are not detected with IVC venography.

Recently, MR venography has shown a great potential in overcoming many of the limitations of IVC venography. MR venography accurately depicts the site and cause of IVC obstruction with clear delineation of IVC both above and below the obstruction **(Fig. 8)**.[25,29] MR is excellent for detection of both intra- and extrahepatic collaterals, portal vein obstruction, and detection of tumor thrombi within the IVC. Incidence of portal vein thrombosis in BCS is 5–20%.[35,36]

Five Types of Collateral Pathways Develop in Budd–Chiari Syndrome[37]

1. Left renal-hemiazygous pathways
2. Vertebrolumbar azygous pathways
3. Intrahepatic collaterals
4. Superficial abdominal wall collaterals
5. Inferior phrenic-pericardiophrenic collaterals.

Intrahepatic collaterals have been noted in 80–93% cases of BCS[36-38] and are seen as comma-shaped bridging venovenous collaterals which reveal flat waveform on color Doppler ultrasound.

ASSESSMENT OF LIVER PARENCHYMA IN BUDD–CHIARI SYNDROME

The hepatic venous or IVC obstruction leads to ischemic damage to the liver cells resulting in severe congestion, centrilobular necrosis followed by fibrosis and cirrhosis. In acute BCS, congestion predominates whereas patients of chronic BCS are more likely to develop cirrhosis and regenerative nodules.[33] Since the obstruction of the HVs is usually asynchronous, liver biopsy may show areas of congestion and hyperplastic enlargement in the recently affected areas and fibrosis with atrophy in the older affected segments. As the distribution of the disease in the liver is inhomogeneous liver biopsy may even be normal.[39]

Development of regenerative nodules in BCS is known to occur in response to focal loss of portal perfusion and hyperarterialization in areas with preserved hepatic venous outflow.[31] Incidence of nodules >5 mm has been documented on histology in up to 40–80% of patients.[36,40] The possibility of malignant transformation of the large regenerative nodule remains unsettled and incidence of HCC is extremely rare in patients of BCS secondary to hepatic venous obstruction alone as compared to patients with IVC obstruction particularly MOVC.[33] The obstruction may make the hepatocytes more susceptible to the action of environment carcinogens. HCC in BCS accounts for 0.7% of all cases of hepatocellular carcinoma.[41] Differentiation of HCC from regenerative nodules is important. The MRI and triphasic CT are investigations of choice.[10,42,43]

Benign regenerative nodules which are hyperintense on T1-weighted image (T1WI) and iso- to hypointense on T2WI are likely to be benign **(Figs. 9A and B)** compared to HCC nodules which are hypointense on T1WI and hyperintense on T2WI **(Figs. 10 A to D)**. Multiple (>10) and small (<4 cm) lesions are suggestive of benignity.[10] On triphasic CT/dynamic contrast MRI evaluation, large regenerative nodules show intense homogeneous hyperenhancement on arterial phase and enhancement persists in the portal venous and late venous phase images unlike HCC which shows washout. On histopathology, these nodules have normal or hyperplastic hepatocytes, arteries extending radially from the center of the nodule, and a central scar in the larger nodules.[40,44] The imaging characteristics of this scar may be similar to those of the scar found in focal nodular hyperplasia on dynamic imaging.[40]

Liver biopsy has been used in the past to differentiate acute from subacute and chronic BCS. A liver biopsy is required only if radiological imaging is inconclusive.[45] Differentiation is important for deciding the plan of treatment. Acute BCS may be treated by infusion of thrombolytic substances at the site of block followed by stenting whereas, chronic BCS requires the creation of a shunt between the HVs and portal vein by transjugular

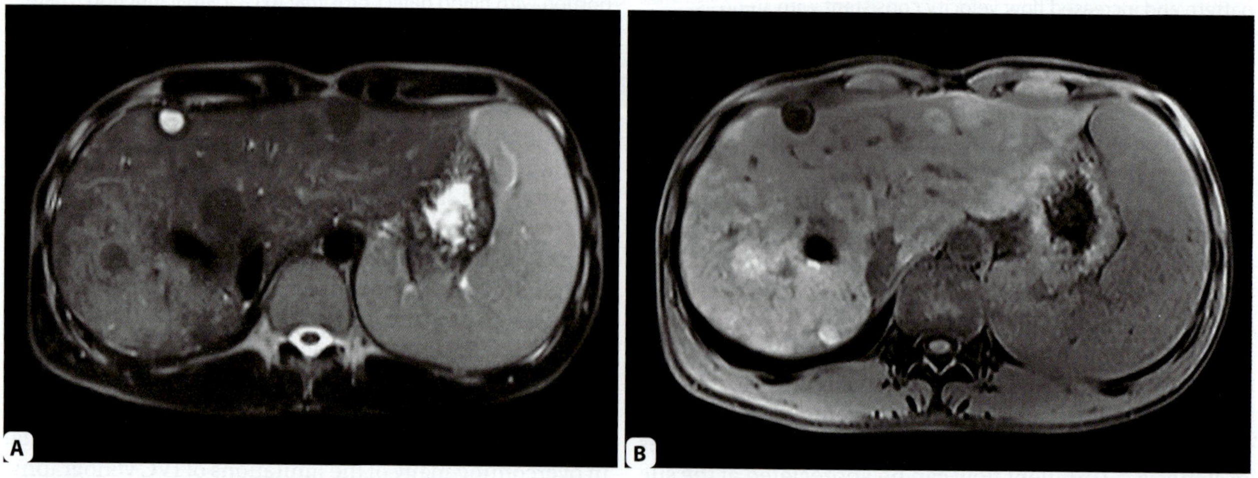

FIGS. 9A AND B: Axial T2W HASTE image shows multiple hypointense nodules of varying sizes in the liver (A). The Axial T1W VIBE image at the same level depicts the hyperintense signal of these nodules (B). The hyperintensity of the nodules on T1WI is suggestive of their benign nature. Note is made of thrombosed mesoatrial shunt and signal drop within the DIPS stent.

(DIPS: direct intrahepatic portosystemic shunt; HASTE: half-Fourier acquisition single- shot turbo spin-echo; T1WI: T1-weighted image; T2W: T2-weighted)

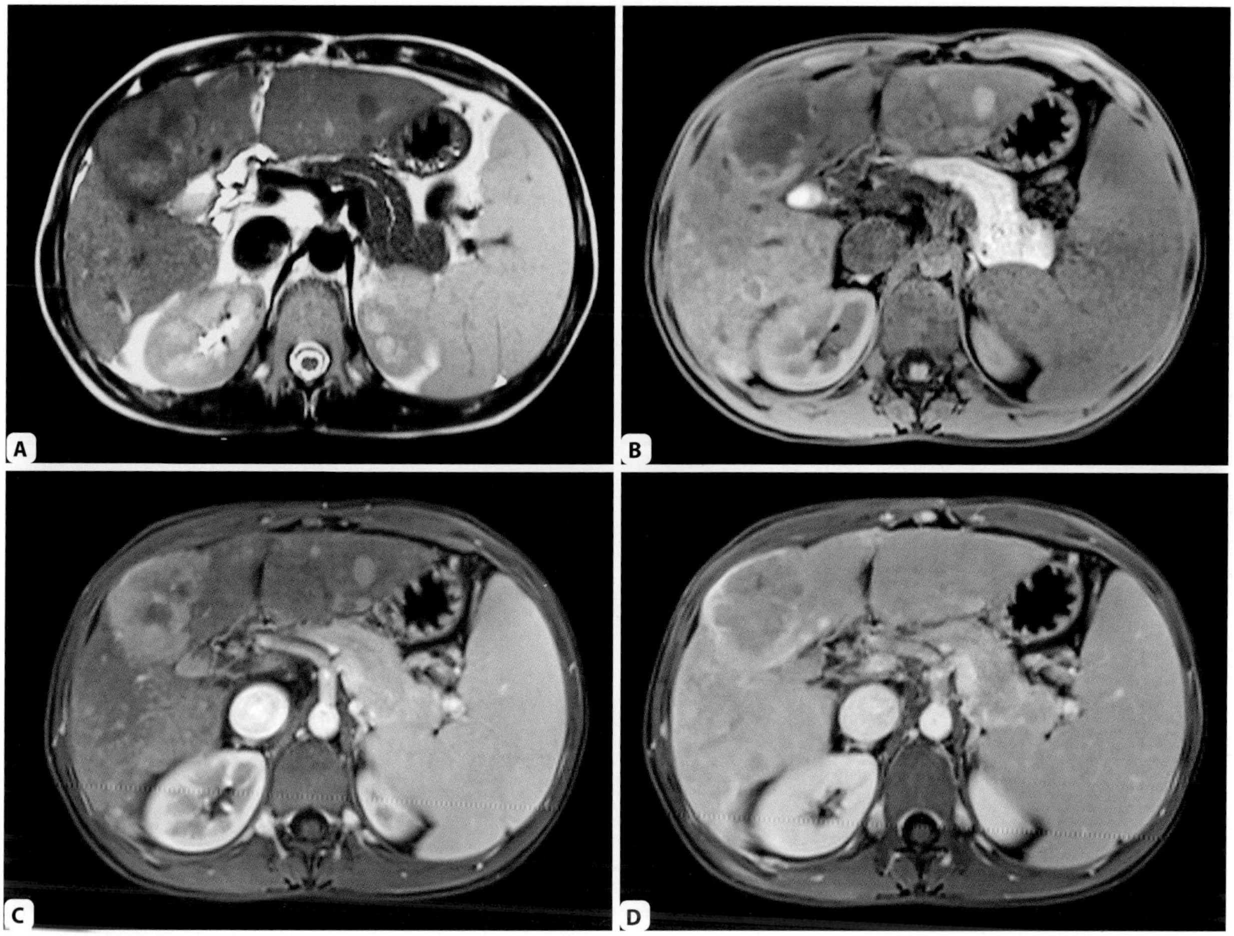

FIGS. 10A TO D: (A) Axial T2W HASTE image shows large heterogeneously hyperintense lesion in segment IV, (B) which appears predominantly hypointense on T1W VIBE MR image. (C) Postcontrast arterial phase image shows arterial hypervascularity with (D) washout and capsular enhancement in the delayed phase images consistent with HCC. Dilated infrahepatic IVC with paravertebral collaterals can be seen. Note made of segment III T2 hypointense, T1 hyperintense lesion with isointense signal on postcontrast delayed phase image suggestive of regenerative nodule.

(HASTE: half-Fourier acquisition single-shot turbo spin-echo; HCC: hepatocellular carcinoma; IVC: inferior vena cava)

intrahepatic portosystemic shunt (TIPS) procedure. MRI and dynamic CT are able to determine the chronicity of the hepatic changes in predominant cases limiting the necessity of liver biopsy.[25,46,47]

The role of MRI in differentiation of acute, subacute, and chronic BCS has been well described by Noone et al.[25] In acute BCS, there is decreased signal intensity on T1WI and heterogeneously increased signal intensity on T2WI peripherally with decreased enhancement of peripheral liver after gadolinium administration **(Figs. 11A to D)**.[48] These changes were attributed to acutely increased tissue pressures and edema in the peripheral portions of the liver because of hepatic venous obstruction thus causing diminished inflow of blood. As the duration of disease increases, there is reversal of flow in the portal vein and development of small collaterals permitting egress of blood. Thus, in subacute BCS, the signal characteristics on T1WI and T2 WI are like those observed in patients with acute disease, however, periphery shows marked heterogeneous enhancement unlike to that seen in acute BCS. Chronic BCS is characterized by changes of fibrosis and absence of parenchymal edema, and hence no differential signal intensity or enhancement is noted between peripheral and central liver. Using these criteria, in a study conducted at our institute 13 out of 20 cases of chronic BCS were correctly diagnosed with MRI **(Figs. 12A and B)**.[49]

Abnormal patterns of parenchymal enhancement have also been reported on triphasic helical CT in different stages of BCS in a study by Camera et al.[47] They found abnormal enhancement of the caudate lobe in the arterial phase, the "fan-shaped pattern", in all cases of acute BCS. Later a "flip-flop" pattern develops in which the central liver becomes hypodense compared to the peripheral liver. On the other hand, "patchy pattern" of enhancement was seen in patients of subacute and chronic BCS.

In conclusion, ultrasound with color flow Doppler imaging is the modality of choice for initial diagnosis of BCS. When combined with MR and magnetic resonance

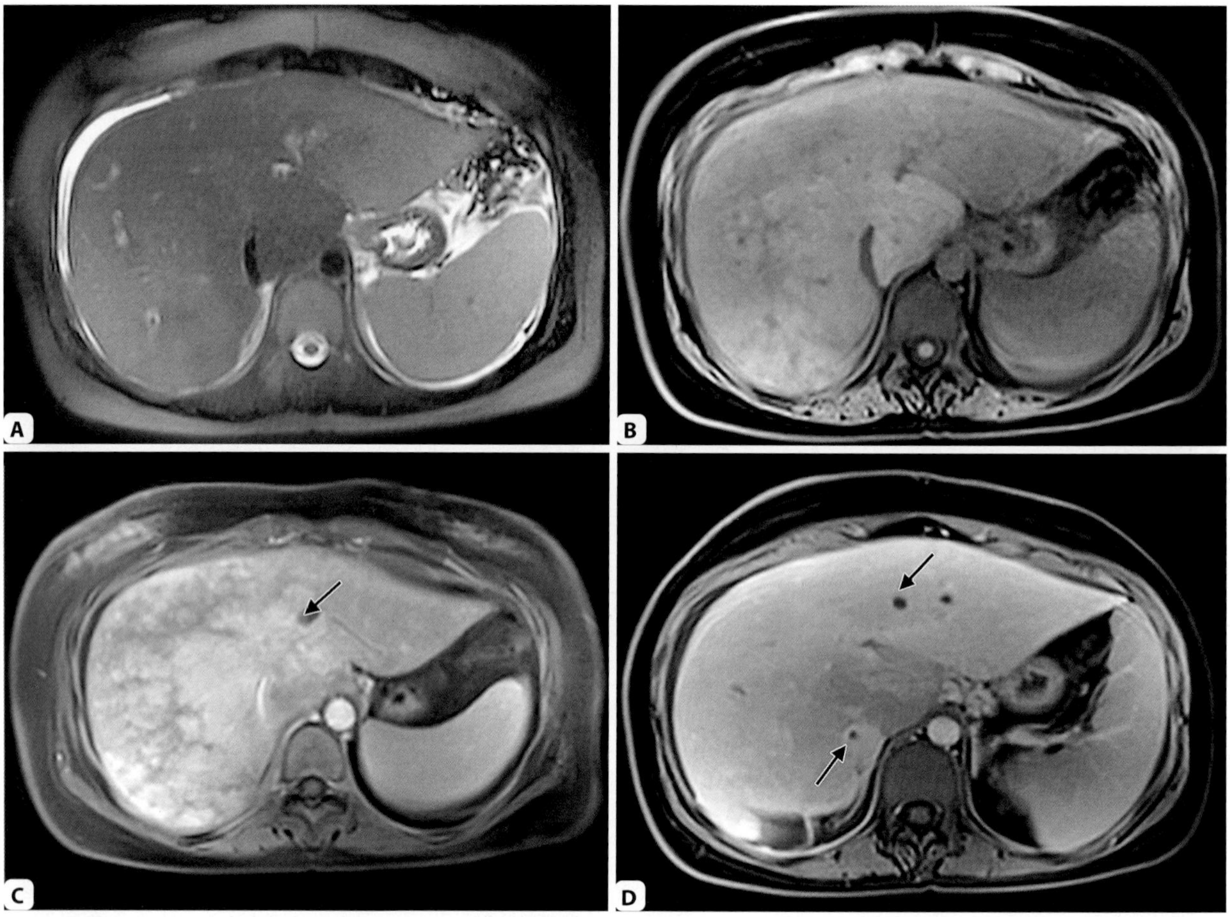

FIGS. 11A TO D: CEMRI abdomen of Acute BCS. (A) T2W axial image showing hypointense caudate and central part of liver with hyperintense periphery. (B) T1W axial image showing hyperintense caudate and central part of liver with hypointense periphery. (C and D) Postcontrast MR images show heterogeneous enhancement of liver with "flip-flop" appearance on delayed images. Hypointense thrombus in LHV and partial thrombus in IVC are noted (arrows).

(BCS: Budd–Chiari syndrome; CEMRI: contrast-enhanced magnetic resonance imaging; LHV: left hepatic vein; IVC: inferior vena cava)

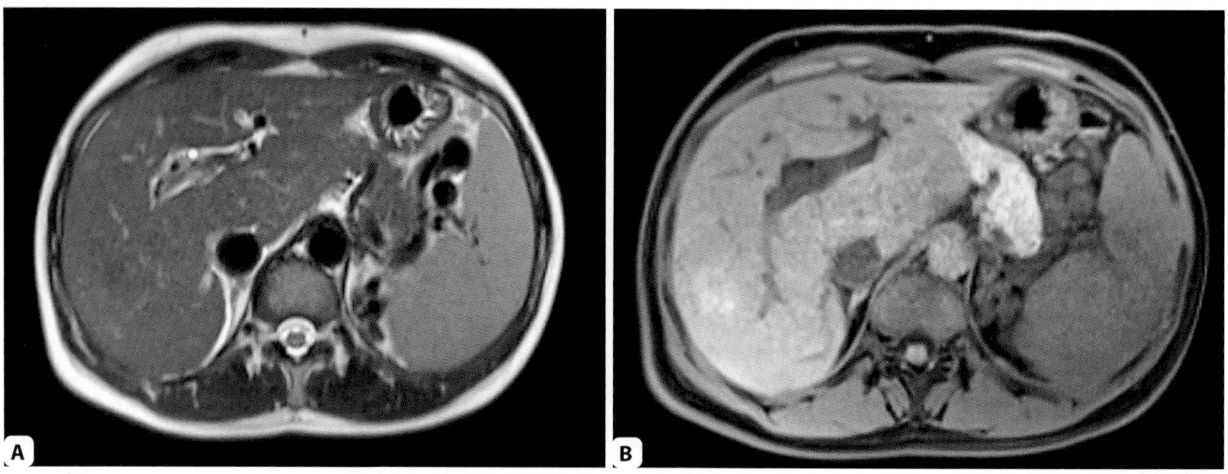

FIGS. 12A AND B: Axial T2W HASTE and T1W VIBE MR images show heterogeneous signal intensity of the liver with hypertrophied caudate lobe and dilated inferior vena cava (IVC). There is no differential SI of the peripheral or central liver seen. A case of chronic Budd–Chiari syndrome (BCS) due to hepatic vein thrombosis and IVC stenosis.

venography (MRV), need for diagnostic IVC venography can be obviated which can be reserved for patients where surgical or radiological intervention is being contemplated.

MANAGEMENT OF BUDD–CHIARI SYNDROME

The medical management or mode of intervention in cases of BCS is determined by the stage of the disease and the status of hepatocyte necrosis. The current recommendations for interventions are based primarily on retrospective studies, few prospective studies and expert guidelines. The management goals are aimed at treating underlying cause of BCS, medical management of portal hypertension complications, and correction of hepatic venous outflow tract obstruction by radiological or surgical interventions. Since BCS is a chronic disorder, presenting at younger age for most of the patients, it is imperative to have individualized, tailored stepwise approach with prioritization of least invasive intervention over more invasive options to achieve good long term results.[50-55]

The medical management includes lifelong anticoagulation, indicated in all patients irrespective of the underlying disease[52-54] and treatment of complications of portal hypertension. The aim of anticoagulation is to achieve recanalization of thrombosed veins and to prevent further progression or formation of thrombus. Currently, unfractionated heparin or low-molecular-weight heparin (LMWH) for the first 5–7 days in the acute setting and vitamin K agonists (VKA) for life-long administration are recommended. In case of acute BCS, systemic thrombolytic therapy has been shown to have varying outcome. Best results are noted by combining systemic thrombolysis with local direct pharmacological and mechanical thrombolysis.[56] The thrombolytic technique depends on the age of thrombus, with pharmacological thrombolysis for hyperacute thrombus and combined pharmacomechanical thrombolysis reserved for subacute to chronic thrombi.[54]

Radiological Interventions

Treatment of BCS by radiological intervention was first described in 1974 by Eguchi et al. who reported the successful balloon membranotomy for obstruction of the IVC.[57] The aim of the radiological interventions is the restoration of hepatic blood outflow by means of repermeation of the obstructed HVs or IVC or by portosystemic shunting. The methods include balloon angioplasty, stent insertion, and TIPS.

Angioplasty and Stenting

Angioplasty is the least invasive intervention, and as a standalone technique it is best suited for short segment stenosis of HVs/IVC and MOVC. Favorable outcomes after angioplasty recanalization have been reported from large series[58,59] with frequent restenosis reported in up to 50% of patients within a year.[60] A RCT comparing angioplasty alone with routine stenting during primary intervention reported a significant reduction in restenosis in patients who underwent routine stenting.[61] Hence, decision for primary stenting depends on length of the stenosis and initial response to angioplasty. Transjugular or percutaneous transhepatic access routes are used for HV recanalization, whereas transfemoral or transjugular route is used for MOVC or segmental IVC stenosis, while a combined approach is used in resistant cases **(Figs. 13 and 14)**. Griffith et al.[62] found restenosis in all 18 patients of angioplasty when followed for longer than 10 months. The use of stents has resulted in better long-term patency rates of the order of 80–90% over a year follow-up period **(Figs. 15A to F)**.[36,63,64] Baijal et al.[65] performed percutaneous angioplasty followed by primary stent placement in their study of nine patients with IVC obstruction. There was residual stenosis of about 9–40% after the procedure. Revascularization was successful in all patients and the IVC remained patent during the follow-up period (3–31 months).

Transjugular Intrahepatic Portosystemic Shunt/Direct Intrahepatic Portosystemic Shunt

Peltzer et al. and Ochs et al. described the successful treatment of BCS with TIPS in 1993.[66,67] This involves the placement of an intrahepatic shunt connecting a HV stump or IVC through the liver to a branch of the portal vein **(Figs. 16A to D)**. The transcaval approach is technically more feasible in BCS due to the enlarged caudate lobe surrounding the intrahepatic IVC providing stability for the transcaval direct intrahepatic portosystemic shunt (DIPS). These shunts may be created using a transjugular approach but a combined percutaneous and transhepatic approach may also be required **(Figs. 17A to E)**. The primary patency rate of these shunts has also increased with the use of polytetrafluoroethylene (PTFE) covered stents. The advantages of TIPS are its minimal invasiveness and the lower mortality rate as compared with surgical shunting. In addition, intrahepatic caval stenosis can also be bypassed by using TIPS which is not possible with the surgical shunts. This essentially functions as a portoatrial shunt. The most frequent complication of TIPS is hepatic encephalopathy which can occur in up to 30% of patients but can be treated medically. Other complications include stenosis or occlusion requiring revision in about 70% of cases by 6 months, intraperitoneal bleed, liver failure, and subcapsular hematomas. The 6- and 12-month patency rates were 100% and 85.7%, respectively for stent graft compared with 16.7% and 0% for bare stents.[68] Surgical options are now usually reserved for patients with failed

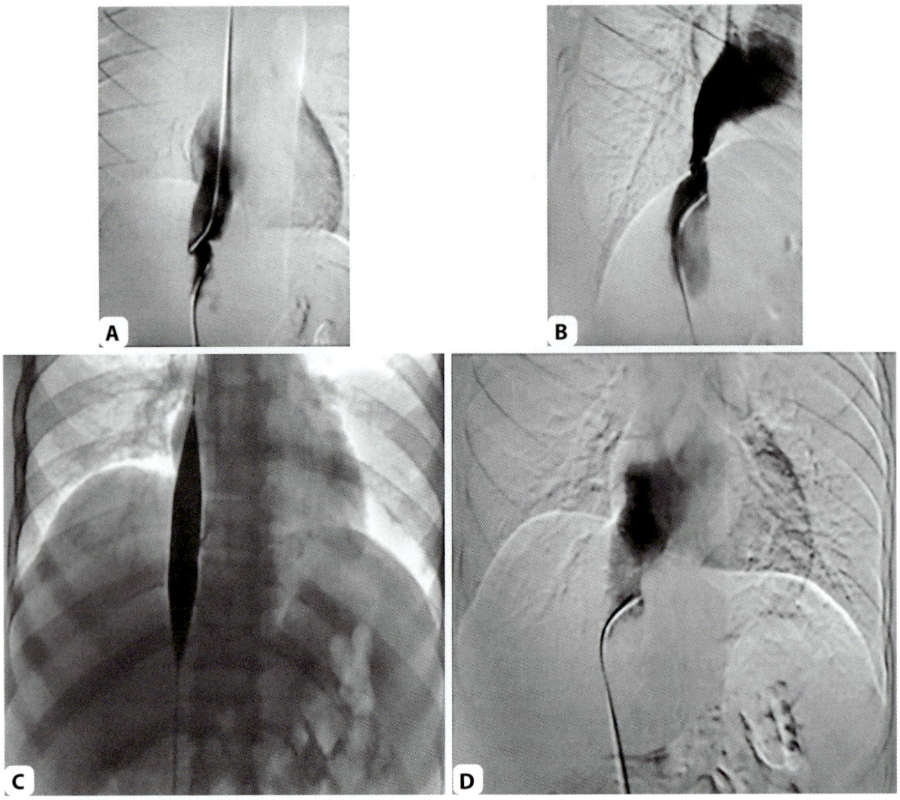

FIGS. 13A TO D: (A) Inferior vena cava (IVC) venography in AP (B) and lateral views with contrast injection from both the jugular and femoral access catheters showing a short segment stenosis of the IVC. The stenosis was crossed with a guidewire from the femoral access. (C) Subsequently a balloon catheter was used for dilatation of the narrowing (C). (D) Contrast injection through the femoral catheter shows no residual stenosis.

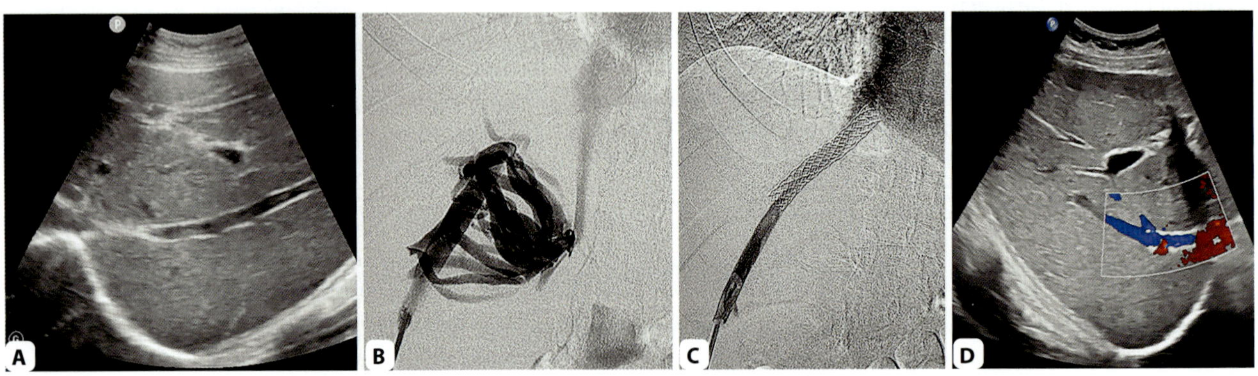

FIGS. 14A TO D: RHV stenting in chronic BCS—(A and B) US and venography with US-guided percutaneous access into RHV shows short segment complete occlusion with collaterals. (C) Post tenting run shows adequate dilatation with good flow into IVC. (D) Color Doppler image 2 months postprocedure shows good flow across the stent.

(BCS: Budd–Chiari syndrome; IVC: inferior vena cava; RHV: right hepatic vein)

radiological interventions. Some studies have suggested that an early use of TIPS in selected cases may have a survival advantage.[69,70] However, a study from India found that angioplasty and not TIPS, is of utility to the majority of BCS patients. The authors also reported that Child class and response to interventional treatment are important predictors of survival in BCS patients.[71]

Surgical Interventions

Surgical management of BCS is indicated in patients with features of congestion, hepatocyte necrosis, and fibrosis on liver biopsy. Decompressive surgical shunts such as portocaval and mesocaval shunts relieve the sinusoidal congestion and thus halt the ongoing hepatocyte necrosis.

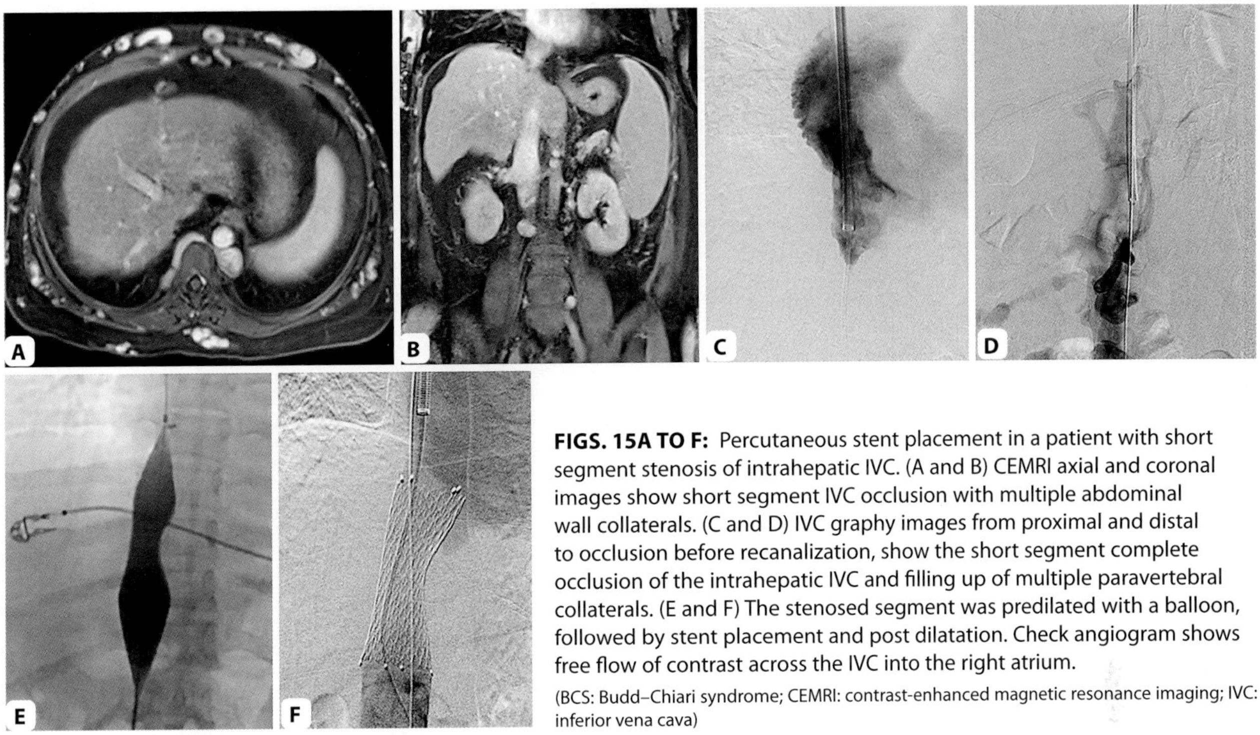

FIGS. 15A TO F: Percutaneous stent placement in a patient with short segment stenosis of intrahepatic IVC. (A and B) CEMRI axial and coronal images show short segment IVC occlusion with multiple abdominal wall collaterals. (C and D) IVC graphy images from proximal and distal to occlusion before recanalization, show the short segment complete occlusion of the intrahepatic IVC and filling up of multiple paravertebral collaterals. (E and F) The stenosed segment was predilated with a balloon, followed by stent placement and post dilatation. Check angiogram shows free flow of contrast across the IVC into the right atrium.

(BCS: Budd–Chiari syndrome; CEMRI: contrast-enhanced magnetic resonance imaging; IVC: inferior vena cava)

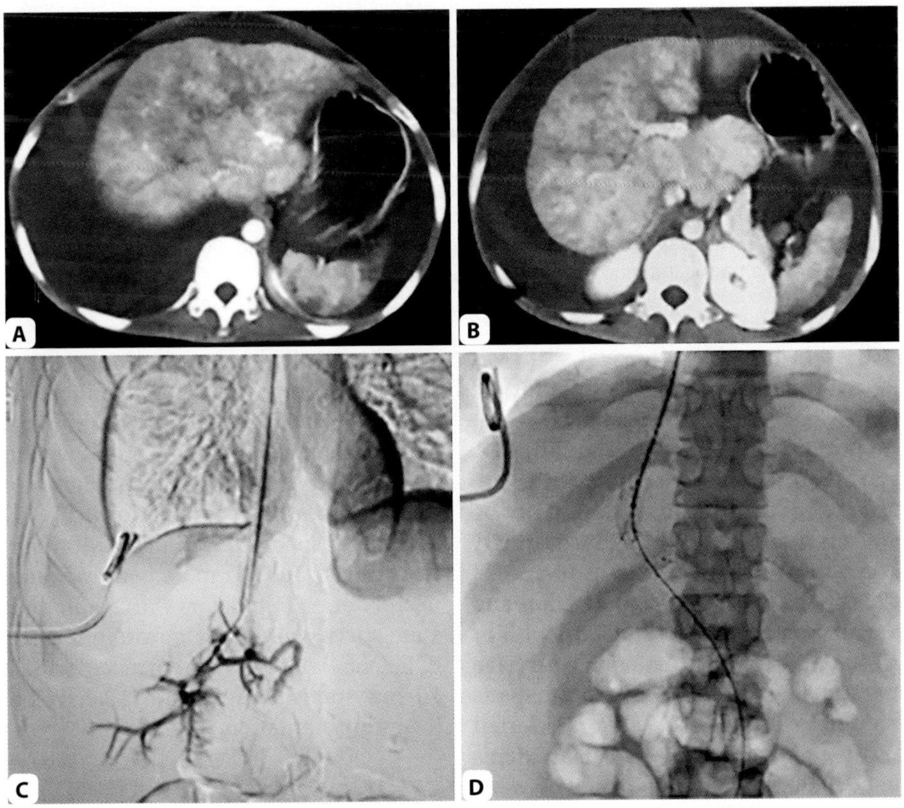

FIGS. 16A TO D: (A and B) Contrast-enhanced CT scan showing mosaic attenuation of liver parenchyma with attenuated hepatic veins and normal caliber portal vein. There is gross ascites and right pleural effusion. Using the transjugular approach the hepatic vein stump was cannulated with a sheath. (C) A puncture needle was advanced through the sheath and the liver parenchyma into the right branch of portal vein. Subsequently a calibrated pigtail catheter was advanced in the track. This was followed by balloon dilatation of the track. (D) The stent was then placed in the track over an exchange guidewire.

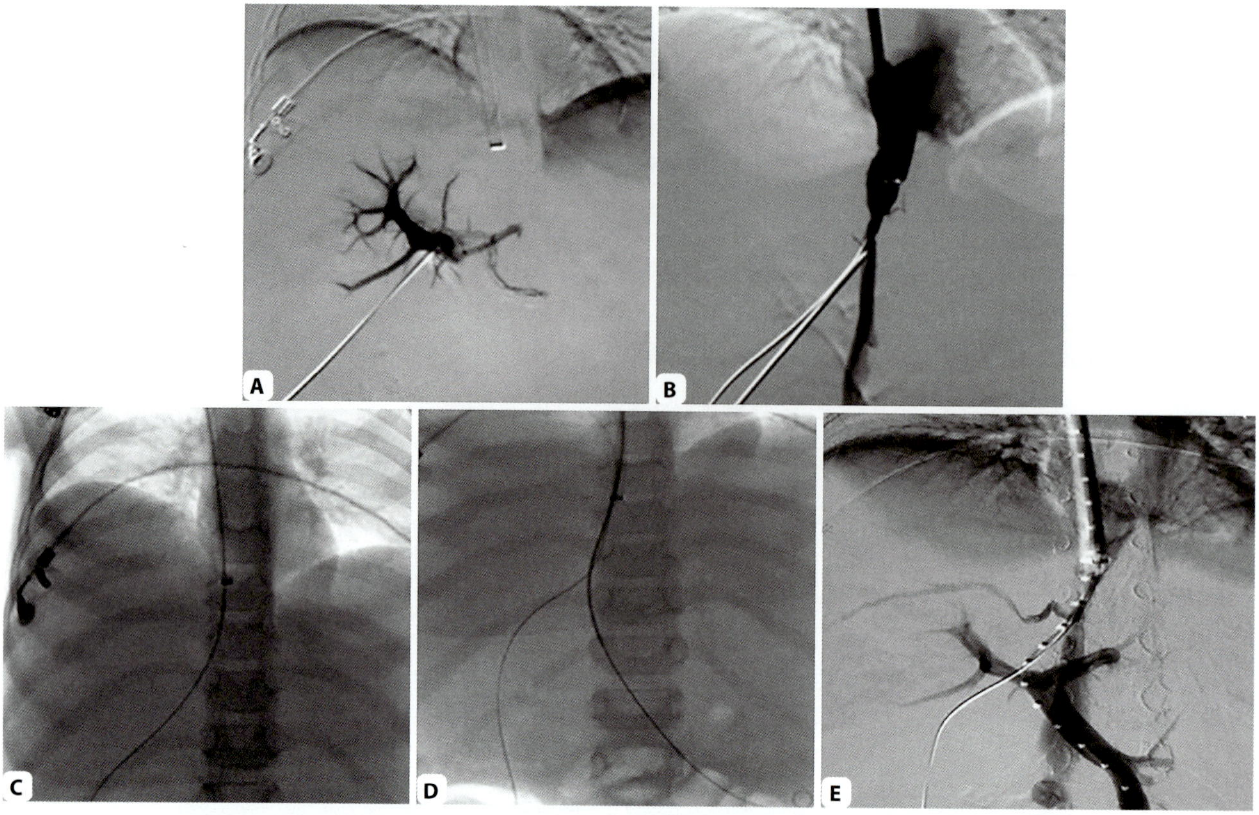

FIGS. 17A TO E: Percutaneous transhepatic puncture was performed using a 17.5 G, 15 cm Chiba needle. (A) The Chiba needle was guided under ultrasound toward the anterior branch of the right portal vein, after which entry into the portal vein was confirmed by injection of contrast material. Without changing the angle of entry, the needle was introduced further toward the IVC, again under the guidance of ultrasound. (B) Entry into the inferior vena cava (IVC) was confirmed by contrast injection. 0.035-inch guidewire was then introduced through the Chiba needle until the right atrium was reached. (C) Through-and-through access was achieved by pulling the tip of the guidewire into the right atrium through the jugular vascular sheath and out using a snare. The vascular sheath was then advanced over the guidewire into the liver parenchyma till the portal vein. (D) Through the vascular sheath another guidewire was maneuvered into the portal vein. (E) This was followed by contrast injection using marking pigtail catheter, balloon dilatation of the track and placement of stent in the track extending from the portal vein till the IVC.

The rationale for the side-to-side portocaval shunts is to transform the portal vein into an outflow tract for the hepatic circulation. A portocaval or mesocaval shunt is successful if the portal vein minus infrahepatic IVC pressure is >10 mm Hg. If this pressure gradient is <10 mm Hg, these infrahepatic surgical shunts should not be done.[30] These shunts are associated with a 25% mortality rate and shunt thrombosis which may occur in 10–25% of patients. Stenosis of the shunt is a late complication and is amenable for percutaneous balloon dilatation with or without stenting **(Figs. 18A to C)**. In patients who have intrahepatic IVC abnormality, these classical infrahepatic portocaval shunts do not work unless a stent is inserted in the IVC to correct the pressure gradient. Such patients require a suprahepatic shunt, i.e., mesoatrial shunt between the superior mesenteric vein (SMV) and the right atrium. The criteria for the mesoatrial shunt are reduction of IVC diameter > 75% or a caval atrial gradient exceeding 20 mm Hg.[72] These shunts are, however, associated with poorer results and a higher incidence of shunt thrombosis.

The first liver transplant for BCS was performed in 1974. Liver transplantation is indicated for patients with fulminant hepatic failure, those who deteriorate after shunt procedure and in cirrhotics with end-stage disease. In fact, orthotopic liver transplantation is considered the only curative treatment for BCS.[63] Significant fibrosis and cirrhosis on liver biopsy with poor hepatocellular reserve can only be managed by transplantation. It is a useful option in patients with a hereditary thrombophilia state such as protein C, protein S, and antithrombin III deficiency which can be corrected with liver replacement. 10-year survival rates up to 75% have been reported after liver transplantation.[36,73]

CONCLUSION

Radiological imaging plays the most crucial role in the diagnosis of BCS, and radiological interventions are the cornerstone in the management. The vascular changes can be well appreciated on Doppler ultrasonography.

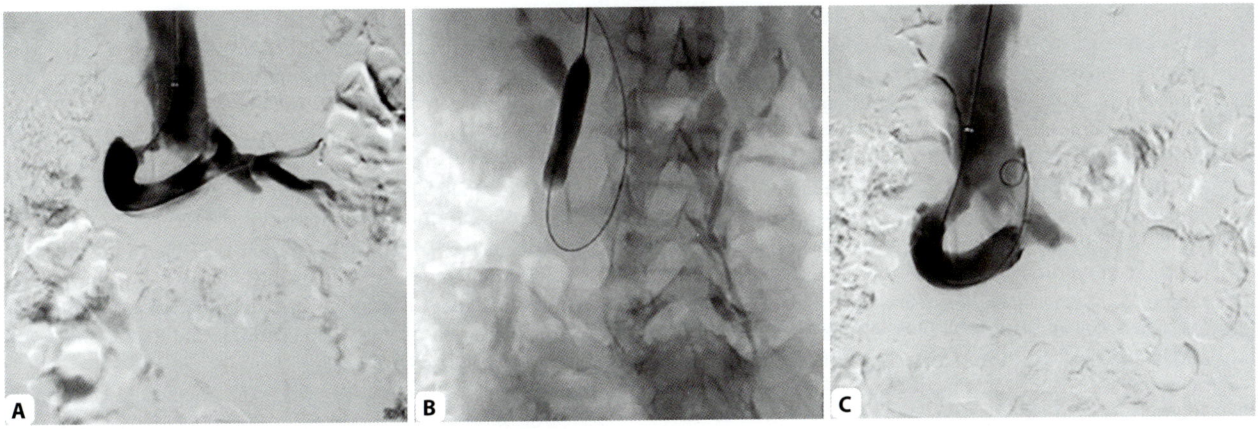

FIGS. 18A TO C: BCS patient with mesocaval stent and recurrence of ascites. (A) Shuntography done from the jugular route shows a short segment stenosis at the caval end of the stent. (B) The narrowed segment was crossed with a guidewire and balloon dilatation of the narrowed segment was done. (C) Shuntography now shows no residual stenosis.

However, cross-sectional imaging especially MRI may be required for the evaluation of the parenchyma and nodules associated with BCS. Radiological interventions adopt a step-wise approach with least invasive angioplasty and stenting as an initial intervention and derivative techniques like DIPS/TIPS reserved for those patients who fail to respond for angioplasty/stenting. Liver transplant being more invasive, is recommended for those who don't respond to medical management or radiological interventions.

REFERENCES

1. Ferral H, Behrens G, Lopera J. Budd-Chiari syndrome. AJR Am J Roentgenol. 2012;199(4):737-45.
2. Li Y, De Stefano V, Li H, Zheng K, Bai Z, Guo X, et al. Epidemiology of Budd-Chiari syndrome: A systematic review and meta-analysis. Clin Res Hepatol Gastroenterol. 2019;43(4):468-74.
3. Parekh J, Matei VM, Canas-Coto A, Friedman D, Lee WM. Budd-Chiari syndrome causing acute liver failure: A multicenter case series. Liver Transpl. 2017;23(2):135-42.
4. Garcia-Pagán JC, Valla DC. Primary Budd-Chiari syndrome. N Engl J Med. 2023;388(14):1307-16.
5. Patil P, Deshmukh H, Popat B, Rathod K. Spectrum of imaging in Budd Chiari syndrome. J Med Imaging Radiat Oncol. 2012;56(1):75-83.
6. Mulholland JP, Fong SM, Kafaghi FA, Fong W. Budd-Chiari syndrome: Diagnosis with ultrasound and nuclear medicine calcium colloid liver scan following non-diagnostic contrasted CT scan. Australas Radiol. 1997;41(1):53-6.
7. Sharma V, Aggarwal A, Singla R, Kalra N, Chawla YK. Giant Hemangioma causing Budd-Chiari syndrome. J Clin Exp Hepatol. 2014;4(4):380-1.
8. Mahmoud A, Elias E. New approaches to the Budd-Chiari syndrome. J Gastroenterol Hepatol. 1996;11(12):1121-3.
9. Eapen CE, Mammen T, Moses V, Shyamkumar NK. Changing profile of Budd Chiari syndrome in India. Indian J Gastroenterol. 2007;26(2):77-81.
10. Vilgrain V, Lewin M, Vons C, Denys A, Valla D, Flejou JF, et al. Hepatic nodules in Budd-Chiari syndrome: Imaging features. Radiology. 1999;210(2):443-50.
11. DeLeve LD, Valla DC, Garcia-Tsao G. Vascular disorders of the liver. Hepatology. 2009;49(5):1729-64.
12. Valla DC. Budd-Chiari syndrome and veno-occlusive disease/sinusoidal obstruction syndrome. Gut. 2008;57(10):1469-78.
13. Bansal V, Gupta P, Sinha S, Dhaka N, Kalra N, Vijayvergiya R, et al. Budd-Chiari syndrome: imaging review. Br J Radiol. 2018;91(1092):20180441.
14. Das CJ, Soneja M, Tayal S, Chahal A, Srivastava S, Kumar A, et al. Role of radiological imaging and interventions in management of Budd-Chiari syndrome. Clin Radiol. 2018;73(7):610-24.
15. Sharma A, Keshava SN, Eapen A, Elias E, Eapen CE. An Update on the Management of Budd-Chiari Syndrome. Dig Dis Sci. 2021;66(6):1780-90.
16. Gupta P, Bansal V, Kumar-M P, Sinha SK, Samanta J, Mandavdhare H, et al. Diagnostic accuracy of Doppler ultrasound, CT and MRI in Budd Chiari syndrome: Systematic review and meta-analysis. Br J Radiol. 2020;93(1109):20190847.
17. Arora A, Sharma MP. Recent trends in the diagnosis and treatment of Budd Chiari syndrome. J Assoc Physicians India. 1992;40(8):533-6.
18. Floyd JL. The radiographic gamut of Budd-Chiari syndrome. Am J Gastroenterol. 1981;76(4):381-7.
19. Menu Y, Alison D, Lorphelin JM, Valla D, Belghiti J, Nahum H. Budd-Chiari syndrome: US evaluation. Radiology. 1985;157(3):761-4.
20. Powell-Jackson PR, Karani J, Ede RJ, Meire H, Williams R. Ultrasound scanning and 99mTc sulphur colloid scintigraphy in diagnosis of Budd-Chiari syndrome. Gut. 1986;27(12):1502-6.
21. Makuuchi M, Hasegawa H, Yamazaki S, Moriyama N, Takayasu K, Okazaki M. Primary Budd-Chiari syndrome: Ultrasonic demonstration. Radiology. 1984;152(3):775-9.

22. Aydinli M, Bayraktar Y. Budd-Chiari syndrome: Etiology, pathogenesis and diagnosis. World J Gastroenterol. 2007;13(19):2693-6.
23. Lupescu IG, Dobromir C, Popa GA, Gheorghe L, Georgescu SA. Spiral computed tomography and magnetic resonance angiography evaluation in Budd-Chiari syndrome. J Gastrointest Liver Dis JGLD. 2008;17(2):223-6.
24. Bargalló X, Gilabert R, Nicolau C, García-Pagán JC, Bosch J, Brú C. Sonography of the caudate vein: value in diagnosing Budd-Chiari syndrome. Am J Roentgenol. 2003;181(6):1641-5.
25. Noone TC, Semelka RC, Siegelman ES, Balci NC, Hussain SM, Kim PN, et al. Budd-Chiari syndrome: Spectrum of appearances of acute, subacute, and chronic disease with magnetic resonance imaging. J Magn Reson Imaging JMRI. 2000;11(1):44-50.
26. Xu K, Ren K, Chen YS. Application and evaluation of non-invasive examination for Budd-Chiari syndrome. Chin Med J (Engl). 2007;120(2):91-4.
27. Ohta M, Hashizume M, Tomikawa M, Ueno K, Tanoue K, Sugimachi K. Analysis of hepatic vein waveform by Doppler ultrasonography in 100 patients with portal hypertension. Am J Gastroenterol. 1994;89(2):170-5.
28. Gupta P, Koshi S, Sinha SK, Sharma V, Mandavdhare H, Samanta J, et al. Contrast-enhanced ultrasound is a useful adjunct to Doppler ultrasound in the initial assessment of patients suspected of Budd-Chiari syndrome. Curr Probl Diagn Radiol. 2021;50(5):646-9.
29. Kane R, Eustace S. Diagnosis of Budd-Chiari syndrome: comparison between sonography and MR angiography. Radiology. 1995;195(1):117-21.
30. Kamath PS. Budd-Chiari syndrome: Radiologic findings. Liver Transpl. 2006;12(11 Suppl 2):S21-2.
31. Brancatelli G, Vilgrain V, Federle MP, Hakime A, Lagalla R, Iannaccone R, et al. Budd-Chiari syndrome: spectrum of imaging findings. AJR Am J Roentgenol. 2007;188(2):W168-76.
32. Datta DV, Saha S, Singh SA, Gupta BB, Aikat BK, Chugh KS, et al. Chronic Budd-Chiari syndrome due to obstruction of the intrahepatic portion of the inferior vena cava. Gut. 1972;13(5):372-8.
33. Dilawari JB, Bambery P, Chawla Y, Kaur U, Bhusnurmath SR, Malhotra HS, et al. Hepatic outflow obstruction (Budd-Chiari syndrome). Experience with 177 patients and a review of the literature. Medicine (Baltimore). 1994;73(1):21-36.
34. Kage M, Arakawa M, Kojiro M, Okuda K. Histopathology of membranous obstruction of the inferior vena cava in the Budd-Chiari syndrome. Gastroenterology. 1992;102(6):2081-90.
35. Bolondi L, Gaiani S, Li Bassi S, Zironi G, Bonino F, Brunetto M, et al. Diagnosis of Budd-Chiari syndrome by pulsed Doppler ultrasound. Gastroenterology. 1991;100(5 Pt 1):1324-31.
36. Valla DC. Hepatic vein thrombosis (Budd-Chiari syndrome). Semin Liver Dis. 2002;22(1):5-14.
37. Cho OK, Koo JH, Kim YS, Rhim HC, Koh BH, Seo HS. Collateral pathways in Budd-Chiari syndrome: CT and venographic correlation. AJR Am J Roentgenol. 1996;167(5):1163-7.
38. Clain D, Freston J, Kreel L, Sherlock S. Clinical diagnosis of the Budd-Chiari syndrome. A report of six cases. Am J Med. 1967;43(4):544-54.
39. Janssen HLA, Garcia-Pagan JC, Elias E, Mentha G, Hadengue A, Valla DC, et al. Budd-Chiari syndrome: A review by an expert panel. J Hepatol. 2003;38(3):364-71.
40. Maetani Y, Itoh K, Egawa H, Haga H, Sakurai T, Nishida N, et al. Benign hepatic nodules in Budd-Chiari syndrome: radiologic-pathologic correlation with emphasis on the central scar. AJR Am J Roentgenol. 2002;178(4):869-75.
41. Tanju S, Erden A, Ceyhan K, Soygür IT, Bozkaya H, Erden I. Contrast-enhanced MR angiography of benign regenerative nodules following TIPS shunt procedure in Budd-Chiari syndrome. Turk J Gastroenterol. 2004;15(3):173-7.
42. Brancatelli G, Federle MP, Grazioli L, Golfieri R, Lencioni R. Benign regenerative nodules in Budd-Chiari syndrome and other vascular disorders of the liver: Radiologic-pathologic and clinical correlation. Radiogr Rev Publ Radiol Soc N Am Inc. 2002;22(4):847-62.
43. Brancatelli G, Federle MP, Grazioli L, Golfieri R, Lencioni R. Large regenerative nodules in Budd-Chiari syndrome and other vascular disorders of the liver: CT and MR imaging findings with clinicopathologic correlation. AJR Am J Roentgenol. 2002;178(4):877-83.
44. Cazals-Hatem D, Vilgrain V, Genin P, Denninger MH, Durand F, Belghiti J, et al. Arterial and portal circulation and parenchymal changes in Budd-Chiari syndrome: A study in 17 explanted livers. Hepatol Baltim Md. 2003;37(3):510-9.
45. Valla DC. Prognosis in Budd Chiari syndrome after re-establishing hepatic venous drainage. Gut. 2006;55(6):761-3.
46. Arita T, Matsunaga N, Kobayashi H. Budd-Chiari syndrome: Peripheral abnormal intensity of the liver on magnetic resonance imaging. Clin Radiol. 2000;55(8):640-2.
47. Camera L, Mainenti PP, Di Giacomo A, Romano M, Rispo A, Alfinito F, et al. Triphasic helical CT in Budd-Chiari syndrome: patterns of enhancement in acute, subacute and chronic disease. Clin Radiol. 2006;61(4):331-7.
48. Chaluvashetty SB, Kalra N, Damarla V, Gupta P, Bhujade H, Gorsi U, et al. (2022). Imaging and Interventions in Budd Chiari syndrome. [online] Available from https://epos.myesr.org/poster/esr/ecr2022/C-14156 [Last accessed July, 2024].
49. Kalra N, Virmani V, Singh P, Kang M, Anand A, Chawla Y, et al. Imaging of Budd-Chiari syndrome (electronic exhibit presented at the 109th Annual Meeting of the American Roentgen Ray Society). Boston, USA: American Roentgen Ray Society; 2009.
50. Plessier A, Sibert A, Consigny Y, Hakime A, Zappa M, Denninger MH, et al. Aiming at minimal invasiveness as a therapeutic strategy for Budd-Chiari syndrome. Hepatol Baltim Md. 2006;44(5):1308-16.
51. Seijo S, Plessier A, Hoekstra J, Dell'era A, Mandair D, Rifai K, et al. Good long-term outcome of Budd-Chiari syndrome with a step-wise management. Hepatol Baltim Md. 2013;57(5):1962-8.
52. Simonetto DA, Singal AK, Garcia-Tsao G, Caldwell SH, Ahn J, Kamath PS. ACG Clinical Guideline: Disorders of the hepatic and mesenteric circulation. Am J Gastroenterol. 2020;115(1):18-40.
53. Hernández-Gea V, De Gottardi A, Leebeek FWG, Rautou PE, Salem R, Garcia-Pagan JC. Current knowledge in pathophysiology and management of Budd-Chiari syndrome and non-cirrhotic non-tumoral splanchnic vein thrombosis. J Hepatol. 2019;71(1):175-99.
54. Shukla A, Shreshtha A, Mukund A, Bihari C, Eapen CE, Han G, et al. Budd-Chiari syndrome: consensus guidance of the Asian Pacific Association for the study of the liver (APASL). Hepatol Int. 2021;15(3):531-67.

55. Northup PG, Garcia-Pagan JC, Garcia-Tsao G, Intagliata NM, Superina RA, Roberts LN, et al. Vascular liver disorders, portal vein thrombosis, and procedural bleeding in patients with liver disease: 2020 Practice Guidance by the American Association for the Study of Liver Diseases. Hepatol Baltim Md. 2021;73(1):366-413.
56. Mukund A, Gamanagatti S. Imaging and interventions in Budd-Chiari syndrome. World J Radiol. 201128;3(7):169-77.
57. Eguchi S, Takeuchi Y, Asano K. Successful balloon membranotomy for obstruction of the hepatic portion of the inferior vena cava. Surgery. 1974;76(5):837-40.
58. Han G, Qi X, Zhang W, He C, Yin Z, Wang J, et al. Percutaneous recanalization for Budd-Chiari syndrome: An 11-year retrospective study on patency and survival in 177 Chinese patients from a single center. Radiology. 2013;266(2):657-67.
59. Eapen CE, Velissaris D, Heydtmann M, Gunson B, Olliff S, Elias E. Favourable medium term outcome following hepatic vein recanalisation and/or transjugular intrahepatic portosystemic shunt for Budd Chiari syndrome. Gut. 2006;55(6):878-84.
60. Valla DC. Primary Budd-Chiari syndrome. J Hepatol. 2009;50(1):195-203.
61. Wang Q, Li K, He C, Yuan X, Luo B, Qi X, et al. Angioplasty with versus without routine stent placement for Budd-Chiari syndrome: a randomised controlled trial. Lancet Gastroenterol Hepatol. 2019;4(9):686-97.
62. Griffith JF, Mahmoud AE, Cooper S, Elias E, West RJ, Olliff SP. Radiological intervention in Budd-Chiari syndrome: techniques and outcome in 18 patients. Clin Radiol. 1996;51(11):775-84.
63. Lopez RR, Benner KG, Hall L, Rösch J, Pinson CW. Expandable venous stents for treatment of the Budd-Chiari syndrome. Gastroenterology. 1991;100(5 Pt 1):1435-41.
64. Pisani-Ceretti A, Intra M, Prestipino F, Ballarini C, Cordovana A, Santambrogio R, et al. Surgical and radiologic treatment of primary Budd-Chiari syndrome. World J Surg. 1998;22(1):48-53;discussion 53-54.
65. Baijal SS, Roy S, Phadke RV, Agrawal DK, Kumar S, Choudhuri G. Management of idiopathic Budd-Chiari syndrome with primary stent placement: early results. J Vasc Interv Radiol JVIR. 1996;7(4):545-53.
66. Peltzer MY, Ring EJ, LaBerge JM, Haskal ZJ, Radosevich PM, Gordon RL. Treatment of Budd-Chiari syndrome with a transjugular intrahepatic portosystemic shunt. J Vasc Interv Radiol JVIR. 1993;4(2):263-7.
67. Ochs A, Sellinger M, Haag K, Nöldge G, Herbst EW, Walter E, et al. Transjugular intrahepatic portosystemic stent-shunt (TIPS) in the treatment of Budd-Chiari syndrome. J Hepatol. 1993;18(2):217-25.
68. Gandini R, Konda D, Simonetti G. Transjugular intrahepatic portosystemic shunt patency and clinical outcome in patients with Budd-Chiari syndrome: covered versus uncovered stents. Radiology. 2006;241(1):298-305.
69. Liu L, Qi XS, Zhao Y, Chen H, Meng XC, Han GH. Budd-Chiari syndrome: current perspectives and controversies. Eur Rev Med Pharmacol Sci. 2016;20(15):3273-81.
70. Mancuso A. Budd-chiari syndrome management: Timing of treatment is an open issue. Hepatol Baltim Md. 2014;59(3):1213.
71. Shalimar , Kumar A, Kedia S, Sharma H, Gamanagatti SR, Gulati GS, et al. Hepatic venous outflow tract obstruction: treatment outcomes and development of a new prognostic score. Aliment Pharmacol Ther. 2016;43(11):1154-67.
72. Orloff MJ, Orloff MS, Daily PO. Long-term results of treatment of Budd-Chiari syndrome with portal decompression. Arch Surg. 1992;127(10):1182-7; discussion 1187-8.
73. Mentha G, Giostra E, Majno PE, Bechstein WO, Neuhaus P, O'Grady J, et al. Liver transplantation for Budd-Chiari syndrome: A European study on 248 patients from 51 centres. J Hepatol. 2006;44(3):520-8.

SECTION

3

Biliary Tree

CHAPTER 15

Anjali Prakash, Sapna Singh, Rashmi Dixit, Deeksha Bhalla

Inflammatory Disorders of Gallbladder and Biliary Tract

INTRODUCTION

Inflammatory conditions of the gallbladder (GB) are a common cause of acute abdomen. Imaging plays a vital role in the early diagnosis and also to detect complications helping to reduce morbidity. The advances in imaging have highlighted the various causes of biliary tract inflammation.

The differential diagnosis of right upper quadrant (RUQ) pain is manifold, including a gamut of pathologies arising from the gallbladder, liver, stomach, pancreas, and adrenal glands as well as the pleural cavity. Among these, GB pathology is most frequently implicated and also the most well recognized, as several clinical signs such as the Murphy's sign and Charcot's triad have been described for acute cholecystitis. Calculous form of cholecystitis is by far the most common, seen in ~90% patients. It could further lead to life-threatening complications such as GB empyema, perforation, or chronic cholecystitis (CC).

It is important to remember the goals of imaging, which are:

- Detection of gallbladder and biliary tract involvement—most commonly in the acute setting
- Monitor treatment response
- Detection of complications in patients with inadequate response or recurrence of symptoms

IMAGING APPROACH

The imaging modality performed as well as its interpretation must be tailored to the clinical presentation of the patient as well as possible differential diagnosis. It is important for radiologists to be aware, therefore, of the strengths and pitfalls of each modality and their role in the imaging algorithm based on the American College of Radiology (ACR) appropriateness criteria.[1,2]

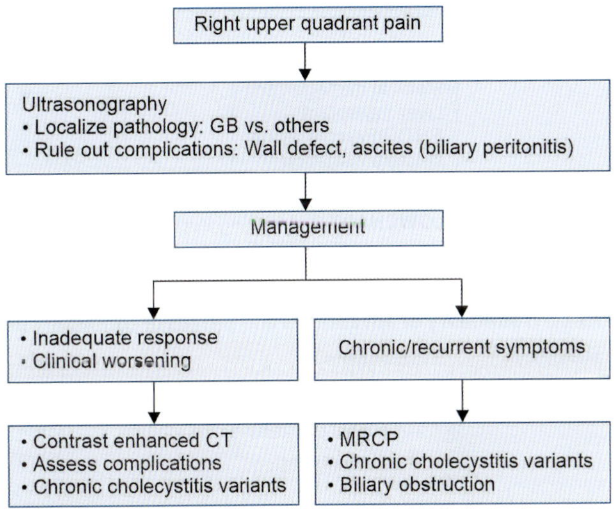

FLOWCHART 1: Imaging approach to a patient with right upper quadrant (RUQ) pain.

The imaging approach is summarized in **Flowchart 1 and 2**. The role of imaging modalities is detailed in **Table 1**.

OTHER RELEVANT INVESTIGATIONS

Hepatic Scintigraphy

Functional imaging of the liver parenchyma can be performed using ^{99m}Tc hydroxy iminodiacetic acid (HIDA). Nonvisualization of GB in delayed scans up to 90 minutes indicates acute cholecystitis. Delayed GB filling or reduced ejection fraction indicates chronic GB dysfunction as in CC. However, these investigations are rarely used for this purpose. The primary role of HIDA scan in adults is for detection of bile leaks, while in children

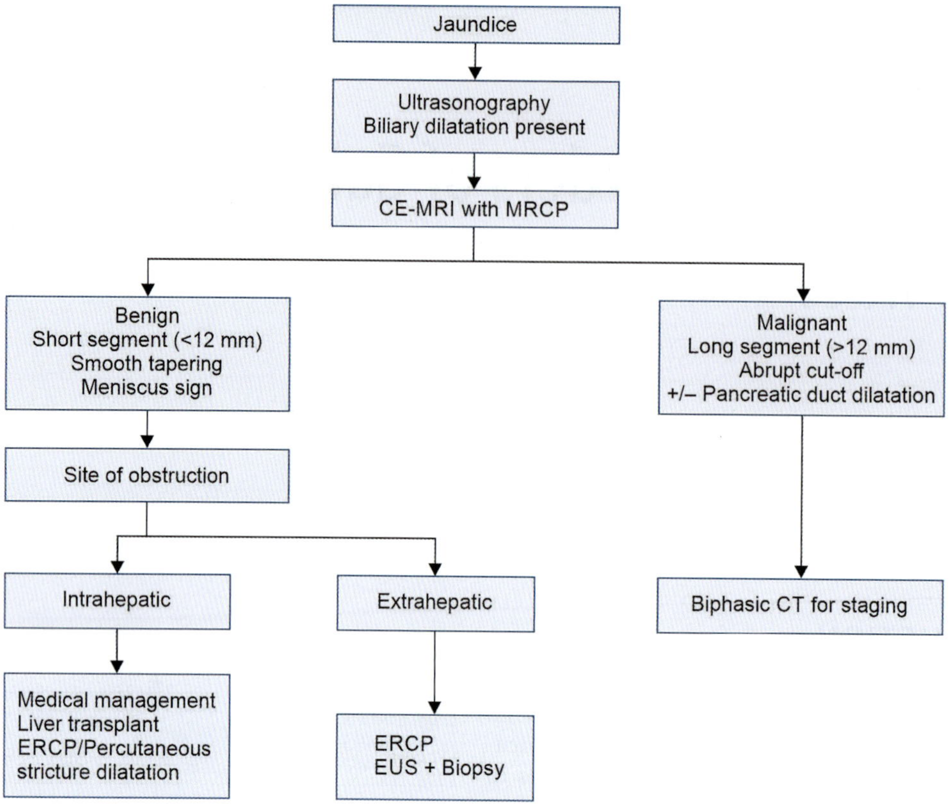

FLOWCHART 2. Imaging approach in a patient with obstructive jaundice.

TABLE 1: Summary of advantages and pitfalls of commonly used imaging modalities.

Modality	Strengths	Pitfalls	Special techniques
Ultrasonography	High sensitivity for cholelithiasis: • GB wall thickening • Biliary dilatation	• Wall echo shadow complex in chronic cholecystitis prevents adequate evaluation • Low sensitivity for bile duct calculi • Inadequate characterization of biliary obstruction • Gas in GB/biliary tree obscures pathology	Contrast enhanced US can be used as an adjunct for definition of GB wall and causes of wall thickening, differentiation of polyps from stones[3]
CT	High sensitivity for: • GB wall thickening • Diagnosis of complicated cholecystitis	• Low sensitivity for gallstones • Depiction of biliary anatomy inferior to MRI • Low sensitivity for bile leaks • Artifacts with metallic stents	DECT generated virtual monochromatic images at 40 keV and 140 keV improve contrast and help in detection of stones in GB, bile duct[4]
MRI	• Excellent soft tissue contrast • Demonstration of gallstones and associated complications • Depiction of GB wall thickening • Delineates details of biliary anatomy including strictures, leaks	• Long examination time, unfavorable in the acute setting • Signal void in pneumobilia, surgical clips • Overlap in MIP images may lead to misinterpretation	• Perfusion MRI for differentiation of benign and malignant GB wall thickening, biliary strictures • Hepatobiliary contrast agents are excreted into the bile. After a variable time interval based on the agent, may be used for contrast-enhanced MRCP

(CT: computed tomography; DECT: dual-energy CT; GB: gallbladder; MIP: maximum intensity projection; MRCP: magnetic resonance cholangiopancreatography; MRI: magnetic resonance imaging) with biliary atresia, it is used to confirm the diagnosis which is established by absence of biliary drainage into bowel.[5]

Endoscopy-based Imaging

Endoscopic Ultrasonography

This is performed via ultrasonography (US) probes mounted on endoscopes. The frequency of these probes ranges between 7.5 and 10 MHz and water balloon technique is used for acoustic coupling. It provides excellent resolution for biliary disorders, including detection of small biliary calculi. Endoscopic ultrasonography (EUS)-guided tissue sampling can also be performed. However, it is highly operator dependent and also does not possess therapeutic ability. It suffers from the same disadvantages as US, the presence of air in the biliary tract may significantly hamper visualization of pathology.

Endoscopic Retrograde Cholangiopancreatography

This has a combined diagnostic and therapeutic role in patients with biliary obstruction. The procedure involves passing of an endoscope, cannulation of the ampulla, and contrast injection to study biliary pathology. Endoscopic retrograde cholangiopancreatography (ERCP) has not just high sensitivity (90–96%), but also excellent specificity (98%) for detection of calculi.[6] However, similar to MRCP, care must be taken to avoid misinterpretation of air bubbles as calculi. The endoscopic access can be used for a variety of interventions including stone clearance from bile duct, biliary stenting, biopsy, and cytology from the duct.

18F-fluorodeoxyglucose Positron Emission Tomography-Computed Tomography

Positron emission tomography-computed tomography (PET-CT) is indicated in the evaluation of GB wall thickening; presenting as a diagnostic dilemma on other modalities. Benign conditions show less standardized uptake value (SUV) than malignant conditions. It also has a role in staging malignant disease.

INFLAMMATORY PATHOLOGY OF GALLBLADDER

Gallstone-associated Disorders

The population prevalence of gallstones is estimated to be around 10%.[7] These may be cholesterol or pigment stones, of which the vast majority are cholesterol stones. The accuracy of US for detection of gallstones is 95%.[8] The detection rate on CT is, however, much lower due to their variable composition, and only 20% stones are homogeneously hyperdense on CT.[9] Magnetic resonance imaging (MRI) is also an excellent modality for depiction of gallstones, which appear uniformly hypointense regardless of composition, and thus are readily detected against the bright background of bile on T2-weighted images.

Hydrops of the Gallbladder

A calculus that is impacted at the GB neck or cystic duct can lead to distension of the GB due to continued mucus production by the mucosa. On ultrasound, the distended GB maintains its rounded shape and is noncompressible. This is called the hydrops sign. On graded compression, the GB bulges into the abdominal wall. The continued increase in pressure may lead to ischemia of the GB wall. Stagnant bile in the GB leads to bacterial infection and acute cholecystitis. Alternately the stone may dislodge leading to reperfusion edema **(Box 1)**.

ACUTE CALCULOUS CHOLECYSTITIS

It is the most common GB pathology, patients present with typical RUQ pain along with tenderness and leukocytosis. In 80–95% cases, occurs secondary to obstruction of the neck or cystic duct by a gallstone.[10] Presence of fever and raised inflammatory markers differentiate acute cholecystitis from hydrops.

On US, there is diffuse GB wall thickening with a stratified pattern. It is important to note that the GB is distended, versus chronic forms where it is often reduced in volume due to fibrosis. Pericholecystic hypoechogenicity is seen suggesting edema. Sonographic Murphy's sign refers to maximum probe tenderness elicited over the GB. The combination of Murphy's sign and gallstones is very specific for acute cholecystitis. The positive predictive value for these is 92%.[11] On CT/MR, there is distension of GB with stratified wall enhancement, pericholecystic edema, and fat stranding. Further, hyperenhancement of the surrounding liver parenchyma may be seen, which is also a specific sign for acute cholecystitis.[7] The management of acute cholecystitis is usually supportive, with hydration and antibiotics. Interval cholecystectomy is usually performed at 4–6 weeks postresolution of inflammation.

Complications of Acute Cholecystitis

An important goal of imaging is to recognize complications that portend a poor prognosis and therefore warrant urgent surgical management.

BOX 1 Ultrasound signs of hydrops of gallbladder.

- Impacted stone in gallbladder neck/cystic duct
- Large distended gallbladder
- Hydrops sign—noncompressibility, rounded shape
- Ultrasound Murphy's positive

Gangrenous Cholecystitis

Gangrenous cholecystitis is a life-threatening complication, which is reported to develop in 15–20% patients of acute cholecystitis.[12] Diabetes is a major risk factor. This develops due to increased intraluminal pressure in the GB during an episode of acute cholecystitis that leads to cut-off of the arterial supply and necrosis of the wall.

The US appearance of an edematous, striated wall is usually not seen but rather replaced by asymmetric wall thickening and poorly defined mucosa, with intraluminal content due to sloughed off membranes.

Similarly, on CT, reduced enhancement of the wall or wall defects are seen with intraluminal membranes. Defects in the GB wall that communicate with pericholecystic fluid are very important to diagnose on CT, since these represent perforation of the GB **(Figs. 1A to C)**. GB perforation can lead to localized pericholecystic abscess, intrahepatic abscess, or even diffuse biliary peritonitis.[13] The "interrupted rim" sign, used to describe defects in the mucosal enhancement, is characteristic.[14]

Suppurative Cholecystitis

Suppurative cholecystitis, also called pyocele or empyema of the gallbladder, is another complication seen in patients with gallstones obstructing the drainage of pus from the lumen.

In this setting, the GB lumen fills up with purulent material.

The degree of GB distension is higher compared to uncomplicated acute cholecystitis, and the mural stratification is often lost. Further, the lumen shows echogenic material on US corresponding to the pus. On MR, heavily T2-weighted sequences may be used to demonstrate a fluid level in the Gb with layering of bile upon the relatively hypointense purulent debris.[15]

Diffusion-weighted imaging (DWI) may also prove useful in distinguishing the purulent material within the lumen that shows restriction **(Figs. 2A to E)**.

Gallbladder empyema is associated with higher rates of conversion of laparoscopic to open cholecystectomy. Percutaneous drainage may be performed in case patients are not fit for surgery.

CHRONIC CHOLECYSTITIS

Chronic cholecystitis is a chronic inflammatory disorder of GB, which is almost always associated with gallstones. Microscopically, chronic inflammation and fibrosis are present which lead to a contracted, shrunken GB on imaging.

On US, the "wall echo shadow" (WES) complex is characteristic, which is seen due to gallstones in a contracted GB causing extensive posterior acoustic shadowing. The "wall" is the thin hyperechoic anterior wall, along with a thin rim of bile which may be seen. The "echo" refers to the near surface of stone beneath the wall and the "shadow" is the extensive posterior shadowing seen due to the stones **(Figs. 3A and B)**.

On CT and MRI, thin wall can be made out with uniform enhancement which is slow and prolonged **(Figs. 4 and 5)**. Irregular thickening in the wall should alert the radiologist to possible development of GB carcinoma.

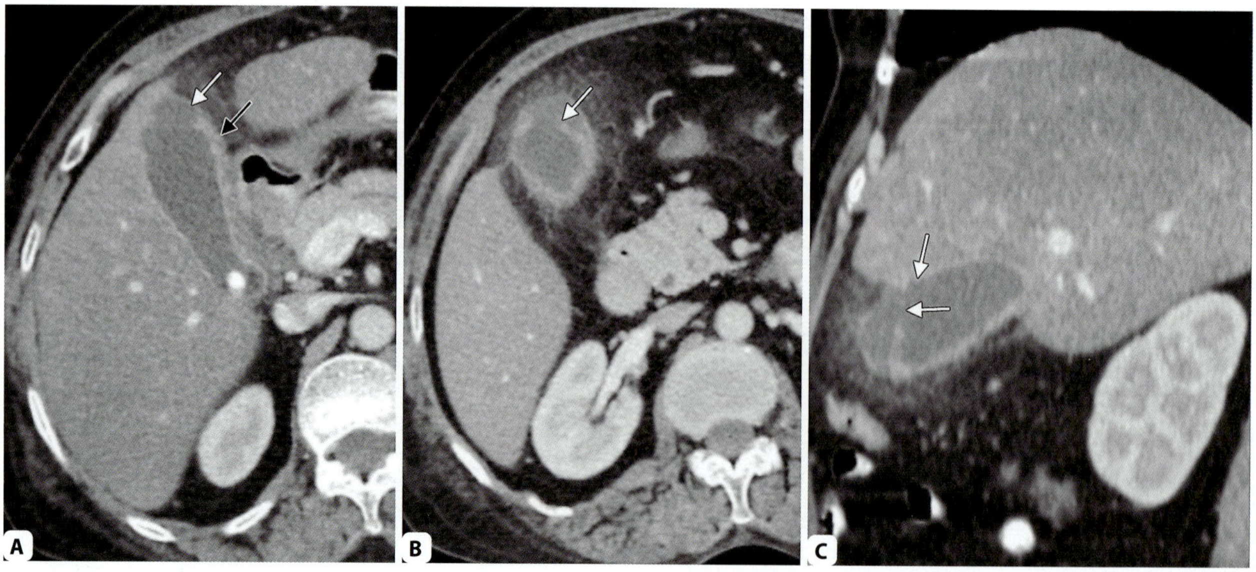

FIGS. 1A TO C: Gangrenous cholecystitis. (A) Diffuse thickening of the gallbladder (GB) wall is seen (black arrow) with focal thinning of the GB wall at the fundus (white arrow). A calculus is seen at the GB neck. (B) A focal defect is seen in the GB wall with pericholecystic collection and extensive fat stranding suggesting perforation. (C) Sagittal section depicts the focal defect in the wall—"interrupted rim" sign.

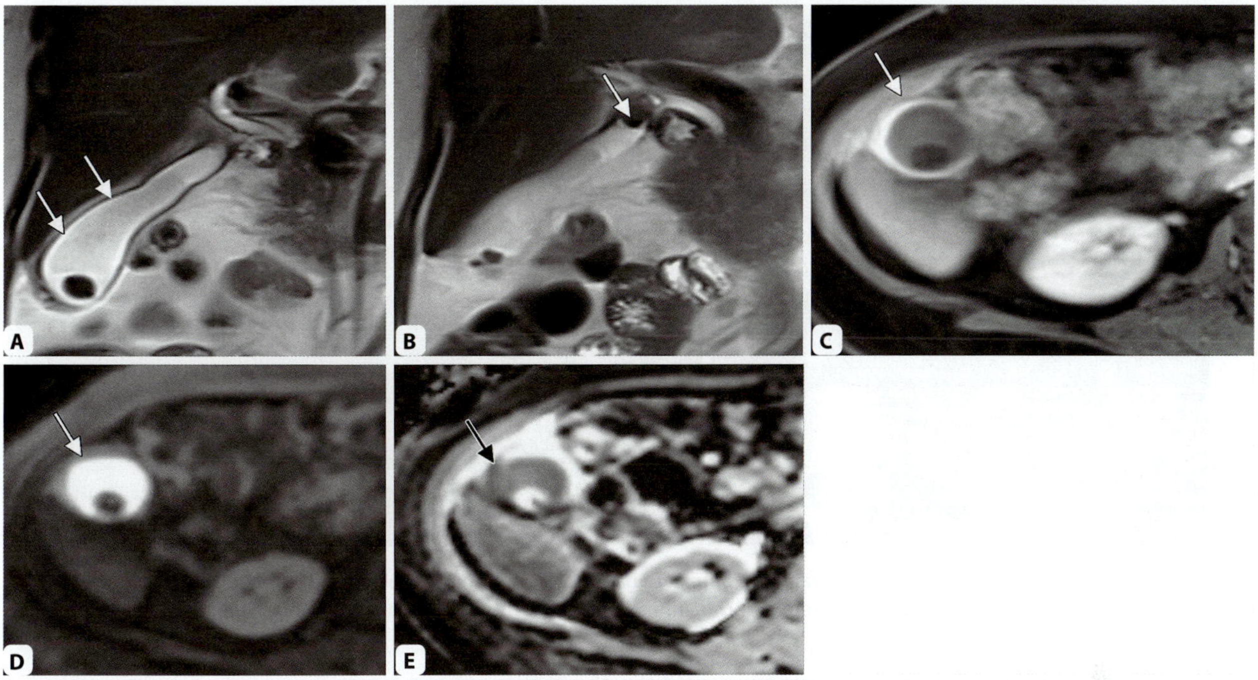

FIGS. 2A TO E: Suppurative cholecystitis. (A) There is an overdistended gallbladder (GB) with wall thickening (arrow) and gallstones. (B) An impacted stone is seen at the neck (arrow). (C) Homogeneous enhancement of the wall is seen. (D and E) Diffusion-weighted imaging (DWI) (D) and apparent diffusion coefficient (ADC) (E) show diffusion restriction within the lumen due to pus.

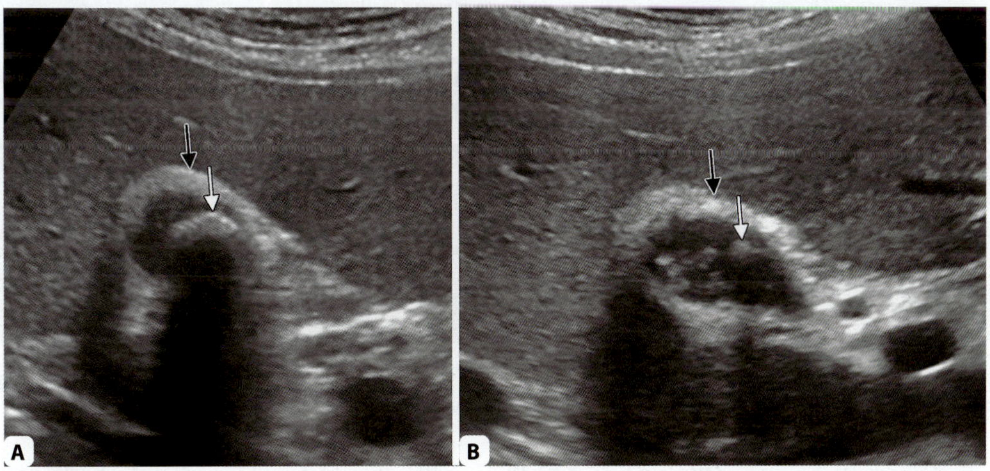

FIGS. 3A AND B: Ultrasound appearance of chronic cholecystitis. (A) The wall echo shadow (WES) complex, showing thickened wall (black arrow), the anechoic bile and anterior surface of gallstone (white arrow). (B) Contracted gallbladder (GB) is seen with wall thickening (black arrow) and small stones in the lumen (white arrow).

Complications of Chronic Cholecystitis

The course of patients with CC may be complicated by superimposed episodes of acute cholecystitis, which present with acute pain and tenderness Further, long-standing CC predisposes to the development of GB carcinoma. As mentioned above, irregular wall thickening showing early enhancement should be viewed with suspicion. Another rare, but important complication is the development of cholecystoenteric fistulae.

Cholecystoenteric Fistula

This refers to migration of a gallstone into the intestinal tract due to a defect in the wall of the GB and bowel. These are most commonly seen as cholecystoduodenal fistula. The most well-recognized complication of this is gallstone ileus. This occurs when the stone gets lodged at the narrow terminal ileum and causes bowel obstruction. It is identified by the Rigler's triad on radiography. This consists of pneumobilia, bowel obstruction,

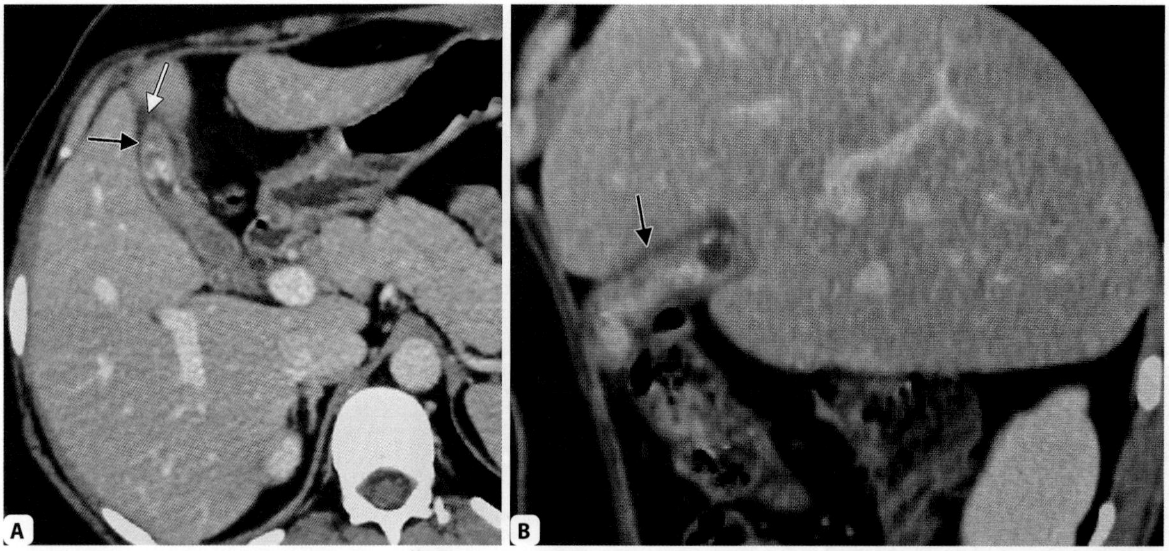

FIGS. 4A AND B: Chronic cholecystitis. (A and B) Contracted gallbladder is seen with calculi in the lumen and regular wall thickening with striated appearance. A hyperenhancing inner wall (black arrow) and hypoenhancing outer wall (white arrow) is seen.

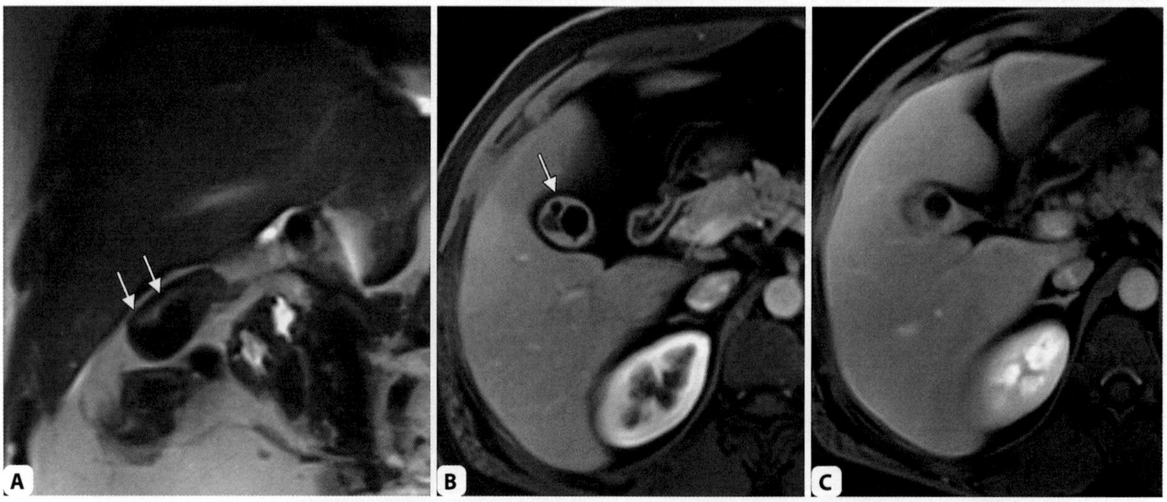

FIGS. 5A TO C: Chronic cholecystitis. (A) T2W coronal image shows a contracted gallbladder (GB) wall-dependent gallstones and wall thickening (white arrows). (B and C) Axial T1W postgad image shows diffuse wall enhancement (arrow).

and a gallstone in ectopic location **(Figs. 6A and B)**.[16] Gallstone ileus is a surgical emergency and carries high mortality if not adequately treated, a large gallstone may get impacted at the fistula to the duodenum which due to secondary inflammatory changes may lead to stenosis.

Due to secondary inflammatory and fibrous tissue, this may eventually lead to stenosis and obstruction and the patient presents as gastric outlet obstruction. This constellation of findings is known as "Bouveret syndrome".

Xanthogranulomatous Cholecystitis

It is a chronic inflammatory disorder which is associated with gallstones in 80% of patients.[17] There is a distinct male predilection (2:1 males to females). The presentation of majority of patients is like chronic cholecystitis, though acute presentation is also possible. Pathologically, it is characterized by accumulation of lipid laden macrophages and inflammatory infiltrates in the wall of the gallbladder. In addition, this inflammation can also involve adjacent organs such as the liver and duodenum, and therefore imaging features often overlap with GB malignancy.

On US, moderate to marked mural thickening of GB is noted. The characteristic finding is hypoechoic nodules with the wall of the GB, which correspond to the xanthogranulomatous deposits. Sometimes, well-defined nodules may not be seen and rather hypoechoic bands are present.[18]

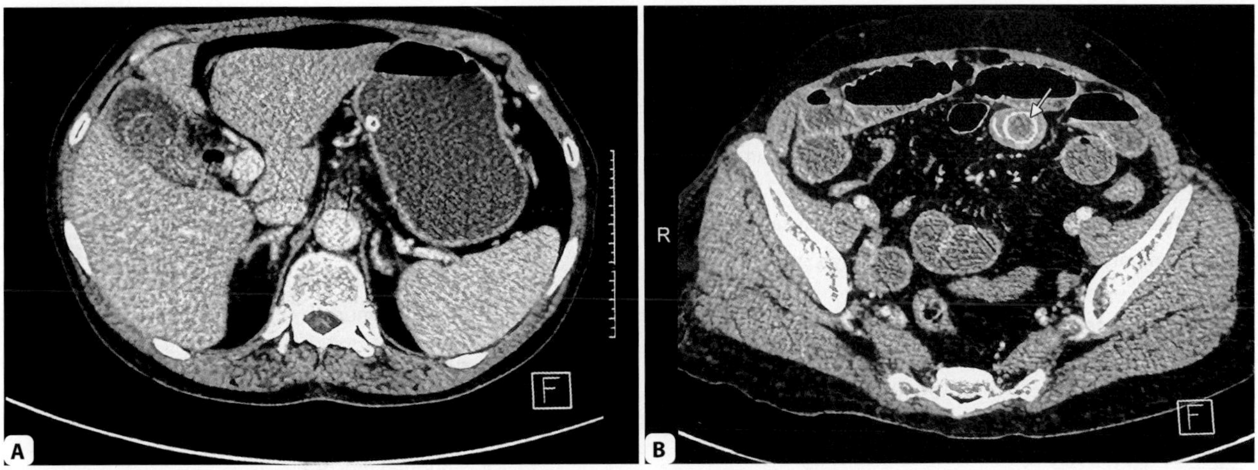

FIGS. 6A AND B: Gallstone ileus—Cholecystoduodenal fistula (A) with ileus and gallstone in the ileum (arrow in B).

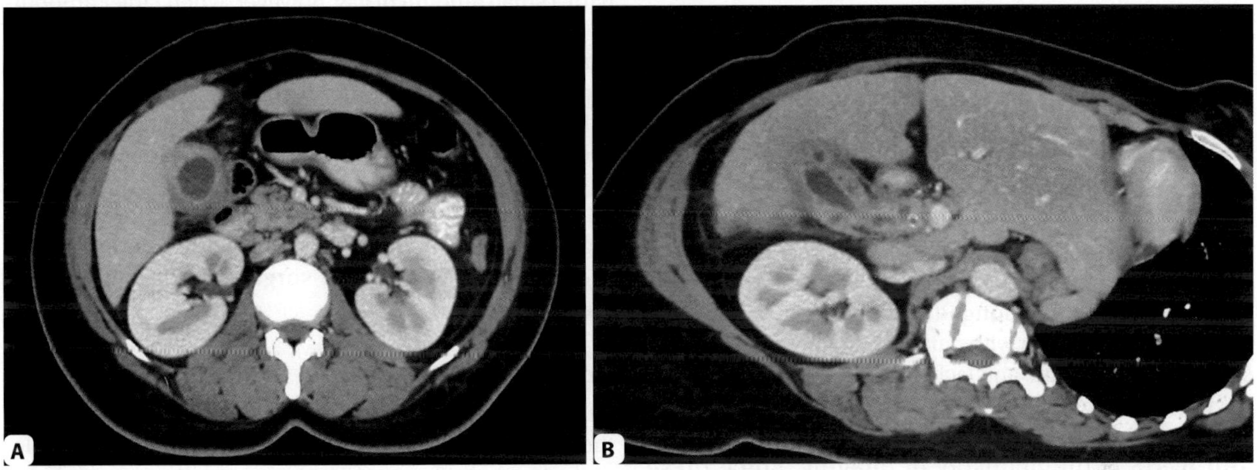

FIGS. 7A AND B: Xanthogranulomatous cholecystitis. (A) Axial and (B) Oblique reformat. There is mural thickening of the gallbladder (GB) wall with hypodense mural nodules. Note the uninterrupted mucosal lining.

In a study by Zhao et al., ~88% patients showed diffuse wall thickening and ~86% patients showed hypoattenuating mural nodules in the wall. Other CT signs which have been described include continuous mucosal lining and luminal surface enhancement, since the pathology is centered in the wall of the GB and therefore mucosal breach is not expected **(Figs. 7A and B)**. Patients with disrupted mucosa have a higher incidence of liver infiltration.[19]

On MRI, similar features of GB wall thickening with T2 hyperintense intramural nodules are noted **(Fig. 8)**. Chemical shift MR may be used to exploit the lipid content in the GB wall, there is signal drop on the opposed phase images compared to in phase. The main differential is from carcinoma GB **(Table 2)**.

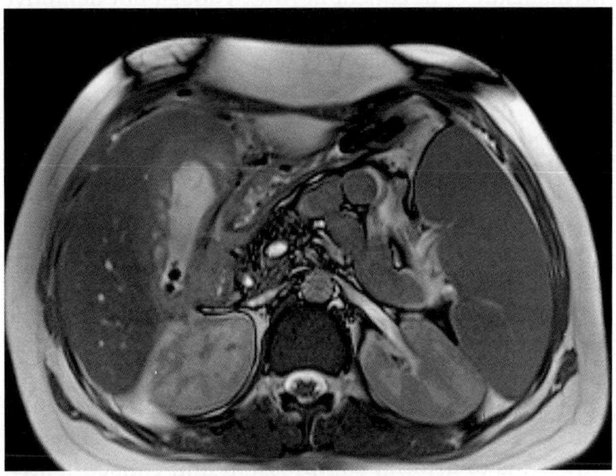

FIG. 8: Xanthogranulomatous cholecystitis. Multiple intramural nodules are seen with preserved mucosal lining on the T2W (T2-weighted) image.

TABLE 2: Differentiating features between carcinoma gall bladder and xanthogranulomatous cholecystitis.

Carcinoma gallbladder	Xanthogranulomatous cholecystitis
Focal asymmetric wall thickening	Diffuse symmetric wall thickening
Disrupted mucosal line	Continuous mucosal line usually
No intramural nodules	Intramural hypoattenuating nodules
May be associated with intrahepatic biliary dilatation	Usually absent biliary dilatation
May have macroscopic hepatic invasion	Absence of macroscopic liver infiltration
Significant loco regional lymphadenopathy and distant metastasis	• Absence of significant lymphadenopathy • Does not show metastasis

NONGALLSTONE-ASSOCIATED DISORDERS

Acute Acalculous Cholecystitis

Acute acalculous cholecystitis (AAC) is much rarer compared to acute calculous cholecystitis, and remains a poorly understood entity. This is usually seen in critically ill patients, such as in association with sepsis, burns, shock, trauma, or prolonged fasting.[20] AAC is a necro-inflammatory disorder with pathophysiology related to bile stasis, hypoperfusion, and ischemia.

Imaging criteria have been proposed for the diagnosis of AAC.[20] These are summarized in **Table 3 and Figs. 9A and B**. US is the mainstay of imaging, since these patients are often critically ill and bedside diagnosis is required. The sensitivity of US ranges between 30 and 90%. Image-guided percutaneous cholecystostomy is the mainstay of treatment in AAC. Though not definitive therapy, it acts as bridge to cholecystectomy for decompression of the gallbladder.

Complications of Acute Acalculous Cholecystitis

Emphysematous Cholecystitis

Emphysematous cholecystitis develops secondary to infection by gas forming bacteria such as *Clostridium perfringens* or *Escherichia coli*. Diabetes mellitus is the most important risk factor. It is most often, but not exclusively associated with acalculous cholecystitis, since high pressure in the biliary system which is seen in acute acalculous cholecystitis is an important risk factor. This leads to arterial compression and consequently, ischemia of the GB wall.[21] This favors the growth of anaerobic organisms which produce gas. US findings vary based on the amount of gas in the GB, echogenic

TABLE 3: Criteria for diagnosis of acalculous cholecystitis. Two major criteria, or a combination of one major and two minor criteria are required for diagnosis.

Imaging modality	Major	Minor
US	1. 4 mm or greater wall thickening 2. Pericholecystic edema 3. Air within GB wall 4. Sloughed mucosa	1. Sludge in gallbladder (GB) 2. Distension > 8 cm longitudinal or >5 cm transverse with clear fluid
CT	1. GB wall thickening 2. Pericholecystic edema 3. Air within GB wall 4. Sloughed mucosa	1. Hyperdense sludge in GB 2. Distension of GB

foci are seen in the GB wall showing reverberation artifact with a small amount of gas, however, when larger amounts of gas are present, the GB may be obscured by a band of shadow. In this setting, it is difficult to differentiate it from the WES complex of complex cholecystitis or a porcelain gallbladder. Therefore, CT remains the imaging modality of choice, which can pinpoint the exact location and extent of the gas **(Fig. 10)**.

Emphysematous cholecystitis has high mortality, with high propensity of development of perforation; therefore prompt identification and surgical management are a must.

Gallbladder Polyps

Gallbladder polyps (GBP) are intraluminal projections of the GB mucosa. These are identified in 2–12% of cholecystectomy specimens.[22] These are usually asymptomatic, and are a common incidental finding on US, identified in 3–7% scans.

These may be neoplastic, which are true adenomatous polyps and have high potential to transform into GB carcinoma, or non-neoplastic. The majority of non-neoplastic polyps are cholesterol polyps. Inflammatory polyps may also be seen secondary to gallstones and chronic inflammation, but these are indistinguishable at imaging.

Ultrasonography is the best modality for diagnosis and follow-up of polyps. These are visualized as rounded, echogenic lesions with smooth contour. The differentiation from gallstones can be made by lack of posterior acoustic shadowing, as well as fixation to the wall. Dynamic scanning with patient placed in supine and left lateral positions is performed, gallstones change position and move to the most dependent location, while polyps do not. A "ball on the wall" sign has been described when the GB wall attachment or stalk is visible; these appear as echogenic balls along the wall **(Fig. 11)**. Doppler scanning may show flow in the polyp; however, it cannot differentiate between a benign and malignant polyp.

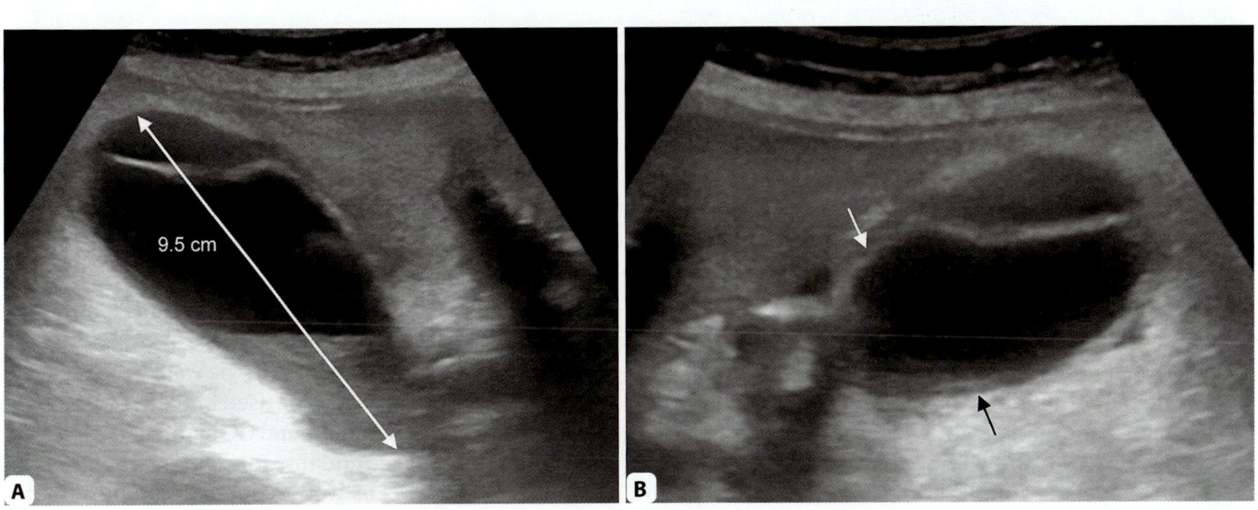

FIGS. 9A AND B: Acute acalculous cholecystitis. (A) On longitudinal scan, there is an overdistended gallbladder (GB) with dependent sludge. Echogenicity of surrounding fat is seen suggesting inflammation. (B) On the axial view, there is wall thickening (arrow), which shows an echogenic inner (white arrow) and hypoechoic outer wall (black arrow).

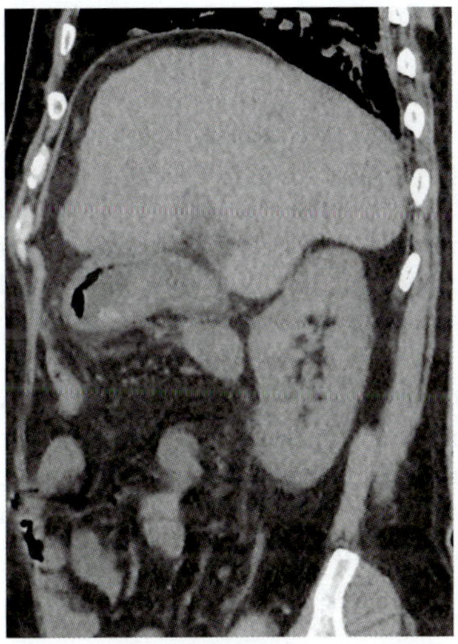

FIG. 10: Emphysematous cholecystitis—gallbladder is distended with diffuse wall thickening with intraluminal air. Hyperdense calculus is also seen in this noncontrast CT.

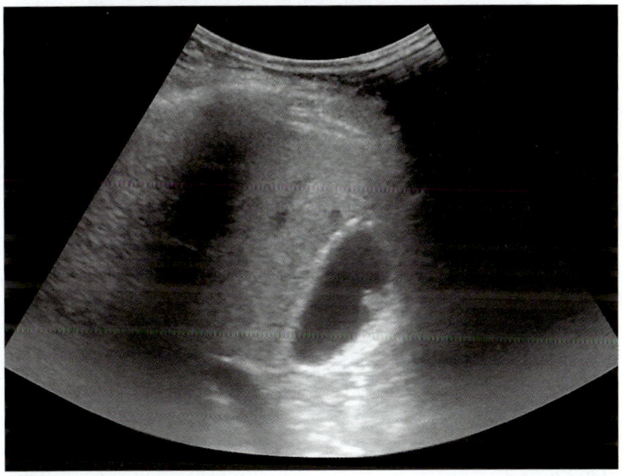

FIG. 11: Gallbladder polyp—an echogenic rounded focus without acoustic shadowing attached to the wall.

Polyps of size >10 mm have high association with malignancy. Single polyps are no more likely to be neoplastic than multiple polyps. Polyp growth rate of <0.6 mm/month is associated with a high negative predictive value for neoplastic polyps.

Risk factors for malignancy in GB polyp are sessile morphology, GB wall thickening >4 mm, cholelithiasis, concomitant primary sclerosing cholangitis (PSC), age of the patient > 50 years, and Indian ethnicity.

Contrast-enhanced US may help to differentiate benign and malignant polyps. Benign polyps show narrow stalks and delayed enhancement, while malignant polyps show wider stalks and arterial hyperenhancement with/without washout.[23] European consensus guidelines advocate cholecystectomy for polyps >10 mm, in symptomatic patients with polyp size <10 mm and for polyps of size 6–9 mm in patients with risk factors. Polyps >6 mm without any risk factors can be followed by ultrasound.

Adenomyomatosis (Adenomyomatous Hyperplasia/Cholecystitis Glandularis Proliferans)

Adenomyomatosis (ADM) is a common benign cause of GB wall thickening. It occurs in up to 9% of cholecystectomy specimens and is associated with gallstones in >90% of cases. Pathologically, it represents intramural invaginations of the mucosa into the muscular layer. These invaginations are called Rokitansky-Aschoff sinuses and often contain cholesterol.[8] Patients are usually asymptomatic. There are three forms of involvement—(1) focal, (2) segmental, and (3) diffuse.

The focal form commonly involves the fundus; the segmental form forms a "ring" of involvement in the body, while the diffuse form involves the entire GB.

On US, tiny echogenic foci are seen in the wall of the GB which show comet tail artifact on gray scale **(Fig. 12)** and twinkling artifact on color Doppler imaging. This is the hallmark of ADM, seen secondary to cholesterol crystals in the Rokitansky–Aschoff sinuses.

On CT, multiple intramural diverticulae are seen which appear hypodense in a thickened GB wall. This is called the "CT rosary" sign.

On MRI, the same is referred to as the "pearl necklace" sign, which are multiple T2 hyperintense foci within the GB wall corresponding to the intramural cystic spaces **(Fig. 13)**. In ADM, the wall is regular and the size of intramural cysts is small and uniform. This helps to differentiate from malignancy, where wall contour is irregular and cysts are larger, even multilobulated. ADM by itself requires no treatment, though it may be seen in association with other inflammatory conditions of the GB.

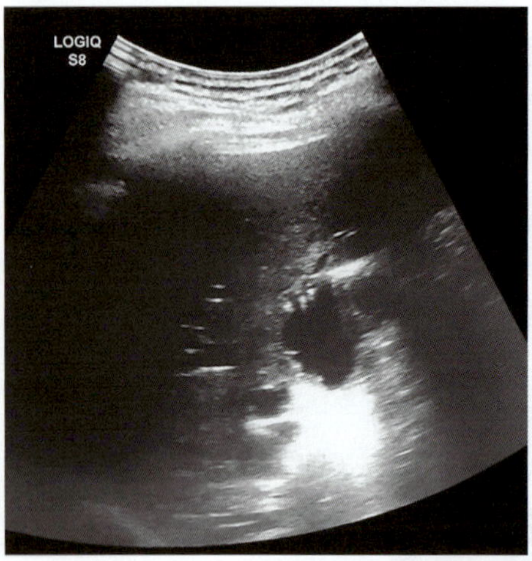

FIG. 12: Adenomyomatosis-tiny echogenic foci with comet tail artifact seen studding the gallbladder wall.

Miscellaneous

Porcelain Gallbladder

Porcelain GB is a chronic inflammatory disorder, which is considered a premalignant condition. The risk of GB malignancy was earlier estimated to be around 60%, though recent studies suggest that the actual risk is <10%.[24]

Calcium encrustation is seen in the wall, which may be focal or diffuse. While US may be used initially, overlapping features with emphysematous and CC hamper its utility. CT is considered the best modality for demonstration of the calcification **(Fig. 14)** as well as depiction of focal mural thickening that may indicate malignant transformation.

Approach to GB Wall Thickening

Thickening of the GB wall can be seen in intrinsic pathology of the GB or may be part of extracholecystic conditions.

Wall thickening may be diffuse or focal. Presence of distended GB with pericholecystic fluid and ultrasound Murphy' sign positive is diagnostic for acute cholecystitis. Absence of probe tenderness with sloughed in intraluminal membranes is noted in gangrenous cholecystitis. A thickened gallbladder wall with "dirty shadowing" like air should raise the possibility of emphysematous cholecystitis whereas a diffusely calcified GB wall is a porcelain GB. Diffusely thick walled GB wall with a mesh-like thickening can be seen in systemic disease or other extrinsic causes like ascites. Acute acalculous cholecystitis is seen in patients who are critically ill and have features like acute cholecystitis but without GB calculus.

Focal thickening of GB wall is often a diagnostic dilemma. The main differential diagnosis are focal ADM,

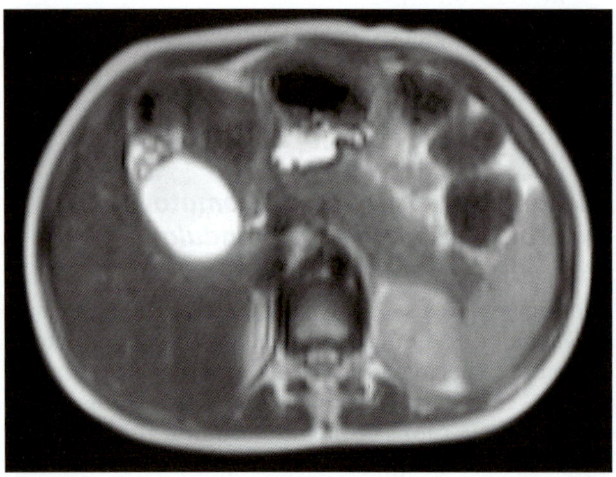

FIG. 13: Multiple tiny cystic spaces seen in the fundus of the gallbladder wall on T2W HASTE (Half fourier Single-shot Turbo spin-Echo) image in a case of focal adenomyomatosis.

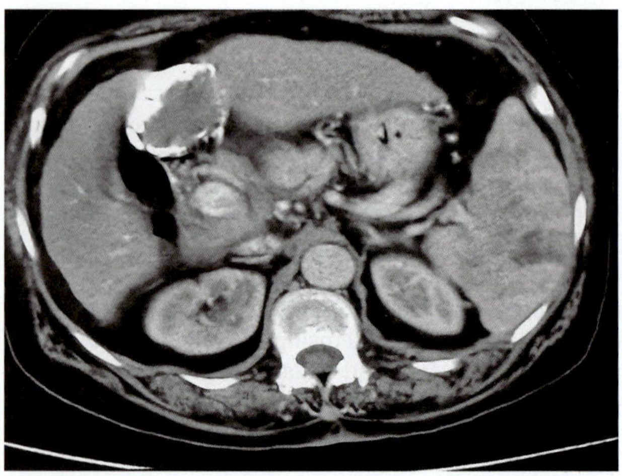

FIG. 14: Porcelain gallbladder. Diffuse calcium encrustation of the wall of a contracted gallbladder (GB).

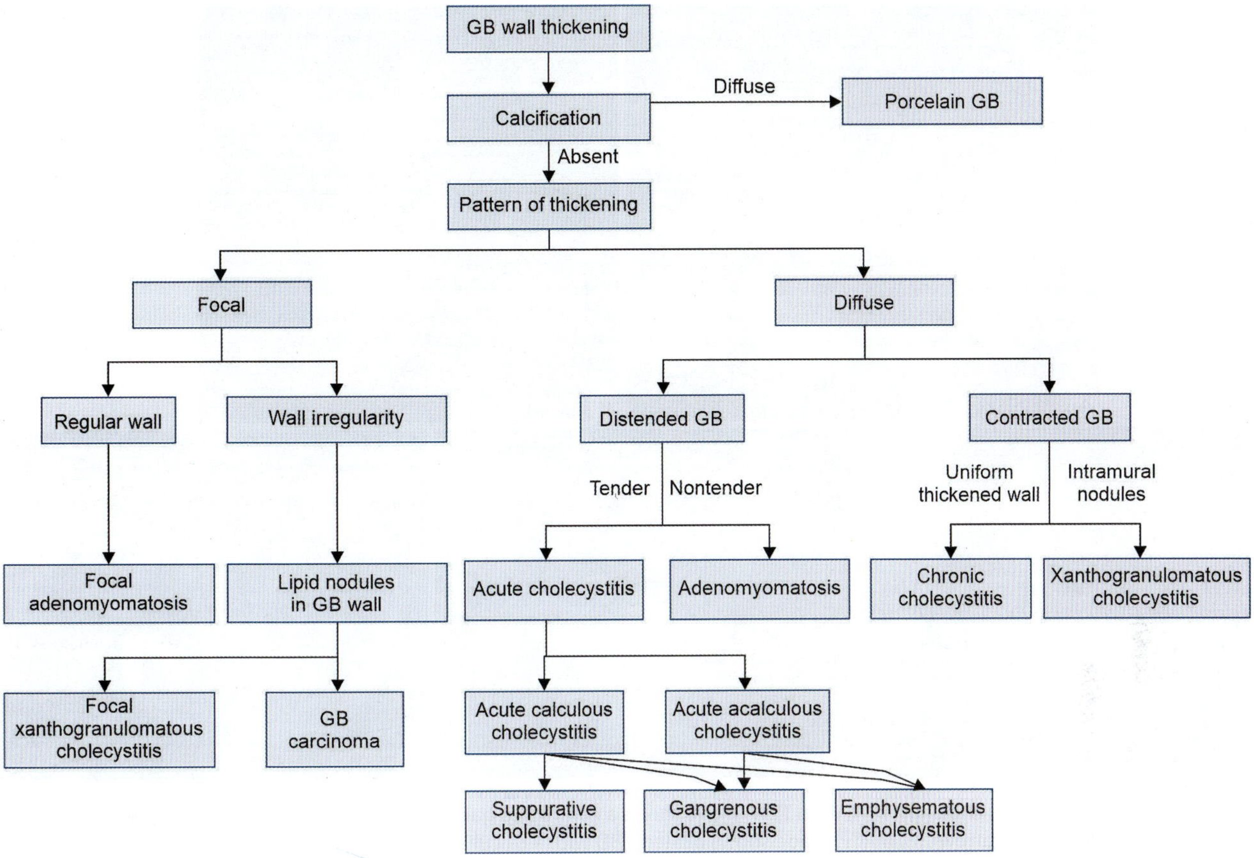

FLOWCHART 3: Algorithmic approach to gallbladder (GB) wall thickening.

xanthogranulomatous cholecystitis, and GB carcinoma. An intact mucosa in a focally thickened GB wall points toward xanthogranulomatous cholecystitis ,whereas an asymmetrical mural thickening with mucosal disruption and liver infiltration is suggestive of carcinoma of GB.

The approach to GB wall thickening[3] is summarized in **Flowchart 3**.

INFLAMMATORY DISORDERS OF BILIARY TREE

Infectious Disorders

Acute Cholangitis

Acute cholangitis or ascending cholangitis is seen due to infection of the biliary usually, by gram negative bacteria, usually *E. coli*. This usually occurs in the setting of biliary obstruction, due to bile stasis and raised intrabiliary pressure. Patients typically present with the Charcot triad of pain, fever, and jaundice.

Acute cholangitis is primarily a clinical diagnosis, so the goal of imaging remains to define the cause of obstruction as well as liver parenchymal complications. Bile duct obstruction by gallstones, or choledocholithiasis remains the most important cause, accounting for up to 80% of cases.[25] The other important causes are malignancy, sclerosing cholangitis, and biliary instrumentation.

On imaging, dilation of the bile ducts is seen proximal to the site of enhancement, which show concentric wall thickening and enhance with intravenous contrast **(Figs. 15A to E)**. Parenchymal complications occur due to spread of infection into the portal triads. The most common among these is hepatic abscess formation (~25%) and portal vein thrombosis (~15%). Altered hepatic enhancement patterns are also seen, peribiliary arterial hyperenhancement is a common pattern.

Acute cholangitis carries a high mortality rate of over 80% if not treated adequately. Emergent biliary drainage must be performed in conjunction with antibiotic therapy since patients typically do not respond to conservative therapy alone.

Recurrent Pyogenic Cholangitis

Recurrent pyogenic cholangitis (RPC), previously known as oriental cholangiohepatitis is characterized by repeated episodes of bacterial cholangitis. There is an association with *Clonorchis sinensis* and *Ascaris lumbricoides* infestation, though their causative role has not been established. It is postulated that the infestation leads to strictures, bile stasis, and pigment stone formation, which predisposes to recurrent infection.

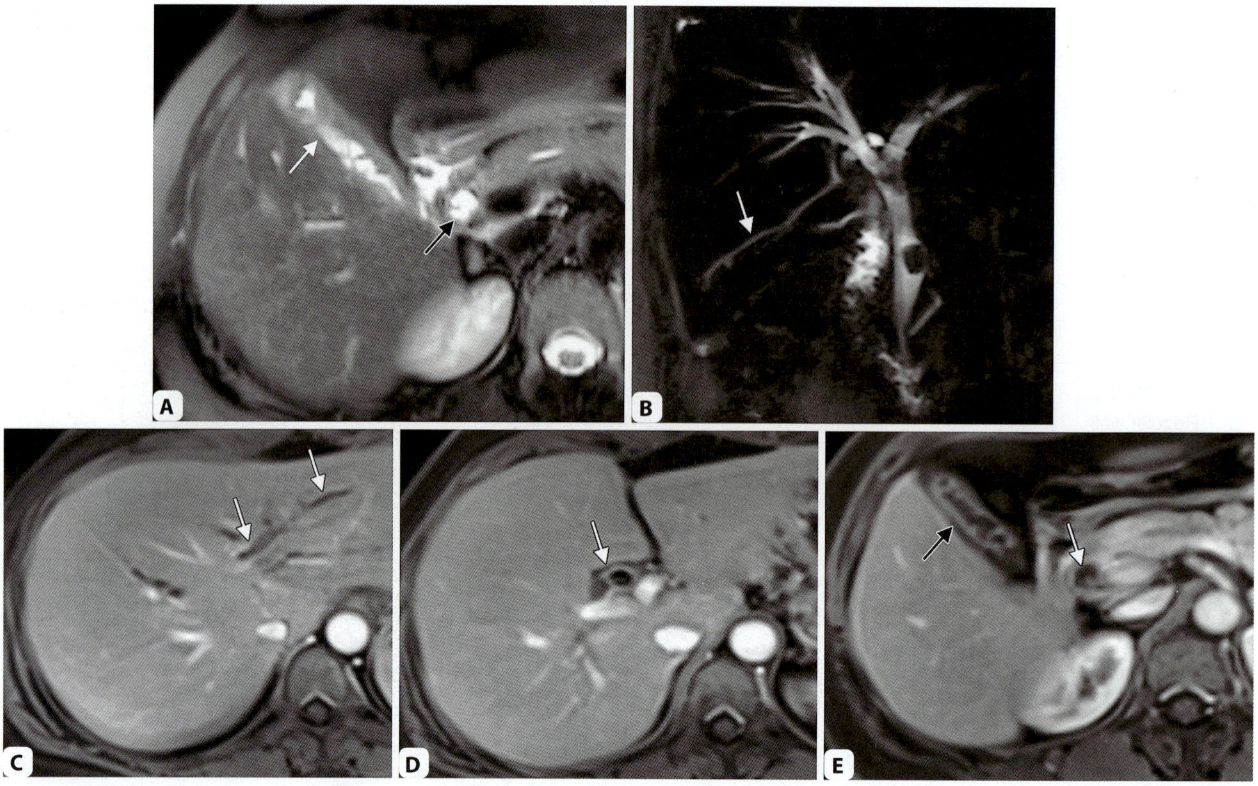

FIGS. 15A TO E: Ascending cholangitis. (A) Axial T2W image shows a contracted gallbladder (GB) with thickened wall (white arrow) and dilated bile duct (black arrow). (B) MRCP image shows dilated CBD with a calculus and contracted GB lumen (arrow). (C to E) Axial T1W enhanced images show enhancement along the bile ductules, CBD (white arrow), and the GB wall (black arrow).

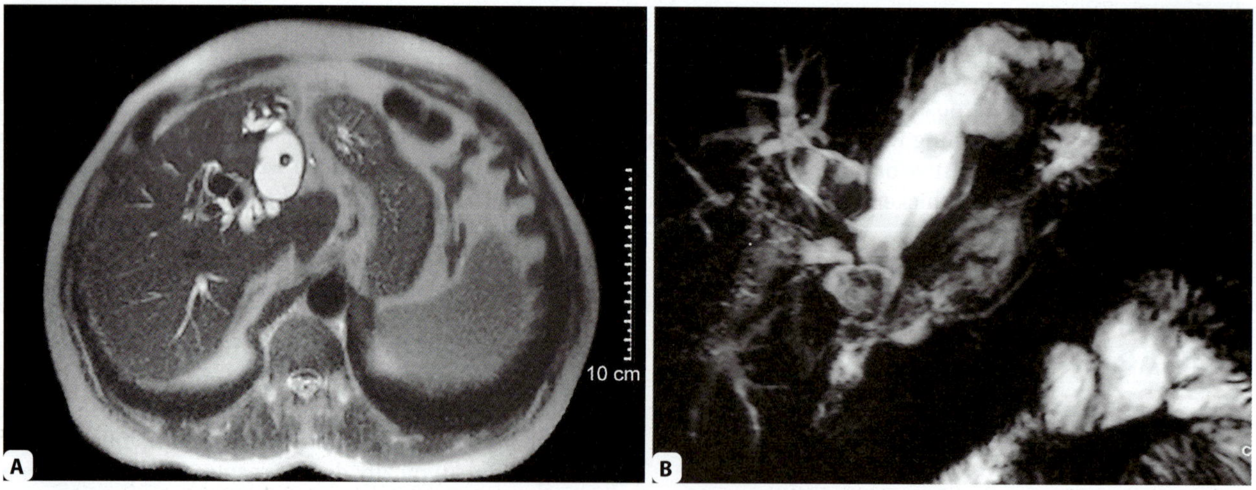

FIGS. 16A AND B: Recurrent pyogenic cholangitis—(A) T2W HASTE and (B) MRCP-disproportionate dilation of the central ducts with intrahepatic ductal dilatation.

The geographic distribution has also widened from its previous predilection for Asian populations. It is increasingly being recognized in Western and Latin American countries as well in lower socioeconomic strata. Patients present with recurrent episodes of pain, fever, and jaundice. Imaging findings include multifocal strictures with intrahepatic ductal dilatation. Pigment calculi are noted within the dilated ducts. The ducts show a decreased arborization and appear to branch in a right angled fashion **(Figs. 16A and B)**.

The extrahepatic biliary system may be dilated disproportionate to stricture/calculi.

The imaging findings are summarized in **Table 4**. RPC predisposes to the development of cholangiocarcinoma, and thus surveillance with MR is advised for early detection.

TABLE 4: Imaging features of recurrent pyogenic cholangitis.

Biliary tree	Hepatic parenchyma
• Strictures in peripheral bile ducts • Pigment calculi in intrahepatic ducts: T1 hyperintense due to proteinaceous content • Reduced branching of intrahepatic ducts, branches arise at right angles ("arrowhead appearance") • Disproportionate dilatation of central ducts, unrelated to obstruction	• *Hepatic atrophy*: Peripheral segments of liver are affected • Cholangiolar abscess may be seen occasionally

Acquired Immunodeficiency Syndrome Cholangitis

The incidence of acquired immunodeficiency syndrome-related cholangiopathy has decreased due to wider availability of antiretroviral drugs. A low CD 4 count (<100 cells/mm^3) and alkaline phosphatase (ALP) five to seven times normal is seen. A long smooth-tapered stricture of the distal common bile duct (CBD) up to the ampulla is seen on imaging.

Autoimmune Disorders

Primary Sclerosing Cholangitis

Primary sclerosing cholangitis is a chronic disorder of the biliary tree characterized by inflammation and fibrosis of both intra and extrahepatic bile ducts. The pathogenesis of PSC is considered to be an exaggerated immune response to cholangiocyte injury. Three subtypes of PSC have been described—classic, small duct type, and an overlapping type with autoimmune hepatitis.

It is associated with inflammatory bowel disease in ~80% of patients.[26] Patients may present with features of cholestasis or may be asymptomatic.

The important complications of PSC are development of cirrhosis and portal hypertension, as well as superimposed acute cholangitis. The risk of cholangiocarcinoma is estimated to be between 5 and 15%. Increase in the risk of developing hepatocellular carcinoma and GB malignancy has also been noted.

The American Association for the study of liver diseases in their guidelines suggests that the diagnosis of PSC is to be made on the cholestatic pattern on biochemistry (elevated serum bilirubin and at least a threefold increase in serum ALP), characteristic biliary changes on MRCP, and after exclusion of secondary causes of sclerosing cholangitis **(Box 2)**.

The MRCP is the recommended imaging modality, with reported sensitivity of 83–100% and specificity of 67–100%.[27] PSC is characterized by biliary strictures involving both intra and extrahepatic biliary ducts; isolated involvement of intrahepatic ducts is also seen.

BOX 2 Diagnostic criteria for primary sclerosing cholangitis (PSC).

- Cholestatic biochemistry (elevated serum bilirubin) 3 times alkaline phosphatase (ALP)
- Characteristic changes on magnetic resonance cholangiopancreatography (MRCP)
- Exclusion of secondary causes of sclerosing cholangitis

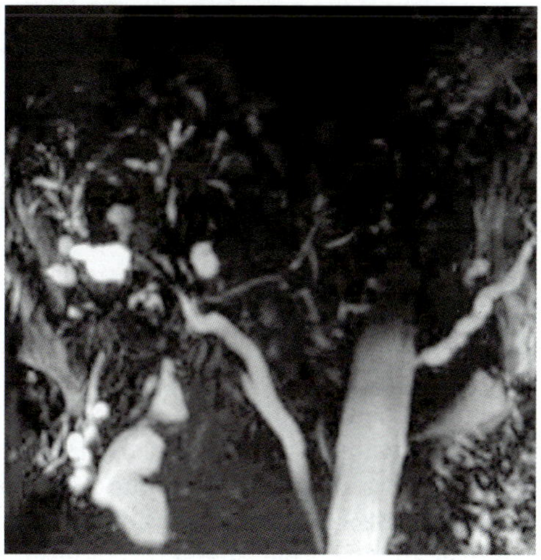

FIG. 17: Primary sclerosing cholangitis—MRCP multifocal stricture of the intrahepatic biliary tree are seen with biliary diverticula.

Intrahepatic strictures are usually multifocal and involve both lobes. A stricture causing >75% luminal narrowing is termed high grade. The length of the strictures may be variable. Diverticula of the biliary ducts are seen. The "beaded" appearance of biliary radicles is characteristic, which arises due to multifocal short segment strictures that alternate with dilated radicles **(Fig. 17)**. Further, a "pruned tree" appearance may be seen in advanced PSC, where there is near obliteration of the peripheral ducts. Liver parenchyma shows changes in morphology in later stages of PSC. Prominent lobulations of the caudate lobe, left lobar atrophy, and regenerative nodules in the medial segments are seen. Peripheral hyperenhancing areas may be noted on late arterial phase indicating an increase in arterial flow to compensate for decreased venous flow in areas where there is biliary obstruction. This pattern denotes transient hepatic attenuation difference (THAD). Periportal T2 hyperintensity (periportal halo) is seen due to inflammatory infiltrate, lymphatics, and fibrosis. In the small duct variant, PSC may not be easily diagnosed as the ducts may not be visualized. Liver biopsy may be required for the diagnosis of PSC.

Enhancement and wall thickening of the bile ducts may suggest the possibility of development of cholangiocarcinoma. A wall thickness of >2 mm is considered abnormal. Cholangiocarcinoma should be suspected in patients with progressive ductal dilatation or a soft tissue nodule. Majority of cholangiocarcinomas are detected within a year of the primary diagnosis of PSC, with an annual risk of 1.5% thereafter.[28] Several MR imaging-based scoring systems are available to predict progression of disease.[29] One of these is ANALI risk score, based on use of MR contrast (ANALI1) and without gadolinium (ANALI 2). MR elastography (MRE) is also being used to measure liver stiffness as a prognostic tool.

Liver transplant is the only definitive treatment. ERCP may also be used for therapeutic purpose for biliary drainage and also balloon dilatation of strictures.

IgG4 Sclerosing cholangitis

IgG4-related sclerosing cholangitis (IgG4-SC) is part of the larger spectrum of IgG4-related disease which presents with multisystem manifestations, the best recognized of which autoimmune pancreatitis. Other common sites of involvement include the salivary glands, lymph nodes, kidney, and periaortic soft. ISC is associated with autoimmune pancreatitis in 90% of cases.[30]

Patients are usually elderly male (M:F 4:1) who present with recurrent cholestatic jaundice. Elevated serum bilirubin, ALP, and aminotransferases are noted. A characteristic finding is elevated levels of IgG4, usually >1.4 g/L and an increased ratio of serum IgG4 to total IgG OF >0.10.

Multiple international societies have evolved diagnostic criteria for IgG4-related disease over the years. The HISORt criteria **(Table 5)** is based on *hi*stological findings, *s*erology, other organ involvement and *r*esponse to steroid therapy.[31] The Japanese criteria, proposed by Ohara et al. divide different diagnostic categories along with diagnostic features.[32] The most recent among these is the American College of Rheumatology and European League against Rheumatism (ACR/EULAR) classification criteria, formulated in 2019.[33] This criterion combines imaging, histopathology, and raised serum IgG4 levels.

TABLE 5: HISORt criteria for diagnosis of IgG4-related sclerosing cholangitis.

Criteria	Description
Histological	Characteristic lymphoplasmacytic infiltration (>10 IgG4-positive plasma cells per high power field), obliterative phlebitis, and storiform fibrosis
Imaging	Single or multiple bile duct strictures (intrahepatic, extrahepatic, and both), fleeting biliary strictures
Serological finding	Elevated serum IgG4 levels (>135 mg/dL)
Other organ involvement	Pancreas (autoimmune pancreatitis), kidneys, retroperitoneum, salivary, or lacrimal gland
Response to steroid therapy	Improvement in liver function tests, bile duct strictures, or both

Imaging Findings

Smooth bile duct wall thickening is noted with a long segment of narrowing, the bile duct lumen remains visible in the thickened ducts, a finding characteristic of ISC. Delayed homogeneous enhancement is noted on administration of contrast on CT/MRI. The duct involvement may be single or multifocal. Liver parenchyma is usually normal, diffuse GB wall thickening is seen in half the patients. Other manifestations may be in the form of ill-defined soft tissue seen at the porta hepatitis, or focal liver lesions known as hepatic pseudotumors. Based on cholangiographic appearance and location of the strictures, ISC has been classified into four types **(Box 3)**. IgG4-SC shows a dramatic response to steroids, such that it forms part of the diagnostic criteria. There is normalization of biochemical parameters and improvement in biliary strictures with steroid therapy.

The main differential diagnoses are PSC and cholangiocarcinoma. The important differentiation from PSC is the older age of patient involvement, longer segments of involvement, and associated pancreatic involvement.[34] Further, a cut-off of 8 mm for the mural thickening has been proposed for differentiation of IgG4-SC from cholangiocarcinoma.[35] Preserved ductal lumen and lesser degree of biliary dilatation (<9 mm) are also differentiators of IgG4-SC from malignancy. CBD wall thickening with continuous long segment involvement of CBD with GB abnormality are seen in IgG4 sclerosing cholangitis and can be used to differentiate from PSC.

The main differentiating features are outlined in **Table 6**.

Primary Biliary Cholangitis

This is an immune-mediated inflammatory disease affecting the small intrahepatic bile ducts. It is a slowly progressive disease leading to chronic cholestasis and cirrhosis. Diffuse hepatosplenomegaly and portal hypertension are noted on imaging. On MRI, periportal hyperintensity may be seen on T2-weighted imaging. The periportal halo sign has also been described, which is T1 and T2 low signal intensity surrounding the portal venous branches. Primary biliary cholangitis typically does not cause strictures of the bile duct.

BOX 3 Classification of IgG4-related sclerosing cholangitis based on cholangiographic features.[34]

- Involvement of lower part of bile duct only
- Involvement of distal bile duct and intrahepatic bile duct with proximal dilatation
- Involvement of distal bile duct and diffuse intrahepatic bile duct without proximal dilatation
- Involvement of distal bile duct and ducts at hepatic hilum
- Involvement of ducts at hepatic hilum only

TABLE 6: Imaging differentiation of ISC, PSC, and cholangiocarcinoma.

Imaging feature	IgG4 sclerosing cholangitis	Primary sclerosing cholangitis	Cholangiocarcinoma
Location	Extrahepatic > Intrahepatic	Extrahepatic plus intrahepatic mostly	Hilar more often than extrahepatic more often than intrahepatic
Length of involvement	Long, continuous	Short, multiple	Short, single
Duct wall thickening	Symmetrical, often >2.5 mm	Symmetrical, usually <2.5 mm	Asymmetrical > 5 mm
Margins of thickening	Sharp and smooth	Fuzzy and smooth	Fuzzy and irregular
Lumen of thickened segment	Often visible	Often occluded	Mostly occluded
Duct dilatation	Less (<9 mm)	Mild	Gross
Contrast enhancement	Single layer Delayed homogeneous	Uniform	Double layer
Skip lesions	Common	Less common	Rare
Liver parenchymal changes	Usually normal, pseudotumors seen in late stages	Common	Rare
Others	Funnel-shaped dilatation	Pruned tree ducts, diverticula	Vascular invasion
Associations	Autoimmune pancreatitis type 1	Inflammatory bowel disease	Usually none
Serum IgG4 level	Elevated in majority	Usually normal	Usually normal
Response to steroids	Good	Poor	No response

Eosinophilic Cholangitis

It is a rare disorder, usually self-limiting, and characterized by eosinophilic infiltration of the biliary tree. Thickening of the CBD wall is noted with a dominant stricture up to the biliary confluence. The condition responds to steroid therapy.

MISCELLANEOUS CHOLANGITIS

Chemotherapy Related

It is seen rarely in patients who had received trans arterial chemoembolization. CBD stricture with intrahepatic biliary duct dilation is seen.

Metastatic Disease

Hepatic metastasis from primary malignancy of pancreas, prostate, or liver among others may cause compression and invasion of biliary ducts leading to biliary obstruction and cholangitis.

Ischemic Cholangitis

The blood supply of the biliary system is the hepatic arteries. Ischemic cholangitis arises when the blood supply is compromised as in hepatic artery thrombosis or stenosis. It is also seen within first 6 months postliver transplant as nonanastomotic biliary strictures in liver allograft. In the acute phase, there is formation of biliary casts which look like calculi and appear hyperintense on T1W images. later there is necrosis, bile leaks, and formation of bilomas. In the chronic phase, multifocal biliary strictures, and indistinguishable from those seen in PSC are seen.

CONCLUSION

There is a myriad of both acute and chronic inflammatory conditions affecting the GB and biliary tract. While some have characteristic imaging appearances that are easy to identify, for others, an algorithmic approach such as has been detailed for GB wall thickening must be employed.

REFERENCES

1. Expert Panel on Gastrointestinal Imaging, Russo GK, Zaheer A, Kamel IR, Porter KK, Archer-Arroyo K, Bashir MR, et al. ACR Appropriateness Criteria® Right Upper Quadrant Pain: 2022 Update. J Am Coll Radiol. 2023;20(5S):S211-23.
2. Expert Panel on Gastrointestinal Imaging:, Hindman NM, Arif-Tiwari H, Kamel IR, Al-Refaie WB, Bartel TB, Cash BD, et al. ACR Appropriateness Criteria® Jaundice. J Am Coll Radiol. 2019;16(5S):S126-40.
3. Gupta P, Marodia Y, Bansal A, Kalra N, Kumar-M P, Sharma V, et al. Imaging-based algorithmic approach to gallbladder wall thickening. World J Gastroenterol. 2020;26(40):6163-81.
4. Ratanaprasatporn L, Uyeda JW, Wortman JR, Richardson I, Sodickson AD. Multimodality Imaging, including dual-energy CT, in the evaluation of gallbladder disease. Radiogr Rev Publ Radiol Soc N Am Inc. 2018;38(1):75-89.

5. Snyder E, Banks KP. Hepatobiliary Scintigraphy. In: StatPearls [Internet]. Treasure Island (FL): StatPearls Publishing; 2024.
6. Jailwala J, Fogel EL, Sherman S, Gottlieb K, Flueckiger J, Bucksot LG, et al. Triple-tissue sampling at ERCP in malignant biliary obstruction. Gastrointest Endosc. 2000;51(4 Pt 1):383-90.
7. Catalano OA, Sahani DV, Kalva SP, Cushing MS, Hahn PF, Brown JJ, et al. MR imaging of the gallbladder: A pictorial essay. Radiogr Rev Publ Radiol Soc N Am Inc. 2008;28(1): 135-55;quiz 324.
8. Yu MH, Kim YJ, Park HS, Jung SI. Benign gallbladder diseases: Imaging techniques and tips for differentiating with malignant gallbladder diseases. World J Gastroenterol. 2020;26(22):2967-86.
9. Gore RM, Thakrar KH, Newmark GM, Mehta UK, Berlin JW. Gallbladder imaging. Gastroenterol Clin North Am. 2010;39(2):265-87.
10. Chang TC, Lin MT, Wu MH, Wang MY, Lee PH. Evaluation of early versus delayed laparoscopic cholecystectomy in the treatment of acute cholecystitis. Hepatogastroenterology. 2009;56(89):26-8.
11. Spence SC, Teichgraeber D, Chandrasekhar C. Emergent right upper quadrant sonography. J Ultrasound Med Off J Am Inst Ultrasound Med. 2009;28(4):479-96.
12. Teefey SA, Dahiya N, Middleton WD, Bajaj S, Dahiya N, Ylagan L, et al. Acute cholecystitis: do sonographic findings and WBC count predict gangrenous changes? AJR Am J Roentgenol. 2013;200(2):363-9.
13. Chawla A, Bosco JI, Lim TC, Srinivasan S, Teh HS, Shenoy JN. Imaging of acute cholecystitis and cholecystitis-associated complications in the emergency setting. Singapore Med J. 2015;56(8):438-43;quiz 444.
14. Pedrosa I, Guarise A, Goldsmith J, Procacci C, Rofsky NM. The interrupted rim sign in acute cholecystitis: A method to identify the gangrenous form with MRI. J Magn Reson Imaging. 2003;18(3):360-3.
15. Smith EA, Dillman JR, Elsayes KM, Menias CO, Bude RO. Cross-sectional imaging of acute and chronic gallbladder inflammatory disease. AJR Am J Roentgenol. 2009;192(1):188-96.
16. Chuah PS, Curtis J, Misra N, Hikmat D, Chawla S. Pictorial review: the pearls and pitfalls of the radiological manifestations of gallstone ileus. Abdom Radiol N Y. 2017;42(4):1169-75.
17. Guzmán-Valdivia G. Xanthogranulomatous cholecystitis in laparoscopic surgery. J Gastrointest Surg Off J Soc Surg Aliment Tract. 2005;9(4):494-7.
18. Singh VP, Rajesh S, Bihari C, Desai SN, Pargewar SS, Arora A. Xanthogranulomatous cholecystitis: What every radiologist should know. World J Radiol. 2016;8(2):183-91.
19. Zhao F, Lu PX, Yan SX, Wang GF, Yuan J, Zhang SZ, et al. CT and MR features of xanthogranulomatous cholecystitis: an analysis of consecutive 49 cases. Eur J Radiol. 2013;82(9): 1391-7.
20. Huffman JL, Schenker S. Acute acalculous cholecystitis: A review. Clin Gastroenterol Hepatol. 2010;8(1):15-22.
21. Sunnapwar A, Raut AA, Nagar AM, Katre R. Emphysematous cholecystitis: Imaging findings in nine patients. Indian J Radiol Imaging. 2011;21(2):142-6.
22. Mellnick VM, Menias CO, Sandrasegaran K, Hara AK, Kielar AZ, Brunt EM, et al. Polypoid lesions of the gallbladder: disease spectrum with pathologic correlation. Radiogr Rev Publ Radiol Soc N Am Inc. 2015;35(2):387-99.
23. Zhang HP, Bai M, Gu JY, He YQ, Qiao XH, Du LF. Value of contrast-enhanced ultrasound in the differential diagnosis of gallbladder lesion. World J Gastroenterol. 2018;24(6): 744-51.
24. Schnelldorfer T. Porcelain gallbladder: A benign process or concern for malignancy? J Gastrointest Surg Off J Soc Surg Aliment Tract. 2013;17(6):1161-8.
25. Catalano OA, Sahani DV, Forcione DG, Czermak B, Liu CH, Soricelli A, et al. Biliary infections: spectrum of imaging findings and management. Radiogr Rev Publ Radiol Soc N Am Inc. 2009;29(7):2059-80.
26. Bali MA, Pezzullo M, Pace E, Morone M. Benign biliary diseases. Eur J Radiol. 2017;93:217-8.
27. Dave M, Elmunzer BJ, Dwamena BA, Higgins PDR. Primary sclerosing cholangitis: meta-analysis of diagnostic performance of MR cholangiopancreatography. Radiology. 2010; 256(2):387-96.
28. O'Brien C, Malik M, Jhaveri K. MR Imaging in Primary Sclerosing Cholangitis and Other Cholangitis. Radiol Clin North Am. 2022;60(5):843-56.
29. Lemoinne S, Cazzagon N, El Mouhadi S, Trivedi PJ, Dohan A, Kemgang A, et al. Simple magnetic resonance scores associate with outcomes of patients with primary sclerosing cholangitis.Clin Gastroenterol Hepatol. 2019; 17(13):2785-92.e3.
30. Naik M, Hesni S, Tamimi A, Hameed M, Tomlinson J, Poo S, et al. Imaging manifestations of IgG4-related disease. Clin Radiol. 2023;78(8):555-64.
31. Ghazale A, Chari ST, Zhang L, Smyrk TC, Takahashi N, Levy MJ, et al. Immunoglobulin G4-associated cholangitis: Clinical profile and response to therapy. Gastroenterology. 2008;134(3):706-15.
32. Ohara H, Okazaki K, Tsubouchi H, Inui K, Kawa S, Kamisawa T, et al; Research Committee of IgG4-related Diseases; Research Committee of Intractable Diseases of Liver and Biliary Tract; Ministry of Health, Labor and Welfare, Japan; Japan Biliary Association. Clinical diagnostic criteria of IgG4-related sclerosing cholangitis 2012. J Hepatobiliary Pancreat Sci. 2012;19(5):536-42.
33. Wallace ZS, Naden RP, Chari S, Choi H, Della-Torre E, Dicaire JF, et al. The 2019 American College of Rheumatology/ European League Against Rheumatism Classification Criteria for IgG4-Related Disease. Arthritis Rheumatol Hoboken NJ. 2020;72(1):7-19.
34. Madhusudan KS, Das P, Gunjan D, Srivastva DN, et al. IgG4-reated sclerosing cholangitis: A clinical and imaging review. AJR. 2019;213:1221231.
35. Naitoh I, Nakazawa T, Ohara H, Ando T, Hayashi K, Tanaka H, et al. Endoscopic transpapillary intraductal ultrasonography and biopsy in the diagnosis of IgG4-related sclerosing cholangitis. J Gastroenterol. 2009;44(11):1147-55.

CHAPTER 16

Pankaj Gupta, Ujjwal Gorsi, Naveen Kalra, Ajay Gulati

Malignant Pathologies of Gallbladder and Biliary Tree

INTRODUCTION

Biliary tract cancers (BTCs) are the second most common hepatobiliary malignancy after hepatocellular carcinoma (HCC).[1] BTCs include gallbladder carcinoma (GBC) and cholangiocarcinomas (CCAs). GBC arises from the gallbladder or the cystic duct. CCA originates from intrahepatic or extrahepatic bile ducts. Patients with BTC present clinically with jaundice and right upper quadrant pain. The clinical presentation and laboratory investigations are nonspecific. Radiological imaging plays a crucial role in the diagnosis and staging. Recently, radiological features that help to guide individualized treatment and predict the prognosis have been identified. However, differentiating benign and malignant biliary tract diseases sometimes poses a considerable challenge to radiologists. Combining radiological and endoscopic imaging techniques improves the characterization of biliary tract lesions. In this chapter, we will discuss the role of radiological imaging techniques in diagnosing and staging BTCs.

GALLBLADDER CARCINOMA

Epidemiology

Gallbladder carcinoma is the 23rd most common cancer in the world, and 6th most common malignancy of the gastrointestinal (GI) tract, and the most common malignant neoplasm of the biliary tree.[2] There is a marked geographic predisposition for GBC.[2-4] Regions with the highest incidence of GBC include South America, the Northern and Northeastern states of India, and mainland China. GBC is more common in females. The prognosis is poor, with a 5-year survival rate of < 20.7%.[5] The incidence and mortality of GBC are expected to increase worldwide in both males and females.[2]

Risk Factors

The most common risk factor of GBC is chronic inflammation caused by gallstones. The risk increases with the larger stones.[6] Primary sclerosing cholangitis (PSC), pancreaticobiliary maljunction (PBM), and gallbladder polyps are also associated with an increased risk of GBC. Other associations include typhoid carrier state, chronic bacterial infections affecting the gallbladder, obesity, exposure to particular carcinogens (including nitrosamines and aflatoxins), and specific genetic syndromes (Gardner syndrome and Peutz–Jeghers syndrome).[6]

Pathological Features, Staging, and Prognosis

Precursor lesions of GBC include pyloric gland adenoma, biliary intraepithelial neoplasm (BilIN), and intracholecystic papillary neoplasm (ICPN).[7] Most GBCs are adenocarcinoma (85–90%) and can be papillary, tubular, mucinous, or signet cell type.[8] Other pathological subtypes include squamous cell carcinoma, undifferentiated, primary hepatoid, and sarcomatoid. The most common locations are fundus (60%), followed by the body (30%) and neck (10%).[9] The gallbladder lacks submucosa and serosa (along the liver surface). In addition, the connective tissue of the gallbladder is continuous with the interlobular connective tissue of the liver.[9] These anatomical features promote early local invasion into the liver.

Gallbladder carcinoma is staged surgically by the depth of invasion, extension of disease into adjacent structures, involvement of lymph nodes, and presence of metastases by the American Joint Committee on Cancer (AJCC) TNM (tumor, node, and metastasis) staging system.[10] The 8th AJCC classification is the latest and includes two significant changes compared to the 7th edition. The T2 disease has been classified into T2a (peritoneal side) and T2b (hepatic side), and nodal staging is now based on the number of lymph nodes rather than the location. The most decisive prognostic factor in GBC is the tumor stage.[11]

Imaging Modalities

Ultrasound (US) is often the initial imaging modality for suspected GBC.[12] Although detecting gallbladder masses is easy, there is a considerable challenge to characterize gallbladder wall thickening and polyps accurately.[13] Endoscopic US (EUS) can accurately assess the depth of tumor invasion and improve the characterization of gallbladder polyps.[14] Multiphasic contrast-enhanced computed tomography (CT) and magnetic resonance imaging (MRI) with magnetic resonance cholangiopancreatography (MRCP) are the most useful imaging modalities for the depiction of tumor morphology and staging.[15] Although CT is the most commonly used radiological imaging for staging, in many cases, MRCP may have a complementary role in assessing the site of biliary invasion. Additionally, MRI has better accuracy in differentiating benign and malignant gallbladder lesions.[16] Diffusion-weighted imaging (DWI) is routinely included in the MRI protocol. Advanced imaging techniques like dual-energy CT, intravoxel incoherent motion MRI (IVIM-MRI), perfusion imaging, and diffusion tensor imaging (DTI) may have a problem-solving role.[17] Positron emission tomography-computed tomography (PET-CT) is increasingly utilized for staging, although there is no recommendation for routine use of PET-CT.

Radiological Findings

Morphological Types of Gallbladder Carcinoma

Conventionally, GBC has been reported to have three morphological types—(1) mass replacing gallbladder, (2) wall thickening, and (3) intraluminal polypoidal form **(Figs. 1A to C)**. Recently, a combined type showing features of both mass and wall thickening with preserved gallbladder lumen was described **(Figs. 2A and B)**.[18]

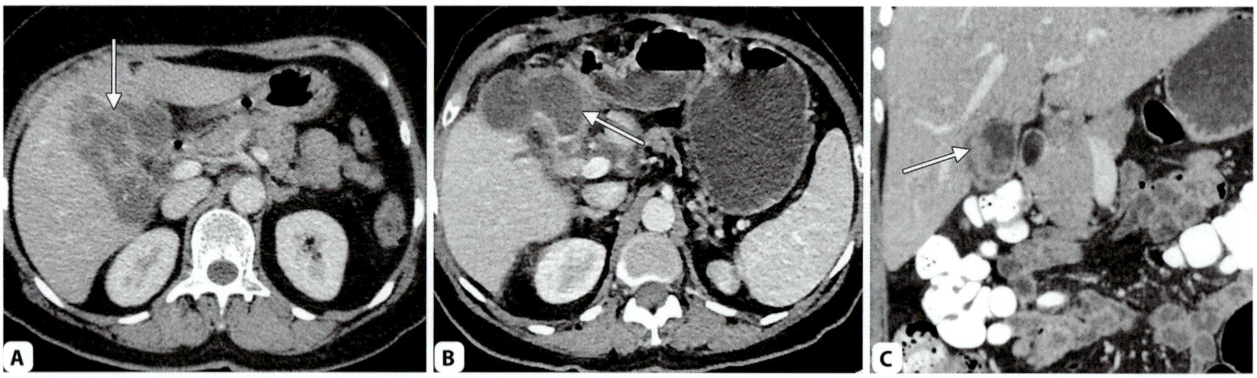

FIGS. 1A TO C: Morphological types of gallbladder carcinoma (GBC). (A) Mass replacing gallbladder. A heterogenous mass is seen in the gallbladder fossa (arrow). Normal gallbladder lumen is not seen. (B) Wall thickening type of gallbladder cancer. There is an asymmetrical mural thickening in the distal gallbladder body and neck (arrow). (C) Intraluminal polypoidal mass. There is a soft tissue mass protruding into the lumen (arrow).

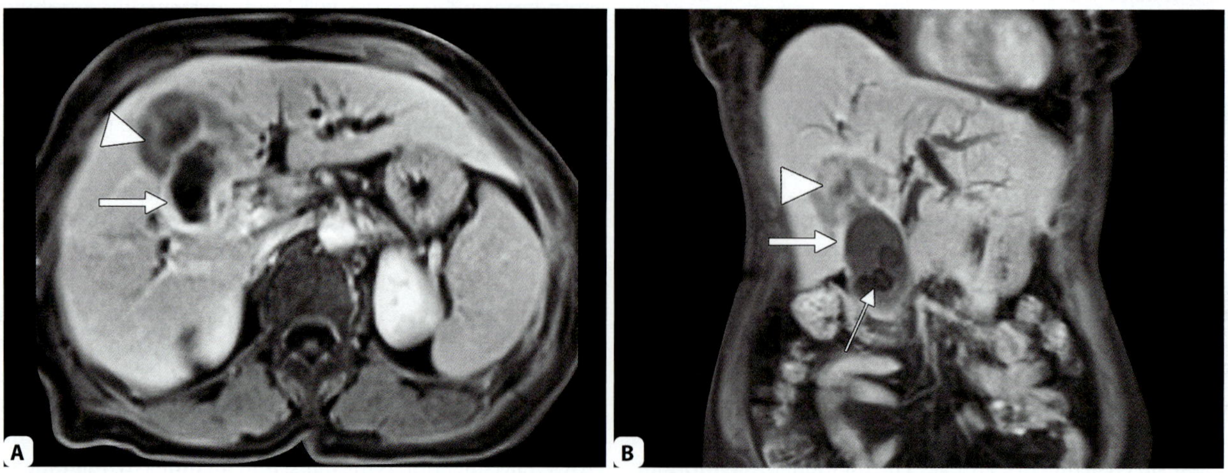

FIGS. 2A AND B: Combined type of gallbladder cancer. Axial (A) and coronal (B) contrast enhanced MRI images show mural thickening at the neck (thick arrow) and a mass extending into the liver parenchyma (arrow head). Note that the gallbladder lumen is preserved and shows calculi (thin arrow, B).

Mass Replacing Gallbladder

The most common presentation of GBC is a large mass obscuring or replacing the gallbladder. This pattern is seen in 40–65%.[19] A large mass in the gallbladder fossa that replaces it and is seen invading the adjacent liver parenchyma is likely to be a GBC. On US, heterogeneous hypoechoic mass is seen in the gallbladder fossa **(Fig. 3)**. Hyperechoic foci may be seen within the mass. These are commonly due to calculi but may also represent porcelain gallbladder or tumor calcifications.

On noncontrast CT (NCCT), GBC is hypodense. GBC is hypo- to isointense on T1-weighted and hyperintense on T2-weighted MR images.[19] In the early arterial phase, the periphery of the mass may show enhancement. During portal venous and delayed phases, the gallbladder mass remains hypodense in most cases **(Fig. 4)**. Marked hypodensity may be due to extensive mucinous contents within the mass **(Fig. 5)**. Less commonly, contrast may be retained in fibrous stromal components in the delayed phase. Rarely, GBCs may show nonrim arterial phase hyperenhancement. Differential diagnoses include intrahepatic CCA (iCCA), metastasis to gallbladder fossa, xanthogranulomatous cholecystitis (XGC), and Immunoglobulin G4 (IgG4)-related sclerosing cholecystitis.[20]

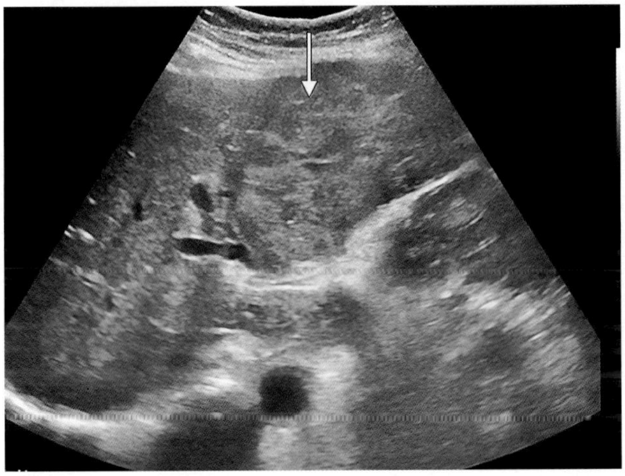

FIG. 3: Mass replacing gallbladder: US. A heterogeneous mass is seen in the gallbladder fossa (arrow). The gallbladder is not visualized.

Mural Thickening Type

This type comprises 20–30% of GBC cases and poses a considerable diagnostic challenge.[21] Gallbladder wall thickening is a nonspecific finding commonly seen in benign gallbladder lesions and may be seen in extracholecystic and systemic causes. US features may help differentiate benign and malignant gallbladder wall thickening.[22] Recently, a gallbladder reporting and data system (GB-RADS) has been proposed to characterize nonacute gallbladder wall thickening accurately.[23] GB-RADS stratifies the gallbladder wall thickening into six categories (GB-RADS 0 to 5) with increasing risk of malignancy. GB-RADS 0 is inconclusive US evaluation due to technical or patient-related factors (e.g., obesity). GB-RADS 1 is normal gallbladder wall (< 3 mm). GB-RADS 2 refers to benign gallbladder wall thickening and is characterized by mural layering or intramural echogenic foci and cysts with distinct liver interface. GB-RADS 3 lesions lack intramural features but the interface of the gallbladder wall with liver parenchyma is distinct. The key feature associated with the likelihood of malignancy (GB-RADS 4) is an indistinct interface with the adjacent liver. GB-RADS 5 is characterized by extramural mass or invasion of biliary or vascular structures **(Figs. 6 and 7)**. A recent study reported moderate intra- and interobserver agreement for GB-RADS. A few studies validated GB-RADS

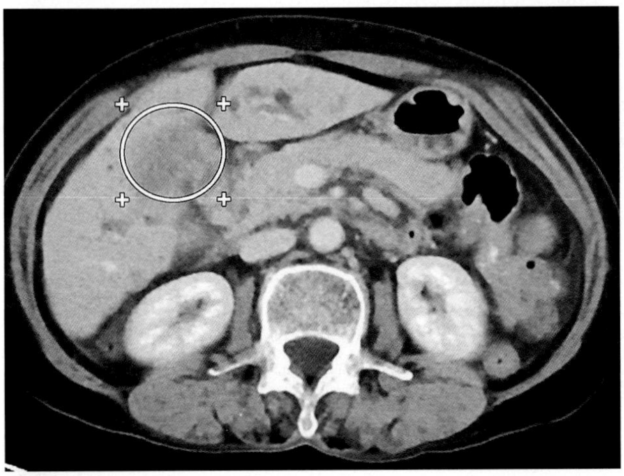

FIG. 4: Mass replacing gallbladder: CT. Axial contrast-enhanced CT in the portal venous phase shows a hypodense mass replacing the gallbladder (circle).

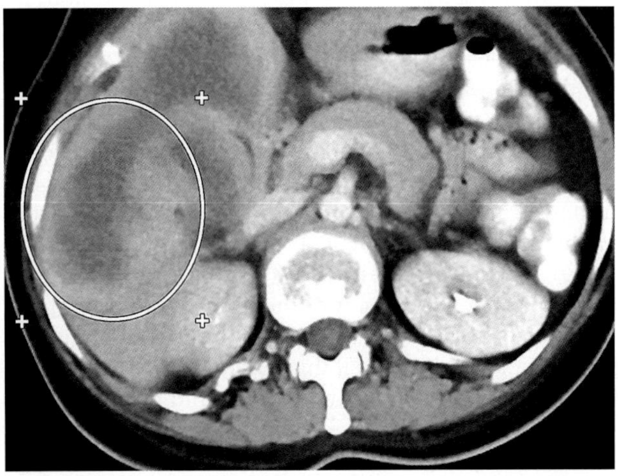

FIG. 5: Mass replacing gallbladder with mucinous change: CT. Axial contrast-enhanced CT in the portal venous phase shows a hypodense mass replacing the gallbladder. Note one of the markedly hypodense regions in the tumor (circle).

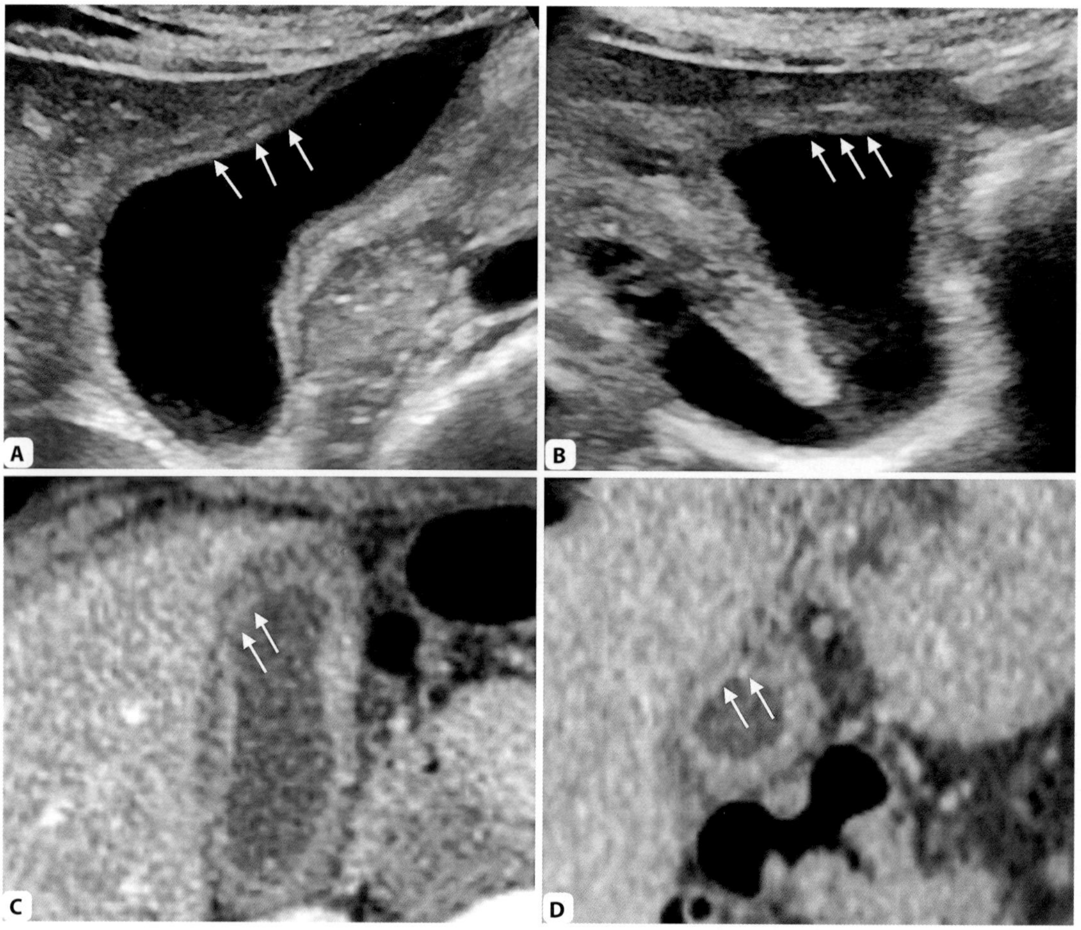

FIGS. 6A TO D: Gallbladder reporting and data system (GB-RADS) category 2 thickening. (A and B) Diffuse gallbladder wall thickening (GWT) with mural layering (arrows). The liver interface is maintained. (C and D) The thickening was confirmed as benign on CT, with the presence of mucosal enhancement, mural stratification, and well-defined liver interface (arrows).

proposed risk of malignancy in each category.[24-26] CT or MRI is recommended for patients with GB-RADS 3–5 lesions for confirming the diagnosis and for staging.[23] US cervix signs have been described to differentiate benign and malignant gallbladder wall thickening.[27] A few studies have reported the value of transabdominal shear wave elastography for the differentiation of benign and malignant gallbladder wall thickening.[28,29] Contrast-enhanced US (CEUS) has also been reported to improve the detection of malignant gallbladder wall thickening.[30]

On contrast-enhanced CT, thick (>2.6 mm) and substantial enhancement of the inner wall and heterogeneous enhancement are associated with malignancy in diffuse gallbladder wall thickening **(Figs. 8A and B)**.[31] Thin, weakly enhancing inner layer, and homogeneous enhancement favor benign gallbladder wall thickening. Focal thickening and indistinct planes with adjacent structures is likely to represent GBC. However, XGC and less likely chronic cholecystitis may have similar appearance. Enhancement patterns favoring malignancy in the focal type of thickening (heterogeneous enhancement of the focal fundal wall thickening without discrete cystic spaces and enhancement of the entire focal fundal thickening) were reported by Corwin et al.[32]

Benign GB wall thickening is hyperintense on T2-weighted MRI and has a smooth appearance.[19] Malignant thickening has an irregular or papillary appearance. Early enhancement on dynamic contrast-enhanced MRI is seen in malignant gallbladder wall thickening.[33] DWI is a valuable adjunct to the other MRI sequences for differentiating malignant and benign GB wall thickening. Malignant gallbladder wall thickening shows diffusion restriction and a lower apparent diffusion coefficient (ADC) than benign gallbladder wall thickening.[34] Recently, Kalage et al. proposed a multiparametric approach to evaluate nonacute gallbladder wall thickening. Combining routine MRI acquisition (and DWI) with IVIM, DTI, and dynamic contrast enhanced MRI, the accuracy in detecting malignant gallbladder wall thickening was better than conventional MRI alone **(Figs. 9A to F)**.[17]

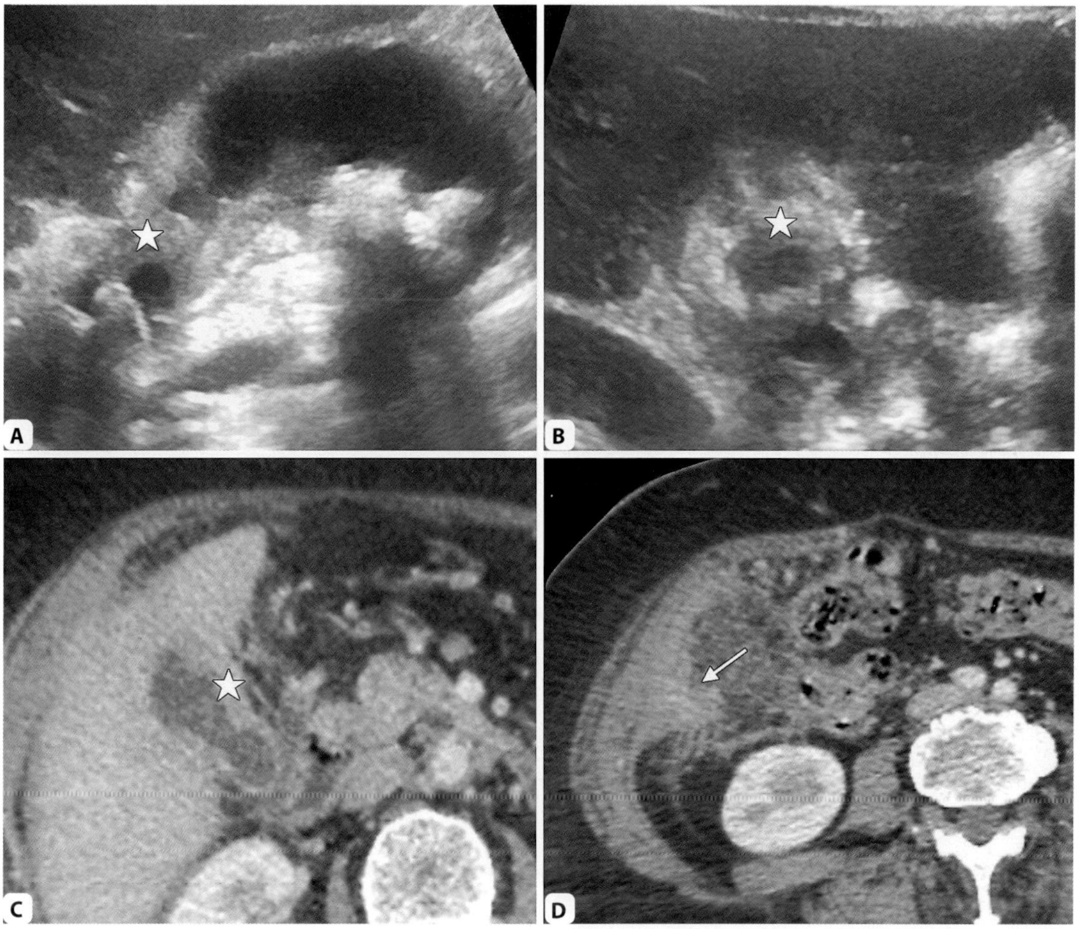

FIGS. 7A TO D: Radiopathological discordance. (A and B). Mural thickening (star) involving the neck of the gallbladder with maintained liver interface and no intramural features. The peritoneal aspect of fundus was inadequately evaluated due to shadowing from calculi. Based on these findings, consensus gallbladder reporting and data system (GB-RADS) category 3 was assigned. (C) At CT, there was asymmetric mural thickening involving the neck and peritoneal aspect of the body of the gallbladder (star). (D) An omental nodule with haziness in the right lumbar region (arrow). Cytological sampling from the nodule was diagnostic of metastatic adenocarcinoma.

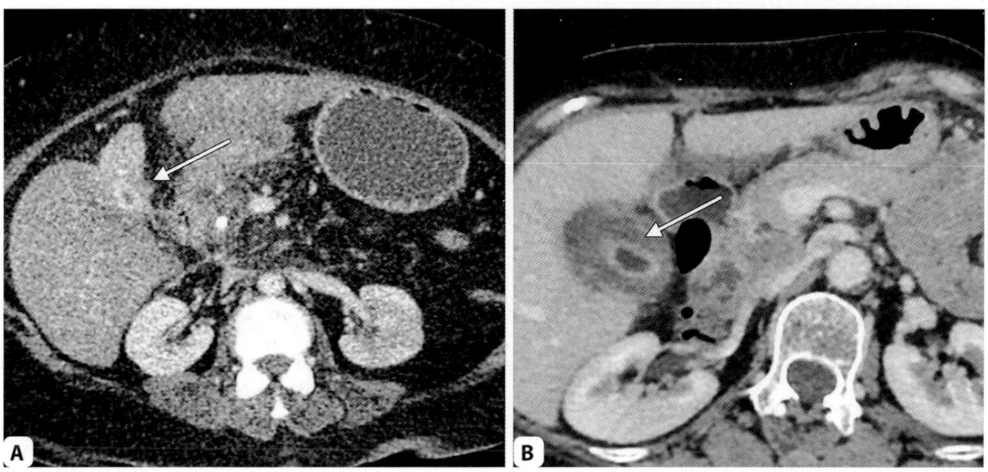

FIGS. 8A AND B: Mural thickening type of gallbladder cancer. Axial CT images in two patients showed a bilayered enhancement pattern with a thick inner layer suggestive of gallbladder cancer.

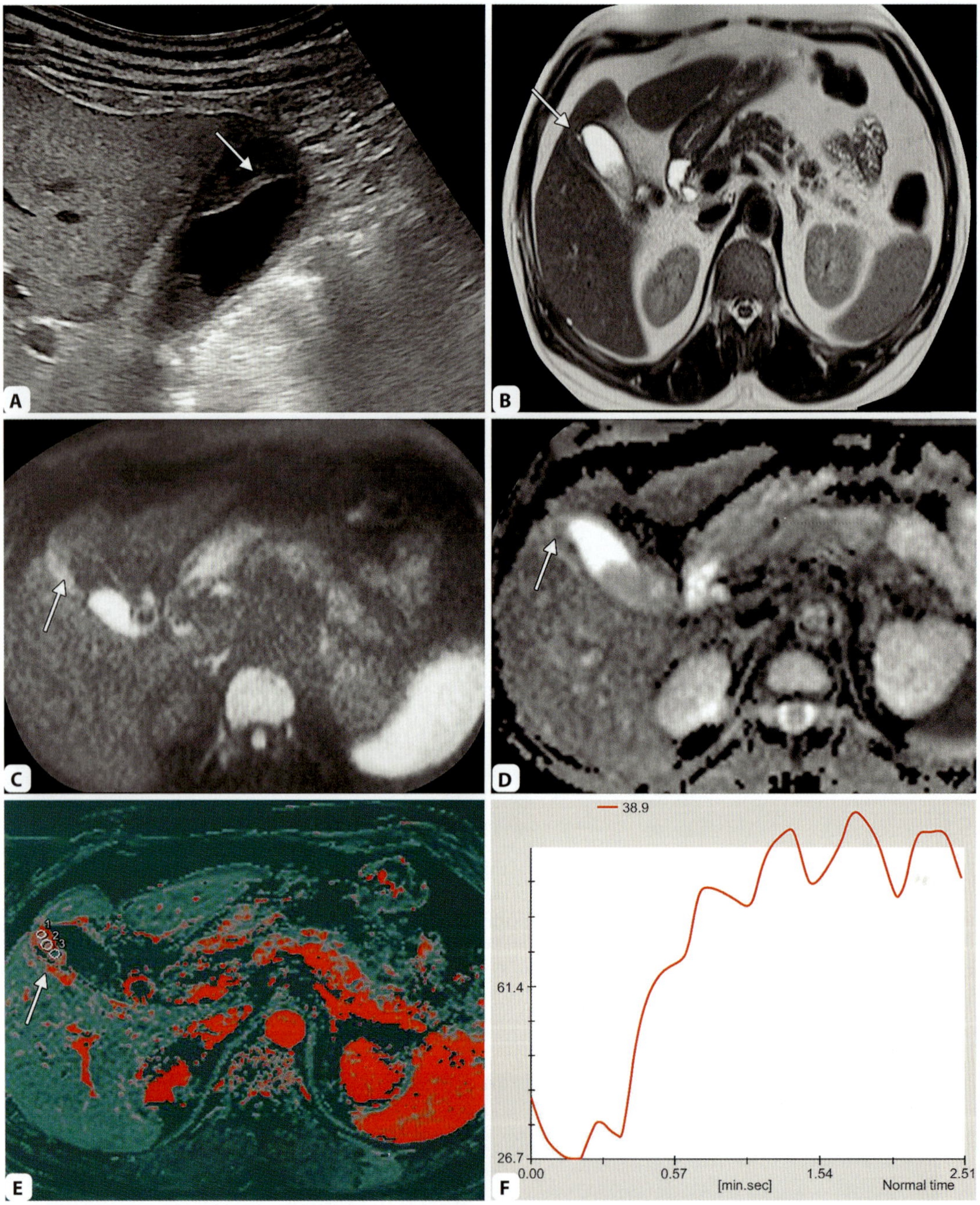

FIGS. 9A TO F: Multiparametric MRI in gallbladder cancer. Ultrasound (A) and MRI (B) images show focal thickening of the gallbladder fundus (arrow). Diffusion-weighted imaging (C) and apparent diffusion coefficient (ADC) map (D) show diffusion restriction. The wash-in map shows increased uptake (E). (F) Time intensity curve shows rapid increase in enhancement.

A recent study reported better accuracy of MRI compared to CT in evaluating gallbladder wall thickening.[16] MRI may give a specific diagnosis in a few cases where CT findings are nonspecific due to better contrast resolution. The cysts in benign gallbladder wall thickening cases are seen better at MRI than CT.[35] Dual-energy CT may have a role in differentiating benign and malignant gallbladder wall thickening **(Figs. 10A to F)**.[36] However, there needs to be more research in this area.

Intraluminal Polypoid Type

Intraluminal polypoidal gallbladder lesions also pose a diagnostic challenge. It is crucial to differentiate non-neoplastic from neoplastic polyps and benign from malignant polyps. Also, it is essential to differentiate tumefactive sludge from true polypoidal lesions. When routine maneuvers like changing patient position and re-examination fail to differentiate sludge from polyp accurately, CEUS may be

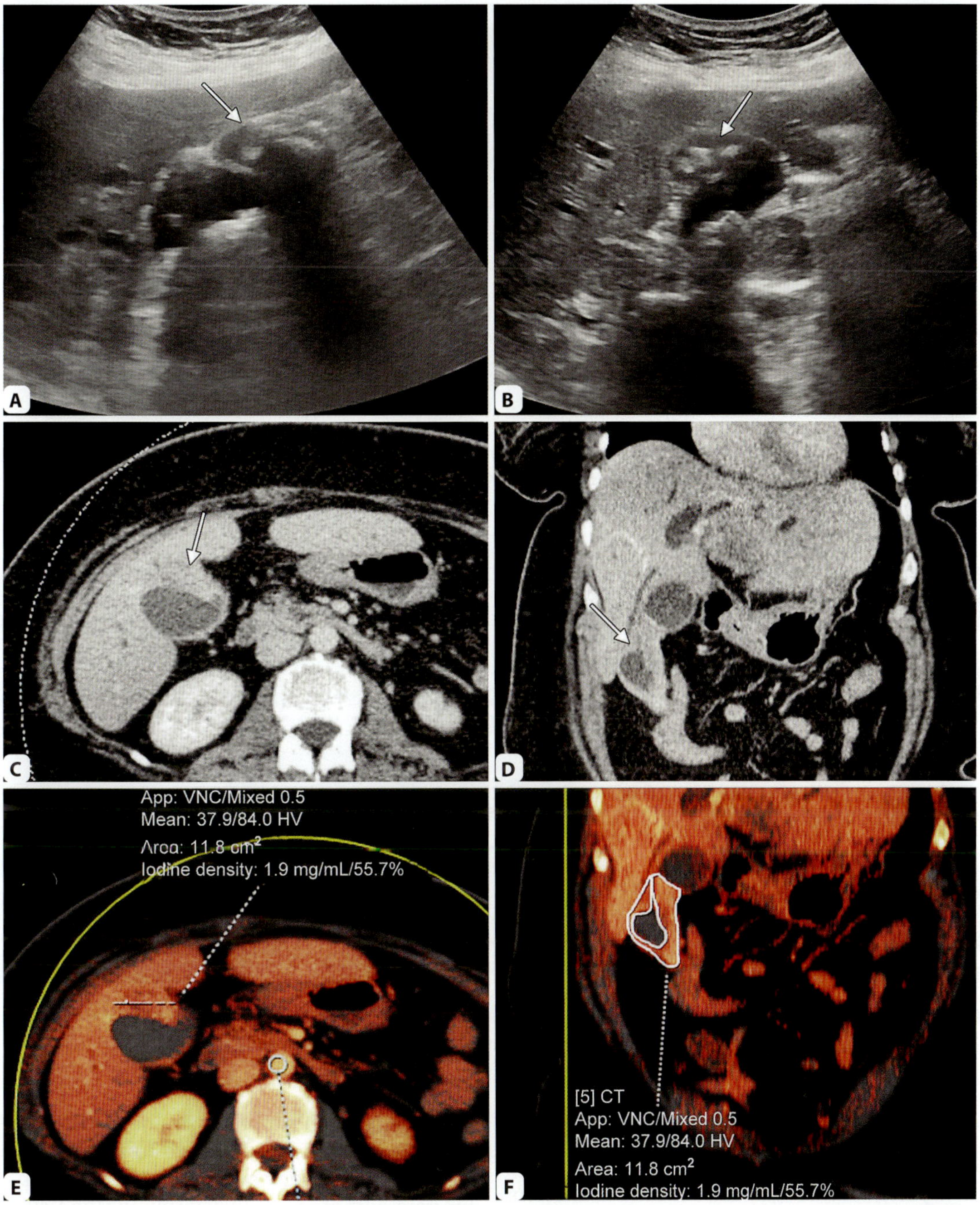

FIGS. 10A TO F: Dual-energy CT (DECT) in a patient with gallbladder carcinoma. Gray scale ultrasound images (A and B) show focal mural thickening involving the fundus and body and gallstones (arrow). Contrast-enhanced computed tomography (CECT) images (C and D) show heterogeneously enhancing focal mural thickening of the fundus and body (arrows). DECT images (E and F) show iodine density and normalized iodine density in the portal venous phase.

used as a problem-solving tool. The significant morphological predictors of risk of malignancy are the polyp's size and shape.[37] A recent consensus proposed the risk stratification of gallbladder polyps into very low-risk, low-risk, and intermediate risk **(Figs. 11A and B)**.[37]

Polypoidal GBCs are usually homogenous and can be hyperechoic, isoechoic, or hypoechoic on sonography and do not cast an acoustic shadow. On contrast-enhanced imaging, these lesions show homogenous enhancement. Necrosis and calcification are rare.

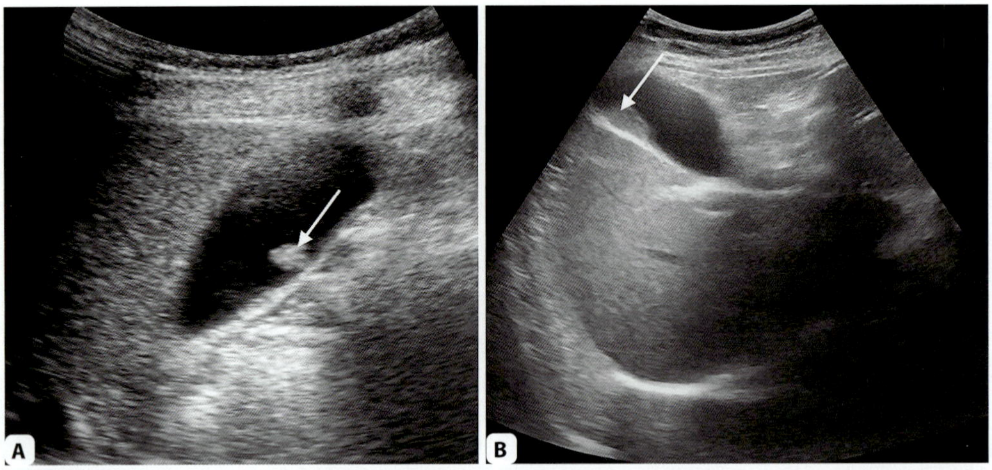

FIGS. 11A AND B: Polyps: US. (A) US image shows a polyp in the body of gallbladder. It has a "ball-on-wall" configuration suggestive of low-risk polyp (arrow). (B) A polyp is seen in the body of gallbladder with associated mural thickening suggestive of intermediate risk polyp.

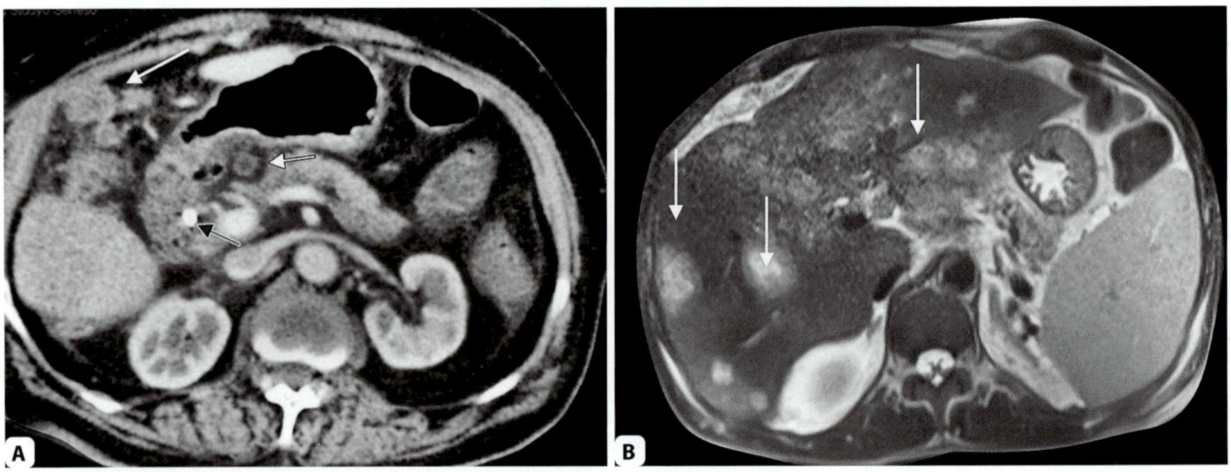

FIGS. 12A AND B: Metastases in gallbladder cancer. Axial CT image in a patient with gallbladder cancer shows multiple omental nodules (arrow). Axial T2-weighted MRI in a patient with gallbladder cancer shows multiple liver lesions.

Pathways of Tumor Spread

Gallbladder carcinoma spread may occur via direct invasion of the liver, hepatoduodenal ligament, duodenum, or colon; lymphatic spread to regional and retroperitoneal lymph nodes; intraductal tumor extension; and hematogenous spread to the liver and peritoneal spread **(Figs. 12A and B)**.[38]

Gallbladder carcinoma spreads most commonly by direct invasion of the liver.[38] Invasion of the gastrohepatic ligament may lead to biliary obstruction at the porta hepatis. Compression of CBD by lymphadenopathy, intraductal tumor growth, and choledocholithiasis are other causes of biliary obstruction in a patient of GBC.[39] Rarely, there may be multifocal involvement causing synchronous or metachronous involvement of the gallbladder and the bile ducts.

There is a rich lymphatic drainage of the gallbladder, which facilitates rapid spread to lymph nodes, most commonly at the porta hepatis as well as in peripancreatic, and para-aortic regions. In determining the T-stage of GBC, multidetector CT (MDCT) has an accuracy of up to 84%.[40] MDCT has an accuracy of 85% in predicting resectability.[41] Sensitivity and specificity of multiphasic MRI with MRCP in detecting hepatic invasion, lymph node metastasis, and bile duct invasion are 87.5% and 86%, 60% and 90%, and 80% and 100%, respectively.[42]

Duodenum and hepatic flexure of the colon are the most common sites of GI involvement. Although, their involvement is not a criterion for unresectability, GI involvement is associated with a poor prognosis.[43] A CT-based classification of GI involvement in GBC was recently reported. Probable involvement, definite involvement, and GI fistulization on staging CT were reported with near-perfect inter-reader agreement.[44] There was no association between the pattern of GI involvement and morphological type.

Perineural invasion (PNI) in GBC occurs in 44–72% of patients and is associated with poor prognosis.[45] A recent study reported that the wall-thickening morphology and soft tissue stranding around the celiac plexus had a sensitivity of 75% and 62.5% and specificity of 81.8% and 100% for PNI, respectively.[45]

OTHER MALIGNANT GALLBLADDER NEOPLASMS

Metastases to the gallbladder are rare, mostly reported from melanoma, breast carcinoma, HCC, and lymphoma.[46] The imaging appearance of a metastatic lesion to the gallbladder is similar to GBC. Other gallbladder malignancies include lymphoma and neuroendocrine tumors.

CHOLANGIOCARCINOMA

Epidemiology

Like GBC, CCA has a poor prognosis.[47] Its incidence also shows distinct geographic variation with the highest prevalence in the Far East and Southeast Asia, where liver fluke infection and choledocholithiasis are common. Men are affected more than women with a male-to-female ratio of 1.3:1. Most of the tumors are diagnosed between 50 and 70 years.

Risk Factors

Risk factors for developing CCA include PSC, choledochal cyst, congenital hepatic fibrosis, hepatolithiasis, familial polyposis, liver flukes, chronic typhoid carriers, and a history of exposure to thorotrast.[48] Cirrhotic patients have a 10-fold higher risk of developing CCA than the general population. Premalignant neoplastic lesions include BilIN, intraductal papillary neoplasms of the bile duct (IPNB), adenofibroma, and mucinous cystic neoplasms.[49]

Pathology and Classification

CCAs are classified based on their anatomical location as intrahepatic or extrahepatic with the latter being more common.[50] A tumor that arises peripheral to the secondary bifurcation of the left or right hepatic duct is considered an iCCA. Extrahepatic CCAs are classified into perihilar CCA (pCCA) and distal CCA (dCCA). pCCAs occur at or near the primary biliary confluence up to the cystic duct insertion, whereas dCCAs arise from the extrahepatic bile duct above the ampulla of Vater. pCCA is the most common type, representing about 50% of CCAs. dCCAs and iCCAs account for 40% and 10% of cases, respectively.[51] The three subtypes of CCA have different epidemiology, risk factors, pathology, clinical features, management, and prognosis.

Histologically, iCCAs have conventional or rare variants.[52] Conventional iCCA can be classified into small and large bile duct iCCA.[53] Small bile duct iCCAs originate from hepatic stem or progenitor cells (HpSCs) and appear as small tubular or acinar adenocarcinomas with nodular growth and no or minimal mucin production.[53] Large bile duct iCCAs originate from columnar mucous cholangiocytes or peribiliary glands and are arranged in a large duct or papillary architecture and are associated with mucin production. Small bile duct iCCAs are associated with isocitrate dehydrogenase (*IDH1, IDH2)* mutations or fibroblast growth factor receptor 2 (*FGFR2*) fusions, and large bile duct iCCAs show a high frequency of *KRAS* and/ or *TP53* gene mutations.[47]

Intrahepatic CCAs show three main growth patterns: (1) mass-forming, (2) periductal-infiltrating, and (3) intraductal-growing. pCCA and dCCA present as flat or poorly defined nodular sclerosing tumors or, less frequently, as intraductal papillary tumors.[54]

Radiological Findings

The imaging features of CCAs depend on tumor location and type.

Intrahepatic Cholangiocarcinoma

Intrahepatic CCAs most commonly present as a mass-forming type. Mass-forming iCCAs appear as well-defined masses with irregular borders.[54] They lack the fibrous capsule found in HCC. Peripheral iCCAs are usually large at presentation because symptoms occur late. US reveals a hypoechoic, isoechoic, or hyperechoic mass, which may be homogenous or heterogeneous. Unenhanced CT reveals a hypodense solitary mass that may have satellite lesions. Focal intrahepatic biliary ductal dilatation, segmental atrophy, and capsular retraction may be seen **(Figs. 13A to C)**. On MRI, iCCA is hypointense on T1-weighted images and hyperintense on T2-weighted images.[55] On contrast-enhanced CT and MRI, the tumor may show a thin rim or thick band of peripheral and patchy enhancement in the arterial phase corresponding to the active tumor growth. The central area of the cancer, due to its fibrous composition, does not enhance in the arterial phase but may show delayed phase enhancement, a feature which may help differentiate it from HCC **(Figs. 13 and 14)**.[56] A targetoid pattern comprising arterial phase rim enhancement, portal venous phase peripheral washout, and delayed central enhancement can also be present in iCCA. CT is considered the standard imaging method for the preoperative assessment of iCCA.[54] CT comprehensively evaluates the primary tumor, the relationship with adjacent structures, and potential thoracic and abdominal spread **(Figs. 15A and B)**.

MRI has accuracy like CT for diagnosis and staging but incorporates specific sequences such as DWI and MRCP.

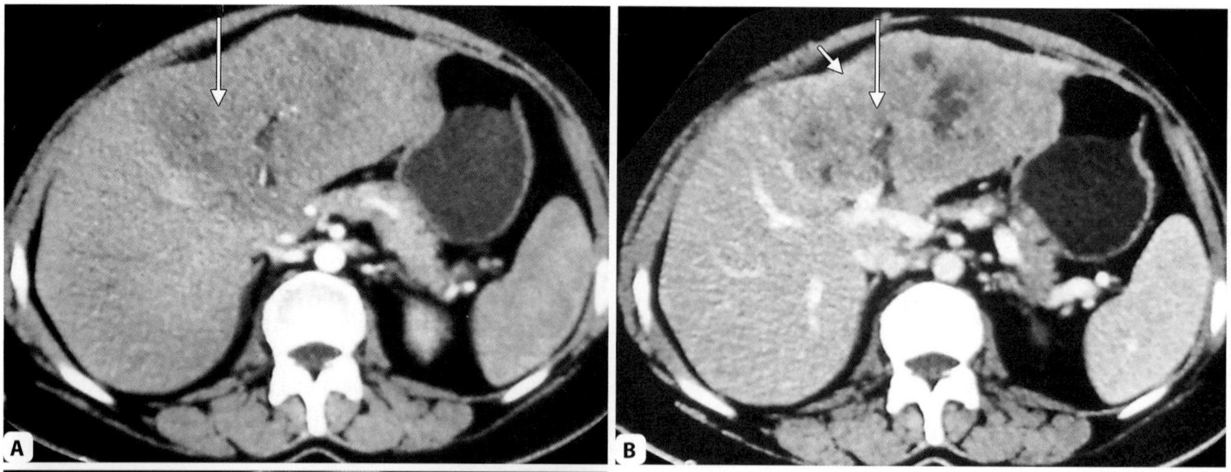

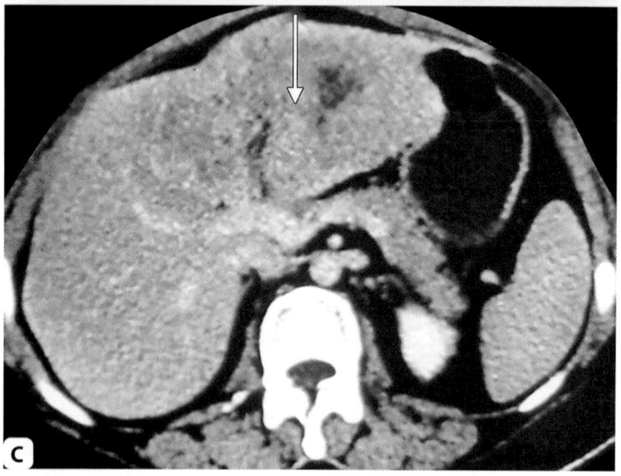

FIGS. 13A TO C: Mass forming intrahepatic cholangiocarcinoma (parenchymal type): Arterial (A), portal venous (B), and delayed phase (C) CT images show a mass in the left lobe of liver that is hypoenhancing on arterial phase and shows progressive enhancement in the delayed phase (arrow). Note the capsular retraction (short arrow, B).

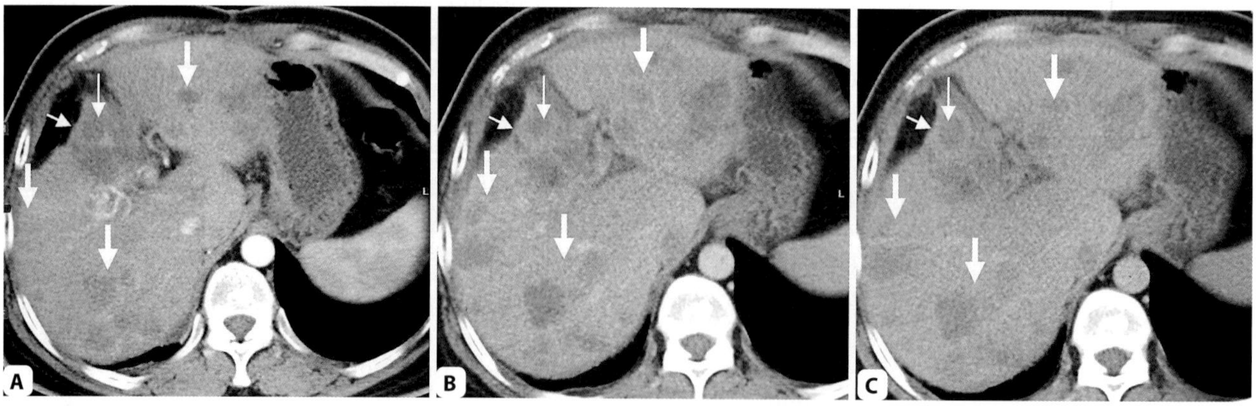

FIGS. 14A TO C: Mass forming intrahepatic cholangiocarcinoma with multiple satellite nodules: Arterial (A) phase CT image shows a mass in the segment five showing subtle peripheral hyperenhancement (arrow). There is progressive enhancement in the portal venous and delayed phases (arrows, B and C). Note the capsular retraction (short arrow), multiple satellite nodule and multiple metastatic lesions in both lobes of liver (thick arrows).

Mass-forming iCCAs are classified into parenchymal and ductal types. Bile duct dilatation and periductal tumor spread characterize ductal-type iCCAs **(Figs. 16A and B)**. Parenchymal-type iCCAs are associated with chronic liver disease, small-duct histology, and better prognosis.[57]

Perihilar Cholangiocarcinoma

pCCAs are usually periductal infiltrating and most often arise at the primary confluence or in the proximal common hepatic duct.[54] US findings include intrahepatic bile ductal dilatation with or without isolation of right and left-sided

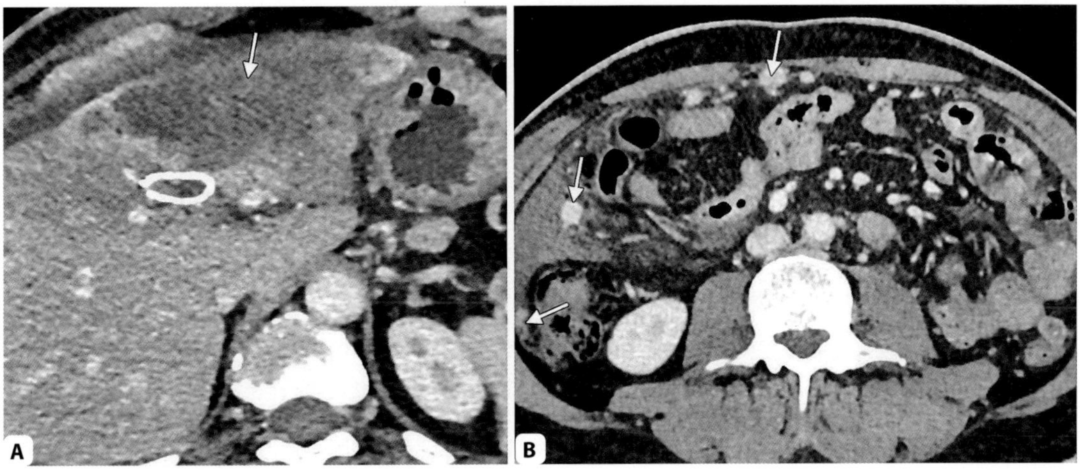

FIGS. 15A AND B: Mass forming intrahepatic cholangiocarcinoma with omental metastases. Axial portal venous phase CT image (A) shows a mass in the left lobe of liver (arrow). (B) There are multiple omental metastases (arrows).

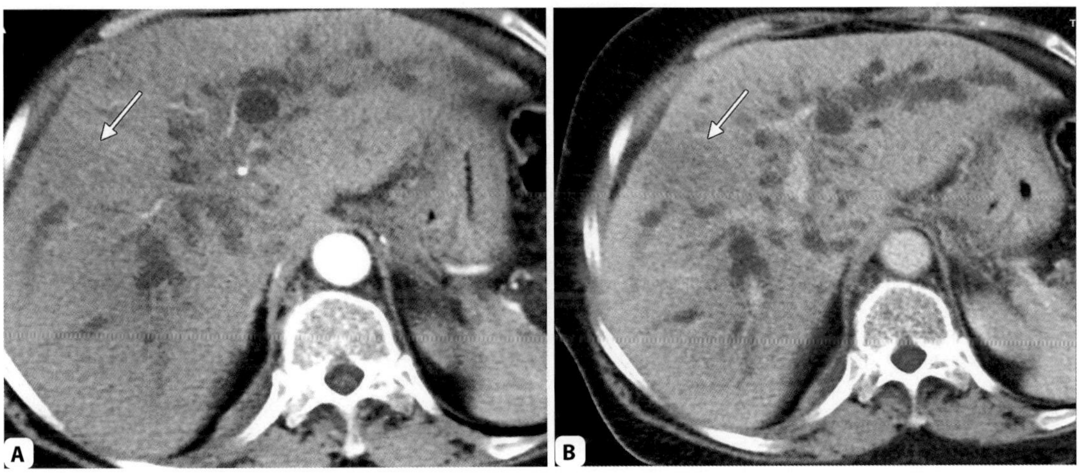

FIGS. 16A AND B: Intrahepatic mass forming cholangiocarcinoma (ductal type). Arterial (A) and portal venous phase (B) CT images show a mass in segment 5 with involvement of primary confluence and bilobar intrahepatic biliary ductal dilatation (arrows).

ducts and lobar atrophy. Definite mass is rarely seen on US, and demonstration of dilated intrahepatic bile ducts without any evidence of extrahepatic biliary dilatation alone should raise the suspicion of pCCA. Sometimes, the tumor may be seen as a bile duct wall thickening and, less commonly, as a polypoidal lesion. The tumors are moderately echogenic, reflecting their fibrous nature. Although the tumor appears hypodense to the liver in both unenhanced and enhanced CT scans, the focally thickened bile duct wall appears hyperenhancing relative to the liver in the arterial and portal venous phase **(Figs. 17 and 18)**. Due to their fibrous-rich stroma, delayed enhancement can be seen. pCCAs are isointense/hypointense on T1-weighted images, while T2-weighted signal intensity varies from markedly hyperintense to mildly increased signal in fibrous tumors. Lobar hepatic atrophy is seen in one-fourth of patients with pCCAs, and this finding with biliary dilatation is strongly suggestive of CCAs. Atrophy from long-standing biliary obstruction or portal venous involvement results in crowding of dilated bile ducts and volume loss. Contiguous invasion of the liver parenchyma and hepatoduodenal ligament is frequent.

Lymph nodal metastases can be seen in the periportal and peripancreatic regions. Retroperitoneal lymphadenopathy and peritoneal dissemination occur in advanced stages. Contrast-enhanced MRI with MRCP provides the most comprehensive tumor staging.[51] EUS with EUS-guided fine needle aspiration is increasingly used for characterizing biliary strictures and assessing the extent of periductal involvement and lymph node metastasis.[58]

pCCAs rarely present as intraductal papillary tumors **(Figs. 19A and B)**. The intraductal tumors are hyperdense on NCCT images and are hypodense on postcontrast images as they lack fibrotic stroma. Multiple tumors can

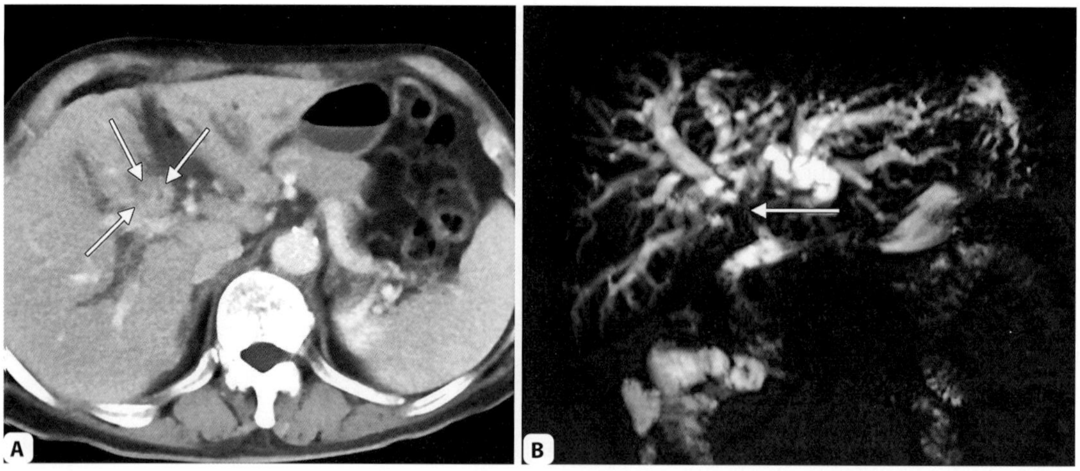

FIGS. 17A AND B: Periductal infiltrating cholangiocarcinoma. (A) Axial portal venous phase CT image shows marked thickening and hyperenhancement of the primary confluence with bilobar intrahepatic biliary dilatation (arrows). (B) Magnetic resonance cholangiopancreatography (MRCP) image confirms the level of biliary involvement at primary confluence (arrow).

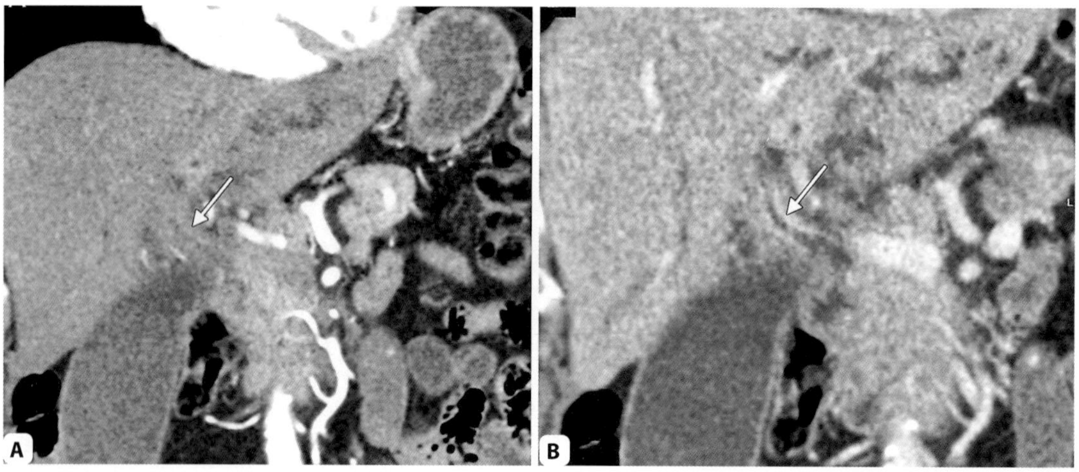

FIGS. 18A AND B: Perihilar infiltrating cholangiocarcinoma. Coronal reformatted arterial (A) and portal venous (B) phase CT images show a hyperenhancing mural thickening at the primary confluence (arrows). Note that the thickening is marked, asymmetric, irregular, and long segment differentiating it from benign biliary stricture.

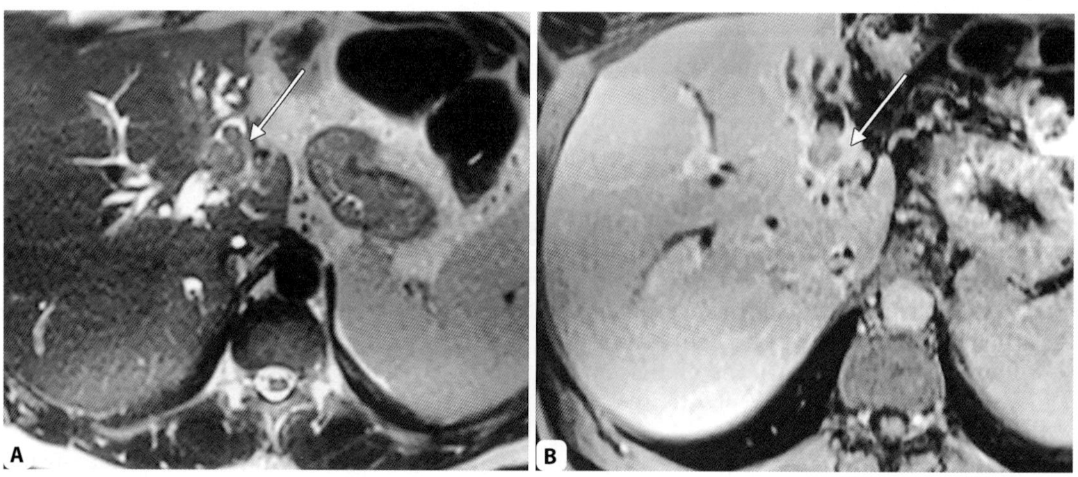

FIGS. 19A AND B: Perihilar intraductal polypoidal cholangiocarcinoma. T2-weighted (A) and contrast-enhanced T1-weighted (B) axial MR images show subtle hyperintense intraluminal lesion in the primary confluence extending into the left hepatic duct (arrow, A). There is marked and irregular ductal enhancement (arrow, B). Note the marked atrophy of the left lobe of liver.

be confused with calculi. Contrast enhancement in these tumors helps in differentiating them from stones.[59]

Several staging systems are used in pCCA.[54] Although the Bismuth-Corlette classification is the most popular, it is based solely on the longitudinal extent of the tumor **(Table 1)**. It does not consider the radial extent, vascular status, lymph node and distant metastases, and future liver remnant volume.[60] TNM system includes a longitudinal and radial extension of the tumor and other features except for the liver remnant volume.[11] Memorial Sloan Kettering Cancer Center system consists of the longitudinal extent, portal venous involvement, and liver remnant volume. Deoliveira et al. proposed a classification system that includes the most important features.[61]

Distal Cholangiocarcinoma

dCCA is the tumor arising from the common bile duct between the cystic duct's origin and Vater's ampulla. Tumors arising from ampulla are not included in dCCA.[62]

TABLE 1: Bismuth–Corlette classification of perihilar cholangiocarcinoma.

Type	Description
1	Tumor not involving the primary confluence of right and left hepatic ducts
2	Tumor involving the primary confluence
3a	Tumor involving the primary confluence and the right hepatic duct
3b	Tumor involving the primary confluence and the left hepatic duct
4	Tumor extending to bilateral hepatic ducts

Source: Modified from Bismuth H, Nakache R, Diamond T. Management strategies in resection for hilar cholangiocarcinoma. Ann Surg. 1992;215(1):31-8.

These are usually small and have better prognosis than pCCA. Imaging features include biliary dilatation proximal to an abrupt obstruction in the distal common bile duct **(Fig. 20)**. No mass is usually demonstrated in imaging. Hence, differentiation from benign strictures is essential. Asymmetric, long (>12 mm) segment stricture with a thick wall (>3 mm), irregularity of lumen, indistinct outer margin, and hyperenhancement relative to the liver in the portal venous phase favor malignant stricture.[63]

Role of Imaging in Predicting Molecular Signatures and Prognosis in CCA

Morphological imaging features that suggest poor prognosis include necrosis, satellite nodules, vascular encasement, hypovascularity in arterial and portal venous phase, a greater degree of enhancement in the delayed phase, and diffusion restriction of less than one-third of the tumor. IDH mutation is associated with intratumoral arteries, rim and internal arterial phase enhancement, and hyperenhancement in the arterial and portal venous phases.[64]

RADIOMICS AND ARTIFICIAL INTELLIGENCE IN BTC

Radiomics refers to the extraction of many quantitative features from images. Selecting valuable features from many extracted features usually relies on machine learning (ML) algorithms. There is extensive literature on radiomics and ML based on all imaging modalities for diagnosing and prognosticating BTCs.[65-67] Recently, deep learning (DL) has also been explored to improve the characterization of biliary tract lesions. DL involves training deep neural networks.[68-70]

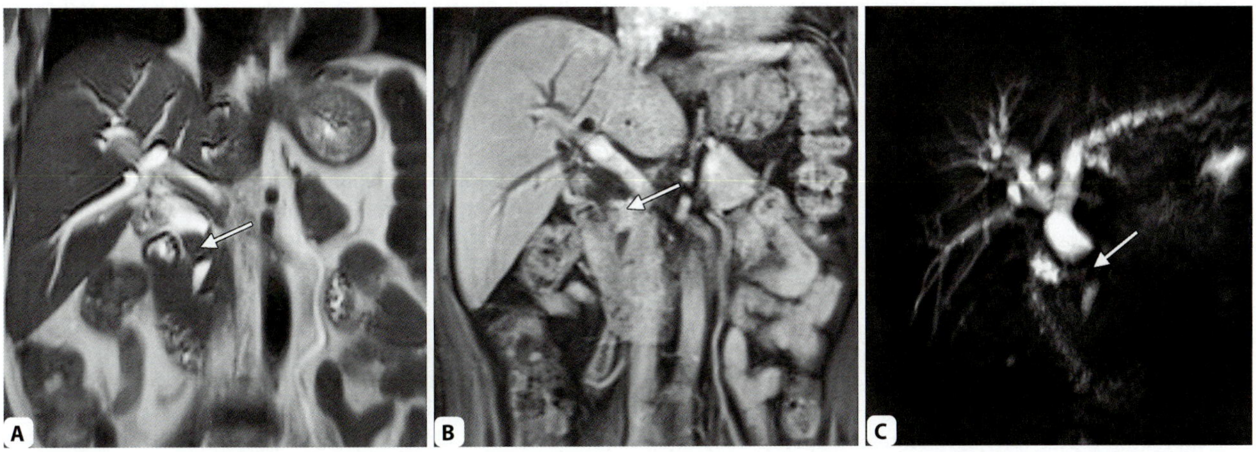

FIGS. 20A TO C: Distal cholangiocarcinoma. Coronal T2-weighted (A), contrast-enhanced T1-weighted (B), and magnetic resonance cholangiopancreatography (MRCP) (C) images show an intraluminal enhancing lesion (arrows A and B), causing upstream biliary dilatation (arrow, C).

CONCLUSION

Biliary tract cancers are often discovered late. US allows risk stratification in gallbladder wall thickening and gallbladder polyps. Multiphasic contrast-enhanced CT is the most commonly employed imaging for staging BTCs. MRI and MRCP are critical for the evaluation of pCCA and dCCA. There are several mimics of BTCs, and a systematic approach should be adopted. The role of imaging has evolved from diagnosis and staging to prognostication and identification of molecular signatures. Radiomics and artificial intelligence are evolving, and in the future, these may be integrated into the routine clinical workflow.

REFERENCES

1. Valle JW, Kelley RK, Nervi B, Oh DY, Zhu AX. Biliary tract cancer. Lancet. 2021;397:428-44.
2. Sung H, Ferlay J, Siegel RL, Laversanne M, Soerjomataram I, Jemal A, et al. Global Cancer Statistics 2020: GLOBOCAN Estimates of Incidence and Mortality Worldwide for 36 Cancers in 185 Countries. CA Cancer J Clin. 2021;71(3):209-49.
3. National Cancer Institute. (2024). SEER*Explorer: an interactive website for SEER cancer statistics. Surveillance Research Program. [online] Available from https://seer.cancer.gov/statistics-network/explorer/application.html?site=1&data_type=1&graph_type=2&compareBy=sex&chk_sex_3=3&chk_sex_2=2&rate_type=2&race=1&age_range=1&hdn_stage=101&advopt_precision=1&advopt_show_ci=on&hdn_view=0&advopt_show_apc=on&advopt_display=2#resultsRegion0 [Last accessed June, 2024].
4. Roa JC, García P, Kapoor VK, Maithel SK, Javle M, Koshiol J. Gallbladder cancer. Nat Rev Dis Primers. 2022;8(1):69. Erratum in: Nat Rev Dis Primers. 2022;8(1):75.
5. Dutta U, Bush N, Kalsi D, Popli P, Kapoor VK. Epidemiology of gallbladder cancer in India. Chin Clin Oncol. 2019;8:33.
6. Rawla P, Sunkara T, Thandra KC, Barsouk A. Epidemiology of gallbladder cancer. Clin Exp Hepatol. 2019;5(2):93-102.
7. Fukumura Y, Rong L, Maimaitiaili Y, Fujisawa T, Isayama H, Nakahodo J, et al. Precursor Lesions of Gallbladder Carcinoma: Disease Concept, Pathology, and Genetics. Diagnostics. 2022;12(2):341.
8. Henson DE, Albores Saavedra J, Corle D. Carcinoma of the gallbladder. Histologic types, stage of disease, grade and survival rates. Cancer. 1992;70:1493-7.
9. Albores Saavedra J, Henson DE. Tumors of the Gallbladder and Extrahepatic Bile Ducts. Atlas of Tumor Pathology, Fascicle 22, 2nd Series. Washington, DC: Armed Forces Institute of Pathology; 1986.
10. Amin MB, Edge SB, Greene FL, Byrd DR, Brookland RK, Washington MK, et al. AJCC Cancer Staging Manual, 8th edition. New York: Springer; 2017.
11. Oven Ustaalioglu BB, Bilici A, Seker M, Kefeli U, Aydin D, Celik S, et al. Prognostic Factors for Operated Gallbladder Cancer. J Gastrointest Cancer. 2019;50(3):451-7.
12. Gupta P, Marodia Y, Bansal A, Kalra N, Kumar-M P, Sharma V, et al. Imaging-based algorithmic approach to gallbladder wall thickening. World J Gastroenterol. 2020;26(40):6163-81.
13. Gupta P, Kumar M, Sharma V, Dutta U, Sandhu MS. Evaluation of gallbladder wall thickening: a multimodality imaging approach. Expert Rev Gastroenterol Hepatol. 2020;14(6):463-73.
14. Hashimoto S, Nakaoka K, Kawabe N, Kuzuya T, Funasaka K, Nagasaka M, et al. The Role of Endoscopic Ultrasound in the Diagnosis of Gallbladder Lesions. Diagnostics (Basel). 2021;11(10):1789.
15. Kalra N, Gupta P, Singhal M, Gupta R, Gupta V, Srinivasan R, et al. Cross-sectional Imaging of Gallbladder Carcinoma: An Update. J Clin Exp Hepatol. 2019;9(3):334-44.
16. Kalage D, Gupta P, Gulati A, Reddy KP, Sharma K, Thakur A, et al. Contrast Enhanced CT Versus MRI for Accurate Diagnosis of Wall-thickening Type Gallbladder Cancer. J Clin Exp Hepatol. 2024;14(5):101397.
17. Kalage D, Gupta P, Gulati A, Yadav TD, Gupta V, Kaman L, et al. Multiparametric MR imaging with diffusion-weighted, intravoxel incoherent motion, diffusion tensor, and dynamic contrast-enhanced perfusion sequences to assess gallbladder wall thickening: a prospective study based on surgical histopathology. Eur Radiol. 2023;33(7):4981-93.
18. Chhabra M, Kalage D, Gupta P, Siddiqui R, Singh S, Yadav TD, et al. Proposal for a new morphological "combined type" of gallbladder cancer: description of radiopathological characteristics and comparison with other morphological types. Abdom Radiol (NY). 2024;49(3):703-9.
19. Lopes Vendrami C, Magnetta MJ, Mittal PK, Moreno CC, Miller FH. Gallbladder Carcinoma and Its Differential Diagnosis at MRI: What Radiologists Should Know. Radiographics. 2021;41(1):78-95.
20. Furlan A, Ferris JV, Hosseinzadeh K, Borhani AA. Gallbladder carcinoma update: multimodality imaging evaluation, staging, and treatment options. AJR Am J Roentgenol. 2008;191(5):1440-7.
21. Soundararajan R, Marodia Y, Gupta P, Rana P, Chhabra M, Kalage D, et al. Imaging patterns of wall thickening type of gallbladder cancer. Clin Exp Hepatol. 2022;8(4):255-66.
22. Rana P, Gupta P, Kalage D, Soundararajan R, Kumar-M P, Dutta U. Grayscale ultrasonography findings for characterization of gallbladder wall thickening in non-acute setting: a systematic review and meta-analysis. Expert Rev Gastroenterol Hepatol. 2022;16(1):59-71.
23. Gupta P, Dutta U, Rana P, Singhal M, Gulati A, Kalra N, et al. Gallbladder reporting and data system (GB-RADS) for risk stratification of gallbladder wall thickening on ultrasonography: an international expert consensus. Abdom Radiol (NY). 2022;47(2):554-65.
24. Soundararajan R, Subramanian P, Gupta P, Rana P, Chhabra M, Singh S, et al. Agreement of Gallbladder Reporting and Data System for Gallbladder Wall Thickening at Ultrasonography: A Multireader Validation Study. J Clin Exp Hepatol. 2024;14(4):101393.
25. Zhu L, Li N, Zhu Y, Han P, Jiang B, Li M, et al. Value of high frame rate contrast enhanced ultrasound in gallbladder wall thickening in non-acute setting. Cancer Imaging. 2024;24(1):7.
26. Kaur M, Gupta P, D S, Rana P, Soundararajan R, Kalage D, et al. An audit of the adequacy of first-time ultrasound reports

in patients with non-acute gallbladder wall thickening: Need for gallbladder reporting and data system. Indian J Gastroenterol. 2023;42(5):741-3.

27. Rana P, Pruthi H, Gupta P, Chhabra M, Soundararajan R, Singh S, et al. Sonographic "Cervix Sign": A New Ancillary Sign of Gallbladder Neck Malignancy. J Clin Exp Hepatol. 2023;13(6):972-6.
28. Soundararajan R, Dutta U, Bhatia A, Gupta P, Nahar U, Kaman L, et al. Two-dimensional Shear Wave Elastography: Utility in Differentiating Gallbladder Cancer From Chronic Cholecystitis. J Ultrasound Med. 2023;42(7):1577-85.
29. Kapoor A, Kapoor A, Mahajan G. Differentiating malignant from benign thickening of the gallbladder wall by the use of acoustic radiation force impulse elastography. J Ultrasound Med. 2011;30(11):1499-507.
30. Boddapati SB, Lal A, Gupta P, Kalra N, Yadav TD, Gupta V, et al. Contrast enhanced ultrasound versus multiphasic contrast enhanced computed tomography in evaluation of gallbladder lesions. Abdom Radiol (NY). 2022;47(2):566-75.
31. Kim SJ, Lee JM, Lee JY, Kim SH, Han JK, Choi BI, et al. Analysis of enhancement pattern of flat gallbladder wall thickening on MDCT to differentiate gallbladder cancer from cholecystitis. AJR Am J Roentgenol. 2008;191(3):765-71.
32. Corwin MT, Khera SS, Loehfelm TW, Yang NT, Fananapazir G. Incidentally Detected Focal Fundal Gallbladder Wall Thickening at Contrast-Enhanced Computed Tomography: Prevalence and Computed Tomography Features of Malignancy. J Comput Assist Tomogr. 2019;43(1):149-54.
33. Tang Z, Wu YP, Tan BG, Chen XQ, Guo WW, Wu KS, et al. Apparent diffusion coefficient and its standard deviation from diffusion-weighted imaging in preoperative predicting liver invasion by T3-staged resectable gallbladder carcinoma. Clin Radiol. 2024;79(2):e247-55.
34. Sato M, Kurita Y, Sakai E, Watanabe S, Sanada H, Shimizu T, et al. Computed diffusion-weighted magnetic resonance imaging with high b-values in the diagnosis of gallbladder lesions. Abdom Radiol (NY). 2022;47(9):3278-89.
35. Bonde AA, Virarkar M, Zahid M, Jaganathan S, Menendez MJ, Calimano L, et al. Imaging update on gallbladder adenomyomatosis and its mimics. Clin Imaging. 2024;105:109997.
36. Pruthi H, Chabbra M, Soundararajan R, Rana P, Gupta P, Dutta U, et al. Role of dual energy computed tomography in evaluation of suspected wall thickening type of gallbladder cancer. Clin Exp Hepatol. 2022;8(1):92-5.
37. Kamaya A, Fung C, Szpakowski JL, Fetzer DT, Walsh AJ, Alimi Y, et al. Management of Incidentally Detected Gallbladder Polyps: Society of Radiologists in Ultrasound Consensus Conference Recommendations. Radiology. 2022;305(2):277-89.
38. Gupta P, Meghashyam K, Marodia Y, Gupta V, Basher R, Das CK, et al. Locally advanced gallbladder cancer: a review of the criteria and role of imaging. Abdom Radiol (NY). 2021;46(3):998-1007.
39. Leigh N, Pletcher E, Solomon D, Sarpel U, Labow DM, Magge DR, et al. The significance of anatomic tumor location in gallbladder cancer. J Surg Oncol. 2021;123(4):932-8.
40. Kim SJ, Lee JM, Lee JY, Choi JY, Kim SH, Han JK, et al. Accuracy of preoperative T-staging of gall bladder carcinoma using MDCT. AJR Am J Roentgenol. 2008;190:74-8.
41. Kalra N, Suri S, Gupta R, Natarajan SK, Khandelwal N, Wig JD, et al. MDCT in the staging of gallbladder carcinoma. AJR Am J Roentgenol. 2006;186(3):758-62.
42. Kaza RK, Gulati M, Wig JD, Chawla YK. Evaluation of gall bladder carcinoma with dynamic magnetic resonance imaging and magnetic resonance cholangiopancreatography. Australas Radiol. 2006;50(3):212-7.
43. Agarwal AK, Mandal S, Singh S, Sakhuja P, Puri S. Gallbladder cancer with duodenal infiltration: is it still resectable? J Gastrointest Surg. 2007;11:1722-7.
44. Soundararajan R, Vanka S, Gupta P, Chhabra M, Rana P, Gulati A, et al. Gastrointestinal involvement in gallbladder cancer: Computed tomography findings and proposal of a classification system. Indian J Gastroenterol. 2023;42(5):708-12.
45. Marodia Y, Kharel J, Saikia UN, Kumar R, Yadav TD, Gupta V, et al. Association of CT Findings With Perineural Invasion in Gallbladder Cancer: Preliminary Assessment. AJR Am J Roentgenol. 2023;220(6):850-1.
46. Choi BI, Lee JM. Neoplasms of the gallbladder and biliary tract. In: Gore RM, Levine MS (Eds). Textbook of Gastrointestinal Radiology, 4th edition. USA: Saunders Elsevier; 2015. pp. 1402-26.
47. Banales JM, Marin JJG, Lamarca A, Rodrigues PM, Khan SA, Roberts LR, et al. Cholangiocarcinoma 2020: the next horizon in mechanisms and management. Nat Rev Gastroenterol Hepatol. 2020;17(9):557-88.
48. Sainani NI, Catalano OA, Holalkere NS, Zhu AX, Hahn PF, Sahani DV. Cholangiocarcinoma: current and novel imaging techniques. Radiographics. 2008;28:1263-87.
49. Komuta M, Govaere O, Vandecaveye V, Akiba J, Van Steenbergen W, Verslype C, et al. Histological diversity in cholangiocellular carcinoma reflects the different cholangiocyte phenotypes. Hepatology. 2012;55(6):1876-88.
50. Rizvi S, Khan SA, Hallemeier CL, Kelley RK, Gores GJ. Cholangiocarcinoma - evolving concepts and therapeutic strategies. Nat Rev Clin Oncol. 2018;15(2):95-111.
51. DeOliveira ML, Cunningham SC, Cameron JL, Kamangar F, Winter JM, Lillemoe KD, et al. Cholangiocarcinoma: thirty-one-year experience with 564 patients at a single institution. Ann Surg. 2007;245(5):755-62.
52. Kendall T, Verheij J, Gaudio E, Evert M, Guido M, Goeppert B, et al. Anatomical, histomorphological and molecular classification of cholangiocarcinoma. Liver Int. 2019;39 Suppl 1:7-18.
53. Aishima S, Kuroda Y, Nishihara Y, Iguchi T, Taguchi K, Taketomi A, et al. Proposal of progression model for intrahepatic cholangiocarcinoma: clinicopathologic differences between hilar type and peripheral type. Am J Surg Pathol. 2007;31(7):1059-67.
54. Joo I, Lee JM, Yoon JH. Imaging Diagnosis of Intrahepatic and Perihilar Cholangiocarcinoma: Recent Advances and Challenges. Radiology. 2018;288(1):7-13.
55. Jhaveri KS, Hosseini-Nik H. MRI of cholangiocarcinoma. J Magn Reson Imaging. 2015;42(5):1165-79.
56. Rimola J, Forner A, Reig M, Vilana R, de Lope CR, Ayuso C, et al. Cholangiocarcinoma in cirrhosis: absence of contrast washout in delayed phases by magnetic resonance imaging avoids misdiagnosis of hepatocellular carcinoma. Hepatology. 2009;50(3):791-8.

57. Sarcognato S, Sacchi D, Fassan M, Fabris L, Cadamuro M, Zanus G, et al. Cholangiocarcinoma. Pathologica. 2021;113(3):158-69.
58. Nguyen K, Sing JT Jr. Review of endoscopic techniques in the diagnosis and management of cholangiocarcinoma. World J Gastroenterol. 2008;14:2995-9.
59. Kim JE, Lee JM, Kim SH, Baek JH, Moon SK, Yu IS, et al. Differentiation of intraductal growing-type cholangiocarcinomas from nodular-type cholangiocarcinomas at biliary MR imaging with MR cholangiography. Radiology. 2010;257(2):364-72.
60. Bismuth H, Corlette MB. Intrahepatic cholangioenteric anastomosis in carcinoma of the hilus of the liver. Surg Gynecol Obstet. 1975;140(2):170-8.
61. Deoliveira ML, Schulick RD, Nimura Y, Rosen C, Gores G, Neuhaus P, et al. New staging system and a registry for perihilar cholangiocarcinoma. Hepatology. 2011;53(4):1363-71.
62. Razumilava N, Gores GJ. Classification, diagnosis, and management of cholangiocarcinoma. Clin Gastroenterol Hepatol. 2013;11:13-21.
63. Katabathina VS, Dasyam AK, Dasyam N, Hosseinzadeh K. Adult bile duct strictures: role of MR imaging and MR cholangiopancreatography in characterization. Radiographics. 2014;34(3):565-86.
64. Katabathina VS, Khanna L, Surabhi VR, Minervini M, Shanbhogue K, Dasyam AK, et al. Morphomolecular Classification Update on Hepatocellular Adenoma, Hepatocellular Carcinoma, and Intrahepatic Cholangiocarcinoma. Radiographics. 2022;42(5):1338-57.
65. Gupta P, Basu S, Arora C. Applications of artificial intelligence in biliary tract cancers. Indian J Gastroenterol. 2024.
66. Gupta P, Kambadakone A, Sirohi B. Editorial: Role of imaging in biliary tract cancer: diagnosis, staging, response prediction and image-guided therapeutics. Front Oncol. 2024;14:1387531.
67. Gupta P, Rana P, Ganeshan B, Kalage D, Irrinki S, Gupta V, et al. Computed tomography texture-based radiomics analysis in gallbladder cancer: initial experience. Clin Exp Hepatol. 2021;7(4):406-14.
68. Basu S, Gupta M, Rana P, Gupta P, Arora C. RadFormer: Transformers with global-local attention for interpretable and accurate Gallbladder Cancer detection. Med Image Anal. 2023;83:102676.
69. Gupta P, Basu S, Yadav TD, Kaman L, Irrinki S, Singh H, et al. Deep-learning models for differentiation of xanthogranulomatous cholecystitis and gallbladder cancer on ultrasound. Indian J Gastroenterol. 2023.
70. Gupta P, Basu S, Rana P, Dutta U, Soundararajan R, Kalage D, et al. Deep-learning enabled ultrasound based detection of gallbladder cancer in northern India: a prospective diagnostic study. Lancet Reg Health Southeast Asia. 2023;24:100279.

CHAPTER 17

Mandeep Kang, Harish Bhujade, Naveen Kalra, Anupam Lal

Biliary Interventions

INTRODUCTION

In past few decades, there has been a revolution in minimally-invasive surgeries and techniques with forefront developments in image-guided interventions. Percutaneous biliary interventions had their origin way back in 1921 when biliary tree was first visualized using direct puncture of the gallbladder. This was followed by reports describing percutaneous direct puncture of the biliary tree. The technique of percutaneous biliary drainage to relieve obstructive jaundice was introduced in the 1970s[1-3] followed by percutaneous cholecystostomy in the 1980s.[4-6] The development of biliary stents has further expanded the scope of percutaneous applications in the management of biliary diseases.[7-11]

Currently, percutaneous biliary interventions include percutaneous transhepatic cholangiography (PTC) and biliary drainage (PTBD) for the diagnosis and management of biliary obstruction and percutaneous cholecystostomy. This route can also be used for percutaneous transhepatic cholangioscopy (PTCS) or biliary ultrasonography (US); biopsy of the biliary duct, cholangioplasty for benign biliary strictures and as an access for the removal of bile duct calculi, the application of intraluminal brachytherapy (ILBT) or radiofrequency ablation, and placement of various biliary stents.

PERCUTANEOUS TRANSHEPATIC CHOLANGIOGRAPHY

Percutaneous transhepatic cholangiography is a diagnostic procedure which involves placement of a fine needle into a peripheral biliary radical under image guidance followed by contrast injection to opacify the biliary tree. Nowadays, the procedure is used as the preliminary step for draining the biliary tree (most common indication).[8,12]

Although PTC has been shown to be an effective technique which reliably demonstrates the level of obstruction, it is more invasive and painful than endoscopic retrograde cholangiopancreatography (ERCP). It also involves the risk of significant complications such as hemoperitoneum and bile peritonitis. Hence, PTC is nowadays reserved for the patients in whom an ECRP is not possible due to anatomy altering surgeries or following unsuccessful cannulation of the common bile duct (CBD).

Preprocedure Evaluation and Preparation

The initial work-up of a patient with obstructive biliopathy includes a clinical evaluation with history taking, physical examination, and relevant blood work-up. Imaging, such as US, CT, and MRI should be performed to provide information about the level and cause of biliary obstruction. Coagulation parameters including prothrombin time, prothrombin time index (>75%), and the international normalized ratio (≤1.5) as well as platelet count (>50–75,000) should be checked prior to the procedure and corrected with fresh frozen plasma or platelets if deranged.

Broad-spectrum antibiotics covering both gram-positive and gram-negative organisms should be started prior to the procedure. A venous access should be secured and an informed-written consent obtained after explaining the procedure completely to the patient and attendants.

Conscious sedation is useful for reasonable pain control. Over sedation should not be done as the patient needs to be instructed to hold the breath during procedure. Nevertheless general anesthesia may be required in selected cases.[12-14]

Technique

Patients need to lie down in supine position on the fluoroscopy table. The upper abdomen is cleaned and draped. The skin puncture area is infiltrated with a local anesthetic agent (2% lidocaine) up to the liver capsule. The dilated peripheral biliary radicals can be punctured under US guidance. If there is no dilatation, the procedure is done under fluoroscopic guidance. Right mid-axillary approach through an intercostal space which is caudal to the costophrenic sulcus is generally used which can be identified on fluoroscopy on deep inspiration. A 15 cm fine (22G) Chiba needle is inserted into the liver aiming for the right lateral aspect of the 12th thoracic vertebral body. After removing the stylet, the needle is slowly withdrawn while injecting a small amount of diluted contrast. Once the biliary radicals opacified, needle withdrawal is stopped and cholangiography performed to delineate the biliary anatomy. A second or third puncture may be used on unsuccessful first attempt by changing the needle angle once the needle tip is near the liver capsule.

The success rates for PTC are reported to be over 90% in a dilated system and 67–80% in a nondilated system. Major complications are seen in 3.5–10% of procedures and include sepsis, cholangitis, bile leak, hemorrhage, or pneumothorax.[12-15]

PERCUTANEOUS TRANSHEPATIC BILIARY DRAINAGE

Percutaneous transhepatic biliary drainage is a therapeutic procedure that consists of sterile puncture of a peripheral biliary radical under image guidance followed by placement of a catheter or stent over the guidewire for internal or external drainage of bile. Percutaneous therapy of bile duct lesions is often a staged procedure, requiring multiple sessions to achieve the therapeutic goals.[8]

Indications for Biliary Drainage

The presence of cholestasis, whether due to benign or malignant etiology, predisposes to biliary infection. Secondly, protracted hyperbilirubinemia causes impairment of the renal function. The surgical morbidity and mortality rates are also high (40–60% and 15–25%, respectively) in the setting of hyperbilirubinemia; therefore, decompression should be done as early as possible in patients with obstructive biliopathy. Malignancy causing biliary obstruction is often unresectable at the time of diagnosis and palliative therapy is the only management option possible. A normalized liver function is also required for the administration of chemotherapy. Biliary drainage thus will not only normalize liver function, restore the physiological drainage of bile into the duodenum, prevent the development of cholangitis, and sepsis but also improve the nutritional status and quality of life of the patient.[7,9,10]

Common causes of benign biliary obstruction include choledocholithiasis, sclerosing cholangitis, and inflammatory conditions such as pancreatitis, iatrogenic causes (postlaparoscopic cholecystectomy, liver transplantation, or anastomotic strictures), and infections such as human immunodeficiency virus (HIV) infection and oriental and parasitic cholangitis.[15] The common causes of malignant biliary obstruction include gallbladder carcinoma, cholangiocarcinoma, carcinoma of the pancreas, and metastatic disease.[10,16]

The indications include:

- To decompress the obstructed biliary tree
- To dilate benign biliary strictures
- To remove bile duct stones
- To divert bile from and stent bile duct defects
- To stent malignant strictures

There are no absolute contraindications for the procedure. Deranged coagulation parameters are a relative contraindication and should be corrected prior to the procedure with platelets or fresh frozen plasma. The presence of gross ascites with presence of perihepatic fluid is also a relative contraindication which requires to be drained before performing a PTBD.[14,16]

PATIENT PREPARATION

The patient preparation and preprocedure work-up are as for PTC. The endoscopic route is preferred for drainage, particularly in lesions involving the mid or distal CBD as it is associated with a decreased complication rate. However, with lesions involving the hilum, the percutaneous approach has a higher success rate and is therefore preferred. In cases of failed ERCP or where ERCP is not possible due to anatomy altering surgeries, PTBD is the approach of choice.[10,11,16,17]

Preprocedure Imaging

Cross-sectional imaging with contrast-enhanced CT (CECT) and MRI with magnetic resonance cholangiopancreatography (MRCP) should be performed prior to the procedure. These will help to identify the level and cause of obstruction and aid in planning the approach to percutaneous management.[7,10] When there is obstruction beyond the hilum of the liver, only one access is required. The left system is accessed from an anterior and subxiphoid approach while the right is accessed from the midaxillary approach using as caudal an intercostal space as possible, well below the costophrenic sulcus. Whether to use a left or right approach is largely a matter of individual or institutional preference, when both sided biliary radicles are adequately dilated. When the drainage is required for a longer period of time, most patients are more comfortable with a subxiphoid catheter rather than a right intercostal catheter. Other advantages of a left approach include a less painful procedure which is technically easier to perform (limited respiratory excursion of the left lobe of liver in comparison to the right and a shorter route to be traversed through the hepatic parenchyma), decreased pleural complication rate, and less likelihood of catheter dislodgment, again due to less respiratory excursion of the left lobe as well as the fact that the patient finds it easier to look after a percutaneous catheter which is in front of his/her eyes rather than on one side of the body. The disadvantage of the left approach is the increased radiation dose to the operator's hands.

In cases of hilar obstruction with isolation of the biliary radicles, careful assessment of the cross-sectional imaging and US has to be done to assess the degree of biliary dilatation. One also has to look for obstruction of the secondary confluence, both right and the left as well as for multilevel isolation which may be present in the setting of metastatic disease. One also has to assess the approach to the segmental duct to be punctured for any mass or cyst in the path of the needle. At least 25–30% of the liver parenchyma should be drained with a single catheter as placement of multiple catheters increases the morbidity and mortality in a patient.[7,10]

If the procedure is done for palliative purposes for the relief of jaundice, drainage of one lobe is enough. However, in the presence of cholangitis, if drainage of one side does not relieve the symptoms, the other side also needs to be drained. The drainage of atrophic segment or lobe is not useful as it is unlikely to improve the hepatic function. In case of segmental isolated obstructions, if the patient is not in cholangitis, one should not drain that segment as once a drainage catheter is placed, it becomes virtually impossible to withdraw the access due to bacterial contamination and the patient will be left with an unneeded, potentially problematic catheter.[7,10,18]

Technique

The procedure is performed under conscious sedation with the patient placed supine on the fluoroscopy table. The initial step of the procedure is performing a PTC as described above. The underlying soft tissues should be dissected free as this will ease the subsequent drainage catheter insertion.[14] In a dilated system, a 18G puncture needle with a diamond tip is used to enter the selected biliary radicle as peripherally as possible.

Allowing a small amount of bile to drain after the puncture before injecting contrast is beneficial as it prevents overdistension of the biliary system which can result in bacteremia and sepsis. A little diluted-contrast is injected to opacify the biliary tree and to confirm that the needle tip is completely within the biliary system. If contrast is seen pooling at the puncture site, it signifies that the tip is within the parenchyma. If contrast is seen entering a tubular system with rapid dissipation, it denotes placement of the needle tip within avascular structure. In both these situations, the needle has to be carefully repositioned. Once there is backflow of bile and contrast injection opacifies the biliary tree, a 0.032 or 0.035 inch hydrophilic guidewire is passed through the needle and manipulated into the biliary tree toward the liver hilum **(Figs. 1A to C)**.[10,14]

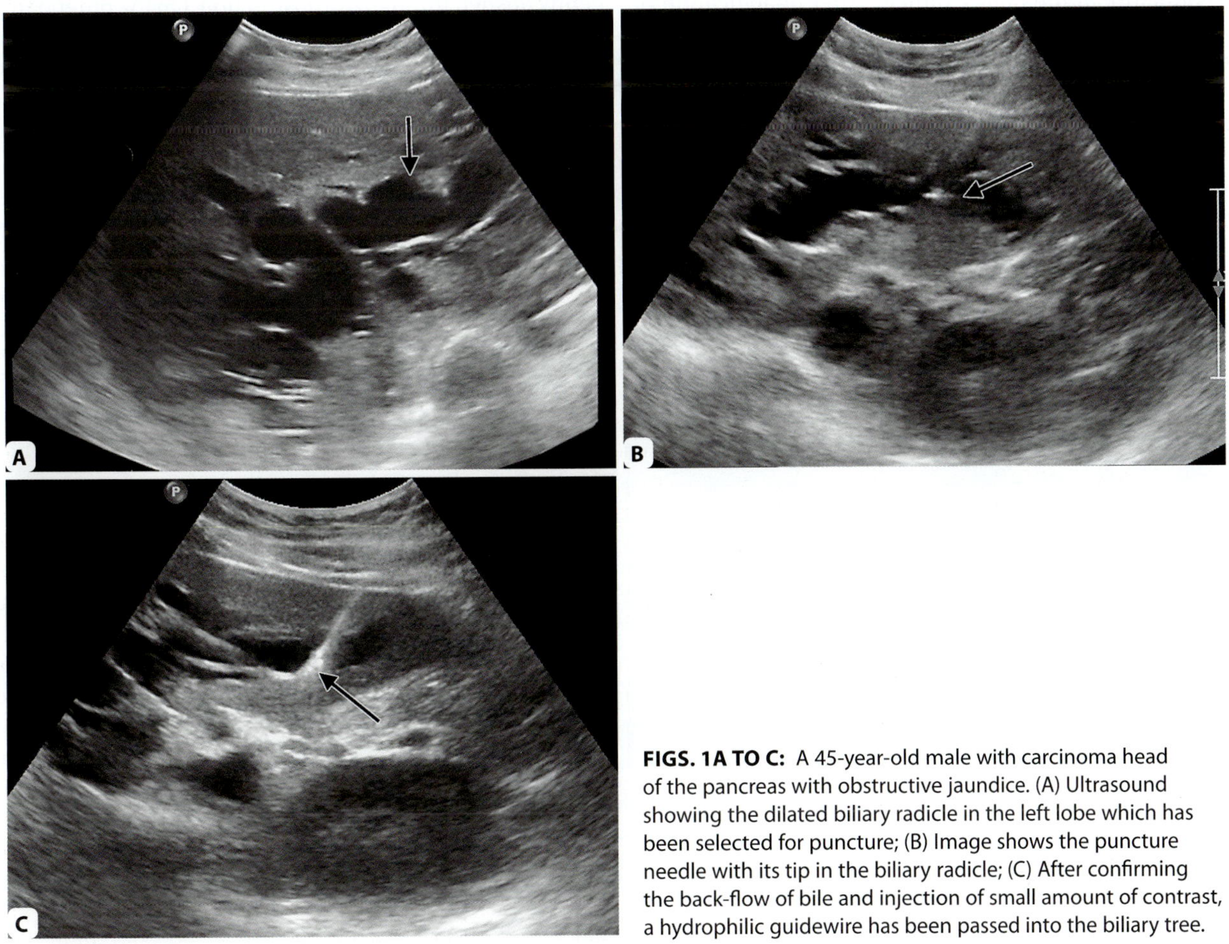

FIGS. 1A TO C: A 45-year-old male with carcinoma head of the pancreas with obstructive jaundice. (A) Ultrasound showing the dilated biliary radicle in the left lobe which has been selected for puncture; (B) Image shows the puncture needle with its tip in the biliary radicle; (C) After confirming the back-flow of bile and injection of small amount of contrast, a hydrophilic guidewire has been passed into the biliary tree.

After safely anchoring the guidewire, the needle is removed and a 4F or 5F sheath or cannula introduced. The hydrophilic guidewire is exchanged with a stiffer (Teflon coated) guidewire over which a 7F or 8F drainage catheter can be placed after dilatation of the tract with fascial dilators **(Figs. 2A and B)**. If the tip of the catheter is in the CBD, a catheter of the pigtail type is placed. If the tip of the catheter is in an intrahepatic duct an angled catheter is selected. A self-locking catheter is usually used to prevent accidental slippage. The catheter should also be secured to the skin surface by using a suture or commercially available skin anchoring devices. The catheter is then attached to a drainage bag and left for gravity drainage.

Fluoroscopic Guidance

Fluoroscopic guidance may be used in patients with or without biliary dilatation for performing PTBD. There are two methods by which the procedure can be done. In the one step method, a 21G Chiba needle is used for the puncture as for PTC. A 0.018" guidewire is then passed through the needle and manipulated into the biliary tree. The needle is then removed and a 4F percutaneous access set introduced over the guidewire. Through the sheath, a 0.035" stiff guidewire is passed and the rest of the procedure is as described under US guidance.[7]

In the two step method, a 22G Chiba needle is used for puncture of the biliary radicle. After opacification of the biliary tree, a second 18G puncture needle is used for repuncture of a suitable biliary radicle.[14] This allows passage of a 0.035 guidewire and the rest of the procedure is as described earlier.

Minimal diluted contrast injection and minimal possible handling should be done on the first day of procedure during placement of an indwelling catheter to avoid overdistension of the biliary tree and cholangiovenous reflux.

Two things should be remembered while doing the procedure. The puncture site of the biliary radical should be as far as possible from the level of obstruction so as to allow safe anchorage of the external drainage catheter. Also, a longer tract makes subsequent internal drainage easier. Secondly, the puncture during deep inspiration should be avoided as the liver will move caudal, which causes a difference in the level between the site of punctures of the skin surface and the liver. Therefore, the puncture should be performed in shallow inspiratory breath-hold.

Internal and External Drainage

Internal drainage should ideally be attempted 48–72 hours after the initial PTBD which helps to decompress the biliary system and therefore, straightening of the course of the wire. Secondly, this time allows to settle the inflammatory changes and edema around the obstructing lesion.[3,10,19] Injection of contrast through the drainage catheter at this stage will show the true picture of the type of obstruction whether beak-shaped, tapered, or flat-shaped. The drainage catheter is replaced with a 4F or 5F angiographic or biliary manipulation catheter with a curved or angled tip over a stiff guidewire. The stiff guidewire is then changed for a soft, angled, or J-tip hydrophilic guidewire. If the site of obstruction is beak-shaped or tapered, the tip of the catheter is wedged into the beak and the soft hydrophilic guidewire is gently pushed through the obstruction. On the other hand, if the site of obstruction is flat or irregular it may be better to keep the catheter a little proximal to the obstruction and gently probe the area with the hydrophilic guidewire, while simultaneously rotating the tip of the angled catheter into different directions.[10,20]

Once the guidewire successfully crosses the obstruction, it is advanced into the duodenal lumen along with the catheter. The hydrophilic guidewire is then exchanged for

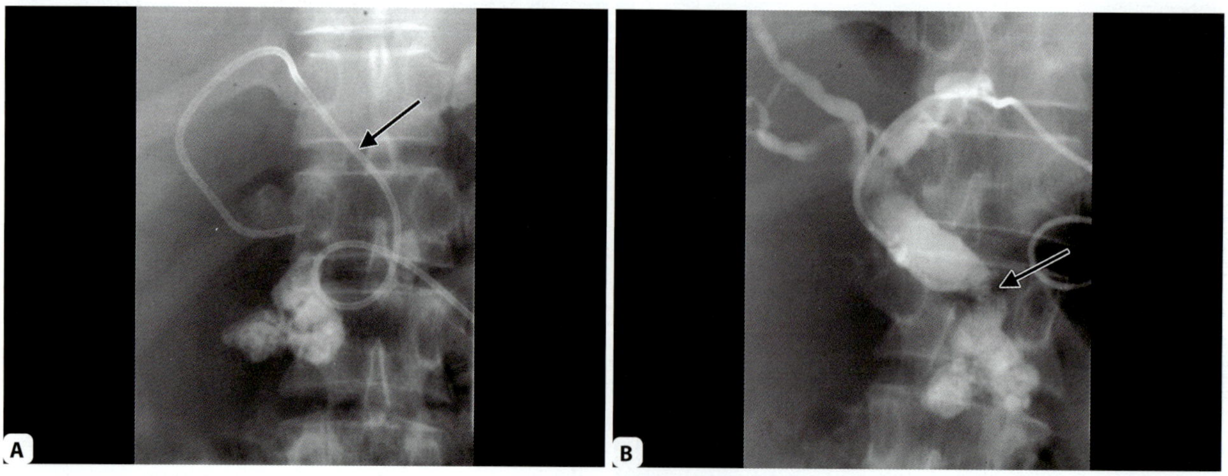

FIGS. 2A AND B: External biliary drainage: A 52-year-old male with chronic calcific pancreatitis with obstructive jaundice. (A) An 8F PTBD catheter has been placed via the left duct approach into the CBD for external drainage; (B) Cholangiogram shows a complete block of the distal CBD.

(CBD: common bile duct; PTBD: percutaneous transhepatic biliary drainage)

a stiff guidewire over which an 8.3F ring biliary catheter or 10F pigtail catheter is placed with the loop in the duodenum **(Fig. 3)**. Contrast injection to check that side-holes are present in both proximal and distal to the obstruction and no side-holes are within the hepatic parenchyma completes the procedure **(Figs. 4A and B)**. The catheter should initially be left to external biliary drainage while ensuring adequate hydration of the patient. It can be capped to allow internal drainage once the bile is clear from blood or debris and the patient is afebrile. Once the "capping test" is successful with no fever, pain, or vomiting, the patient can be discharged to home with the instruction to open the cap and attach an external drainage bag in the event of any of the above complications, and to report back to the hospital as soon as possible.

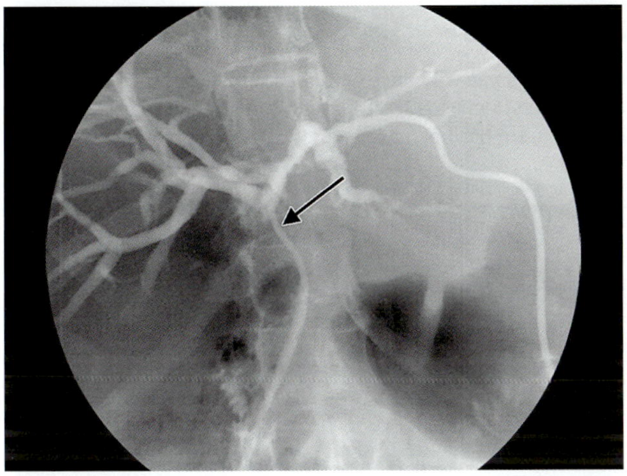

FIG. 3: External-internal biliary drainage: A 55-year-old female with carcinoma gallbladder with obstructive jaundice. Cholangiogram shows complete block of the common hepatic duct just distal to the confluence. An external-internal drainage has been instituted with the distal catheter tip placed in the second part of duodenum.

Postprocedure Management

Patients who have undergone biliary drainage procedures require inpatient admission for at least 24 hours following the procedure. The patient needs to be closely monitored as the procedures can cause bacteremia and sepsis. Vital signs should be checked every 15 minutes for 1 hour, every 30 minutes for 2 hours, hourly thereafter for 4 hours, and then 6 hourly for 4 hours. Biliary output can range from 400 to 800 mL every 24 hours, so adequate hydration needs to be taken care of. Adequate analgesics need to be administered for controlling the postprocedural pain. Appropriate antibiotics also need to be continued for at least 48 hours after the procedure.[14]

Follow-up of Biliary Catheters

After PTBD procedures, patients require close monitoring and regular follow-up to identify catheter dislodgment or obstruction at an early stage. Biliary output, color, and body temperature should be recorded daily. The serum bilirubin and amylase levels should be checked regularly. The usual daily biliary output of bile is 400–800 mL which is clear and yellow in color. Any decrease in the output, change in color, or increased turbidity are signs of cholangitis. Regular US examination to look for any dilated intrahepatic radicles which denote undrained ducts or development of catheter obstruction should be performed. Some interventionists advice daily, gentle, forward flushing of the catheter with 5–10 mL of normal saline or sterile water to avoid clogging of lumen. Pericatheter leakage is usually due to occlusion of the catheter or dislodgment and requires fluoroscopic

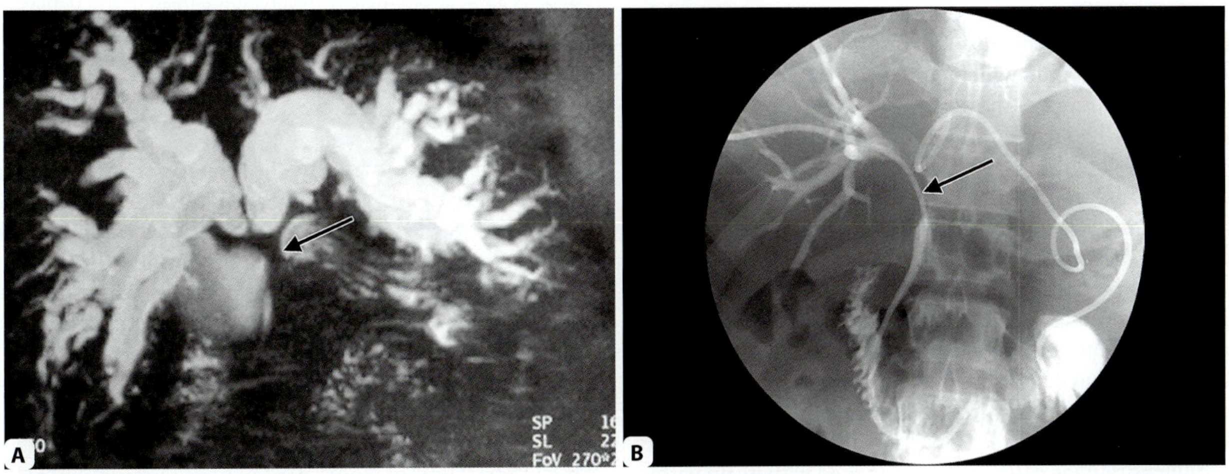

FIGS. 4A AND B: A 45-year-old male with carcinoma gallbladder with obstructive jaundice. (A) MRCP MIP image shows a hilar block with isolation of the biliary radicles; (B) An external-internal catheter has been placed in the right ductal system with its tip in the third part of duodenum. Check cholangiogram after the procedure confirms that side-holes are present both above and below the strictured segment. An external drainage catheter is seen in the left ductal system with its tip lying just proximal to the confluence.
(MIP: maximum intensity projection; MRCP: magnetic resonance cholangiopancreatography)

evaluation and correction of the problem. Catheter blockage will also cause the serum bilirubin values to rise. Catheters should ideally be exchanged every 2–3 months to avoid blockage or breakage.[14]

Biliary Stenting

Biliary stents can be various kinds of either plastic or metallic stents. An external drainage tube can be uncomfortable or of psychological disadvantage to the patient particularly in cases of malignant obstruction. An internal stent also prevents the complications of pericatheter biliary leakage or slippage. The disadvantage of stents is the need for performing a new procedure (PTBD or ERCP) in case of stent obstruction.

Metallic stents are used almost exclusively for the palliative management of unresectable biliary malignant obstruction. The major advantage of metallic stents is that they can be inserted in a contracted state through a small caliber tract and can achieve a large lumen (up to 10 mm) following expansion **(Fig. 5)**. They are available as self-expanding metallic stents (SEMS) or balloon-mounted stents. These stents are less prone to displacement and show a better patency rate than plastic stents.[7,21,22] Metallic stents can be covered or uncovered. The covered stents has better patency compared to uncovered stent as stent mesh may get occluded in uncovered stents. The disadvantages of metallic stents include the high cost and difficulty in removal, whereas plastic stents are cheap but have many disadvantages including early occlusion, frequent migration, and a traumatic insertion procedure due to the large tract size required **(Fig. 6)**. Because of the large caliber, endoscopic insertion is done more frequently than the percutaneous route.[23,24]

Most physicians prefer to allow internal drainage for a few days prior to stent placement. However, if the passage through the stricture has been relatively atraumatic without significant hemorrhage or debris, stenting can be done in the same sitting as the internal-external drainage.[25]

A super-stiff guidewire is passed through the internal-external drainage catheter and securely looped in the duodenum. The catheter is removed and an appropriate introducer sheath placed. If a SEMS is being used, some workers prefer to balloon dilate the stricture prior to stent deployment.[14] It is advisable to overstent the stricture with the proximal and distal end of the stent at least 1-1.5 cm beyond the strictures limits.[21] Once the stent is at the appropriate site, as evidenced by the position of the radiopaque markers at the ends of the stent, it is deployed. Since SEMS have a thermal memory, they will gradually expand to their maximum width within 24 hours after deployment once they achieve body temperature. A safety 8F biliary drainage catheter is then placed with its tip within the stent and the guidewire removed **(Figs. 7A to E)**. The external drain is capped after 24 hours and if the patient tolerates the "capping", a check cholangiogram is performed to confirm adequate drainage through the stent, following which the external catheter is removed.[9,14]

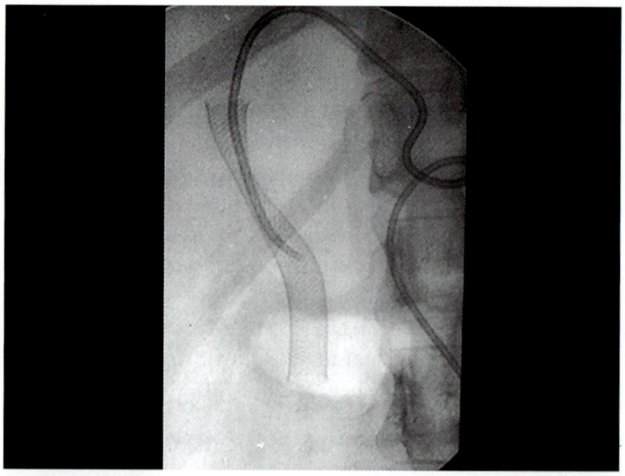

FIG. 5: A 63-year-old male with carcinoma head of the pancreas causing obstructive jaundice. A single and self-expanding metallic stent has been placed in the common bile duct.

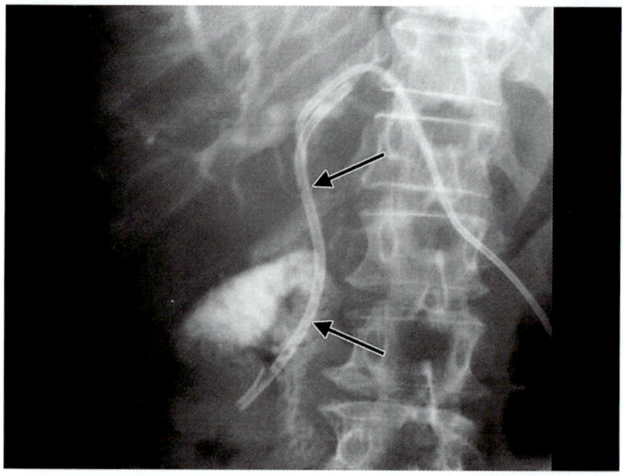

FIG. 6: A 58-year-old male with carcinoma head of the pancreas. A single plastic biliary stent has been placed across the stricture. An external drainage catheter has been left in place as a safety measure in the immediate postprocedure period.

A single stent normally suffices for short segment strictures in the CBD. For longer strictures, one may need to place two telescoped stents (one stent overlapping with the other). In cases of hilar obstruction, bilateral stents may be required which can be placed in either a "T" or "Y" configuration. When placing in a "Y" configuration, it is advisable to place the lower ends of the stents at the same level in the CBD **(Figs. 8A and B)**.[7,26] This parallel arrangement may prevent complete expansion of the stents at the level of the liver hilum, so other workers advocate using a "stent within stent" deployment technique. In this technique, the second stent is placed through the mesh of the first stent.[27] This technique is also said to prevent displacement of the stents. The advantage of "T" stenting is that only a single percutaneous access is required thereby decreasing the complication rate **(Figs. 9A and B)**. However,

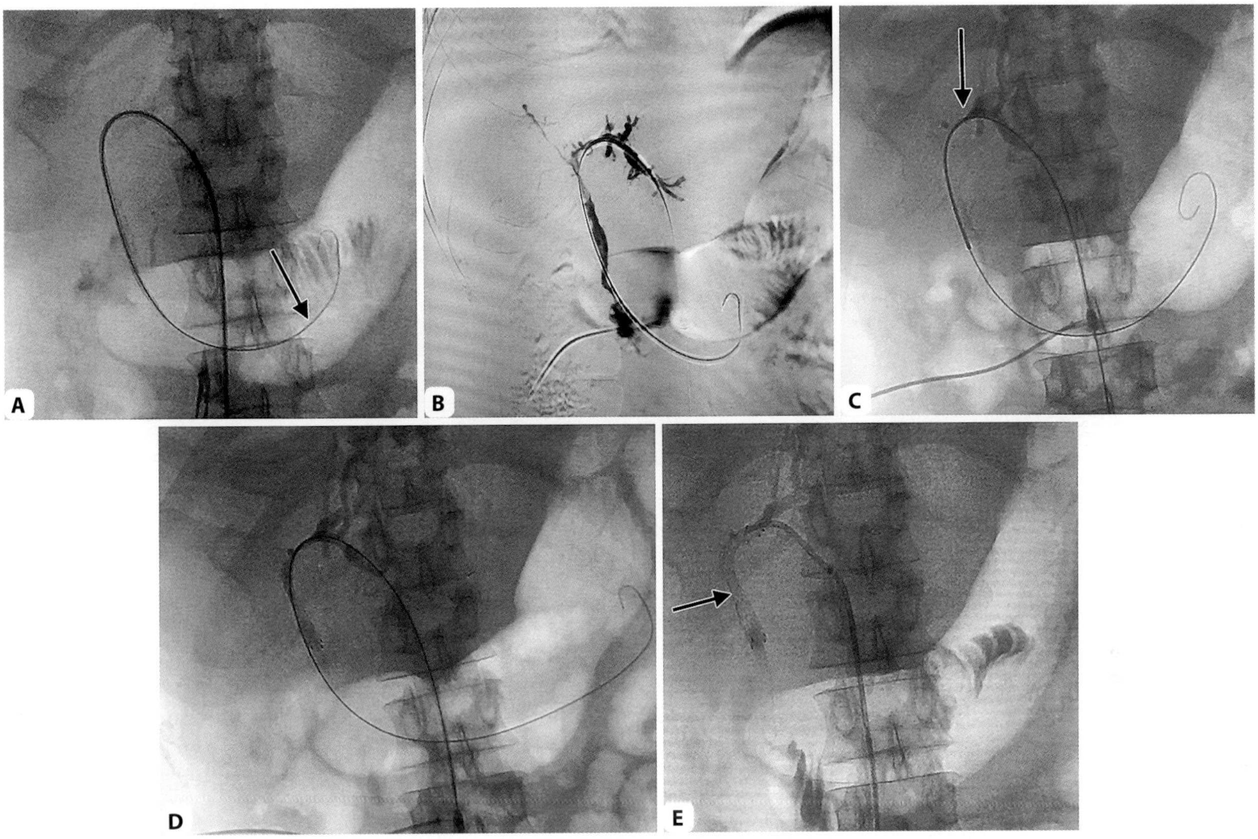

FIGS. 7A TO E: Biliary stenting: (A) Fluoroscopic image shows that a super-stiff guidewire has been passed through the internal-external catheter into the duodenum; (B) Contrast injection to check the exact location and length of stricture; (C) The stent has been placed across the stricture with the help of the radiopaque markers (arrow); (D) The stent is being deployed; and (E) The stent has been fully deployed. A safety external drain has been placed with its tip within the proximal end of the stent.

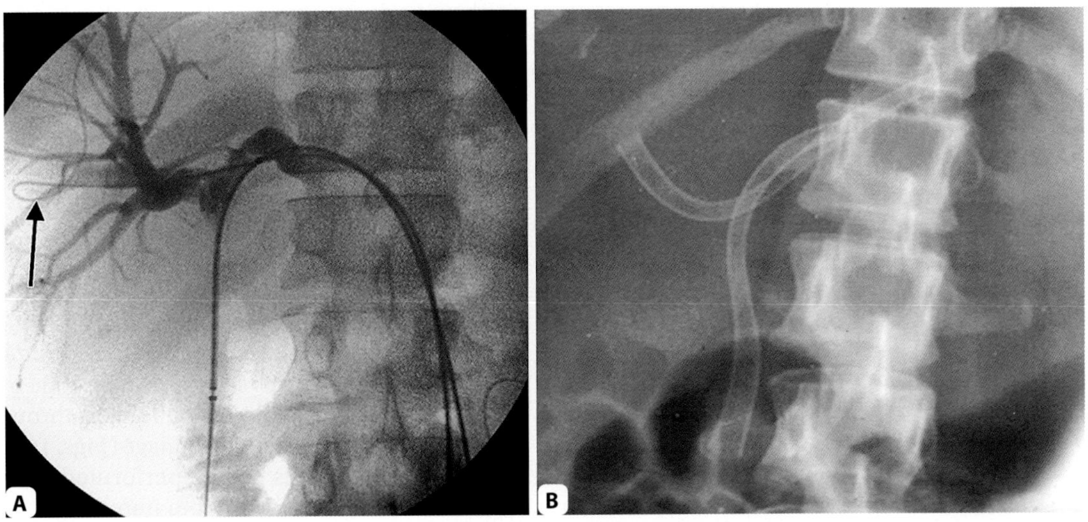

FIGS. 8A AND B: T-stenting in a 38-year-old female with hilar block due to carcinoma gallbladder. (A) An internal-external drain is present on the left side along with a left-to-right drain. A stiff guidewire (arrow) has been anchored in the right ductal system and a stent placed across the hilar stricture into the duodenum; (B) Two metallic stents have been placed across the hilar stricture in a "T" configuration.

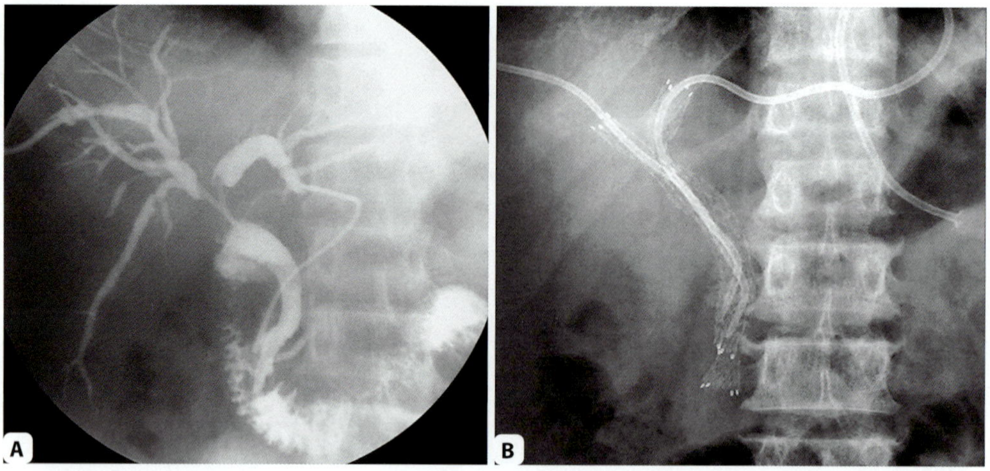

FIGS. 9A AND B: Y-stenting in a 58-year-old male with hilar obstruction due to cholangiocarcinoma. (A) Cholangiogram shows an internal-external drainage catheter placed via left and right ductal systems; (B) Two metallic stents have been placed parallel to each other in a "Y" configuration.

at times the stricture cannot be crossed to the contralateral side, thereby necessitating the second puncture.[28] No significant difference has been reported between using the "T" or the "Y" configurations in terms of rates of technical success, complications or stent patency.[28] Multiple stents may be required in cases of involvement of the secondary confluences (Bismuth type III or IV strictures).[7]

The reported patency rate for palliative metallic stents in malignant obstructions is about 50% at 6 months.[17] Stent blockage occurs because of tumor ingrowth through the mesh of the stent or tumor overgrowth at the ends of the stent, biliary sludge, and debris.[10,17] In an effort to limit tumor ingrowth, covered stents coated with polyurethane, silicone, or expanded polytetrafluoroethylene (ePTFE) were developed. These stents are not integrated within the biliary wall, and therefore, are prone for migration. Secondly, the openings of the side branches or cystic duct may be blocked by the stent, resulting in a higher complication rate of cholangitis, cholecystitis, or pancreatitis.[29] Stent obstruction requires a repeat procedure with either placement of an internal-external drain or a fresh stent through the lumen of the obstructed stent.

Results and Complications of Biliary Drainage

Successful biliary drainage is defined as placement of a drainage tube or stent to provide continuous drainage of bile. The reported rates are 95% in dilated ducts and 70% in nondilated ducts for placement of external drainage catheters. Of these, about 90% of cases successfully undergo internal-external drain placement.[8]

The complication rate for PTBD can be substantial and depends upon the preprocedure patient status and diagnosis. The rate is more often in patients with malignant strictures, cholangitis, or deranged coagulogram. Major complications include bleeding, shock due to injection of contrast medium or acute biliary decompression, sepsis, and biliary peritonitis due to displacement of catheter. The hemorrhage may be due to venous or arterial injury. Hemobilia following the procedure is common and usually resolves within 48–72 hours but may require clamping of the catheter or change to a larger bore catheter.[25] If hemobilia persists, a CT angiogram should be done. If the scan shows a pseudoaneurysm or active extravasation of contrast, it can be managed with embolization. Pancreatitis may occur after internalization of catheter and can be due to edema of the CBD wall or obstruction of the main pancreatic duct by the catheter. Pneumothorax or pleural effusion may occur due to inadvertent transpleural puncture. Cholangitis can develop if there is blockage of the catheter or if any intrahepatic ducts remain undrained. The reported rate of major complications is 2.5–10% while the reported mortality is 0–3%.[7]

INTRALUMINAL PROCEDURES THROUGH PERCUTANEOUS TRANSHEPATIC BILIARY DRAINAGE

Various procedures can be performed using the access available through the percutaneous biliary drainage route. Diagnostic procedures include endobiliary tissue sampling for histopathological analysis. This can be done by using a cytological brush or endoluminal forceps through an 8F sheath after internal-external drainage **(Figs. 10A to C)**.[30]

Palliative therapies can be performed through the PTBD access route in an effort to improve the quality of life, life expectancy, and stent patency. These include brachytherapy, radiofrequency ablation, and photodynamic therapy. High-dose rate ILBT using Iridium-192 can be delivered selectively to the tumor while avoiding the side effect of external radiotherapy. This treatment can be offered in patients who have a single tumor with an overall stricture

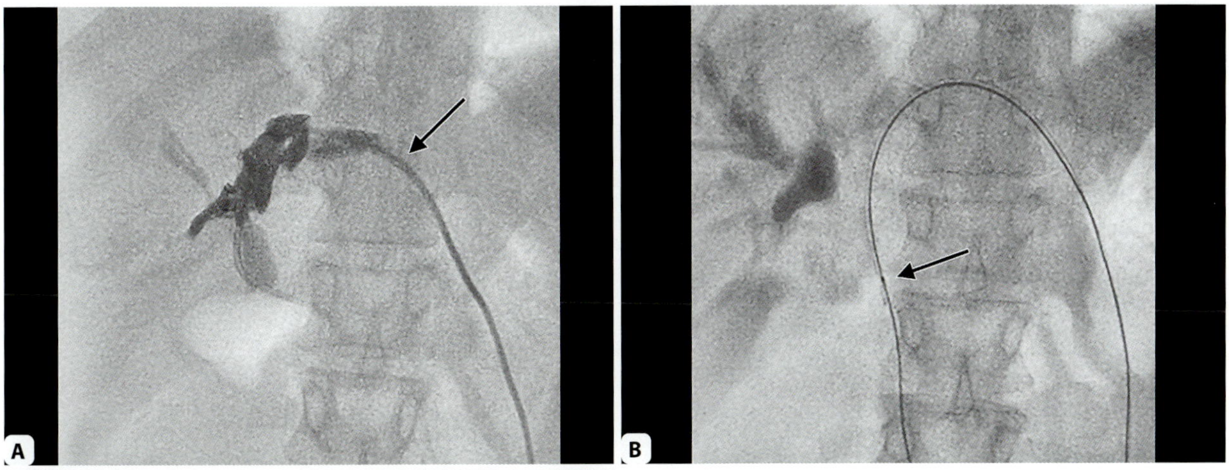

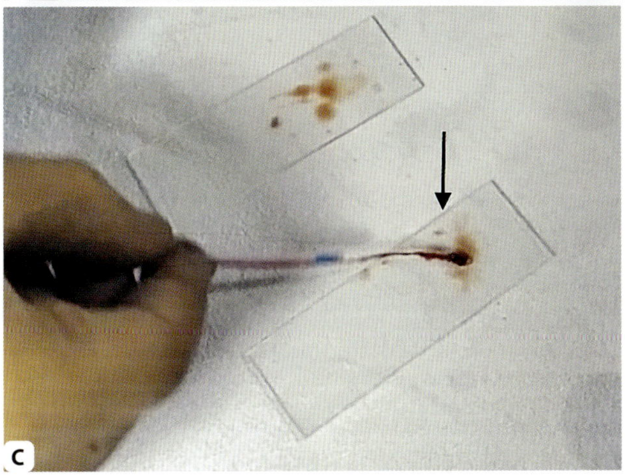

FIGS. 10A TO C: Percutaneous biliary brushing. (A) Cholangiogram via percutaneous transhepatic biliary drainage (PTBD) (arrow) showing biliary obstruction. (B) Biliary cytology brush (arrow) is advanced across the obstruction over guide-wire. (C) Smear (arrow) can be made from the materials obtained from the brush.

length of <6 cm and the absence of distant disease. The drainage catheter is replaced by the brachytherapy catheter over a stiff guidewire and positioned with its tip 1 cm beyond the distal end of the stricture. The unit is programmed to treat the stricture length and 1 cm beyond and proximal to the stricture **(Figs. 11A and B)**. Studies have shown a significant improvement in the quality of life when ILBT is combined with PTBD with improved stent patency.[31,32]

Similarly, a radiofrequency probe can be introduced through a sheath and the active part placed across the stricture **(Figs. 12A to C)**. Radiofrequency energy is applied in the range of 8–15 watts for 2 minutes at each level. The procedure has been shown to be safe, whether it results in improved stent patency requires further larger studies to be done.[33] Photodynamic therapy using laser has also been described.[34]

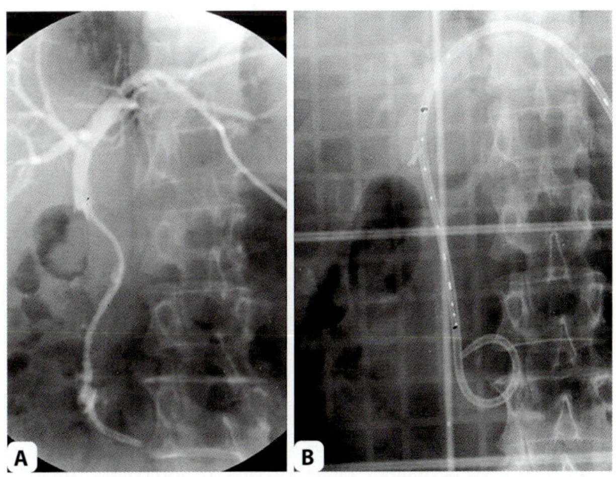

FIGS. 11A AND B: Intraluminal brachytherapy in a 41-year-old female with carcinoma gallbladder. (A) Cholangiogram after internal-external drainage demonstrates a 4 cm stricture in the mid common bile duct (CBD); (B) A 10F pigtail catheter has been placed with it's tip in the duodenum. Simulator film shows placement of the brachytherapy catheter within the pigtail catheter with its distal end 1 cm beyond the distal end of the stricture.

Percutaneous Transhepatic Cholangioplasty

Biliary enteric anastomoses are commonly performed for most of the benign biliary strictures. However, there is considerable recurrence of the stricture after surgery

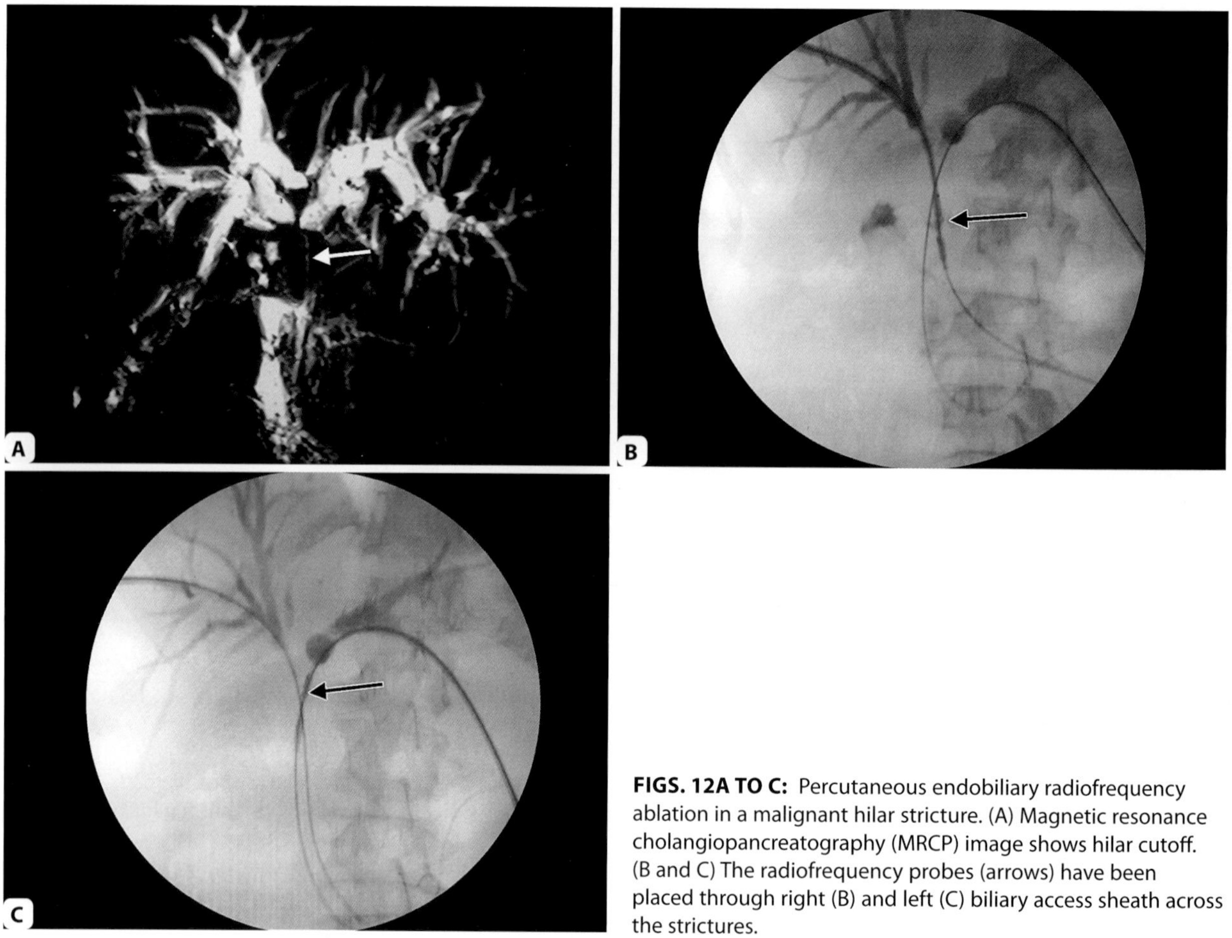

FIGS. 12A TO C: Percutaneous endobiliary radiofrequency ablation in a malignant hilar stricture. (A) Magnetic resonance cholangiopancreatography (MRCP) image shows hilar cutoff. (B and C) The radiofrequency probes (arrows) have been placed through right (B) and left (C) biliary access sheath across the strictures.

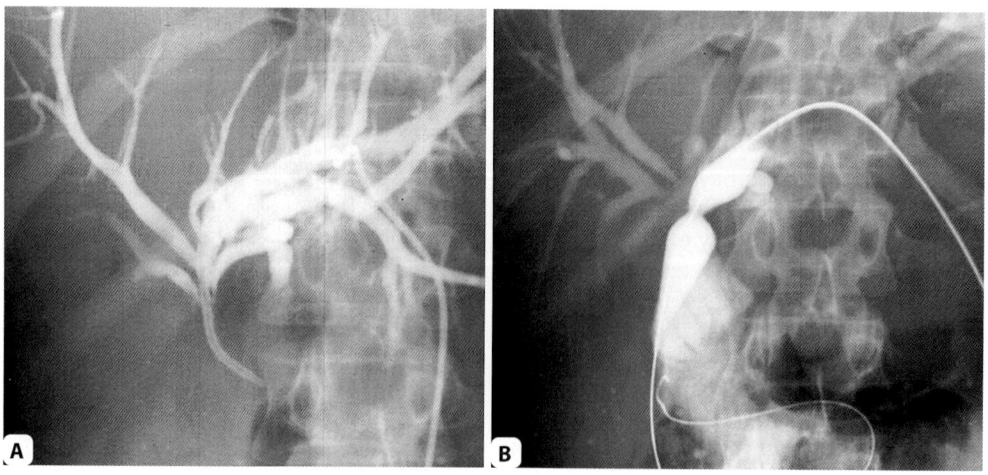

FIGS. 13A AND B: Balloon dilatation of a benign biliary stricture in a case of postoperative choledochojejunostomy stricture. (A) An 8F drainage catheter has been placed across the stricture with its tip in the jejunal loop from the left duct approach; (B) Balloon catheter has been placed over the stricture and inflated. Note the "waist" formation in the balloon due to the tight stricture.

and these are even more difficult to explore surgically. Percutaneous balloon dilatation can be a therapeutic choice for benign biliary strictures **(Figs. 13A and B)**. The technique consists of replacing the internal-external drainage catheter with a balloon catheter. The stricture is inflated with an 8–10 mm balloon for at least 10 minutes and a large diameter catheter is placed across the stricture to induce nonstenosed fibrosis **(Figs. 14A to C)**. It is recommended that 3–6 balloon inflations be performed at intervals of 3 weeks with upsizing of the drainage catheter at

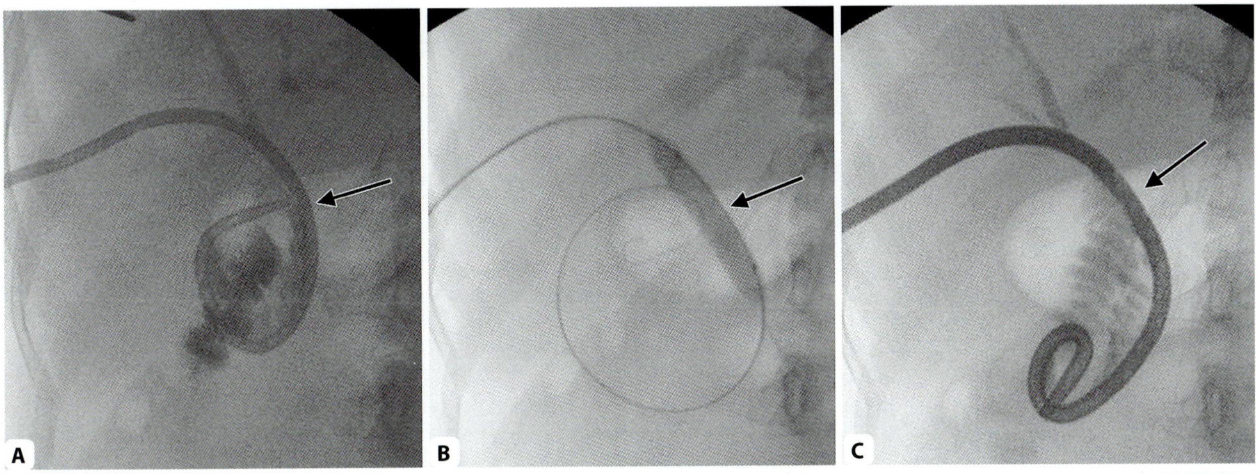

FIGS. 14A TO C: Percutaneous cholangioplasty with serial dilatation. (A) A 10F drainage catheter (arrow) has been placed across the stricture with its tip in the jejunal loop from the right duct approach; (B) Balloon catheter (arrow) has been placed over the stricture and inflated. (C) New 14F catheter (arrow) is placed across the stricture after cholangioplasty.

each sitting. Once cholangiograms show free flow of contrast across the stricture, the catheter is retracted proximal to the stricture and capped. The patient is monitored for a few days to ensure that the bile is flowing internally. The external catheter is removed if the patient remains asymptomatic. Success rates of 70–93% have been reported in literature.[15,35]

Biodegradable Biliary Stents

Development of the biodegradable biliary self-expanding stent has shown a revolutionary management of anastomotic biliary strictures. There are a few case reports and case series of percutaneously placed self-expanding biodegradable polydioxanone stents in benign biliary strictures which have shown promising result. These stents get degraded in a few to several months.

PERCUTANEOUS CHOLECYSTOSTOMY

Percutaneous cholecystostomy may be used as a temporary measure in patients of acute cholecystitis who are critically ill and therefore cannot undergo surgery.[4-6,36] After the patient's condition is stabilized, cholecystectomy as the definitive treatment will still be required. However, in acalculous cholecystitis, percutaneous drainage may be the only treatment required. Cholecystostomy can also provide a means of accessing the biliary tree in patients with obstructive jaundice in whom the bile ducts are not dilated and the level of obstruction is distal to the insertion of the cystic duct.

Technique

Two approach routes are available for US-guided puncturing the gallbladder. The transhepatic route is usually preferred as the transperitoneal approach carried a greater risk of biliary leak with bile peritonitis. Using the transhepatic route, the gallbladder is punctured where it is fixed to the liver, generally at the junction between the cephalic and middle third of the body. In the transperitoneal approach, the gallbladder is punctured at the point where it lies closest to the anterior abdominal wall. The trocar technique is generally used for direct puncture while the Seldinger technique is preferred for the transhepatic route.

An 18G needle is used to puncture the gallbladder and sample collected for Gram staining and culture. A small amount of contrast is then injected to opacify the gallbladder for the subsequent steps for which fluoroscopic guidance is used. A J-shaped soft tip guidewire is then inserted through the needle and coiled within the lumen. After dilating the tract, a 7F or 8F catheter having an anchor mechanism or of the pigtail type is placed within the gallbladder lumen and sutured to the skin. The catheter is left to drain by gravity **(Figs. 15A to C)**.

If surgery is not considered as in acalculous cholecystitis, the catheter can be removed once the patient's signs and symptoms resolve and a sufficient time has elapsed for the tract to mature. This is said to be at least 2 weeks when the transhepatic route is used and 3 weeks when the transperitoneal approach is used. Removal of the catheter before tract maturation may result in leakage of bile and peritonitis.[37,38] Percutaneous cholecystostomy can be used for cystic duct embolization and subsequent chemical ablation of gallbladder when surgery is contraindicated in patients with recurrent cholecystitis.[39]

Complications

The complications which can occur following percutaneous cholecystostomy include bile peritonitis, hemobilia, and gallbladder perforation. Vasovagal reaction due to tube placement can be managed with atropine. Hemorrhage can at times be fatal. Minimal manipulation should be

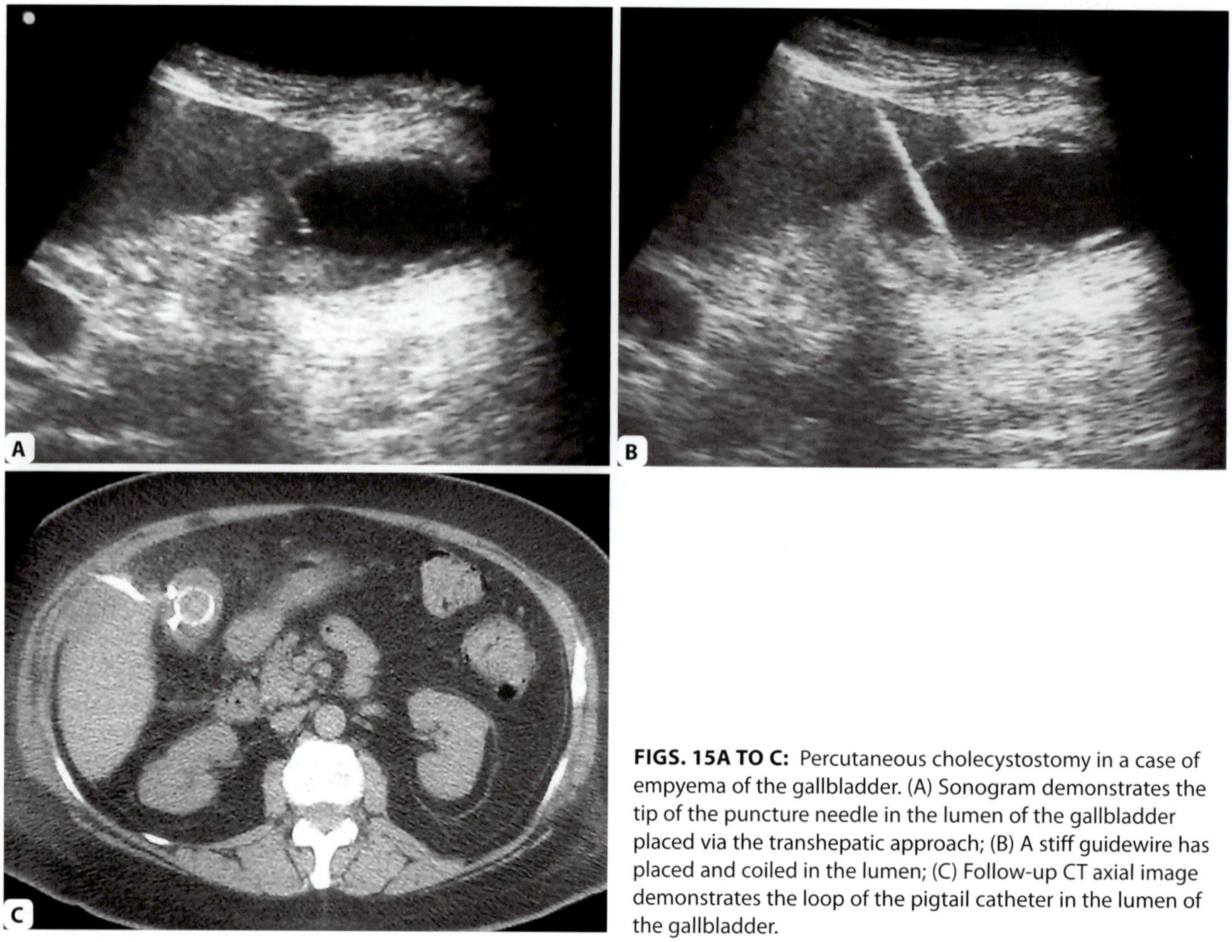

FIGS. 15A TO C: Percutaneous cholecystostomy in a case of empyema of the gallbladder. (A) Sonogram demonstrates the tip of the puncture needle in the lumen of the gallbladder placed via the transhepatic approach; (B) A stiff guidewire has placed and coiled in the lumen; (C) Follow-up CT axial image demonstrates the loop of the pigtail catheter in the lumen of the gallbladder.

done at the time of initial drainage to avoid complications.[40] Reported mortality rates range from 3 to 36% depending on the comorbid conditions.[14]

Percutaneous Transhepatic Cholangioscopy

Percutaneous transhepatic cholangioscopy involves direct visualization of biliary tree. Recent literature has suggested that it is safe, feasible, and useful for the visualization and assessment of undetermined biliary pathologies and in difficult biliary anatomy.[41,42] It helps to evaluate the biliary tree, obtaining samples of suspected malignant lesions, and lithotripsy.

The cholangioscopic visualization of the bile duct for malignancy has a sensitivity of 91–95% and specificity of 80–86% and for guided-biopsy has a sensitivity of approximately 70% and specificity of 98%.

For PTCS, the PTBD tract needs dilation of at least 12F. A guidewire is advanced into the bowel lumen via PTBD catheter. After removal of catheter, the scope is advanced into the bile duct beside the guidewire. Through the scope, various diagnostic as well as therapeutic procedures can be done. Complications of PTCS include hemobilia, ductal injuries, catheter migration, and cholangitis with overall incidence are 5–50%.[43]

CONCLUSION

Percutaneous biliary procedures are well-established methods of management of patients with obstructive jaundice. PTBD and stenting offer a safe and effective method for the palliative treatment of malignant biliary obstruction. Newer intraluminal palliative techniques hold the promise of improvement in the patient's quality of life and improved stent patency rates. Percutaneous cholangioplasty is a safe and effective therapeutic procedure for benign biliary strictures. Percutaneous cholecystostomy is a lifesaving management option in critically ill patients.

REFERENCES

1. Molnar W, Stockum AC. Relief of obstructive jaundice through percutaneous transhepatic catheter—a new therapeutic method. AJR. 1974;122:356-67.
2. Ferrucci JT Jr, Mueller PR, Harbin WP. Percutaneous transhepatic biliary drainage: technique, results and applications. Radiology. 1980;135:1-13.
3. Mueller PR, Van Sonnenberg E, Ferrucci JT Jr. Percutaneous biliary drainage: Technical and catheter related problems in 200 procedures. AJR. 1982;138:17-23.
4. Hamy A, Visset J, Likholatnikov D, Lerat F, Gibaud H, Savigny B, et al. Percutaneous cholecystostomy for acute cholecystitis in critically ill patients. Surgery. 1997;121:398-404.
5. Lee KT, Wong SR, Cheng JS, Ker CG, Sheen PC, Liu YE. Ultrasound guided percutaneous cholecystostomy as an initial treatment for acute cholecystitis in elderly patients. Dig Surg. 1998;15:328-32.
6. Davis CA, Landercasper J, Gundrsen LH, Lambert PJ. Effective use of percutaneous cholecystostomy in high risk surgical patients: techniques, tube management, and results. Arch Surg. 1999;134:727-31.
7. van Delden OM, Laméris JS. Percutaneous drainage and stenting for palliation of malignant bile duct obstruction. Eur Radiol. 2008;18:448-56.
8. Saad WEA, Wallace MJ, WojakJC, Kundu S, Cardella JF. Quality improvement guidelines for percutaneous transhepatic cholangiography, biliary drainage, and percutaneous cholecystostomy. J Vasc Interv Radiol. 2010;21:789-95.
9. Tapping CR, Byass OR, Cast JEI. Percutaneous trans-hepaticbiliary drainage (PTBD) with or without stenting—complications, restentrate and a new risk stratification score. Eur Radiol. 2011;21:1948-55.
10. Madhusudan KS, Gamanagatti S, Srivastava DN, Gupta AK. Radiological interventions in malignant biliary obstruction. World J Radiol. 2016;8(5):518-29.
11. PuL ZCT, SinghR, Loong CK, de Moura EGH. Malignant biliary obstruction: Evidence for best practice. Gastroenterol Res Pract. 2016;2016:3296801.
12. Devane AM, Annam A, Brody L, Gunn AJ, Himes EA, Patel S, et al. Society of Interventional Radiology Quality Improvement Standards for Percutaneous Cholecystostomy and Percutaneous Transhepatic Biliary Interventions. J Vasc Interv Radiol. 2020;31(11):1849-56.
13. Feldman M, Friedman LS, Brandt LJ. Sleisenger and Fordtran's Gastrointestinal and Liver Disease, 9th edition. Philadelphia, PA: WB Saunders; 2010. pp. 323-35.
14. Rosenblatt M, Aruny JE, Kandarpa K. Transhepatic cholangiography, biliary decompression, endobiliary stenting and cholecystectomy. In: Kandarpa K, Aruny JE (Eds). Handbook of Interventional Radiologic procedures, 3rd edition. Philadelphia, PA: Lippincott Williams and Wilkins; 2002.
15. Fidelman N. Benign biliary strictures: Diagnostic evaluation and approaches to percutaneous treatment. Tech Vasc Interv Radiol. 2015;18(4):210-7.
16. Baijal SS, Dhiman RK, Gupta S, Sharma BC, Roy S, Agarwal DK, et al. Percutaneous transhepatic biliary drainage in the management of obstructive jaundice. Trop Gastroenterol. 1997;18:167-71.
17. Tsetis D, Krokidis M, Negru D, Prassopoulos P. Malignant biliary obstruction: the current role of interventional radiology. Ann Gastroenterol. 2016;29:33-6.
18. Shim DJ, Gwon DI, Han K, Kim Y, Ko GY, Shin JH, et al. Percutaneous Metallic Stent Placement for Palliative Management of Malignant Biliary Hilar Obstruction. Korean J Radiol. 2018;19(4):597-605.
19. Madhusudan KS, Gamanagatti S, Gupta AK. Imaging and interventional in hilar cholangiocarcinoma: A review. World J Radiol. 2015;7:28-44.
20. Kücükay F, Okten RS, Yurdakal M, Ozdemir E, Parlak E, Olçer T, et al. Percutaneous management of malignant biliary disease: factors influencing the ability to overcome the stricture. Diagn Interv Radiol. 2011;17:169-73.
21. Krokidis M, Hatzidakis A. Covered biliary stents with proximal bare stent extension for the palliation of malignant biliary disease: can we reduce tumour overgrowth rate? Ann Palliat Med. 2017;6(Suppl 1):58-S64.
22. Moss AC, Morris E, Mac Mathuna P. Palliative biliary stents for obstructing pancreatic carcinoma. Cochrane Database Syst Rev. 2006;CD004200.
23. Moss AC, Morris E, Leyden J, MacMathuna P. Do the benefits of metal stents justify the costs? A systematic review andmeta-analyses of trials comparing endoscopic stents for malignant biliary obstruction. Eur J Gastroenterol Heaptol. 2007;19:1119-24.
24. Mukai T, Yasuda I, Nakashima M, Doi S, Iwashita T, Iwata K, et al. Metallic stents are more efficacious than plastic stents in unresectable malignant hilar biliary strictures: a randomized controlled trial. J Hepatobiliary Pancreat Sci. 2013;20(2): 214-22.
25. Inal M, Akgül E, Aksungur E, Demiryürek H, Yağmur O. Percutaneous self-expandable uncovered metallic stents in malignant biliary obstruction. Complications, follow-up and re-interventions in 154 patients. Acta Radiol. 2003;44:139-46.
26. Sohn SH, Park JH, Kim KH, Kim TN. Complications and management of forgotten long-term biliary stents. World J Gastroenterol. 2017;23(4):622-8.
27. Gwon D, Ko G, Kim JH, Shin JH, Kim KA, Yoon HK, et al. Percutaneous bilateral metallic stent placement using a stent-in-stent deployment technique in patients with malignant hilar biliary obstruction. AJR. 2013;200:909-14.
28. Kim CW, Park AW, Won JW, Kim S, Lee JW, Lee SH. T-configured dual stent placement in malignant biliary hilar obstructionswith a newly designed stent. J Vasc Interv Radiol. 2004;15:713-7.
29. Gwon DI, Ko GY, Yoon HK, Kim YJ, Kim TH, Lee WH, et al. Safety and efficacy of percutaneous Y-configured covered stent placement for malignant hilar biliary obstruction: a prospective, pilot study. J Vasc Interv Radiol. 2012;23(4):528-34.
30. Xing GS, Geng JC, Han XW, Dai JH, Wu CY. Endobiliary brush cytology during percutaneous transhepatic cholangio drainage in patients with obstructive jaundice. Hepatobiliary Pancreat Dis Int. 2005;4:98-103.
31. Aggarwal R, Patel FD, Kapoor R, Kang M, Kumar P, Sharma S. Evaluation of high-dose rate intraluminal brachytherapy by percutaneous transhepatic biliary drainage in the palliative

management of malignant biliary obstruction—a pilot study. Brachytherapy. 2013;12:162-70.
32. Chen Y, Wang XL, Yan ZP, Cheng JM, Wang JH, Gong GQ, et al. HDR-192Ir intraluminal brachytherapy in treatment of malignant obstructive jaundice. World J Gastroenterol. 2004;10(23):3506-10.
33. Mizandari M, Pai M, Xi F, Valek V, Tomas A, Quaretti P, et al. Percutaneous intraductal radiofrequency ablation is a safe treatment for malignant biliary obstruction: feasibility and early results. Cardiovasc Intervent Radiol. 2013;36(3):814-9.
34. Lee TY, Cheon YK, Shim CS. Current status of photodynamic therapy for bile duct cancer. Clin Endosc. 2013;46:38-44.
35. Gwon DI, Ko GY, Ko HK, Yoon HK, Sung KB. Percutaneous transhepatic treatment using retrievable covered stents in patients with benign biliary strictures: mid-term outcomes in 68 patients. Dig Dis Sci. 2013;58(11):3270-9.
36. Boggi U, Di Candio G, Campatelli A, Oleggini M, Pietrabissa A, Filipponi F, et al. Percutaneous cholecystostomy for acute cholecystitis in critically ill patients. Hepatogastroenterology. 1999;46(25):121-5.
37. Kiviniemi H, Mäkelä JT, Autio R, Tikkakoski T, Leinonen S, Siniluoto T, et al. Percutaneous cholecystostomy in acute cholecystitis in high-risk patients: an analysis of 69 patients. Int Surg. 1998;83(4):299-302.
38. Hatjidakis AA, Karampekios S, Prassopoulos P, Xynos E, Raissaki M, Vasilakis SI, et al. Maturation of the tract after percutaneous cholecystostomy with regard to the access route. Cardiovasc Intervent Radiol. 1998;21(1):36-40.
39. Atar E, Khasminsky V, Friehmann T, Choen A, Bachar GN. Cystic Duct Embolization with Chemical Gallbladder Ablation for the Treatment of Acute Calculous Cholecystitis in High-Risk Patients: A Prospective Single-Center Study. J Vasc Interv Radiol. 2020;31(4):644-8.
40. Pang KW, Tan CH, Loh S, Chang KY, Iyer SG, Madhavan K, et al. Outcomes of Percutaneous Cholecystostomy for Acute Cholecystitis. World J Surg. 2016;40(11):2735-44.
41. Derdeyn J, Laleman W. Current role of endoscopic cholangioscopy. Curr Opin Gastroenterol. 2018;34:301-8.
42. Colombi D, Bodini FC, Morelli N, Aragona G, Ciatti C, Maniscalco P, et al. Spyglass percutaneous transhepatic lithotripsy of symptomatic recurrent lithiasis of the intrahepatic bile duct with distal stenosis. Acta Biomed. 2022;93(1):e2022020.
43. Gerges C, Vázquez AG, Tringali A, Verde JM, Dertmann T, Houghton E, et al. Percutaneous transhepatic cholangioscopy using a single-operator cholangioscope (pSOC), a retrospective, observational, multicenter study. Surg Endosc. 2021;35(12):6724-30.

SECTION

4

Pancreas

CHAPTER 18

Ankur Goyal, Sanchita Gupta, Raju Sharma

Acute Pancreatitis: Imaging and Interventions

INTRODUCTION

Acute pancreatitis (AP) is one of the most common indications for emergent hospital admissions globally[1] and has an incidence of 5–80 per 100,000 population worldwide. There is significant regional heterogeneity in the incidence of AP; however, a definite increasing trend globally has been seen over the past few years.[2] The clinical course of pancreatitis varies and can range from mild to severe life-threatening illness. Early diagnosis of AP and its associated complications can help reduce the morbidity and mortality associated with pancreatitis.

The revised Atlanta classification (RAC) was introduced in 2012 to clarify the ambiguities of the 1992 original Atlanta classification for AP. It defines the criteria for diagnosing AP, differentiates the types of AP [interstitial edematous pancreatitis (IEP) and necrotizing pancreatitis], classifies the disease based on severity, and defines the morphology of pancreatic and peripancreatic collections. Previously (mis)used and ambiguous terms such as pancreatic abscess, acute pseudocyst, and phlegmon have been discarded by the new classification and replaced by standard terminology.

The radiologist is a core multidisciplinary team member managing AP. Knowledge of current clinical terminology, associated complications, and interventional techniques is essential for appropriate and timely disease management.

ETIOLOGY AND PATHOPHYSIOLOGY

Gallstones account for the majority of cases (40%) of AP globally, followed by regular excessive alcohol consumption (30%). Hypertriglyceridemia is the third most common cause. Less frequent causes of AP are postendoscopic retrograde cholangiopancreatography (ERCP), hypercalcemia, tumors, drugs, pancreas divisum, and hereditary causes. Up to 20% of cases of AP may have no identifiable cause and are termed "idiopathic pancreatitis", the majority of which are a result of microliths. Addressing the etiological factor is essential to prevent recurrent attacks of AP. Certain gene mutations like those of cationic trypsinogen (PRSS1), pancreatic secretory trypsin inhibitor (PSTI/SPINK1), and cystic fibrosis transmembrane conductance regulator (CFTR) may lead to recurrent attacks of pancreatitis.[3]

Increased ductal pressure due to obstruction and acinar cell injury (due to alcohol, drugs, and toxins) leads to intracellular activation of trypsinogen and other proteolytic enzymes within acinar cells (instead of the pancreatic duct), which is the main inciting event for the development of AP. Destructive enzymes lead to local complications of pancreatic necrosis, while the release of inflammatory mediators leads to systemic complications.

CLINICAL PERSPECTIVE

Diagnosis

The RAC requires two out of the following three criteria to be present for establishing a diagnosis of AP:[4]

1. Persistent epigastric abdominal pain radiating to the back
2. Raised serum amylase and/or lipase more than three times upper limit of normal (ULN) and
3. Typical findings on imaging

Serum lipase is more specific for diagnosing AP than amylase due to its relative organ specificity. Moreover, blood lipase levels remain elevated for up to 2 weeks from symptom onset (compared to 3–5 days for serum amylase) **(Fig. 1)**. Serum amylase levels may be falsely low in patients with alcoholic pancreatitis, hypertriglyceridemia, and delayed presentation. This results in greater diagnostic sensitivity of blood lipase for diagnosing AP than a similar

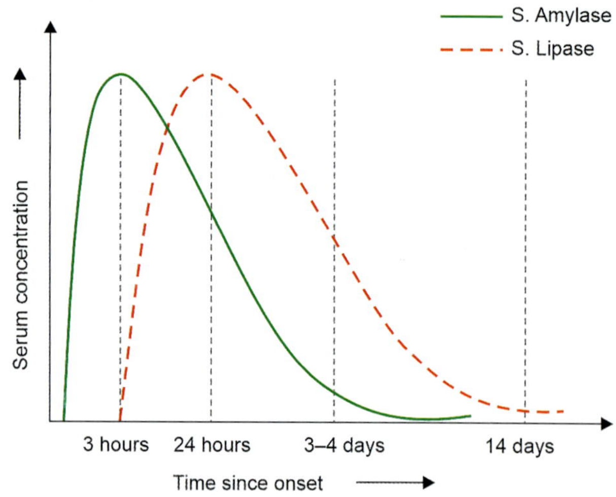

FIG. 1: Serum concentration of pancreatic enzymes with time since onset of symptoms.

TABLE 1: Causes of falsely elevated pancreatic enzymes.

False elevation of pancreatic enzymes	
Reduced clearance	• Renal impairment • Macrolipase • Complex formation with IgG and IgA
Intra-abdominal diseases	• Bowel perforation • Cholangitis • Post-ERCP • Intra-abdominal hemorrhage • Neoplasms • Nonpathological pancreatic hyperenzymemia
Critical illness	• Traumatic brain injury • Multisystem trauma
Drugs	• Alcohol • Morphine

(ERCP: endoscopic retrograde cholangiopancreatography; IgA: immunoglobulin A)

elevation of amylase (64–100% vs. 45–87%).[5] Pancreatic enzymes may be falsely elevated in various clinical scenarios **(Table 1)**. However, elevation in such cases is generally less than three times the ULN.

Stages

The *early stage* of AP is less than a week from symptom onset, while *late AP* is more than a week from the onset of symptoms. The cytokine cascade is activated in the early stage, and thus, the treatment involves supportive care and management of organ failure. Imaging findings do not correlate well with the clinical severity in the early stage of the disease.

The late stage can last for weeks and occurs only in patients with moderately severe AP (MSAP) or severe AP (SAP). Imaging is an essential determinant of patient management in this stage.

Recurrent AP is described as two or more well-documented separate attacks of AP with complete resolution of symptoms in between with an interval of >3 months between the attacks. Up to 20% of patients with AP may develop RAP, and >30% of the latter may go on to develop chronic pancreatitis.[6]

Subtypes (Based on the Presence of Necrosis)

Acute pancreatitis is divided into two subtypes—(1) IEP and (2) necrotizing pancreatitis, depending on the presence of necrosis. Early and accurate categorization of AP is essential for management and prognostication. IEP is a mild, self-limiting disease, whereas necrotizing pancreatitis is an ominous condition associated with significant morbidity and occasional mortality.

Subtypes (Based on Severity)

As per RAC, AP can be divided into three categories based on severity:

1. *Mild AP*: No organ failure and no local/systemic complications are seen in this category.
2. *Moderately severe AP*: Transient organ failure (lasting < 48 hours) and/or local/systemic complications are associated with this type. Local complications are defined as one of the following—peripancreatic fluid collections, pancreatic and peripancreatic necrosis (sterile or infected), pseudocyst, walled-off necrosis (WONs) (sterile or infected), gastric outlet dysfunction, splenic and portal vein thrombosis, and colonic necrosis. Pancreatitis-related collections usually develop in the second week (late phase) and are suspected in patients with unrelenting pain, rising pancreatic enzymes, organ dysfunction, and sepsis. Systemic complications include pleural effusion, acute respiratory distress syndrome, hyperglycemia, hypocalcemia, coagulopathy, encephalopathy, sepsis, and multiorgan failure along with worsening of comorbidities (such as coronary artery disease or chronic obstructive pulmonary disease) that is precipitated by AP.
3. *Severe AP*: Persistent organ failure (>48 hours) and/or local/systemic complications are the features of this type.

Organ failure can be assessed by the modified Marshall multiple organ dysfunction score (MODS) or sequential organ failure assessment (SOFA) score.

Mild cases of AP show rapid recovery with conservative management and early discharge, frequently within a week. Severe cases are associated with high morbidity and mortality with a requirement for early intensive care. Body mass index (>25 kg/m^2) and hyperglycemia (blood glucose level higher than 200 mg/dL) have been linked with a risk of severe disease.[7]

TABLE 2: Systemic inflammatory response syndrome (SIRS) criteria.

Two or more of the following criteria		
Body temperature	–	>38°C or < 36°C
Tachypnea	–	Respiratory rate > 20 breaths/min or, $PaCO_2$ < 32 mm Hg
Heart rate	–	>90 beats/min
WBC count	–	>12,000/mm^3, or <4,000/mm^3, or >10% immature neutrophils (band forms)

The determinant-based classification (DBC) of AP was developed in 2012 and is similar to the RAC; however, it is less commonly used. It classifies AP as mild, moderate, severe, or critical based on local determinants (sterile or infected necrosis) and/or systemic determinants (transient or persistent organ failure).[8]

Several different scoring systems, such as Ranson's score, modified Glasgow score, bedside index for severity in AP (BISAP), harmless AP score (HAPS), and acute physiology and chronic health evaluation II (APACHE II), have been developed over the years to determine the severity of AP. However, most of these scoring systems are time-consuming and complex, limiting usage in an emergency. The International Association of Pancreatology (IAP)/American Pancreatic Association (APA) guidelines recommend using the presence of persistent SIRS (systemic inflammatory response syndrome) criteria **(Table 2)** at admission and at 48 hours of hospitalization for predicting severe AP.[9] All of the other complex scoring systems show no definite superiority over the presence of persistent SIRS for predicting the severity of AP.

IMAGING

The diagnosis of AP is predominantly clinical—typical abdominal pain with raised amylase and lipase levels. However, an ultrasound is always done in a suspected case of AP to rule out other causes. Atypical abdominal pain or borderline elevated amylase and lipase levels in the presence of nondiagnostic ultrasound may require a contrast-enhanced CT (CECT) to confirm the diagnosis **(Flowcharts 1 and 2)**.

Imaging helps to:

- Exclude other causes of acute abdominal pain in atypical clinical scenarios
- It can help determine the etiology of pancreatitis.
- Assess severity [modified CT severity index (CTSI)]
- Assess for any complications
- In cases that fail to respond to conservative treatment/show clinical worsening/or are planned for invasive intervention.

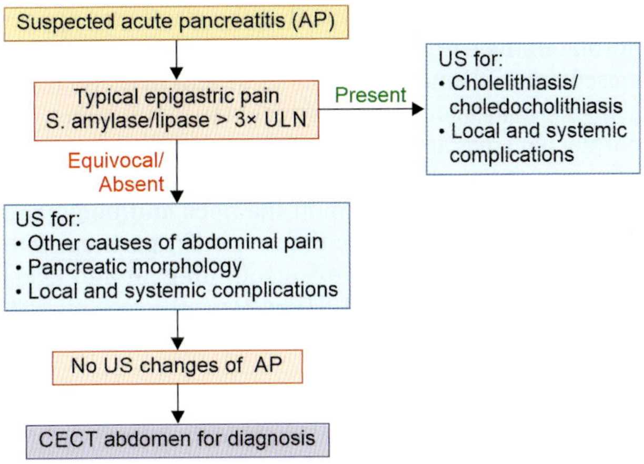

FLOWCHART 1: Algorithm for imaging during an episode of suspected acute pancreatitis.

(CECT: contrast-enhanced computed tomography; ULN: upper limit of normal)

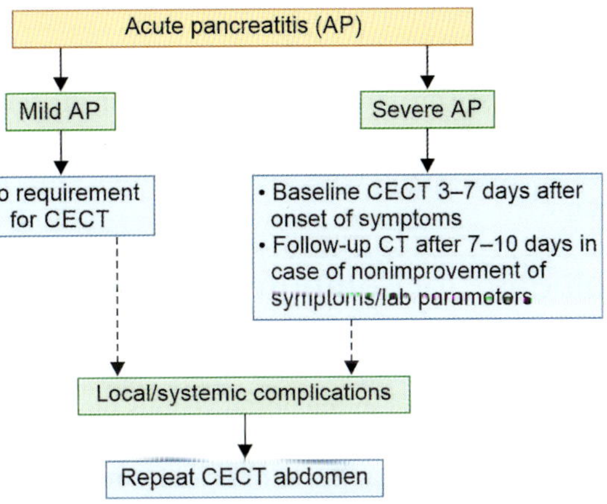

FLOWCHART 2: Role of imaging in the management of acute pancreatitis.

(CECT: contrast-enhanced computed tomography)

Radiographs

Conventional radiographs are neither sensitive nor specific for the diagnosis of AP. However, they may be performed in the emergency for patients presenting with acute abdominal pain. Local inflammation during AP may lead to focal ileus of a jejunal loop in the upper abdomen (sentinel loop sign) or air in the duodenal C-loop or the colon at the splenic flexure (colon cut off), appearing as a distended proximal bowel loop with abrupt termination of bowel gas distal to the site of inflammation. Loss of the left psoas shadow, ascites, or a gasless abdomen may also be seen on abdominal radiographs. Pleural effusion especially left-sided with adjacent atelectasis may also be seen in severe cases of AP on chest radiographs.[10] Radiographs help assess the position of ductal stents and any calcified gallstones.

Ultrasound

It is generally the first-line imaging modality for evaluating acute abdominal pain. The role of US in detecting the early stages of the AP is limited as the gland may appear normal in the early or mild cases of AP.[11] Panniculitis of mesenteric and omental fat with focal ileus may also result in poor visualization of the pancreas in such situations. The normal pancreas appears isoechoic to slightly hypoechoic compared to the adjacent hepatic parenchyma, measuring <3 cm at the head, <2.5 cm at the neck and body, and <2 cm at the tail.[12] Focally or diffusely bulky pancreas with a hypoechoic (compared to surrounding fat and liver) edematous appearance on US **(Fig. 2)** may be seen in ~20% of cases of AP.[13] Extrapancreatic fluid collections may be seen on US later in the disease.

Most importantly, ultrasound can help evaluate the presence of cholelithiasis and choledocholithiasis, which are responsible for most AP cases. Complications of pancreatitis, such as acute collections, ascites, and pleural effusion, may be seen. Pleural effusions may be seen in >30% of cases of AP and are more extensive in SAP.[14] Splenic or portal vein thrombosis can also be seen on Doppler ultrasound.

The percentage of debris within necrotic collections can be assessed on ultrasound which helps in the selection of either plastic stent (<30% debris) or lumen-apposing metal stents (LAMS) (>30% debris) during endoscopic therapy.[15]

Multidetector Computer Tomography

Contrast-enhanced multidetector CT (MDCT) is the workhorse of imaging in AP. A single-phase CECT with intravenous contrast in the portal venous phase (60–70s) is sufficient for diagnosing AP and assessing pancreatic necrosis and local complications. Additional pancreatic phase is recommended in a few guidelines; however, it may overestimate necrosis.[9] Dual-phase CECT in the arterial and portal venous phase may be required in cases of gastrointestinal (GI) bleeding or bleeding from drainage catheters for assessment of additional vascular complications. CT is also recommended to exclude malignancy if the first episode of pancreatitis occurs in patients >40 years of age without any identifiable cause. An optimal choice may be the pancreatic phase (40s from the start of contrast injection or 20s after trigger) of the upper abdomen for arterial complications and pancreatic necrosis/tumors, followed by portal venous phase (65s from the start of contrast injection or 20s after the first acquisition) of the entire abdomen and pelvis.

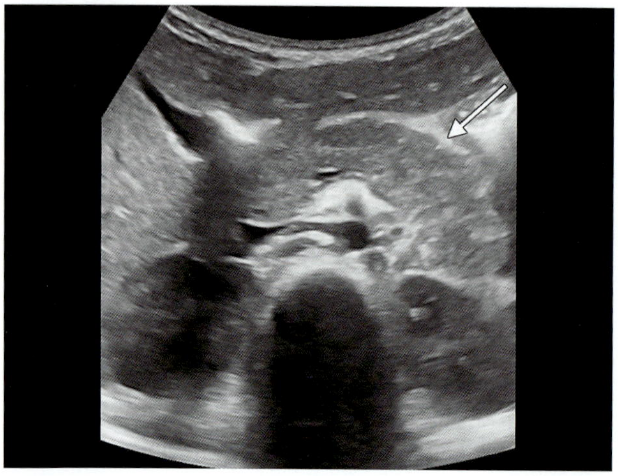

FIG. 2: *Appearance of acute pancreatitis on ultrasound.* Transverse US image demonstrates a hypoechoic, bulky, and edematous pancreatic body and tail (white arrow) with loss of pancreatic lobulations and mild peripancreatic fluid.

The CECT for grading the severity of AP (in cases of SAP) may be performed only after 72 hours have elapsed from the onset of symptoms (even better if performed after 5–7 days of the onset of symptoms).[13] An early CECT may underestimate the extent of necrosis (as necrosis evolves and becomes more demarcated and confluent as time progresses). Also, the fluid collections generally form in the second week. Moreover, the internal heterogeneity of a acute necrotic collections (ANCs) may be better appreciated in the second week. If the diagnosis is uncertain, CECT may be performed at the presentation, mainly to rule out other causes of acute abdomen. In case of SAP, CT may be repeated after a week to grade the severity of pancreatitis.

Interstitial Edematous Pancreatitis

It is more common and represents inflammation of the pancreas without any associated necrosis. On CECT, focal or diffuse enlargement of the pancreas is seen with homogenous enhancement without focal areas of hypoenhancement **(Figs. 3A and B)**. Due to edema, the inflamed pancreas may enhance less avidly than the normally expected enhancement, but there are no areas of necrosis (nonenhancement). Peripancreatic inflammatory changes usually track along the pancreatic tail and left pararenal space and appear as fat stranding, thickening of anterior and posterior perinephric fascia, and free fluid. Loss of surface lobulations may be the only sign of mild forms of IEP. Peripancreatic changes are more pronounced compared to the pancreatic changes in IEP.

Necrotizing Pancreatitis

It can be seen in up to 20% of patients with AP. There are three subtypes of necrotizing pancreatitis based on the site of necrosis:

1. Pancreatic parenchymal necrosis only—5%
2. Extrapancreatic necrosis only—20%
3. Both pancreatic and extrapancreatic necrosis—most common (75%)

Pancreatic necrosis appears as nonenhancing areas (<30 HU) within the parenchyma. These become better demarcated and more hypodense after the first week of illness, thus becoming easier to identify. In contrast, extrapancreatic necrosis is seen as nonenhancing heterogeneous collections in the peripancreatic region with a propensity to accumulate in the lesser sac and the anterior pararenal space. Extrapancreatic necrosis refers to

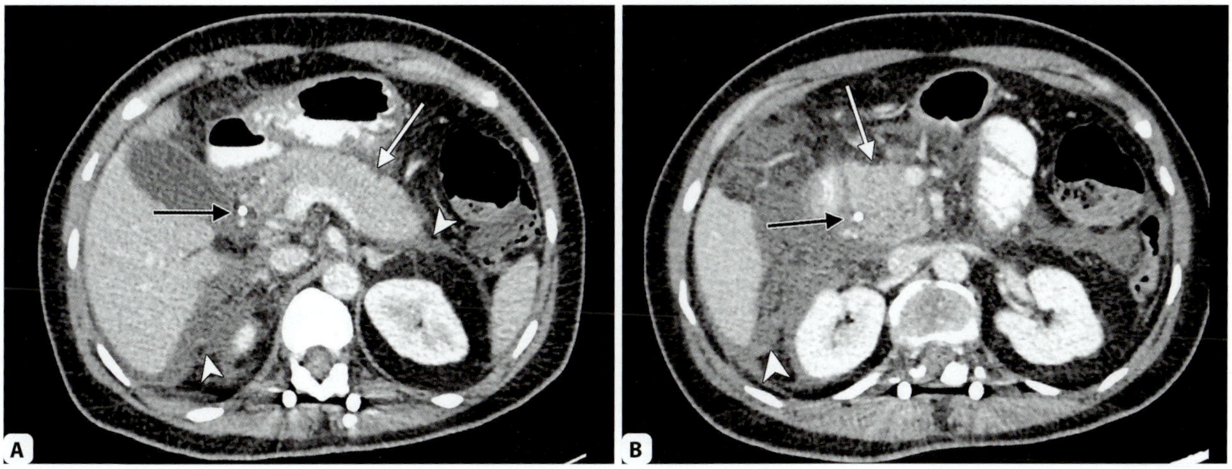

FIGS. 3A AND B: Acute interstitial pancreatitis on CECT abdomen. Axial CECT images in the portal venous phase in a 32-year-old female with post-ERCP pancreatitis show a bulky and edematous pancreas (white arrows) with acute peripancreatic fluid collection (APFC) in the retroperitoneum (white arrowheads). Note made of common bile duct (CBD) stent in situ (black arrows).

the areas of fat and tissue necrosis in the surroundings and may extend into the paracolic gutters and the pelvis **(Figs. 4A to D)**.

Balthazar developed the CTSI as a 10-point scoring system to assess the severity of pancreatitis based on CT findings.[16] Poor interobserver agreement, noninclusion of organ failure, and extrapancreatic complications along with no difference in mortality between patients > 50% and between 30 and 50% led to the development of the modified CTSI by Mortele et al., which is a simplified extension of the CTSI.[17] The *modified CTSI* incorporates organ failure and extrapancreatic complications and gives a total score out of 10 **(Table 3)**. The quantification of pancreatic necrosis may be based on the rough guide that the head constitutes 50% while the body and tail constitute 25% of the pancreatic parenchyma each. Another scoring system relies on assessing extrapancreatic inflammation on (noncontrast) CT (EPIC), based on the evaluation of pleural effusion, ascites, and retroperitoneal fluid collections to predict mortality due to AP.[18]

The CT must be used judiciously since many patients with severe pancreatitis are exposed to radiation doses of >24–30 millisieverts in a single admission. This is because they are imaged at multiple time points for severity assessment, image-guided interventions, and multiphasic examinations are commonly performed.[19]

Magnetic Resonance Imaging (MRI)

While CT is the primary modality for assessing AP, magnetic resonance imaging (MRI) with MRCP may be a helpful alternative/adjunct to CT in the following situations:

- Noncontrast MRI scans have a similar sensitivity for the detection of pancreatic and peripancreatic necrosis and hemorrhage compared to CECT, a valuable attribute in patients with renal failure or contrast allergy.[20] Necrosis is seen as T2 dark areas, whereas fluid is T2 bright.
- MRI may be better in detecting early/mild interstitial pancreatitis (loss of typical T1 hyperintensity and presence of T2 hyperintensity and diffusion restriction). Reduced/absent enhancement may better identify areas of necrosis **(Figs. 5A to D)**.
- MRI provides a radiation-free method for evaluating patients requiring repeat imaging for follow-up, especially in the pediatric age group.
- MRCP can help evaluate the biliary system (especially the distal bile duct for choledocholithiasis) and the pancreatic duct morphology (pancreatic divisum, abnormal pancreaticobiliary junction)—identifying the etiology of the AP.

In the acute setting, MRCP may help to determine the patients needing urgent ERCP for clearance of lower common bile duct (CBD) calculus. Urgent ERCP is recommended in cases of biliary pancreatitis with biliary obstruction and/or cholangitis.[21,22] ERCP can detect calculi only in approximately 50% of patients with biliary dilatation on US/CT. This may be because obstruction is usually transient and gets resolved spontaneously. MRCP and endoscopic ultrasound (EUS) are more accurate than US/CT for detecting choledocholithiasis.

- Diffusion-weighted MR imaging may help in the detection of early inflammation and infection.[23,24]

The MR severity index (MRSI) assesses peripancreatic inflammation and pancreatic necrosis similar to CTSI by Balthazar et al. and is comparable to the CTSI for determining the severity of AP.[25]

New Techniques for Diagnosis of Acute Pancreatitis

Diffusion-weighted imaging (DWI) measures the diffusion of water molecules within biological tissue. Pancreatic and

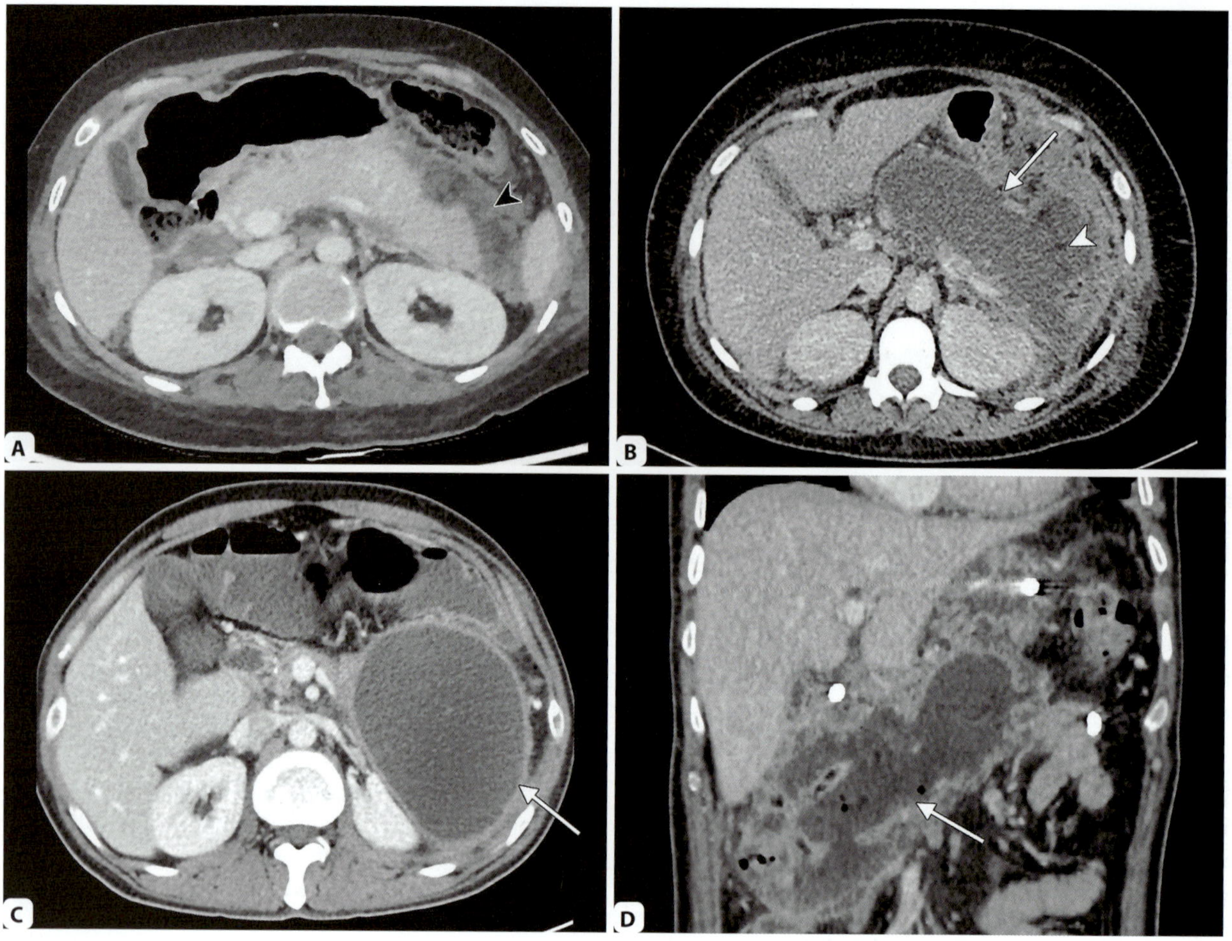

FIGS. 4A TO D: CECT appearance of collections associated with acute pancreatitis. (A) Axial CECT image in the portal venous phase in a 40-year-old male with alcohol-related acute pancreatitis shows acute peripancreatic necrotic collection (black arrowhead). (B) Axial CECT image in the portal venous phase in a 44-year-old male with alcohol-related acute pancreatitis shows near complete replacement of the pancreatic body and tail with an ill-defined acute necrotic pancreatic collection (ANPC) extending into the lesser sac. Note the ill-defined areas of fat attenuation (arrowhead) within the collection consistent with peripancreatic fat necrosis; (C) Axial CECT image in the portal venous phase in a 34-year-old female with gallstone-associated acute pancreatitis shows a well-defined, encapsulated hypodense collection in the region of the pancreatic tail suggestive of pseudocyst (arrow). (D) Coronal CECT image in the venous phase in a 44-year-old male demonstrates a well-encapsulated, heterogeneous collection in the peripancreatic region (arrow) suggestive of walled-off necrosis (WON). Numerous foci of air are also seen within the collection implying secondary infection.

TABLE 3: Modified CT severity index (CTSI).

	0	2	4
Pancreatic inflammation	Normal pancreas	Intrinsic pancreatic abnormality ± peripancreatic fat inflammation	Pancreatic/peripancreatic fluid collection or peripancreatic fat necrosis
Pancreatic necrosis	None	≤30%	≥30%
Extrapancreatic complications*	Absent	Present	
Mild pancreatitis: Modified CTSI score 0–2			
Moderate pancreatitis: Modified CTSI score 4–6			
Severe pancreatitis: Modified CTSI score 8–10			

*Pleural effusion, ascites, vascular complications, parenchymal complications, and gastrointestinal tract involvement.

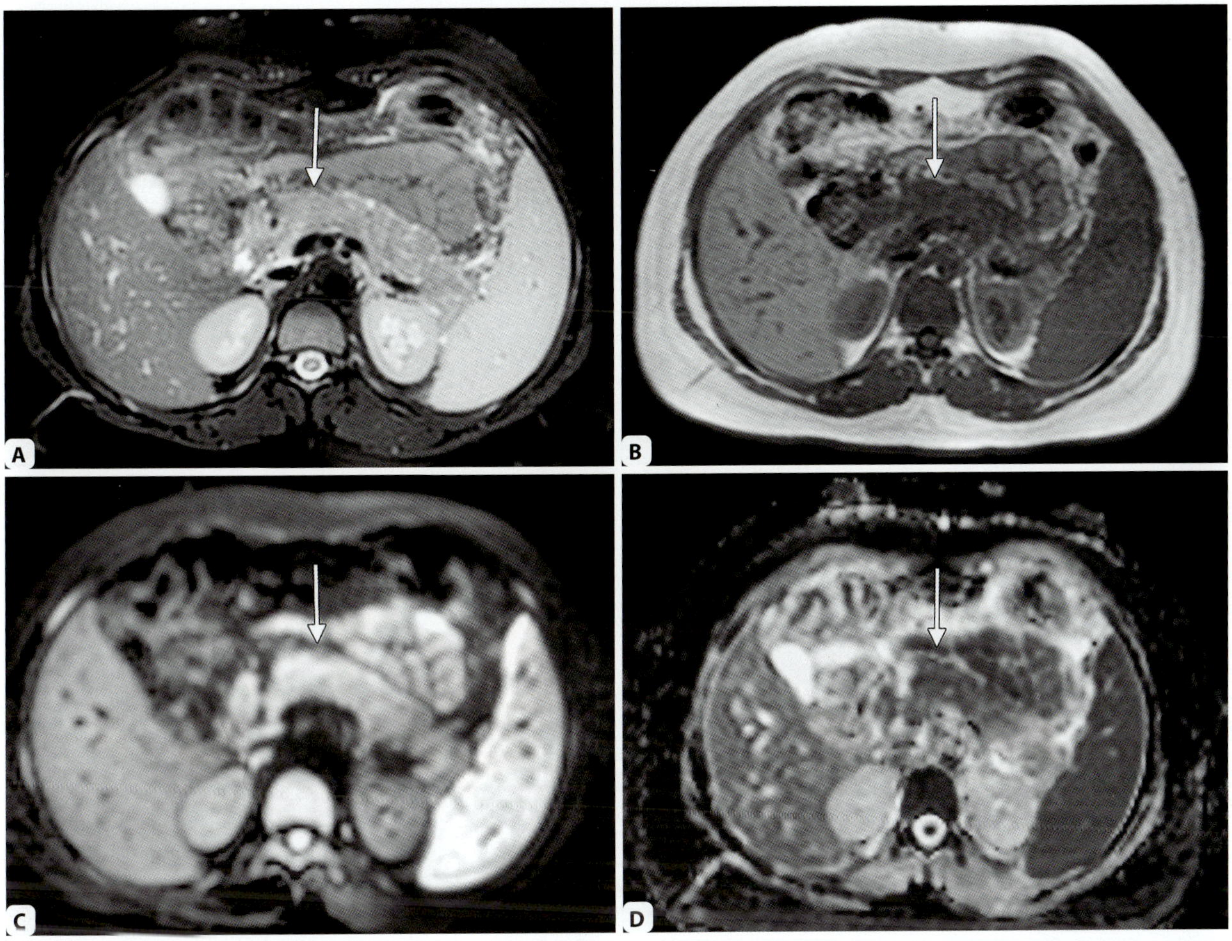

FIGS. 5A TO D: MR appearance of acute interstitial pancreatitis. T2W MR image (A) in a 32-year-old female with gallstone-induced acute pancreatitis demonstrates a hyperintense and bulky pancreatic head and body (arrow on all images), which appear hypointense on T1WI (B) showing restricted diffusion on DWI (C) and ADC images (D).

peripancreatic inflammation in AP restricts this movement, consequently increasing the signal on DWI and low values on apparent diffusion coefficient (ADC) compared to normal pancreas. It can help determine areas of pancreatic necrosis in severely ill patients with contraindications to IV contrast. Infected collections also show more restricted diffusion and lower ADC values than sterile collections.[24]

Contrast-enhanced US (CEUS) shows higher diagnostic accuracy compared to conventional US for the diagnosis of AP and SAP, with results comparable to those of CECT for the detection of necrosis. It may be used as a nonionizing and safe imaging alternative.[26] However, nonvisualization of the entire pancreas due to bowel gas is a deterrent.

Unlike conventional CT, which frequently underestimates the presence of pancreatic necrosis during the early stages of AP, perfusion defects on perfusion CT show a high sensitivity and specificity of 87.5% and 100%, respectively, for predicting the development of pancreatic necrosis in scans done within 72 hours of symptom onset **(Figs. 6A to F)**.[27]

New research evaluating the role of T1 and T2 mapping in chronic pancreatitis and autoimmune pancreatitis is underway, which may aid in the diagnosis and prognostication of AP.

Radiomics and the development of artificial neural networks may help identify additional features for diagnosing and prognosticating AP that the human eye may not appreciate. Multiple radiomics models based on imaging have been developed to predict the severity of AP during the early disease process,[24] the possibility of the development of new complications,[25] and the risk of recurrence of AP after the first episode.[28]

COMPLICATIONS OF ACUTE PANCREATITIS

Pancreatic and Peripancreatic Collections

These are the most common complications associated with AP. Collections refer to fluid accumulations which

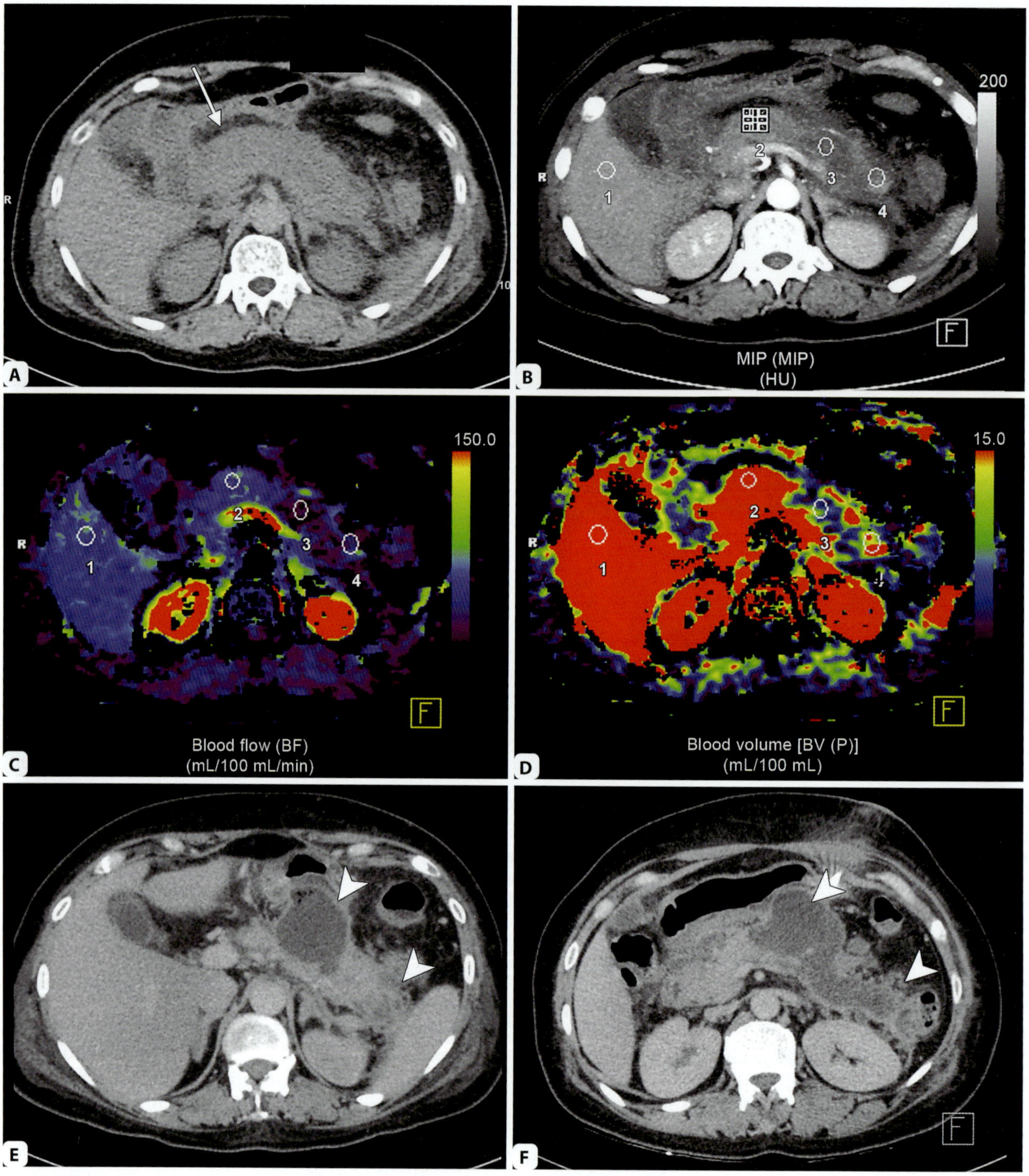

FIGS. 6A TO F: Early prediction of pancreatic necrosis using perfusion CT. Axial CT image (A) in a 45-year-old female with acute pancreatitis at <72 hours of symptom onset shows a diffusely bulky pancreas (white arrow) with surrounding inflammatory changes. MIP (B), blood flow (C) and blood volume (D) images of the pancreas show multiple perfusion defects throughout the pancreatic parenchyma (ROIs 2-4 in pancreas, ROI 1 in liver). Follow-up CECT at 3 weeks (E) and 6 weeks (F) demonstrates development of extensive pancreatic necrosis (arrowheads) in the corresponding areas of perfusion defects.

are different from fat stranding. The common sites include the lesser sac, anterior pararenal space, paracolic gutters, transverse mesocolon, and mesentery. The RAC differentiates collections based on the presence or absence of necrotic debris within and time since the onset of symptoms (<4 weeks or >4 weeks) because the latter corresponds to the formation of a wall around these collections **(Figs. 7A to D and Table 3)**. The time limit of 4 weeks serves as an important guide, but the actual morphology is more important, and the presence of a

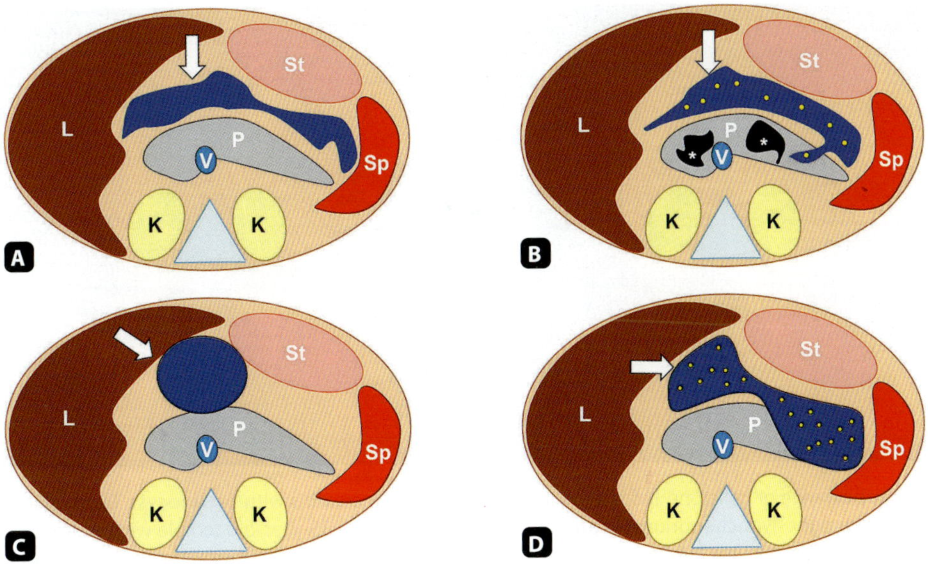

FIGS. 7A TO D: Collections associated with acute pancreatitis. (A) Acute peripancreatic fluid collection (APFC) (arrow) with no definite wall formation. (B) Acute necrotizing fluid collection (ANFC) (arrow) with no definite wall and areas of intrapancreatic pancreatic necrosis (asterisk); (C) Pseudocyst with a well-defined capsule. (D) Walled-off necrosis (WON) (arrow) with internal debris (yellow dots) and replacing the pancreatic tail.

(L: liver; Sp: spleen; St: stomach; P: pancreas; V: portal vein; K: kidney)

well-formed wall on CT/MRI is more definitive for the distinction of these collections.

Less than 4 weeks:

- *Acute fluid collection*: Associated with acute edematous pancreatitis, with no well-defined wall
- *Acute necrotic fluid collection*: Associated with necrotic pancreatitis, with no well-defined wall

More than 4 weeks:

- *Pseudocysts*: Associated with acute edematous pancreatitis, with a well-defined wall
- *Walled-off necrosis (WON)*: Associated with necrotizing pancreatitis, with a well-defined wall

Acute peripancreatic fluid collection (APFC) may develop in patients with IEP in the first 4 weeks. On CECT, they appear as ill-defined hypodense homogeneous fluid collections with no obvious wall formation or internal debris. Most APFCs are sterile and resolve without any intervention.

Nonresolution of APFCs beyond 4 weeks can result in the development of *pseudocysts*, which are well-defined fluid collections with a conspicuous capsule surrounding the collections. Most APFCs (>50%) and pseudocysts resolve spontaneously. When persistent, symptoms may develop due to secondary infection, hemorrhage within the collection, mass effect, or rupture. APFC and pseudocysts, by definition, are extrapancreatic, and any intrapancreatic collection is considered to be necrotic. The only exception is when the pancreatic duct is disrupted since pancreatic juice leakage can also form intrapancreatic pseudocyst **(Figs. 8A and B)**.[29]

Unusual extensions of pancreatic pseudocysts: Pseudocysts are mainly found in the retroperitoneum due to leakage of pancreatic enzymes. These pseudocysts may extend into the mediastinum through the aortic or esophageal hiatus leading to the formation of a posterior mediastinal mass lesion. Dissection of a pancreatic pseudocyst into the splenic hilum may result in an intrasplenic pseudocyst **(Figs. 9A and B)**.

Acute necrotic collections (ANC) are seen within the first 4 weeks of necrotizing pancreatitis. They are ill-defined, heterogeneous collections with no obvious capsule formation. The presence of hyperdensity, heterogeneity, linear stranding, and interspersed fat attenuation (due to fat necrosis) within the collection may help differentiate ANC from APFCs. This internal heterogeneity is better perceived in the second week of illness. Even the homogeneous-appearing peripancreatic collections, in the presence of pancreatic necrosis, should be labelled as ANC. These heterogeneity criteria for diagnosing peripancreatic collections as acute necrotic ones are subjective and not uniform.[30] Sometimes, the distinction between APFC and ANC may not be definitive, especially in the early phase, and the term "indeterminate peripancreatic collections" may be used for such scenarios. Repeat imaging after a week may better achieve this distinction.

Peripancreatic necrotic collections can be classified into limited and diffuse. Limited refers to small collections < 5 cm confined to the peripancreatic region, while "diffuse" suggests extension into paracolic gutters and pelvis or three or more regions.[31]

The ANCs develop into *WONs* after 4 weeks of illness. WONs are organized collections with a thick enhancing

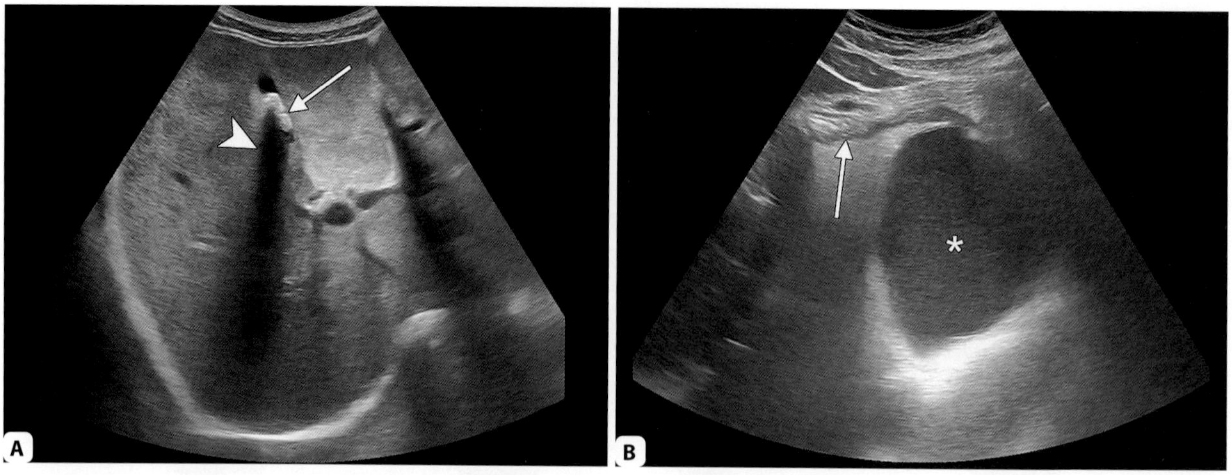

FIGS. 8A AND B: US appearance of gallstone-associated acute interstitial pancreatitis with pseudocyst. Transverse US images with the curvilinear probe at the right hypochondrium (A) and the epigastrium (B) in a 35-year-old female with acute pancreatitis in the 5th week of illness. (A) An echogenic calculus (white arrow) with posterior acoustic shadowing (arrowhead) in the contracted gallbladder lumen. (B) A well-defined fluid collection with posterior acoustic enhancement (asterisk) and no internal debris is seen in the lesser sac abutting the posterior wall of the stomach (white arrow in B) suggestive of pseudocyst.

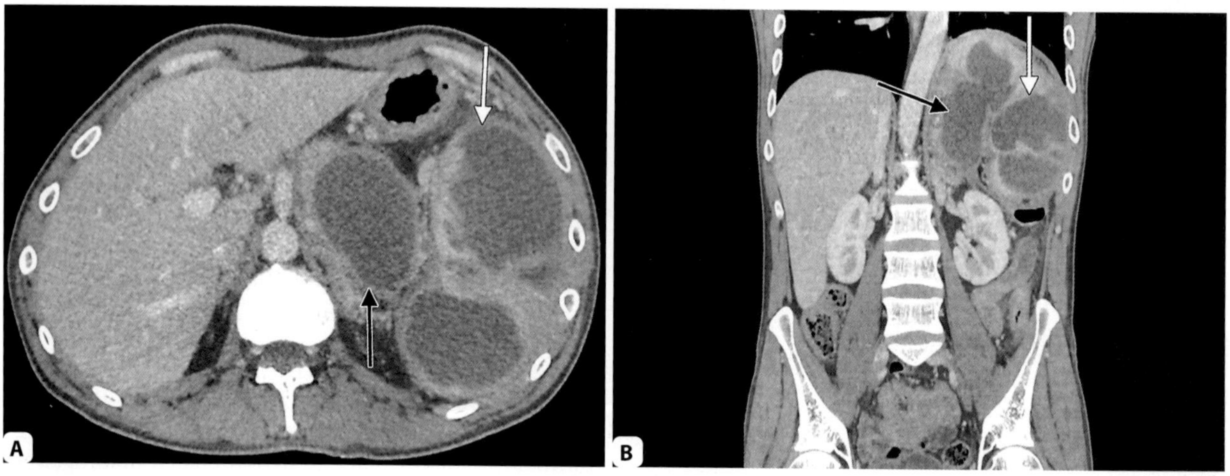

FIGS. 9A AND B: Intrasplenic extension of pancreatic pseudocyst. CECT images of the abdomen in the axial (A) and coronal (B) plane in a 35-year-old patient with acute on chronic pancreatitis show a thick-walled fluid attenuation collection abutting the pancreatic tail and splenic hilum (black arrows) suggestive of a pseudocyst. Multiple similar fluid attenuation collections are also seen extending within splenic parenchyma (white arrows).

capsule and internal debris in the pancreatic parenchyma or the peripancreatic region. WONs may appear as homogenous collections on CT, which may underestimate the associated internal debris and solid components. The presence or absence of pancreatic necrosis at the onset of pancreatitis may help differentiate WONs from pseudocysts **(Figs. 10 to 13)**.[32] Imaging features favoring WON over pseudocyst include presence of any solid/fat component, increase in size, irregular borders, pancreatic involvement, and extension to paracolic regions.[32] Pancreatic ductal dilatation (>3 mm) favors pseudocyst over WON. MRI and US are better for quantifying internal debris prior to percutaneous or endoscopic drainage. The areas of necrosis appear as echogenic debris and hypointense debris within the T2 hyperintense fluid collections.

Secondary infection of peripancreatic fluid collections: Necrotic collections [acute necrotizing pancreatitis (ANP) and WON] are more prone to superadded infections compared to APFCs and pseudocysts. Clinical signs of infection such as fever, raised leukocyte counts, and persistently high SIRS are useful. Imaging is not sensitive since the only sign of infection on CECT is the presence of mottled air foci **(Figs. 14A and B)**. Air foci may also be seen within a collection due to an enteric communication or postdrainage. Serum procalcitonin is the most sensitive laboratory test with a high negative predictive value for detecting pancreatic infections.[22]

Fine needle aspiration cytology (FNAC) may be performed for microbiological analysis of infected collections in cases of nonresponse to empirical antibiotics; however,

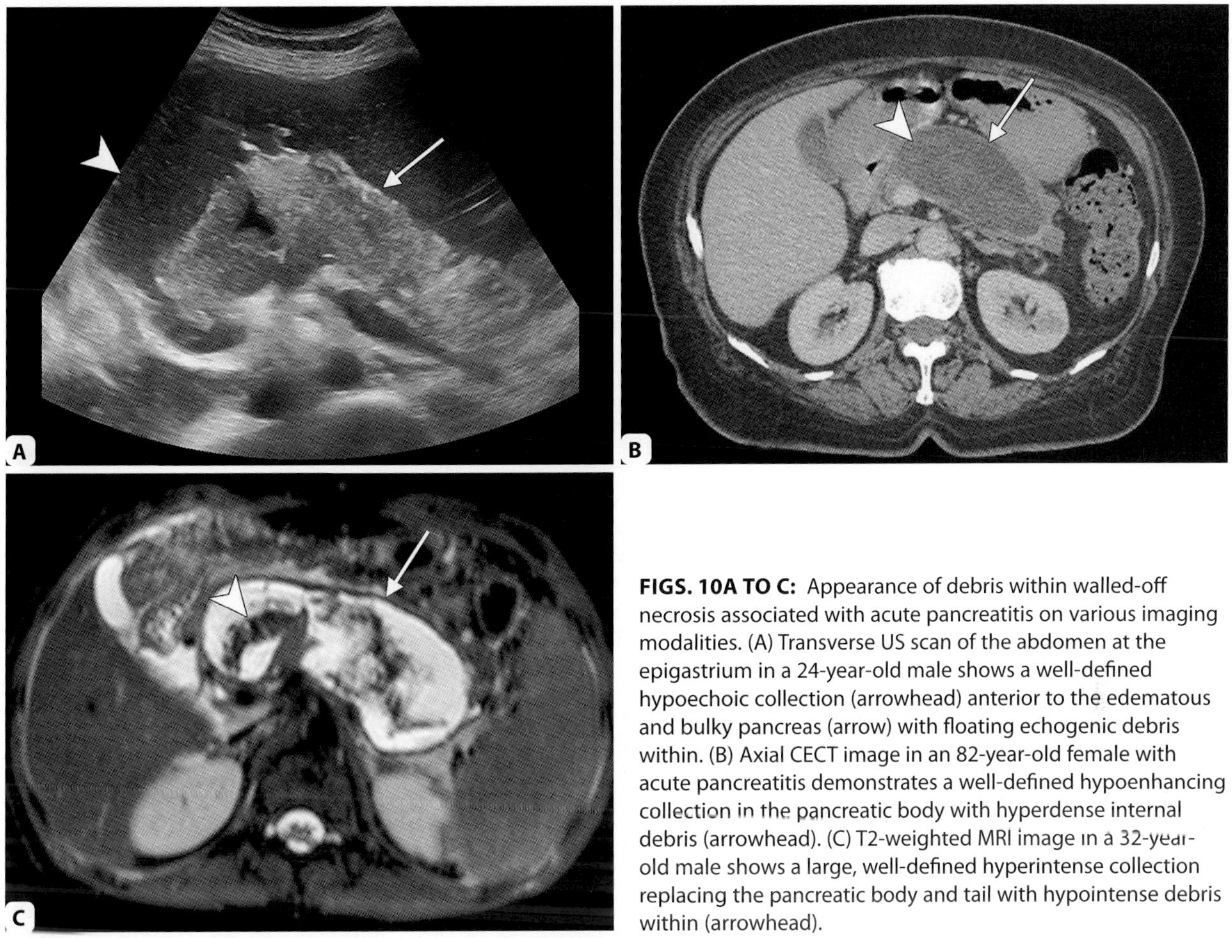

FIGS. 10A TO C: Appearance of debris within walled-off necrosis associated with acute pancreatitis on various imaging modalities. (A) Transverse US scan of the abdomen at the epigastrium in a 24-year-old male shows a well-defined hypoechoic collection (arrowhead) anterior to the edematous and bulky pancreas (arrow) with floating echogenic debris within. (B) Axial CECT image in an 82-year-old female with acute pancreatitis demonstrates a well-defined hypoenhancing collection in the pancreatic body with hyperdense internal debris (arrowhead). (C) T2-weighted MRI image in a 32-year-old male shows a large, well-defined hyperintense collection replacing the pancreatic body and tail with hypointense debris within (arrowhead).

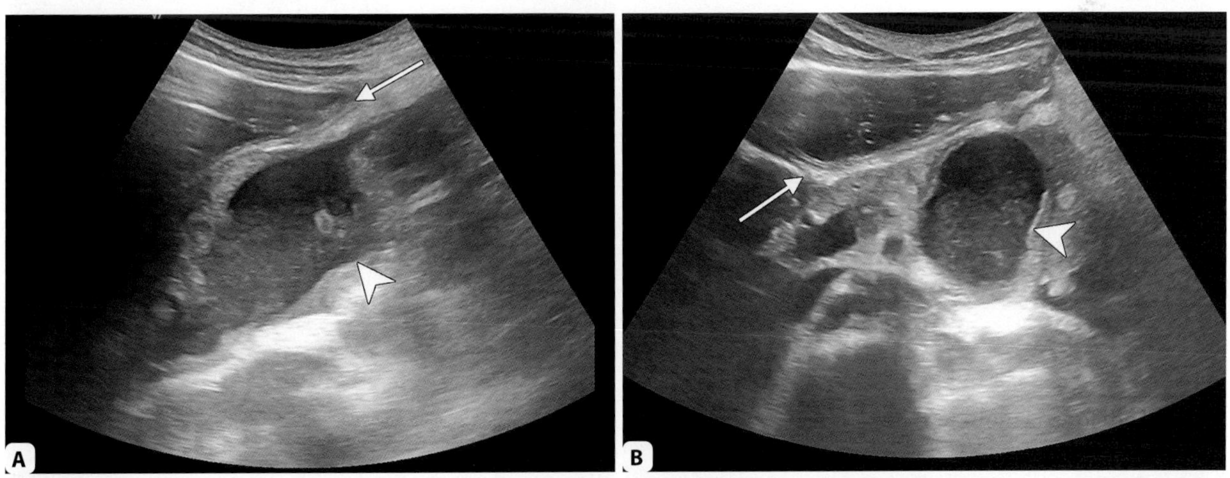

FIGS. 11A AND B: US appearance of acute necrotizing pancreatitis with walled-off necrosis. Transverse US images with a curvilinear probe at the epigastrium in a 36-year-old female with acute necrotizing pancreatitis demonstrate a thick-walled, fluid collection (arrowheads) with >30% internal debris involving the proximal body of the pancreas extending into the lesser sac, in close apposition with the posterior wall of the stomach (white arrows).

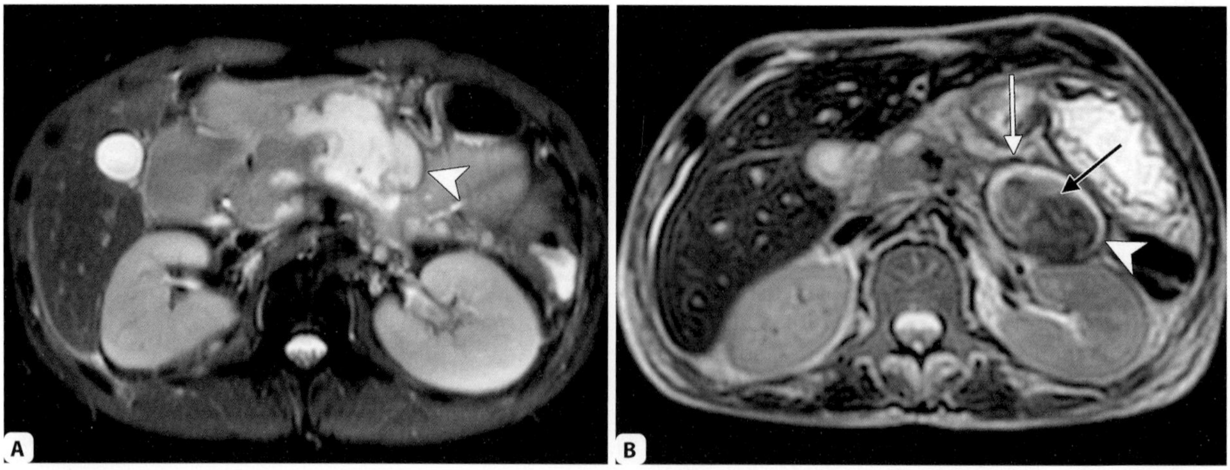

FIGS. 12A AND B: MRI appearance of acute necrotic collection (ANC) and walled off necrosis (WON). (A) Axial T2-weighted MRI image of the abdomen of a 20-year-old with post-traumatic acute pancreatitis demonstrates an ill-defined acute necrotic collection involving the pancreatic body extending into the lesser sac with few hypointense internal debris. (B) Axial T2-weighted MRI image of the abdomen of a 56-year-old male with acute necrotizing pancreatitis demonstrates walled-off necrosis in the pancreatic tail (arrowhead). The wall of the WON appears as a T2 hypointense rim surrounding the collection (white arrow), with internal debris appearing heterogeneously hypointense (black arrow) against the T2 hyperintense fluid within the collection.

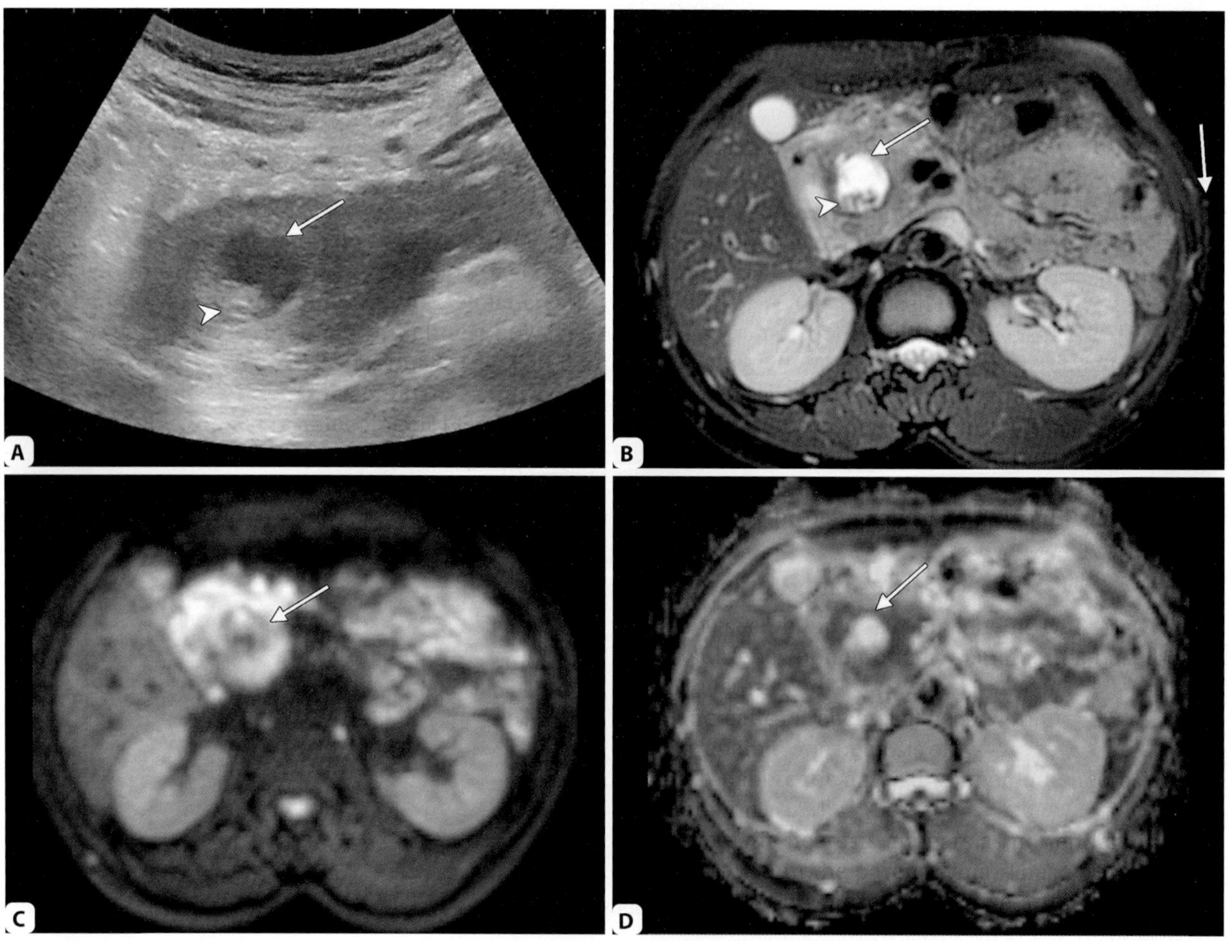

FIGS. 13A TO D: Intrapancreatic walled off necrosis US image (A) in a 32-year-old female with gallstone-induced acute pancreatitis shows a well-defined hypoechoic lesion in the pancreatic head (marked with arrow on all images) with dependent hyperdense debris (marked with arrowhead on all images). T2W MRI image (B) demonstrates a well-defined T2 hyperintense lesion (arrow) with dependent hypodense debris (arrowhead) within a bulky pancreatic head showing no evidence of any diffusion restriction on DWI (C) and ADC images (D).

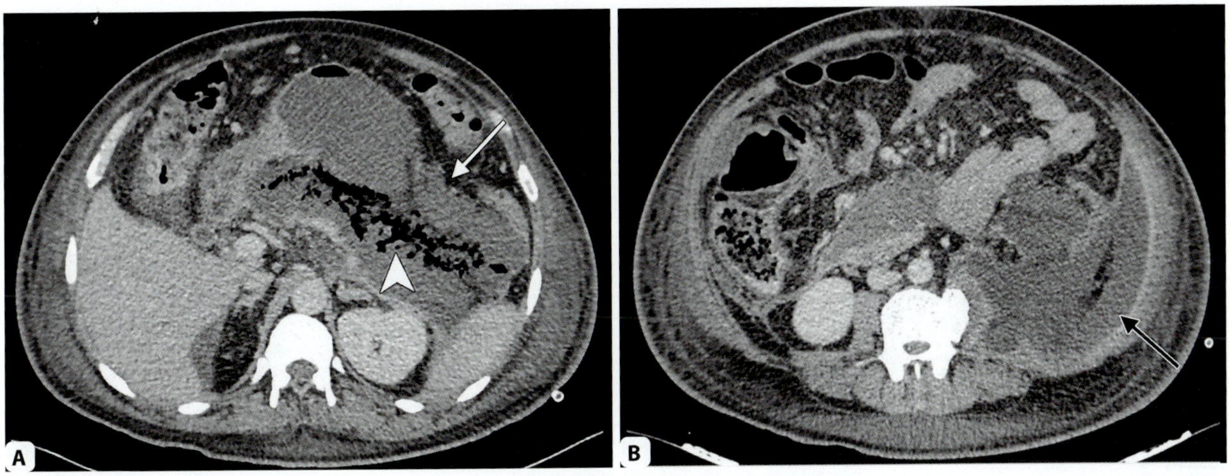

FIGS. 14A AND B: Infected walled-off necrosis in a 44-year-old male with alcohol-related acute pancreatitis with persistent SIRS. Axial CECT image in the portal venous phase at the level of the pancreas (A) and lower (B) demonstrates multiple air foci (arrowhead) within a walled-off necrosis (WON) nearly completely replacing the pancreas and extending into the lesser sac (white arrow) indicating superadded infection. The collection also extends along the left paracolic gutter (black arrow). Endoscopic drainage is not possible in such laterally placed collections, and thus percutaneous drainage is the procedure of choice.

it is seldom done due to the possibility of false negatives and the increased risk of introducing infection in sterile collections.

Bowel Complications

In AP, the bowel may be affected either by the direct effect of pancreatic enzymes or by fluid collections caused by AP.

- *Inflammation*: The release of pancreatic enzymes results in inflammation of the adjacent bowel loops especially the transverse colon and the splenic flexure of the colon due to their proximity to the distal pancreatic body and tail. It appears as segments of circumferential stratified bowel wall thickening and enhancement with stranding of adjacent fat.
- *Ischemia*: As enzymes track along mesenteric vasculature, they may cause thrombosis which is amplified by systemic hypercoagulability associated with pancreatitis. This leads to ischemia of the bowel loops supplied by these vessels.
- *Perforation*: Inflammation and ischemia of the bowel wall may result in thinning and rupture of the wall, especially the splenic flexure of the colon. The presence of pneumoperitoneum or pneumoretroperitoneum should alert the radiologist to the presence of a perforation. Leakage of oral/rectal positive contrast during CECT is definite evidence of perforation **(Figs. 15A to C)**. Infrequently, direct visualization of a colonic wall discontinuity may also be seen.
- *Obstruction*: Paralytic ileus (functional obstruction without a structural abnormality) frequently develops in patients with AP. On CT, it appears as dilatation of small and large bowel loops with no definite transition point.

Focal strictures may develop at the splenic flexure in the later course of the disease as a sequela to bowel wall inflammation and necrosis. Large pseudocysts may compress any part of the GI tract and lead to features of obstruction. Gastric outlet obstruction is commonly seen due to involvement of the second and third parts of the duodenum (due to their proximity to the pancreatic head).

Disconnected Pancreatic Duct Syndrome

Disconnected pancreatic duct syndrome (DPDS) is an important but potentially overlooked complication of ANP, occurring in up to 50% of patients.[33] Focal pancreatic duct disruption due to central gland necrosis leads to disconnection of the upstream viable pancreatic parenchyma from the proximal main pancreatic duct. The disconnected viable pancreatic parenchyma continues its exocrine secretion outside the GI tract, resulting in persistent peripancreatic fluid collections, pancreatic ascites, and pancreatocutaneous fistula. The diagnosis is suspected in case of persistent drainage of amylase-rich fluid.

A confident diagnosis of DPDS requires the fulfilment of the following criteria:

- Extensive intrapancreatic collection or area of focal necrosis resulting in nonvisualization of the pancreatic duct for at least 2 cm.
- Normal signal/enhancing pancreatic parenchyma consistent with viable pancreatic tissue seen distal to the disrupted duct (in the body/tail).
- The dilated distal pancreatic duct enters the collection at ~ 90° on CECT/MRI.
- Extravasation of contrast material injected into the main pancreatic duct at pancreatography.[34]

All intra- or peripancreatic collections do not signify duct disconnection. Large collections may compress pancreatic parenchyma, which may appear as areas of focal pancreatic necrosis. Multiplanar reconstructions should be analyzed for any thin bridge of compressed viable pancreatic tissue in suspicious areas. Moreover, in cases of compression by collection, the pancreatic duct is displaced and enters at oblique angles into the wall of the collection (cf 90° entry in DPDS) **(Figs. 16 to 19)**.

Endoscopic stent placement into the pancreatic duct can help overcome this leak and reduce output from the disconnected duct. In patients who do not respond to

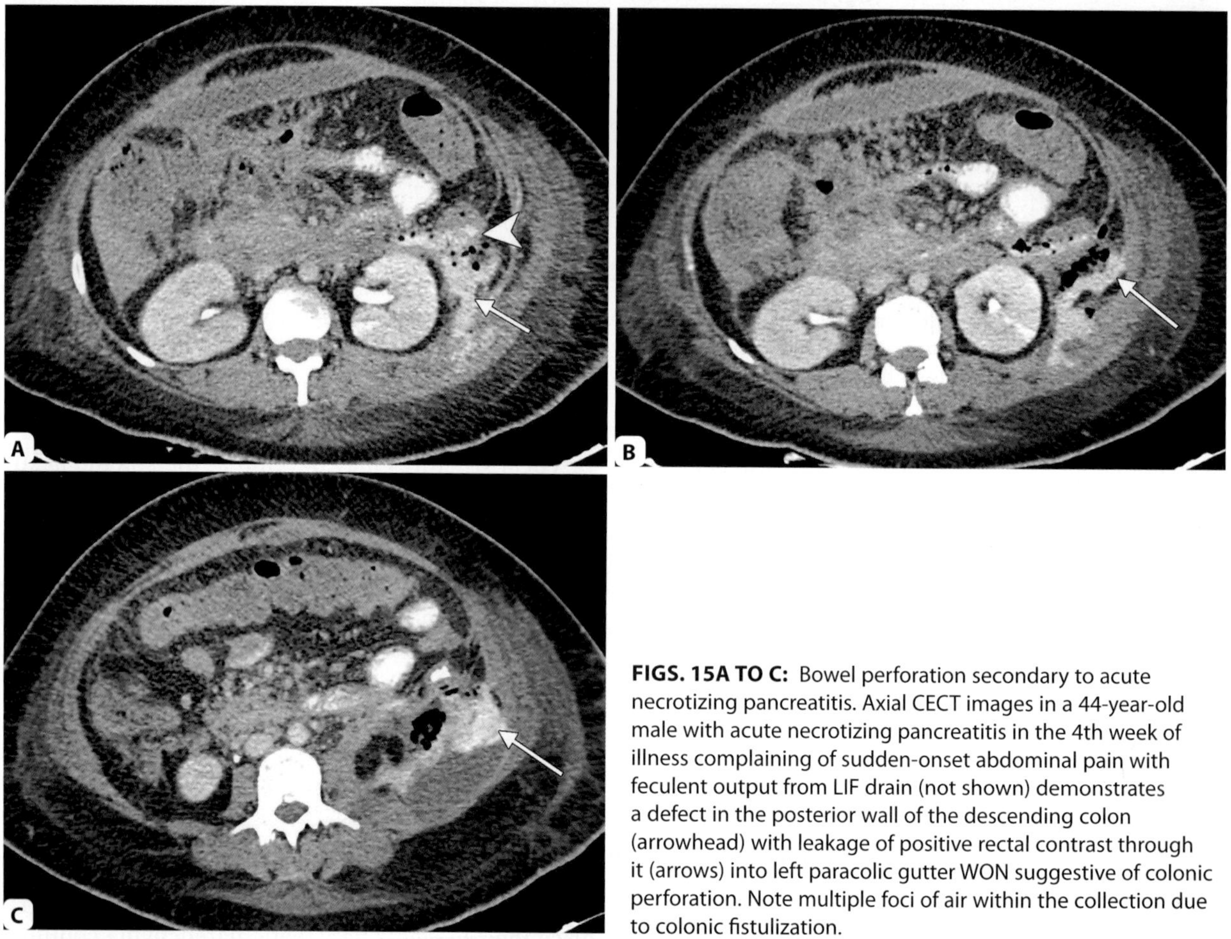

FIGS. 15A TO C: Bowel perforation secondary to acute necrotizing pancreatitis. Axial CECT images in a 44-year-old male with acute necrotizing pancreatitis in the 4th week of illness complaining of sudden-onset abdominal pain with feculent output from LIF drain (not shown) demonstrates a defect in the posterior wall of the descending colon (arrowhead) with leakage of positive rectal contrast through it (arrows) into left paracolic gutter WON suggestive of colonic perforation. Note multiple foci of air within the collection due to colonic fistulization.

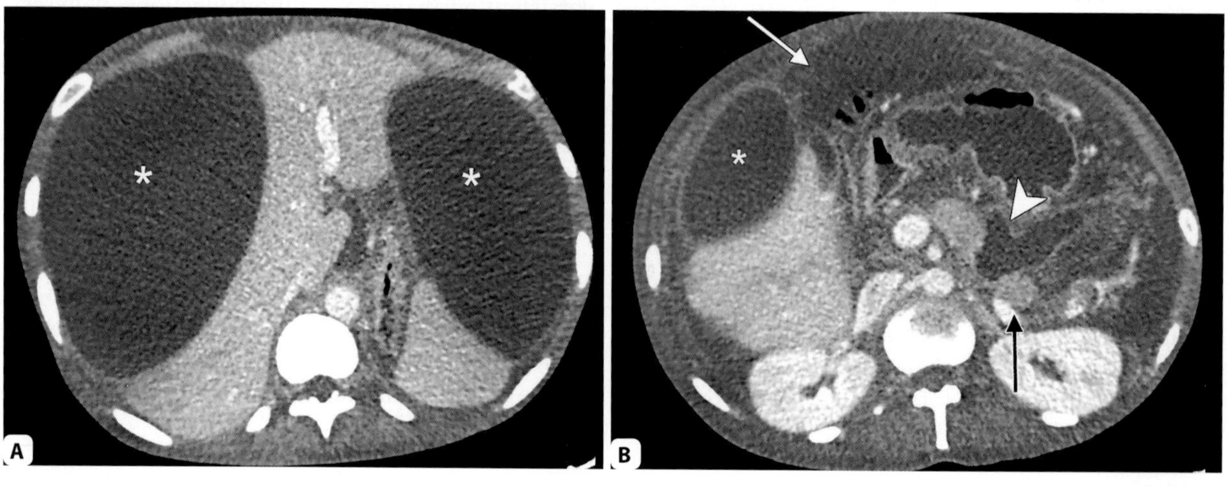

FIGS. 16A TO D: *Continued*

Continued

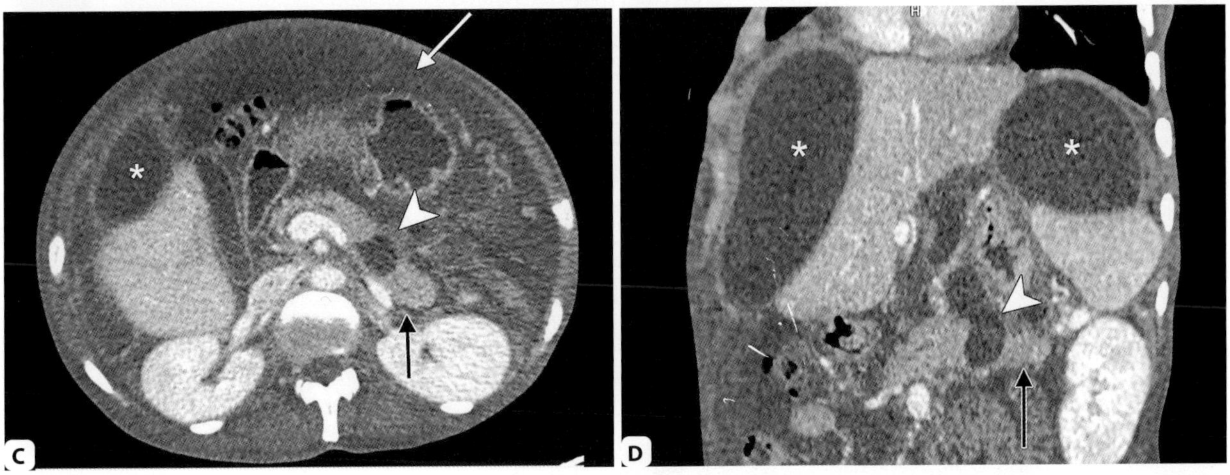

FIGS. 16A TO D: Disconnected pancreatic duct syndrome (DPDS). CECT images in the axial (A to C) and coronal plane (D) in a 34-year-old male with increasing abdominal girth after an episode of acute necrotizing pancreatitis show a complete defect in the pancreatic parenchyma (arrowheads) with viable distal pancreatic parenchyma (black arrows) with multiple hepatic subcapsular collections (asterisks) and pancreatic ascites (white arrows).

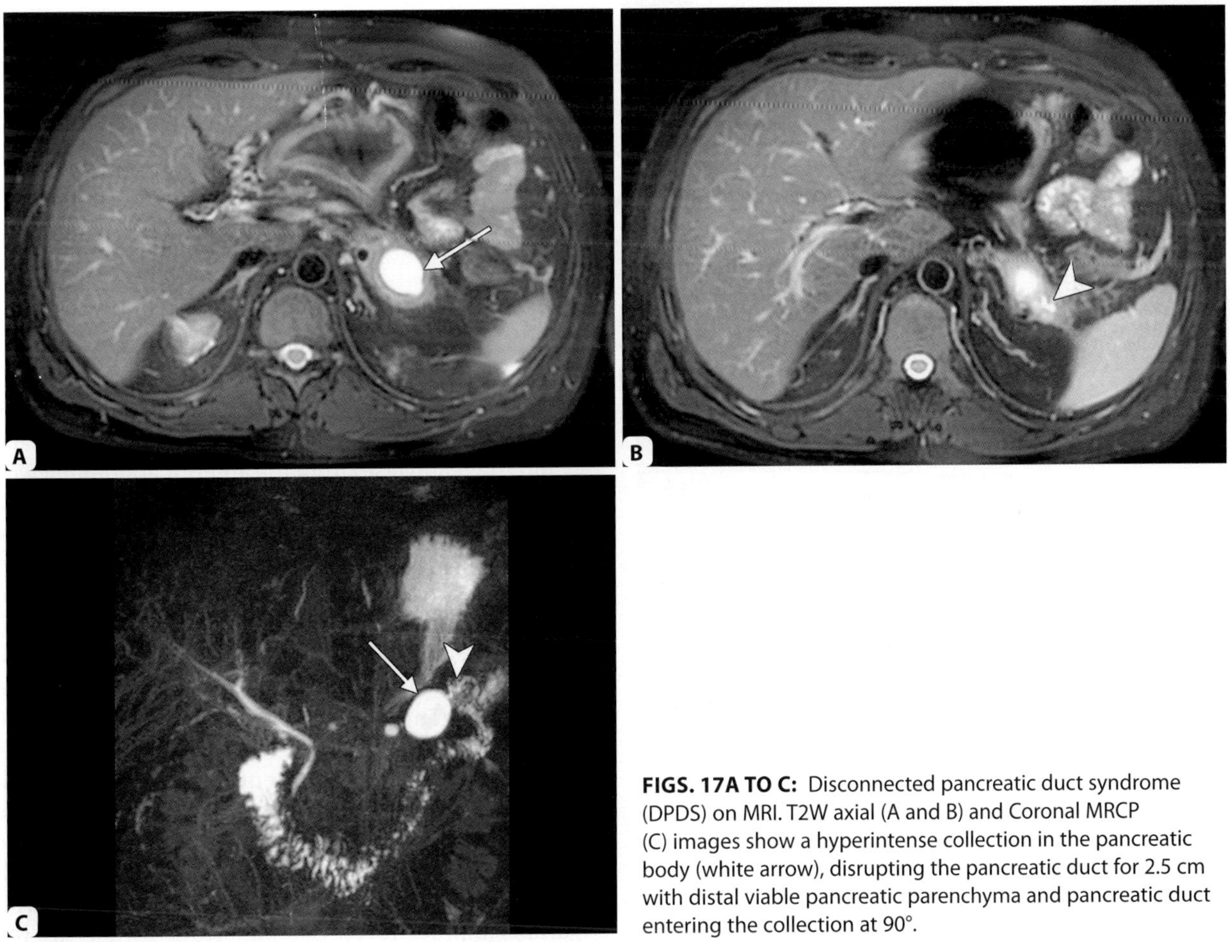

FIGS. 17A TO C: Disconnected pancreatic duct syndrome (DPDS) on MRI. T2W axial (A and B) and Coronal MRCP (C) images show a hyperintense collection in the pancreatic body (white arrow), disrupting the pancreatic duct for 2.5 cm with distal viable pancreatic parenchyma and pancreatic duct entering the collection at 90°.

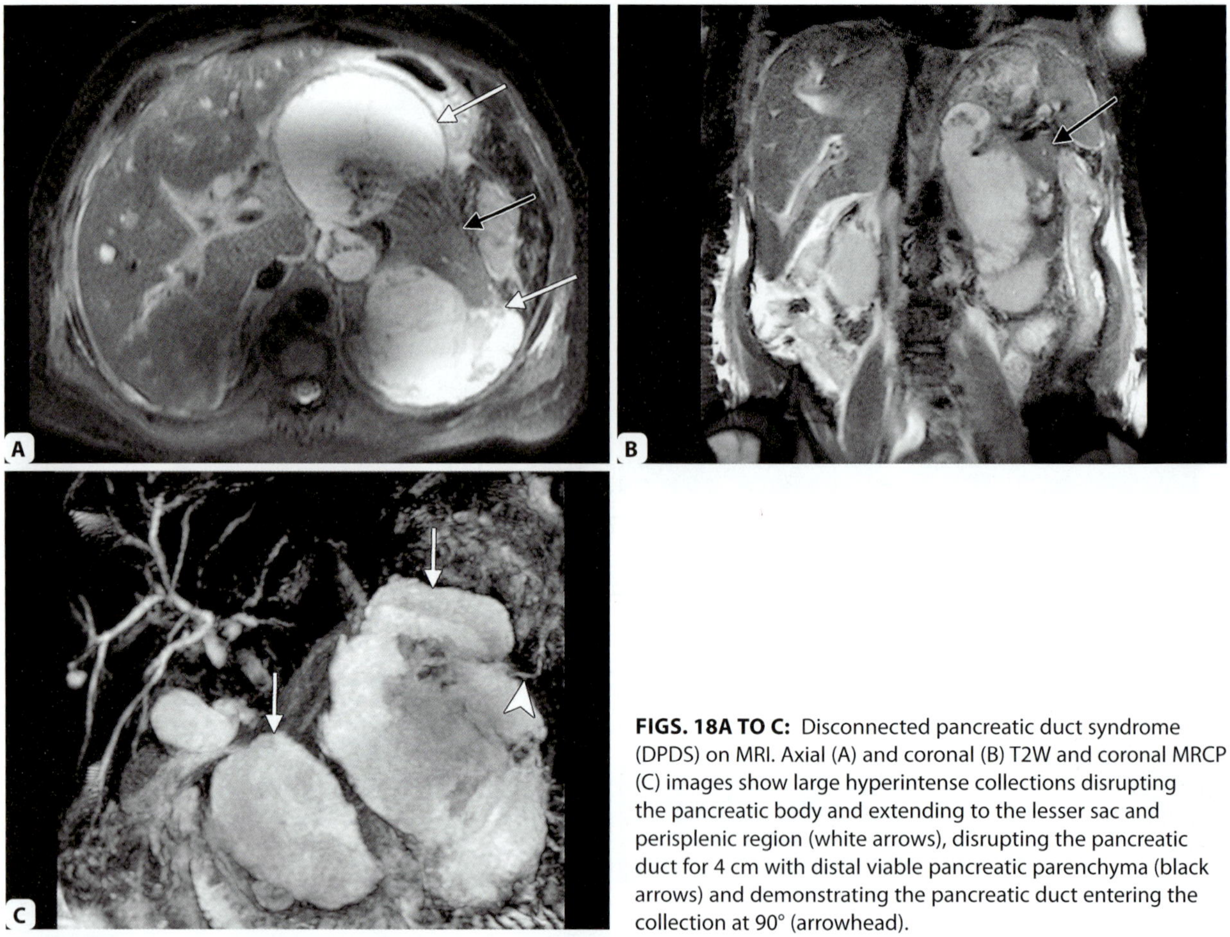

FIGS. 18A TO C: Disconnected pancreatic duct syndrome (DPDS) on MRI. Axial (A) and coronal (B) T2W and coronal MRCP (C) images show large hyperintense collections disrupting the pancreatic body and extending to the lesser sac and perisplenic region (white arrows), disrupting the pancreatic duct for 4 cm with distal viable pancreatic parenchyma (black arrows) and demonstrating the pancreatic duct entering the collection at 90° (arrowhead).

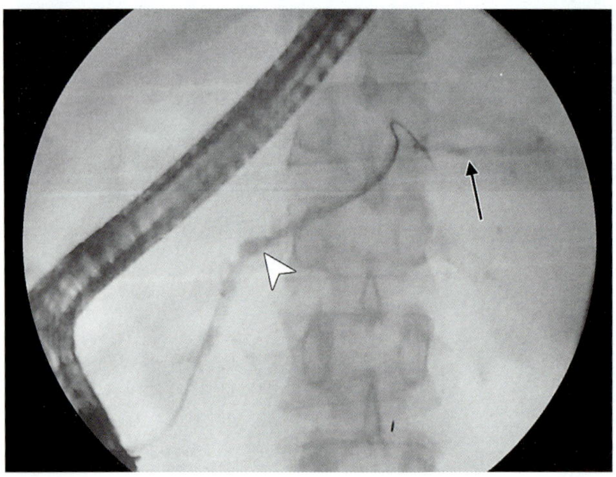

FIG. 19: Disconnected pancreatic duct syndrome (DPDS). A spot image of a pancreatogram shows contrast leak (black arrow) from the distal end of the pancreatic duct (arrowhead).

stent placement, surgical removal of the isolated segment followed by a median segment pancreatojejunostomy may be done. If the viable parenchyma distal to leak is small, a distal pancreatectomy may be considered.

Fistula

Pancreatic fistulae can be classified as either external or internal.

- *Pancreaticocutaneous fistula*: An external pancreatic fistula is described as persistent drainage of pancreatic fluid (high amylase) from the anterior abdominal wall or drainage site for >7 days. It is most commonly a complication of percutaneous drainage of pancreatic collections. A fistulogram through the cutaneous opening or from the pancreatic drain shows communication with a peripancreatic collection. There is an increased risk of pancreaticocutaneous fistula development in cases of DPDS.
- *GI fistulas*: These are common complications of AP which result in increased morbidity and mortality because of the high incidence of hemorrhage and secondary bacterial infections. Fistulization with the bowel occurs mainly due to the action of proteolytic enzymes on the gut walls combined with bowel wall ischemia. Fistulae may also develop as a result of drainage procedures. Colopancreatic fistulas are the most common sites of fistulization. Clinical features of a GI fistula formation are GI bleeding, persistent collections, or sepsis. Frank feculent output from a

percutaneous drain is seen in cases of colopancreatic fistula. On CECT, multiple mottled foci of air may be seen leading from the bowel loop to the pancreatic collection. Frank extravasation of oral or rectal contrast into collections may be seen in cases of duodenal and colopancreatic fistulas, respectively.

Pancreatic Ascites

Early AP may present with small quantities of reactive ascites that do not require active intervention. Pancreatic ascites develops later during the disease, with increasing abdominal distension and pain, and is associated with duct disruption. It is a low serum albumin-ascites gradient (SAAG) ascites with high levels of amylase (>1,000 U/L).[35]

Pancreatitis, Panniculitis, and Polyarthritis Syndrome

It is a rare syndrome associated with pancreatitis, where the release of large amounts of pancreatic lipase into the systemic circulation leads to multiple extrapancreatic sites of fat necrosis.[36] It usually affects middle-aged men with a history of chronic alcohol abuse. Abdominal symptoms of pancreatitis are absent in most cases of pancreatitis, panniculitis, and polyarthritis (PPP), resulting in a delayed diagnosis.[37] Persistently high levels of serum amylase and lipase are seen with subcutaneous fat necrosis leading to the development of multiple painful and nodular skin lesions of panniculitis. The periarticular bone marrow around the knee, wrist, and ankle joints also undergoes fat necrosis and appears as intramedullary infarcts on MR images. Polyarthritis develops due to the release of fatty acids into joints during fat autodigestion **(Figs. 20A to D)**.

Vascular Complications

Vascular complications are more common in acute exacerbations of chronic pancreatitis and are associated with a high overall mortality rate.[38]

- *Venous thrombosis* is the most common vascular complication of AP. The pancreas is closely related to

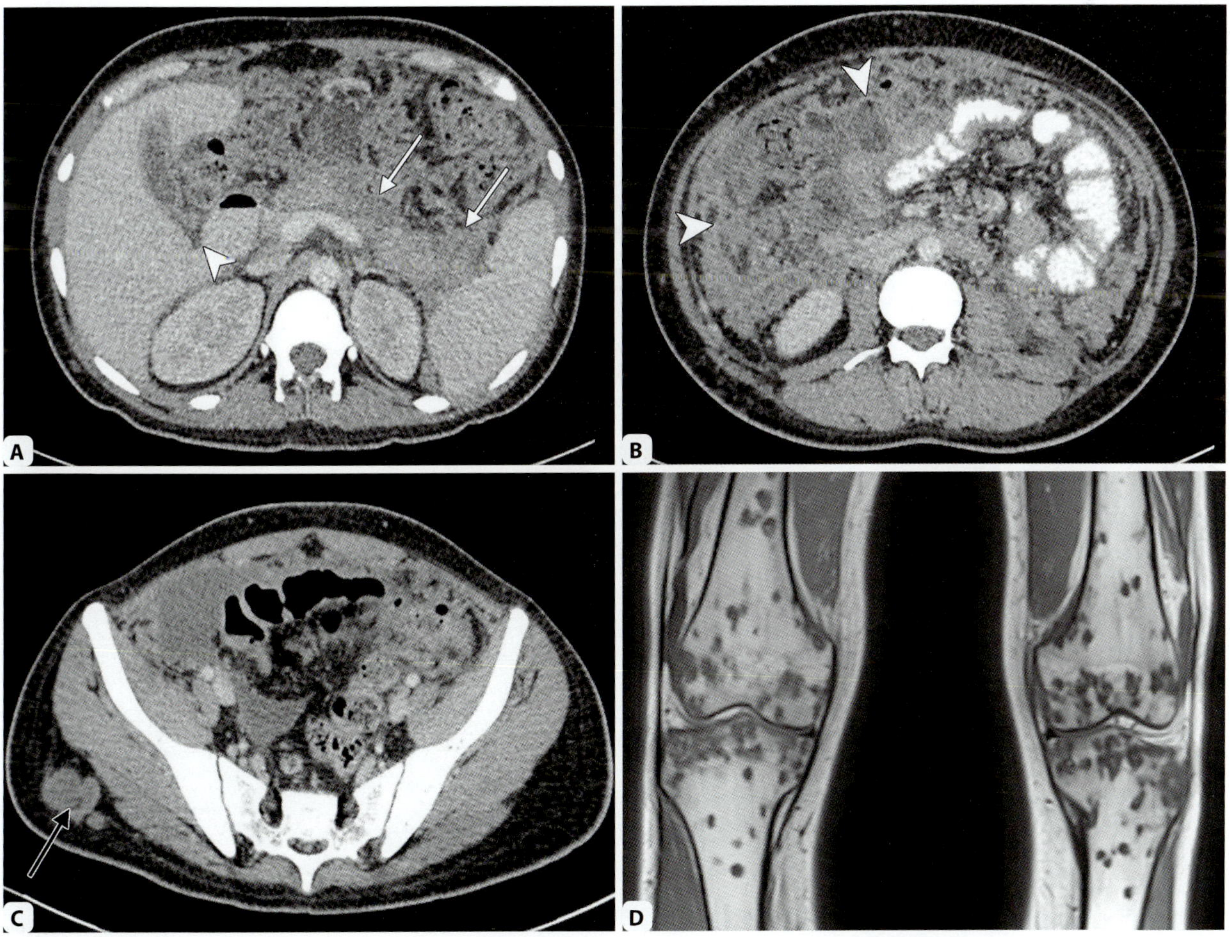

FIGS. 20A TO D: Pancreatitis, panniculitis, and polyarthritis syndrome. CECT images in the axial plane (A to C) in an 18-year-old male demonstrate pancreatic (white arrows) and extensive extrapancreatic fat necrosis (arrowheads). Subcutaneous fat necrosis is seen in the right gluteal region (black arrow). (D) Coronal T1w MRI image shows associated multiple geographic and rounded hypointense lesions replacing the hyperintense bone marrow in the bilateral distal femur and proximal tibia.

the portal venous system. Local inflammation due to AP and compression of the veins due to peripancreatic fluid collections may result in venous thrombosis. The splenic vein is the most commonly involved, resulting in the development of sinistral portal hypertension (left-sided portal hypertension). The superior mesenteric and portal vein may also get thrombosed.

- *Pseudoaneurysms*: They are uncommon but catastrophic vascular complications associated with AP. The release of proteolytic pancreatic enzymes may cause erosion and the resultant weakening of the vessel wall leading to the development of pseudoaneurysms. The splenic and gastroduodenal arteries are the most frequently involved, followed by pancreaticoduodenal, hepatic, and left gastric arteries.
  - Pseudoaneurysms are prone to rupture and may lead to massive intraperitoneal or retroperitoneal bleeding. Communication with the bowel may lead to the development of melena or hematochezia.
  - Pseudoaneurysms appear as well-defined, round, anechoic structures on ultrasound, with a "yin-yang" sign on color Doppler and a pulsatile arterial waveform on pulsed wave Doppler. On CT, pseudoaneurysms appear as defined, saccular outpouchings with arterial phase hyperenhancement that maintains its shape and persists in the venous phase, paralleling the enhancement of vessels.
- *Active contrast extravasation*: Erosion of the arterial wall due to pancreatic enzymes may also lead to uncontained arterial extravasation that appears as a focal area of increased attenuation within the hematoma/cavity that enlarges on delayed images. The presence of contrast extravasation on CT is consistent with clinically significant active arterial bleeding, and it may be associated with hemodynamic instability that requires urgent life-saving interventions **(Figs. 21A to D)**.
- *Pancreatic portal vein fistula*: Rarely, a pancreatic pseudocyst may rupture into the portal vein, resulting in the development of a pancreatic portal vein fistula **(Figs. 22A to C)**. These usually occur in alcohol-related AP, predominantly in male patients.

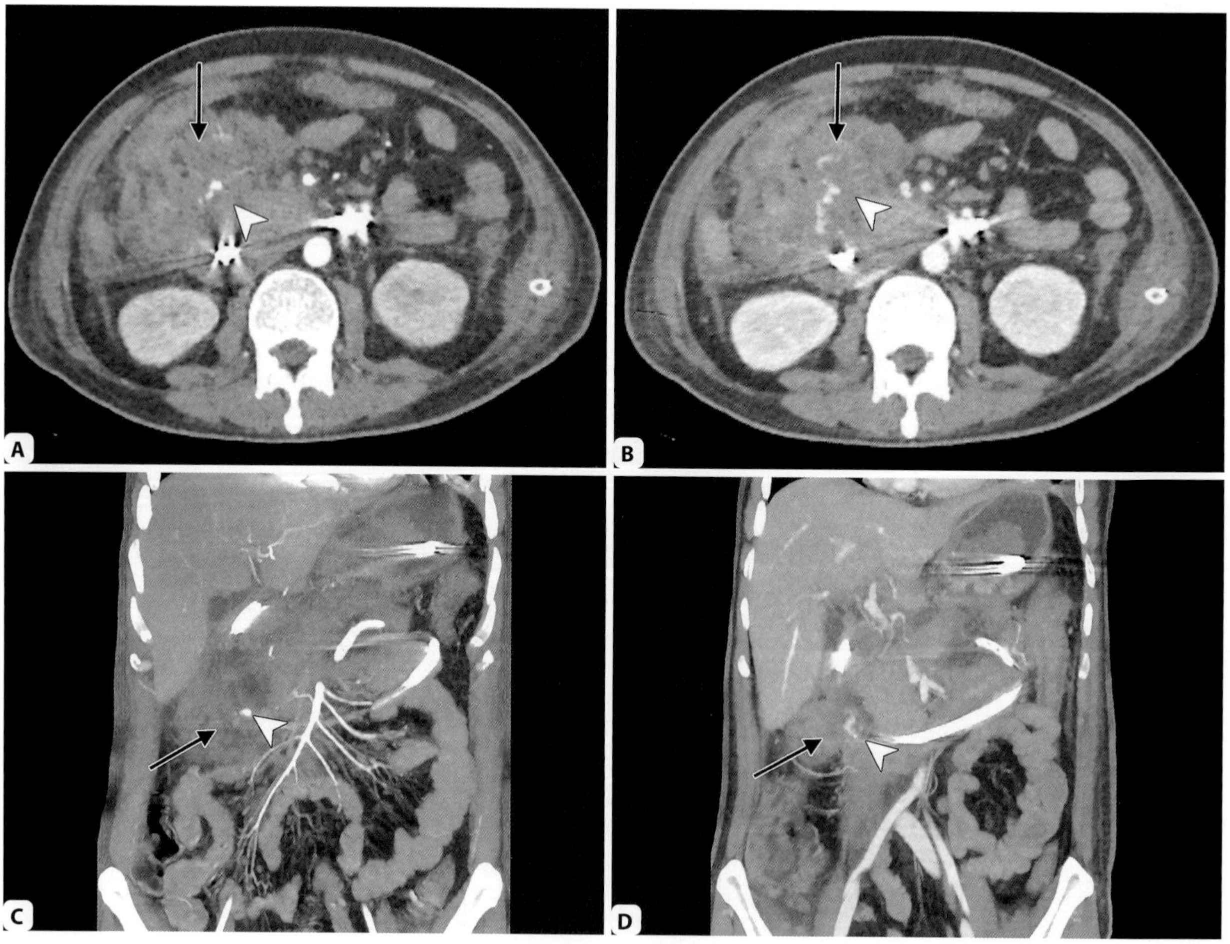

FIGS. 21A TO D: Active contrast extravasation in a 44-year-old male with acute necrotizing pancreatitis with sudden onset hypovolemic shock. CECT images of the abdomen in the axial plane (A and B) and coronal MIP images (C and D) demonstrate contrast extravasation (arrowheads) within a peripancreatic acute necrotic collection (black arrows), which increases in size from the arterial (A and C) to the venous phase (B and D).

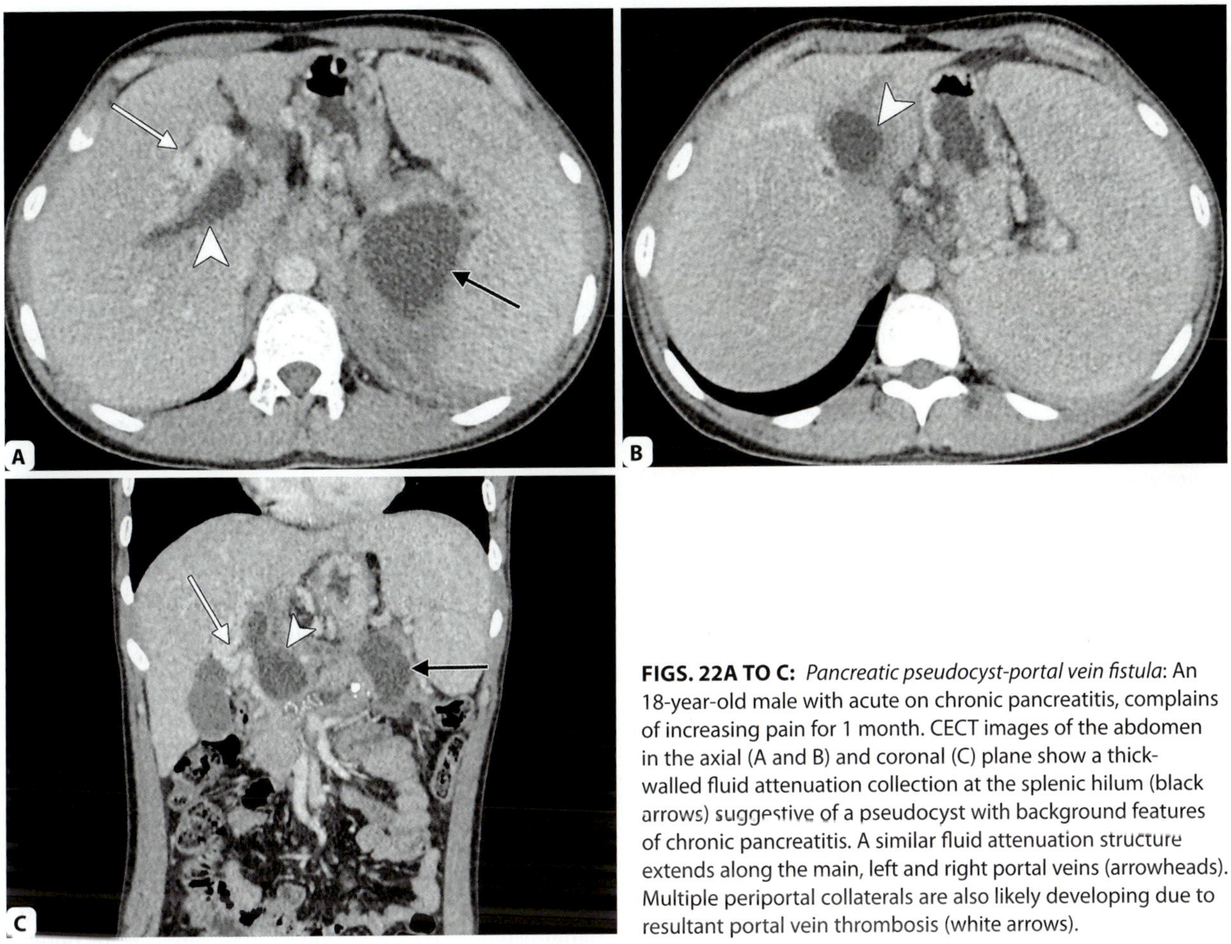

FIGS. 22A TO C: *Pancreatic pseudocyst-portal vein fistula*: An 18-year-old male with acute on chronic pancreatitis, complains of increasing pain for 1 month. CECT images of the abdomen in the axial (A and B) and coronal (C) plane show a thick-walled fluid attenuation collection at the splenic hilum (black arrows) suggestive of a pseudocyst with background features of chronic pancreatitis. A similar fluid attenuation structure extends along the main, left and right portal veins (arrowheads). Multiple periportal collaterals are also likely developing due to resultant portal vein thrombosis (white arrows).

- *Pulmonary embolism* is a rare, life-threatening complication of AP. The release of pancreatic enzymes damages the vascular endothelium and results in a hypercoagulable state. The systemic inflammatory response also releases mediators that damage the endothelium.

Thus, reporting of pancreatitis should not only grade the severity but also comprehensively list out the complications and the possible etiology **(Table 4)**.[39] PANCODE (PAncreatic Nonenhancement COllection DEscription) acronym has also been proposed to enhance structured reporting of pancreatitis.[40]

IMAGE-GUIDED INTERVENTIONS IN ACUTE PANCREATITIS

Treatment of pancreatitis requires a tailored, multidisciplinary treatment plan discussed between the interventional radiologist, endoscopist, and surgeons.

Indications for Drainage of a Pancreatic Collection

Most acute collections resolve spontaneously, especially APFC; thus, drainage is unnecessary. Instead, there is a risk

TABLE 4: Reporting template for acute pancreatitis.

Pancreatic inflammation	
Site	Head/body/tail/diffuse
Bulkiness/enlargement	Absent/focal/diffuse
Surface lobulations	Preserved/lost
Enhancement	Homogenous/heterogenous
Necrosis (%)	<30 or 30–50 or >50%
Peripancreatic inflammation	
Fat stranding	Present/absent
Fascial thickening	Present/absent
Systemic inflammation	
Pleural effusion	Present/absent, mild/moderate/severe unilateral/bilateral
Ascites	Present/absent
Fluid collections	
Location	Intrapancreatic/extrapancreatic (EP)
	EP—lesser sac/paracolic gutter/subhepatic/anterior pararenal/pelvic/mesenteric root

Continued

Continued

Fluid collections	
Size (largest diameter)	
Type	APFC/ANC/pseudocyst/WON
Debris	Present/absent, % of debris
Hemorrhage	Present/absent
Gas	Present/absent
Vascular	
Venous thrombosis	Present/absent, SV/MPV/SMV
	Presence of collaterals
Pseudoaneurysm/contrast extravasation	Present/absent, artery involved
Underlying pathology	
Cholelithiasis	Present/absent
Choledocholithiasis	Present/absent
Pancreatic mass lesion	Present/absent
Pancreatic divisum	Present/absent
Abnormal pancreaticobiliary junction	Present/absent
Interventions	
Stent	Location/type
Drain	Location/type
Other complications	
Bowel communication	

(ANC: acute necrotic collection; APFC: acute peripancreatic fluid collection; MPV: main portal vein; SMV: superior mesenteric vein; SV: splenic vein; WON: walled-off necrosis)

of iatrogenic infection in sterile collections. Thus, drainage is indicated in the following scenarios:

- Infected collections preferably after the formation of a wall (>4 weeks since onset). Infection may be suspected based on clinical signs (fever, raised leukocyte counts, and persistently high SIRS) or the presence of gas on imaging **(Flowchart 3)** without a history of prior intervention or any apparent bowel communication.
- Clinical deterioration or ongoing organ failure.
- Symptomatic large sterile collection with features of gastric outlet/biliary/bowel obstruction, persistent pain, vomiting, and nutritional failure.[9]

The presence of mesenteric ischemia, bowel communication, and abdominal compartment syndrome (as a direct consequence of AP) may represent absolute indications for early open surgical intervention.

Timing of Drainage

Drainage of a pancreatic fluid collection during the early phase of AP (<2 weeks) is associated with high morbidity and mortality due to systemic inflammation along with a high risk of bleeding. Drainage of infected pancreatic collections, radiological, or endoscopic, is usually delayed for up to 3–4 weeks since symptom onset to allow for encapsulation of these collections since no difference is seen between immediate versus delayed drainage of collections (POINTER trial).[41]

Percutaneous catheter drainage may be considered in patients with infected or symptomatic collections between 2 and 4 weeks in cases where organ failure is persistent and medical management alone is insufficient.[21]

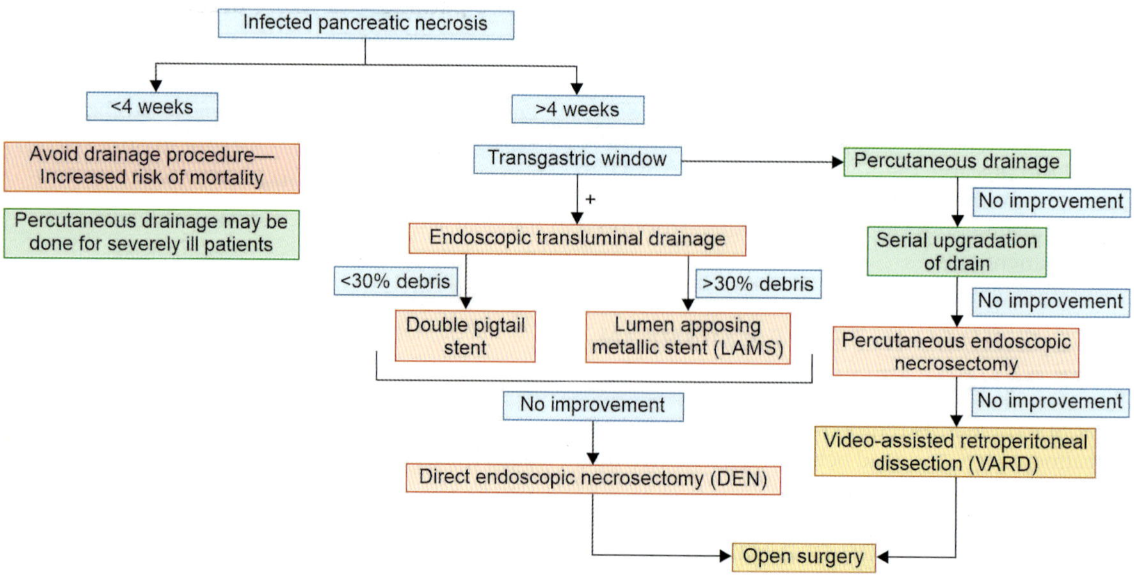

FLOWCHART 3: Protocol for management of infected pancreatic necrosis.

Endoscopic Drainage—Cystogastrostomy

Infected pancreatic necrosis is associated with high morbidity and mortality. Emergent drainage becomes necessary in these situations. Minimally invasive endoscopic drainage of centrally placed WONs is the procedure of choice. The development of a wall around the infected collection is a prerequisite before any endoscopic procedure. Endoscopic drainage saves the patient from the discomfort of an external catheter and the risk of enterocutaneous fistula.

Endoscopic insertion of LAMS **(Figs. 23A and B)** or plastic stents **(Figs. 24A and B)** can be done depending on the percentage of debris within the WONs. LAMS is preferred in collections with >30% debris; however, they are associated with increased complications like bleeding and perforation.[15]

Percutaneous Drainage

Image-guided percutaneous drainage is considered the primary therapy for drainage of infected necrotic collection in sick patients. It may also be used as an adjunct to endoscopic or surgical procedures for any residual infected collections. The overall success rate is 55–64%,[42] and the complication rate is 20–25%.[43] A multiphase CECT is required before drainage to look for the location of collection, its relationship to the colon, and any vascular abnormality (pseudoaneurysm). Any infected collection with hemorrhage **(Figs. 21A to D)** needs special attention to exclude underlying vascular abnormality before attempting drainage.

Drainage of pancreatitis-associated collections is preferably done under CT guidance (if patient can be shifted to CT suite) since these are deep-seated, and CT

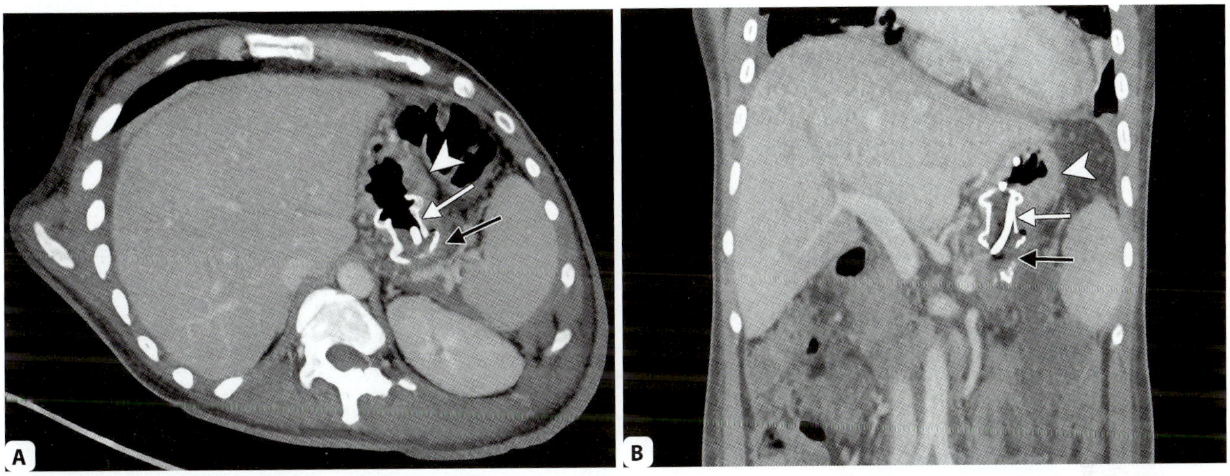

FIGS. 23A AND B: Endoscopically placed lumen apposing metallic stent in walled-off necrosis. Oblique axial (A) and coronal (B) CECT image in the portal venous phase in a 46-year-old with alcohol-related acute pancreatitis shows a LAMS (white arrows) placed via endoscopic cystogastrostomy between the posterior wall of the stomach (arrowheads) and walled off necrosis in the lesser sac (black arrows).

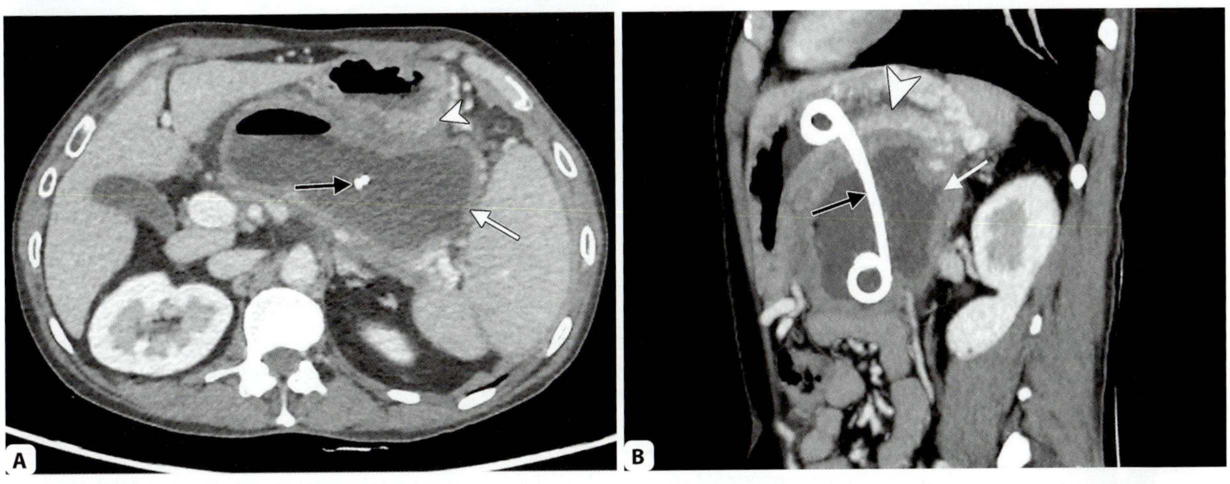

FIGS. 24A AND B: Endoscopically placed double pigtail plastic stent in a pseudocyst. Axial (A) and Sagittal (B) CECT image in the portal venous phase in a 34-year-old male with acute pancreatitis demonstrates a large pseudocyst in the lesser sac (white arrows) abutting the greater curvature of the stomach. Double pigtail stents (black arrows) were inserted into the pseudocyst via endoscopic cystogastrostomy. Follow-up US at 2 months demonstrated complete resolution of lesser sac pseudocyst.

guidance avoids transgressing bowel loops and allows easier retroperitoneal approach with hydrodissection (if needed). Bedside drainage may be required for sick patients who cannot be shifted to the CT room (because of life support lines and ventilators). Depending upon the collection location, a retroperitoneal or transgastric approach may be employed under ultrasonography guidance.

Low-dose CT protocols and smaller fields of view must be used during interventions to minimize radiation to the patient due to multiple scans. The shortest and safest route into the collection, remote from the intestine or large vessels, is chosen, and a 12–14 Fr-sized drainage catheter (using Seldinger or trocar technique) is inserted under local anesthesia. An 18-G Chiba needle may also be used for aspiration from collections when avoiding percutaneous drain placement.

Catheters with a minimum diameter of 12–14 Fr and multiple side holes or Malecot catheters are preferred to allow debris to drain. The maximum length of the catheter with side holes should be placed within the collection. Large or multiloculated necrotic collections may even require multiple catheters.

Laterally placed collections often require additional drainage and are easily accessible by the percutaneous route. A retroperitoneal approach through the lateral flank is preferred. Anterior routes through the liver or stomach (due to sterile gastric acid content) can also be used; however, we should avoid traversing the colon, small bowel, spleen, and kidney. Pancreatic tail collections can be drained through the left anterior pararenal space, while the pancreatic head collections can be drained through the right anterior or posterior pararenal space **(Figs. 25 to 30)**.

The left retroperitoneal route is the most commonly used route for drain placement as it avoids bowel loops, prevents peritoneal dissemination of infection, and provides access for minimally invasive surgery in the future. After the diagnosis of infected pancreatic/peripancreatic necrosis is made by either CT or clinical status, a 12–14 Fr drainage tube is inserted percutaneously into the collection via the Seldinger technique through a left retroperitoneal approach (posterior to the spleen). Serial upgradation of the percutaneous drainage tube up to 24 Fr is frequently done to allow for drainage of viscous and thick necrotic debris.

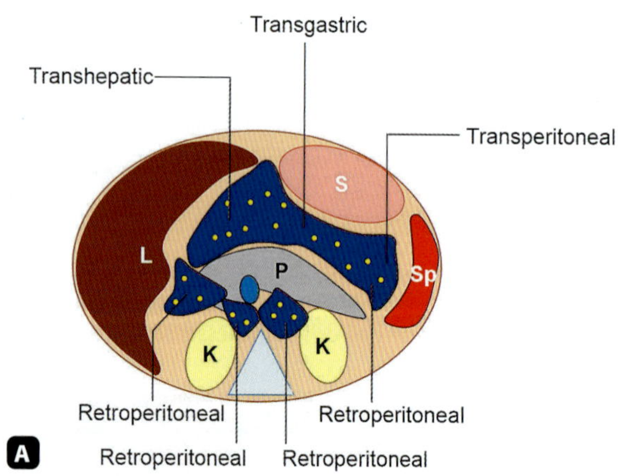

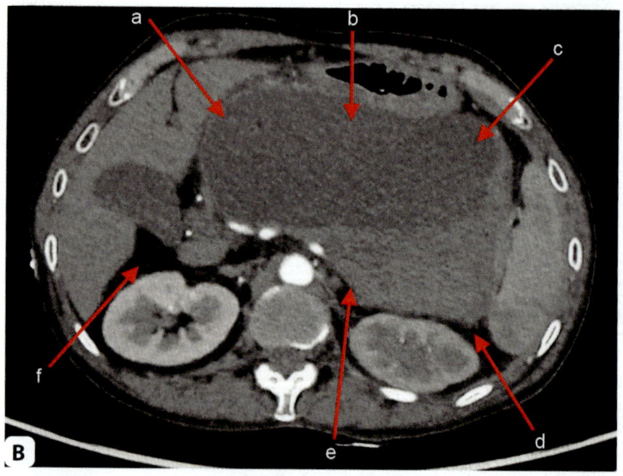

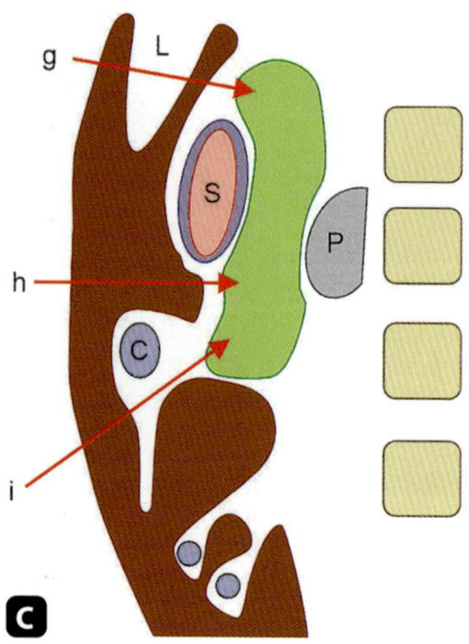

FIGS. 25A TO C: Approach for percutaneous drainage of pancreatic and peripancreatic collections. (A) Schematic diagram shows the various access routes for drainage of pancreatitis-related collections. (B) Axial CT image showing access routes in axial plane. Arrows labeled (a) Transhepatic approach; (b) Transgastric approach; (c) Gastrosplenic approach; (d) Left anterior pararenal approach; (e) Paravertebral approach; (f) Right anterior pararenal approach. (C) Schematic diagram showing access routes in sagittal plane. (g) Transhepatic approach; (h) Gastrocolic ligament approach; (i) Infra colic lesser sac approach.

(L: liver; Sp: spleen; S: stomach; P: pancreas; K: kidney; C: Colon)

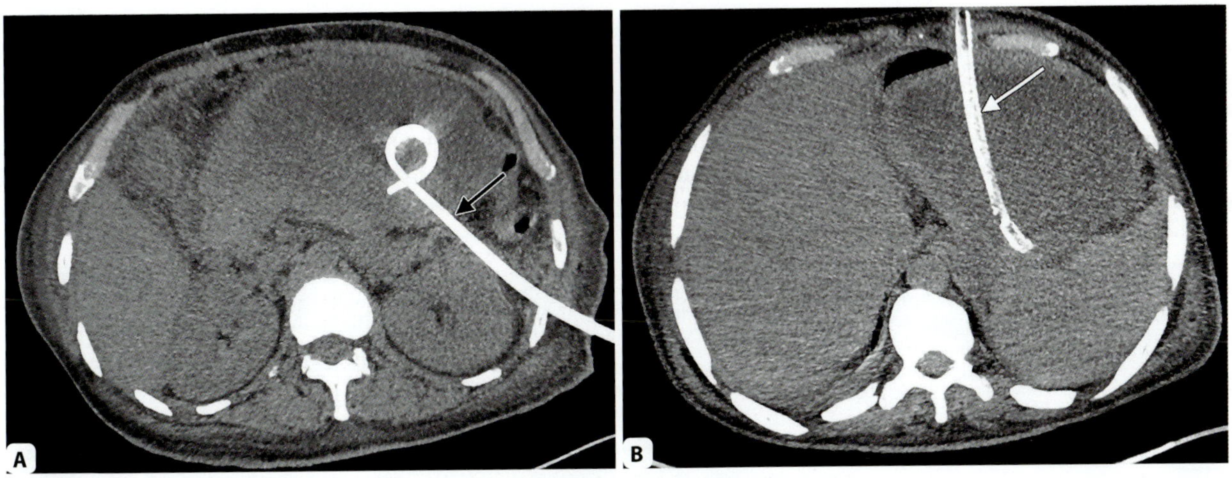

FIGS. 26A AND B: Percutaneous routes for drainage of collections associated with acute pancreatitis. (A) Axial NCCT MIP image in a 44-year-old male with idiopathic acute pancreatitis demonstrates a percutaneous drainage tube placement using a *retroperitoneal approach* (black arrow). (B) Axial NCCT MIP image in a 37-year-old male with alcohol-induced acute pancreatitis shows a percutaneous drainage tube inserted via the *transgastric approach* (white arrow).

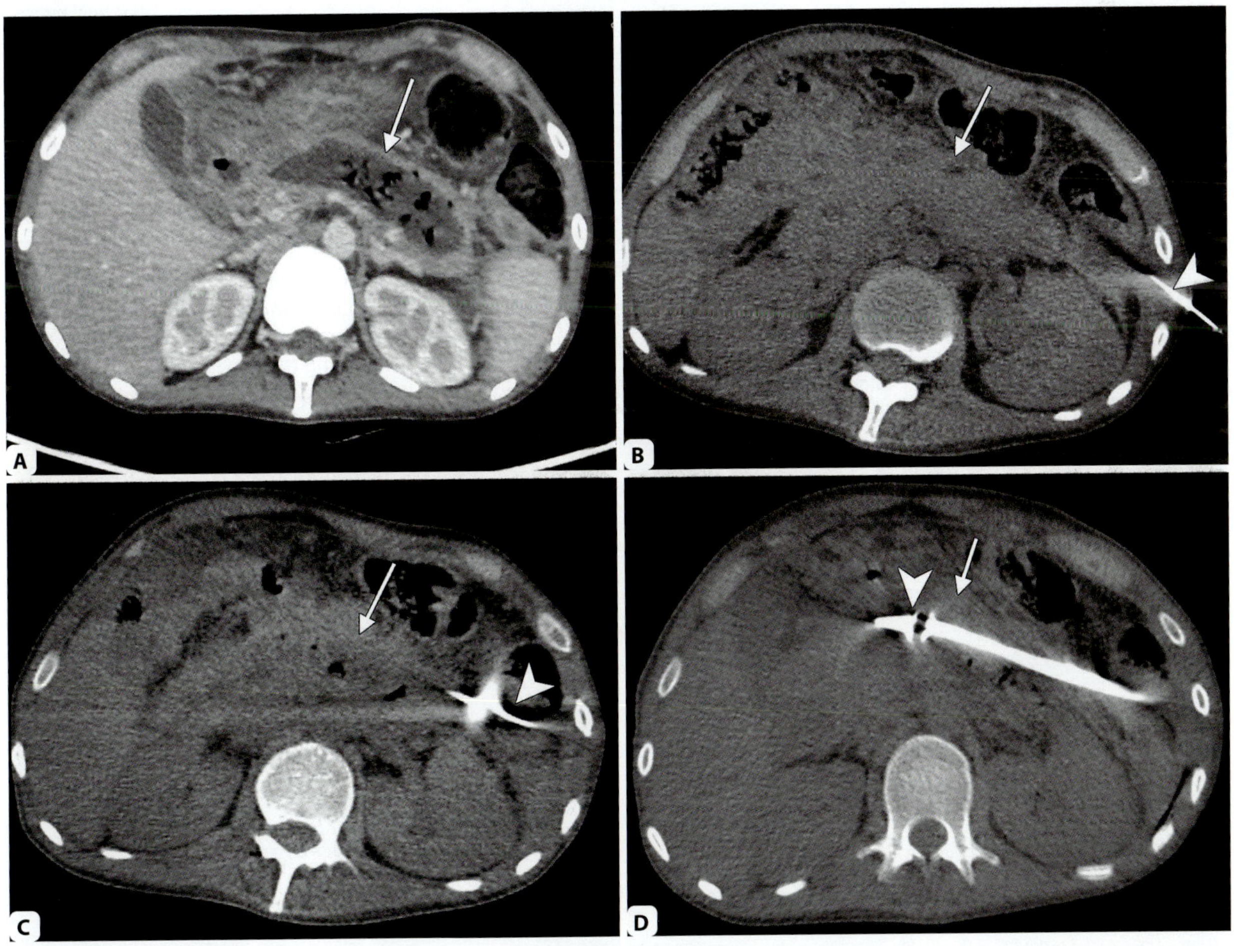

FIGS. 27A TO D: Left anterior pararenal intercostal approach for WON associated with acute pancreatitis. (A) Axial CECT image shows a well-encapsulated hypoenhancing collection with multiple foci of air completely replacing the pancreatic body and tail-infected WON (white arrow on all images). (B) Axial NCCT image shows an 18-G puncture needle (arrowhead) inserted along the left anterior pararenal space. (C) Axial NCCT image shows the insertion of stiff guidewire (arrowhead) through puncture needle into the collection. (D) Axial NCCT image shows a 16 Fr Malecot catheter (arrowhead) within the pancreatic collection.

The development of pancreatic-cutaneous fistulas is one of the major complications associated with percutaneous drain placement in pancreatitis. If there is suspicion of bleeding into the pancreatic collection, such as hemoglobin drop, hemodynamic instability, or bleeding from the drain site, interventional radiology (IR) management of arterial injury should be undertaken first before attempting drainage of hematoma since the latter may remove the tamponade effect and precipitate blood loss.

In the postprocedure period, the catheter should be connected to a low-pressure closed-suction drainage system and flushed with 10–20 mL of sterile saline three times daily. In cases where drainage is inadequate, and patient's condition is not improving, the tube position

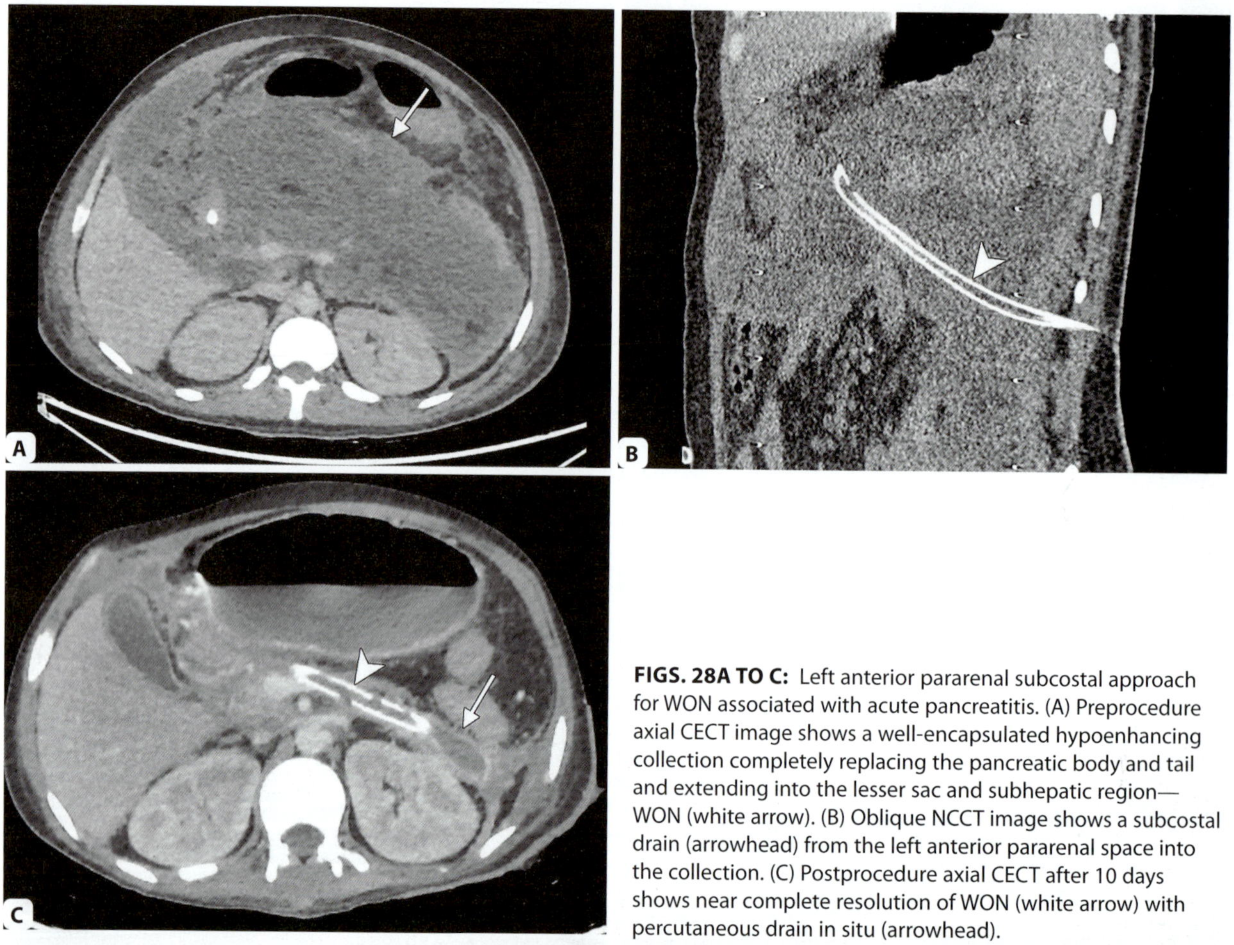

FIGS. 28A TO C: Left anterior pararenal subcostal approach for WON associated with acute pancreatitis. (A) Preprocedure axial CECT image shows a well-encapsulated hypoenhancing collection completely replacing the pancreatic body and tail and extending into the lesser sac and subhepatic region—WON (white arrow). (B) Oblique NCCT image shows a subcostal drain (arrowhead) from the left anterior pararenal space into the collection. (C) Postprocedure axial CECT after 10 days shows near complete resolution of WON (white arrow) with percutaneous drain in situ (arrowhead).

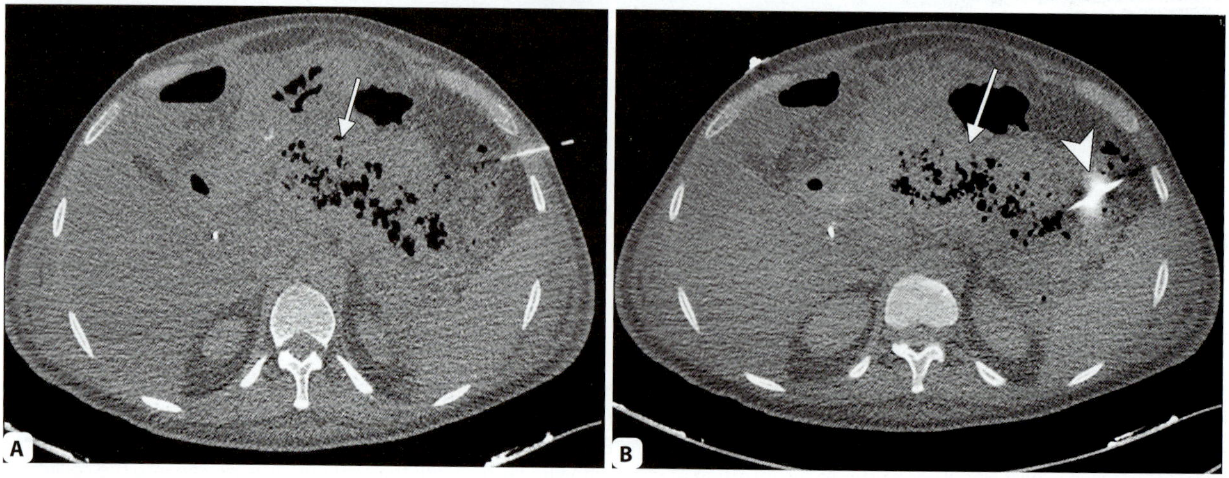

FIGS. 29A TO D: *Continued*

Continued

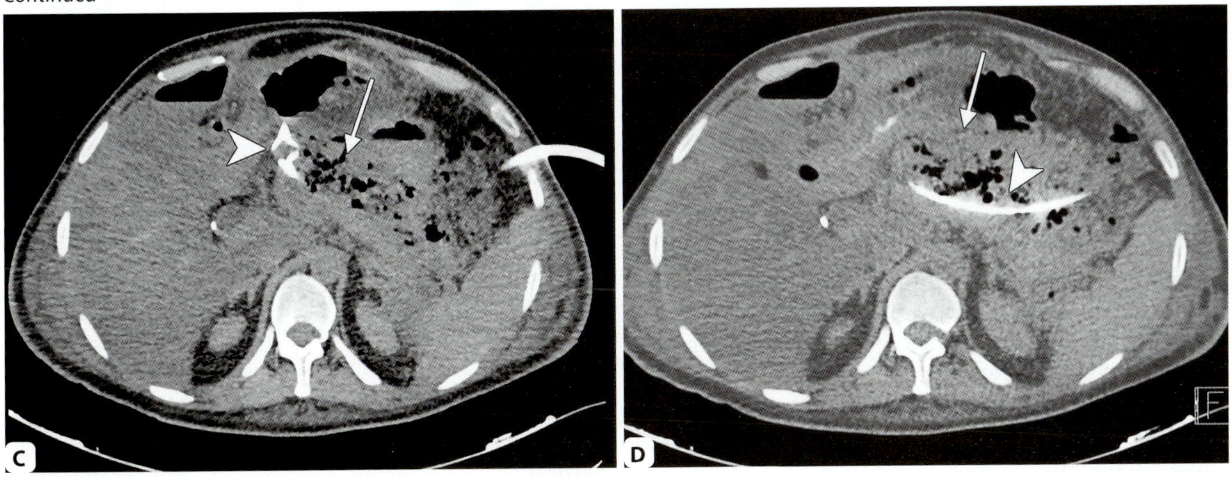

FIGS. 29A TO D: Transperitoneal approach for WON associated with acute pancreatitis. (A) Axial NCCT image shows a poorly encapsulated collection with multiple foci of air completely replacing the pancreatic body and tail extending to the lesser sac-infected acute necrotizing fluid collection (white arrow on all images). (B) Axial NCCT image shows an 18-G puncture needle (arrowhead) inserted transperitoneally into the collection. (C and D) Axial NCCT images show a 12 Fr Malecot catheter (arrowheads) within the pancreatic collection.

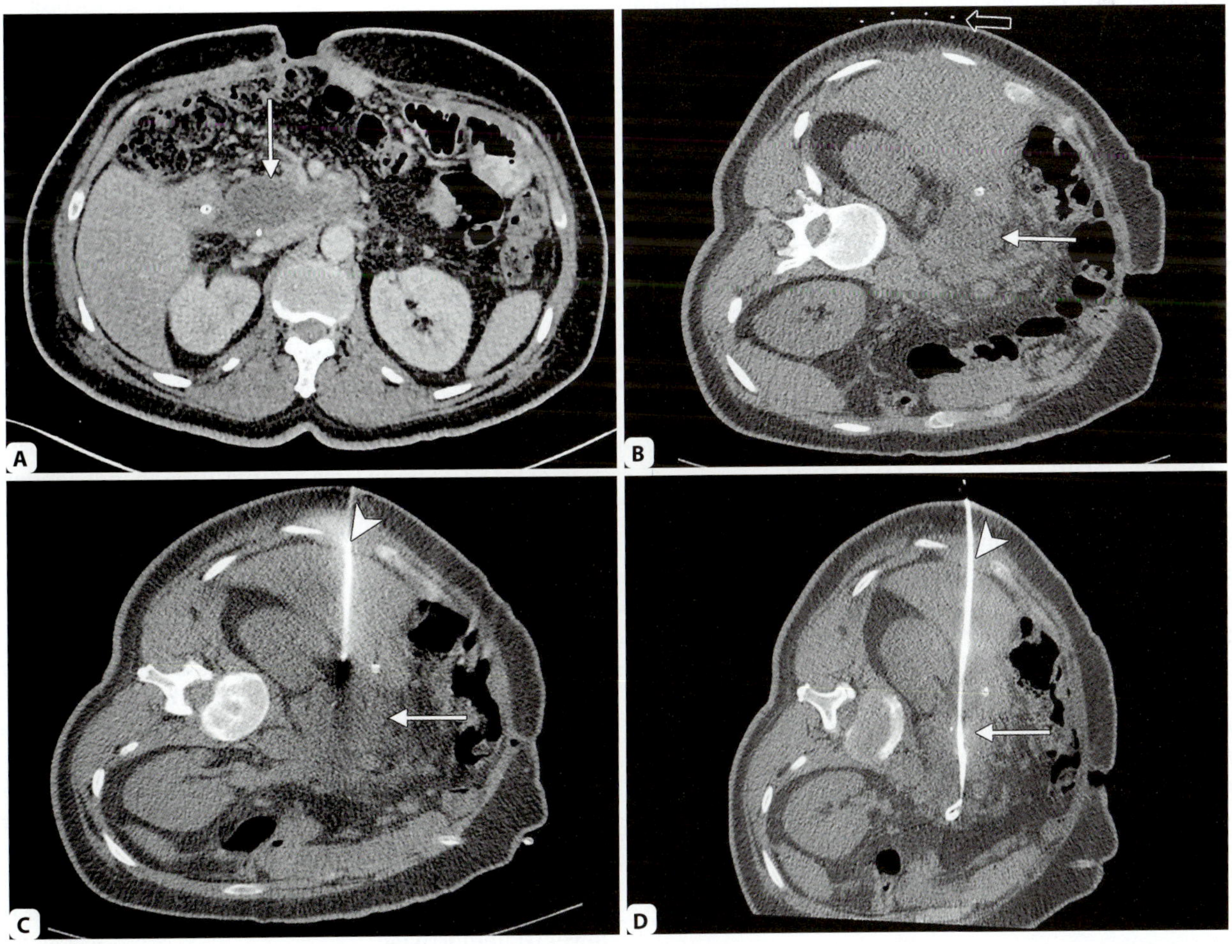

FIGS. 30A TO D: Transhepatic approach for WON associated with acute pancreatitis. (A) Axial CECT image shows a well-encapsulated hypoenhancing collection replacing the pancreatic head and uncinate process posterior to the 2nd part of the duodenum (white arrow on all images). (B) Axial NCCT image in the left decubitus positions shows a needle grid (black arrow) for localizing the site of the skin puncture. (C and D) Axial NCCT image in the left decubitus positions shows a transhepatically inserted 12 Fr pigtail catheter (arrowheads) within the pancreatic collection.

must be assessed. If the tube is malpositioned, it must be repositioned, or a secondary tube must be inserted. If the tube is in the correct position, it may be serially upgraded with a Malecot drainage tube up to 16/18F/20F/24F/28F after 48–72 hours. The step-up approach may be considered if patient's condition is not improving even after upgradation.

Step-up Approach

Multiple studies have established the superiority of a minimally invasive step-up approach over open necrosectomy in cases of infected pancreatic necrosis (PANTER trial).[44] The step-up approach comprises initial retroperitoneal percutaneous drainage followed by minimally invasive retroperitoneal necrosectomy, if clinically required.

If this does not lead to clinical improvement, endoscopic necrosectomy is attempted. Surgical intervention is considered necessary if both drainage and endoscopic necrosectomy do not lead to clinical improvement. Both endoscopic necrosectomy and surgical necrosectomy are performed after the development of a mature wall around the collection (usually ~ 4 weeks after disease onset).

- *Endoscopic step-up approach*: A cystoenterostomy (usually the posterior gastric wall or medial duodenal wall) is created, followed by double pigtail plastic stents or LAMS insertion under EUS guidance. Using this fistula, the endoscope is negotiated into the cyst cavity, and necrotic debris is removed, a procedure called *direct endoscopic necrosectomy (DEN)*.
- *Surgical step-up approach*: It is the technique of debridement of infected necrosis using a flexible endoscope via a mature tract along the percutaneous catheter insertion site—*percutaneous endoscopic necrosectomy (PDEN)*.

Laparoscopic Cystogastrostomy

It is a minimally invasive surgical approach preferred over open surgery for internal drainage of symptomatic pancreatic pseudocyst/WON due to its less invasive nature, faster postoperative recovery, and less postoperative pain. Both laparoscopic cystogastrostomy and endoscopic cystogastrostomy show similar success rates for drainage of peripancreatic collections. Laparoscopic drainage may be performed in patients when endoscopic cystogastrostomy is not possible or feasible, WON containing significant necrotic debris (>50%) and associated gallbladder stones so that cholecystectomy may also be done in the same setting.[45]

Video-assisted Retroperitoneal Dissection

It is a minimally invasive surgical procedure for infected pancreatic necrosis, currently the first-line surgical procedure after failure of percutaneous drainage and endoscopic necrosectomy. During video-assisted retroperitoneal dissection (VARD), a subcostal incision is made in the left lumbar region close to the exit point of the percutaneous drain. The percutaneous drain is used to guide port placement into the retroperitoneal collection. Loose necrosis is removed with long grasping forceps combined with irrigation and suction for improved visualization of the cavity. Postprocedure, the percutaneous drain is replaced with two large bore drains in the deep and shallow parts of the cavity, and continuous postoperative lavage is performed for 24 hours till the effluent is clear.

Open Necrosectomy

Open surgery is associated with high mortality in the setting of AP. However, certain situations may warrant open necrosectomy:

- Failed step-up approach
- Inability to control bleeding after endovascular treatment
- Bowel perforation
- Disconnected pancreatic duct syndrome
- Widespread areas of necrosis

Prognostic Factors

Recently, clinical, endoscopic, and imaging-based QNI (number of abdominal **Q**uadrants involved, percentage **N**ecrosis, and presence of **I**nfection) classification has been proposed to stratify the patients of WON and decide optimal management. Patients with higher QNI may need more endoscopic/other drainage procedures and a longer time for the resolution of WON.[46]

Numerous biomarkers have been studied as potential early predictors of the severity of AP. C-reactive protein ≥150 mg/L on the third day can be used as a prognostic marker for SAP. Serum Urea ≥ 20 mg/dL is an independent predictor of mortality.[22]

Endovascular Management of Pseudoaneurysms

Pancreatitis-related pseudoaneurysms are associated with significant morbidity and mortality without appropriate management. These may present with bleeding inside the collection or within the gut lumen.

Bleeding inside the collection presents with a sudden fall in blood pressure, tachycardia, and a fall in hemoglobin or frank blood draining through the drainage tube if it was placed earlier.

Bleeding within the gut may present as upper GI or lower GI hemorrhage.

All pseudoaneurysms associated with AP, irrespective of size, need treatment due to their thin wall and consequent high risk of rupture. Endovascular embolization is the intervention of choice for the management of pancreatitis-associated pseudoaneurysms.

Drainage or debridement is contraindicated in the presence of pseudoaneurysms, and the latter are to be dealt with first (otherwise, the hematoma's tamponade effect will be lost, resulting in bleeding).

Acquiring a dual-phase CECT is important for diagnosing pseudoaneurysms and planning endovascular interventions for their embolization. CT angiography images can help identify pseudoaneurysms, contrast extravasation, culprit artery, bony landmarks for origin or arteries, and any variant arterial anatomy.

Transarterial embolization of mesenteric vessel pseudoaneurysms is considered a high-risk procedure for bleeding as per the Society of Interventional Radiology guidelines,[47] and routine evaluation of the prothrombin time/international normalized ratio (PT/INR) and platelets is recommended. If deranged, the INR is corrected to ≤1.5–1.8 and platelet count to > 50 × 10^9/L.

Technique

The right common femoral artery is punctured, followed by the insertion of a 6 French arterial sheath. The culprit artery is selectively catheterized using RC1 or SIM1 catheters (5 Fr), and angiography is performed to delineate the pseudoaneurysm site. Microcatheters (<3 Fr) are then utilized to reach the site of pseudoaneurysm or contrast extravasation super selectively. Permanent embolization is usually performed by coils and glue.

Coil embolization is preferred due to better control and lower risk of distal ischemia (compared to glue). The diameter of the selected coil should be 20–30% larger than the size of the artery to allow adequate packing. Distal migration of coil can occur due to the smaller size of coil and straight deployment can occur due to an oversized coil. The sandwich technique is preferred in splenic pseudoaneurysms as collateral blood inflow is highly likely. These collaterals may cause incomplete embolization and recurrence of pseudoaneurysm. In this technique, the occlusion is done distal, across, and proximal to the neck of the pseudoaneurysm blocking both the efferent and afferent arteries (back door and front door closure) **(Figs. 31 and 32)**.

N-butyl cyanoacrylate glue is a permanent embolizing agent that polymerizes to form a cast when it encounters blood. It is generally mixed with lipiodol contrast agent for fluoroscopic visibility and as a carrier. The concentration of glue in the glue-lipiodol mixture determines the polymerization rate. Dextrose (5%) is used to flush the catheter before and after the administration of glue to prevent its polymerization within the catheter. The glue embolization technique is usually used if the vessels are tortuous (making it difficult to reach for coil deployment), there is persistence or recurrence after coil embolization, or if coagulation factors are deranged. Its use requires expertise to prevent nontarget embolization and catheter trapping.

If distal flow needs to be preserved, as in cases of proximal large parent vessel pseudoaneurysms, stenting can also be done. It is also done in cases where pseudoaneurysms have a wide neck, as the latter carries a higher risk of embolic agent migration.

Percutaneous Embolization of Pseudoaneurysms

Percutaneous embolization of pseudoaneurysms can also be done if endovascular management fails. It is done under US or CT guidance. Lyophilized thrombin is available in powder form and is reconstituted with a calcium chloride solution. Thrombin activates the coagulation cascade, polymerizing fibrinogen that forms a fibrin clot. The pseudoaneurysm is punctured using a 22-G Chiba needle and the tip of the needle is kept away from the neck to prevent the risk of nontarget embolization. These agents are slowly injected under guidance until thrombosis ensues. This technique, however, carries a higher risk of recurrence and nontarget embolization.

PREVENTION OF RECURRENT ATTACKS

In cases of acute biliary pancreatitis, cholecystectomy is recommended in the same initial hospital admission, especially in nonsevere cases, to prevent attacks of recurrent AP.[21] In the presence of collections, cholecystectomy may be deferred until their resolution/stability/encapsulation and resolution of acute inflammation. Smoking and alcohol abuse show a synergistic and dose-dependent association with recurrent AP and its progression to chronic pancreatitis.[48]

CONCLUSION

Acute pancreatitis is a complex disease process that requires a multidisciplinary approach for appropriate management. The radiologist plays a key role in both the diagnosis and the management of pancreatitis and its complications. Percutaneous pancreatic drainage is the cornerstone of the treatment of infected pancreatic necrosis using the step-up approach. Endovascular management of life-threatening bleeding from ruptured pseudoaneurysm secondary to pancreatitis is associated with a significant reduction in mortality from pancreatitis.

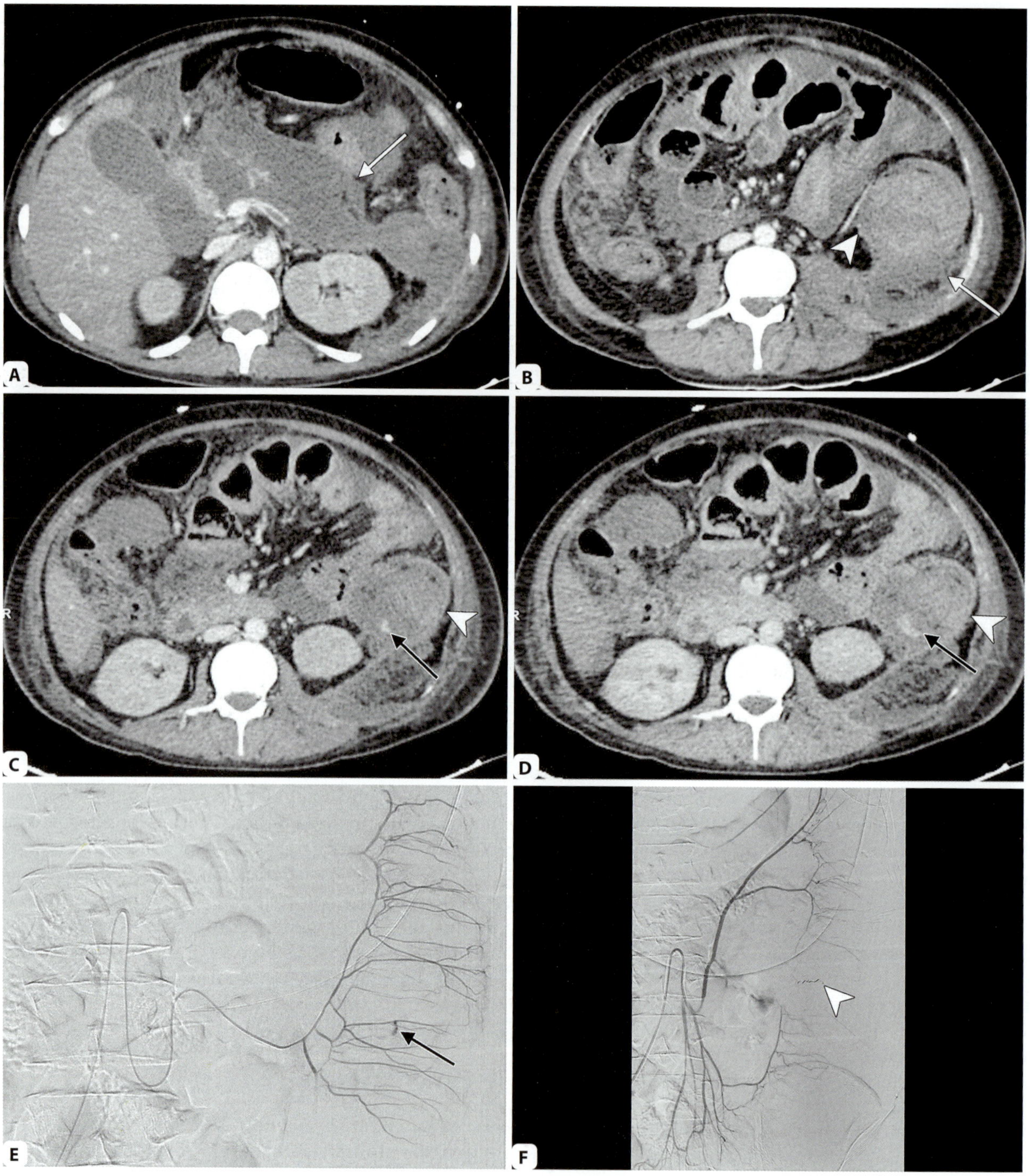

FIGS. 31A TO F: Active contrast extravasation in acute necrotizing pancreatitis managed by transarterial coil embolization. CECT abdomen images in the venous (A to C) and delayed (D) phase in a 29-year-old male with acute pancreatitis in the 5th week of illness show a large well-encapsulated collection with areas of fat necrosis in the lesser sac and along the left paracolic gutter (white arrows). A hyperdense clot is seen within the left paracolic gutter collection (arrowheads) with associated focal contrast extravasation (black arrow) increasing in size from the venous (C) to the delayed (D) phase. (E) DSA images of the same patient show contrast extravasation from the vasa recta of the left colic artery (black arrow). A single microcoil (18-3-2) was deployed in the culprit vasa recta (arrowhead). (F) Postprocedure angiogram shows resolution of the contrast extravasation.

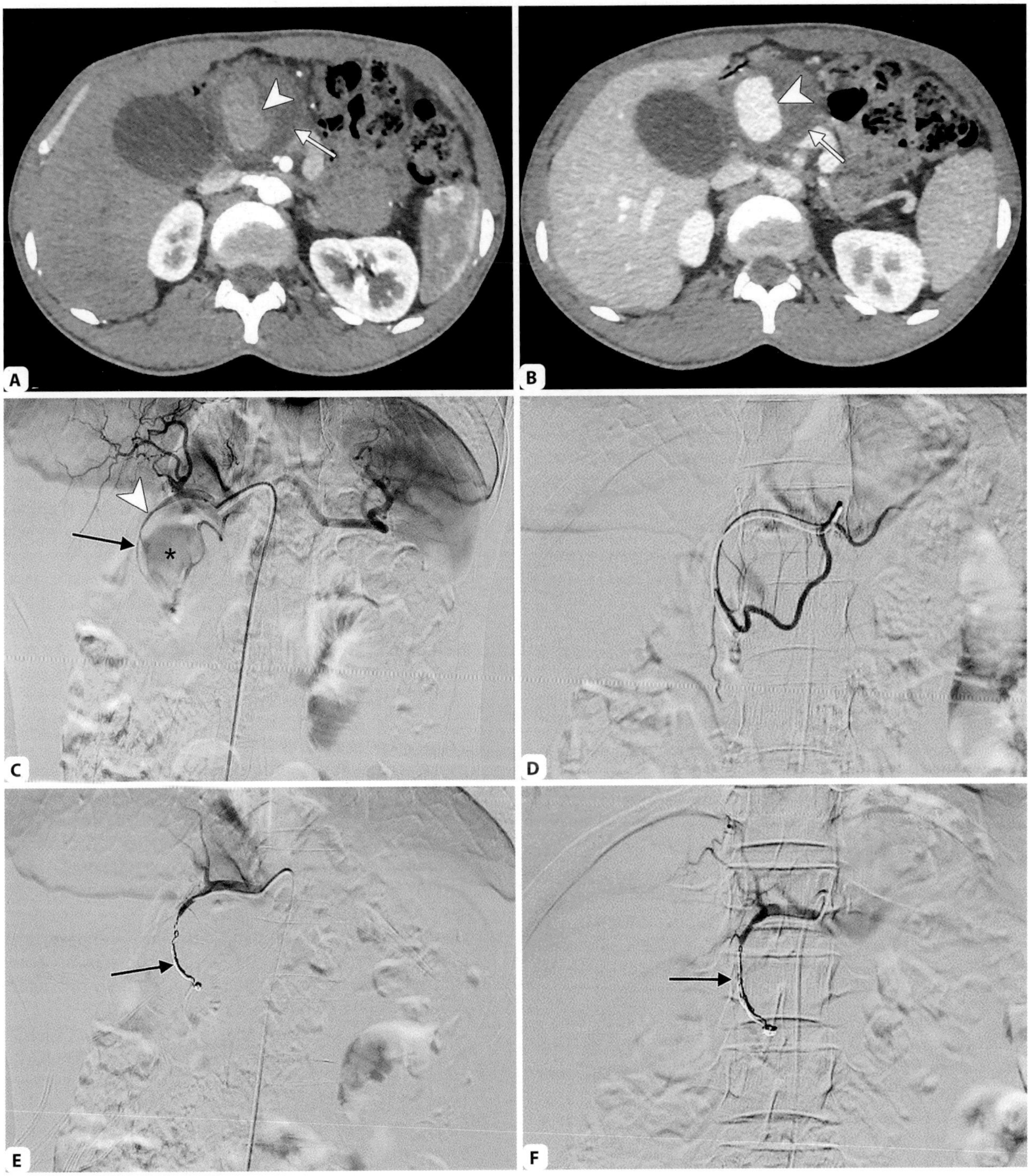

FIGS. 32A TO F: Pseudoaneurysm of the gastroduodenal artery treated by transarterial coil embolization. CECT abdomen images in the arterial (A) and venous (B) phase in a 36-year-old male with acute necrotizing pancreatitis in the 6th week of illness demonstrate a well-defined area of contrast enhancement (arrowhead) in the arterial phase (A) which maintains its shape while increasing contrast attenuation in the venous phase (B) suggestive of a pseudoaneurysm. Note made of hypodense hematoma (arrow) surrounding the pseudoaneurysm. (C) Pre-embolization DSA image (A) in the same patient demonstrates a saccular outpouching (asterisk) with a narrow neck (black arrow) arising from the gastroduodenal artery (arrowhead). The microcatheter is advanced distal to the neck of the pseudoaneurysm in image (D). Post-embolization check angiograms (E and F) show coils across the neck of the pseudoaneurysm in the gastroduodenal artery (black arrow) with no filling of the pseudoaneurysm.

KEY LEARNING POINTS

- US must be done in all suspected cases of AP. It serves to rule out other diseases, identify fluid collections, and identify biliary calculi as the cause of pancreatitis.
- CT is not required in all suspected cases of AP. CT may help diagnose cases where clinical presentation and/or amylase/lipase elevation is equivocal and rule out other causes of acute abdomen.
- CT should be done at least 3 days and preferably 5–7 days after the onset of symptoms to assess the severity and extent of pancreatitis.
- MRI may be useful in the acute setting to identify biliary calculi (warranting urgent ERCP) and better detect acute interstitial pancreatitis.
- US and MRI are more accurate than CT in quantifying necrosis/debris in pancreatitis-related collections.
- Endoscopic cystogastrostomy is the drainage procedure of choice for collections located in the lesser sac, while percutaneous drainage is helpful for collections located in the paracolic gutter.
- Drainage is usually done after 4 weeks to reduce the risk of iatrogenic infection and because early drainage is unlikely to be clinically beneficial.

REFERENCES

1. Krishna SG, Kamboj AK, Hart PA, Hinton A, Conwell DL. The Changing epidemiology of acute pancreatitis hospitalizations: A decade of trends and the impact of chronic pancreatitis. Pancreas. 2017;46(4):482-8.
2. Iannuzzi JP, King JA, Leong JH, Quan J, Windsor JW, Tanyingoh D, et al. Global incidence of acute pancreatitis is increasing over time: A systematic review and meta-analysis. Gastroenterology. 2022;162(1):122-34.
3. Seppänen H, Puolakkainen P. Classification, severity assessment, and prevention of recurrences in acute pancreatitis. Scand J Surg. 2020;109(1):53-8.
4. Banks PA, Bollen TL, Dervenis C, Gooszen HG, Johnson CD, Sarr MG, et al. Classification of acute pancreatitis—2012: revision of the Atlanta classification and definitions by international consensus. Gut. 2013;62(1):102-11.
5. Alter D, Koch DD. A review of acute pancreatitis. JAMA. 2021;325(23):2402.
6. Brizi MG, Perillo F, Cannone F, Tuzza L, Manfredi R. The role of imaging in acute pancreatitis. Radiol Med (Torino). 2021;126(8):1017.
7. Alves JR, Ferrazza GH, Nunes Junior IN, Teive MB. The acceptance of changes in the management of patients with acute pancreatitis after the revised Atlanta classification. Arq Gastroenterol. 2021;58:17-25.
8. Dellinger EP, Forsmark CE, Layer P, Lévy P, Maraví-Poma E, Petrov MS, et al. Determinant-based classification of acute pancreatitis severity: an international multidisciplinary consultation. Ann Surg. 2012;256(6):875-80.
9. IAP/APA evidence-based guidelines for the management of acute pancreatitis. Pancreatology. 2013;13(4):e1-15.
10. Merkle EM, Görich J. Imaging of acute pancreatitis. Eur Radiol. 2002;12(8):1979-92.
11. Burrowes DP, Choi HH, Rodgers SK, Fetzer DT, Kamaya A. Utility of ultrasound in acute pancreatitis. Abdom Radiol. 2020;45(5):1253-64.
12. Kreel L, Haertel M, Katz D. Computed tomography of the normal pancreas. J Comput Assist Tomogr. 1977;1(3):290-9.
13. Expert Panel on GYN and OB Imaging; Robbins JB, Sadowski EA, Maturen KE, Akin EA, Ascher SM, Brook OR, et al. ACR Appropriateness Criteria® Abnormal Uterine Bleeding. J Am Coll Radiol JACR. 2020;17(11S):S336-45.
14. Zeng T, An J, Wu Y, Hu X, An N, Gao L, et al. Incidence and prognostic role of pleural effusion in patients with acute pancreatitis: a meta-analysis. Ann Med. 2023;55(2):2285909.
15. Angadi S, Mahapatra SJ, Sethia R, Elhence A, Krishna A, Gunjan D, et al. Endoscopic transmural drainage tailored to quantity of necrotic debris versus laparoscopic transmural internal drainage for walled-off necrosis in acute pancreatitis: A randomized controlled trial. Pancreatology. 2021;21(7):1291-8.
16. Balthazar EJ, Robinson DL, Megibow AJ, Ranson JH. Acute pancreatitis: value of CT in establishing prognosis. Radiology. 1990;174(2):331-6.
17. Mortele KJ, Wiesner W, Intriere L, Shankar S, Zou KH, Kalantari BN, et al. A Modified CT severity index for evaluating acute pancreatitis: improved correlation with patient outcome. Am J Roentgenol. 2004;183(5):1261-5.
18. De Waele JJ, Delrue L, Hoste EA, De Vos M, Duyck P, Colardyn FA. Extrapancreatic inflammation on abdominal computed tomography as an early predictor of disease severity in acute pancreatitis: Evaluation of a new scoring system. Pancreas. 2007;34(2):185-90.
19. Gupta P, Jain R, Koshi S, Gulati A, Samanta J, Mandavdhare H, et al. Radiation dose from computed tomography in patients with acute pancreatitis: An audit from a tertiary care referral hospital. Abdom Radiol N Y. 2020;45(5):1517-23.
20. Viremouneix L, Monneuse O, Gautier G, Gruner L, Giorgi R, Allaouchiche B, et al. Prospective evaluation of nonenhanced MR imaging in acute pancreatitis. J Magn Reson Imaging JMRI. 2007;26(2):331-8.
21. Baron TH, DiMaio CJ, Wang AY, Morgan KA. American Gastroenterological Association Clinical Practice Update: Management of Pancreatic Necrosis. Gastroenterology. 2020;158(1):67-75.e1.
22. Leppäniemi A, Tolonen M, Tarasconi A, Segovia-Lohse H, Gamberini E, Kirkpatrick AW, et al. 2019 WSES guidelines for the management of severe acute pancreatitis. World J Emerg Surg. 2019;14(1):1-20.
23. Sureka B, Rai B, Varshney VK, Nag VL, Garg MK, Garg P, et al. Diffusion-weighted magnetic resonance imaging is an ideal imaging method to detect infection in pancreatic collections: A brief primer for the gastroenterologists. Cureus. 2022;14(1):e21530.

24. Abuzeid HM, Yassin A, Kamel OF, Sabry KA. Role of diffusion-weighted MR imaging in diagnosis of acute pancreatitis. Egypt J Radiol Nucl Med. 2020;51(1):1-9.
25. Arvanitakis M, Delhaye M, De Maertelaere V, Bali M, Winant C, Coppens E, et al. Computed tomography and magnetic resonance imaging in the assessment of acute pancreatitis. Gastroenterology. 2004;126(3):715-23.
26. Cai D, Parajuly SS, Wang H, Wang X, Ling W, Song B, et al. Accuracy of contrast-enhanced ultrasound compared with conventional ultrasound in acute pancreatitis: Diagnosis and complication monitoring. Exp Ther Med. 2016;12(5): 3189-3194.
27. Yadav AK, Sharma R, Kandasamy D, Bhalla AS, Gamanagatti S, Srivastava DN, et al. Perfusion CT: can it predict the development of pancreatic necrosis in early stage of severe acute pancreatitis? Abdom Imaging. 2015;40(3):488-99.
28. Chen Y, Chen TW, Wu CQ, Lin Q, Hu R, Xie CL, et al. Radiomics model of contrast-enhanced computed tomography for predicting the recurrence of acute pancreatitis. Eur Radiol. 2019;29(8):4408-17.
29. Foster BR, Jensen KK, Bakis G, Shaaban AM, Coakley FV. (2016). Revised Atlanta Classification for Acute Pancreatitis: A Pictorial Essay. [online] Available from https://pubs.rsna.org/doi/10.1148/rg.2016150097 [Last accessed July, 2024].
30. Sternby H, Verdonk RC, Aguilar G, Dimova A, Ignatavicius P, Ilzarbe L, et al. Significant inter-observer variation in the diagnosis of extrapancreatic necrosis and type of pancreatic collections in acute pancreatitis—An international multicenter evaluation of the revised Atlanta classification. Pancreatol Off J Int Assoc Pancreatol IAP Al. 2016;16(5):791-7.
31. Rana SS, Sharma V, Sharma RK, Chhabra P, Gupta R, Bhasin DK. Clinical significance of presence and extent of extrapancreatic necrosis in acute pancreatitis. J Gastroenterol Hepatol. 2015;30(4):794-8.
32. Takahashi N, Papachristou GI, Schmit GD, Chahal P, LeRoy AJ, Sarr MG, et al. CT findings of walled-off pancreatic necrosis (WOPN): differentiation from pseudocyst and prediction of outcome after endoscopic therapy. Eur Radiol. 2008;18(11): 2522-9.
33. Vanek P, Urban O, Trikudanathan G, Freeman ML. Disconnected pancreatic duct syndrome in patients with necrotizing pancreatitis. Surg Open Sci. 2023;11:19.
34. Sandrasegaran K, Tann M, Jennings SG, Maglinte DD, Peter SD, Sherman S, et al. Disconnection of the pancreatic duct: An important but overlooked complication of severe acute pancreatitis. RadioGraphics. 2007;27(5):1389-400.
35. Bush N, Rana SS. Ascites in acute pancreatitis: Clinical implications and management. Dig Dis Sci. 2022;67(6):1987-93.
36. Narváez J, Bianchi MM, Santo P, de la Fuente D, Ríos-Rodriguez V, Bolao F, et al. Pancreatitis, panniculitis, and polyarthritis. Semin Arthritis Rheum. 2010;39(5):417-23.
37. Castro JP, Atanásio G, Canelas MA, Ferreira A, Barbosa AR, Barbedo M, et al. A case report of pancreatitis-panniculitis-polyarthritis syndrome—an unusual but serious presentation of pancreatic disease. Scott Med J. 2019;65(1):19-23.
38. Popa D, Grigorescu B, Hoffner S, Copotoiu C. Vascular complications—poor prognostic factors in severe acute pancreatitis. Acta Medica Marisiensis. 2011;57:74-6.
39. Khurana A, Nelson LW, Myers CB, Akisik F, Jeffrey BR, Miller FH, et al. Reporting of acute pancreatitis by radiologists-time for a systematic change with structured reporting template. Abdom Radiol N Y. 2020;45(5):1277.
40. van Santvoort HC, Bollen TL, Besselink MG, Banks PA, Boermeester MA, van Eijck CH, et al. Describing Peripancreatic Collections in Severe Acute Pancreatitis Using Morphologic Terms: An International Interobserver Agreement Study. Pancreatology. 2008;8(6):593-9.
41. Boxhoorn L, van Dijk SM, van Grinsven J, Verdonk RC, Boermeester MA, Bollen TL, et al. Immediate versus postponed intervention for infected necrotizing pancreatitis. N Engl J Med. 2021;385(15):1372-81.
42. Singh AK, Samanta J, Gulati A, Gautam V, Bhatia A, Gupta P, et al. Outcome of percutaneous drainage in patients with pancreatic necrosis having organ failure. HPB. 2021;23(7): 1030-8.
43. Ke L, Li J, Hu P, Wang L, Chen H, Zhu Y. Percutaneous catheter drainage in infected pancreatitis necrosis: A systematic review. Indian J Surg. 2016;78(3):221-8.
44. Besselink MG, van Santvoort HC, Nieuwenhuijs VB, Boermeester MA, Bollen TL, Buskens E, et al. Minimally invasive "step-up approach" versus maximal necrosectomy in patients with acute necrotising pancreatitis (PANTER trial): design and rationale of a randomised controlled multicenter trial [ISRCTN13975868]. BMC Surg. 2006;6:6.
45. Garg PK, Meena D, Babu D, Padhan RK, Dhingra R, Krishna A, et al. Endoscopic versus laparoscopic drainage of pseudocyst and walled-off necrosis following acute pancreatitis: A randomized trial. Surg Endosc. 2020;34(3):1157-66.
46. Baroud S, Chandrasekhara V, Storm AC, Law RJ, Vargas EJ, Levy MJ, et al. Novel classification system for walled-off necrosis: a step toward standardized nomenclature and risk-stratification framework. Gastrointest Endosc. 2023;97(2): 300-8.
47. Dariushnia SR, Redstone EA, Heran MKS, Cramer HR, Ganguli S, Gomes AS, et al. Society of Interventional Radiology Quality Improvement Standards for Percutaneous Transcatheter Embolization. J Vasc Interv Radiol. 2021;32(3):476.
48. Szentesi A, Farkas N, Sipos Z, Mátrai P, Vincze Á, Izbéki F, et al. Alcohol consumption and smoking dose-dependently and synergistically worsen local pancreas damage. Gut. 2022; 71(12):2601-2.

CHAPTER 19

Pankaj Gupta, Anupam Lal, Manphool Singhal, Mandeep Kang

Chronic Pancreatitis and Its Variants

INTRODUCTION

Chronic pancreatitis (CP) is a progressive fibroinflammatory disease of the pancreas. CP impairs the quality of life due to chronic pain and exocrine and endocrine insufficiency. The highest prevalence in India has been reported to be 125/100,000 population.[1] Acute complications of CP include fluid collections, internal fistulae (leading to pancreatic ascites and pleural effusions), and vascular complications.[2] Long-term complications of CP are diabetes mellitus and pancreatic cancer.[2] There has been significant evolution in the understanding of the pathophysiology of CP. Consequently, the clinicopathological definitions of CP have been replaced by a mechanistic definition.[3] Noninvasive imaging studies most commonly employed in investigating patients with suspected CP include magnetic resonance imaging (MRI) and magnetic resonance cholangiopancreatography (MRCP), endoscopic ultrasound (EUS), and computed tomography (CT).[2] Despite advances in imaging, diagnosis of early CP remains challenging. CP is one of the most important predisposing factors for pancreatic ductal adenocarcinoma (PDAC).[4] In this chapter, we discuss the definitions of CP, pathophysiology, risk factors, and role of various imaging modalities in diagnosing CP. We also discuss variants of the classic CP and conundrum of inflammatory mass versus malignant mass in the setting of CP.

DEFINITION OF CHRONIC PANCREATITIS

Chronic pancreatitis was traditionally defined using a clinicopathologic approach that attempted to link typical signs and symptoms to chronic inflammation and irreversible fibrosis. However, this definition not only led to a delay in diagnosis but also failed to identify the underlying etiology, could not predict the disease course, and allowed only supportive care. In 2016, a mechanistic definition of CP was proposed, and was adopted by the major pancreas societies.[3] This definition proposes a "progressive model of CP to organize risk factors, clinical scenarios, disease biomarkers, sequential and progressive features, and individual variables within a lifetime". Besides affirming the characteristics of end-stage disease "as pancreatic atrophy, fibrosis, pain syndromes, duct distortion and strictures, calcifications, pancreatic exocrine dysfunction, pancreatic endocrine dysfunction, and dysplasia", it also addressed the disease mechanism as "a pathologic fibroinflammatory syndrome of the pancreas in individuals with genetic, environmental, and/or other risk factors who develop persistent pathologic responses to parenchymal injury or stress."

The progressive model identifies five stages: (i) at risk, (ii) acute pancreatitis (AP)-recurrent AP (RAP), (iii) early CP, (iv) established CP, and (v) end-stage CP.[5]

Definition of Early Chronic Pancreatitis

Early CP was previously defined based on the morphological changes in the Rosemont criteria (RC) for CP.[6] However, it was realized that most of the parenchymal changes in RC do not correlate with histological changes.[7] The Japan Pancreas Society (JPS) in 2019 defined early CP more comprehensively and included risk factors, clinical features, and morphological changes as identified by imaging studies.[8]

ETIOPATHOGENESIS

The established risk factors for CP are alcohol use, smoking, certain gene mutations, and recurrent episodes of AP.[9] The disease is idiopathic in 28% of patients. Alcohol use and smoking have a synergistic effect. CP is more common in men.[10] Genetic mutations most commonly associated with CP include cystic fibrosis transmembrane conductance regulator (CFTR), serine protease inhibitor kazal type 1 (SPINK1), or chymotrypsin C (CTRC).[11] These cases manifest as sporadic early-onset CP or may be associated with hereditary pancreatitis. Hereditary pancreatitis is a rare autosomal dominant disease mostly caused by cationic trypsinogen (*PRSS1*) gene mutation.[10]

Recent studies have identified a change in the phenotype of CP in India.[12] Genetic susceptibility due to genetic mutations is the most common risk factor for idiopathic CP compared to conventional risk factors including malnutrition or dietary toxins, suggesting that the term "tropical pancreatitis" is a misnomer. A recent systematic review reported similar demographic characteristics across cohorts from the East and the West including age, prevalence among males and females, and predominant etiology.[13]

Acute Pancreatitis as a Risk Factor

About 60% of CP cases evolve from AP and RAP. The progression to CP is faster with alcoholic etiologies.[14,15] In a recent study of 1,184 patients with AP (with a median follow-up of 9 years), recurrent acute pancreatitis (RAP) and CP developed in 25% and 6% patients, respectively.[16] Nonbiliary etiology, RAP, prior pancreatic interventions, smoking, and male sex were independently associated with CP. Another recent study reported the prevalence of CP in AP, RAP (2 episodes), RAP (3 episodes), RAP (4 episodes), and RAP (5+ episodes) to be 0%, 1%, 16%, 50%, and 47%, respectively. The authors concluded that three or more episodes of AP is a strong risk factor for CP.[17]

CLASSIFICATION OF CHRONIC PANCREATITIS

In contrast to AP, there are no globally accepted classification or severity scores in CP. Although 11 original scores and 6 modified scores for CP were identified in a recent systematic review, it was concluded that none of the scores reflect the recent advances in the understanding of CP.[18] TIGAR-O system classifies CP according to major predisposing risk factors as (1) toxic-metabolic, (2) idiopathic, (3) genetic, (4) autoimmune, (5) recurrent and severe acute pancreatitis, or (6) obstructive.[19]

DIAGNOSIS

American College of Gastroenterology guidelines for diagnosis of CP

CT or MRI are recommended for the first-line diagnosis of CP. EUS is recommended only if the diagnosis of CP is in question after CT and MRI, due to its invasive nature and interobserver variability. Secretin-enhanced MRCP (s-MRCP) is recommended when the diagnosis of CP is not confirmed with cross-sectional imaging or EUS and the clinical suspicion remains high. Pancreatic function testing is considered complementary to imaging for diagnosing CP. Histological examination is suggested in "high-risk patients when the clinical and functional evidence of CP is strong, but imaging modalities are inconclusive".[20]

IMAGING MODALITIES IN CHRONIC PANCREATITIS DIAGNOSIS

Abdominal Radiographs

Abdominal radiographs are not recommended for the diagnosis of CP. Abdominal radiographs have a role for guiding extracorporeal shock wave lithotripsy (ESWL) treatment of pancreatic ductal calcifications **(Fig. 1)**.[21]

Endoscopic Retrograde Cholangiopancreatography

Endoscopic retrograde cholangiopancreatography (ERCP) is considered the gold standard for the diagnosis of CP because of its superior spatial resolution and its ability to depict the ductal system in a distended state. Side branch abnormalities in early CP can be detected. However, owing to complications and the availability of noninvasive imaging, ERCP is no longer recommended for the diagnosis of CP.[22] ERCP is mostly for therapeutic interventions. On ERCP, diameter of normal main pancreatic duct (MPD) varies with the region of pancreas—up to 4 mm in head, 3 mm in body, and 2 mm in tail region.[19] Side branches join the MPD at right angles in alternating fashion. In early CP, there is irregularity and dilatation of side branches **(Fig. 2)**.

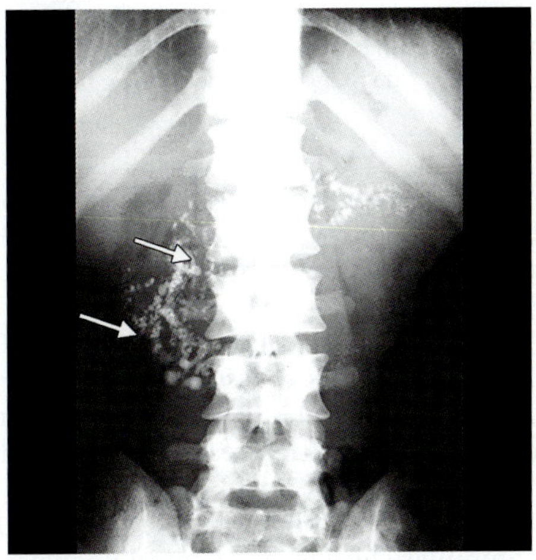

FIG. 1: Chronic pancreatitis: Plain radiograph abdomen shows calcifications along the course of pancreas. Note a pancreatic stent in situ (arrows).

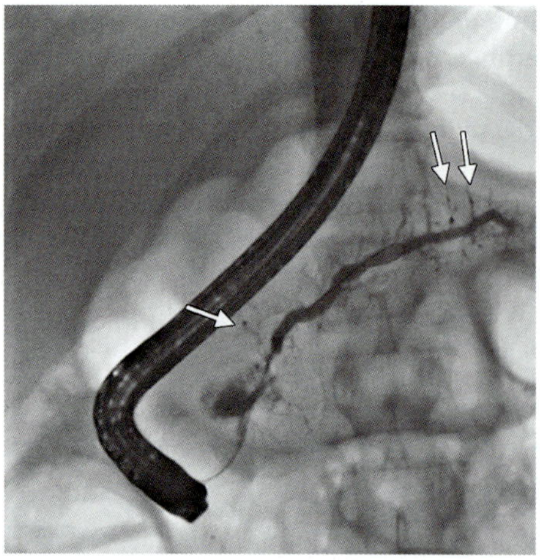

FIG. 2: Endoscopic retrograde cholangiopancreatography in chronic pancreatitis: Changes in early chronic pancreatitis include mild irregularity of side branches (arrows). Main pancreatic duct is not dilated.

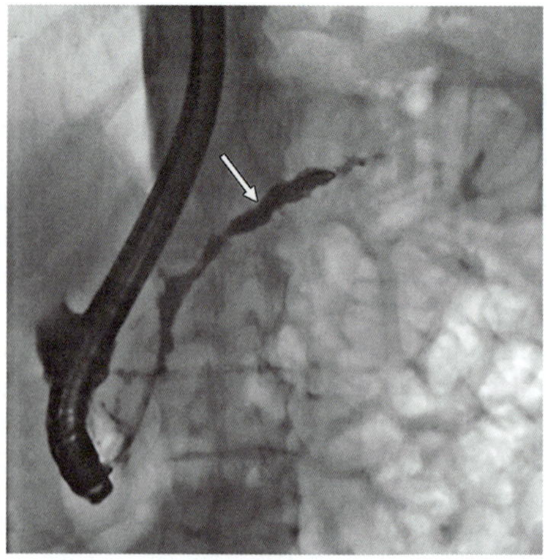

FIG. 4: Endoscopic retrograde cholangiopancreatography in chronic pancreatitis: Main pancreatic duct (arrow) shows multiple strictures and irregular dilatation with truncated and abnormal side branches.

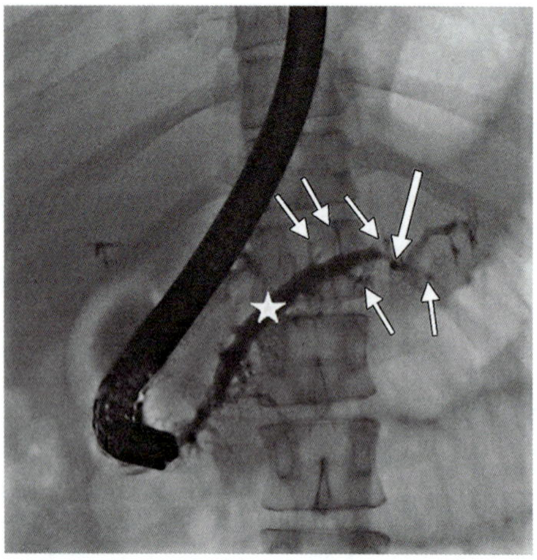

FIG. 3: Endoscopic retrograde cholangiopancreatography in chronic pancreatitis: Main pancreatic duct is dilated (star). Note narrowing of main pancreatic duct in tail region (long arrow) and multiple abnormal side branches (arrows).

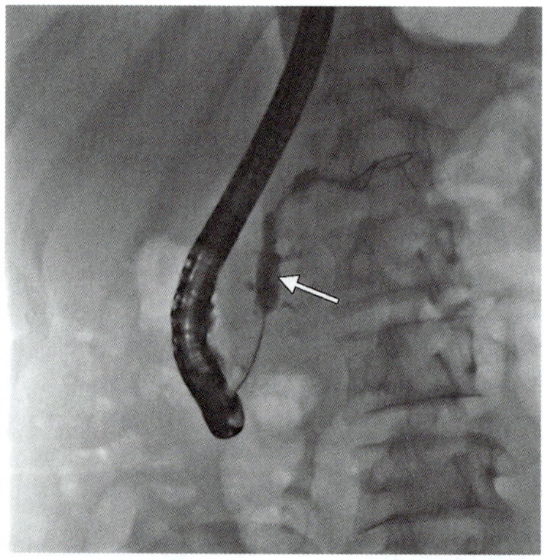

FIG. 5: Endoscopic retrograde cholangiopancreatography in chronic pancreatitis: Multiple strictures of MPD (chain of lakes appearance). Note abnormally dilated side branches in head region and nonopacification of side branches in body and tail region.

As the disease progresses, these changes become more marked **(Fig. 3)**. In advanced stages, alternate dilatation and stenosis of MPD can give the appearance of chain of lakes **(Figs. 4 and 5)**.

The Cambridge classification of CP based on ERCP is used to group patients into equivocal, mild, moderate, or marked type. The status of MPD, side branches, presence of calculi, and ductal strictures are considered in the Cambridge classification **(Box 1)**.[23]

ERCP may diagnose other cause of MPD obstruction such as ampullary lesions, intraductal neoplasms, and congenital anomalies such as pancreatic divisum **(Fig. 6)** or annular pancreas.

Ultrasonography

Transabdominal sonography (TAS): It is usually the initial imaging modality for evaluating patients with clinically suspected CP.[20] TAS evaluation is often challenging due to obscuration of pancreas by bowel gases. Maneuvers such as distending the stomach with water, changing position of patient, and visualizing the tail of pancreas through splenic window are helpful.[24] TAS findings vary with the stage of CP. In early stage, pancreatic echotexture is normal in up to 40% of the patients.[25] In rest of the patients, pancreas appears heteroechoic **(Fig. 7)**. In moderate-to-severe stages, the changes become more marked and

BOX 1 Cambridge classification of CP.

- *Normal:* Quality imaging study visualizing whole gland without any abnormality
- *Equivocal:* Less than 3 abnormal branches at ERCP with one of the US and CT features
- *Mild:* 3 or more abnormal branches at ERCP with two or more US and CT features
- *Moderate:* More than 3 abnormal main pancreatic duct (MPD) and branches at ERCP with two or more US and CT features
- *Severe:* Features of moderate plus one or more at ERCP: large cavities >10 mm, gland enlargement (>2 times normal), intraductal filling defects or calculi, duct obstruction (stricture), duct dilatation or irregularity, and contiguous organ invasion
- *Features at US and CT:* MPD <4 mm, pancreatic enlargement (>2 times normal), cavities <10 mm, duct irregularity, focal pancreatitis, parenchymal heterogeneity, increased duct wall echogenicity, and irregular head and body contour

(CP: chronic pancreatitis; CT: computed tomography; ERCP: endoscopic retrograde cholangiopancreatography, US: ultrasound)

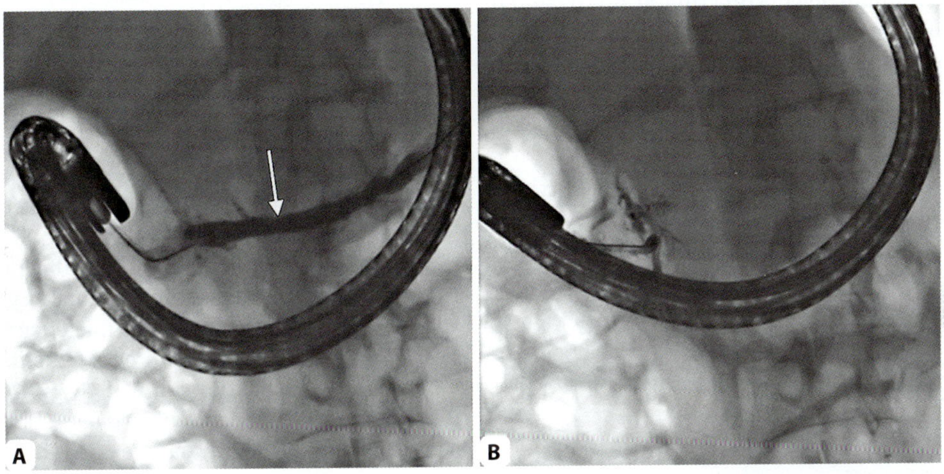

FIGS. 6A AND B: Endoscopic retrograde cholangiopancreatography (ERCP) in pancreatic divisum. ERCP images (A and B). Cannulation of minor papilla (A) shows opacification of entire dorsal duct which is mildly dilated (arrow) with truncation of some side branches. Cannulation of major papilla shows only part of ventral duct draining, part of head, and uncinate process of pancreas. Also note the long route taken by the endoscope required for cannulation of minor papilla.

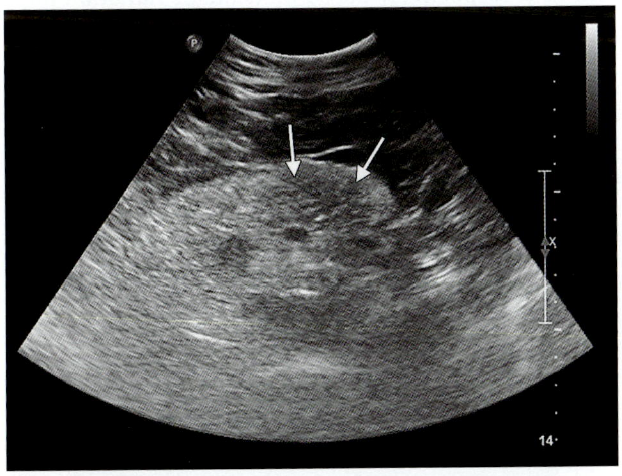

FIG. 7: Early chronic pancreatitis: Transabdominal ultrasound image showing subtle ill-defined hypoechoic areas in pancreatic body (arrows).

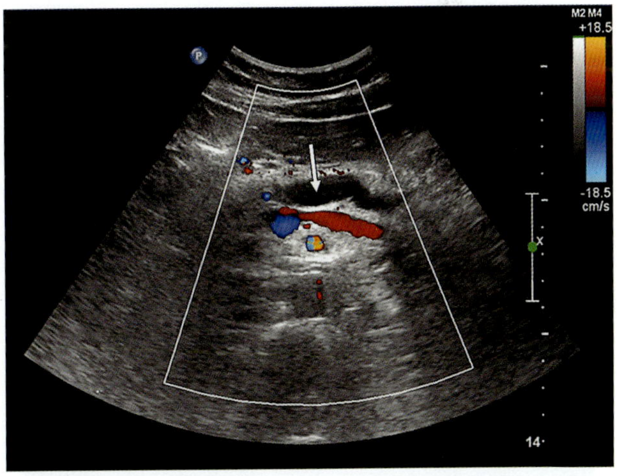

FIG. 8: Advanced chronic pancreatitis: Transabdominal ultrasound with Doppler shows dilated main pancreatic duct (arrow) with atrophy of pancreas.

include irregular dilated MPD with parenchymal and intraductal calculi and associated atrophy of pancreas **(Fig. 8)**. TAS is useful to detect complications like pseudocysts and venous thrombosis.

Endoscopic ultrasound: EUS allows high-resolution imaging of the pancreas without interference by the bowel gas. EUS may detect changes of early CP.[26] These include lobularity (well-circumscribed reticulated areas ≥5 mm in size with a hyperechoic rim) with and without honeycombing (at least three lobules located contiguously), hyperechoic foci without shadowing (≥3 mm, at least three in number), stranding (hyperechoic lines), cysts, dilatation of side branches, and hyperechoic margins of the MPD (Japan Pancreas Society criteria 2019) **(Figs. 9 to 11)**.[8] The other commonly used criterion for diagnosis of CP on EUS is the RC.[6] In the RC, the ductal and parenchymal changes are classified into major A criteria (hyperechoic foci with shadowing and MPD calculi), major B criteria (lobularity with honeycombing), and minor criteria ("hyperechoic strands, hyperechoic foci without shadowing, lobularity without honeycombing, cyst, MPD dilatation, irregular MPD contour, dilated side branch, and hyperechoic MPD margin"). According to the RC, EUS findings are classified as "consistent with CP," "suggestive of CP," "indeterminate for CP," or "normal". Several studies have reported lack of interobserver agreement for qualitative assessment using RC and lack of association between RC and exocrine/endocrine function and pathological changes.[27,28]

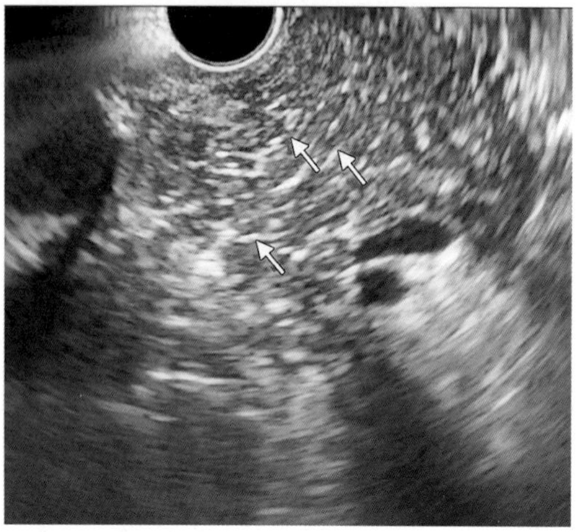

FIG. 9: Early chronic pancreatitis: Endoscopic ultrasound image shows echogenic foci (without posterior acoustic shadowing and echogenic strands) (arrows).

Elastography: Assessment of pancreatic stiffness is a useful adjunct to other imaging tests for diagnosis of CP. Retroperitoneal location of pancreas and proximity to aorta (effect of aortic pulsations) may hinder pancreatic elastography. However, the elastography technology has significantly improved allowing its increased utilization for detection of early CP. EUS-based elastography is the technique of choice for assessment of pancreatic stiffness. EUS elastography may alleviate the subjective assessment of B-mode EUS.[26] Elastography may be qualitative (color-coded strain distribution), semiquantitative (strain histogram and strain ratio), or quantitative [shear-wave elastography (SWE)]. Strain elastography is operator-dependent and the results are affected by the position and size of the region of interest **(Fig. 12)**. SWE gives an absolute stiffness value. Yamashita et al. reported 100% sensitivity and 94% specificity for the diagnosis of CP using EUS SWE. EUS SWE measurements have a good correlation with exocrine and endocrine insufficiency in CP patients.[29] Few other studies have also reported similar results.[30,31] Due to limited availability of EUS SWE, TAS elastography may also be utilized. Choudhry et al. reported the normal stiffness values of healthy pancreas in Indian subjects.[32] The pancreatic stiffness values were correlated with age and fatty change in the liver. TAS SWE has been reported to be positively correlated with histological grade of pancreatic fibrosis.[33] Yashima et al. reported a cut-off value of 1.40 m/s to diagnose CP with a sensitivity and specificity of 75% and 72%, respectively based on acoustic radiation force impulse (ARFI) and based on SWE.[34] Few other studies have also reported high diagnostic performance of the TAS SWE for diagnosis of CP.[35,36]

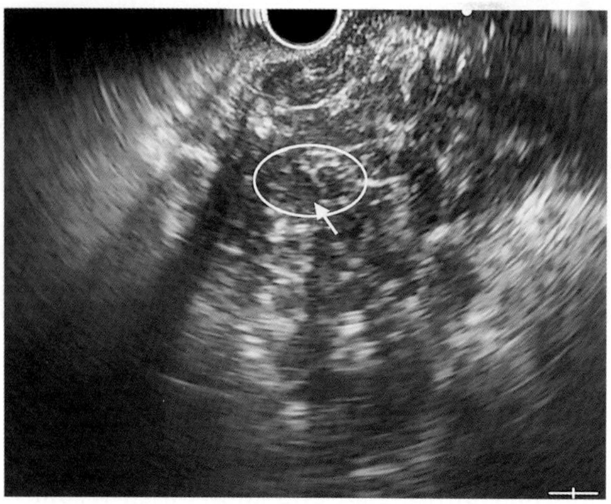

FIG. 10: Early chronic pancreatitis: Endoscopic ultrasound image shows lobularity (arrow) with honey combing (circle).

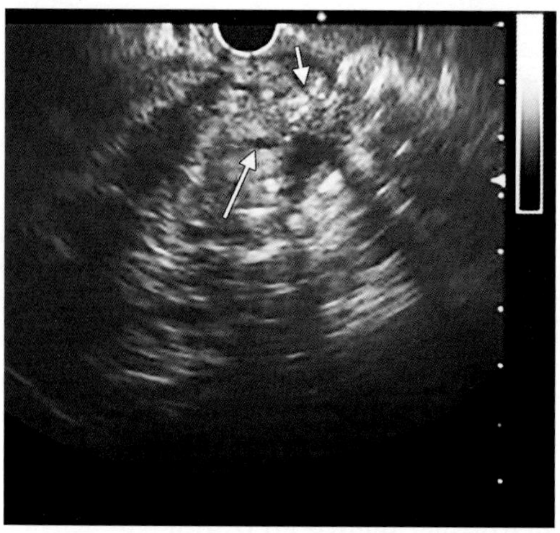

FIG. 11: Advanced chronic pancreatitis: Endoscopic ultrasound image shows calcifications (arrow) in pancreatic head and mildly dilated main pancreatic duct (long arrow).

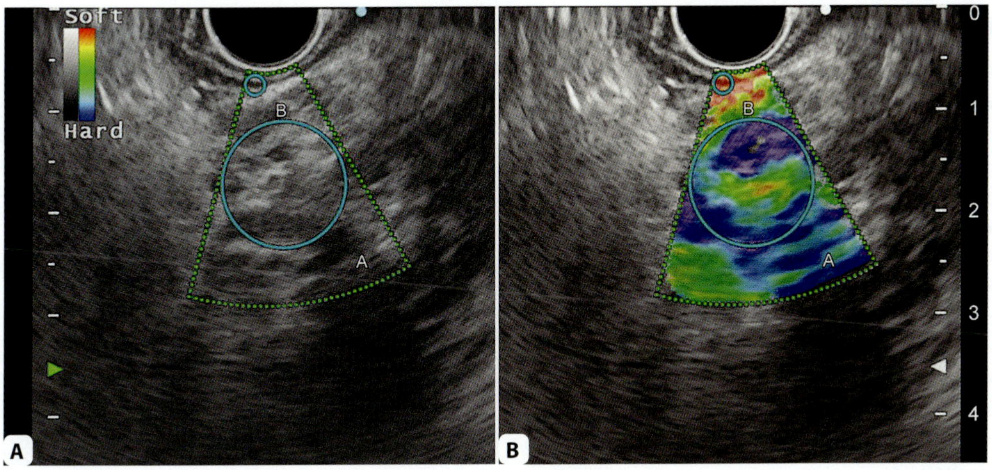

FIGS. 12A AND B: Endoscopic ultrasound strain elastography: Elastography image shows heterogenous soft to hard pattern with strain ratio of 7.89 suggestive of chronic pancreatitis.

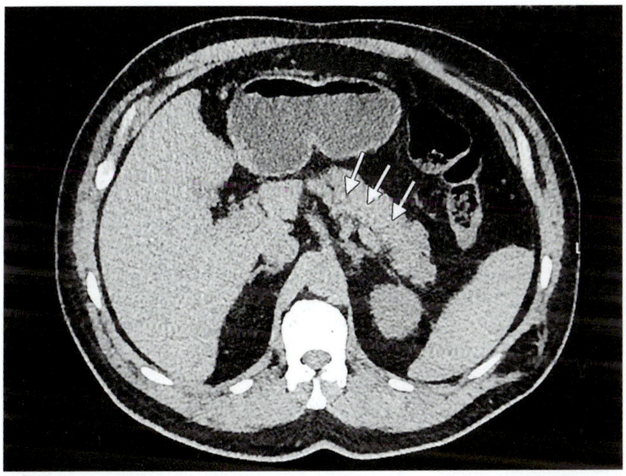

FIG. 13: Noncontrast computed tomography image showing subtle pancreatic calcifications (arrows) in pancreatic body and tail region.

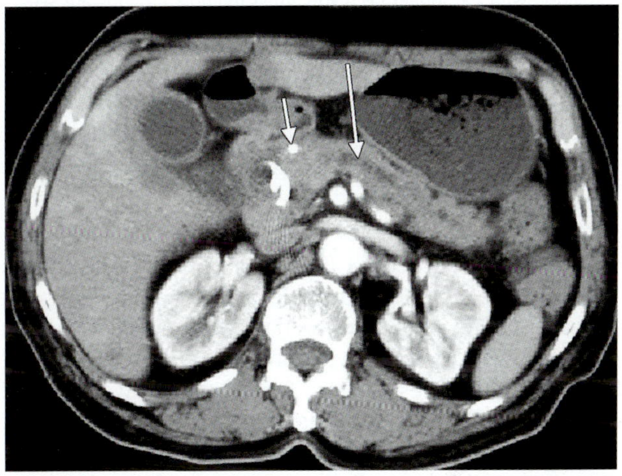

FIG. 14: Pancreatic parenchymal phase computed tomography image shows calcification (arrow) and dilated main pancreatic duct (long arrow). An inflammatory mass is seen in head region obstructing the main pancreatic duct. Note biliary stents in situ.

Computed Tomography

CT is the imaging modality of choice for the evaluation of CP.

CT protocol: A typical CT protocol for CP comprises noncontrast CT (NCCT), pancreatic parenchymal (late arterial phase at 40–45 seconds after initiation of contrast injection), and portal venous phases (at 60–70 seconds).[37] There is emerging literature on the use of dual-energy CT (DECT) in CP. DECT can be used to generate virtual nonenhanced (VNE) images and reduce the radiation dose.[38] The pancreatic calcifications are best seen on NCCT **(Fig. 13)**. Pancreatic parenchymal phase is used to assess alterations in pancreatic parenchymal enhancement, focal pancreatic lesions, and arterial complications **(Fig. 14)**. The portal venous phase allows assessment of the progression of pancreatic enhancement, other organs, and the splenoportal axis.

CT findings of CP: Normal pancreas on CT appears as a homogeneous structure with smooth lobulated borders. Inflammation in pancreas leads to focal or diffuse hypodensity and surrounding fat stranding. In a meta-analysis, CT had a sensitivity and specificity of 75% and 91%, respectively for detection of CP.[39] The characteristic CT features of CP are atrophy of pancreas, ductal dilatation, and multiple parenchymal and intraductal calcifications **(Box 2)**. In early CP, the MPD and side branches changes are not identified on CT and the contrast enhancement is also relatively homogeneous. With disease progression, multifocal fibrotic changes lead to heterogeneity of enhancement as the normal parenchyma enhances earlier than the fibrotic areas. The pancreatic head is the most common location of parenchymal calcifications. The calcification can vary in size and morphology. Calcifications develop early in alcoholic CP and certain hereditary pancreatitis as

BOX 2 CT features of CP.

*Common findings**
- Ductal dilatation (68%)
- Parenchymal atrophy (54%)
- Parenchymal/ductal calcifications—most specific feature (50%)
- Collections (30%)
- Glandular enlargement due to interlobular and periductal fibrosis (30%)
- Bile duct dilatation (29%)
- Peripancreatic fat stranding (16%)

Complications
- Fluid collections
- Pseudoaneurysms
- Biliary obstruction
- Venous thrombosis
- Pancreatic-pleural fistulae (pleural effusion)#
- Pancreatic ascites#

*Diagnosis of CP should be made when multiple findings are seen rather than based on a single finding.

#Hallmark of nonvascular complications of CP is pancreatic ductal disruption that is diagnosed more confidently on MRI/MRCP.

(CP: chronic pancreatitis; CT: computed tomography; MRCP: magnetic resonance cholangiopancreatography; MRI: magnetic resonance imaging)

compared to obstructive CP. In patients with cystic fibrosis having CFTR mutations, the calcifications appear late and they are smaller when compared to other genetic mutation. The stones in hereditary pancreatitis are usually round or oval measuring >15 mm. On CT, they have atypical appearance with hypodense center and hyperdense periphery which is due to the lack of calcium in the center. It is often referred to as Bull's eye stone.[40] These stones are usually arranged linearly within the dilated MPD. MPD dilatation is commonly associated with CP. The MPD may show segments of stenosis alternating with dilatation containing multiple calculi of varying sizes and irregular morphology **(Fig. 15)**. Another important role of CT is to evaluate the cause for MPD obstruction such as pancreatic adenocarcinoma, periampullary carcinoma, and rarely nonfunctioning neuroendocrine tumors that can cause repeated attacks of pancreatitis eventually presenting as CP **(Fig. 16)**.

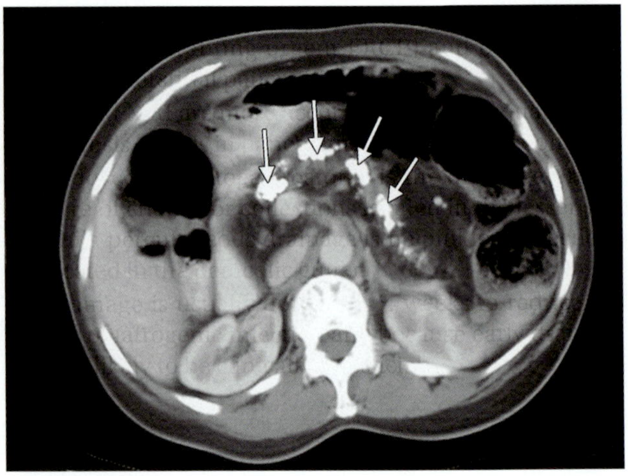

FIG. 15: Portal venous phase computed tomography image shows large pancreatic ductal calculi (arrows) with atrophy and fatty replacement of pancreas.

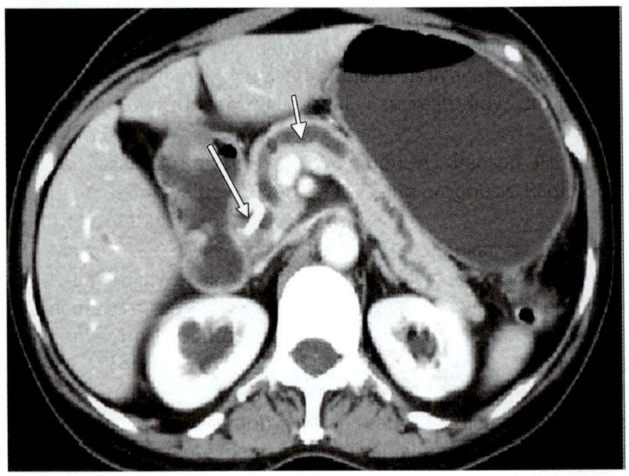

FIG. 16: Portal venous phase computed tomography image showing ill-defined hypoenhancing lesion at ampulla (periampullary carcinoma) obstructing the main pancreatic duct (arrow). Note biliary stents in situ (long arrow).

CT imaging of complications: CT is the imaging modality of choice to detect the complications of CP. Fluid collections/pseudocysts are seen in 20–40%. Pancreatic pseudocysts most commonly arise in patients with alcoholic CP (70–78%). Pseudocysts are cystic lesions with a well-formed wall.[2] They can be seen in peripancreatic region, intraperitoneal, retroperitoneal or even in remote locations such as chest. In CP, pseudocysts are generally formed during the evolution of peripancreatic fluid collections after an episode of pancreatitis **(Fig. 17)**. Pseudocysts along with peripancreatic inflammation can involve the venous structures in the vicinity leading to phlebitis and thrombosis. These complications can involve splenic, superior mesenteric, and portal vein and are seen as filling defects or occlusion on contrast-enhanced CT.[41] The resulting portal hypertension which is usually limited to left side (segmental portal hypertension) can lead to the development of multiple collaterals. When the inflammation involves the arteries in the vicinity, it can cause formation of pseudoaneurysms **(Fig. 18)**. Gastroduodenal, pancreaticoduodenal, and splenic arteries are the most commonly involved.[42] Pseudoaneurysms can rupture and bleed into peritoneal cavity, bowel, or biliary system and present as gastrointestinal bleeding and shock. Sometimes, pseudoaneurysms may be detected at CT in asymptomatic patients. Pseudoaneurysms are best seen on the arterial phase/pancreatic parenchymal phase when the concentration of contrast in arteries is at its peak. They

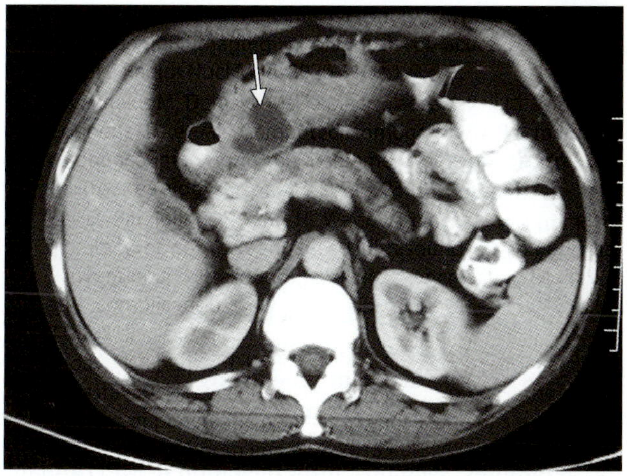

FIG. 17: Contrast-enhanced computed tomography image shows a duodenal intramural pseudocyst (arrow). Changes of chronic pancreatitis in the form of main pancreatic ductal dilatation and pancreatic atrophy are evident.

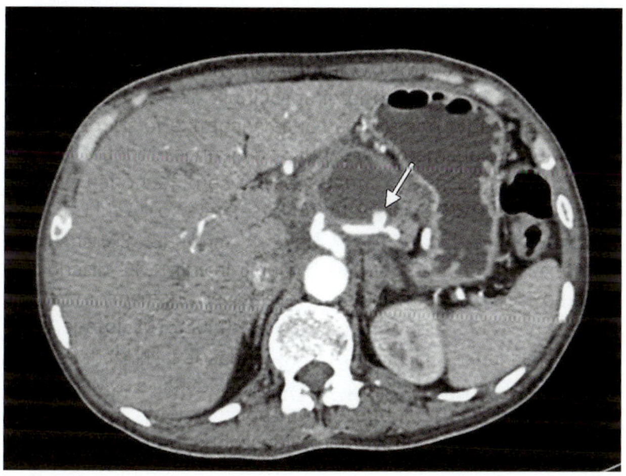

FIG. 18: Arterial phase image shows splenic artery pseudoaneurysm (arrow) projecting into peripancreatic pseudocyst.

can be missed on routine portal venous scan which makes the arterial phase acquisition important in this scenario. Pancreatic fistula can develop with the peritoneal cavity or even pleural cavity.[43] These can occur secondary to rupture of pseudocyst. On CT, they are seen as ascites or pleural effusion; however, the actual fistula site may not be demonstrated on CT scans.[44] MRI and MRCP are better at detecting pancreatic ductal disruption and fistulae. Patients with CP are at increased risk of pancreatic cancer.[4] Pancreatic carcinoma in patients with CP can mimic inflammatory mass, focal AIP, and groove pancreatitis. Reliable distinction between these lesions on imaging is quite challenging and is discussed later in this chapter.

Limitations of CT: CT leads to exposure to ionizing radiation (several patients may need repeated imaging studies). CT is poor at visualizing subtle parenchymal and ductal changes causing lower sensitivity for early CP. Some of these limitations may be addressed by advances in imaging.

Dual-energy CT: VNE images can be used to replace the true NCCT images and hence reduce the radiation dose. Low-keV images improve the visualization of vessels and pancreatic duct. High-keV images and metal artifact reduction algorithms can reduce stent-related artifacts.[45] DECT can also help detect radiolucent or mixed calculi (comprising 5–8% calculi in CP) that are not detected on conventional CT.[46] DECT can also help improve the diagnostic performance of CT in differentiating inflammatory masses from PDAC. Mean normalized iodine concentration is significantly lower in PDAC than normal pancreas.[47] A recent study reported a strong correlation between DECT parameters and MR-derived extracellular volume fractions (ECVs) in predicting pancreatic fibrosis.[48]

Perfusion CT (PCT): A few studies have reported the utility of PCT in assessing patients with CP. Normal parenchyma is characterized by rapid enhancement and rapid washout.[49] The time-density curve of pancreas generated from PCT in CP has been reported to be significantly different from those of normal pancreas and PDAC.[50] PCT has also been shown to discriminate patients with and without exocrine insufficiency.[51] However, due to high radiation exposure, PCT is not routinely utilized in CP.

Magnetic Resonance Imaging

MRI has excellent contrast resolution. MRCP has replaced ERCP for the evaluation of pancreatic ducts. Normal pancreas is the most T1-weighted hyperintense organ in abdomen due to rich proteinaceous secretion **(Fig. 19)**.[52] Thus, pancreatic inflammation and fibrosis in CP may be diagnosed based on hypointensity on T1-weighted fat saturated sequence.[53] Objective assessment of the pancreas

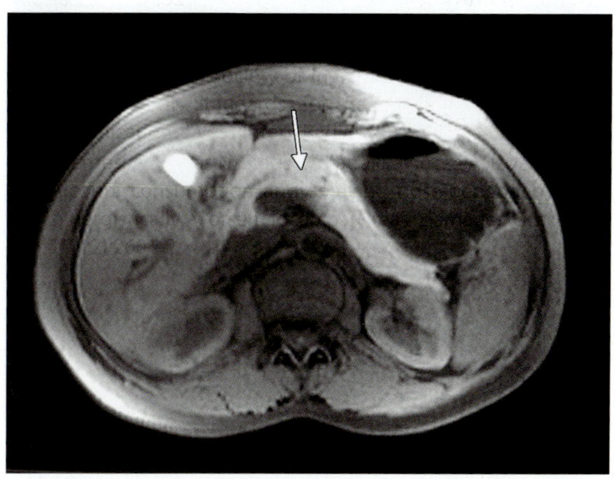

FIG. 19: Axial T1-weighted fat saturated magnetic resonance image showing homogeneous hyperintense signal of pancreas (arrow).

on T1-weighted images relies on comparing the signal to a reference organ, either spleen or paraspinal muscle and calculating the signal intensity ratio (SIR = SI pancreas/SI reference).[51] CP is associated with decreased SIR of the pancreas which correlates with the degree of fibrosis and loss of normal acinar cells.[54] SIR has also been shown to be positively correlated with the pancreatic fluid bicarbonate level.[55] Studies have also shown that T1-weighted imaging may diagnose early CP even when no ductal changes are seen at MRCP. The sensitivity and specificity of T1-weighted MRI to detect parenchymal changes in CP is 77% and 83%, respectively.[2] On contrast-enhanced MRI, there is delayed heterogeneous enhancement due to fibrosis. A study reported the performance of T1-weighted SIR (T1 score), arterial-to-venous enhancement ratio (AVR), pancreatic volume, and diameter for differentiating normal pancreas from CP. CP patients had significantly lower mean T1 score, AVR, volume, and diameter.[56]

The ductal changes are better seen on MRCP compared to CT. However, compared to ERCP, subtle side branch changes can be missed. The ductal findings of early disease range from normal MPD to mild irregularity of MPD and side branches **(Fig. 20)**. With progression of disease, there is irregular dilatation of both MPD and side branches with development of strictures giving the appearance of chain of lakes on MRCP. MRI has high sensitivity in depicting the associated complications such as pseudocysts and fistula.[43] Intraductal calcifications are seen as filling defects. The sensitivity of MR for small calcification is poor compared to CT. MR is excellent at detecting ductal variations such as pancreatic divisum **(Fig. 21)** and any solid or cystic focal lesions causing obstruction to MPD. MRI can also differentiate CP from other mimics like intraductal papillary mucinous neoplasms and variants of CP such as groove pancreatitis and autoimmune pancreatitis (AIP). MRI may help differentiate mass-forming CP from pancreatic adenocarcinoma (discussed later).

Secretin-enhanced MRCP: One of the major limitations of MRCP in the evaluation of CP is the lack of functional information and inability to image the ductal system in distended state. This drawback can be overcome by using secretin and acquiring serial MR images. Secretin causes transient increase in the tone of sphincter of Oddi and increased secretion of bicarbonate-rich pancreatic fluid. Patient should be fasting for 4–6 hours and a negative oral contrast is administered 30 minutes before the study to suppress the signals from preexisting fluid in the duodenum.[57] Baseline images are acquired and secretin is injected. T2-weighted images are acquired every 30 seconds for 15 minutes. Secretin causes dilatation of MPD and the maximum dilatation occurs at 2–5 minutes after which the sphincteric tone decreases and MPD diameter returns to baseline after 10 minutes. The pancreatic secretions in the duodenum can be graded in quantitative or semiquantitative manner and reflect the exocrine function of the pancreas. The MPD should increase at least 1 mm compared to baseline in patients with normal sphincter. Lack of dilatation implies impaired ductal compliance.[58] In normal pancreas, the side branches are not visualized after secretin, whereas in patient with early CP, the side branches show dilatation.[59] The exocrine function can be graded as follows: fluid confined to duodenal bulb (grade 1), fluid confined to first and second parts of duodenum (grade 2), and fluid reaching the third part (grade 3). Grade 3 is considered normal and grades 1 and 2 imply impaired exocrine function. Duodenal filling grade has a sensitivity and specificity of 72% and 87% to assess exocrine function.[58] Duodenal filling grade has also been found to correlate with fecal elastase 1 values.[60]

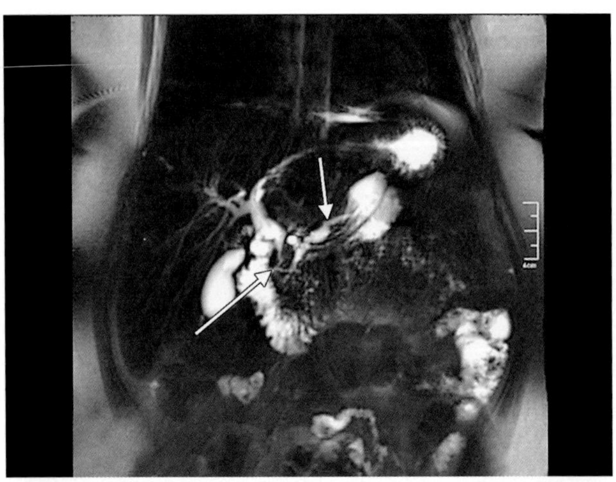

FIG. 20: Ductal changes in chronic pancreatitis: Magnetic resonance cholangiopancreatography image showing multiple strictures (arrow) with irregular dilatation of main pancreatic duct (arrow). Note stricture at lower end of common bile duct (long arrow).

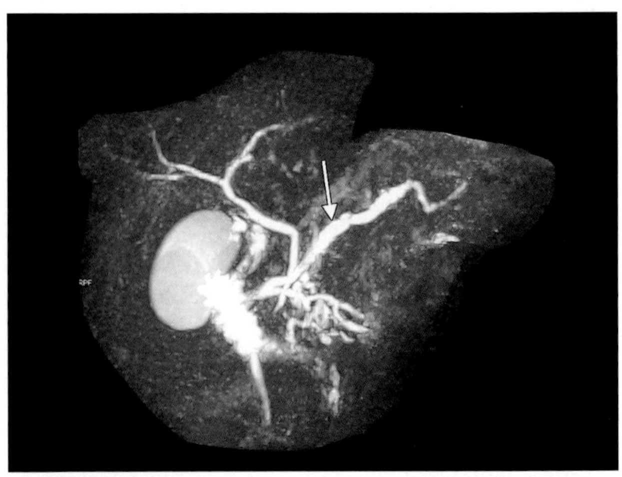

FIG. 21: Pancreatic divisum: Magnetic resonance cholangiopancreatography image showing the main pancreatic duct (arrow) crossing the CBD horizontally and opening into minor papilla.

Thus s-MRCP provides structural as well as functional information. MRCP uses Cambridge classification designed for ERCP for diagnosis and severity grading of CP, which has shown poor sensitivity for the detection of early CP.[61]

Diffusion-weighted imaging (DWI): DWI and apparent diffusion coefficient (ADC) values are useful adjunct to conventional MRI for the evaluation of CP.[62] ADC values of pancreas are lower in patients with CP than in normal subjects. It is because of the decreased exocrine reserve of pancreas leading to decreased water diffusion and fibrosis. ADC values can potentially be used as an indicator of fibrosis and its extent in patients with CP. DWI may be combined with s-MRCP to assess impact of secretin on ADC. ADC values of pancreas should increase in normal subjects due to increased secretion and higher water diffusion.[63]

T1 mapping, ECV, magnetic resonance elastography (MRE), and proton-density fat fraction (PDFF) map: T1 mapping is a quantitative MRI (Q-MRI) technique that allows measurement of T1 relaxation time of the tissues. T1 mapping may be a more reliable and objective method than T1-weighted images. Several methods are used to acquire T1-maps including variable flip angle, modified look-locker inversion recovery, inversion recovery, and saturation recovery single-shot acquisition.[64] ECV is another Q-MRI technique capable of assessing changes to the extracellular matrix that occur secondary to tissue fibrosis. ECV relies on tissue and blood plasma concentration of gadolinium to dichotomize the tissues into intra- and extracellular spaces.

Thresholds of T1 and ECV for differentiating normal pancreas from CP have been reported in a few recent studies. A cut-off of 900–950 ms for T1 has been reported to have a reasonable sensitivity and specificity for detection of CP.[65,66] The feasibility of MRE of pancreas has been reported.[67,68] The mean shear stiffness was reported to be 1.15 ± 0.17 kPa at 40 Hz in a recent study.[67] CP is associated with higher pancreatic fat fraction.[69] PDFF allows objective assessment of pancreatic fat fraction that has been shown to improve the diagnostic performance of MRI for CP.

Multiparametric quantitative MRI: Recently, many studies have investigated MRI protocols comprising several advanced MRI techniques and shown feasibility, reproducibility, and excellent diagnostic performance of multiparametric MRI approach in assessing patients with CP. As a part of the PROCEED (Prospective Evaluation of Chronic Pancreatitis for Epidemiologic and Translational Studies) study (NCT03099850), 101 patients were recruited for Q-MRI on 1.5T MRI scanners at seven US centers. T1 relaxation time, ECV, ADC, and fat signal fraction were compared between the control ($n = 50$) and CP ($n = 51$) groups. A combined Q-MRI score was proposed. The T1 relaxation time, ECV fraction, and pancreatic fat signal fraction were significantly higher in the CP group compared to controls.[70] There was no significant difference in the ADC values between the control and CP group. Another recent study reported significant differences in pancreatic volume, T1 relaxation times, MRE-derived stiffness, and PDFF between controls and CP group. T1 mapping and MRE showed the highest area under the curve (AUC) for distinguishing mild CP group from the control group as well as detecting the presence of any stage of CP.[71] The same group reported the utility of pancreatic volume, MPD diameter, T1 relaxation time, MRE-derived stiffness, and intravoxel incoherent motion DWI to categorize patients into those with preserved pancreatic function, partial pancreatic insufficiency (exocrine insufficiency or diabetes), and complete pancreatic insufficiency (exocrine insufficiency and diabetes). T1 relaxation time and MRE showed the highest performance for detecting patients with early CP (preserved pancreatic function).[72]

Positron Emission Tomography-Computed Tomography

The role of 18F-fluorodeoxyglucose (FDG)-PET-CT in CP is to evaluate patients in whom there is a possibility of an alternate diagnosis, e.g., AIP and PDAC.[73] The pattern of uptake on FDG-PET-CT may suggest the correct diagnosis in conjunction with biochemical tests and serum tumor markers.

REPORTING STANDARDS FOR CP USING CT, MRI, AND MRCP

A consensus on standardized reporting for CP was published in 2018 by the Consortium for the Study of Chronic Pancreatitis, Diabetes, and Pancreatic Cancer (CPDPC). The consensus gave recommendations regarding the CT and MRI protocols and defined the imaging findings and items that should be reported.[74]

VARIANTS OF CHRONIC PANCREATITIS

Autoimmune Pancreatitis

AIP comprises ~10% of the cases of CP.[75] Based on the current understanding, AIP has two distinct subtypes. Type 1 is known as lymphoplasmacytic sclerosing pancreatitis (LPSP), which is characterized by elevated serum immunoglobulin G4 (IgG4) levels, abundant infiltration with IgG4 positive cells, and extrapancreatic involvement.[76] On histology, lymphoplasmacytic infiltration is seen around the veins and ducts sparing the arterioles.[77] Type 2 is known as idiopathic duct centric pancreatitis (IDCP). LPSP is more common in Eastern countries while IDCP is more common in the Western world. Typical feature of IDCP is the presence of granulocyte epithelial lesions.[78] Type I AIP usually affects men (male to female ratio ~3) >60 years. Type 2 has a younger age of onset. Unlike type 1, IDCP usually does not have elevated serum levels of IgG4 and infiltration by IgG4-positive cells. In addition, extrapancreatic involvement is not seen in IDCP except that it can be associated with inflammatory bowel disease. Recurrence is common in LSPS but rare in IDCP.

Three patterns of involvement have been described in AIP. Diffuse, segmental/focal, and multifocal.[79] The imaging features are similar in both type 1 and 2 AIP. However, focal involvement is more commonly seen in type 2 AIP. CT and MRI are the most common imaging modalities for diagnosis. A triphasic protocol comprising pancreatic parenchymal, portal venous, and delayed phases (3-minute) is commonly employed. Diffuse pattern which is the most common type is seen as featureless or sausage-like pancreas because of the loss of lobular architecture **(Figs. 22 to 24)**. The involved pancreas shows reduced enhancement in the parenchymal and portal venous phase and delayed homogenous enhancement.[80] The MPD is either nondilated or diffusely narrowed which is a characteristic finding in AIP. Calcification or intraductal calculi are rare unlike other types of CP. There can be a hypoattenuating rim (30–40% cases) with associated fat stranding and foreshortening of pancreatic tail. The rim has a capsule-like appearance and shows a characteristic delayed enhancement. MRI can show a mildly enlarged pancreas with reduced signal intensity on T1-weighted images and mild hyperintensity on T2-weighted images. After contrast administration, the involved part of the pancreas shows delayed enhancement. The rim around the pancreas is hypointense on both T1- and T2-weighted images and shows delayed enhancement. The characteristic ductal findings of AIP are focal, segmental or diffuse narrowing, and irregularity of MPD.[81]

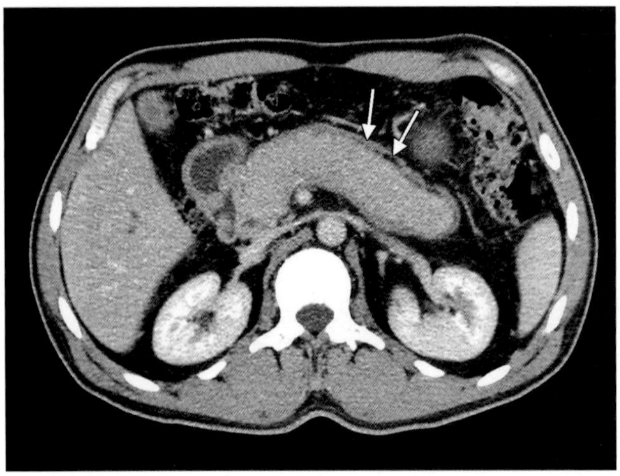

FIG. 22: Autoimmune pancreatitis: Axial computed tomography image showing diffusely enlarged pancreas with loss of lobulations and peripheral hypoenhancing rim (arrows).

The focal type of AIP presents as a focal mass mimicking PDAC. Even the clinical presentation may simulate PDAC, as some of these patients may have elevated carcinoembryonic antigen and carbohydrate antigen 19–9 levels. Focal type can also present with upstream dilatation of MPD. However, the dilatation is less severe compared to PDAC.[79] Delayed enhancement in AIP is another feature which differentiates it from PDAC. Multifocal form is rare.

Various extrapancreatic systems may be involved in AIP type 1.[79] Biliary system involvement occurs in 68–88% cases and presents as smooth strictures. The intrapancreatic bile duct is most commonly involved. Strictures of proximal bile ducts are less common and may resemble primary sclerosing cholangitis. Other manifestations include bowel involvement (about 17%) (most commonly, ulcerative colitis), sialadenitis (12–16%), renal lesions (4–35%), and retroperitoneal fibrosis (3–8%). Renal parenchymal involvement occurs in the form of small peripheral cortical nodules, round lesions,

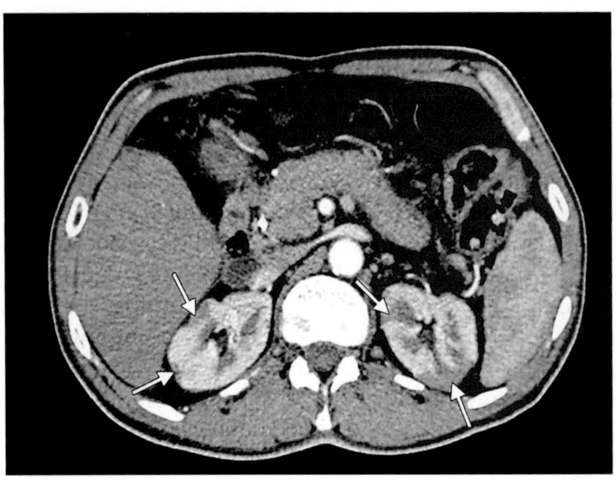

FIG. 23: Renal lesions in autoimmune pancreatitis: Axial computed tomography image showing multiple hypoenhancing wedge-shaped lesions in both kidneys (arrows).

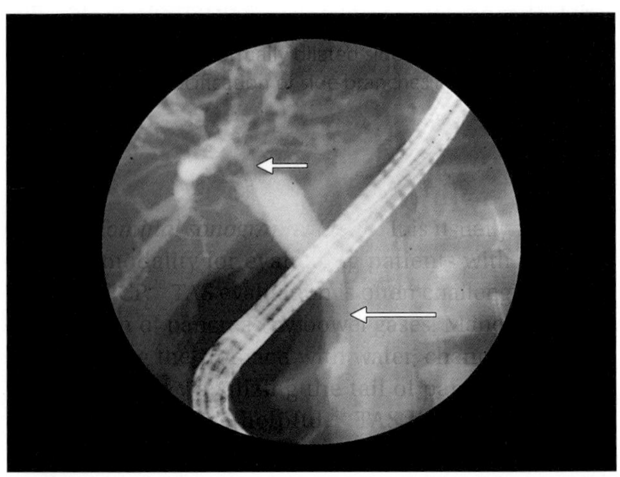

FIG. 24: Autoimmune pancreatitis with cholangiopathy: Endoscopic retrograde cholangiopancreatography image showing a hilar (short arrow) and lower common bile duct (long arrow) stricture.

well-defined wedge-shaped lesions, or diffuse patchy involvement.[82]

A recent systematic review reported the performance of various CT findings to diagnose AIP.[83] Seven CT features suggesting AIP were diffuse pancreatic enlargement (highest diagnostic odds ratio), delayed homogeneous enhancement, capsule-like rim, multiple pancreatic masses, renal lesions, retroperitoneal fibrosis, and bile duct involvement. Delayed homogeneous enhancement had a pooled sensitivity and specificity of 83% and 85%, respectively. The same group conducted a systematic review of the MRI findings and reported features favoring AIP.[84] Besides the diffuse enlargement, delayed homogeneous enhancement, capsule-like rim, and multiple parenchymal masses also reported on CT, multiple MPD strictures, low ADC value, speckled enhancement, tapered narrowing of MPD, and penetrating duct sign were additional features favoring AIP at MRI. The findings favoring PDAC were target type enhancing discrete pancreatic mass, upstream MPD dilatation, peripancreatic fat infiltration, upstream parenchymal atrophy, and vascular involvement. The diagnostic performance of MRI is reported to be better than CT for distinguishing nondiffuse-type AIP from PDAC.[85]

The diagnosis of AIP is based on a combination of various parameters. There is elevation of serum IgG and IgG4. Elevation of IgG4 twice the upper limit of normal (>280 mg/dL) is highly specific.[86] The International Consensus Diagnostic Criteria are based on a combination of histological features, imaging findings, serological parameters, other organ involvement, and response to steroid therapy (HISORt).[86]

FDG-PET-CT can be useful, if other features are equivocal, to differentiate focal AIP from PDAC. On PET-CT, AIP demonstrates heterogeneous pattern with multifocal uptake in the pancreas.[87] Extrapancreatic uptake in lachrymal or salivary gland, biliary system, retroperitoneal space, or prostate gland provides an important clue to the diagnosis.

Paraduodenal Pancreatitis

Paraduodenal pancreatitis (also known as groove pancreatitis) is a rare type of CP which is localized to the pancreaticoduodenal groove. Although the exact etiology is not known, one of the most commonly proposed mechanisms is repeated inflammation in the ectopic pancreas in the medial wall of the duodenum.[88] Two forms of groove pancreatitis have been recognized: pure and segmental. The former involves only groove and the pancreatic head is spared while the later involves the head of pancreas. Patients usually present with duodenal and biliary obstruction. Biliary strictures are common (50% of cases). On imaging, a plaque like crescentic soft-tissue density is seen in the pancreaticoduodenal groove that shows delayed enhancement (fibrosis).[89] Small cystic lesions (in the medial wall of the duodenum) and duodenal thickening are also commonly seen **(Fig. 25)**. MRI is superior to CT for characterization of parenchymal and ductal changes. Paraduodenal pancreatitis (especially the segmental form) may mimic PDAC. Displacement of gastroduodenal artery toward pancreatic head, cystic changes of duodenal wall, and tapered narrowing of the MPD favor groove pancreatitis while encasement of the pancreaticoduodenal artery, infiltration of adjacent organs, and abrupt cut-off of MPD favor PDAC.[89] The venous deformity may be seen in both. One of the pitfalls of relying solely on the presence of cysts for diagnosing paraduodenal pancreatitis is that cysts are also associated with PDAC.[90] A study reported that if focal thickening and abnormal enhancement of the second part of the duodenum and cystic changes in the region of minor papilla are seen in combination, the differentiation of paraduodenal pancreatitis from PDAC is highly accurate.[91]

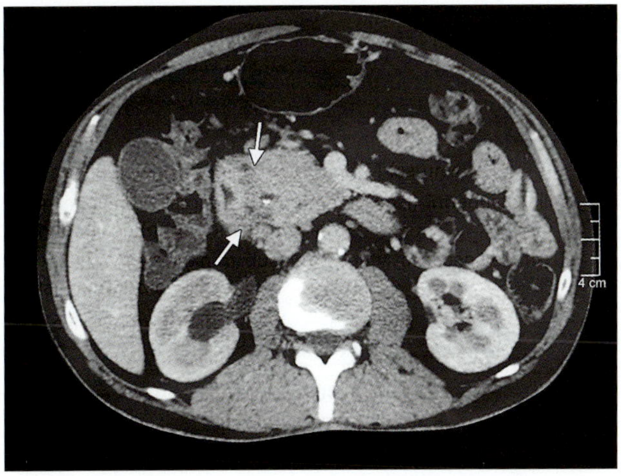

FIG. 25: Groove pancreatitis: Axial computed tomography axial image showing hypoenhancing sheet-like soft tissue in pancreaticoduodenal groove (arrows). Note presence of tiny cysts within this soft tissue and mildly bulky head of pancreas.

CHRONIC PANCREATITIS IN CYSTIC FIBROSIS

The *CFTR* gene mutation in cystic fibrosis leads to dysfunction of chloride channels which fail to add enough fluid in pancreatic glandular secretions causing inspissation of secretions and obstruction to the flow within pancreatic ducts.[92] In pediatric population, cystic fibrosis is the most common cause of exocrine pancreatic insufficiency with incidence of 1 in 2,500 children.[93] Clinical presentation includes failure to thrive, fat intolerance, abdominal pain, bloating, and flatulence. Glucose intolerance is quite common (seen in up to 50% of cases); however, overt diabetes mellitus is noted in only 13% of these patients.[94] The severity of exocrine dysfunction usually correlates with degree of pancreatic fatty infiltration.

Pancreatic calcifications indistinguishable from those in other forms of CP may be seen. TAS may show atrophic pancreas with increased echogenicity secondary to fatty replacement. On CT, fat replacement with or without pancreatic atrophy is the most common and characteristic finding **(Figs. 26 and 27)**.[95] Other findings include calcifications, cysts and ductal strictures, beading, and dilatations. Pancreatic cystosis is a rare manifestation of cystic fibrosis, where the entire pancreas is replaced by multiple cysts of varying sizes. MRI is preferred in children due to lack of exposure to ionizing radiations.

HEREDITARY PANCREATITIS

Hereditary pancreatitis is an autosomal dominant disease that occurs due to mutation of the cationic trypsinogen gene (*PRSS1*) that leads to increased autoactivation of trypsinogen. Other gene mutations including those of *SPINK1, CFTR,* and *CTRC* genes are less commonly implicated.[96] Hereditary pancreatitis should be considered in children with recurrent episodes of pancreatitis, a family history among first- or second-degree relatives, and lack of etiologic factors for pancreatitis.[97] The disease is characterized by RAP in first two decades and early progression to CP. Most of the imaging features of hereditary pancreatitis are nonspecific and similar to the more common forms of pancreatitis. Pancreatic atrophy, ductal dilatation, pseudocysts, and calcifications are commonly seen. The ductal calculi in hereditary pancreatitis are larger (often ≥15 mm in diameter) and have central lucency (bull's-eye appearance).[40] *PRSS1* gene mutation is also associated with lipomatous atrophy of the pancreas. Hereditary pancreatitis is associated with >50-fold increased risk of pancreatic cancer.[98]

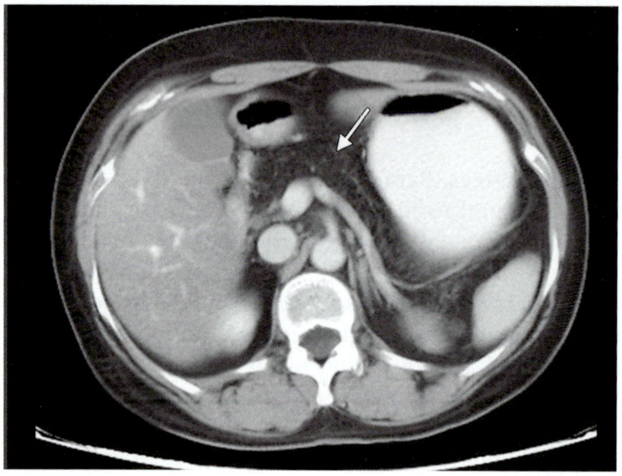

FIG. 26: Chronic pancreatitis in cystic fibrosis: Computed tomography image showing diffuse lipomatous transformation of pancreas (arrow).

CHRONIC PANCREATITIS AND PANCREATIC DUCTAL ADENOCARCINOMA

The standardized incidence rates of pancreatic cancer in patients with CP have been reported to be 7.6-68.1%.[4] Factors associated with PDAC in CP include age, parenchymal calcification, pancreatic duct stricture, and serum CA 19-9 level. Age over 60 years and serum CA 19-9 levels >100 U/mL were reported as independent risk factors for PDAC in one study.[4] The cumulative risk is much higher in hereditary pancreatitis.[98] On imaging, it is challenging to differentiate a focal mass of CP from pancreatic carcinoma **(Fig. 28)**.[99] Inflammatory masses of CP have a "parenchymographic" enhancement similar to the rest of the pancreas in most cases. Masses in PDAC, on the

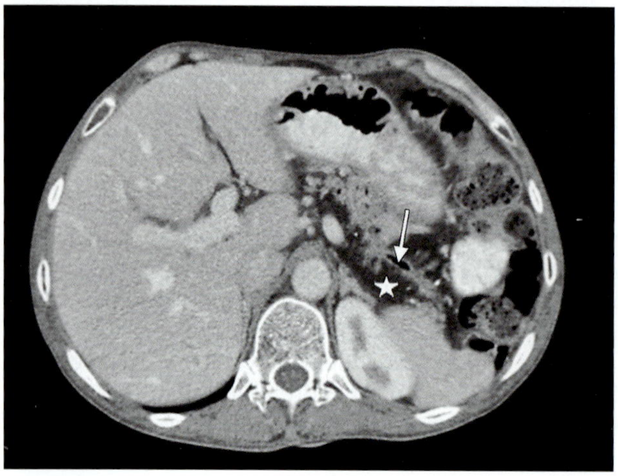

FIG. 27: Chronic pancreatitis in cystic fibrosis: CT image showing focal dilatations of main pancreatic duct (arrow) and fatty transformation of pancreas (star).

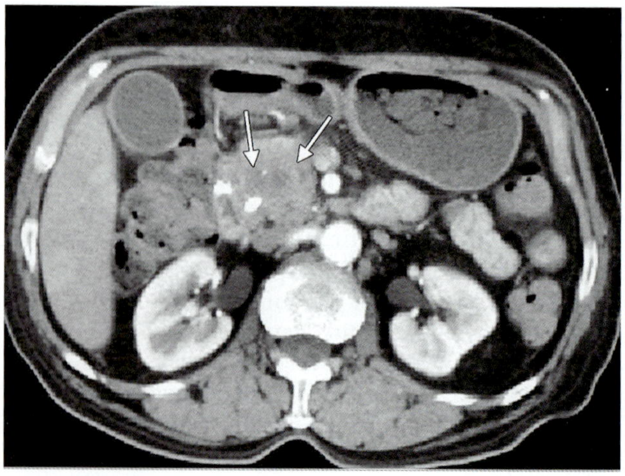

FIG. 28: Malignant change in chronic pancreatitis: Pancreatic head shows multifocal calcifications consistent with chronic pancreatitis. There is marked atrophy of pancreatic body and tail and contour deformity of head. An ill-defined hypodense lesion (arrows) is seen in pancreatic head which was confirmed to be adenocarcinoma on cytology.

other hand, are hypoenhancing in all phases. In advanced cases of CP when there is extensive fibrosis in the mass and enhancement pattern similar to PDAC may be seen.[100] PDAC can also be isoenhancing to the rest of the pancreas in a small proportion of the patients. The ductal changes are better seen at MRCP. Abrupt MPD cut-off, marked dilatation, and marked parenchymal atrophy favor PDAC while tapered narrowing and duct penetrating through the mass favor inflammatory mass.[100] EUS is a useful adjunct to CT and MRI as it allows high-resolution imaging of the duct and the parenchyma. Contrast-enhanced EUS or contrast-enhanced US (CEUS) (transabdominal) may provide additional clues to differentiate inflammatory mass from PDAC. A recent study reported that the lack of central vessels on CEUS was significantly associated with PDAC diagnosis on multivariate analysis.[101] Locoregional or distant lymphadenopathy, metastases, and vascular encasement or invasion are imaging findings of locally advanced PDAC.

Pancreatic perfusion imaging can generate quantitative perfusion parameters that help distinguish inflammatory mass from PDAC.[102] The blood flow and blood volume are much lower in carcinoma than in inflammatory mass. DWI is also helpful as PDAC shows marked diffusion restriction and lower ADC values compared to inflammatory masses.[103] FDG-PET-CT is a problem-solving tool and PDAC shows marked FDG avidity.[104] PET-CT is also more sensitive to the detection of extrapancreatic metastatic lesion that may aid in differential diagnosis.

ACKNOWLEDGMENTS

Professor SK Sinha and Dr Jimil Shah, Department of Gastroenterology, Postgraduate Institute of Medical Education and Research, Chandigarh, India for contributing ERCP and EUS images.

CONCLUSION

Recent insights into the pathophysiology of CP have led to its better definition. Imaging is critical to diagnose and manage CP. CT, MRI, and EUS have a complementary role. Advanced imaging techniques aid in the diagnosis of early CP. Radiologists must be aware of the variants and mimics of CP.

REFERENCES

1. Tandon RK, Garg PK. Tropical pancreatitis. Dig Dis. 2004; 22(3):258-66.
2. Kamat R, Gupta P, Rana S. Imaging in chronic pancreatitis: State of the art review. Indian J Radiol Imaging. 2019;29(2): 201-10.
3. Whitcomb DC, Frulloni L, Garg P, Greer JB, Schneider A, Yadav D, et al. Chronic pancreatitis: An international draft consensus proposal for a new mechanistic definition. Pancreatology. 2016;16:218-24.
4. Kim HS, Gweon TG, Park SH, Kim TH, Kim CW, Chang JH. Incidence and risk of pancreatic cancer in patients with chronic pancreatitis: defining the optimal subgroup for surveillance. Sci Rep. 2023;13(1):106.
5. Whitcomb DC. Peering into the "Black Box" of the complex chronic pancreatitis syndrome. Pancreas. 2016;45(10):1361-4.
6. Catalano MF, Sahai A, Levy M, Romagnuolo J, Wiersema M, Brugge W, et al. EUS-based criteria for the diagnosis of chronic pancreatitis: the Rosemont classification. Gastrointest Endosc. 2009;69(7):1251-61.
7. Albashir S, Bronner MP, Parsi MA, Walsh RM, Stevens T. Endoscopic ultrasound, secretin endoscopic pancreatic function test, and histology: correlation in chronic pancreatitis. Am J Gastroenterol. 2010;105(11):2498-503.
8. Masamune A, Kikuta K, Kume K, Hamada S, Tsuji I, Takeyama Y, et al. Nationwide epidemiological survey of chronic pancreatitis in Japan: introduction and validation of the new Japanese diagnostic criteria 2019. J Gastroenterol. 2020;55(11):1062-1071.
9. Vege SS, Chari ST. Chronic Pancreatitis. N Engl J Med. 2022; 386(9):869-78.
10. Singh VK, Yadav D, Garg PK. Diagnosis and management of chronic pancreatitis: a review. JAMA. 2019;322:2422-34.
11. Hegyi P, Párniczky A, Lerch MM, Sheel ARG, Rebours V, Forsmark CE, et al. International Consensus Guidelines for Risk Factors in Chronic Pancreatitis. Recommendations from the working group for the international consensus guidelines for chronic pancreatitis in collaboration with the International Association of Pancreatology, the American Pancreatic Association, the Japan Pancreas Society, and European Pancreatic Club. Pancreatology. 2020;20(4):579-85.
12. Garg PK, Narayana D. Changing phenotype and disease behaviour of chronic pancreatitis in India: evidence for gene-environment interactions. Glob Health Epidemiol Genom. 2016;1:e17.
13. Desai N, Kaura T, Singh M, Willingham FF, Rana S, Chawla S. Epidemiology and characteristics of chronic pancreatitis-do the East and West meet? Gastro Hep Adv. 2022;1:942-9
14. Yadav D, O'Connell M, Papachristou GI. Natural history following the first attack of acute pancreatitis. Am J Gastroenterol. 2012;107:1096-103.
15. Kumar S, Ooi CY, Werlin S, Abu-El-Haija M, Barth B, Bellin MD, et al. Risk factors associated with pediatric acute recurrent and chronic pancreatitis: Lessons from INSPPIRE. JAMA Pediatr. 2016;170(6):562-9.
16. de Rijk F, Sissingh NJ, Boel TT, Timmerhuis HC, de Jong M, Pauw HS, et al. Development of pancreatic diseases during long-term follow-up after acute pancreatitis: a post-hoc analysis of a prospective multicenter cohort. J Gastroenterol Hepatol. 2024;39(4):674-84.
17. Hegyi PJ, Soós A, Tóth E, Ébert A, Venglovecz V, Márta K, et al. Evidence for diagnosis of early chronic pancreatitis after three episodes of acute pancreatitis: a cross-sectional multicentre international study with experimental animal model. Sci Rep. 2021;11(1):1367.

18. Rahman A, O'Connor DB, Gather F, Koscic S, Gilgan J, Mockler D, et al. Clinical Classification and Severity Scoring Systems in Chronic Pancreatitis: A Systematic Review. Dig Surg. 2020;37(3):181-91.
19. Etemad B, Whitcomb DC. Chronic pancreatitis: diagnosis, classification, and new genetic developments. Gastroenterology. 2001;120(3):682-707.
20. Gardner TB, Adler DG, Forsmark CE, Sauer BG, Taylor JR, Whitcomb DC. ACG Clinical Guideline: Chronic Pancreatitis. Am J Gastroenterol. 2020;115(3):322-39.
21. Tandan M, Talukdar R, Reddy DN. Management of Pancreatic Calculi: An Update. Gut Liver. 2016;10(6):873-80.
22. Beyer G, Habtezion A, Werner J, Lerch MM, Mayerle J. Chronic pancreatitis. Lancet. 2020;396:499-512.
23. Sarner M, Cotton PB. Definitions of acute and chronic pancreatitis. Clin Gastroenterol. 1984;13(3):865-70.
24. Zamboni GA, Ambrosetti MC, D'Onofrio M, PozziMucelli R. Ultrasonography of the pancreas. Radiol Clin North Am. 2012;50(3):395-406.
25. Alpern MB, Sandler MA, Kellman GM, Madrazo BL. Chronic pancreatitis: ultrasonic features. Radiology. 1985;155(1):215-9.
26. Shah J, Chatterjee A, Kothari TH. The role of Endoscopic Ultrasound in early Chronic Pancreatitis. Diagnostics. 2024; 14(3):298.
27. Zubarik R, Ganguly E. The rosemont criteria can predict the pain response to pancreatic enzyme supplementation in patients with suspected chronic pancreatitis undergoing endoscopic ultrasound. Gut Liver. 2011;5(4):521-6.
28. Trikudanathan G, Munigala S, Barlass U, Malli A, Han Y, Sekulic M, et al. Evaluation of Rosemont criteria for non-calcific chronic pancreatitis (NCCP) based on histopathology - A retrospective study. Pancreatology. 2017;17(1):63-9.
29. Yamashita Y, Tanioka K, Kawaji Y, Tamura T, Nuta J, Hatamaru K, et al. Utility of Elastography with Endoscopic Ultrasonography Shear-Wave measurement for diagnosing Chronic Pancreatitis. Gut Liver. 2020;14(5):659-64.
30. Yamashita Y, Yamazaki H, Shimokawa T, Kawaji Y, Tamumra T, Hatamaru K, et al. Shear-wave versus strain elastography in endoscopic ultrasound for the diagnosis of chronic pancreatitis. Pancreatology. 2023;23(1):35-41.
31. Yamashita Y, Tanioka K, Kawaji Y, Tamura T, Nuta J, Hatamaru K, et al. Endoscopic ultrasonography shear wave as a predictive factor of endocrine/exocrine dysfunction in chronic pancreatitis. J Gastroenterol Hepatol. 2021;36(2): 391-6.
32. Choudhry SR, Verma M, Gupta P, Singh H, Sharma V, Kochhar R. Ultrasound Shear Wave Elastography of Normal Pancreas in Adult Subjects. J Gastrointest Abdom Radiol. 2023;6(2):148-53.
33. Kuwahara T, Hirooka Y, Kawashima H, Ohno E, Sugimoto H, Hayashi D, et al. Quantitative evaluation of pancreatic tumor fibrosis using shear wave elastography. Pancreatology. 2016;16(6):1063-8.
34. Yashima Y, Sasahira N, Isayama H, Kogure H, Ikeda H, Hirano K, et al. Acoustic radiation force impulse elastography for noninvasive assessment of chronic pancreatitis. J Gastroenterol. 2012;47:427-32.
35. Llamoza-Torres CJ, Fuentes-Pardo M, Alvarez-Higueras FJ, Alberca-de-Las-Parras F, Carballo-Alvarez F. Usefulness of percutaneous elastography by acoustic radiation force impulse for the non-invasive diagnosis of chronic pancreatitis. Rev Esp Enferm Dig. 2016;108:450-6.
36. Pozzi R, Parzanese I, Baccarin A, Giunta M, Conti CB, Cantù P, et al. Point shear-wave elastography in chronic pancreatitis: a promising tool for staging disease severity. Pancreatology. 2017;17:905-10.
37. Zamboni GA, Ambrosetti MC, Pezzullo M, Bali MA, Mansueto G. Optimum imaging of chronic pancreatitis. Abdom Radiol. 2020;45(5):1410-9.
38. Mileto A, Mazziotti S, Gaeta M, Bottari A, Zimbaro F, Giardina C, et al. Pancreatic dual-source dual-energy CT: is it time to discard unenhanced imaging? Clin Radiol. 2012; 67(4):334-9.
39. Issa Y, Kempeneers MA, van Santvoort HC, Bollen TL, Bipat S, Boermeester MA. Diagnostic performance of imaging modalities in chronic pancreatitis: a systematic review and meta-analysis. Eur Radiol. 2017;27(9):3820-44.
40. Graziani R, Frulloni L, Cicero C, Manfredi R, Ambrosetti MC, Mautone S, et al. Bull's-eye pattern of pancreatic-duct stones on multidetector computed tomography and gene-mutation-associated pancreatitis (GMAP). Radiol Med. 2012; 117(8):1275-86.
41. Walia D, Saraya A, Gunjan D. Vascular complications of chronic pancreatitis and its management. World J Gastrointest Surg. 2023;15(8):1574-90.
42. Sagar S, Soundarajan R, Gupta P, Praveen Kumar M, Samanta J, Sharma V, et al. Efficacy of endovascular embolization of arterial pseudoaneurysms in pancreatitis: A systematic review and meta-analysis. Pancreatology. 2021;21(1):46-58.
43. Chhabra M, Gupta P, Shah J, Samanta J, Mandavdhare H, Sharma V, et al. Imaging diagnosis and management of Fistulas in Pancreatitis. Dig Dis Sci. 2024;69(2):335-48.
44. Kumar P, Gupta P, Rana S. Thoracic complications of pancreatitis. JGH Open. 2018;3(1):71-9.
45. Morgan DE. Dual-energy CT of the abdomen. Abdom Imaging. 2014;39(1):108-34.
46. Aslan S, Camlidag I, Nural MS. Lower energy levels and iodine-based material decomposition images increase pancreatic ductal adenocarcinoma conspicuity on rapid kV-switching dual-energy CT. Abdom Radiol. 2019;44(2):568-75.
47. Uyeda JW, Richardson IJ, Sodickson AD. Making the invisible visible: improving conspicuity of noncalcified gallstones using dual-energy CT. Abdom Radiol. 2017;42(12):2933-9.
48. Sun S, Huang B, Li Q, Wang C, Zhang W, Xu L, et al. Prediction of pancreatic fibrosis by dual-energy CT-derived extracellular volume fraction: Comparison with MRI. Eur J Radiol. 2024; 170:111204.
49. Arikawa S, Uchida M, Kunou Y, Kaida H, Uozumi J, Hayabuchi N, et al. Assessment of Chronic Pancreatitis: Use of Whole Pancreas Perfusion With 256-Slice Computed Tomography. Pancreas. 2012;41(4):535-40.
50. Yadav AK, Sharma R, Kandasamy D, Pradhan RK, Garg PK, Bhalla AS, et al. Perfusion CT - Can it resolve the pancreatic carcinoma versus mass forming chronic pancreatitis conundrum?. Pancreatology. 2016;16(6):979-87.
51. Parakh A, Tirkes T. Advanced imaging techniques for chronic pancreatitis. Abdom Radiol. 2020;45(5):1420-38.
52. Winston CB, Mitchell DG, Outwater EK, Ehrlich SM. Pancreatic signal intensity on T1-weighted fat saturation MR images: clinical correlation. J Magn Reson Imaging. 1995;5(3):267-71.

53. Sica GT, Miller FH, Rodriguez G, McTavish J, Banks PA. Magnetic resonance imaging in patients with pancreatitis: evaluation of signal intensity and enhancement changes. J Magn Reson Imaging. 2002;15(3):275-84.
54. Watanabe H, Kanematsu M, Tanaka K, Osada S, Tomita H, Hara A, et al. Fibrosis and postoperative fistula of the pancreas: correlation with MR imaging findings-preliminary results. Radiology. 2014;270(3):791-9.
55. Tirkes T, Fogel EL, Sherman S, Lin C, Swensson J, Akisik F, et al. Detection of exocrine dysfunction by MRI in patients with early chronic pancreatitis. Abdom Radiol. 2017;42(2):544-51.
56. Tirkes T, Yadav D, Conwell DL, Territo PR, Zhao X, Persohn SA, et al. Diagnosis of chronic pancreatitis using semi-quantitative MRI features of the pancreatic parenchyma: results from the multi-institutional MINIMAP study. Abdom Radiol (NY). 2023;48(10):3162-73.
57. Matos C, Metens T, Devière J, Nicaise N, Braudé P, Van Yperen G, et al. Pancreatic duct: morphologic and functional evaluation with dynamic MR pancreatography after secretin stimulation. Radiology. 1997;203(2):435-41.
58. Cappeliez O, Delhaye M, Devière J, Le Moine O, Metens T, Nicaise N, et al. Chronic pancreatitis: evaluation of pancreatic exocrine function with MR pancreatography after secretin stimulation. Radiology. 2000;215(2):358-64.
59. Manfredi R, Costamagna G, Brizi MG, Maresca G, Vecchioli A, Colagrande C, et al. Severe chronic pancreatitis versus suspected pancreatic disease: dynamic MR cholangiopancreatography after secretin stimulation. Radiology. 2000; 214(3):849-55.
60. Manfredi R, Perandini S, Mantovani W, Frulloni L, Faccioli N, Pozzi Mucelli R. Quantitative MRCP assessment of pancreatic exocrine reserve and its correlation with faecal elastase-1 in patients with chronic pancreatitis. Radiol Med. 2012;117(2):282-92.
61. Conwell DL, Lee LS, Yadav D, Longnecker DS, Miller FH, Mortele KJ, et al. American Pancreatic Association Practice Guidelines in Chronic Pancreatitis: evidence-based report on diagnostic guidelines. Pancreas. 2014;43(8):1143-62.
62. Akisik MF, Aisen AM, Sandrasegaran K, Jennings SG, Lin C, Sherman S, et al. Assessment of chronic pancreatitis: utility of diffusion-weighted MR imaging with secretin enhancement. Radiology. 2009;250(1):103-9.
63. Erturk SM, Ichikawa T, Motosugi U, Sou H, Araki T. Diffusion-weighted MR imaging in the evaluation of pancreatic exocrine function before and after secretin stimulation. Am J Gastroenterol. 2006;101(1):133-6.
64. Tirkes T, Zhao X, Lin C, Stuckey AJ, Li L, Giri S, et al. Evaluation of variable flip angle, MOLLI, SASHA, and IR-SNAPSHOT pulse sequences for T_1 relaxometry and extracellular volume imaging of the pancreas and liver. MAGMA. 2019;32(5): 559-66.
65. Tirkes T, Lin C, Fogel EL, Sherman SS, Wang Q, Sandrasegaran K. T_1 mapping for diagnosis of mild chronic pancreatitis. J Magn Reson Imaging. 2017;45(4):1171-6.
66. Tirkes T, Lin C, Cui E, Deng Y, Territo PR, Sandrasegaran K, et al. Quantitative MR Evaluation of Chronic Pancreatitis: Extracellular Volume Fraction and MR Relaxometry. AJR Am J Roentgenol. 2018;210(3):533-42.
67. Shi Y, Glaser KJ, Venkatesh SK, Ben-Abraham EI, Ehman RL. Feasibility of using 3D MR elastography to determine pancreatic stiffness in healthy volunteers. J Magn Reson Imaging. 2015;41(2):369-75.
68. Kolipaka A, Schroeder S, Mo X, Shah Z, Hart PA, Conwell DL. Magnetic resonance elastography of the pancreas: Measurement reproducibility and relationship with age. Magn Reson Imaging. 2017;42:1-7.
69. Tirkes T, Jeon CY, Li L, Joon AY, Seltman TA, Sankar M, et al. Association of Pancreatic Steatosis with Chronic Pancreatitis, Obesity, and Type 2 Diabetes Mellitus. Pancreas. 2019;48(3):420-6.
70. Tirkes T, Yadav D, Conwell DL, Territo PR, Zhao X, Persohn SA, et al. Quantitative MRI of chronic pancreatitis: results from a multi-institutional prospective study, magnetic resonance imaging as a non-invasive method for assessment of pancreatic fibrosis (MINIMAP). Abdom Radiol (NY). 2022; 47(11):3792-805.
71. Steinkohl E, Olesen SS, Hansen TM, Drewes AM, Frøkjær JB. T1 relaxation times and MR elastography-derived stiffness: new potential imaging biomarkers for the assessment of chronic pancreatitis. Abdom Radiol. 2021;46(12):5598-608.
72. Olesen SS, Steinkohl E, Hansen TM, Drewes AM, Frøkjær JB. Single- and multiparameter magnetic resonance imaging for diagnosing and severity grading of chronic pancreatitis. Abdom Radiol. 2023;48(2):630-41.
73. Sahani DV, Bonaffini PA, Catalano OA, Guimaraes AR, Blake MA. State-of-the-art PET/CT of the pancreas: current role and emerging indications. Radiographics. 2012;32(4): 1133-60.
74. Tirkes T, Shah ZK, Takahashi N, Grajo JR, Chang ST, Venkatesh SK, et al. Reporting Standards for Chronic Pancreatitis by Using CT, MRI, and MR Cholangiopancreatography: The Consortium for the Study of Chronic Pancreatitis, Diabetes, and Pancreatic Cancer. Radiology. 2019;290(1):207-15.
75. Yadav D, Notahara K, Smyrk TC, Clain JE, Pearson RK, Farnell MB, et al. Idiopathic tumefactive chronic pancreatitis: clinical profile, histology, and natural history after resection. Clin Gastroenterol Hepatol. 2003;1(2):129-35.
76. Proctor RD, Rofe CJ, Bryant TJ, Hacking CN, Stedman B. Autoimmune pancreatitis: an illustrated guide to diagnosis. Clin Radiol. 2013;68(4):422-32.
77. Chari ST, Kloeppel G, Zhang L, Notohara K, Lerch MM, Shimosegawa T, et al. Histopathologic and clinical subtypes of autoimmune pancreatitis: the Honolulu consensus document. Pancreas. 2010;39(5):549-54.
78. Shinagare S, Shinagare AB, Deshpande V. Autoimmune pancreatitis: a guide for the histopathologist. Semin Diagn Pathol. 2012;29(4):197-204.
79. Khandelwal A, Inoue D, Takahashi N. Autoimmune pancreatitis: an update. Abdom Radiol. 2020;45(5):1359-70.
80. Kwon JH, Kim JH, Kim SY, Byun JH, Kim HJ, Lee MG, et al. Differentiating focal autoimmune pancreatitis and pancreatic ductal adenocarcinoma: contrast-enhanced MRI with special emphasis on the arterial phase. Eur Radiol. 2019; 29(11):5763-71.
81. Park SH, Kim MH, Kim SY, Kim HJ, Moon SH, Lee SS, et al. Magnetic resonance cholangiopancreatography for the diagnostic evaluation of autoimmune pancreatitis. Pancreas. 2010;39(8):1191-8.

82. Takahashi N, Kawashima A, Fletcher JG, Chari ST. Renal involvement in patients with autoimmune pancreatitis: CT and MR imaging findings. Radiology. 2007;242(3):791-801.
83. Yoon SB, Jeon TY, Moon SH, Shin DW, Lee SM, Choi MH, et al. Differentiation of autoimmune pancreatitis from pancreatic adenocarcinoma using CT characteristics: a systematic review and meta-analysis. Eur Radiol. 2023;33(12):9010-21.
84. Yoon SB, Jeon TY, Moon SH, Lee SM, Kim MH. Systematic review and meta-analysis of MRI features for differentiating autoimmune pancreatitis from pancreatic adenocarcinoma. Eur Radiol. 2022;32(10):6691-701.
85. Lee S, Kim JH, Kim SY, Byun JH, Kim HJ, Kim MH, et al. Comparison of diagnostic performance between CT and MRI in differentiating non-diffuse-type autoimmune pancreatitis from pancreatic ductal adenocarcinoma. Eur Radiol. 2018; 28(12):5267-74.
86. Shimosegawa T, Chari ST, Frulloni L, Kamisawa T, Kawa S, Mino-Kenudson M, et al. International consensus diagnostic criteria for autoimmune pancreatitis: guidelines of the International Association of Pancreatology. Pancreas. 2011; 40(3):352-8.
87. Kamisawa T, Takum K, Anjiki H, Egawa N, Kurata M, Honda G, et al. FDG-PET/CT findings of autoimmune pancreatitis. Hepatogastroenterology. 2010;57(99-100):447-50.
88. Rezvani M, Menias C, Sandrasegaran K, Olpin JD, Elsayes KM, Shaaban AM. Heterotopic Pancreas: Histopathologic Features, Imaging Findings, and Complications. Radiographics. 2017;37(2):484-99.
89. Bello HR, Sekhar A, Filice RW, Radmard AR, Davarpanah AH. Pancreaticoduodenal Groove: Spectrum of Disease and Imaging Features. Radiographics. 2022;42(4):1062-80.
90. Ishigami K, Tajima T, Nishie A, Kakihara D, Fujita N, Asayama Y, et al. Differential diagnosis of groove pancreatic carcinomas vs. groove pancreatitis: usefulness of the portal venous phase. Eur J Radiol. 2010;74(3):e95-e100.
91. Kalb B, Martin DR, Sarmiento JM, Erickson SH, Gober D, Tapper EB, et al. Paraduodenal pancreatitis: clinical performance of MR imaging in distinguishing from carcinoma. Radiology. 2013;269(2):475-81.
92. Witt H. Chronic pancreatitis and cystic fibrosis. Gut. 2003; 52(Suppl 2):ii31-41.
93. Gore MD, Fernbach SK. Pancreatic insufficiency and cystic fibrosis. In: Gore RM, Levine MS, Laufer I (Eds). Textbook of Gastrointestinal Radiology. Philadelphia, PA: Saunders; 1994. pp. 2187-92.
94. De Boeck K, Weren M, Proesmans M, Kerem E. Pancreatitis among patients with cystic fibrosis: correlation with pancreatic status and genotype. Pediatrics. 2005;115(4): e463-9.
95. Soyer P, Spelle L, Pelage JP, Dufresne AC, Rondeau Y, Gouhiri M, et al. Cystic fibrosis in adolescents and adults: fatty replacement of the pancreas—CT evaluation and functional correlation. Radiology. 1999;210(3):611-5.
96. Raphael KL, Willingham FF. Hereditary pancreatitis: current perspectives. Clin Exp Gastroenterol. 2016;9:197-207.
97. Ellis I, Lerch MM, Whitcomb DC; Consensus Committees of the European Registry of Hereditary Pancreatic Diseases, Midwest Multi-Center Pancreatic Study Group, International Association of Pancreatology. Genetic testing for hereditary pancreatitis: guidelines for indications, counselling, consent and privacy issues. Pancreatology. 2001;1(5):405-15.
98. Howes N, Lerch MM, Greenhalf W, Stocken DD, Ellis I, Simon P, et al. Clinical and genetic characteristics of hereditary pancreatitis in Europe. Clin Gastroenterol Hepatol. 2004; 2(3):252-61.
99. Schima W, Böhm G, Rösch CS, Klaus A, Függer R, Kopf H. Mass-forming pancreatitis versus pancreatic ductal adenocarcinoma: CT and MR imaging for differentiation. Cancer Imaging. 2020;20(1):52.
100. Wolske KM, Ponnatapura J, Kolokythas O, Burke LMB, Tappouni R, Lalwani N. Chronic Pancreatitis or Pancreatic Tumor? A Problem-solving Approach. Radiographics. 2019; 39(7):1965-82.
101. Gupta P, Rana P, Marodia Y, Samanta J, Sharma V, Sinha SK, et al. Contrast-enhanced ultrasound of solid pancreatic head lesions: a prospective study. Eur Radiol. 2022;32(10): 6668-77.
102. Siddiqui N, Vendrami CL, Chatterjee A, Miller FH. Advanced MR Imaging Techniques for Pancreas Imaging. Magn Reson Imaging Clin N Am. 2018;26(3):323-44.
103. Wang Y, Miller FH, Chen ZE, Merrick L, Mortele KJ, Hoff FL, et al. Diffusion-weighted MR imaging of solid and cystic lesions of the pancreas. Radiographics. 2011;31(3):E47-64.
104. Pu Y, Wang C, Zhao S, Xie R, Zhao L, Li K, et al. The clinical application of ^{18}F-FDG PET/CT in pancreatic cancer: a narrative review. Transl Cancer Res. 2021;10(7):3560-75.

CHAPTER 20

Ankur Goyal, Raju Sharma, Amarinder Singh Malhi, Dipin Sudhakaran

Pancreatic Cancer Imaging

INTRODUCTION

Pancreatic cancer is an aggressive malignancy with a dismal prognosis. Strategically located deep in the retroperitoneum, it can potentially involve many crucial arteries, veins, and nerves supplying the liver, spleen, stomach, and bowel.[1] Ductal adenocarcinoma is the most common nonendocrine pancreatic malignancy and accounts for >85% of all pancreatic malignancies. After colorectal malignancy, pancreatic carcinoma is the second most common malignancy of the gastrointestinal tract. Because of its sharply rising incidence, pancreatic adenocarcinoma is anticipated to emerge as the second leading cause of cancer-related deaths in the US by 2030, even surpassing breast cancer.[2]

The broad term is malignant exocrine pancreatic tumors and includes neoplasms arising from or showing ductal differentiation (epithelial) and acinar cell differentiation. Progenitor cell differentiation (pancreatoblastoma) also comes under this umbrella term and so does solid pseudopapillary epithelial neoplasm (SPEN).[3] Malignant intraductal papillary mucinous neoplasms (IPMNs) and malignant mucinous cystic neoplasms (MCNs) also come under malignant exocrine pancreatic tumors. There have been a lot of advances in the imaging and surgical management of pancreatic malignancies. Nevertheless, patient survival is dismal owing to early lymphatic and perineural spread.[4] Pancreatic carcinoma has a propensity to spread via celiac and mesenteric neural plexus and this results in preclinical dissemination.

The clinical presentation is vague, leading to a delay in diagnosis. The patients usually present with abdominal pain, anorexia, weight loss, nausea, and jaundice. The age of presentation is middle age or elderly. Jaundice is a common presenting symptom in tumors of the pancreatic head region whereas lesions of the body and tail present with abdominal pain and weight loss. Pancreatic carcinoma should be suspected in diabetic patients with unusual manifestations (such as late age of onset, abdominal symptoms, and continuing weight loss), first episode of pancreatitis after the age of 40 years without an identifiable etiology and in patients with chronic pancreatitis when there is change in the character of pain.[5] It is important to differentiate ampullary cancers from ductal adenocarcinomas, since the former have a much better prognosis and longer survival.[6] The serum levels of carbohydrate antigen CA 19-9 are often elevated. Levels greater than 37 units/mL in symptomatic patients are associated with high-risk of pancreatic malignancy and levels higher than 130 units/mL are associated with unresectable disease.[7,8] Carcinoembryonic antigen (CEA) may also be elevated; however, has lower sensitivity compared to CA 19-9. Activating mutations in K-Ras oncogene are present in >90% of cases.[9] Several genetic syndromes (such as Peutz-Jeghers, familial pancreatitis, cystic fibrosis, Lynch syndrome, and BRCA-associated hereditary breast ovarian cancer syndromes) are associated with high risk of pancreatic cancer.

The risk factors for pancreatic cancer include cigarette smoking, alcohol, high body mass index, chronic pancreatitis, and occupational exposure to chemicals. In recent years, the molecular biology of the disease has been better understood. R0 surgical resection (microscopically negative margins) is the only treatment modality which can prolong survival in these patients; though even with surgery, mean patient survival is only 2 years. Moreover, only 15–20% of patients are suitable for surgery at the time of diagnosis. Whipple surgery is a major intervention and is associated with postoperative morbidity. Thus, imaging is very important to diagnose malignancy and to assess resectability. Accurate preoperative staging is essential for optimal management.

IMAGING MODALITIES

Multidetector computed tomography (MDCT) is the investigation of choice for diagnosis and staging of pancreatic cancer.[10] Thin sections, multiplanar reformation, and high spatial resolution enable accurate delineation of tumor extent on MDCT. Transabdominal sonography may also detect larger lesions and depict local invasion; however, the accuracy is much less. Magnetic resonance imaging (MRI), endoscopic ultrasound (EUS), and positron emission tomography-computed tomography (PET-CT) are also useful in the diagnostic assessment of pancreatic malignancy.

Sonography

Ultrasound (US) is the most commonly used initial imaging modality for the evaluation of abdominal pain and jaundice. It not only diagnoses obstructive jaundice but also localizes the level of obstruction and helps in suggesting the cause. Common benign diseases such as cholelithiasis and choledocholithiasis may be easily diagnosed. Though small pancreatic lesions (<3 cm) may be missed on US, larger lesions can usually be seen and secondary evidence such as pancreatic ductal dilatation may also be evident. The US can also provide real-time guidance for percutaneous sampling; although an endoscopic route is preferred. Disadvantages are operator dependence and proper evaluation of the pancreas may not be feasible because of obesity or bowel gas.

Multidetector Computed Tomography

Helical CT on a scanner with multiple rows of detector (preferably 64 or more) is the workhorse for workup of patients with suspected pancreatic cancer. Thinnest slice thickness possible (<3 mm) is used. A dedicated protocol is essential to accurately detect and stage pancreatic cancers **(Flowchart 1)**. Imaging should be done prior to endoscopic retrograde cholangiopancreatography (ERCP) stenting to avoid missing the smaller lesions (stent may cause artifacts masking the small lesions and may induce inflammatory changes which may mimic or mask malignancy). The examination starts with neutral oral contrast given over 15–30 minutes for gastroduodenal distension. This enables proper visualization of the pancreas and ampullary region. Intravenous nonionic iodinated contrast is injected via rapid bolus at 3–5 mL/second using a pressure injector and a biphasic breath-hold acquisition is done.

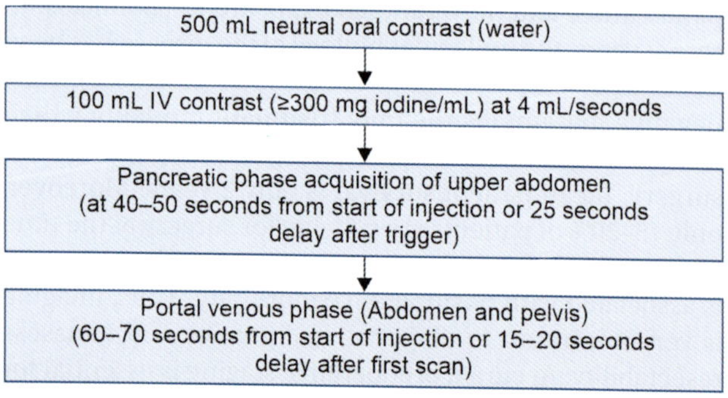

FLOWCHART 1: Multidetector computed tomography (MDCT) protocol for pancreatic cancer imaging.

The first acquisition is done in the pancreatic phase, usually 40–50 second(s) from the start of contrast injection. If contrast triggering is used, then typically a delay of 20–25 seconds is optimal, after the threshold attenuation is reached in the region of interest (ROI) (descending thoracic aorta in this case). The rapid contrast injection produces intense enhancement of the normal pancreas in this phase and thus the hypovascular ductal carcinomas are demonstrated well. The pancreatic phase scan should include the liver and pancreas (upper abdomen). Hypervascular lesions [like neuroendocrine tumors (NETs)], hypervascular liver metastases, as well as flow-related phenomena (arterial hyperenhancement in case of pancreatic cancer liver metastases) are well seen in the late arterial phase. Subtle surrounding perivascular infiltration and arterial anatomy is also well seen.[11]

The second acquisition is the portal venous phase at 65–70 seconds from the start of contrast injection and covers the entire abdomen and pelvis. The portal venous system is well opacified and the splanchnic viscera show homogeneous parenchymal contrast enhancement (CE). Former enables assessment of vascular involvement while the latter enables detection of hypoenhancing liver metastases. The scan coverage in this phase should include the chest also for complete staging.

Careful analysis of thin sections and three-dimensional (3D) reconstructions on a workstation is key to accurate imaging assessment. Coronal and curved multiplanar reformations help to evaluate the status of common bile duct and pancreatic duct in relation to the tumor **(Figs. 1A to D)**. Postprocessing of the volumetric dataset serves to highlight local invasion along blood vessels.

A split-bolus single phase CT has also been advocated with simultaneous acquisition of pancreatic and portal venous phases to improve lesion visualization and reduce radiation exposure.[10]

Magnetic Resonance Imaging

Magnetic resonance imaging has similar accuracy to MDCT in staging of pancreatic cancers with the advantage of absence of radiation exposure.[12] The excellent contrast resolution more than makes up for the lower spatial resolution than MDCT. High-resolution fast imaging of pancreas has become feasible owing to multichannel coils, parallel imaging, higher magnetic field strength (3T) and other advancements in MRI technology.

Fat-suppressed (FS) T1-weighted (T1W) images demonstrate the normally hyperintense pancreatic parenchyma very well. Pancreatic cancers are hypointense on T1W, intermediate signal on T2W and show diffusion restriction on diffusion-weighted MRI (DW-MRI). The latter manifests as retained high signal on the high b-value

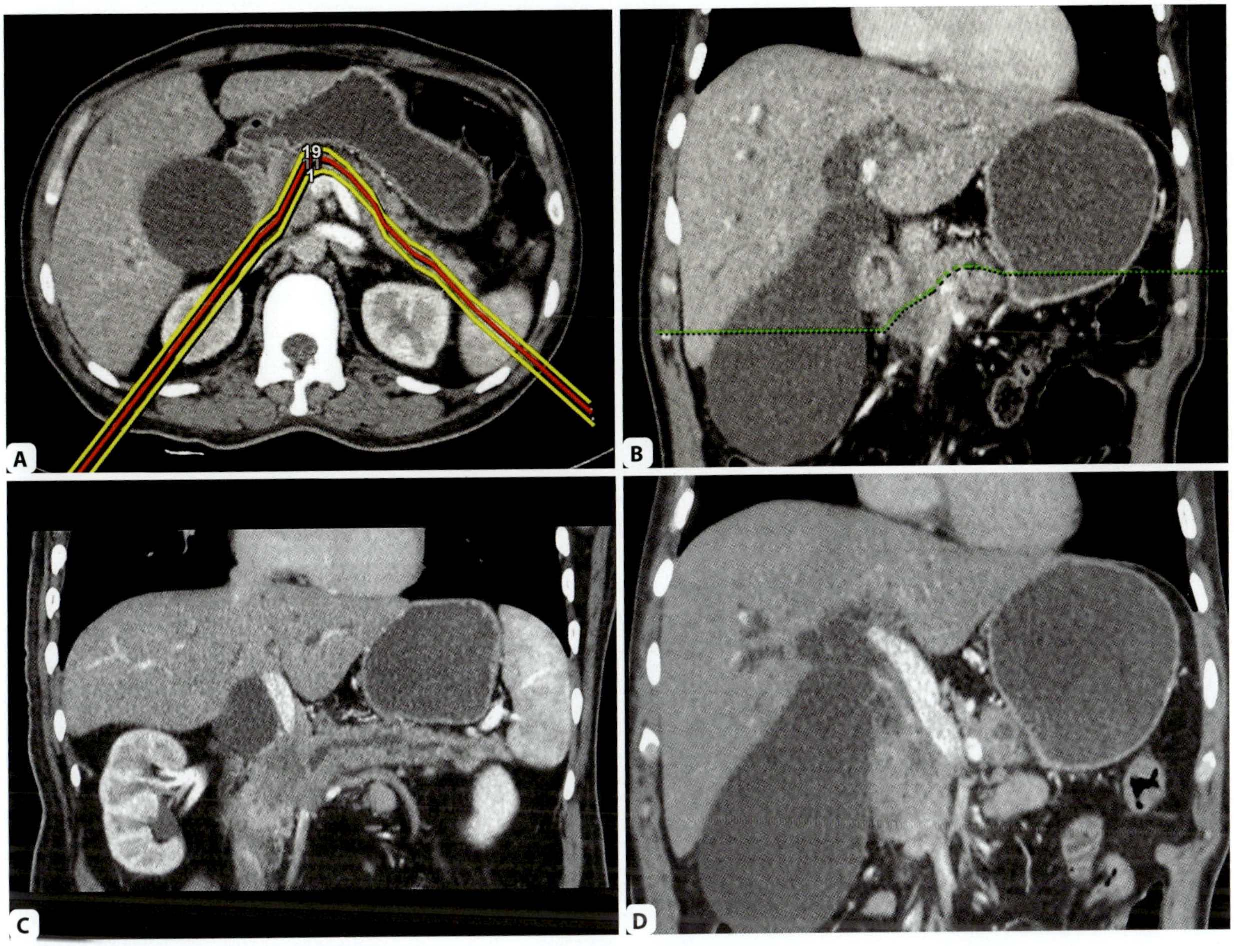

FIGS. 1A TO D: Utility of curved multiplanar reformations (MPRs). Axial (A) and coronal (B) CT (computed tomography) images demonstrate the planning of curved MPR along the pancreas. Resultant image (C) depicts the hypodense mass in the head with abrupt cut-off and upstream dilatation of pancreatic duct. Curved MPR better delineates the mass in relation to pancreatic duct in a single image compared to orthogonal coronal image (D).

image and dark signal on the apparent diffusion coefficient (ADC) map. ADC map also enables quantification and pancreatic carcinoma is associated with lower ADC values compared with rest of parenchyma.[13] Heavily T2-weighted (T2W) sequences like HASTE employed in magnetic resonance cholangiopancreatography (MRCP) enable exquisite demonstration of pancreatic and biliary ducts enabling detection of subtle areas of narrowing/ obstruction. Similar to CT, multiphasic scanning after contrast administration enables detection of pancreatic cancer in the late arterial phase and accurate staging in the portal venous phase. Pancreatic tumors show delayed enhancement at 3–5 minute postcontrast injection. Ideally, MRI for evaluation of pancreatic cancer should include postcontrast multiphasic acquisition. However, non-contrast MR sequences can provide sufficient information in majority of the cases; and thus, MRI is the modality of choice in patients with renal insufficiency where contrast administration is undesirable or in cases with contrast allergy.

Magnetic resonance imaging is also a problem-solving modality in case of small lesions and when CT is indeterminate for liver metastases. The latter are best detected on DWI-MRI **(Figs. 2A and B)**. DW-MRI is useful in detection of small lesions as well as post-therapy response assessment. Absence of exposure to ionizing radiation is another advantage of MRI. Disadvantages include high cost, limited availability, and long examination time.

Endoscopic Techniques

Side-viewing endoscopy is often employed for evaluation of periampullary malignancies, especially when small mass is not visible on CT or MRI, but there is ductal dilatation.

Endoscopic ultrasound may aid in detection of small lesions, may depict subtle vascular involvement and nodal spread, as well as guide sampling **(Figs. 3A and B)**. EUS-guided biopsy is preferable to a CT/US-guided biopsy (especially in patients with nonmetastatic disease) because of better diagnostic yield, safety, and potentially lower risk of

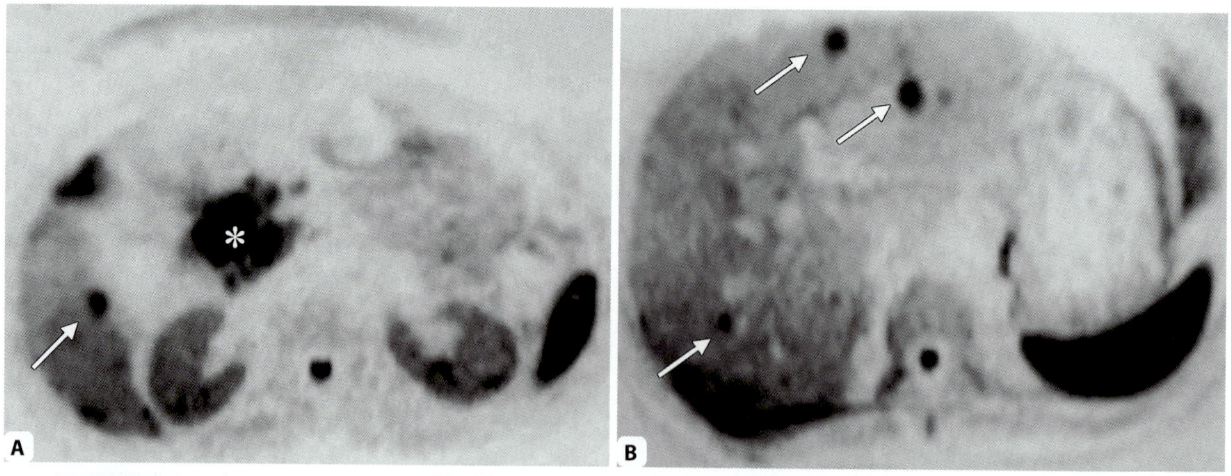

FIGS. 2A AND B: Utility of diffusion-weighted (DW) MRI in detecting small liver metastases. Contrast-inverted high b-value (1,000 s/mm^2) axial DW images (A and B) depict marked restriction of diffusion in the pancreatic head mass (asterisk) and multiple small liver metastases (arrows).

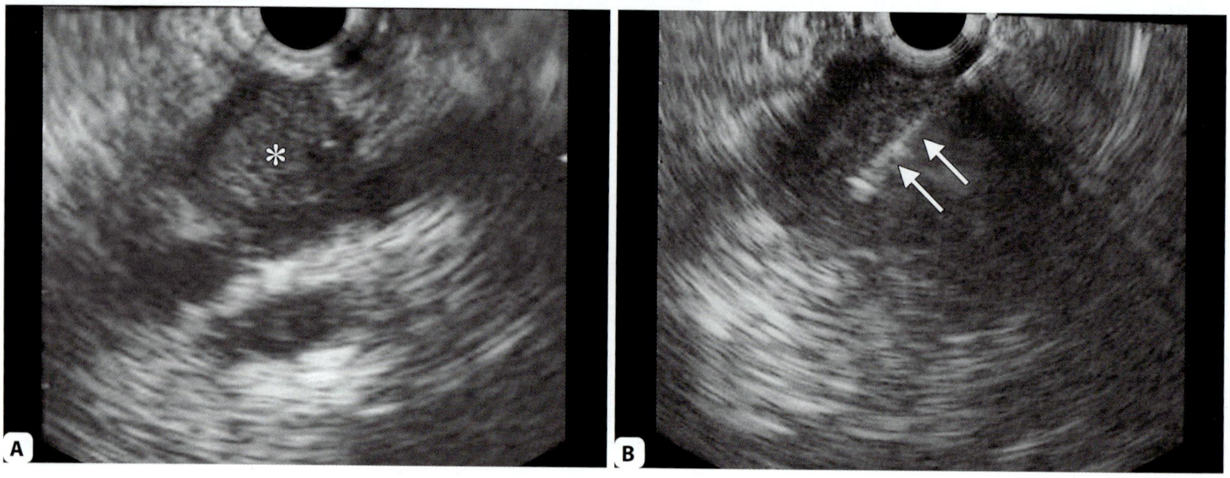

FIGS. 3A AND B: Endoscopic ultrasound (EUS) in evaluation of pancreatic carcinoma. EUS image (A) clearly shows the pancreatic head mass (asterisk) and (B) depicts sampling using EUS guidance (arrows denote the needle).

peritoneal seeding when compared with the percutaneous approach. The role of EUS is complementary to CT for staging.[5] However, it is invasive, not widely available and not recommended as a routine staging tool. For screening in high-risk individuals (those with hereditary syndromes or with presence of worrisome criteria in IPMN and MCN), EUS has the highest sensitivity, followed by MRI and CT in the detection of small (<2 cm) solid lesions.[14]

Endoscopic retrograde cholangiopancreatography with brush cytology is indicated when no mass is seen on imaging and stenting is to be done for palliation. Nowadays, ERCP is done only for the purpose of biliary decompression.

Positron Emission Tomography-Computed Tomography

Positron emission tomography imaging may be used as per institutional preference, in high-risk patients to detect extrapancreatic metastases; but it is not a substitute for diagnostic CT/MRI for staging.[5] PET/CT scan before and after initiation of a neoadjuvant therapy is useful in assessing response to systemic therapy and for restaging. It may also prove useful in identifying unexpected sites of recurrence. However, the exact role of this modality in evaluation of pancreatic carcinoma is still evolving.

Recent Advances

Ultrasound elastography is a new technique which may be employed for detection of pancreatic cancers. Owing to deep location and small size of pancreas, elastography has been considered difficult and less reliable. However, it is a promising modality for distinction between benign and malignant lesions and for screening in high-risk patients.[15] It can be performed through transabdominal or endoscopic routes. Contrary to shear-wave elastography (SWE), strain elastography requires application of external pressure. Manual compression is however not effective for pancreas and strain generated by aortic pulsations is used instead. Thus, it requires the probe, pancreas, and aorta to be in the same line.[15] Also, pancreatic body can be well evaluated but not head and tail regions. SWE can be performed for the entire pancreas but is not currently available via endoscopic route.[16] Pancreatic adenocarcinoma appears as hard heterogeneous lesion while chronic pancreatitis is soft and heterogeneous.[15,16] NETs are seen as hard homogeneous lesions.

Contrast-enhanced ultrasonography (CEUS) employs microbubble contrast media which are excreted via lungs and thus can be used in patients with renal dysfunction. This is especially useful along with EUS to confirm areas of abnormality. Ductal adenocarcinoma commonly appears as hypoenhancing lesion relative to the surrounding pancreas.[17] Mass-forming chronic pancreatitis (MFCP) is isoenhancing or hyperenhancing while NETs are hyperenhancing.[17]

Perfusion CT involves scanning the ROI (pancreas) multiple times over a short span after rapid bolus contrast injection. In addition to color-coded maps, many quantitative parameters, such as blood flow, blood volume, mean transit time, and time to peak are generated which are more representative of the contrast kinetics and vascularity of the lesion. This technique has a potential role in detection of small isodense pancreatic lesions **(Figs. 4A to D)**[18] and in assessment of post-therapy response. The basis of the latter use is that chemotherapeutic agents target tumor neoangiogenesis and thus reduction in vascularity indicates response to therapy. Perfusion CT parameters (especially blood flow) may also help to differentiate adenocarcinoma from MFCP.[19] The main drawback is increased radiation exposure.

Dual-energy CT scanners enable generation of virtual noncontrast images from a single acquisition. Also, lower keV dataset can be generated which offers superior contrast resolution while higher keV images have better signal-to-noise ratio (SNR) **(Figs. 5A to C and 6A to D)**.[20]

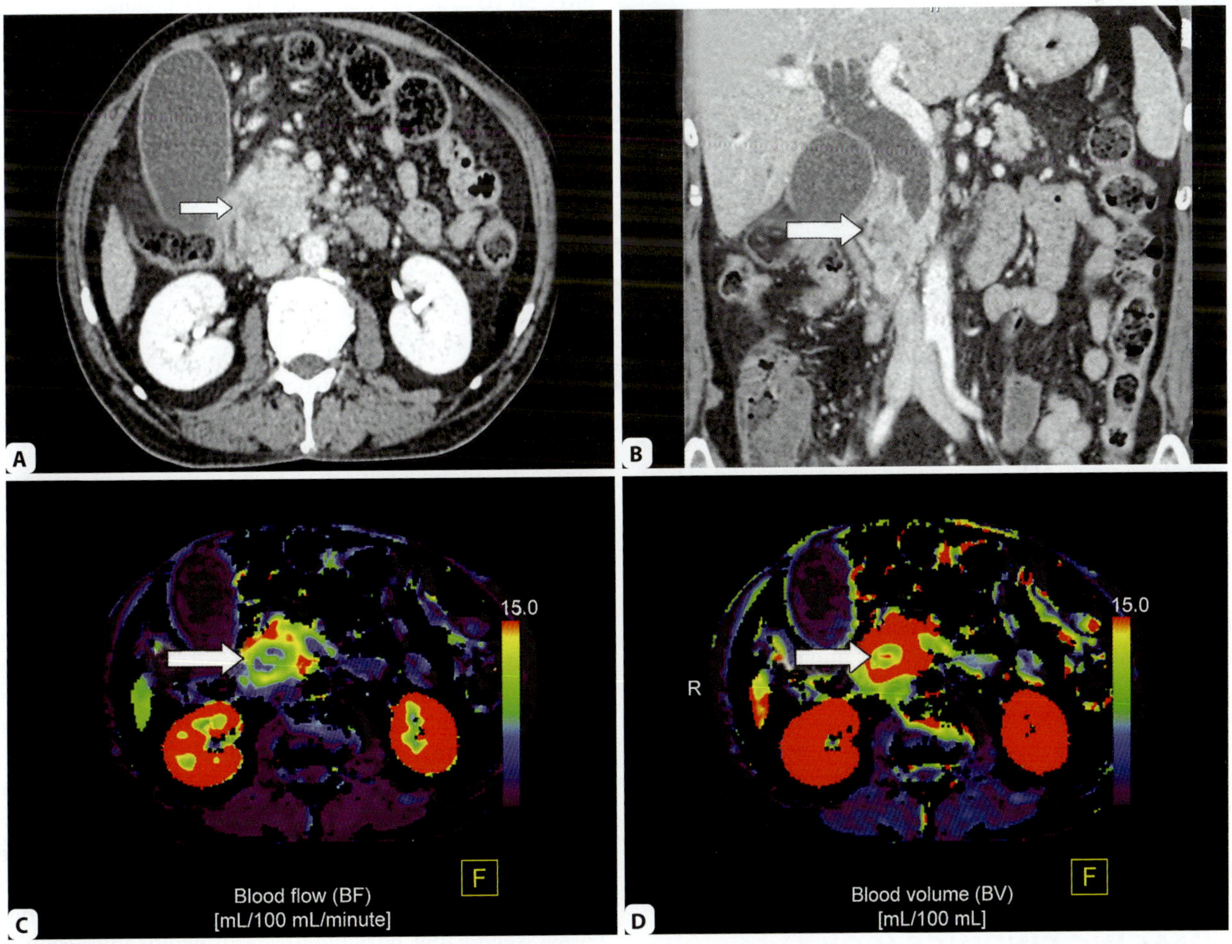

FIGS. 4A TO D: Role of perfusion CT (computed tomography) in isodense masses. Axial (A) and coronal (B) contrast-enhanced CT images show an ill-defined mass in the pancreatic head, which is mildly hypodense to the surrounding parenchyma (solid arrows) with dilated common bile duct. Axial blood flow (C) and blood volume (D) color maps (derived from perfusion CT) enable a much clearer depiction of hypovascular mass, distinct from adjacent parenchyma (solid arrows).

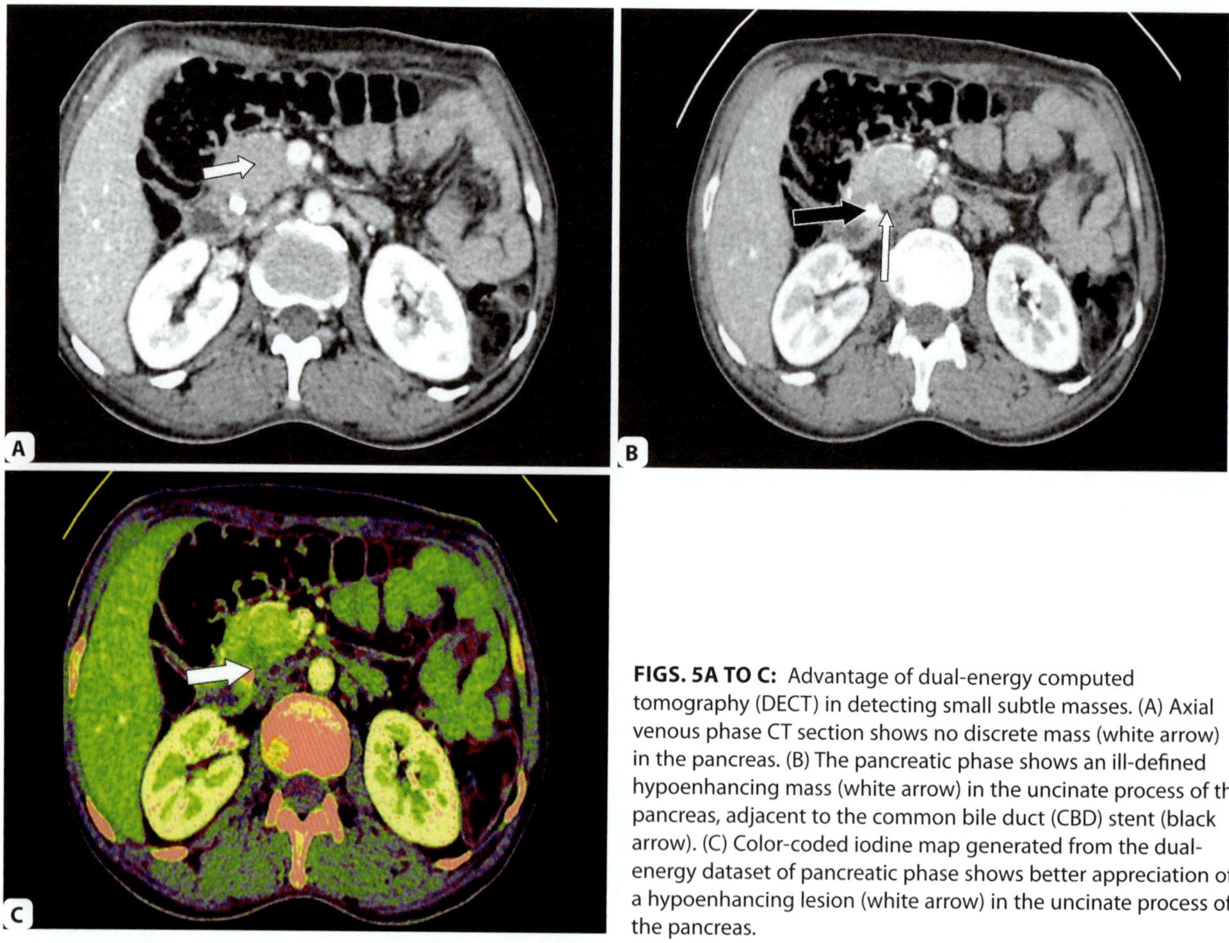

FIGS. 5A TO C: Advantage of dual-energy computed tomography (DECT) in detecting small subtle masses. (A) Axial venous phase CT section shows no discrete mass (white arrow) in the pancreas. (B) The pancreatic phase shows an ill-defined hypoenhancing mass (white arrow) in the uncinate process of the pancreas, adjacent to the common bile duct (CBD) stent (black arrow). (C) Color-coded iodine map generated from the dual-energy dataset of pancreatic phase shows better appreciation of a hypoenhancing lesion (white arrow) in the uncinate process of the pancreas.

Diffusion-weighted MRI is now part of routine abdominal MR protocols in most of the institutions worldwide. The simple way of quantifying the diffusion restriction is based on the monoexponential model which generates a single ADC value based on combination of both diffusion and perfusion effects. Recently, biexponential-based estimation of the intravoxel incoherent motion (IVIM) parameters has been employed with generation of separate diffusion and perfusion metrics. Perfusion fraction (f) has been shown to be markedly reduced in pancreatic ductal adenocarcinomas (PDACs)[21-23] and postulated to be superior than diffusion in differentiating from MFCP.[21,22] Another method which has been proposed is the non-Gaussian kurtosis model, which takes into account tissue heterogeneity (kurtosis effects).[13] Corrected diffusion coefficient (Dk) has been found to have highest accuracy for differentiation of adenocarcinoma and remaining pancreatic parenchyma.[13]

IMAGING FINDINGS (BOX 1)

Pancreatic cancers are solid scirrhous tumor with reduced perfusion compared to normal parenchyma. They are infiltrative and incite surrounding inflammation and desmoplastic reaction. These lesions tend to obstruct and constrict the ductal structures, causing jaundice and pancreatitis. Pancreatic head is the most common location (60–70% cases) and thus biliary obstruction is frequent in pancreatic adenocarcinomas. Head is the part of pancreas to the right of superior mesenteric vein (SMV) while body is to the left of SMV up to the left border of aorta. Distal to that is the tail. Also, head lesions are detected at a relatively earlier stage because of biliary obstruction, whereas body and tail lesions may grow large before producing significant symptoms. Thus, lesions in the body and tail region are large at presentation and have areas of necrosis/hemorrhage within. Pancreatic carcinoma commonly metastasizes to the liver, peritoneum, lungs, and bones.

Pancreatic cancers are usually solid hypoechoic on ultrasound and upstream ductal dilatation (diameter of pancreatic duct >3 mm) may be seen **(Figs. 7A to D)**. Margins are ill-defined and irregular. On color Doppler examination, no significant internal vascularity is seen. Larger lesions may have necrosis within and show infiltration of surrounding structures. Lesions in the pancreatic head often result in biliary dilatation **(Figs. 7A to D)**.

On the late arterial phase CT or MRI, the masses are hypodense in >90% cases **(Figs. 8A to D)**.[24] In addition

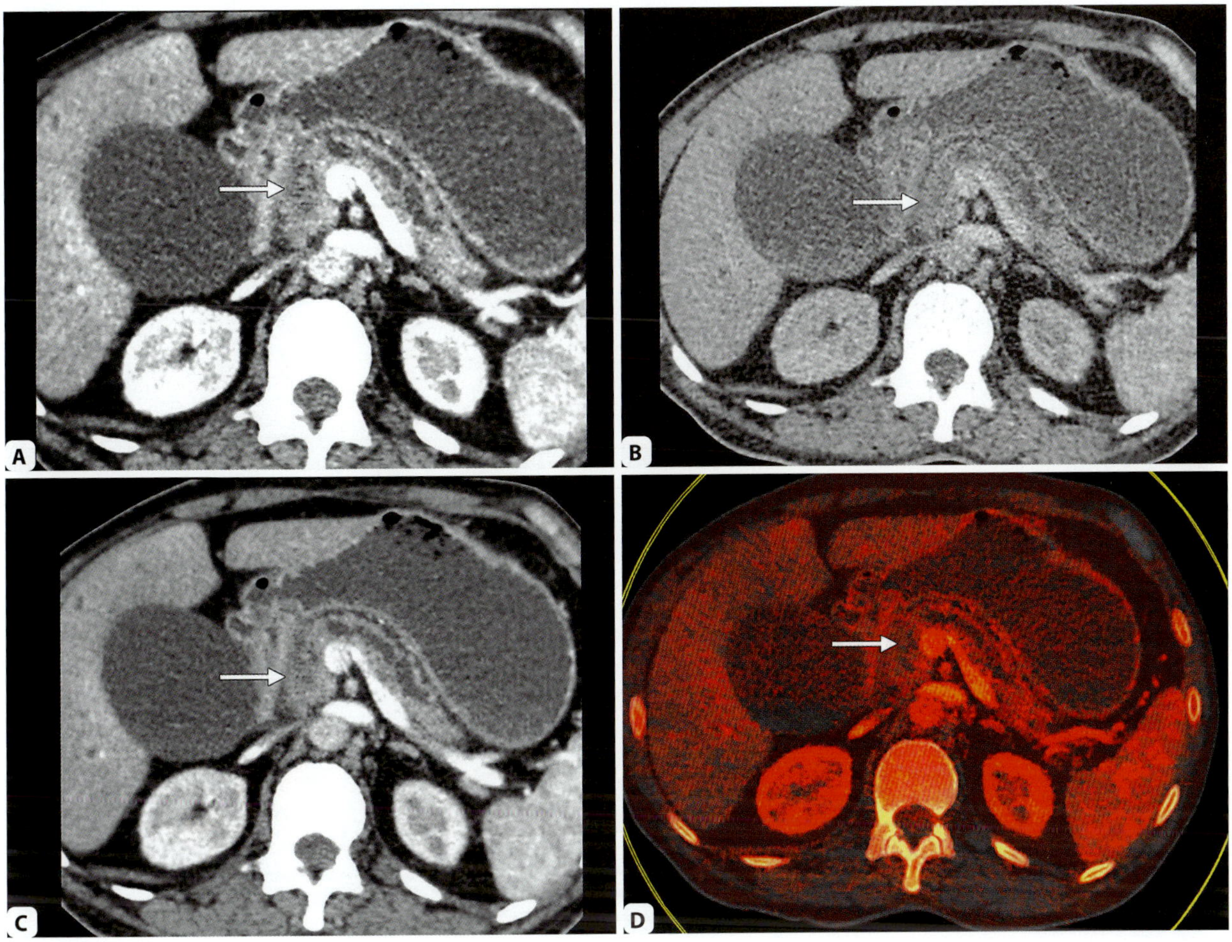

FIGS. 6A TO D: Dual-energy computed tomography (DECT) in pancreatic mass evaluation. Axial monochromatic contrast-enhanced CT (CECT) images generated from dual-energy dataset: 70 keV image (A) gives better demonstration of mass (arrow in all images) compared to 100 keV image (B), however is noisy. Optimal contrast image (C) derived by mixing of the datasets yields high contrast as well as low noise. Iodine map (D) depicts the hypodense mass distinct from the enhancing parenchyma as well as cut-off of pancreatic duct.

BOX 1 Imaging features of pancreatic carcinoma.

- *Sonography*:
  - Solid
  - Hypoechoic
  - Irregular ill-defined margins
  - Usually no demonstrable internal vascularity
- *CT*:
  - Mildly enhancing lesion which appears hypodense relative to brightly enhancing normal pancreatic parenchyma
  - Contour bulge
- *MRI*:
  - T1 hypointense mass against background hyperintense pancreas
  - Diffusion restriction
  - Mass enhances less than surrounding parenchyma in pancreatic phase
- *Secondary signs*:
  - Upstream pancreatic ductal dilatation with/without atrophy
  - Contour bulge (in larger lesions)
  - Local infiltration
  - Biliary dilatation in head lesions

to the attenuation difference, larger masses also produce a contour bulge of the pancreas **(Figs. 8A to D)** and the fat planes with adjacent structures may be lost. 5–10% of the pancreatic carcinomas are isodense to the surrounding parenchyma **(Figs. 8A to D)** and thus difficult to detect based on attenuation values.[25] The problem is further compounded because these isodense cancers are frequently small (<2 cm) and may not deform the pancreatic contour.

Magnetic resonance imaging is useful in such cases with lesion being hypointense on T1W FS images, against background hyperintense parenchyma. MRI may visualize up to 79% of isodense pancreatic lesions **(Figs. 9A to D)**.[24] T2W images depict the mass as having intermediate signal intensity and are not much helpful in demonstrating the mass; but heavily T2W images depict ductal dilatation and obstruction quite well. Calcification, cystic component, and multiplicity are atypical features of pancreatic adenocarcinoma and seen in <10% cases.[26] Pancreatic adenocarcinomas show heterogeneous diffusion restriction on DW-MRI and their ADC values are lower

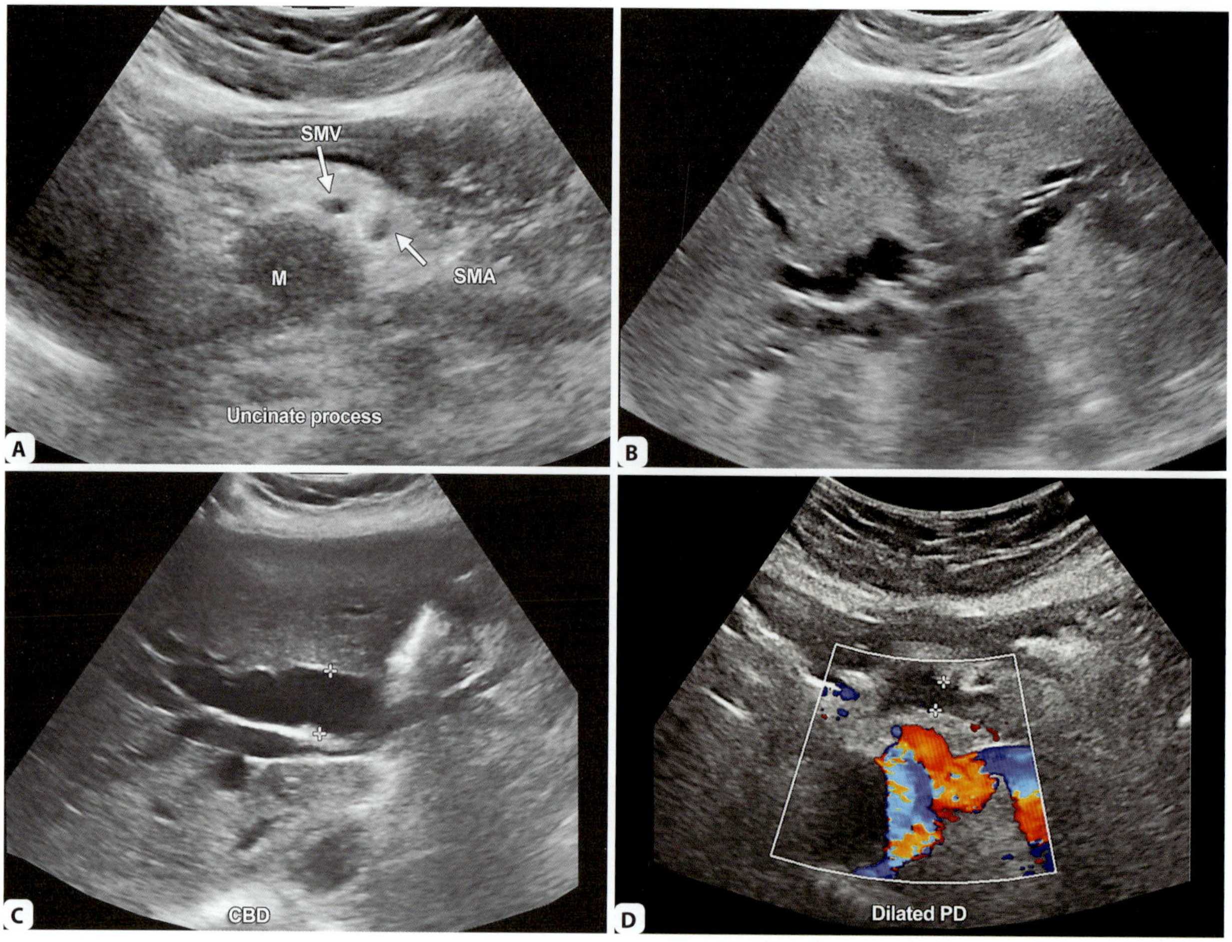

FIGS. 7A TO D: Sonography in pancreatic cancer. Gray-scale ultrasound image (A) shows solid hypoechoic mass lesion in the head and uncinate process of pancreas (M) with irregular margins. Superior mesenteric vessels are seen separately. USG image (B) shows bilobar intrahepatic biliary radical dilatation and (C) depicts dilated common bile duct (cursors). Color Doppler image (D) shows dilated pancreatic duct (cursors).

(CBD: common bile duct: SMA: superior mesenteric artery; SMV: superior mesenteric vein; USG: ultrasonography)

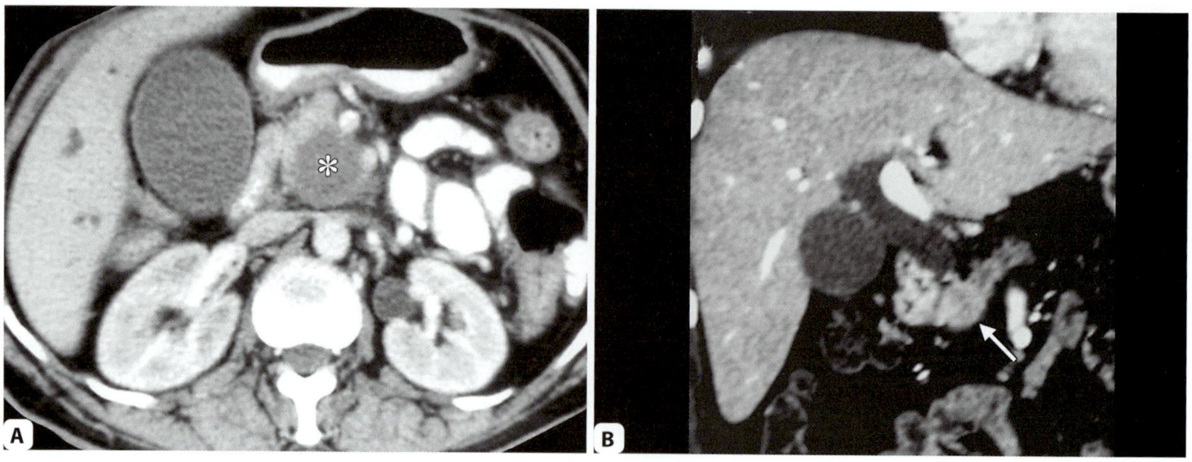

FIGS. 8A TO D: *Continued*

Continued

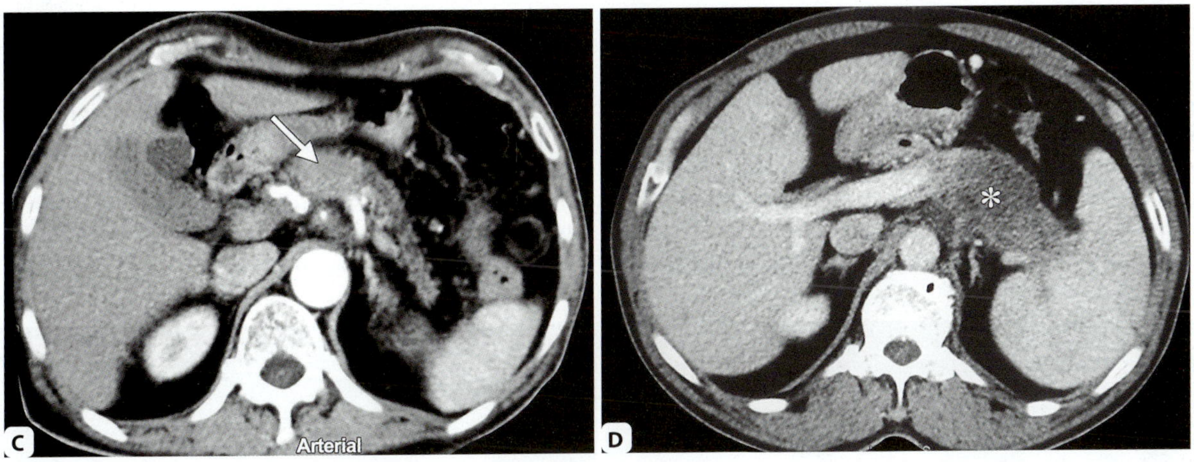

FIGS. 8A TO D: Computed tomography (CT) images of different patients showing pancreatic carcinoma with variable morphology in different locations. Axial contrast-enhanced CT (CECT) image (A) shows a hypodense mass lesion in the uncinate process of pancreas (asterisk), abutting the superior mesenteric artery. Coronal CECT image (B) shows isodense mass lesion in the pancreatic head (arrow) with atrophy of distal pancreatic parenchyma and pancreatic ductal prominence. Axial CECT image (C) demonstrates isodense mass in the neck of pancreas (arrow) without contour bulge, but with pancreatic ductal dilatation. Axial CECT image (D) shows large hypodense mass lesion in the distal body and tail of pancreas with areas of necrosis within (asterisk).

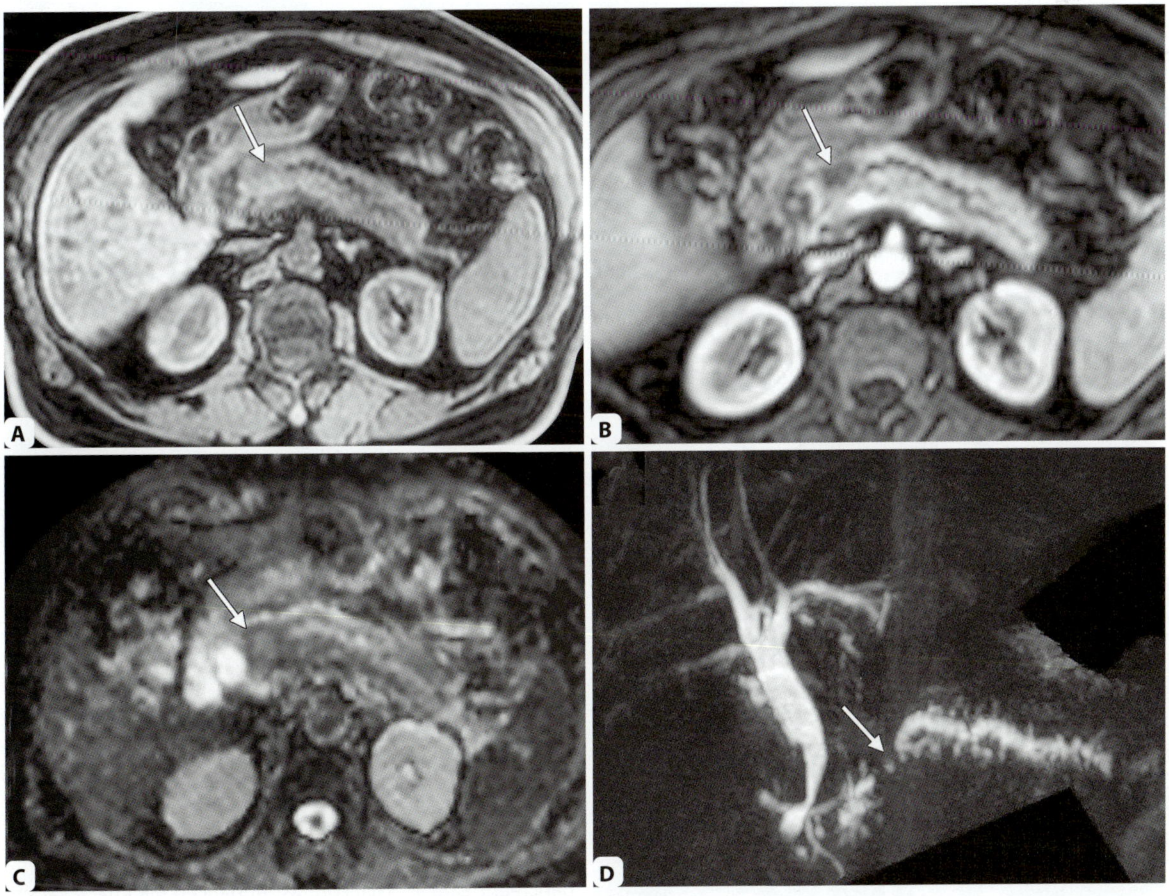

FIGS. 9A TO D: Utility of MRI in small lesions. Axial T1-weighted (T1W) fat-suppressed (FS) image (A) shows an ill-defined small isointense mass in the pancreatic head-neck region (arrow) which is hypoenhancing compared to rest of parenchyma on postcontrast pancreatic phase imaging (B) with pancreatic ductal dilatation. Axial apparent diffusion coefficient (ADC) map (C) shows the lesion is dark (arrow), suggesting restricted diffusion. Projectional magnetic resonance cholangiopancreatography (MRCP) image (D) depicts abrupt cut-off of the main pancreatic duct (arrow). There is diffuse irregular dilatation of main pancreatic duct and side branches due to background chronic pancreatitis.

than surrounding parenchyma **(Figs. 10A to E)**. Addition of DWI to conventional sequences increases the sensitivity of detection of pancreatic cancer **(Figs. 11A to D)**.[27]

The secondary findings include dilatation of the pancreatic duct with or without biliary dilatation **(Figs. 12A to D)**. Biliary dilatation occurs in case of lesions located in the pancreatic head and may occur due to metastatic lymph node enlargement compressing the suprapancreatic part of the common bile duct. The pancreatic duct may be abruptly cut off with upstream dilatation and may be the only clue to diagnosing small isodense and noncontour deforming lesions **(Figs. 12A to D)**.[28] *Double-duct sign* is seen in cancers located in the pancreatic head and represents dilatation of both pancreatic and biliary ducts due to obstruction of both main pancreatic duct (MPD) and adjacent intrapancreatic part of common bile duct **(Figs. 12A to D and 13A and B)**. Long-standing lesions may cause distal parenchymal atrophy as well. Perivascular soft tissue is also an indirect sign of pancreatic malignancy.

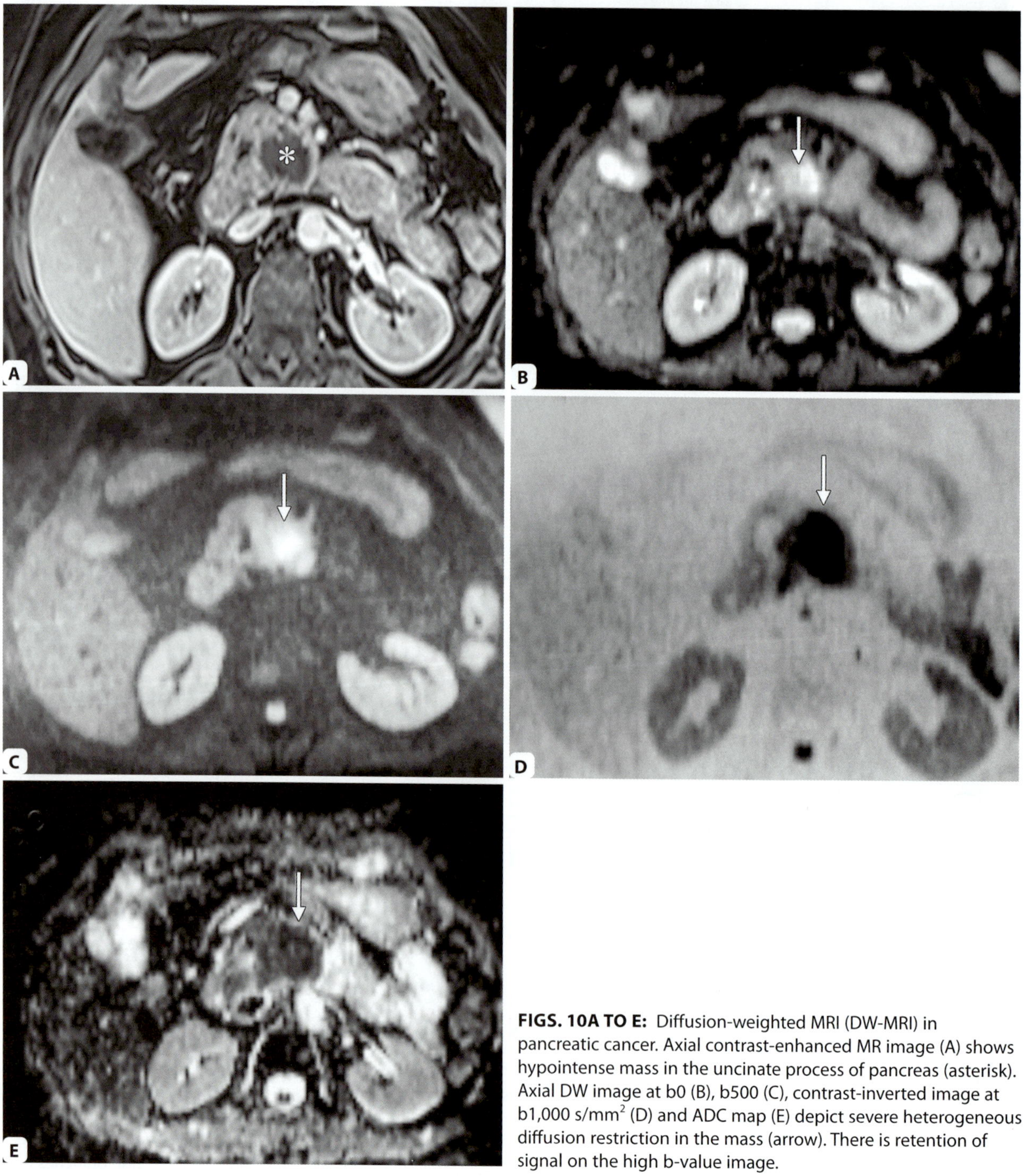

FIGS. 10A TO E: Diffusion-weighted MRI (DW-MRI) in pancreatic cancer. Axial contrast-enhanced MR image (A) shows hypointense mass in the uncinate process of pancreas (asterisk). Axial DW image at b0 (B), b500 (C), contrast-inverted image at b1,000 s/mm^2 (D) and ADC map (E) depict severe heterogeneous diffusion restriction in the mass (arrow). There is retention of signal on the high b-value image.

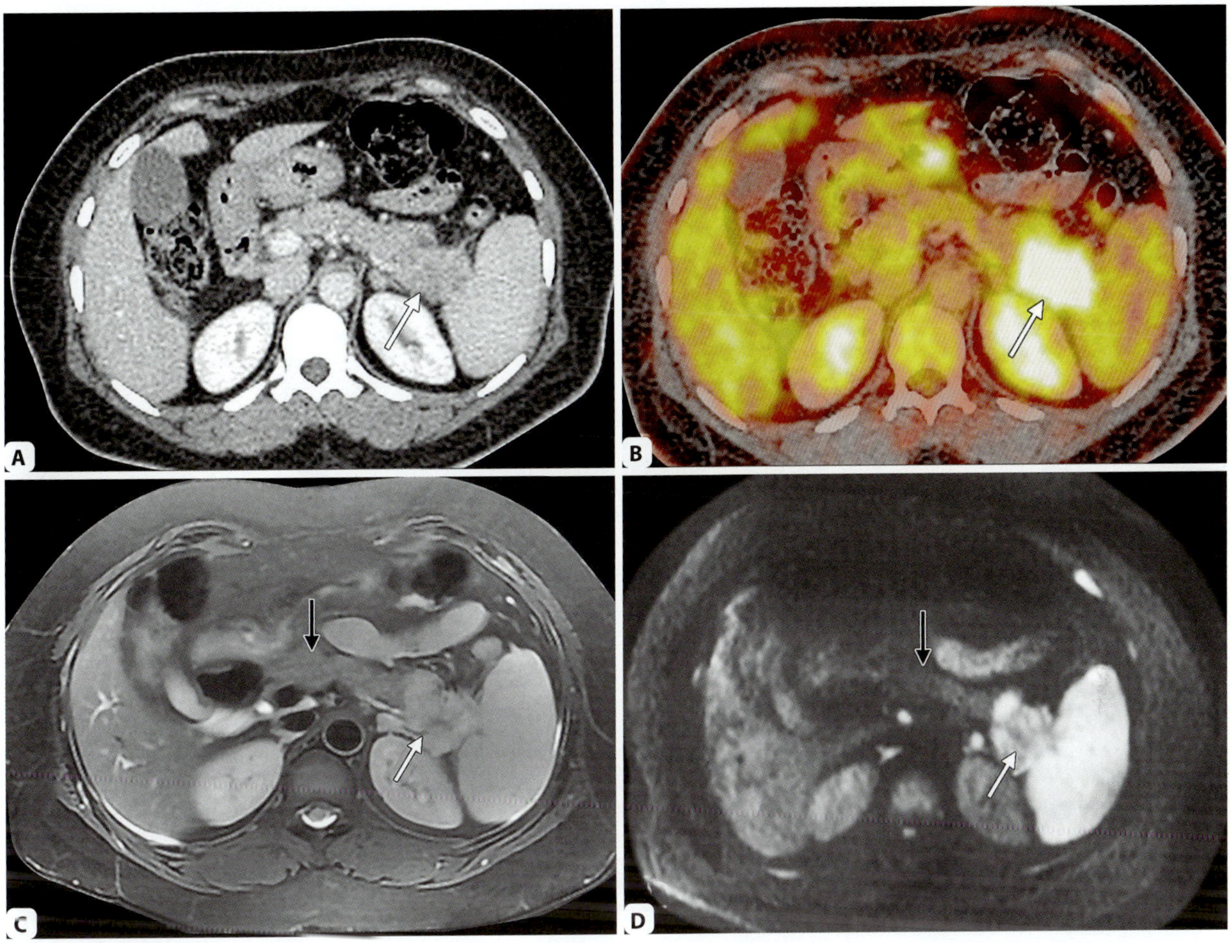

FIGS. 11A TO D: Utility of positron emission tomography (PET) scan and MRI. (A) Contrast-enhanced computed tomography (CECT) axial section shows an ill-defined isohypoenhancing lesion (white arrow in all images) in the tail of pancreas with adjacent fat stranding. (B) PET-CT increases the diagnostic confidence by showing increased focal uptake in the lesion. (C) T2 fat-suppressed axial image shows a well-defined T2 hyperintense lesion (white arrow) in comparison to normal parenchyma (black arrow). (D) Diffusion-weighted imaging (DWI) shows the same lesion (white arrow) showing significant diffusion restriction in comparison to the normal pancreatic parenchyma (black arrow). Thus PET-CT and MRI better depicted the lesion in contrast to the background parenchyma.

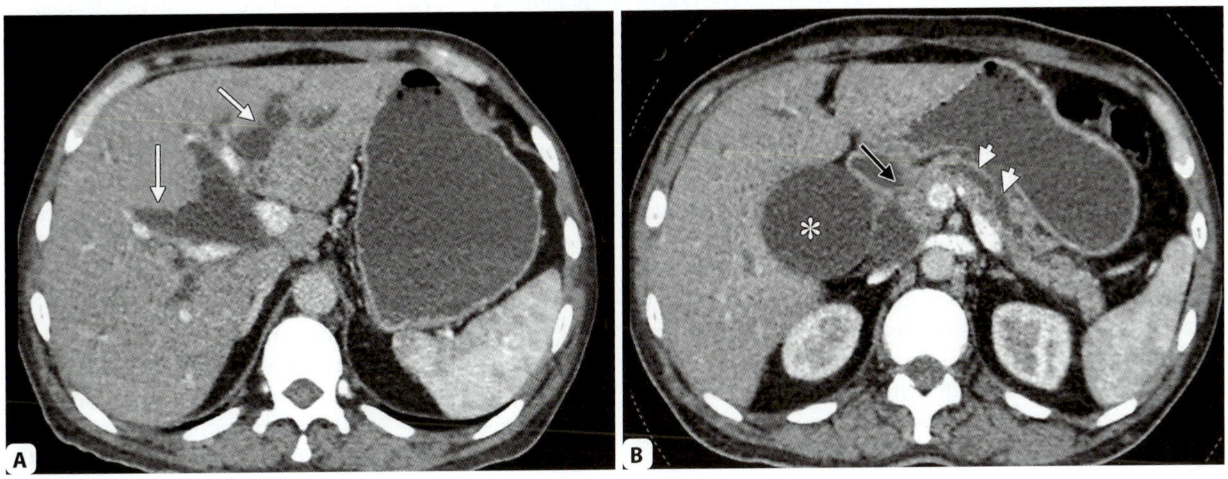

FIGS. 12A TO D: *Continued*

Continued

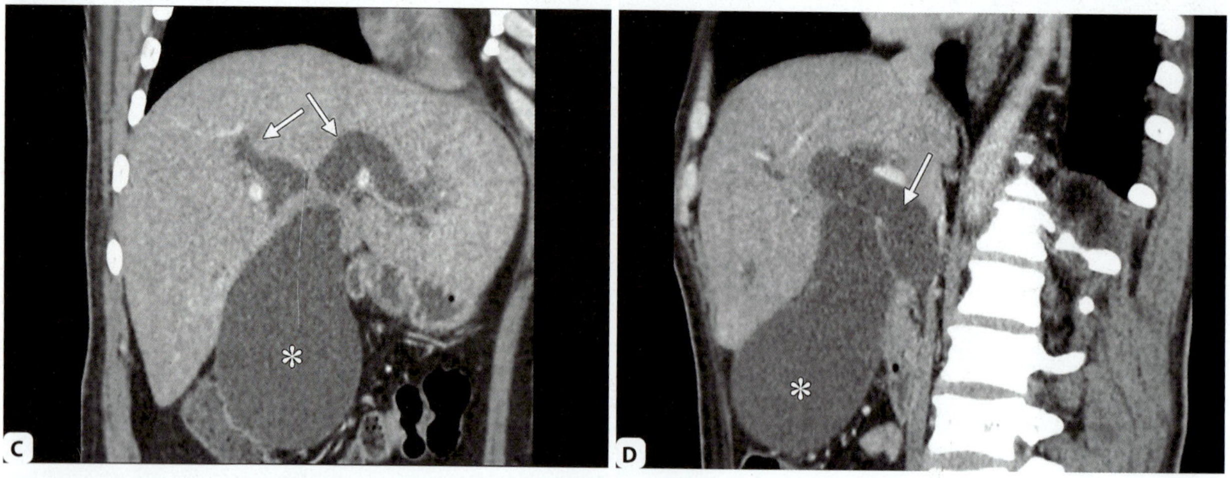

FIGS. 12A TO D: Secondary findings in pancreatic cancer. Axial (A and B), oblique coronal (C), and oblique sagittal (D) CT images in the pancreatic phase show dilatation of intrahepatic biliary radicals (solid arrows), common bile duct (white arrows), gallbladder (asterisk), and pancreatic duct (arrowheads). These secondary signs help in the detection of small isodense mass in the pancreatic head (black arrow).

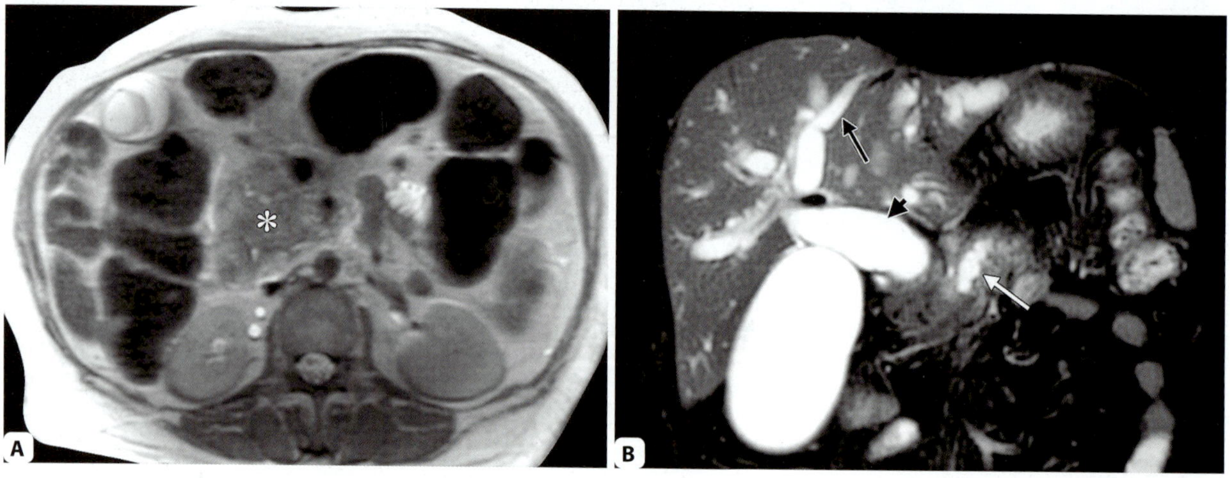

FIGS. 13A AND B: *Double-duct sign.* (A) T2-weighted (T2W) axial image shows a bulky head and uncinate process of pancreas (asterisk). (B) Coronal T2W image shows dilatation of bilobar intrahepatic biliary radicals (black arrow), common bile duct (black arrowhead), and main pancreatic duct (white arrow) giving rise to a double-duct sign.

Rarely, pancreatic cancer may present as single or multiple episodes of acute pancreatitis, secondary to ductal obstruction.[29] In these cases, inflammatory changes predominate and may mask the underlying lesion. Disproportionate enlargement of the head, significant dilatation of the pancreatic duct with abrupt change in caliber, focal pancreatitis distal to obstruction, and recurrent pancreatitis in the absence of risk factors may raise the suspicion of an underlying malignancy **(Figs. 14A and B)**. The lesion may often be diagnosed only on follow-up scans when the inflammatory changes have subsided.[29]

The early features of pancreatic carcinoma include focal pancreatic atrophy, faint parenchymal enhancement, and unifocal changes in the caliber of main pancreatic duct (MPD). Owing to the location, uncinate process masses have a propensity for early invasion of superior mesenteric artery (SMA) and SMV and ductal dilatation may become apparent later. Perineural and duodenal invasion are also more common in tumors occurring in this location.[30]

Both pancreatic phase and venous phase images are important for accurate assessment of staging. A characteristic feature of liver metastases from pancreatic adenocarcinomas is flow-related phenomenon, seen on the late arterial phase images **(Figs. 15A to D)**. This can either be in the form of thin peripheral CE around hypodense metastases or perfusion abnormalities like transient hepatic

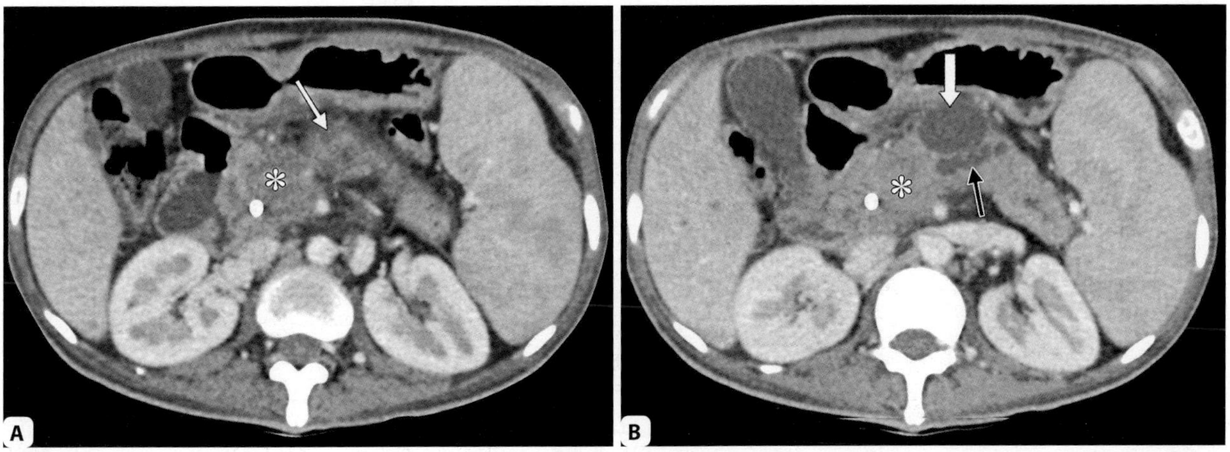

FIGS. 14A AND B: Pancreatic cancer causing acute pancreatitis with biliary stent in situ. Axial contrast-enhanced computed tomography (CECT) images depict bulky heterogeneous mass in the pancreatic head region (asterisk) with heterogeneity in the proximal body (white arrow). Former was ductal adenocarcinoma while latter was focal pancreatitis secondary to obstruction. Note is made of peripancreatic fat stranding in (A), peripancreatic fluid collection (solid arrow) and pancreatic ductal dilatation (black arrow) in (B).

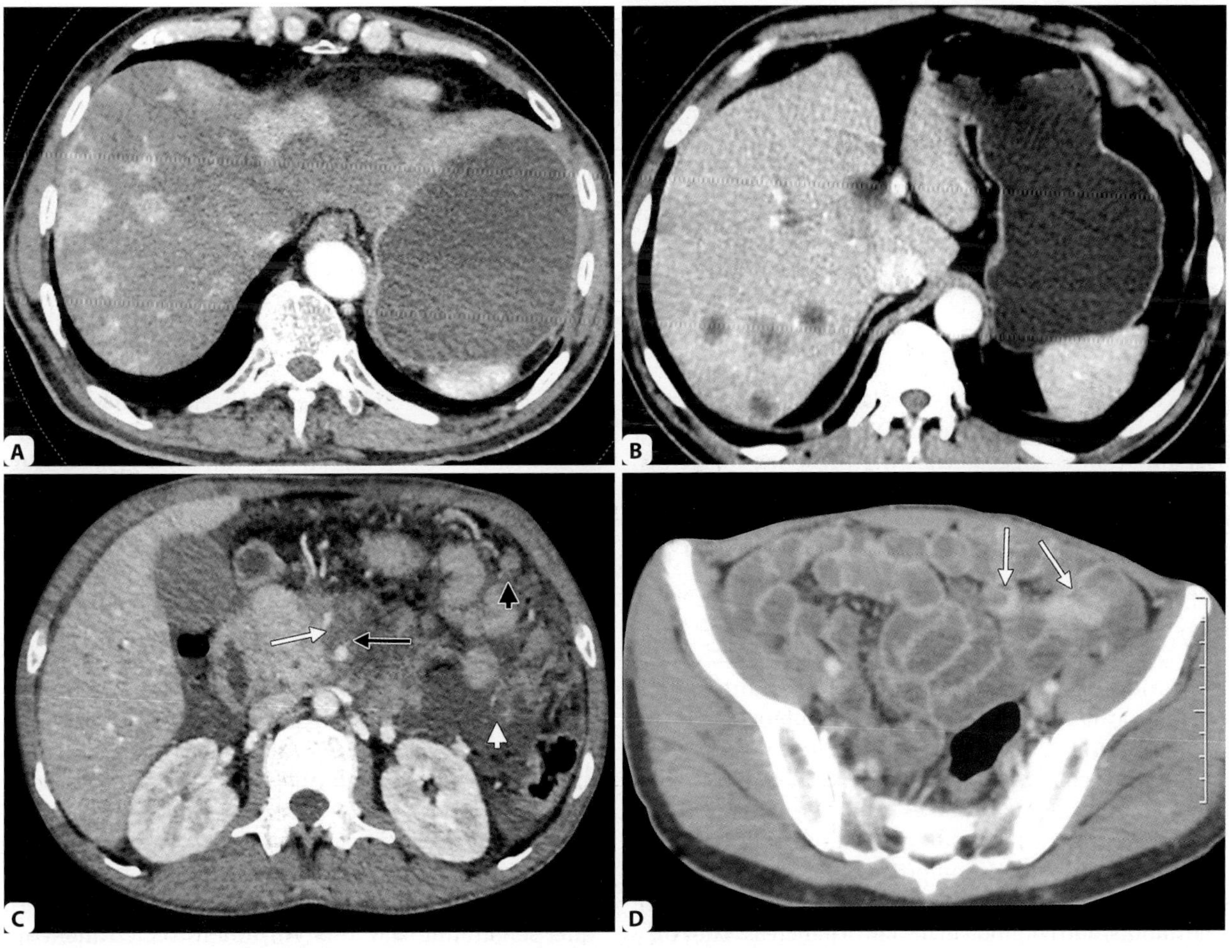

FIGS. 15A TO D: Liver and peritoneal metastases in pancreatic carcinoma. Late arterial phase axial computed tomography (CT) image (A) shows multiple liver lesions with surrounding hyperenhancement and transient hepatic enhancement difference. Axial CT image (B) shows multiple hypodense liver metastases in the venous phase. Axial contrast-enhanced CT (CECT) scan of upper abdomen in a different patient (C) shows an ill-defined hypoenhancing lesion (white arrow) in the neck of pancreas with complete encasement of superior mesenteric artery (black arrow) and vein, moderate free fluid (white arrowhead) in peripancreatic location, and omental thickening and nodularity (black arrowhead). Different patient (D) of pancreatic carcinoma showed multiple areas of eccentric bowel wall thickening (arrows), suggesting serosal metastases (peritoneal dissemination).

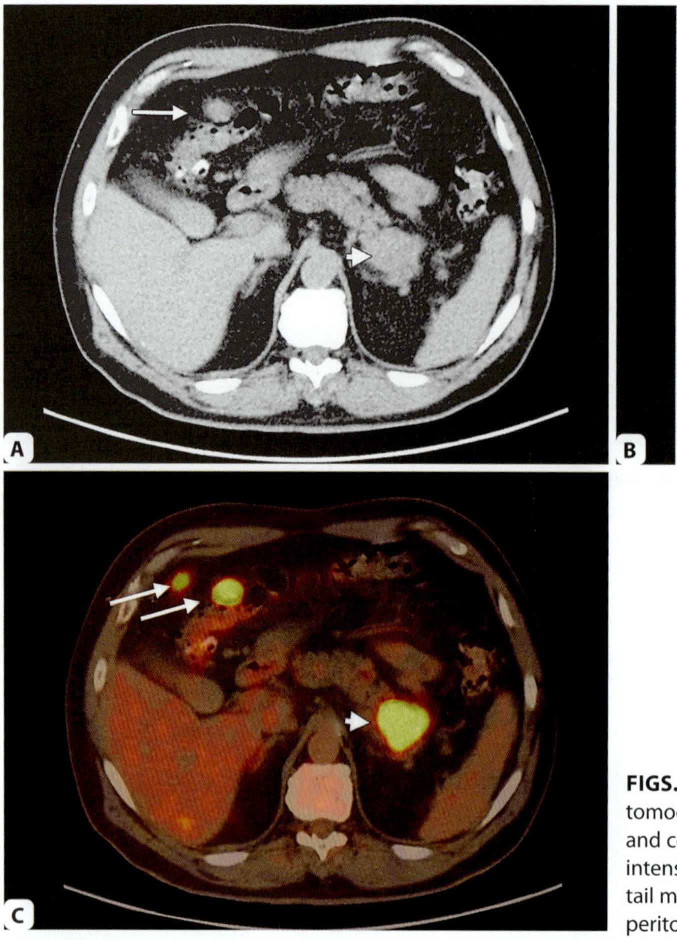

FIGS. 16A TO C: Positron emission tomography-computed tomography (PET-CT) in pancreatic cancer. Axial CT image (A) and corresponding PET (B) and hybrid PET-CT images (C) depict intense fluorodeoxyglucose (FDG) uptake in the pancreatic tail mass (arrowhead) and peritoneal nodules (arrows). Small peritoneal nodules may be difficult to detect on CT.

enhancement difference. Liver metastases are best detected on T2W and diffusion-weighted MR sequences. Peritoneal dissemination is suggested by the presence of ascites, omental thickening, and peritoneal nodularity. Peritoneal nodules are better visualized on DW-MRI and PET-CT **(Figs. 16A to C)**.

PANCREATIC CANCER VARIANTS

Other than PDAC, there are few rare variants which constitute around 10% of the pancreatic tumors.[31] **Table 1** summarizes the salient features.

Mucinous colloid carcinoma also has better prognosis than adenocarcinoma. It shows T2 hyperintensity owing to mucin within. Adenosquamous carcinoma has both glandular and squamous components and is a histological diagnosis with worse prognosis. Anaplastic carcinomas are large tumors, and common in the tail of pancreas. They may show marked CE and have central areas of necrosis, and thus may mimic NETs. These are aggressive lesions which usually present with lymphadenopathy and metastases.

Acinar cell carcinoma is also a malignant epithelial tumor with slightly better prognosis and has a propensity to metastasize to lymph nodes and liver. Jaundice is usually not seen. These tumors are solid, can reach large size, and do not cause ductal dilatation even in advanced stage. Like adenocarcinomas, these are hypoenhancing; but in contrast, they show well-defined margins.

DIFFERENTIAL DIAGNOSES

Focal pancreatitis (including autoimmune type) is an important diagnostic consideration especially because secondary changes of upstream ductal dilatation or atrophy may be seen.[32] *Mass-forming chronic pancreatitis* is chronic inflammation usually involving the pancreatic head. History of repeated episodes of acute abdomen and presence of calcifications indicates underlying chronic calcific pancreatitis. Pancreatic duct in the latter shows a long smooth narrowing or irregular beaded appearance. The "duct penetrating sign" refers to nonobstructed attenuated duct, which traverses the mass instead of getting cut-off and is used to differentiate an inflammatory pancreatic mass from malignancy **(Figs. 17A to D)**.[33] Also, chronically inflamed pancreas demonstrates greater enhancement than tumor in the pancreatic phase imaging. Ratio of

TABLE 1: Pancreatic cancer variants.

Histologic subtype	Key clinical features	Key radiologic features
Conventional PDAC	• Most common • Older adults • Male predominance • Most patients present at an advanced tumor stage	• Indistinct, poorly enhancing • Indirect signs of PDAC: Ductal obstruction, pancreatitis, segmental atrophy, and contour abnormalities
Adenosquamous carcinoma	Less favorable outcome than PDAC	• Smooth margins • Progressive ring enhancement; extensive central tumor necrosis • High signal intensity at T2-weighted MRI
Mucinous colloid carcinoma	More favorable long-term survival after surgical resection	• Cystic imaging appearance *(D/D: IPMN)* • Lobulated contour; Indiscrete margins • High T2 signal intensity with "salt and pepper" appearance • Poorly but gradually enhancing
Hepatoid carcinoma	• Younger patients • Early hematogenous metastasis and lymph node invasion	• Exophytic, well-defined hypointense tumor • Arterial hyperenhancement and washout in the portal venous phase
Medullary carcinoma of pancreas	• Interlinked with hereditary nonpolyposis colorectal cancer (HNPCC) • Better prognosis than that of conventional PDAC	–
Signet-ring cell carcinoma	Unconventional sites of metastasis (bone and leptomeninges)	–
Undifferentiated carcinoma	Less favorable outcome than that with conventional PDAC	• May appear cystic in up to 50% of cases • Aggressive mass with direct invasion to adjacent structures • Peripheral enhancement
Undifferentiated carcinoma with osteoclast-like giant cells	• Slight female predominance • Lymph node metastasis and perineural invasion are not common • Treatment of choice: Surgical en bloc resection	• Low signal intensity at T2- and T2*-weighted MRI due to hemorrhage • Well-defined hypoenhancing and low-signal-intensity rim at T2-weighted MRI calcifications

(D/D: differential diagnosis; IPMN: intraductal papillary mucinous neoplasm; PDAC: pancreatic ductal adenocarcinoma)

the diameter of dilated pancreatic duct to the maximum width of the abnormal part of gland >0.5 favors carcinoma. DW-MRI and perfusion CT can also help to differentiate focal chronic pancreatitis from malignancy.[19,34] Peripheral displacement of the calcifications favors development of malignancy in the background of chronic pancreatitis. EUS may be helpful in these cases and guided sampling may be done.

Autoimmune pancreatitis is characterized by elevated serum immunoglobulin G4 (IgG4) levels and is treated with steroids and does not require surgery. The focal form can mimic malignancy on imaging. Absence of pancreatic duct dilatation, diffuse involvement, halo-like peripancreatic smooth hypodensity, and extrapancreatic manifestations of IgG4-related sclerosing disease may help in differentiating from carcinoma.[34] The pancreatic and biliary ducts may show multifocal long segment (>3 cm) irregular wall thickening and enhancement.[35] Homogeneous enhancement (similar to surrounding parenchyma) and duct penetrating sign may help in differentiating mass-forming autoimmune pancreatitis from carcinoma.[36] Diffusion restriction with low ADC values can be seen in autoimmune pancreatitis also (due to dense lymphoplasmacytic infiltration) and thus ADC values may overlap or be even lower than that of pancreatic malignancy.[36] Low CA 19-9 (<74 units/mL) and elevated IgG4 levels (>1.0 g/L) favor the diagnosis of autoimmune pancreatitis.[37]

Paraduodenal/groove pancreatitis is a type of chronic focal inflammation localized to the space between the pancreatic head and the second part of duodenum. It is seen more often in middle-aged men with history of alcohol overconsumption. Imaging appearance is in

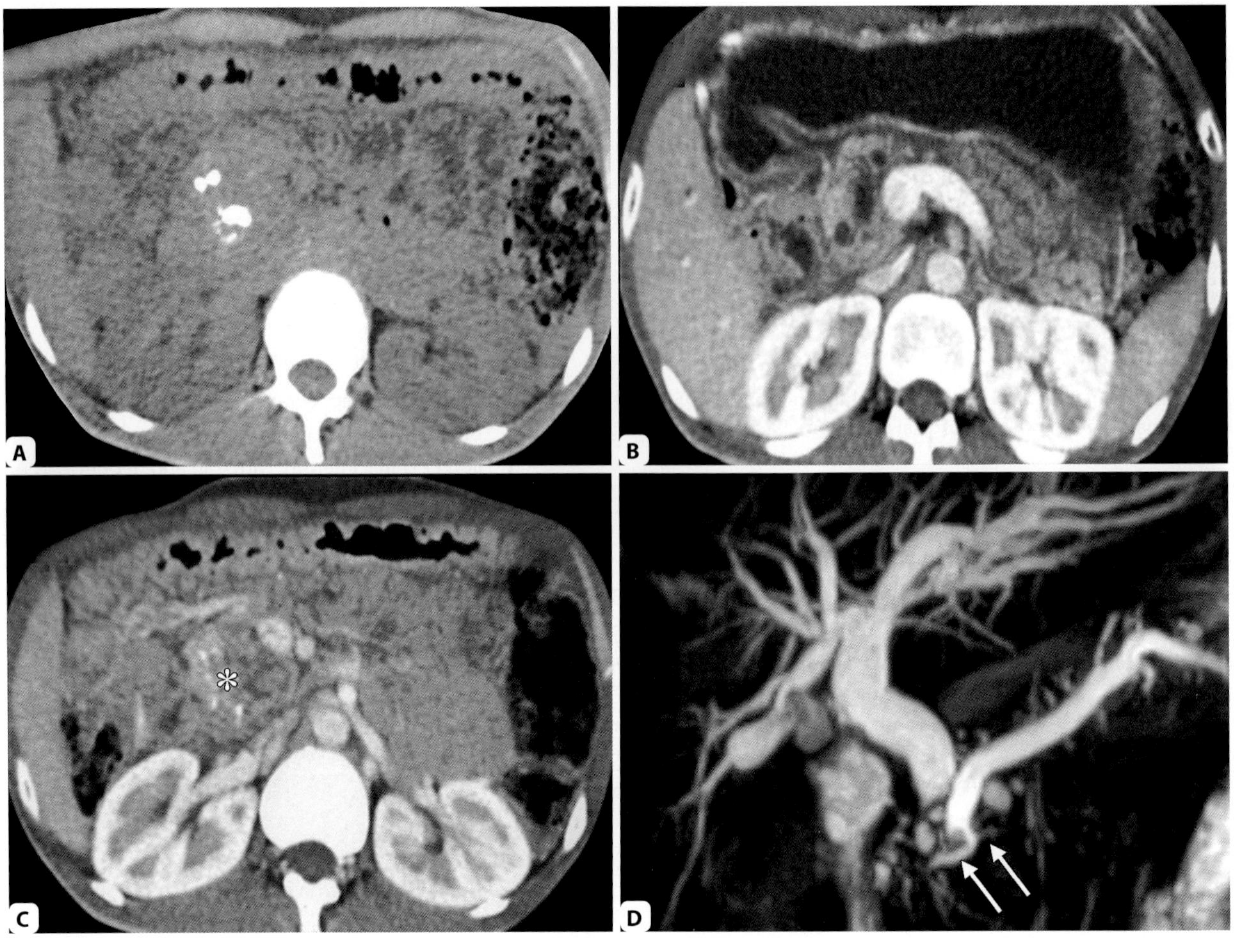

FIGS. 17A TO D: Mass-forming chronic pancreatitis. Axial noncontrast CT image (A) depicts multiple foci of calcification in the region of pancreatic head. Axial contrast-enhanced computed tomography (CECT) images (B and C) show bulky heterogeneously enhancing head (asterisk) with dilated pancreatic and common bile ducts. However, there is no abrupt cut-off of the ducts, and the narrowed pancreatic duct can be seen to course through the head region (arrows in D), suggesting duct penetrating sign. EUS sampling confirmed focal chronic pancreatitis.

the form of ill-defined sheet-like thickening and bulky pancreatic head with delayed enhancement. There is a pure form which affects only the pancreatoduodenal groove and a segmental form which affects the groove and may extend medially to involve the pancreatic head. Cystic changes may be seen especially in the medial duodenal wall along with duodenal wall thickening **(Figs. 18A to D)**.[38] Thus, it comes in the differential diagnosis of periampullary and pancreatic head malignancies. Pancreatic and biliary ductal dilatation is usually not seen. Medial displacement of the gastroduodenal artery and abnormal enhancement of the (medial) wall of the second part of duodenum favor groove pancreatitis over malignancy of pancreatic head.

Despite all imaging advancements and even with sampling, focal pancreatitis may be difficult to differentiate from carcinoma and they may occasionally coexist. Relatively spared pancreatic parenchyma in the background of atrophic gland in chronic pancreatitis may also mimic pancreatic malignancy.

Neuroendocrine tumors are usually small in size, T2 hyperintense, and show hypervascularity on the pancreatic phase imaging. Up to 40% NETs may be hypovascular and thus may be difficult to diagnose. Even in such cases the enhancement is more than PDAC (attenuation >50 HU and tumor-to-pancreas enhancement ratio > 0.53 in early phase). Moreover delayed CE is a feature of PDAC [enhancement ratio: (PV-arterial)/(arterial-NC) is higher in PDAC].[26] Ductal dilatation is uncommon, as opposed to pancreatic carcinomas. Well-defined margins and presence of cystic component favor NET over PDAC. Nonfunctional NETs are large and heterogeneous with areas of necrosis and calcification within **(Figs. 18A to D)**. They may appear similar to ductal adenocarcinomas in the body and tail region because the latter also have large heterogeneous appearance. A particular subtype of pancreatic NETs (serotonin producing) may be associated with desmoplastic response. Thus, they may mimic adenocarcinomas because they lead to ductal dilatation

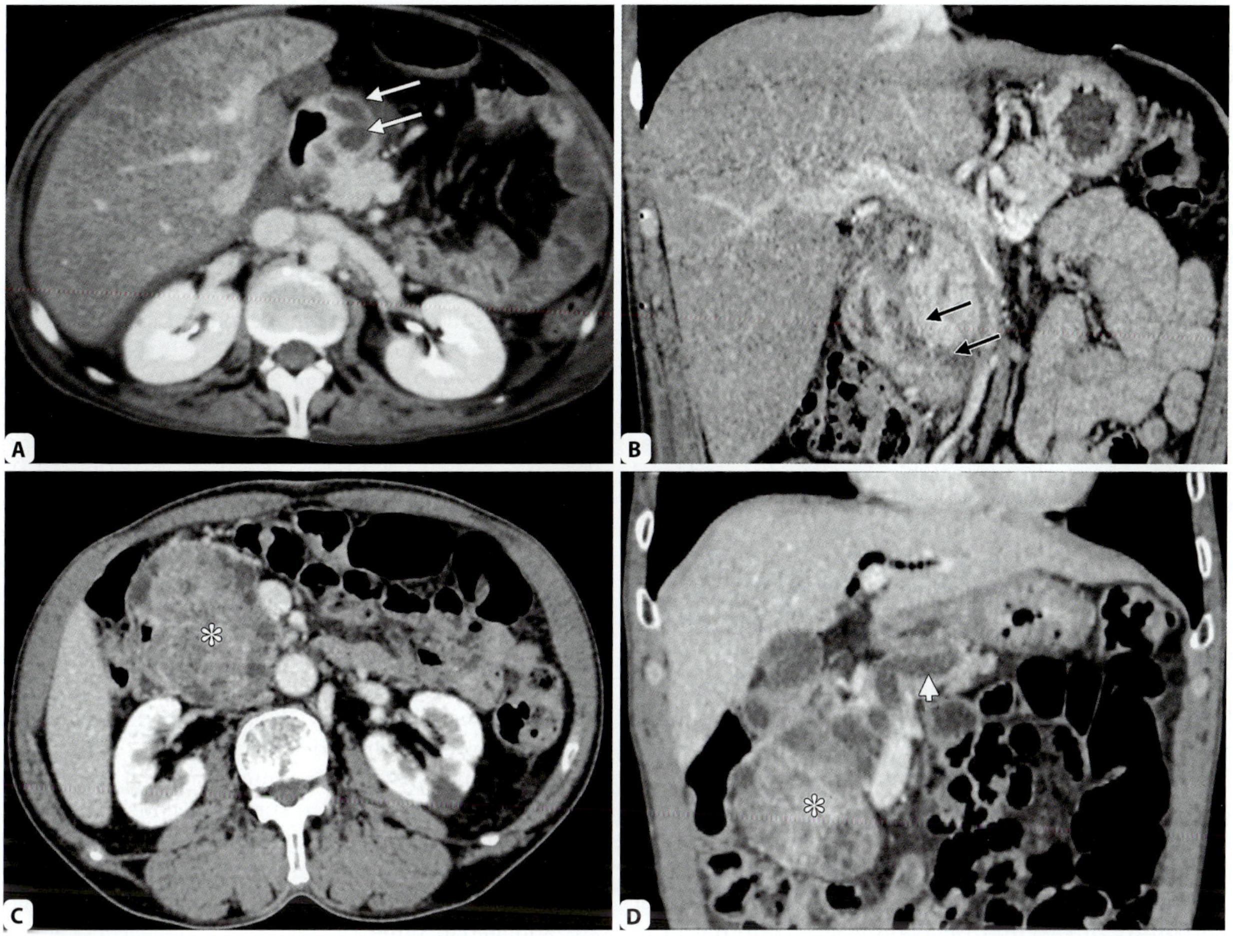

FIGS. 18A TO D: Differential diagnoses of pancreatic cancer. Axial (A) and coronal (B) contrast enhanced computed tomography (CECT) images show ill-defined sheet-like hypodense thickening (black arrows in B) in the pancreatoduodenal groove with cystic change (white arrows in A) and thickening of medial duodenal wall, suggesting groove pancreatitis. Axial (C) and coronal CECT (D) images demonstrate a large mixed solid-cystic mass lesion in the pancreatic head region (asterisk) showing hyperenhancement with ductal dilatation (arrowhead). This was a nonfunctioning neuroendocrine tumor on histopathology.

and atrophy early in the course of disease.[26,39] *Cystic pancreatic tumors* also come in the list of differentials in this scenario.

Metastases to pancreas are not common and most of these patients have metastatic lesions elsewhere in the body also. Primary malignancies which can metastasize to the pancreas include lung, breast, and renal carcinomas and melanomas. Metastases can be solitary, multiple or diffuse infiltrating. Usually, they are multiple and well-defined but may mimic pancreatic carcinoma when they occur singly. Enhancement characteristics are similar to the primary lesion (hypervascular in renal carcinomas and melanomas).

Lymphomatous involvement of the pancreas occurs frequently by direct infiltration from adjacent enlarged lymph nodes and is more common in non-Hodgkin lymphoma. Other manifestations include single/multiple homogeneous focal masses showing little CE. Ductal dilatation is infrequent, as is necrosis and calcification. Pancreatic head is commonly involved, and diffuse involvement of the entire pancreas may also occur.

Occasionally, *gastrointestinal tumors* from the stomach and duodenum may also mimic the imaging appearance of pancreatic cancer. *Tuberculosis* is another confounder, especially in areas where it is endemic.

STAGING OF PANCREATIC CANCER

After diagnosis, the next step is to assess the resectability of the lesion and also the patient's suitability for pancreaticoduodenectomy. Surgery is beneficial only if R0 resection (negative margins on pathology) is possible. Thus, it is important to avoid unnecessary laparotomy in the rest of the patients since there is little survival benefit. The criteria to determine resectability rely more on specificity than sensitivity to avoid denying the benefit of surgery to potentially resectable patients. CT and MRI are equally accurate in the staging of pancreatic cancers.

The spread of pancreatic cancer depends on its location. Anteriorly located head lesions spread toward gastroduodenal and common hepatic arteries while posterior lesions cause early involvement of SMV-PV and replaced/accessory right hepatic arteries (arising from SMA). SMV is more commonly involved in head lesions, compared to SMA. This is because SMV is nearer to the head and also because arteries have thick muscular walls compared to thin walls of veins. Tumors located in the uncinate process have a propensity to grow along jejunal branches of SMA and SMV and thus perineural spread is common. Tumors located in the body and tail region have a tendency to infiltrate splenic vessels and hilum of the spleen. In advanced cases, stomach, gallbladder, and duodenum may also get involved.

There are four categories as per the National Comprehensive Cancer Network (NCCN) 2024 criteria: resectable, borderline resectable, locally advanced, and metastatic disease **(Table 2)**.[5,40] Borderline resectable means that the chance of achieving R0 surgical resection is low; thus upfront surgery is not done even though the lesions appear resectable. Neoadjuvant (chemotherapy ± radiotherapy) therapy is initially started followed by surgery in case no progression is there.

Location of the tumor and vascular involvement are the important determining factors for categorization. It is important to note that arterial encasement (contact >180° or half the arterial circumference in cross-section) is an important criterion of unresectability of the pancreatic mass.[41] Less than 180° contact with a vessel is referred to as abutment, provided there is no contour irregularity or narrowing. Encasement is associated with a much higher probability of vascular invasion (~80%) compared to abutment (~40%). Infiltration of the surrounding structures (stomach, transverse colon, spleen, etc.) does not make the tumor unresectable, though surgery becomes more extensive.[40]

The lesion is *resectable* **(Figs. 19A and B)** if there is neither extrapancreatic infiltration nor distant metastases. Thus, there is a clear fat plane separating the tumor from main arteries [celiac axis (CA), common hepatic artery (CHA), and SMA]. The contact with the surrounding veins (SMV and portal vein PV) is also absent or there is just abutment (≤180° contact without contour irregularity). No venous encasement or tumor thrombus is seen.

Unresectable tumors **(Figs. 20A to F)** either have distant metastases (including nonregional lymphadenopathy) or local invasion. The recent NCCN guidelines have dropped the term "unresectable"; rather have introduced the categories of locally advanced and metastatic disease. Liver and peritoneal cavity are the common sites of metastases. Arterial invasion is in the form of encasement (contact >180° circumference) of SMA, CA, and aorta. Unresectable venous involvement includes unreconstructible SMV-PV due to infiltration/occlusion (which can be due to tumor or bland thrombus also).

Borderline resectability **(Figs. 21A to C)** in terms of venous involvement includes encasement or abutment of short-segment SMV-PV with contour irregularity or venous thrombosis but amenable to surgical reconstruction. The prerequisite for reconstruction is that the two venous ends should have single lumen and thus branches cannot be attached to a single lumen.[1] Arterial involvement criteria are tabulated in **Table 2**.

TABLE 2: Imaging criteria of resectability of pancreatic carcinoma [National Comprehensive Cancer Network (NCCN) guidelines, 2024].

	Arterial	Venous
Resectable	No arterial contact with tumor [celiac axis (CA), superior mesenteric artery (SMA), or common hepatic artery (CHA)]	No tumor contact with the superior mesenteric vein (SMV) or portal vein (PV) or ≤180° contact without vein contour irregularity
Borderline resectability	Pancreatic head/uncinate process: • Tumor contact with CHA without extension to CA proximally or hepatic artery bifurcation distally (so as to allow for surgical reconstruction) • Tumor contact with the SMA of ≤180° • Variant arterial anatomy with tumor contact (e.g., accessory right hepatic artery, replaced right hepatic artery, replaced CHA, and the origin of replaced or accessory artery) Pancreatic body/tail: • Tumor contact with the CA of ≤180°	• Tumor contact with the SMV or PV of >180°, contact of ≤180° with contour irregularity of the vein or thrombosis of the vein but with suitable vessel proximal and distal to the site of involvement allowing for safe and complete resection and vein reconstruction • Tumor contact with • inferior vena cava (IVC)
Locally advanced disease	Head/uncinate process: Tumor contact >180° with the SMA or CA Pancreatic body/tail: • Tumor contact of >180° with the SMA or CA • Tumor contact with the CA and aortic involvement	Unreconstructible SMV/PV due to tumor involvement or occlusion (can be due to tumor or bland thrombus)
Distant metastases, including nonregional lymphadenopathy also make the disease unresectable		

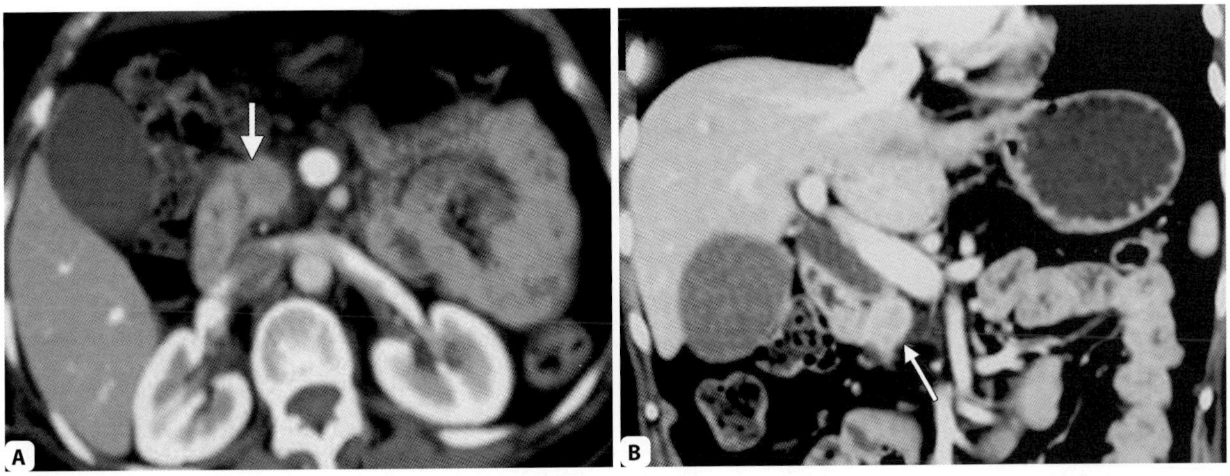

FIGS. 19A AND B: Resectable pancreatic cancer. Axial (A) and coronal contrast-enhanced computed tomography (CECT) images (B) shows small pancreatic head mass (arrows) with clearly maintained fat planes with superior mesenteric vessels.

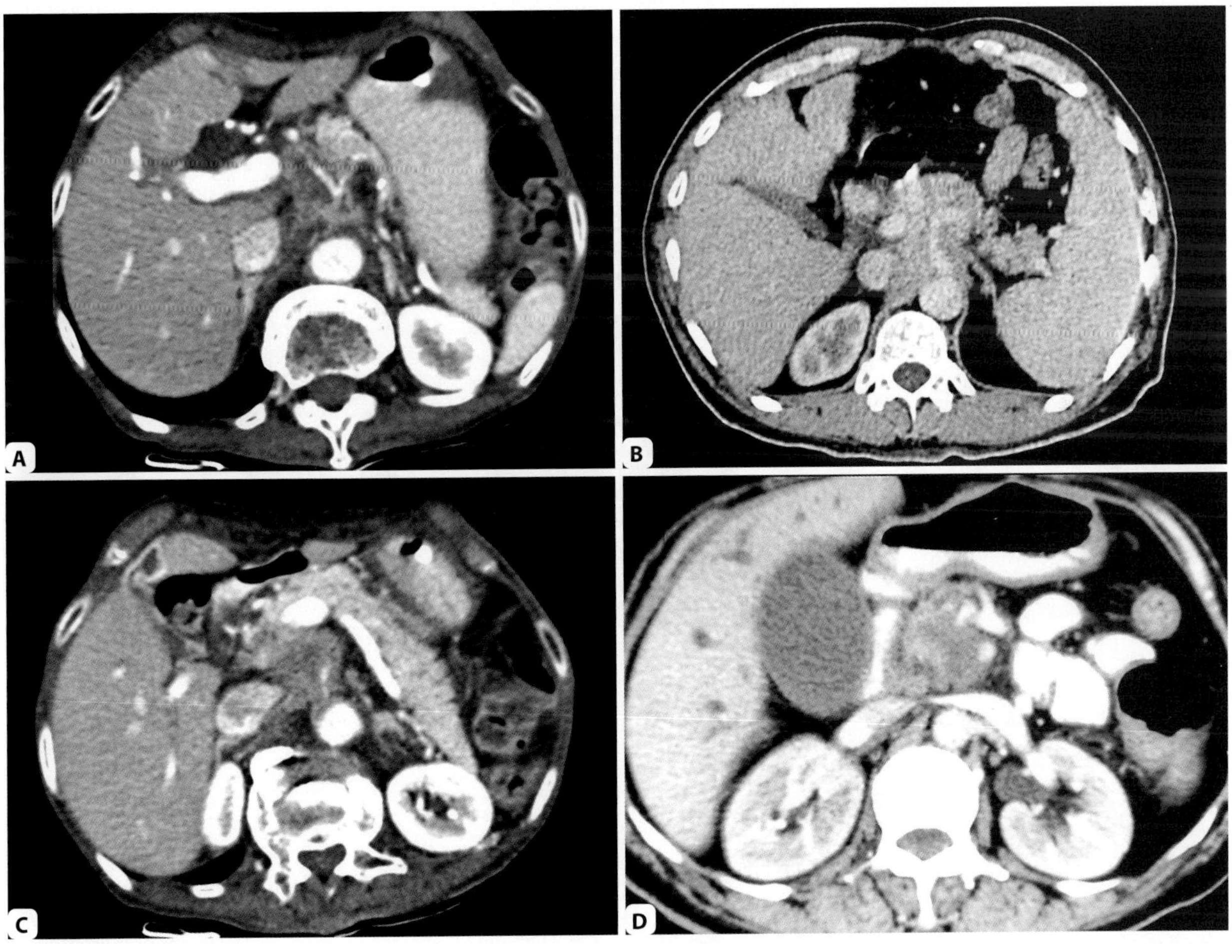

FIGS. 20A TO F: *Continued*

Continued

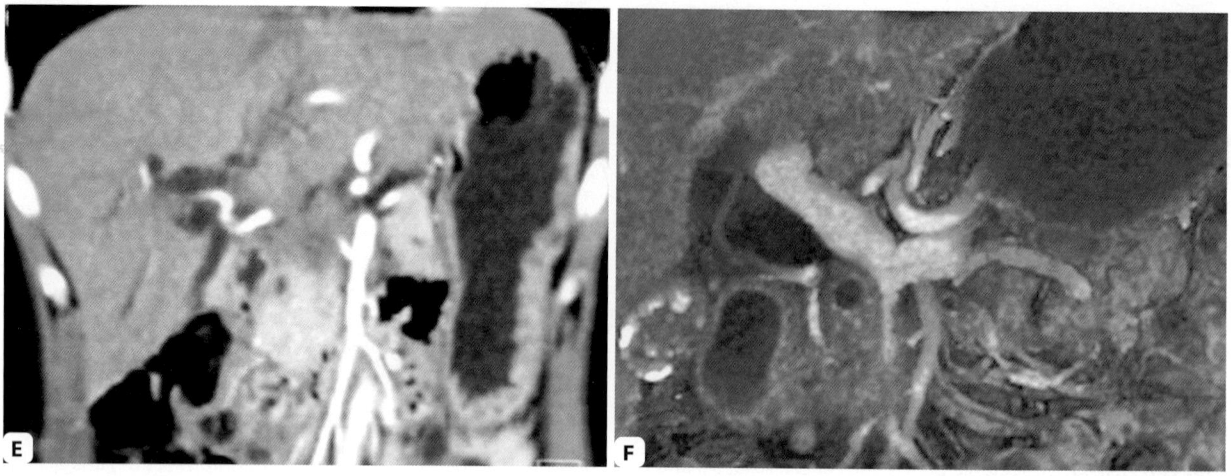

FIGS. 20A TO F: Unresectable (locally advanced) pancreatic cancer. Axial contrast-enhanced computed tomography (CECT) images depict encasement of celiac artery and common hepatic artery (A), encasement of celiac trunk and contact with aorta (B), encasement and irregular narrowing of superior mesenteric artery (SMA) (C) and encasement of both SMA and superior mesenteric vein (SMV) (D). Coronal CECT image, maximal intensity projection (MIP) in late arterial phase (E) depicts tumor encasement of replaced right hepatic artery (arising from SMA). Coronal MIP image generated from postcontrast MR images (F) shows encasement with irregularity of SMV with extension up to the jejunal branch, precluding surgical reconstruction.

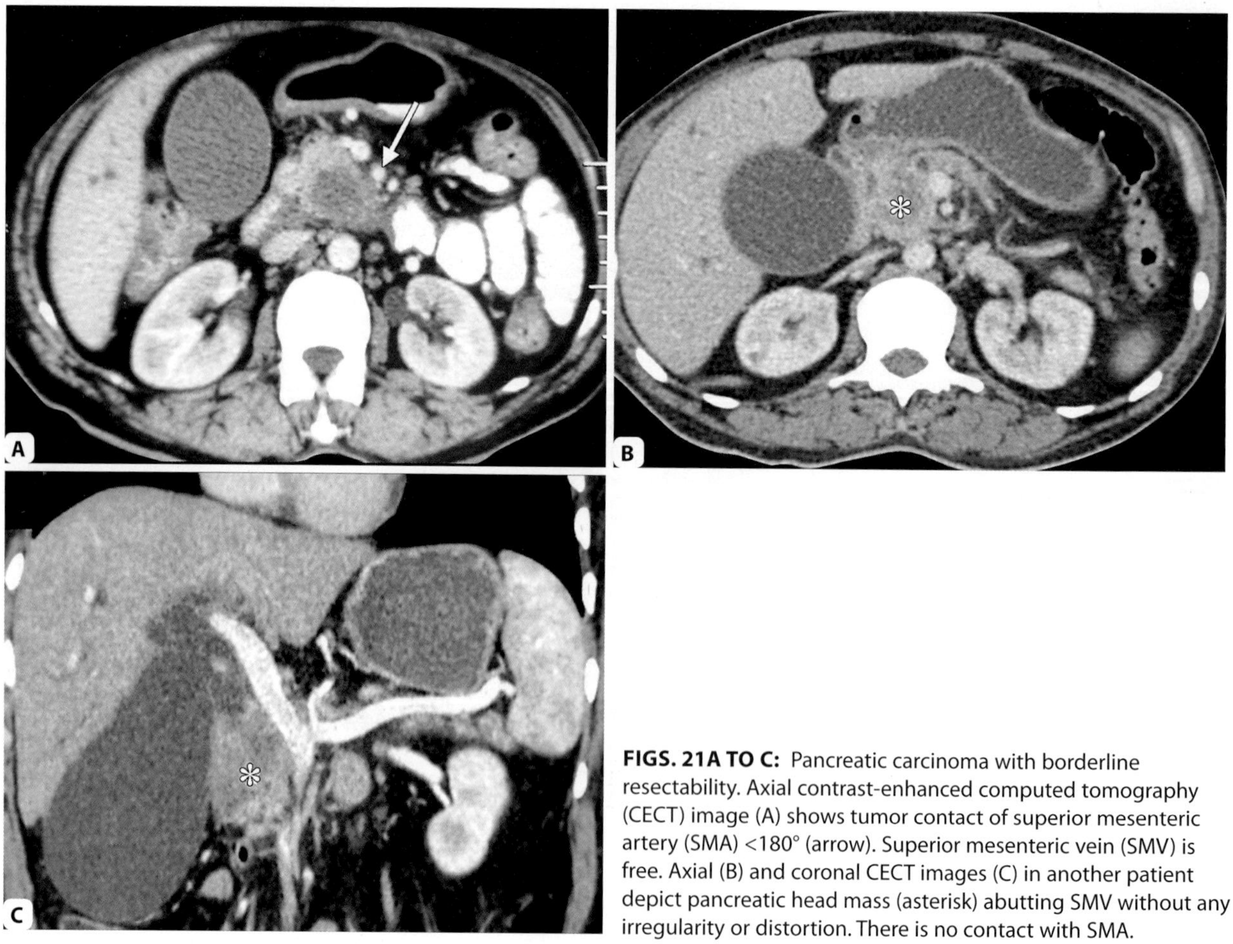

FIGS. 21A TO C: Pancreatic carcinoma with borderline resectability. Axial contrast-enhanced computed tomography (CECT) image (A) shows tumor contact of superior mesenteric artery (SMA) $<180°$ (arrow). Superior mesenteric vein (SMV) is free. Axial (B) and coronal CECT images (C) in another patient depict pancreatic head mass (asterisk) abutting SMV without any irregularity or distortion. There is no contact with SMA.

The borderline resectable group has been subdivided into three categories by the MD Anderson Cancer Center (MDACC) group. BR-A includes fulfillment of anatomic imaging criteria while BR-B includes presence of biomarkers for extrapancreatic disease (like elevated CA 19–9 ≥1,000 U/mL, biopsy-proven nodal metastases and indeterminate liver lesions). BR-C considers patient related comorbidities (Age >80 years and poor performance status) which preclude surgical resection.[42]

Identifying variant vascular anatomy is also important and should be conveyed to the surgeon. Tumor contact with variant vessels (replaced right hepatic artery from SMA, accessory right hepatic artery, replaced CHA, and the origin of replaced or accessory artery) can make resection/reconstruction difficult.[43]

Few authors have tried to correlate the appearance of venous contact of the tumor to the likelihood of successful R0 resection.[44-46] Latter is successful in those having smooth mass effect or unilateral focal mass effect with narrowing of SMV-PV. Patients with bilateral narrowing and circumferential encasement have high probability of positive surgical margins. Encasement of SMV leads to "tear-drop" shape of the vein and suggests unresectability **(Figs. 22A to D)**.[47] Dilated peripancreatic vessels has been suggested to indicate surrounding local invasion.[48]

Invasion of the mesenteric root and transverse mesocolon may complicate the surgical procedure or even completely preclude it. The involvement of first jejunal branches of SMA/SMV may suggest mesenteric root involvement and may occur in the tumors of the uncinate process. Transverse mesocolon involvement may entail additional hemicolectomy. This can be predicted on imaging based on the involvement of the gastrocolic trunk, formed by the confluence of middle colic vein and right gastroepiploic vein (anteriorly draining most proximal vein with respect to SMV).

Metastatic lymph nodes can be identified by size criteria (>1 cm in short axis), morphology (round shape), and/or presence of central hypodensity (necrosis). Unequivocal lymph node enlargement beyond the extent of Whipple resection (i.e., except CA) makes the mass unresectable. For lesions in the pancreatic head and

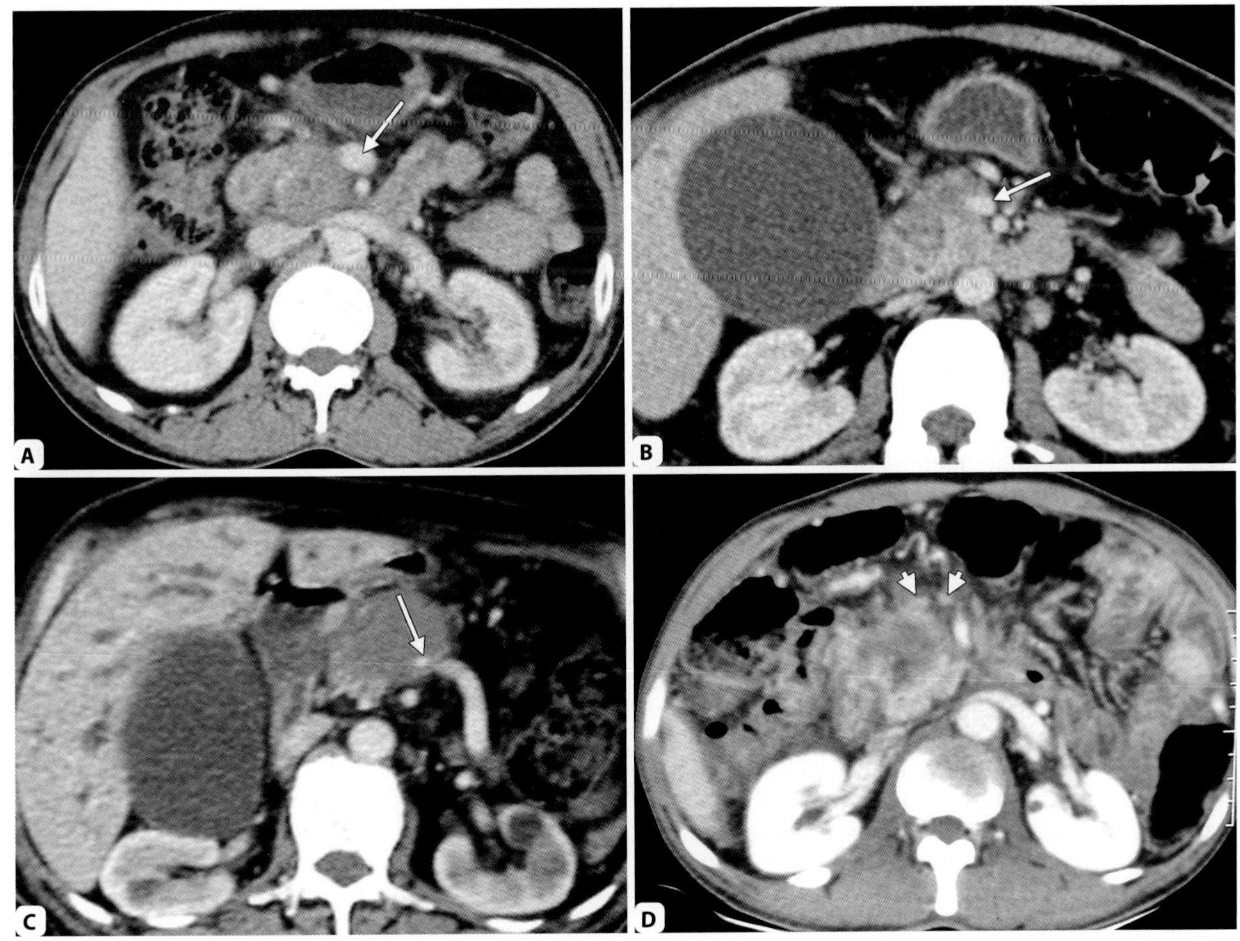

FIGS. 22A TO D: Spectrum of superior mesenteric vein (SMV) involvement in pancreatic carcinoma. Axial contrast-enhanced computed tomography (CECT) images show abutment of SMV (arrow) (A), encasement of SMV (arrow) with deformed contour (B), irregular narrowing of SMV (arrow) due to complete encasement (C), and nonvisualization of SMV (D) due to complete thrombosis and presence of collaterals (arrowheads).

neck, nodes along CA, peripancreatic, and periportal regions can be removed during surgery.[49] For body and tail cancers, nodes along CHA, celiac trunk, splenic vessels, and splenic hilum come in the operative field. If nodal involvement is confirmed at surgery, then adjuvant chemotherapy is indicated. Lymph nodes in the para-aortic location and to the left of SMA are nonregional and considered metastatic.

The overall accuracy of MDCT in predicting resectability of pancreatic cancer is 88–93%.[50] The problem areas include microscopic peritoneal implants and metastases to normal-sized lymph nodes.[51] Former are even more difficult to detect in the absence of ascites. Some centers routinely perform laparoscopy just prior to surgery to detect these peritoneal metastases. In cases of mismatch between surgery and imaging, metastases were found to be the most common cause of unresectability, rather than local invasion.[1] CT is very accurate in diagnosing unresectable disease (89–100% positive predictive value); however, accuracy is lower for predicting resectability (45–79%).[52]

Whipple procedure (pancreatoduodenectomy) or pylorus-preserving pancreatoduodenectomy is the surgical procedure done for pancreatic cancers of the head and uncinate. For body and tail lesions, a distal pancreatectomy with en bloc splenectomy is done. For tumors of the neck (anterior to SMV), either extended Whipple procedure (extending to left of SMV) or extended distal pancreatectomy (extending to the right of the SMV) may be done. In case lesion is found to be unresectable at surgery, then surgical biliary bypass (for alleviation of jaundice) and gastrojejunostomy are recommended, in addition to taking biopsies. Pancreatic body and tail ductal adenocarcinomas often have vascular invasion of the CA at the time of diagnosis. The modified Appleby procedure (distal pancreatectomy with en bloc splenectomy and CA resection) allows for tumor-free margin resection of such tumors. It relies on the presence of collateral arterial circulation via an intact pancreaticoduodenal arcade and the gastroduodenal artery to maintain hepatic and gastric arterial flow.[53] Celiac plexus neurolysis may also be considered for pain relief. Preoperative detection of celiac artery stenosis (due to median arcuate ligament or atherosclerosis) is important because it entails a postoperative risk of hepatic ischemia (due to ligation of the collaterals flow from SMA to CA branches).[54]

Certain features have been found to be associated with high risk of metastases in pancreatic cancer. These include large tumors, bulky nodes, indeterminate imaging findings, markedly elevated CA 19-9 (>100 units/mL), marked weight loss, and severe pain. In the absence of these features, resectable disease on imaging may be managed with upfront surgery or neoadjuvant therapy followed by surgery.

Perineural invasion is a hallmark of ductal adenocarcinomas, although it may be seen in ampullary cancers and cholangiocarcinoma as well.[55] Perineural invasion may be suggested on CT when there is direct soft-tissue infiltration along a known perineural pathway and has poor prognosis **(Figs. 23A to D)**. The most common route of spread is along the plexus pancreaticus capitalis for cancers of the pancreatic head and uncinate process.[56] Plexus pancreaticus capitalis 1 (posterior hepatic plexus) extends from the right celiac ganglion, courses behind the portal vein up to upper medial border of uncinate process.[56] This is involved in pancreatic head lesions. Plexus pancreaticus capitalis 2 extends from SMA plexus, courses along posteroinferior pancreaticoduodenal artery and jejunal trunk of SMV, reaching up to the uncinate process. This plexus is usually involved in cancers of the uncinate process. Anteriorly located tumors of the head region may infiltrate along gastroduodenal artery plexus (anterior pathway), extend to plexus of CHA and hepatoduodenal ligament, and reach the right celiac ganglion and SMA plexus **(Figs. 24A and B)**.[31] Literature regarding radiologic-pathologic correlates of perineural invasion is lacking but this has the potential to become an important criterion of unresectability.

The celiac plexus block is an interventional technique used to manage intractable abdominal pain due to pancreatic carcinoma which does not respond to oral analgesic medications. This block targets visceral afferent pain fibers from abdominal organs. Both anterior and posterior para-aortic approaches have been described. In the posterior approach, the patient is in a prone position. A 20–24G spinal needle is inserted bilaterally in CT guidance into the paravertebral fascia anterior to the aorta and diaphragmatic crura at T12-L1 level and posterior to the stomach. 7.5–15 mL of neurolytic (50–100% ethanol) is injected on each side.[57,58] The needle is flushed with 2–5 mL normal saline to prevent inadvertent retrograde tracking. Although a low-risk procedure, most patients (90%) experience a local back pain which usually lasts for <72 hours. Postprocedural diarrhea and transient hypotension which usually lasts for 2 days are also reported in about 50% patients due to unopposed parasympathetic activity.

Tumor node metastasis (TNM) staging system is not widely used since management depends on the resectability criteria as delineated above. However, it is used to assess the clinical prognosis and generate survival data.[40] The latest TNM staging system is shown in **Box 2** [American Joint Committee on Cancer (AJCC), 8th edition].

The EUS may also be helpful in suggesting vascular invasion. The features suggesting vascular invasion include loss of normally hyperechoic vessel wall, vessel irregularity/occlusion, and direct visualization of intravascular thrombus.[59]

SAMPLING

The EUS-guided fine-needle aspiration (FNA) or biopsy is preferred over CT/USG-guided percutaneous sampling because of better yield, lesser risk of bleeding/infection, and lower risk of peritoneal seeding. In addition, local staging

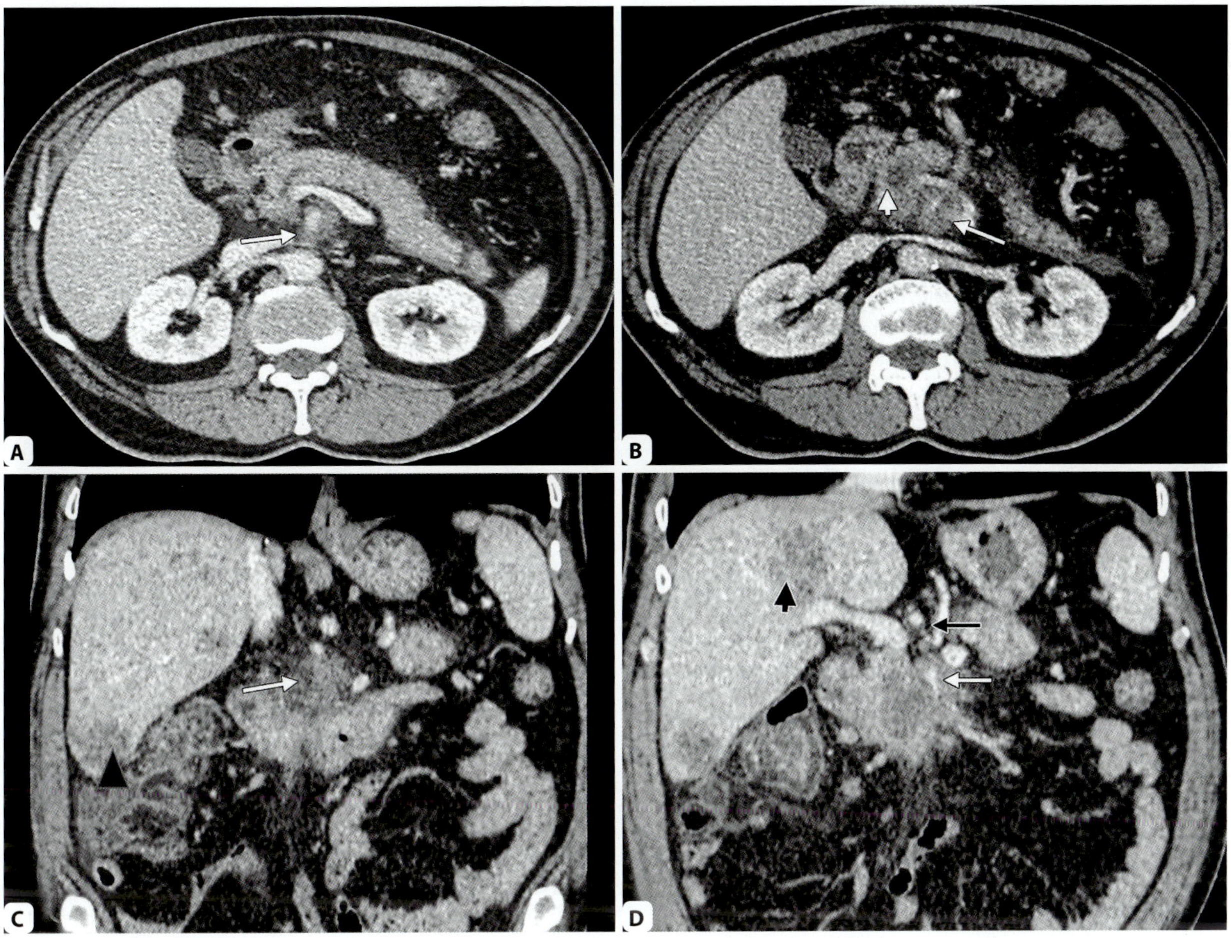

FIGS. 23A TO D: Perineural spread. Axial computed tomography (CT) venous phase image (A) shows ill-defined soft tissue encasement and spread along the superior mesenteric artery (white arrow). Axial CT image at a lower level (B) shows ill-defined hypoenhancing mass in the uncinate process of pancreas (white arrowhead) with complete encasement of the superior mesenteric artery (white arrow). (C and D) Coronal venous phase images show the perineural spread of pancreatic cancer along both superior mesenteric artery (white arrow) and celiac artery (black arrow). Note made of multiple hypoenhancing liver lesions (black arrowhead) suggestive of metastases.

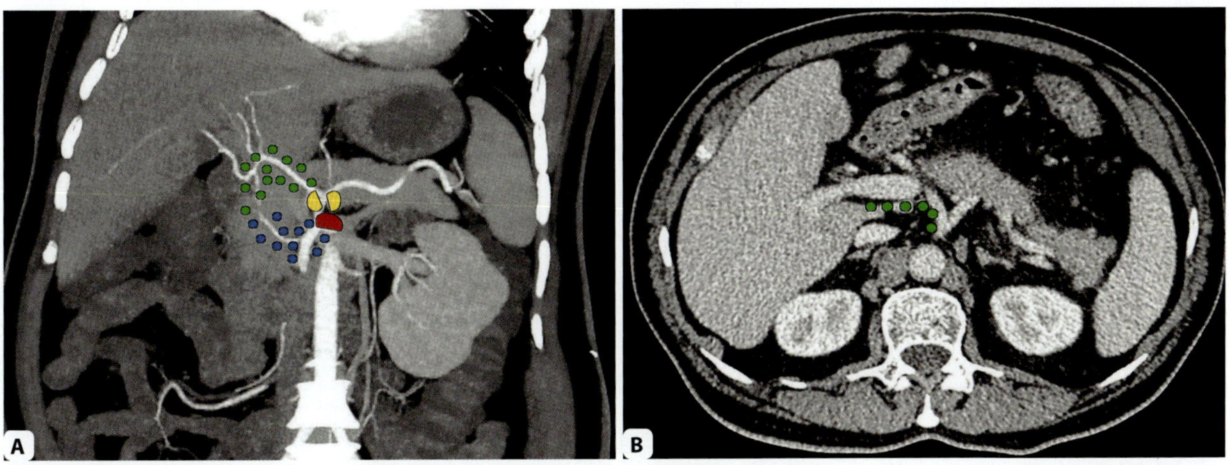

FIGS. 24A AND B: Schematic overlay of peripancreatic plexus on computed tomography (CT) images. CT angiography coronal maximal intensity projection (MIP) image (A) shows celiac ganglion (yellow hemisphere) and mesenteric ganglia (red hemisphere). The PPC1 (plexus pancreaticus capitalis 1) fibers run along the common hepatic artery and gastroduodenal artery into the medial margin of the head (green dots). The PPC-2 fibers run along the superior mesenteric artery and posterior inferior pancreaticoduodenal artery into the medial margin of the uncinate process (blue dots). Axial venous phase image (B) shows the perineural spread pathway of PPC-1 (green dots) which runs posterior to the main portal vein.

BOX 2 **TNM staging (AJCC, 8th edition) of pancreatic carcinoma.**

- *T-stage*:
  - TX: Primary tumor cannot be assessed
  - T0: No evidence of primary tumor
  - Tis: Carcinoma in situ. This includes high-grade pancreatic intraepithelial neoplasia, intraductal papillary mucinous neoplasm with high-grade dysplasia, intraductal tubulopapillary neoplasm with high-grade dysplasia, and mucinous cystic neoplasm with high-grade dysplasia
  - T1: Tumor is 2 cm or less in the greatest dimension
    - T1a: Tumor is ≤0.5 cm in greatest dimension
    - T1b: Tumor is >0.5 cm and <1 cm in greatest dimension
    - T1c: Tumor is 1–2 cm in greatest dimension
  - T2: Tumor is >2 cm and ≤4 cm in the greatest dimension
  - T3: Tumor is >4 cm in greatest dimension
  - T4: Tumor involves the celiac axis, superior mesenteric artery, and/or common hepatic artery, regardless of size
- *N-stage*:
  - Nx: Regional lymph nodes cannot be assessed
  - N0: No regional lymph node metastasis
  - N1: Metastasis in one to three regional lymph nodes
  - N2: Metastasis in four or more regional lymph nodes
- *M-stage*:
  - MX: Distant metastasis cannot be assessed
  - M0: No distant metastasis
  - M1: Distant metastasis
- *Stage 0*: Tis N0 M0
- *Stage IA*: T1 N0 M0
- *Stage IB*: T2 N0 M0
- *Stage IIA*: T3 N0 M0
- *Stage IIB*: T1–3 N1 M0
- *Stage III*: T1–3 N2 M0; T4 Any N M0
- *Stage IV*: Any T Any N M1

(AJCC: American Joint Committee on Cancer; TNM: tumor node metastasis)

can also be done using EUS at the same time **(Figs. 25A and B)**. When clinicoradiologic findings are typical, then biopsy proof is not mandatory, and an equivocal biopsy should not delay surgery in patients suspected to have pancreatic cancer. Nevertheless, tissue diagnosis is necessary before neoadjuvant therapy and in patients with locally advanced disease. In case of negative/equivocal results, one repeat biopsy is warranted. In case of metastatic disease, biopsy from the site of metastasis is recommended. Sampling of equivocal lymph nodes can also be done under EUS guidance. Staging laparoscopy may be beneficial in patients deemed resectable by CT but otherwise at increased risk for dissemination. The additional lesions (usually peritoneal metastases) detected on preoperative laparoscopy may alter the management in 4–15% patients.[60]

BIOMARKERS

Many tumor-associated antigens have been studied in connection with pancreatic adenocarcinoma including CEA, pancreatic anti-oncofetal antigen, tissue polypeptide antigen, CA 125, and CA 19-9. The most validated, studied, and the only Food and Drug Administration (FDA) approved biomarker is CA 19-9, but is nonspecific, being elevated in multiple hepatobiliary and pancreatic malignancies. It may also be elevated in biliary obstruction and infections. However, the degree of increase in CA 19-9 levels may be useful in differentiating pancreatic adenocarcinoma from inflammatory conditions of the pancreas. CA 19-9 has potential uses in diagnosis, in screening, in staging, and in determining resectability as a prognostic marker after resection and as a predictive marker for response to chemotherapy.[61]

Transcriptomic biomarker tissue inhibitor of metalloproteinase-1 (TIMP-1) has emerged as a novel biomarker with promising results and can be considered

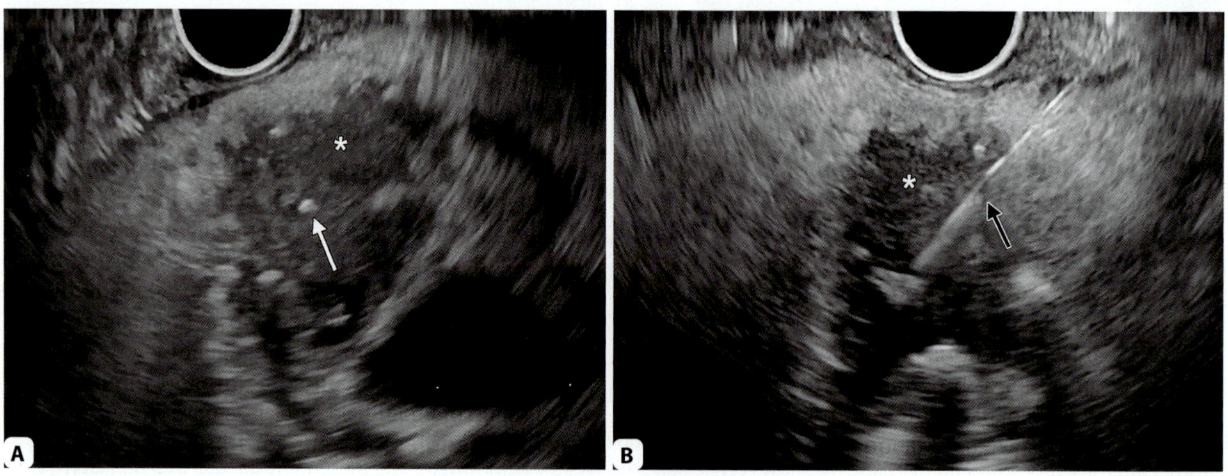

FIGS. 25A TO B: (A) Endoscopic ultrasound (EUS) spot shows an ill-defined hypoechoic mass (asterisk) in pancreatic head with few calcific foci (white arrow). (B) Shows EUS-guided biopsy (black arrow) of the same (asterisk denoting the mass).

as a part of the biomarker panel for PDAC. Another marker which can be used alongside in the biomarker panel is inflammatory protein leucine-rich alpha-2-glycoprotein 1 (LRG1). This combined panel exceeded the accuracy of CA 19-9 alone by over 10% in differentiating PDAC from benign pathologies and other cancers in recent meta-analyses. S100 calcium-binding protein P (S100P) is another biomarker with good results and currently under evaluation.[61] *K-Ras* gene mutations are common in patients with pancreatic carcinoma and are associated with poor prognosis.[62] Detection of K-Ras mutations in the peripheral blood may indicate tumor burden and serve as prognostic biomarker.[62] NCCN guidelines 2024 recommends a next-generation sequencing (NGS)-based array for evaluation of potentially actionable somatic findings including, fusions (ALK, NRG1, NTRK, ROS1, FGFR2, and RET), mutations (BRAF, BRCA1/2, KRAS, and PALB2), amplifications (HER2), microsatellite instability (MSI), mismatch repair deficiency (dMMR), or tumor mutational burden (TMB).

Texture analysis of CT and MR images can not only aid in the distinction between pancreatic cancer and its mimics, but also help to predict survival. Radiomic features of heterogeneity like entropy, gray-level co-occurrence matrix (GLCM) along with iodine density and diffusion parameters have been shown to have prognostic value.[63]

FOLLOW-UP IMAGING

Clinical follow-up is recommended every 3–6 months for the first 2 years after surgery and annually thereafter. CA 19-9 and CT can be done annually for detection of recurrence. For locally advanced or metastatic disease on treatment (chemotherapy and/radiotherapy), serial CT follow-up is advised. Routine portal venous phase acquisition is sufficient, unless surgery is contemplated; for which dedicated pancreatic protocol is required.[5] Conventionally, size of the target lesions has been the main criterion of response evaluation.[31] Whether the lesion has become resectable comes next.

Early detection of nonresponders (to chemotherapy and/radiotherapy) is the key research area, considering the cost and toxicity associated with these therapies. This becomes even more relevant because change in size takes considerable time. Functional imaging modalities like PET-CT, perfusion CT/MRI, and diffusion MRI may have a role in early response assessment. Treatment induces necrosis, and thus is expected to reduce the metabolic activity [indicated by standardized uptake values (SUVs)] on PET scan, reduce the perfusion parameters, and increase the ADC values on DW-MRI. However, differentiating post-treatment changes from viable tumor is difficult. This becomes even more challenging because treatment induces inflammatory changes which may mimic tumor infiltration on conventional imaging and also show increased metabolic uptake. DW-MRI and perfusion imaging may have a role in this scenario. Comparison with previous imaging is also of paramount importance in these cases.

Assessment of resectability postneoadjuvant therapy is difficult because post-treatment inflammation and fibrosis may mimic local vascular infiltration. Thus, the imaging accuracy decreases in detecting resectable disease.[49] This poses a practical problem in patients who receive neoadjuvant therapy after being diagnosed to have borderline resectable disease on initial CT. It has been found that radiological downstaging to resectable disease is rare (0.8%), though a significant proportion (66%) of such patients are actually found to have resectable disease at surgery.[64] Thus International Study Group of Pancreatic Surgery (ISGPS) recommends that in all patients with neoadjuvant therapy, exploratory laparotomy/diagnostic laparoscopy with attempted resection should be done, provided there is no progression on follow-up imaging.[65] Halo sign (thin hypodense periarterial rim without any solid tissue) has been described to be a predictor of pathological response in cases of arterial encasement who receive neoadjuvant therapy.[66] Thus, rather than recategorizing the lesion as resectable/borderline resectable/locally advanced, the report impression should comment on whether the disease has worsened/improved/is stable. Any reduction in tumor size (RECIST 1.1), tumor-vascular contact, and replacement of perivascular soft tissue with halo suggest response to treatment.

STRUCTURED REPORTING

Following a structured format for reporting pancreatic multiphasic CT examinations enables better evaluation of pancreatic cancer and optimal surgical planning.[67] Surgeons find it easier to understand the objective terms used in structured reporting format and are more likely to have all the information needed for surgical planning from these structured reports.[67] A sample structured reporting template for reporting suspected pancreatic malignancies is given in **Table 3**. The main problem with narrative reporting is that some of the key descriptors may be missing and the standardized lexicon may not be used, thus contributing to ambiguity in management.

ROLE OF ARTIFICIAL INTELLIGENCE

Artificial intelligence (AI) models have made significant progress in the recent past. They can be used in detection, segmentation, and classification of the pancreatic malignancies. To increase the patient's survivability in pancreatic adenocarcinoma, the main key is to detect the tumor at a resectable stage. For the same, AI models can be implemented using low-dose screening noncontrast CT or MRI in high-risk patients.[68] Analysis of the CT and MRI radiomics features with correlation of them with the presence of different genes or mutations will improve the management of the patients. Tailor made chemo-/radiotherapy can be devised for patients, especially for borderline cases.[68] With the pace of progress, we may see algorithms that will be implemented in clinical settings.

TABLE 3: Structured reporting format for suspected pancreatic malignancy.

Pancreatic lesion present: Y/N	• Location—head/neck/body/tail • Size • Enhancement relative to pancreas (in pancreatic phase)—hypo/iso/hyper • Miscellaneous—necrosis/calcification/none • Contour bulge—yes/no • Confined to pancreas with clear fat planes—yes/no • PD dilatation—yes with atrophy/yes without atrophy/no • Biliary dilatation—yes/no • GB status • Diagnosis—adenocarcinoma/others (specify differentials)
Status of arteries	• Arterial contact—yes/no • Focal narrowing or contour irregularities • Celiac axis—no contact/abutment/encasement • CHA—no contact/abutment/encasement • Surgically reconstructible—yes/no • SMA—no contact/abutment/ encasement • Surgically reconstructible—yes/no • Contact with first jejunal branch of SMA—yes/no • Aorta—involved/free • Variant arterial anatomy with tumor contact—yes/no • Significant atherosclerosis/narrowing at origin of celiac axis/SMA—yes/no
Status of veins	• Venous contact—yes/no • Focal narrowing or contour irregularities • SMV—no contact/abutment/encasement • Surgically reconstructible—yes/no • MPV—no contact/abutment/encasement • Surgically reconstructible—yes/no • Length of venous involvement • Thrombus within the vein (tumor or bland) • Contact with IVC—yes/no • Venous collaterals—yes/no; location—around pancreatic head/porta hepatis/root of mesentery
• Adjacent structure infiltration • Adenopathy—yes/no (site) • Metastases—yes/no (liver/peritoneal/others—specify) • Ascites—yes/no	
Advise: Endoscopic ultrasound (EUS) +/– sampling/MRI	

(CHA: common hepatic artery; GB: gallbladder; IVC: inferior vena cava; MPV: main portal vein; PD: pancreatic duct; SMA: superior mesenteric artery; SMV: superior mesenteric vein)

CONCLUSION

Early detection, accurate characterization, and staging are essential for optimal management of pancreatic cancer, and imaging plays a crucial role. Sonography is frequently performed as the first investigation for evaluation of these patients. Both MDCT and MRI perform equally well in the detection and staging of pancreatic malignancies with CT being the most validated modality owing to faster acquisition and high spatial resolution. MRI is equally accurate and may have an edge in case of smaller lesions, demonstrating relationship with ducts and in cases where intravenous contrast cannot be given. DW-MRI is very sensitive in detection of liver metastases. EUS provides limited but detailed information and plays a role in image-guided sampling. **Flowchart 2** shows imaging and management algorithm in a patient suspected to have pancreatic malignancy. Structured reporting improves evaluation and provides accurate assessment of the status of vessels and better communication with the surgeon.

The National Comprehensive Cancer Network panel recommends that all diagnostic and surgical management decisions must involve multidisciplinary consultations in high-volume centers. Imaging also plays a role in post-therapy response assessment and this is the field of active research, especially on newer and functional imaging modalities.

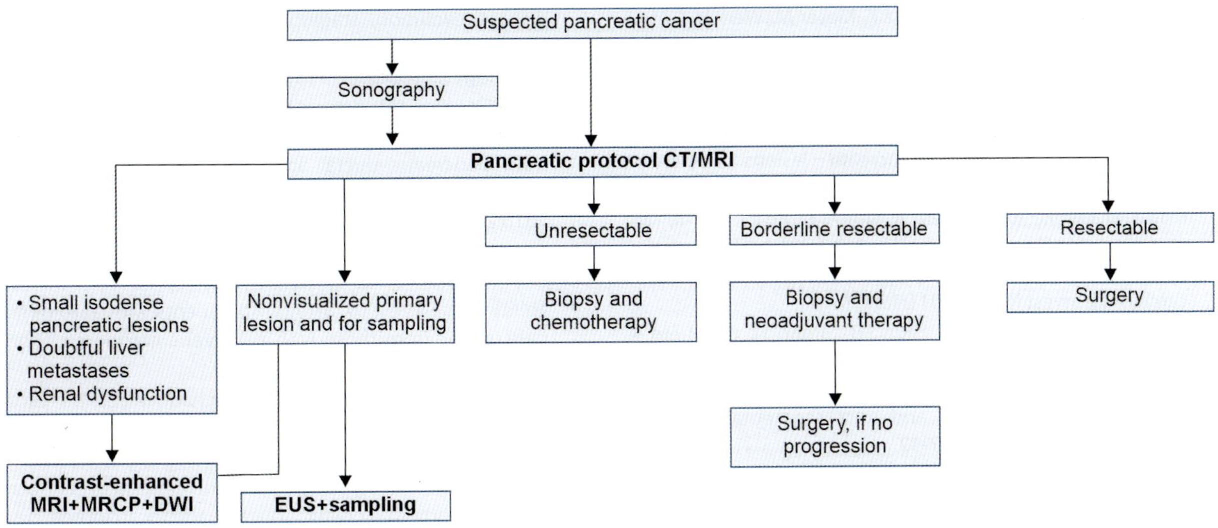

FLOWCHART 2: Imaging and management protocol in a patient suspected to have pancreatic malignancy.
(DWI: diffusion-weighted imaging; EUS: endoscopic ultrasound; MRCP: magnetic resonance cholangiopancreatography)

REFERENCES

1. Tamm EP, Balachandran A, Bhosale PR, Katz MH, Fleming JB, Lee JH, et al. Imaging of pancreatic adenocarcinoma: update on staging/resectability. Radiol Clin North Am. 2012;50(3):407-28.
2. Franck C, Müller C, Rosania R, Croner RS, Pech M, Venerito M. Advanced Pancreatic Ductal Adenocarcinoma: Moving Forward. Cancers (Basel). 2020;12(7):1955.
3. Luchini C, Grillo F, Fassan M, Vanoli A, Capelli P, Paolino G, et al. Malignant epithelial/exocrine tumors of the pancreas. Pathologica. 2020;112(3):210-26.
4. Jeffrey RB. Pancreatic cancer: radiologic imaging. Gastroenterol Clin North Am. 2012;41(1):159-77.
5. NCCN. (2024). NCCN Clinical Practice Guidelines in Oncology. Pancreatic Adenocarcinoma. Version 2.2024. [online] Available from https://www.nccn.org/guidelines/category_1 [Last accessed July, 2024].
6. Allema JH, Reinders ME, van Gulik TM, van Leeuwen DJ, Verbeek PC, de Wit LT, et al. Results of pancreaticoduodenectomy for ampullary carcinoma and analysis of prognostic factors for survival. Surgery. 1995;117(3):247-53.
7. Goonetilleke KS, Siriwardena AK. Systematic review of carbohydrate antigen (CA 19-9) as a biochemical marker in the diagnosis of pancreatic cancer. Eur J Surg Oncol. 2007;33:266.
8. Maithel SK, Maloney S, Winston C, Gönen M, D'Angelica MI, Dematteo RP, et al. Preoperative CA 19-9 and the yield of staging laparoscopy in patients with radiographically resectable pancreatic adenocarcinoma. Ann Surg Oncol. 2008;15:3512-20.
9. Almoguera C, Shibata D, Forrester K, Martin J, Arnheim N, Perucho M. Most human carcinomas of the exocrine pancreas contain mutant c-K-ras genes. Cell. 1988;53(4):549-54.
10. Brook OR, Gourtsoyianni S, Brook A, Siewert B, Kent T, Raptopoulos V. Split-bolus spectral multidetector CT of the pancreas: assessment of radiation dose and tumor conspicuity. Radiology. 2013;269(1):139-48.
11. Kaneko OF, Lee DM, Wong J, Kadell BM, Reber HA, Lu DSK, et al. Performance of multidetector computed tomographic angiography in determining surgical resectability of pancreatic head adenocarcinoma. J Comput Assist Tomogr. 2010;34(5):732-8.
12. Schima W, Ba-Ssalamah A, Goetzinger P, Scharitzer M, Koelblinger C. State-of-the-art magnetic resonance imaging of pancreatic cancer. Top Magn Reson Imaging. 2007;18(6):421-9.
13. Kartalis N, Manikis GC, Loizou L, Albiin N, Zöllner FG, Del Chiaro M, et al. Diffusion-weighted MR imaging of pancreatic cancer: A comparison of mono-exponential, bi-exponential and non-Gaussian kurtosis models. Eur J Radiol Open. 2016;3:79-85.
14. Canto MI, Hruban RH, Fishman EK, Kamel IR, Schulick R, Zhang Z, et al. Frequent detection of pancreatic lesions in asymptomatic high-risk individuals. Gastroenterology. 2012;142(04):796-804; quiz e14-e15.
15. Kawada N, Tanaka S. Elastography for the pancreas: Current status and future perspective. World J Gastroenterol. 2016;22(14):3712-24.
16. Iglesias-Garcia J, Larino-Noia J, Abdulkader I, Forteza J, Dominguez-Munoz JE. EUS elastography for the characterization of solid pancreatic masses. Gastrointest Endosc. 2009;70(6):1101-8.
17. Gonçalves B, Soares JB, Bastos P. Endoscopic Ultrasound in the diagnosis and staging of pancreatic cancer. GE Port J Gastroenterol. 2015;22(4):161-71.
18. Klauss M, Stiller W, Fritz F, Kieser M, Werner J, Kauczor HU, et al. Computed tomography perfusion analysis of pancreatic carcinoma. J Comput Assist Tomogr. 2012;36(2):237-42.
19. Yadav AK, Sharma R, Kandasamy D, Pradhan RK, Garg PK, Bhalla AS, et al. Perfusion CT—Can it resolve the pancreatic carcinoma versus mass forming chronic pancreatitis conundrum? Pancreatology. 2016;16(6):979-87.

20. Klauss M, Stiller W, Pahn G, Fritz F, Kieser M, Werner J, et al. Dual-energy perfusion-CT of pancreatic adenocarcinoma. Eur J Radiol. 2013;82(2):208-14.
21. Kang KM, Lee JM, Yoon JH, Kiefer B, Han JK, Choi BI. Intravoxel incoherent motion diffusion-weighted MR Imaging for characterization of focal pancreatic lesions. Radiology. 2013;270(2):444-53.
22. Klauss M, Lemke A, Grünberg K, Simon D, Re TJ, Wente MN, et al. Intravoxel incoherent motion MRI for the differentiation between mass forming chronic pancreatitis and pancreatic carcinoma. Invest Radiol. 2011;46(1):57-63.
23. Re TJ, Lemke A, Klauss M, Laun FB, Simon D, Grünberg K, et al. Enhancing pancreatic adenocarcinoma delineation in diffusion derived intravoxel incoherent motion f-maps through automatic vessel and duct segmentation. Magn Reson Med. 2011;66(5):1327-32.
24. Kim JH, Park SH, Yu ES, Kim MH, Kim J, Byun JH, et al. Visually isoattenuating pancreatic adenocarcinoma at dynamic-enhanced CT: frequency, clinical and pathologic characteristics, and diagnosis at imaging examinations. Radiology. 2010;257(1):87-96.
25. Prokesch RW, Chow LC, Beaulieu CF, Bammer R, Jeffrey RB. Isoattenuating pancreatic adenocarcinoma at multi-detector row CT: secondary signs. Radiology. 2002;224(3):764-8.
26. Miller FH, Vendrami CL, Hammond NA, Mittal PK, Nikolaidis P, Jawahar A. Pancreatic Cancer and Its Mimics. Radiographics. 2023;43(11):e230054.
27. Park MJ, Kim YK, Choi S, Rhim H, Lee WJ, Choi D. Preoperative detection of small pancreatic carcinoma: value of adding diffusion-weighted imaging to conventional MR imaging for improving confidence level. Radiology. 2014;273(2):433-43.
28. Goodman M, Willmann JK, Jeffrey RB. Incidentally discovered solid pancreatic masses: imaging and clinical observations. Abdom Imaging. 2012;37(1):91-7.
29. Shanbhogue AKP, Fasih N, Surabhi VR, Doherty GP, Shanbhogue DKP, Sethi SK. A clinical and radiologic review of uncommon types and causes of pancreatitis. Radiographics. 2009;29(4):1003-26.
30. Toshima F, Watanabe R, Inoue D, Yoneda N, Yamamoto T, Sasahira N, et al. CT abnormalities of the pancreas associated with the subsequent diagnosis of clinical stage I pancreatic ductal adenocarcinoma more than 1 year later: a case-control study. AJR Am J Roentgenol. 2021;217(6):1353-64.
31. Sharma R, Kandasamy D. Imaging of pancreatic cancer. In: Garg PK (Ed). ECAB Clinical Update—Pancreatic Tumors. Gurugram: Elsevier India; 2014.
32. Lee H, Lee JK, Kang SS, Choi D, Jang KT, Kim JH, et al. Is there any clinical or radiologic feature as a preoperative marker for differentiating mass-forming pancreatitis from early-stage pancreatic adenocarcinoma? Hepatogastroenterology. 2007;54(79):2134-40.
33. Ichikawa T, Sou H, Araki T, Arbab AS, Yoshikawa T, Ishigame K, et al. Duct-penetrating sign at MRCP: usefulness for differentiating inflammatory pancreatic mass from pancreatic carcinomas. Radiology. 2001;221(1):107-16.
34. Coakley FV, Hanley-Knutson K, Mongan J, Barajas R, Bucknor M, Qayyum A. Pancreatic imaging mimics: Part 1, imaging mimics of pancreatic adenocarcinoma. AJR. 2012;199(2):301-8.
35. Sahani DV, Sainani NI, Deshpande V, Shaikh MS, Frinkelberg DL, Fernandez-del Castillo C. Autoimmune pancreatitis: disease evolution, staging, response assessment, and CT features that predict response to corticosteroid therapy. Radiology. 2009;250(1):118-29.
36. Choi SY, Kim SH, Kang TW, Song KD, Park HJ, Choi YH. Differentiating mass-forming autoimmune pancreatitis from pancreatic ductal adenocarcinoma on the basis of contrast-enhanced MRI and DWI findings. Am J Roentgenol. 2016;206(2):291-300.
37. van Heerde MJ, Buijs J, Hansen BE, de Waart M, van Eijck CH, Kazemier G, et al. Serum level of Ca 19-9 increases ability of IgG4 test to distinguish patients with autoimmune pancreatitis from those with pancreatic carcinoma. Dig Dis Sci. 2014;59:1322-9.
38. Blasbalg R, Baroni RH, Costa DN, Machado MCC. MRI features of groove pancreatitis. AJR. 2007;189(1):73-80.
39. Ren S, Chen X, Wang Z, Zhao R, Wang J, Cui W, Wang Z. Differentiation of hypovascular pancreatic neuroendocrine tumors from pancreatic ductal adenocarcinoma using contrast-enhanced computed tomography. PLoS One. 2019;14(2):e0211566.
40. Al-Hawary MM, Francis IR, Chari ST, Fishman EK, Hough DM, Lu DS, et al. Pancreatic ductal adenocarcinoma radiology reporting template: consensus statement of the Society of Abdominal Radiology and the American Pancreatic Association. Radiology. 2014;270(1):248-60.
41. Callery MP, Chang KJ, Fishman EK, Talamonti MS, William Traverso L, Linehan DC. Pretreatment assessment of resectable and borderline resectable pancreatic cancer: expert consensus statement. Ann Surg Oncol. 2009;16(7):1727-33.
42. Denbo JW, Fleming JB. Definition and management of borderline resectable pancreatic cancer. Surg Clin North Am. 2016;96:1337-50.
43. Lall CG, Howard TJ, Skandarajah A, DeWitt JM, Aisen AM, Sandrasegaran K. New concepts in staging and treatment of locally advanced pancreatic head cancer. AJR. 2007;189(5):1044-50.
44. Ishikawa O, Ohigashi H, Imaoka S, Furukawa H, Sasaki Y, Fujita M, et al. Preoperative indications for extended pancreatectomy for locally advanced pancreas cancer involving the portal vein. Ann Surg. 1992;215(3):231-6.
45. Raptopoulos V, Steer ML, Sheiman RG, Vrachliotis TG, Gougoutas CA, Movson JS. The use of helical CT and CT angiography to predict vascular involvement from pancreatic cancer: correlation with findings at surgery. AJR. 1997;168(4):971-7.
46. Chun YS, Milestone BN, Watson JC, Cohen SJ, Burtness B, Engstrom PF, et al. Defining venous involvement in borderline resectable pancreatic cancer. Ann Surg Oncol. 2010;17(11):2832-8.
47. Hough TJ, Raptopoulos V, Siewert B, Matthews JB. Teardrop superior mesenteric vein: CT sign for unresectable carcinoma of the pancreas. AJR. 1999;173(6):1509-12.
48. McNulty NJ, Francis IR, Platt JF, Cohan RH, Korobkin M, Gebremariam A. Multidetector row helical CT of the pancreas: effect of contrast-enhanced multiphasic imaging on enhancement of the pancreas, peripancreatic vasculature, and pancreatic adenocarcinoma. Radiology. 2001;220(1):97-102.
49. Pietryga JA, Morgan DE. Imaging preoperatively for pancreatic adenocarcinoma. J Gastrointest Oncol. 2015;6(4):343-57.

50. Li H, Zeng MS, Zhou KR, Jin DY, Lou WH. Pancreatic adenocarcinoma: the different CT criteria for peripancreatic major arterial and venous invasion. J Comput Assist Tomogr. 2005;29(2):170-5.
51. Sai M, Mori H, Kiyonaga M, Kosen K, Yamada Y, Matsumoto S. Peripancreatic lymphatic invasion by pancreatic carcinoma: evaluation with multidetector row CT. Abdom Imaging. 2010;35(2):154-62.
52. Brennan DDD, Zamboni GA, Raptopoulos VD, Kruskal JB. Comprehensive preoperative assessment of pancreatic adenocarcinoma with 64-section volumetric CT. Radiogr Rev Publ Radiol Soc N Am Inc. 2007;27(6):1653-66.
53. Latona JA, Lamb KM, Pucci MJ, Maley WR, Yeo CJ. Modified Appleby Procedure with Arterial Reconstruction for Locally Advanced Pancreatic Adenocarcinoma: A Literature Review and Report of Three Unusual Cases. J Gastrointest Surg. 2016;20(2):300-6.
54. Elbanna KY, Jang HJ, Kim TK. Imaging diagnosis and staging of pancreatic ductal adenocarcinoma: a comprehensive review. Insights Imaging. 2020;11(1):58.
55. Makino I, Kitagawa H, Ohta T, Nakagawara H, Tajima H, Ohnishi I, et al. Nerve plexus invasion in pancreatic cancer: spread patterns on histopathologic and embryological analyses. Pancreas. 2008;37(4):358-65.
56. Deshmukh SD, Willmann JK, Jeffrey RB. Pathways of extrapancreatic perineural invasion by pancreatic adenocarcinoma: evaluation with 3D volume-rendered MDCT imaging. AJR Am J Roentgenol. 2010;194(3):668-74.
57. John RS, Dixon B, Hendrix JM, Shienbaum R. Celiac Plexus Block. In: StatPearls [Internet]. Treasure Island (FL): StatPearls Publishing; 2024.
58. Cornman-Homonoff J, Holzwanger DJ, Lee KS, Madoff DC, Li D. Celiac Plexus Block and Neurolysis in the Management of Chronic Upper Abdominal Pain. Semin Intervent Radiol. 2017;34(4):376-86.
59. Yusoff IF, Mendelson RM, Edmunds SEJ, Ramsay D, Cullingford GL, Fletcher DR, et al. Preoperative assessment of pancreatic malignancy using endoscopic ultrasound. Abdom Imaging. 2003;28(4):556-62.
60. Pisters PW, Lee JE, Vauthey JN, Charnsangavej C, Evans DB. Laparoscopy in the staging of pancreatic cancer. Br J Surg. 2001;88(3):325-37.
61. Kane LE, Mellotte GS, Mylod E, O'Brien RM, O'Connell F, Buckley CE, et al. Diagnostic Accuracy of Blood-based Biomarkers for Pancreatic Cancer: A Systematic Review and Meta-analysis. Cancer Res Commun. 2022;2(10):1229-43.
62. Tao L, Zhang L, Xiu D, Yuan C, Ma Z, Jiang B. Prognostic significance of K-ras mutations in pancreatic cancer: a meta-analysis. World J Surg Oncol. 2016;14:146.
63. Koch V, Weitzer N, Dos Santos DP, Gruenewald LD, Mahmoudi S, Martin SS, et al. Multiparametric detection and outcome prediction of pancreatic cancer involving dual-energy CT, diffusion-weighted MRI, and radiomics. Cancer Imaging. 2023;23(1):38.
64. Katz MHG, Fleming JB, Bhosale P, Varadhachary G, Lee JE, Wolff R, et al. Response of borderline resectable pancreatic cancer to neoadjuvant therapy is not reflected by radiographic indicators. Cancer. 2012;118(23):5749-56.
65. Bockhorn M, Uzunoglu FG, Adham M, Imrie C, Milicevic M, Sandberg AA, et al. Borderline resectable pancreatic cancer: a consensus statement by the International Study Group of Pancreatic Surgery (ISGPS). Surgery. 2014;155(6):977-88.
66. Soloff EV, Al-Hawary MM, Desser TS, Fishman EK, Minter RM, Zins M. Imaging Assessment of Pancreatic Cancer Resectability After Neoadjuvant Therapy: AJR Expert Panel Narrative Review. AJR Am J Roentgenol. 2022;218(4):570-81.
67. Brook OR, Brook A, Vollmer CM, Kent TS, Sanchez N, Pedrosa I. Structured reporting of multiphasic CT for pancreatic cancer: potential effect on staging and surgical planning. Radiology. 2015;274(2):464-72.
68. Anghel C, Grasu MC, Anghel DA, Rusu-Munteanu GI, Dumitru RL, Lupescu IG. Pancreatic Adenocarcinoma: Imaging Modalities and the Role of Artificial Intelligence in Analyzing CT and MRI Images. Diagnostics (Basel). 2024;14(4):438.

CHAPTER 21

Jyoti Kumar, Alpana Manchanda, Swati Gupta

Cystic Pancreatic Tumors and Neuroendocrine Tumors of Pancreas

CYSTIC PANCREATIC TUMORS

INTRODUCTION

Cystic pancreatic tumors are a diverse group of lesions with varied clinical presentation, histology, biologic behavior, and prognostic implications. Imaging plays a key role in stratifying the risk in these patients, and hence, deciding on the treatment options and appropriate follow-up strategy. The increasing use of cross-sectional imaging techniques and their improved resolution have led to a marked increase in the incidental detection of these lesions, which has in turn led to an increase in surgery for these tumors. In many instances, these resected lesions turn out to be benign and the surgery is not justifiable. Hence, the distinction between these lesions of varying malignant potential is essential.[1] Many societies have developed guidelines for diagnosis and surveillance, which are continuously evolving to accommodate emerging medical evidence. The concept of field defect, whereby pancreatic adenocarcinoma develops at a site different from the site of the pancreatic cystic tumor, necessitates a broader approach to surveillance, even in the absence of concerning features within the cyst itself.[2] Imaging plays a key role in detection and characterization of these lesions as well as in follow-up and surveillance.

IMAGING MODALITIES

Both multidetector computed tomography (MDCT) and magnetic resonance imaging (MRI) are widely used in characterizing the cystic lesions of pancreas. Pancreatic protocol MDCT offers high spatial and temporal resolution. Its wide availability and ease of interpretation are the other advantages. CT also shows calcification within lesions to a greater advantage. In various studies, the accuracy of MDCT (56–85%) has been found to be comparable to MRI in characterizing cystic pancreatic lesions.[3]

Magnetic resonance imaging (MRI), on the other hand, has superior soft tissue and contrast resolution. Hence, it is an excellent technique to assess internal morphological features of cystic tumors (enhancing mural nodule/internal septations), especially small cystic tumors measuring <3 cm.[4] Three-dimensional magnetic resonance cholangiopancreaticography (MRCP) is an effective tool in detecting communication of the lesion with the pancreatic duct. Sainini et al. showed a higher accuracy of MR in revealing ductal communication as compared to CT (100% vs. 75% sensitivity).[4] Secretin-enhanced MRCP improves the distention and visibility of pancreatic duct and can aid the visualization of this communication. However, its high cost remains prohibitive.[3] As MR does not involve radiation, it is the preferred modality for follow-up of patients with cystic pancreatic tumors.[5]

Endoscopic ultrasound (EUS) is used as an adjunct when there are clinical or imaging features of concern. It is an excellent technique to depict internal morphology of cystic lesions, showing internal septations and nodularity to a greater advantage, and hence assessing the aggressiveness of the pathology. Contrast-enhanced EUS can aid in distinguishing mural nodules from mucin clots. EUS also enables fluid aspiration for cytopathological examination, detection of extracellular mucin and analysis of biochemical and genetic markers.[6] EUS-guided tissue acquisition using micro forceps is an investigational technique for obtaining samples from the cyst wall/mural nodule for histopathology.[3] The limitations of EUS include its invasive nature, operator dependance, and limited evaluation of the pancreatic tail.

CLINICAL PRESENTATION

Many pancreatic cystic tumors are picked up incidentally during work-up for other nonrelated conditions.[6] Symptomatic cystic tumors mostly present with abdominal lump and pain. Pancreatitis may result from pancreatic ductal obstruction. Jaundice, weight loss, and diabetes may be seen in patients with malignant lesions.[1,6]

CLASSIFICATION

Although cystic tumors of pancreas are uncommon tumors of pancreas, they may be classified into 'relatively common' tumors and 'rare' tumors **(Box 1)**. The relatively common cystic tumors include serous cystadenoma (SCA), mucinous cystic neoplasm (MCN), intraductal papillary mucinous neoplasm (IPMN), and solid pseudopapillary neoplasm (SPN). The rare cystic tumors include cystic teratoma, cystic paraganglioma, cystic pancreatic neuroendocrine tumor (PNET), cystic ductal adenocarcinoma, acinar cell cystic neoplasm (ACCN), cystic hamartoma, and cystic pancreatoblastoma.

BOX 1 Classification of cystic pancreatic tumors.

`Relatively common' cystic tumors:
- Serous cystadenoma (SCA)
- Mucinous neoplasms:
  - Mucinous cystic neoplasm (MCN)
  - Intraductal papillary mucinous neoplasm (IPMN)
    - Main duct intraductal papillary mucinous neoplasm (MD-IPMN)
    - Branch duct intraductal papillary mucinous neoplasm (BD-IPMN)
    - Mixed type
- Solid pseudopapillary neoplasm (SPN)

Rare cystic tumors:
- Cystic teratoma
- Cystic paraganglioma
- Cystic pancreatic neuroendocrine tumor (PNET)
- Cystic ductal adenocarcinoma
- Acinar cell cystic neoplasm (ACCN)
- Cystic hamartoma
- Cystic pancreatoblastoma

Morphological Classification

On the basis of imaging morphology, pancreatic cystic lesions may be unilocular in appearance, microcystic, macrocystic, or cysts with solid component. In addition, there may be communication with the main pancreatic duct (MPD) **(Figs. 1A to F) (Box 2)**.

- Unilocular cysts include cysts with no internal septation, calcification, or nodularity. Although inflammatory pseudocysts are the prototype example, cystic tumors that may uncommonly have a unilocular appearance are MCNs and SCAs. Since pseudocysts are the most common cystic lesions of pancreas, correlation with history of acute or chronic pancreatitis is of paramount importance.
- Microcystic lesions are cysts with internal septations resulting in formation of mutiple tiny cysts which are usually >6 in number and <2 cm in size. The main example of a microcystic lesion is SCA.
- Macrocystic (oligocystic) lesions are multilocular cysts with fewer loculi (<6) which are larger in size (>2 cm). The characteristic examples of macrocystic lesions are MCNs and BD-IPMNs.

BOX 2 Morphological classification of cystic pancreatic tumors.

- Unilocular
- Microcystic
- Macrocystic
- Cystic lesions with solid component
- Cysts communicating with the main pancreatic duct
- Dilated main pancreatic duct

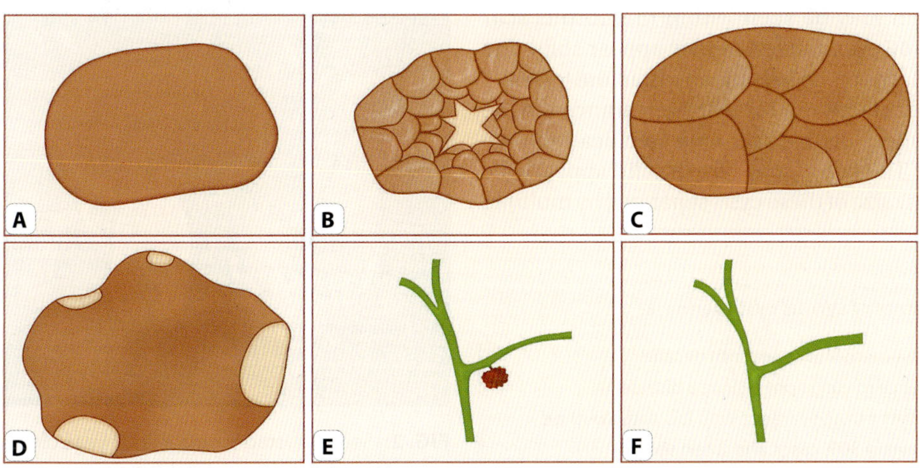

FIGS. 1A TO F: Morphological classification of cystic lesions. (A) Unilocular cyst with no internal septations. (B) Microcystic appearance with formation of multiple small cysts (>6 in number and <2 cm in size). (C) Macrocystic lesion with larger and fewer cysts. (D) Cyst with solid mural nodule. (E) Cysts communicating with the main pancreatic duct. (F) Diffusely dilated main pancreatic duct.

- Cysts communicating with the MPD are seen in branch duct-intraductal papillary mucinous neoplasms (BD-IPMNs). The more common nonneoplastic lesions which show communication with the MPD are pseudocysts and walled-off necrosis. Main duct intraductal papillary mucinous neoplasms (MD-IPMNs) may be seen as diffuse or segmental dilatation of the MPD.
- Cystic lesions with a solid component may be unilocular or multilocular. MCNs or IPMNs may have this appearance. Mixed solid and cystic lesions can also be SPNs and PNETs.

Serous Cystadenoma (Box 3)

Serous cystadenomas account for 1–2% of all pancreatic tumors and 10–15% of cystic pancreatic lesions. About 80% of these lesions occur in older women, with a peak incidence in fifth to seventh decades of life ("grandmother" lesions).[2,7,8] There is a slight preponderance of these tumors in the head region, but they are seen to occur throughout the pancreas. These lesions are mostly asymptomatic, and hence can become large at presentation. The larger lesions may result in mass effect and nonspecific abdominal discomfort. In cases of von Hippel–Lindau disease, there is an increased incidence of SCAs.[9]

Serous cystadenomas are typically microcystic lesions showing a honey-comb appearance on gross inspection. The other morphologic appearances include macrocystic, mixed microcystic—macrocystic and solid varieties.

Microcystic SCAs are well-circumscribed lesions with lobulated outline and are not encapsulated. These fine external lobulations result from the larger cysts in the periphery of the lesion in this microcystic tumor. These lesions may have a central scar with or without stellate calcification. Although seen in only 30% of SCAs, the scar is considered pathognomonic when present.[6]

On ultrasound, these lesions are seen as lobulated lesions with hypoechoic cysts and hyperechoic central scar. Calcification may be seen within the fibrous scar when present. However, the lesion may appear solid due to multiple interfaces of the septations within the lesion.[1]

On CT, the lobulated microcystic appearance can be appreciated. Central stellate scar with calcification may be seen **(Fig. 2)**. The lesion may have a solid appearance because of the tiny size of these cysts separated by multiple septations. On contrast administration, the septae and scar enhance avidly with persistent enhancement on delayed images. Absence of ductal obstruction or invasion of surrounding structures confirms the benign nature of these lesions as these tumors displace surrounding structures rather than invade them.

MRI aids in delineating the microcystic appearance of these tumors to a greater advantage **(Figs. 3A to C)**. The fibrous component is seen as hypointense on T1-weighted images and T2-weighted images. On contrast administration, the scar and septae show intense enhancement on the arterial phase with persistent enhancement on the delayed images, which help to differentiate these tumors from hypervascular neuroendocrine tumors of pancreas which show washout on delayed images.[1]

Cyst fluid aspirated from these tumors on EUS is usually clear and thin and may sometimes be hemorrhagic. On cyst fluid analysis, these tumors depict low carcino-embryonic antigen (CEA), low amylase, and high vascular endothelial growth factor (VEGF). The low CEA levels help to differentiate them from mucin secreting tumors such as MCNs and IPMNs. A cut-off of 192 ng/mL has been accepted by the current guidelines.[10-12] Low amylase distinguishes these from pseudocysts and IPMNs which have high amylase levels owing to pancreatic ductal communication.

Uncommonly, SCAs may have a macrocystic or oligo-cystic appearance (in <10% of cases) **(Fig. 4)**.[7,13] In these cases, MCN is a close differential. In a study by Cohen-Scali et al., presence of a combination of any three of the following imaging features could help to distinguish these two entities with a specificity of 100%—location in head region, lobulated outline, wall thickness < 2 mm and absence of wall enhancement. These findings favor the

BOX 3	Key points of serous cystadenoma.

- Mostly in older women; fifth to seventh decade
- Increased incidence in von Hippel–Lindau disease
- Typically, microcystic in appearance with lobulated outline
- Central scar is seen in 30% cases and when seen is pathognomonic
- No communication with main pancreatic duct
- Benign tumor with no malignant potential

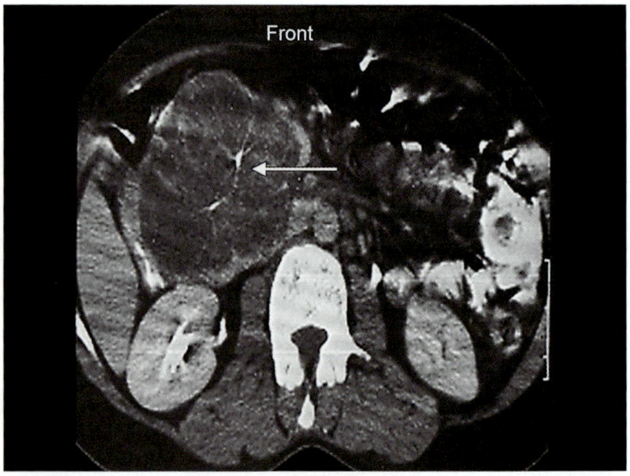

FIG. 2: Serous cystadenoma in a 62-year-old woman. Axial contrast-enhanced computed tomography (CECT) image reveals a microcystic lesion with lobulated outline in the pancreatic head region. Central scar with stellate calcification (arrow) is seen in this case which is pathognomonic for the lesion.

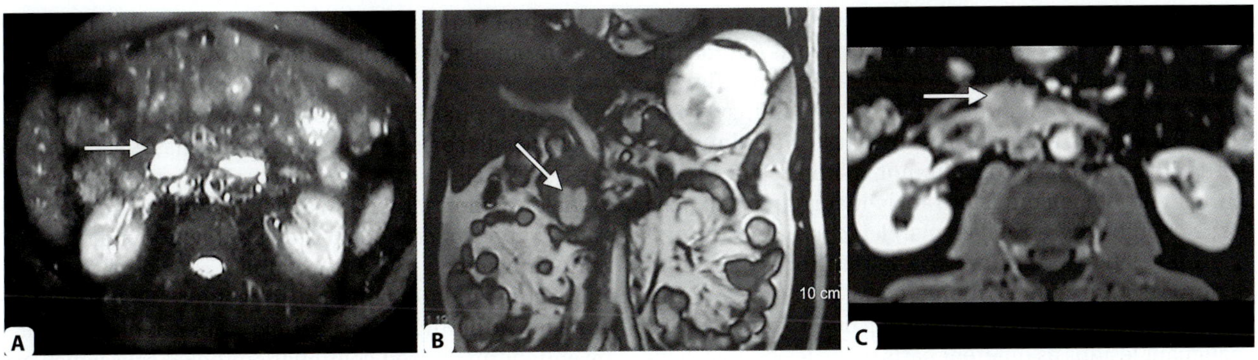

FIGS. 3A TO C: Serous cystadenoma in a 60-year-old male. A microcystic lesion with lobulated outline (arrows) is seen on axial HASTE (A) and coronal True FISP images (B) with internal septations within. Postcontrast arterial phase image (C) reveals subtle enhancement of the septae.

(HASTE: half-fourier acquisition single-shot turbo spin-echo; True FISP: true fast imaging with steady state precession)

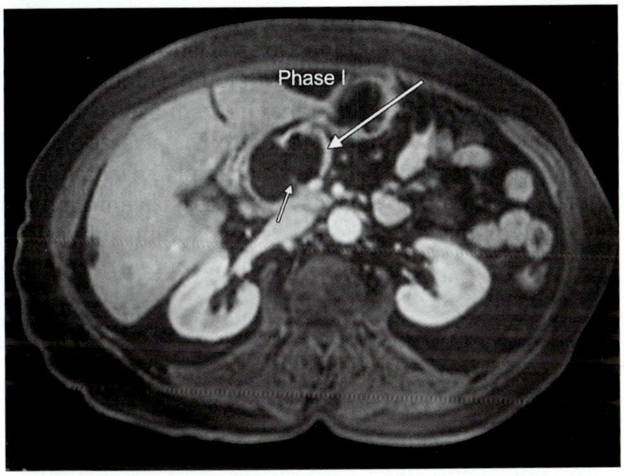

FIG. 4: Macrocystic serous cystadenoma in a 55-year-old woman. A lobulated macrocystic lesion (long arrow) with thin septal enhancement (short thin arrow) is seen in the head region of pancreas on this axial T1-weighted postgadolinium MR image.

diagnosis of oligocystic SCA.[14] The differential diagnoses of SCAs are given in the **Table 1**.

When a confident diagnosis of SCA is made, no surveillance is indicated as the malignant potential of these masses is practically nonexistent. However, surgery is recommended if the size is large enough to result in symptomatology related to compression of adjacent organs.[3]

Mucinous Cystic Neoplasm (Box 4)

Mucinous cystic neoplasms account for approximately 10% of cystic pancreatic lesions.[13] MCNs are most frequently encountered in middle-aged women with a peak incidence in fourth to fifth decade ("mother" lesions), slightly lesser than that of SCAs. These are known to occur almost exclusively in women with a frequency of approximately 99.7%.[1,2]

TABLE 1: Differential diagnoses of serous cystadenoma.

MCN	Oligocystic SCA mimics MCN. Features such as location in head region, lobulated outline, wall thickness < 2 mm, and absence of wall enhancement favor the diagnosis of SCA
PNET	SCAs and PNETs are hypervascular cystic lesions. Solid areas and calcification within SCAs may mimic PNET. On dynamic imaging, while there is persistent enhancement in SCAs, PNETs depict washout on delayed images. PNETs may also show thick enhancing walls
SPN	As SPN is frequently hemorrhagic, SCA with intratumoral hemorrhage mimics SPN. However, hemorrhage within SCA is not very common. The typical age of presentation of both these lesions is also different
BD-IPMN	BD-IPMNs are cystic lesions communicating with pancreatic duct while SCAs show no communication with the duct. When communication with pancreatic duct is not visualized in BD-IMPNs, the distinction with SCAs may be difficult

(BD-IPMN: branch duct intraductal papillary mucinous neoplasm; MCN: mucinous cystic neoplasm; PNET: pancreatic neuroendocrine tumor; SCAs: serous cystadenomas; SPN: solid pseudopapillary neoplasm)

BOX 4 Key points of mucinous cystic neoplasm.

- Almost exclusively in women
- Fourth to fifth decade; slightly lesser than SCA
- Body and tail of pancreas are the most common sites involved
- Typically, macrocystic in appearance with smooth outline
- Peripheral calcification can be seen, which is best appreciated on CT
- There is no ductal communication
- Thick wall, mural, or septal calcification and internal enhancing soft-tissue component are predictive of malignancy

(SCA: serous cystadenoma)

Patients may be symptomatic due to mass effect caused by the neoplasm although they are asymptomatic in 75% cases.[15-17] These neoplasms have a malignant potential ranging from 10 to 17%.[18] On histology, these could range from benign mucinous cystadenoma, borderline mucinous cystic tumor, mucinous neoplasm with carcinoma in situ to a frankly malignant mucinous cystadenocarcinoma. The stromal elements of these tumors are similar to ovarian stroma unlike IPMNs which have ductal origin stroma. Sampling of the lesion may not be an accurate method of differentiating between benign and malignant lesions as different parts of the lesion may have different configuration of epithelium.[19]

These neoplasms are most commonly macrocystic in appearance. On ultrasound, a well-circumscribed multicystic mass is often seen which may have septations, mural nodules or calcification **(Fig. 5)**. Rarely, debris or hemorrhage may be seen within these cysts.[1]

On CT, these are well-defined encapsulated lesions with a smooth outline **(Fig. 6)**. They may have a "cyst within a cyst" appearance. Calcification may be seen along the septae or wall of the lesion **(Fig. 7)**. This may be seen in approximately 15% of cases. On contrast administration, the wall is seen to enhance along with septae and mural nodules.

MR can better delineate the internal morphology of the lesion. On T2WI, the lesion is usually seen as a hyperintense fluid-filled multiloculated lesion with hypointense wall. The signal intensity of the cyst, however, may be variable due to proteinaceous contents of the cyst. The wall and septations enhance on contrast administration, more so on the delayed images due to fibrous nature of the wall **(Figs. 8A and B)**. If the lesion results in pancreatic ductal obstruction, concomitant pancreatitis may result which may be seen as glandular atrophy, ductal dilatation, and decreased parenchymal signal on T1WI with delayed enhancement.[1,20]

The imaging features predictive of malignancy are local invasion, lymph nodal and distant metastases, large lesion size (cyst > 4 cm), thick irregular wall, mural calcification, internal enhancing soft-tissue component, mural nodule and pancreatic ductal dilatation.[21-23] MCN in male gender is also more likely to be malignant.[2]

The cyst fluid contains thick and viscous mucus in these tumors. High CEA levels are noted as these tumors are lined by endoderm derived columnar epithelial cells which are

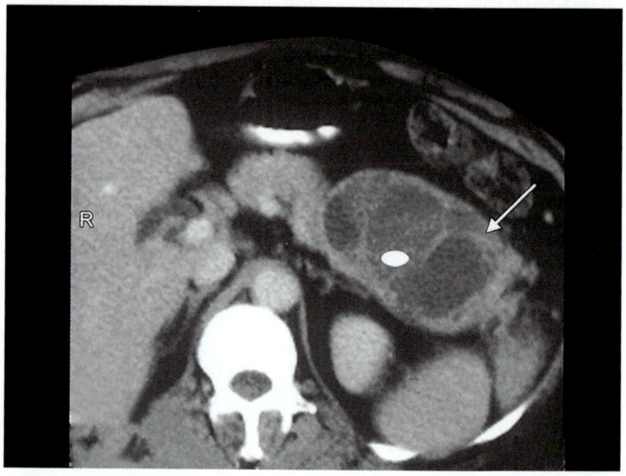

FIG. 6: Mucinous cystic neoplasm in a 51-year-old woman. Axial contrast-enhanced computed tomography (CECT) image depicts a well-circumscribed macrocystic lesion in pancreatic tail (arrow) with variable attenuation of the internal contents of the cyst (dot) which could be due to proteinaceous contents.

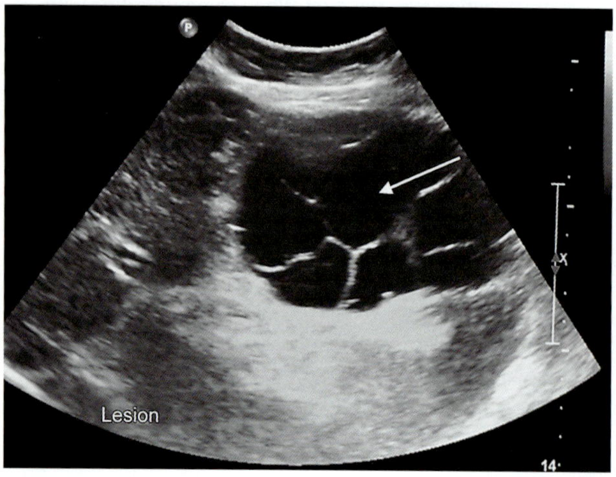

FIG. 5: Mucinous cystic neoplasm in a 52-year-old woman. US images show a well-marginated macrocystic mass (arrow) arising from the pancreatic tail.

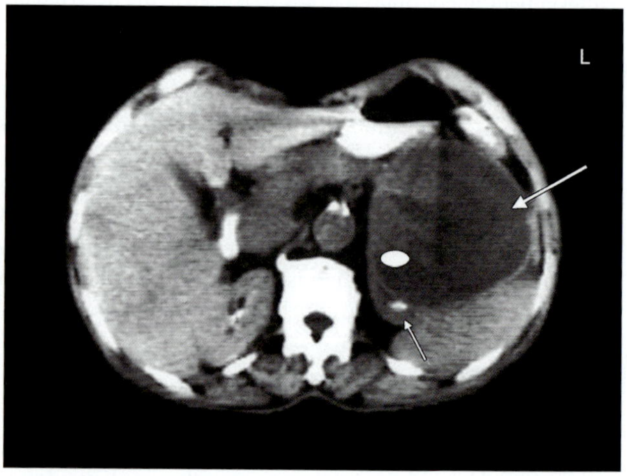

FIG. 7: Mucinous cystic neoplasm in a 48-year-old woman. Contrast-enhanced computed tomography (CECT) image showing a unilocular thin-walled cystic mass in the pancreatic tail (arrow) with small peripheral calcification in the inferior part of the cyst (short thin arrow).

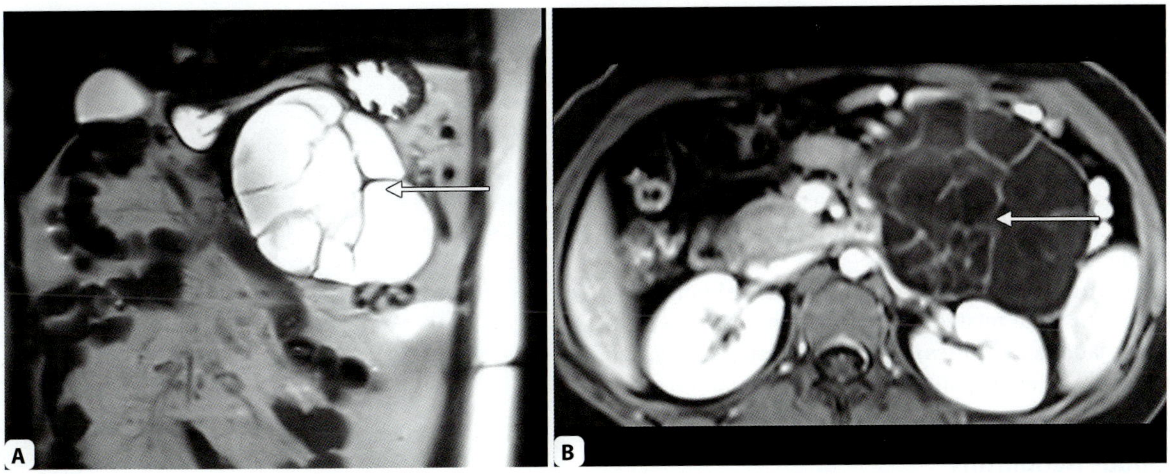

FIGS. 8A AND B: Macrocystic neoplasm in a 52-year-old woman. Coronal HASTE (A) and axial postgadolinium (B) images reveal a well-circumscribed macrocystic neoplasm in the tail region of pancreas with enhancing septae (arrows).

TABLE 2: Differential diagnoses of mucinous cystic neoplasms.

SCA	SCAs are microcystic lesions with external lobulations. However, oligocystic serous cystadenomas may mimic MCN
BD-IPMN	Communication with the pancreatic duct is the classical feature of BD-IPMN which is not seen in MCN

(BD-IPMN: branch duct intraductal papillary mucinous neoplasm; MCN: mucinous cystic neoplasm; SCA: serous cystadenoma)

capable of secreting CEA. Nonmucinous cysts on the other hand are lined by simple cuboidal epithelium not derived from endoderm and hence secrete little or no CEA. The amylase levels have been found to be variable in MCNs.[3]

Branch duct IPMNs are a close-imaging differential diagnosis. Patient demographics and absence of ductal communication in MCNs can help in differentiating the two entities. Although they do not communicate with ductal system, they can result in ductal obstruction, especially when aggressive. MCNs are most commonly encountered in body and tail region of pancreas whereas the uncinate process is the typical location of branch duct IPMN.[6,19] The differential diagnoses of MCNs are enumerated in **Table 2**.

Various guidelines differ in their respective management recommendations of MCNs. While 2015 American gastroenterological association (AGA)[24] and 2017 International Association of Pancreatology (IAP)[10] recommend resections for all MCNs irrespective of size, the 2018 European guidelines[11] recommend resection for MCNs only when size ≥40 mm, when symptomatic or when there is a concerning feature (i.e., mural nodule) irrespective of size.

Intraductal Papillary Mucinous Neoplasm (Box 5)

Intraductal papillary mucinous neoplasms are one of the most common cystic pancreatic neoplasms accounting for 20–50% of these tumors.[25,26] These are mucinous tumors arising from ductal epithelium and may be main duct, branch duct or mixed type. These are encountered equally in men and women with a peak incidence in sixth to seventh decades of life.[2]

These lesions have a variable degree of aggressiveness with risk of malignancy being higher in main duct (mean 61.6%) and mixed type IPMNs than branch duct IPMNs (mean 25.5%).[27,28] IPMNs have been shown to have a unique feature of predisposition to pancreatic ductal adenocarcinoma elsewhere within the pancreas. This suggests the presence of diffuse parenchymal involvement in these patients known as the "field defect" discussed later in the chapter. The pathological spectrum ranges from benign adenomas to invasive carcinomas. Dysplastic grades are classified as low-, intermediate-, or high-grade dysplasia (HGD) and invasive carcinoma.

Four histopathological subtypes of IPMN have been described with distinct clinicopathological behavior. These include gastric, intestinal, oncocytic, and pancreaticobiliary subtypes. The gastric subtype accounts for

BOX 5 Key points of intraductal papillary mucinous neoplasm.

- Equally seen in men and women, sixth to seventh decade
- Can be main duct, branch duct, or combined type
- BD-IPMNs present as cystic pancreatic lesions
- Uncinate process is the classical site of BD-IPMNs, although can be seen throughout the pancreas
- Communication with pancreatic duct is pathognomonic of this cystic tumor
- Copious mucin extruding from bulging papilla on endoscopy is highly suggestive
- Main duct dilatation > 10 mm, large enhancing mural nodule (>5 mm) and obstructive jaundice are high-risk features

(BD-IPMNs: branch duct intraductal papillary mucinous neoplasms) the majority of BD-IPMNs and is less likely to develop into carcinoma. If a carcinoma develops in this setting, it usually behaves like a conventional pancreatic ductal adenocarcinoma. The intestinal subtype contributes to a significant proportion of MD-IPMNs and can have invasive carcinoma which is relatively indolent. The pancreaticobiliary subtype is the least common and the invasive carcinoma associated with this form is usually quite aggressive.[13]

Intraductal papillary mucinous neoplasms may present with meal related epigastric pain, loss of weight, vomiting, jaundice, features of pancreatic insufficiency, and, occasionally, as acute pancreatitis/recurrent pancreatitis.

Branch Duct Intraductal Papillary Mucinous Neoplasms

Branch duct intraductal papillary mucinous neoplasms generally present as unifocal/multifocal pleomorphic cystic lesions (often arranged in grape-like clusters separated by thin septae) communicating with the pancreatic duct. The cystic lesion is actually the mucin distended branch duct which is affected by the pathology. Communication with pancreatic duct is the key diagnostic imaging feature, best depicted on MRCP, which is not seen in other cystic pancreatic neoplasms.[19] When multifocal cystic lesions are present, it helps in suggesting the correct diagnosis of BD-IPMNs.

On ultrasound, a well-defined cystic mass may be seen. However, communication of the cystic lesion with pancreatic duct cannot be appreciated on ultrasound in most cases. Other ancillary features such as mural nodularity, mucin globules or septations may be seen on ultrasound depending on the aggressive nature of the lesion.[1,19]

On CT, a branch duct IPMN appears as a pleomorphic cystic lesion most often in the uncinate process, which is the classical site. Communication with pancreatic duct may be seen on curved multiplanar reformatted images.

MRI with MRCP remains the modality of choice to depict communication of the lesion with the pancreatic duct. The branch duct lesion is seen as hyperintense on T2WI and hypointense on T1WI. When communication with MPD is not clearly depicted, the differential diagnoses include pseudocyst, MCN and SCN in case of a unifocal BD-IPMN and the rare ACCN in case of a multifocal BD-IPMN.[13]

Main Duct and Mixed Type Intraductal Papillary Mucinous Neoplasms

Main duct intraductal papillary mucinous neoplasms do not strictly fall into the category of a cystic pancreatic neoplasm and mainly present as diffuse or segmental dilatation of the pancreatic duct **(Figs. 9 and 10)**. The criteria for dilatation of pancreatic duct is >5 mm as per Fukuoka guidelines[10] and 7 mm according to the American College of Radiology.[18] Septations and filling defects may be seen within the dilated duct **(Figs. 11A to C)**. The filling defects seen within the lesion may either be mucin globules or soft-tissue component associated with a more aggressive

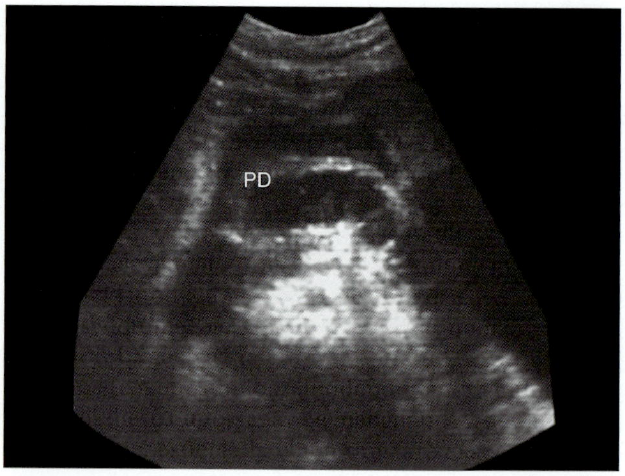

FIG. 9: Main duct intraductal papillary mucinous neoplasm (IPMN) in a 63-year-old male. US image depicts a markedly dilated main pancreatic duct (PD) with few-filling defects within.

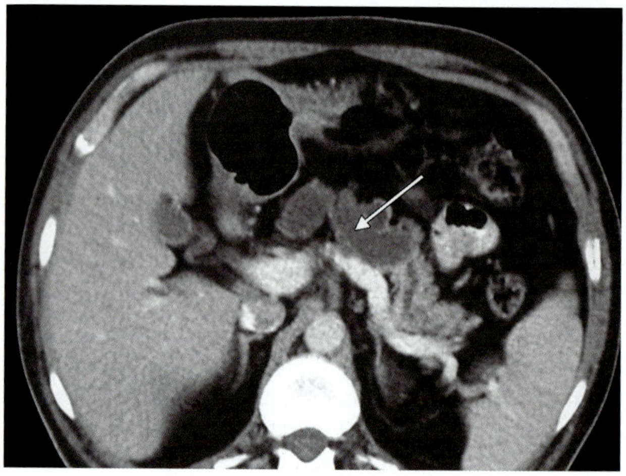

FIG. 10: Main duct intraductal papillary mucinous neoplasm (IPMN) in a 63-year-old male. There is segmental dilatation of the main pancreatic duct (arrow) in the pancreatic body region in this case of segmental main duct IPMN.

lesion; these may be differentiated using contrast-enhanced imaging, where soft tissue enhances and mucin globules do not enhance.[1,19] These nodules are better seen on EUS and may be difficult to detect on CT/MR. Segmental MD-IPMNs may appear as cystic lesions if a very short segment of the MPD is involved. These may result in upstream dilatation of MPD and then be mistaken for diffuse MD-IPMNs.

Parenchymal atrophy is frequently seen in MD-IPMN and the duct is dilated with no obvious obstructive lesion or narrowing. Papillary bulging may be evident due to copious mucin production by the tumor. Copious mucin extruding from a bulging papilla seen on correlative endoscopic examination is considered highly suggestive of the diagnosis.[29]

Mixed-type IPMNs **(Figs. 12A to E)** are seen as dilatation of both MPD and its branch ducts. When a suspected

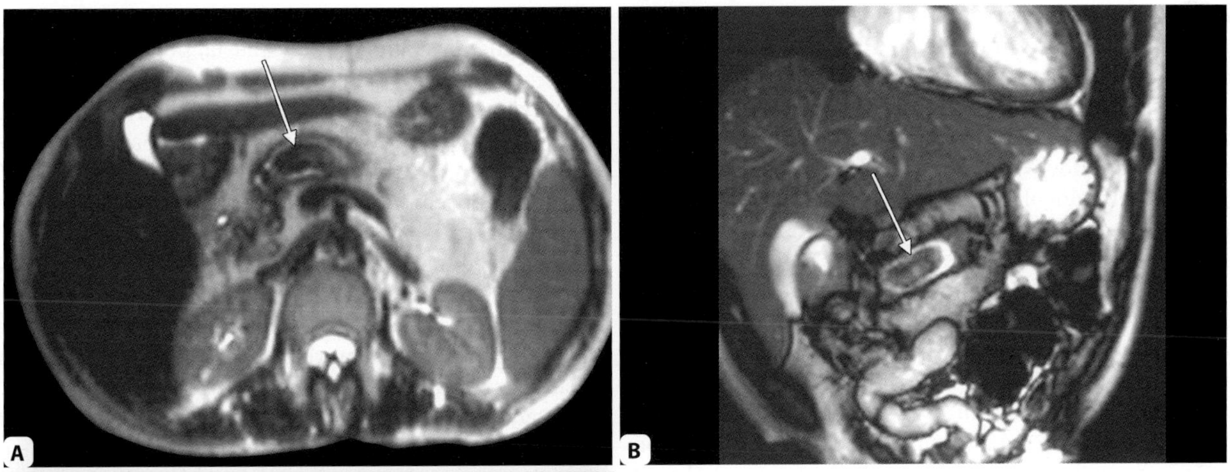

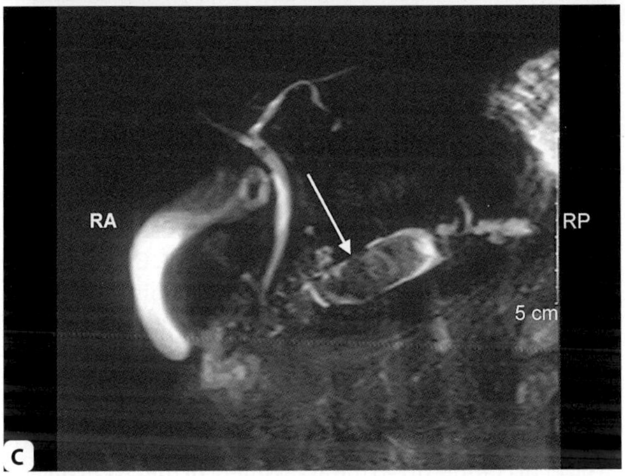

FIGS. 11A TO C: Intraductal papillary mucinous neoplasm (IPMN) in a 65-year-old male. Axial (A) and coronal true-fast imaging with steady state precession (FISP) MR images (B) depicts the filling defects (arrows) in the dilated pancreatic duct. These are also well depicted on magnetic resonance cholangiopancreaticography (MRCP) image (C). These were nonenhancing mucin globules.

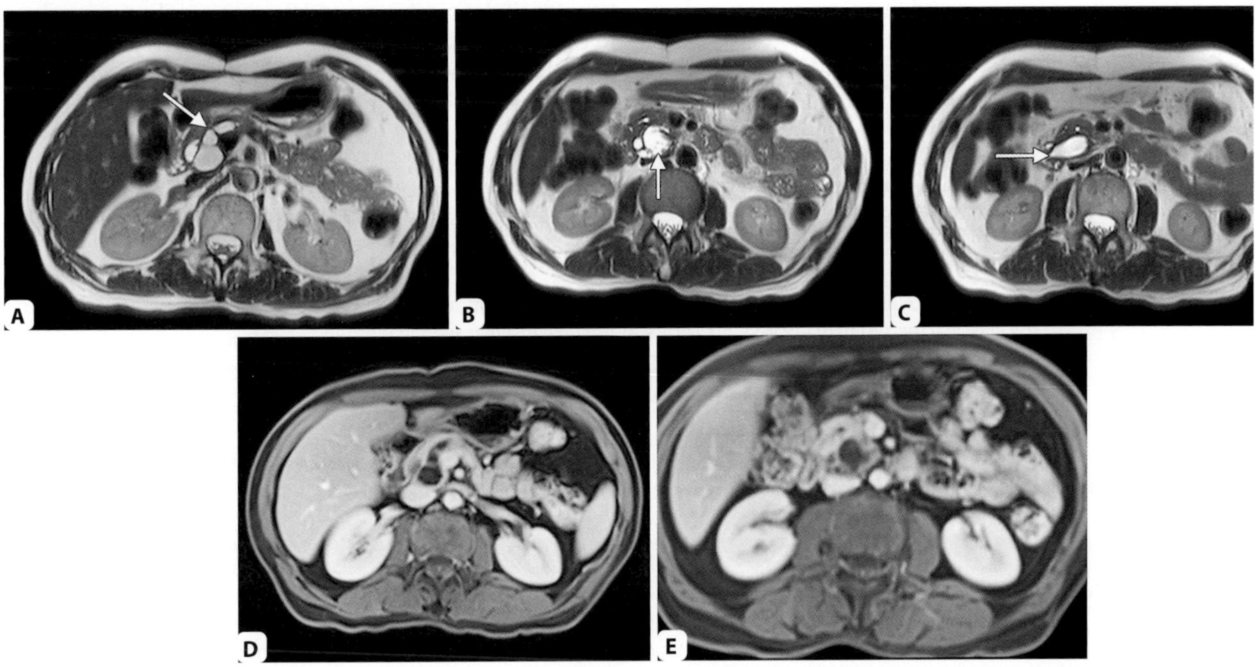

FIGS. 12A TO E: Mixed intraductal papillary mucinous neoplasm (IPMN) in a 62-year-old male. T2-weighted axial images (A to C) of the abdomen show a pleomorphic intrapancreatic cystic lesion in the uncinate process of pancreas (arrow in B) with dilated main (arrow in A) and branch ducts and bulging duodenal papilla (arrow in C). Postcontrast axial images (D and E) show absence of any enhancing soft-tissue component.

BD-IPMN is being evaluated, the main duct must also be assessed to rule out a mixed type IPMN as the latter has a higher risk of malignancy than BD-IPMNs.

Examination of the cyst fluid depicts viscous mucus and high CEA levels. Elevated amylase levels are also seen owing to communication with pancreatic duct.

The International Association of Pancreatology (Revised 2017 Fukuoka consensus)[10] has established two-tier criteria for predicting malignancy in IMPNs. The first tier, known as "worrisome features", encompasses imaging findings suggestive of potential malignancy that could evolve in this lesion, indicating the need for further evaluation through EUS and rigorous follow-up. The worrisome features include cyst size exceeding 3 cm, thickened or enhancing cyst walls, moderate MPD dilatation (5–9 mm), small enhancing mural nodules (<5 mm), abrupt changes in MPD caliber with distal pancreatic atrophy, lymphadenopathy, a rapid rate of cyst growth (>5 mm/2 years) and elevated serum CA 19-9 levels.

The second tier, termed "high-risk stigmata", comprises imaging features indicative of a possibly malignant lesion, necessitating surgical intervention in suitable candidates. High-risk stigmata encompass obstructive jaundice, larger enhancing mural nodules (≥5 mm), and MPD diameter exceeding 10 mm.[10]

Patients with IPMN exhibiting high-risk stigmata warrant prompt surgical resection if fit for surgery. Young patients with worrisome features may also undergo resection due to their long life expectancy and heightened cumulative risk of malignant progression. For patients deemed unfit for surgery or lacking worrisome features or high-risk stigmata, regular surveillance is essential, involving clinical assessments, serum CA 19-9 monitoring, and imaging studies such as MRI and/or EUS at specified intervals.[10]

The 2018 European guidelines[11] delineate absolute and relative indications for surgery in patients with IPMNs. Absolute indications for surgery include positive cytology for malignancy/high grade dysplasia, presence of a solid mass, tumor-related jaundice, enhancing mural nodules ≥ 5 mm, or MPD dilatation ≥ 10 mm. Relative indications for surgery are growth rate ≥ 5 mm/year, serum CA 19-9 levels > 37 U/mL in the absence of jaundice, MPD diameter between 5 and 9.9 mm, cyst diameter ≥ 40 mm, presence of enhancing mural nodule < 5 mm, new onset of diabetes mellitus, or acute pancreatitis attributed to IPMN.

Although these guidelines are highly comprehensive, the treatment decision may be based on individual factors like life expectancy, operative risk, comorbidities, and extent of surgery required.

In addition, surveillance in the case of IMPNs is needed not only for early detection of malignant transformation of the primary mass but also for the detection of concomitant pancreatic ductal adenocarcinoma as discussed earlier.

Main duct IPMN can be confused with chronic pancreatitis, which can also have duct dilatation and parenchymal atrophy. Presence of irregular beaded appearance of duct with stricture formation and presence of ductal calculi favor the diagnosis of chronic pancreatitis. The other causes of ductal dilatation such as a pancreatic mass, ductal stone or stricture also need to be excluded. Bulging papilla and enhancing nodules within the lesion are pointers to the diagnosis of IPMN. The differential diagnoses are enumerated in **Table 3**.

Field Defect

The concept of field defect in pancreatic cystic tumors adds a layer of complexity to the assessment of the risk of invasive cancer development. Similar to how cirrhosis predisposes to hepatocellular carcinoma and Barret's esophagus may lead to esophageal carcinoma, IPMN in pancreas may indicate underlying parenchymal abnormalities. Few studies have highlighted an increased prevalence of synchronous and

TABLE 3: Differential diagnoses of intraductal papillary mucinous neoplasm.

BD-IPMN	
SCA	Oligocystic SCAs may mimic unifocal BD-IPMNs where pancreatic duct communication is not well visualized
MCN	BD-IPMNs and MCNs both show presence of mucin on aspiration. Communication with the pancreatic duct is the classical feature of BD-IPMNs. MCNs are almost exclusively seen in women
Pseudocyst	Both IPMNs and pseudocysts show communication with the pancreatic duct. Prior history of pancreatitis suggests the correct diagnosis. Cyst fluid amylase levels > 250 U/L is considered specific for the diagnosis of a pseudocyst
Acinar cell cystic neoplasm (ACCN)	ACCN is a rare neoplasm that can mimic multifocal BD-IPMNs. Clustered peripheral small cysts, cyst calcifications, and absence of communication with the main pancreatic duct can suggest the diagnosis of ACCN
MD-IPMN	
Chronic pancreatitis	Regular duct dilatation without strictures, bulging ampulla, nodule within the dilated duct and grape-like secondary duct dilatation are features suggestive of diffuse MD-IPMN whereas irregular ductal dilatation with strictures, presence of ductal calculi and side branch ectasia with noncystic appearance are features specific for chronic pancreatitis

(BD-IPMN: branch duct intraductal papillary mucinous neoplasm; MCN: mucinous cystic neoplasm; MD-IPMN: main duct intraductal papillary mucinous neoplasm; SCA: serous cystadenoma)

metachronous invasive adenocarcinoma (9.3%) in patients with IPMNs, emphasizing the importance of thorough examination of the entire pancreatic tissue during follow-up. Notably, factors such as age over 70 years, newonset or worsening diabetes mellitus, abnormal serum carbohydrate antigen 19-9 (CA 19-9) levels, and multifocal pancreatic cysts have been associated with an increased risk of invasive carcinoma in IPMN patients. Even after resection of IPMNs, there remains a heightened risk of invasive carcinoma, including cases with low-grade dysplasia, making the surveillance of IPMNs challenging.[2,30-32]

Acinar Cell Cystic Neoplasm

Acinar cell cystic neoplasm is an uncommon cystic neoplasm, distinguished by its serous content and distinct acinar cell differentiation, which develops independently of the major ductal system. Initially labeled as "acinar cystic transformation", subsequent research has leaned toward its neoplastic nature, although further studies are warranted for definitive clarification. Typically presenting as multilocular cysts, ACCN exhibits a diverse age distribution with a notable predominance in females, often manifesting as abdominal pain. Diagnosing ACCN preoperatively poses a challenge due to its radiological similarities with other cystic pancreatic lesions. While the imaging features of unilocular ACCNs can often resemble those of MCN and macrocystic SCN, multilocular ACCNs can mimic IPMNs. However, a combination of two or three of the following imaging findings—presence of five or more cysts, clustered peripheral small cysts, cyst calcifications, and absence of communication with the MPD can help to diagnose ACCN.[33] Since no malignant transformation has been reported and ACCNs can be managed conservatively, accurate diagnosis remains crucial. Surgical biopsy with frozen section examination is often necessary for definitive diagnosis, as the lining cells of ACCN may mimic normal acinar cells on fine-needle aspiration. Close long-term monitoring is advised due to the ambiguous nature of ACCN.

Solid Pseudopapillary Neoplasm (Box 6)

Solid pseudopapillary neoplasms, also known as solid pseudopapillary epithelial neoplasms, are rare pancreatic tumors which account for 1–2% pancreatic exocrine neoplasms.[13] They are seen to occur mostly in young women with a peak incidence in second to fourth decades of life. They are seen most often in the body/tail region of pancreas, but can be seen anywhere in the pancreas.[2]

BOX 6 Key points of solid pseudopapillary neoplasm.

- Mostly seen in young women, second to fourth decade
- Encapsulated lesion
- Combination of solid and cystic components
- Areas of hemorrhage commonly seen
- Low-grade malignant neoplasm with a favorable prognosis after resection

Solid pseudopapillary neoplasms are mostly asymptomatic and usually detected when large in size. Larger masses may present with symptoms due to mass effect.

On imaging, SPN is a well-demarcated encapsulated lesion. Ultrasound features are nonspecific with a large complex attenuation mass with or without through transmission **(Fig. 13)**.

On CT, these are seen as well-defined encapsulated masses which have a combination of solid and cystic components **(Fig. 14)**. Areas of hemorrhage are commonly seen. The tumors may have peripheral and punctate calcifications within. The capsule and solid component enhance on contrast administration.

Areas of hemorrhage can be better seen on MRI, appearing hypointense on T2WI and hyperintense on T1WI.

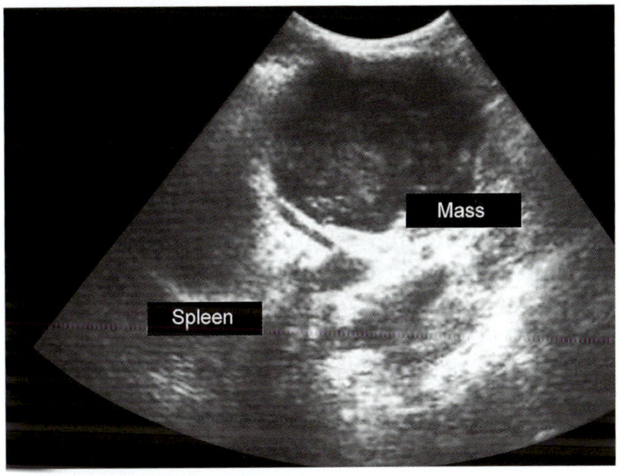

FIG. 13: Solid papillary epithelial neoplasm in a 32-year-old woman. Transverse sonogram image showing a mixed solid cystic mass in the pancreatic tail.

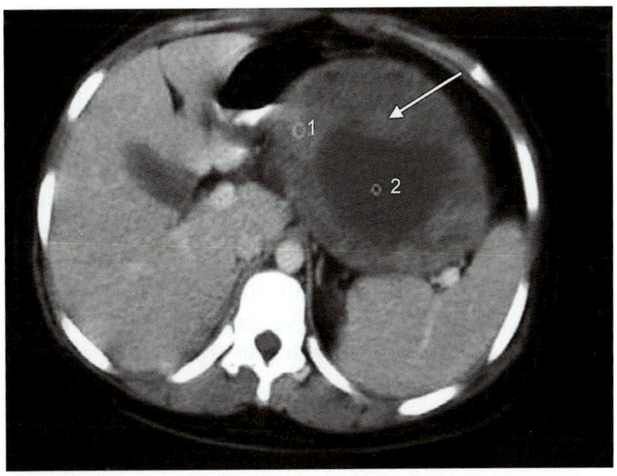

FIG. 14: Solid pseudopapillary neoplasm in a 35-year-old woman. Axial contrast-enhanced computed tomography (CECT) image depicts a large well-circumscribed heterogeneous mass (arrow) with peripheral solid (1) internal necrotic (2) component in the region of pancreatic tail.

Hemorrhagic and cystic degeneration is mostly seen in the central part of the lesion while solid component is seen at the periphery. Presence of hemorrhage helps in pointing toward this diagnosis especially when the tumor is seen in the appropriate demographic group of young women. On contrast administration, solid portions are seen to progressively enhance.

Cyst fluid analysis reveals low CEA and low amylase levels and can show necrotic debris.

These are tumors with low malignant potential and 80% of these tumors are benign.[34] Vascular invasion and metastatic disease can be seen in aggressive cases. Malignant SPNs are more likely to exhibit features such as size larger than 5–6 cm, focal discontinuity of the capsule, and liver lesions suggestive of metastases. The other rare sites of metastasis may be lymph nodes, peritoneum, or lungs. Treatment is generally surgery and prognosis is favorable after resection. The 5-year survival rates are in the range of 71–97%.[35]

Surveillance of Cystic Pancreatic Tumors

The gradual progression of IPMNs and MCNs to invasive cancers offers a window for early detection and potential surgical intervention. Although the effectiveness of surveillance for pancreatic cysts is uncertain, surveillance should be considered for surgically fit patients with asymptomatic cysts presumed to be IPMN or MCN without concerning features. The guidelines vary regarding the optimal modality and frequency of surveillance.[3]

The timing of surveillance intervals for IPMNs depends on cyst size according to IAP[10] guidelines, while AGA[24] and European[11] guidelines recommend surveillance regardless of cyst size. While European guidelines recommend follow-up of asymptomatic patients with MCN < 40 mm without mural nodule, AGA, and IAP recommend resection of all MCNs.

Surveillance is generally not recommended for asymptomatic patients with SCA due to their low malignant potential and slow growth rate.

MRI with MRCP is the modality of choice for surveillance due to its lack of radiation and superior pancreatic duct delineation. EUS may be considered for patients unable to undergo MRI. Surveillance should continue as long as the patient remains suitable for surgery and willing to undergo resection, if necessary, with some guidelines suggesting discontinuation after a period of stability. Individualized surveillance protocols based on initial cyst size and growth rate are likely to be most effective.[3]

Postresection Surveillance

Patients with surgically excised MCN exhibiting low-grade, borderline, or high grade dysplasia do not require surveillance. Surveillance guidelines of IPMNs after partial pancreatectomy have been variably laid down by different societies. The European[11] guidelines recommend 6-month follow-up until 2 years, followed by annual surveillance, for IPMN with high grade dysplasia or main duct involvement after resection. The IAP[10] guidelines recommend follow-up every 6 months in patients with a family history of pancreatic cancer, IPMN with high grade dysplasia, and IPMN of the nonintestinal subtype. Surveillance should be done as long as the patient remains suitable for surgery and consents to potential reresection if indicated. However, MCNs and IPMNs with invasive cancer should be followed up like pancreatic adenocarcinoma after partial pancreatectomy.

UNCOMMON CYSTIC PANCREATIC TUMORS

Cystic Metastases

Cystic metastases to pancreas most often arise from renal cell carcinoma and lung carcinoma. These are usually seen in late stages of disease when hematogenous metastases are also found at multiple other sites. An exception here is metastases from renal carcinoma where isolated pancreatic metastases have been encountered.[36]

Cystic Teratoma

Cystic teratoma is a very rare tumor with only few cases reported in literature. They can have varied imaging appearances as they can be composed of up to three germinal layers. Teratomas are generally well-defined lesions with a variable internal appearance. These could range from predominantly cystic to mixed cystic solid to pure solid masses. They may have fatty elements and areas of calcification. Various studies have shown that although these masses may abut vascular or biliary structures, they generally do not result in invasion or obstruction of these structures.[37,38] Definitive treatment is complete surgical resection.[39]

Cystic Hamartoma

Cystic Hamartoma is a rare benign tumor and imaging diagnosis may be difficult. The lesion is usually mixed solid and cystic with well-defined margins and progressive enhancement. It is isointense to hyperintense on T2-weighted MRI with absence of restriction of diffusion. Progressive enhancement pattern and absence of diffusion are features that aid in distinguishing this lesion from the more ominous pancreatic tumors.[40-42]

PANCREATIC NEUROENDOCRINE NEOPLASMS (BOX 7)

Pancreatic neuroendocrine neoplasms (paNENs) are rare tumors and account for only 1–2% of pancreatic neoplasms.[43] These are mostly seen between 40 and 60 years of age.[44] They may be sporadic or associated with various syndromes such as multiple endocrine neoplasia (MEN)-I, Von Hippel–Lindau syndrome, neurofibromatosis, and tuberous sclerosis.[45]

Pancreatic neuroendocrine neoplasms arise from pluripotent cells within the exocrine pancreas that undergo differentiation similar to neuroendocrine cells.[46] They have heterogenous biologic behavior ranging from indolent to aggressive. Though the final diagnosis may often require histopathologic evaluation, morphologic imaging using ultrasound, CT, and MRI and functional imaging using somatostatin receptor scintigraphy and positron emission tomography are essential for characterization, staging, surveillance, and therapy monitoring.

These tumors may or may not be associated with symptoms due to hormone production, and hence, may be termed functioning and nonfunctioning, respectively. About 30% of paNENs are functioning type. The common functioning tumors are insulinoma, gastrinoma, glucagonoma, VIPoma, and somatostatinoma. They are diagnosed early because of symptoms produced by them.[44] Nonfunctioning tumors are more common than functioning tumors. These may secrete pancreatic polypeptide, but have no associated hormonal symptoms. Historically, these presented when large in size with features of mass effect or systemic metastases. However, these are being increasingly detected incidentally as small masses owing to improved imaging techniques.[47]

BOX 7 **Key points of pancreatic neuroendocrine neoplasms (paNENs).**

- Rare tumors, mostly seen between 40 and 60 years of age
- May be functioning or nonfunctioning
- Functional tumors are mostly hypervascular tumors which enhance brightly on arterial phase images
- Calcification may be seen and is more frequent in nonfunctioning tumors
- Cystic paNEN is a distinct entity and has an indolent behavior
- Peripancreatic nodes and liver metastases are pointers toward malignancy
- Metastases are also hypervascular in nature

Pancreatic neuroendocrine neoplasms are seen evenly distributed throughout the pancreas. They can have varied morphology, appearing solid or cystic and can demonstrate calcification.[44,48]

As per the World Health Organization (WHO) 2019 classification system, paNENs are stratified according to cellular differentiation and cellular proliferation as depicted in **Flowchart 1**. These are classified as well-differentiated pancreatic neuroendocrine tumors (pNETs), poorly differentiated pancreatic neuroendocrine carcinomas (pNECs) and mixed neuroendocrine/nonneuroendocrine neoplasms (MiNENs) of the pancreas. Well-differentiated paNENs also known as pNETs, typically have an organoid architecture, and are classified into three grades according to the Ki-67 proliferation index and/or mitotic index—low grade with a Ki-67 index of <3% and/or a mitotic count of <2 mitoses/2 mm^2, intermediate grade with Ki-67 index between 3 and 20% or a mitotic count between 2 and 20 mitoses/2 mm^2, while high-grade pNET is identified by a high proliferation index (Ki-67 > 20% and/or mitotic rate > 20/2 mm^2).[49,50] Staging of well-differentiated pNET is based on 8th edition American Joint Committee TNM system as discussed in **Table 4**.[51] Staging of poorly differentiated paNEN, also known as pNEC, is similar to the staging for pancreatic ductal adenocarcinoma.

About 7–17% of resected paNENs have been found to be cystic. Originally, cystic degeneration was attributed to necrosis and hemorrhage in a previously large solid neuroendocrine neoplasm. However, small cystic pNETs are being increasingly detected on modern cross-sectional imaging techniques and are now considered a distinct entity, often seen in pancreatic body and tail. They are typically nonfunctioning and less aggressive with lower rate of metastases and risk of recurrence.[52]

On US examination, paNENs may be seen as well-defined hypoechoic masses. The larger tumors may be more heterogeneous. Presence of peripancreatic nodes and liver metastases are pointers toward malignancy. Due to low sensitivity and specificity of transabdominal ultrasound in detecting paNENs, its role is limited to detecting liver metastases. EUS, on the other hand, can detect small lesions. On contrast administration, rapid and

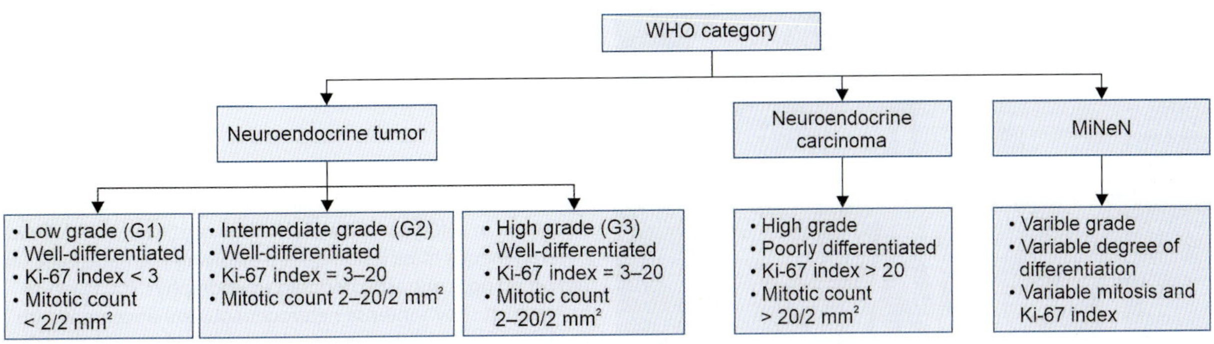

FLOWCHART 1: 2019 WHO classification of pancreatic neuroendocrine neoplasms.

(MiNeN: mixed neuroendocrine/nonneuroendocrine neoplasms; WHO: World Health Organization)

early enhancement is seen in arterial phase.[44] Sampling via fine-needle aspiration and follow-up in syndromic patients are other uses of EUS.

At CT, paNENs can have varied imaging appearance ranging from few millimeters to many centimeters. The margins of the tumor can be round and well-defined or ill-defined and infiltrative. Typical paNENs are well-circumscribed, hypervascular tumors which enhance brightly on late arterial phase images **(Figs. 15A to C)**. However, they may not always be hypervascular, especially the nonfunctioning tumors.[53] In various studies, it has been shown that late arterial phase images have a higher sensitivity for detecting paNENs (83–89%) than venous phase images (11–76%).[54,55] However, some tumors may only be seen on venous phase images.[44] Calcification may also be seen in paNENs and is more frequent in non-functioning tumors.[51] Vascular and ductal obstruction may sometimes be seen, simulating pancreatic ductal adenocarcinoma. Atypical imaging features also include intravascular and intraductal growth pattern. Cystic pNETs can be differentiated from other cystic lesions of pancreas on the basis of the hypervascular nature of the peripheral rim.

On MRI, paNENs appear hypointense to the pancreatic parenchyma on T1WI and hyperintense on T2WI. Tumors with more fibrous content may have intermediate or hypointense signal on T2WI. paNENs are generally seen as hypervascular masses with homogeneous, heterogeneous, or rim enhancement. Heterogeneous enhancement is seen in necrotic tumors. Liver metastases are hypointense

TABLE 4: The American Joint Committee on Cancer (AJCC) 8th edition TNM staging of well-differentiated pancreatic neuroendocrine neoplasms (pNETs).

AJCC stage	TNM stage	Description
I	T1N0M0	Tumor <2 cm localized to pancreas, no nodal or distant metastases
II	T2N0M0 or T3N0M0	Tumor 2–4 cm (T2) or >4 cm (T3) localized to pancreas, can invade duodenum or common bile duct (T3), no nodal or distant metastases
III	T4N0M0 or any TN1M0	Tumor invades adjacent organs or blood vessels (T4), can spread to nearby lymph nodes(N1), no distant metastases
IV	Any T any N M1	Distant metastases present

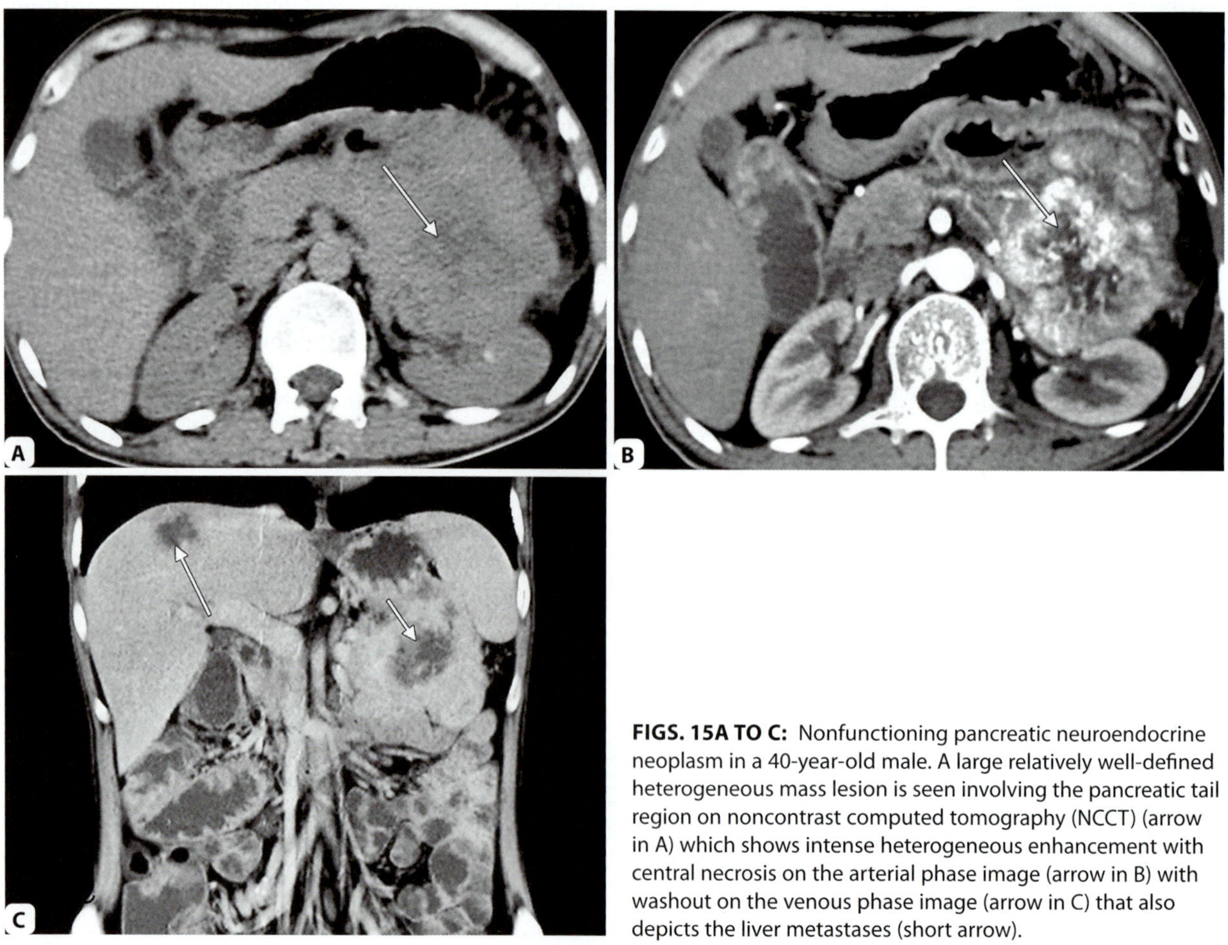

FIGS. 15A TO C: Nonfunctioning pancreatic neuroendocrine neoplasm in a 40-year-old male. A large relatively well-defined heterogeneous mass lesion is seen involving the pancreatic tail region on noncontrast computed tomography (NCCT) (arrow in A) which shows intense heterogeneous enhancement with central necrosis on the arterial phase image (arrow in B) with washout on the venous phase image (arrow in C) that also depicts the liver metastases (short arrow).

on T1- and hyperintense on T2WI. Liver and lymph node metastases may also show prominent enhancement. With liver specific contrast agents, these metastases are seen as hypointense lesions on hepatocyte phase imaging.[44,56] Furthermore, MRI may have a potential role in the surveillance of patients with syndromic lesions.

The size and shape of tumor, pattern of enhancement, presence of metastases, involvement of vasculature, and findings on diffusion imaging can help in predicting the grade of tumors on imaging. An ADC cut-off value of $< 1.21 \times 10^{-3}$ mm^2/sec can be used to predict grade 2 and grade 3 tumors.[56]

If these cross-sectional modalities are unable to depict these tumors, then endoscopic US and nuclear imaging studies may be performed. Sensitivity with endoscopic US may be as high as 94%, although it has poorer performance in the tail region of pancreas.[57]

The majority of paNENs (about 70%), with the exception of insulinomas and poorly differentiated neoplasms, have lots of somatostatin receptors (SSRs) along the cell membrane, and this is the reason why functional imaging with somatostatin analogs is able to clearly show these neoplasms. Nuclear medicine studies can depict the primary tumor, evaluate metastases, and also receptor status for planning therapy. Octreotide is the most commonly used somatostatin analog. Octreotide is conjugated with the chelator tetra-azacyclododecanetetra-acetic acid (DOTA) and is used for imaging as well as therapy of paNENs. Ga^{68} DOTA-TOC (DOTA-tyrosine-3-octreotide), ^{68}Ga-DOTATATE, and Ga^{68} DOTANOC (DOTA-1-NaI-octreotide) are the most frequently used analogs.[44] Octreotide scans have the highest sensitivity for gastrinomas and the lowest sensitivity for insulinomas depending upon the expression of somatostatin receptors.[53]

Scintigraphy techniques using octreotide include planar imaging as well as single-photon emission computed tomography (SPECT).[53] PET scan has better spatial resolution than scintigraphy.

Apart from somatostatin receptors, PET-CT may also be performed using the ^{18}F-FDG and its uptake has been found to be inversely correlated with prognosis.[58] Poorly differentiated neuroendocrine cancers exhibit poor expression of somatostatin receptors and have higher uptake of ^{18}F-FDG. PET/MRI utilizes the advantages of both molecular imaging and superior contrast resolution of MRI to optimize detection of metastatic disease, particularly in the abdomen and pelvis. Poorly differentiated neuroendocrine cancers are extremely rare tumors and carry a prognosis much worse than well-differentiated tumors. The tumors usually are fatal within a year of detection. They are mostly seen in elderly men and in the pancreatic head region. On imaging, they are ill-defined masses with local invasion and distant metastases at presentation.

The differential diagnoses for solid well-differentiated pNET are given in **Table 5**.

TABLE 5: Differential diagnoses for solid pancreatic neuroendocrine tumor (pNET).

Differential diagnosis	Features
Metastases	Hypervascular metastases, e.g., from renal cell carcinoma can mimic solid pNETs
Intrapancreatic splenunculus	Well-defined lesion located in pancreatic parenchyma, with similar enhancing phases as splenic parenchyma
Mostly solid serous cystadenoma	May be difficult to distinguish from pNETs on imaging alone. On dynamic imaging, while there is persistent enhancement in SCAs, PNETs depict washout on delayed images
Gastrointestinal stromal tumor	Origin of tumor arises from stomach or duodenum, fat plane usually preserved with pancreas

According to current North America NeuroEndocrine Tumor Society (NANETS) and European Neuroendocrine Tumor Society guidelines, nonfunctioning paNENs < 2 cm in size are likely benign and can be kept under follow-up. For functional tumors, surgery is advised for relief of symptoms regardless of size. The first line of treatment in larger paNENs is radical surgery. In cases where the disease has reached advanced stages, multidisciplinary approach is needed in addition to surgery.[59,60]

The patients are advised to follow up for a long duration. Morphological imaging and somatostatin analog-PET/CT are recommended 3–6 months after surgery, followed by morphological imaging every 6–12 months for 5 years, then every 12–24 months for 10 years and then every 5 years.[61]

SPECIFIC FEATURES OF FUNCTIONING PANCREATIC NEUROENDOCRINE NEOPLASMS (BOX 8)

Functioning paNENs result in symptoms related to hormone production. Functional tumors are generally indolent and have a good prognosis.

Insulinomas are the most common functioning tumors and account for >40% of functioning endocrine tumors of pancreas. These are usually smaller than other functioning as well as nonfunctioning tumors of pancreas due to the dramatic clinical symptomatology associated with these tumors. Most of these tumors (90%) are <2 cm in size and 40% are even smaller than 1 cm **(Fig. 16)**.[62] Since they are discovered early, they also usually carry the best prognosis. The characteristic Whipple's triad of their presentation includes the following symptoms: low blood glucose level, symptoms of hypoglycemia and relief of symptoms on administering glucose.[63] These are evenly distributed through the head, body, and tail region of pancreas. Multiple lesions may be seen with MEN-1 syndrome.[44]

Gastrinomas are the second most common functioning tumors after insulinomas. These are mostly encountered in pancreatic head region and have an average size of 3–4 cm. These are most often seen in the gastrinoma triangle region, which is bounded by the following three points—junction of cystic and common bile duct, junction of second and third parts of duodenum and junction of neck and body of pancreas **(Fig. 17)**. Their somatostatin receptor concentration is also high and hence these are more readily depicted on nuclear imaging techniques than insulinomas. Gastrin levels in these patients are usually markedly elevated to >1,000 pg/mL resulting in increased gastric acid production and peptic ulcer disease. Zollinger–Ellison syndrome refers to a triad of a gastrinoma, increased secretion of gastric acid and peptic ulcers in unusual locations (e.g., postbulbar duodenum and jejunum). Up to 60% of these tumors may be malignant.[44] They are often multicentric, especially when they are associated with MEN-1. On contrast-enhanced images, gastrinomas often show a delayed enhancement due to presence of fibrosis.

Glucagonomas are the third most common functioning neuroendocrine neoplasms. These are usually large at presentation with an average size of 5–6 cm. These are most often seen in pancreatic body and tail region. Most of these tumors are malignant. Clinically, they present with 4D syndrome which includes dermatitis, diabetes, deep vein thrombosis, and depression.[44]

VIPomas are rare tumors that can be pancreatic or extrapancreatic in origin. Extrapancreatic tumors may arise from sympathetic ganglia of the retroperitoneum or mediastinum and even from stomach, small bowel, colon, and liver. Symptoms result from excessive production of vasoactive intestinal peptide (VIP), a hormone that is not normally secreted by the pancreas. VIP prevents intestinal reabsorption and promotes intestinal secretion of water and electrolytes and these patients then present with watery diarrhea, hypokalemia, and achlorhydria (WDHA syndrome). Most of these tumors are seen in tail region and are malignant tumors with an average size of approximately 5 cm.[44]

BOX 8 Functioning pancreatic neuroendocrine neoplasms (paNENs).

- *Insulinomas*:
  - Most common functioning tumors
  - Characteristic Whipple's triad with low blood glucose, symptoms of hypoglycemia, and relief of symptoms on administering glucose
  - Evenly distributed through head, body, and tail region
  - Multiple lesions in MEN-1 syndrome
- *Gastrinomas*:
  - Second most common
  - Most often seen in gastrinoma triangle
  - Zollinger–Ellison syndrome constitutes a triad of gastrinoma, increased gastric acid production and peptic ulcers in unusual locations
- *Glucagonomas*:
  - Third most common
  - Mostly in pancreatic body and tail region
  - Present with 4D syndrome—dermatitis, deep vein thrombosis, diabetes, and depression
- *VIPomas*:
  - Rare tumors; pancreatic or extrapancreatic in origin
  - Mostly seen in tail region
  - WDHA syndrome—watery diarrhea, hypokalemia, and achlorhydria
- *Somatostatinoma*:
  - Rare tumors
  - Can present with diabetes mellitus, diarrhea, steatorrhea, and weight loss

(MEN: multiple endocrine neoplasia-1)

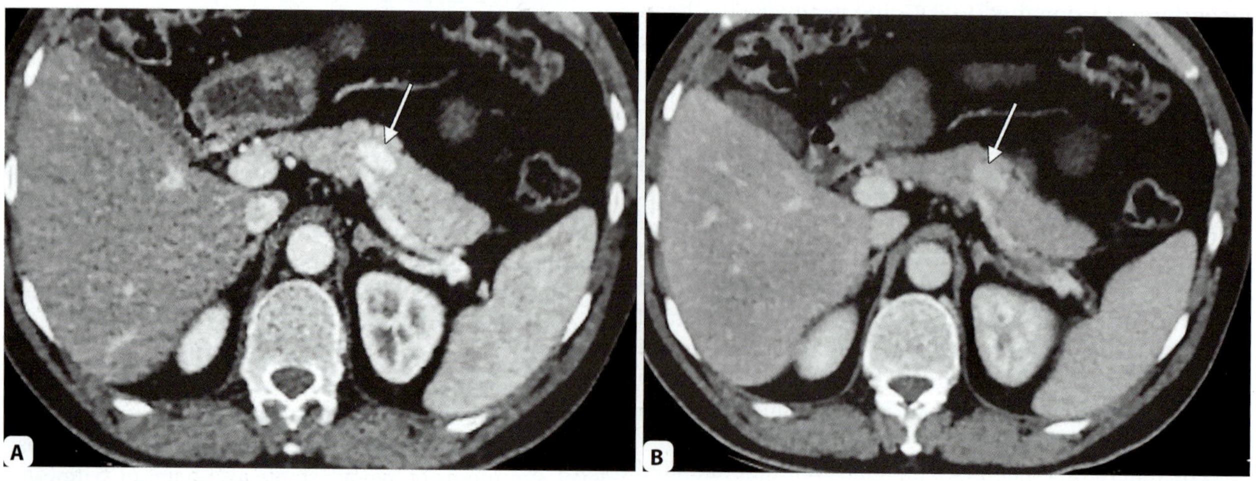

FIGS. 16A AND B: Insulinoma in a 40-year-old male. Axial CT images in arterial (A) and portal venous (B) phases show a hypervascular small well-defined lesion within the body of pancreas (arrows).

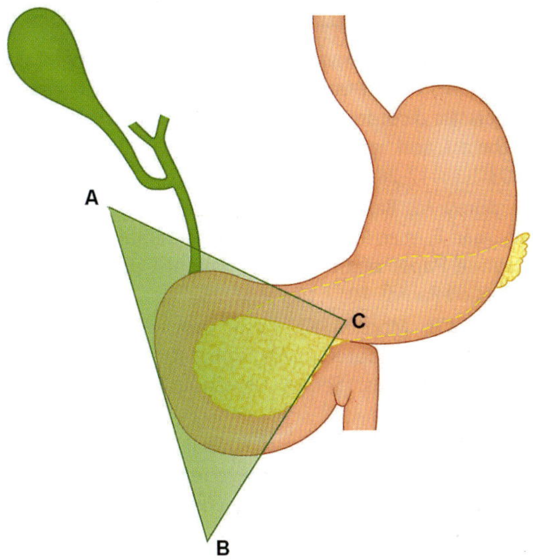

FIG. 17: Gastrinoma triangle region. This region is bounded by the following three points—junction of cystic and common bile duct (A), junction of second and third parts of duodenum (B), and junction of neck and body of pancreas (C).

Somatostatinomas are rare tumors which can present with diabetes mellitus, steatorrhea, diarrhea, and weight loss. Other hormones that may very rarely be produced by these functioning pancreatic neoplasms are adrenocorticotropic hormone, serotonin, growth hormone, and calcitonin.[44]

The differentiating features of various cystic pancreatic neoplasms are given in **Table 6**.

CONCLUSION

Cystic tumors of pancreas as well as pancreatic neuroendocrine neoplasms are heterogeneous groups of tumors with varying aggressiveness and prognosis. It is crucial to characterize them for appropriate planning of therapeutic and follow-up strategies. Morphological and functional imaging techniques play a key role in characterization of these tumors. However, these techniques may still not provide all the answers. There is ongoing research on computer augmented diagnostics using radiomics, based on quantitative evaluation of objective features "hidden" inside radiological images, that may further optimize characterization of these tumors.

TABLE 6: Differentiating features of cystic pancreatic neoplasms.

	SCA	MCN	IPMN	SPN	Cystic paNEN
Demographics	• Elderly women • Fifth to seventh decade (Grandmother lesion)	• Middle-aged women • Fourth to fifth decade (Mother lesion)	• Men = Women • Sixth to seventh decade	• Young women • Second to fourth decade (Daughter lesion)	• Men = Women • Fifth to sixth decade
Common site	Head	Body and tail	• MD: All parts • BD: Uncinate	All parts	Body and tail
Morphology	Microcystic (honeycomb) (>6 cysts, <2 cm)	Macrocystic (<6 cysts, >2 cm)	• MD: Dilatation of MPD • BD: Cluster of cysts (grape-like) communicating with pancreatic duct	• Solid and cystic areas • Areas of hemorrhage and necrosis	Cystic and solid
Calcification	Central scar (Stellate calcification) 30–40%	Wall/septal calcification 25%	May be seen due to mucinous contents	Peripheral, punctate calcification 30%	May be present
Communication with pancreatic duct	No	No	Yes	No	No
Cyst fluid analysis	• Low CEA • Low amylase • High VEGF	• High CEA • Variable amylase	• High CEA • High amylase	• Low CEA • Low amylase	• Low CEA • Low amylase
Molecular markers	VHL positive	• KRAS, RNF3 positive • GNAS negative	• KRAS, RNF43 positive • GNAS positive	CTNNB1 positive	MEN1, DAXX, ATRX positive

(BD: branch duct; CEA: carcinoembryonic antigen; IPMN: intraductal papillary mucinous neoplasm; MCN: mucinous cystic neoplasm; MD: main duct; MPD: main pancreatic duct; paNENs: pancreatic neuroendocrine neoplasms; SCA: serous cystadenoma; SPN: solid pseudopapillary neoplasm; VEGF: vascular endothelial growth factor)

REFERENCES

1. Dewhurst CE, Mortele KJ. Cystic tumors of the pancreas: imaging and management. Radiol Clin North Am. 2012;50(3):467-86.
2. Miller FH, Vendrami CL, Recht HS, Wood CG, Mittal P, Keswani RN, et al. Pancreatic Cystic Lesions and Malignancy: Assessment, guidelines, and the Field Defect. Radiographics. 2022;42(1):87-105.
3. Van Huijgevoort NCM, Del Chiaro M, Wolfgang CL, Van Hooft JE, Besselink MG. Diagnosis and management of pancreatic cystic neoplasms: current evidence and guidelines. Nat Rev Gastroenterol Hepatol. 2019;16(11):676-89.
4. Chang MK, Kyung SK, Jin SC, Kim H, Woo JL, Byong RK. Solid pseudopapillary tumor of the pancreas suggesting malignant potential. Pancreas. 2006;32(3):276-80.
5. Jani N, Bani Hani M, Schulick RD, Hruban RH, Cunningham SC. Diagnosis and management of cystic lesions of the pancreas. Diagn Ther Endosc. 2011;2011:478913.
6. Sahani DV, Kambadakone A, Macari M, Takahashi N, Chari S, Fernandez-del Castillo C. Diagnosis and management of cystic pancreatic lesions. AJR Am J Roentgenol. 2013;200(2):343-54.
7. Jais B, Rebours V, Malleo G, Salvia R, Fontana M, Maggino L, et al. Serous cystic neoplasm of the pancreas: a multinational study of 2622 patients under the auspices of the International Association of Pancreatology and European Pancreatic Club (European Study Group on Cystic Tumors of the Pancreas). Gut. 2016;65(2):305-12.
8. Horvath KD, Chabot JA. An aggressive resectional approach to cystic neoplasms of the pancreas. Am J Surg. 1999;178(4): 269-74.
9. Kanno A, Satoh K, Hamada S, Hirota M, Masamune A, Motoi F, et al. Serous cystic neoplasms of the whole pancreas in a patient with von Hippel–Lindau disease. Intern Med. 2011; 50(12):1293-8.
10. Tanaka M, Fernández-Del Castillo C, Kamisawa T, Jang JY, Levy P, Ohtsuka T, et al. Revisions of international consensus Fukuoka guidelines for the management of IPMN of the pancreas. Pancreatology. 2017;17(5):738-53.
11. European Study Group on Cystic Tumours of the Pancreas. European evidence-based guidelines on pancreatic cystic neoplasms. Gut. 2018;67(5):789-804.
12. Dumonceau JM, Deprez PH, Jenssen C, Iglesias-Garcia J, Larghi A, Vanbiervliet G, et al. Indications, results, and clinical impact of endoscopic ultrasound (EUS)-guided sampling in gastroenterology: European Society of Gastrointestinal Endoscopy (ESGE) Clinical Guideline—Updated January 2017. Endoscopy. 2017;49(7):695-714.
13. Morana G, Ciet P, Venturini S. Cystic pancreatic lesions: MR imaging findings and management. Insights Imaging. 2021;12(1):115.
14. Cohen-Scali F, Vilgrain V, Brancatelli G, Hammel P, Vullierme MP, Sauvanet A, et al. Discrimination of unilocular macro-cystic serous cystadenoma from pancreatic pseudocyst and mucinous cystadenoma with CT: initial observations. Radiology. 2003;228(3):727-33.
15. Sarr MG, Murr M, Smyrk TC, Yeo CJ, Fernandez-del-Castillo C, Hawes RH, et al. Primary cystic neoplasms of the pancreas. Neoplastic disorders of emerging importance-current state-of-the-art and unanswered questions. J Gastrointest Surg. 2003;7(3):417-28.
16. Megibow AJ, Baker ME, Morgan DE, Kamel IR, Sahani DV, Newman E, et al. Management of Incidental Pancreatic Cysts: A White Paper of the ACR Incidental Findings Committee. J Am Coll Radiol. 2017;14(7):911-23.
17. Sidden CR, Mortele KJ. Cystic tumors of the pancreas: ultrasound, computed tomography, and magnetic resonance imaging features. Semin Ultrasound CT MR. 2007;28(5): 339-56.
18. Zhong N, Zhang L, Takahashi N, Shalmiyev V, Canto MI, Clain JE, et al. Histologic and imaging features of mural nodules in mucinous pancreatic cysts. Clin Gastroenterol Hepatol. 2012;10(2):192-8.
19. Procacci C, Carbognin G, Accordini S, Biasiutti C, Guarise A, Lombardo F, et al. CT features of malignant mucinous cystic tumors of the pancreas. Eur Radiol. 2001;11(9):1626-30.
20. Nilsson LN, Keane MG, Shamali A, Millastre Bocos J, Marijinissen van Zanten M, Antila A, et al. Nature and management of pancreatic mucinous cystic neoplasm (MCN): A systematic review of the literature. Pancreatology. 2016;16(6):1028-36.
21. Ahmad M, Maegawa FB, De La Rosa E, Davis B, Tyroch A, Konstantinidis IT. Mucinous cystic neoplasms of the pancreas in the modern era. Experience with 707 patients. Am J Surg. 2020;220(6):1433-7.
22. Vege SS, Ziring B, Jain R, Moayyedi P; Clinical Guidelines Committee; American Gastroenterology Association. American gastroenterological association institute guideline on the diagnosis and management of asymptomatic neoplastic pancreatic cysts. Gastroenterology. 2015;148(4):819-quize13.
23. Yoon WJ, Brugge WR. Pancreatic cystic neoplasms: diagnosis and management. Gastroenterol Clin North Am. 2012;41(1):103-18.
24. Sahani DV, Lin DJ, Venkatesan AM, Sainani N, Mino-Kenudson M, Brugge WR, et al. Multidisciplinary approach to diagnosis and management of intraductal papillary mucinous neoplasms of the pancreas. Clin Gastroenterol Hepatol. 2009;7(3):259-69.
25. Machado NO, Al Qadhi H, Al Wahibi K. Intraductal Papillary Mucinous Neoplasm of Pancreas. N Am J Med Sci. 2015;7(5): 160-75.
26. Tanaka M, Fernández-del Castillo C, Adsay V, Chari S, Falconi M, Jang JY, et al. International consensus guidelines 2012 for the management of IPMN and MCN of the pancreas. Pancreatology. 2012;12(3):183-97.
27. Barral M, Soyer P, Dohan A, Laurent V, Hoeffel C, Fishman EK, et al. Magnetic resonance imaging of cystic pancreatic lesions in adults: an update in current diagnostic features and management. Abdom Imaging. 2014;39(1):48-65.
28. Uehara H, Nakaizumi A, Ishikawa O, Iishi H, Tatsumi K, Takakura R, et al. Development of ductal carcinoma of the

pancreas during follow-up of branch duct intraductal papillary mucinous neoplasm of the pancreas. Gut. 2008;57(11):1561-5.
29. Ingkakul T, Sadakari Y, Ienaga J, Satoh N, Takahata S, Tanaka M. Predictors of the presence of concomitant invasive ductal carcinoma in intraductal papillary mucinous neoplasm of the pancreas. Ann Surg. 2010;251(1):70-5.
30. Ikegawa T, Masuda A, Sakai A, Toyama H, Zen Y, Sofue K, et al. Multifocal cysts and incidence of pancreatic cancer concomitant with intraductal papillary mucinous neoplasm. Pancreatology. 2018;18(4):399-406.
31. Delavaud C, d'Assignies G, Cros J, Ruszniewski P, Hammel P, Levy P, et al. CT and MR imaging of multilocular acinar cell cystadenoma: comparison with branch duct intraductal papillary mucinous neoplasia (IPMNs). Eur Radiol. 2014;24(9): 2128-36.
32. Coleman KM, Doherty MC, Bigler SA. Solid-pseudopapillary tumor of the pancreas. Radiographics. 2003;23(6):1644-8.
33. Hao EIU, Hwang HK, Yoon DS, Lee WJ, Kang CM. Aggressiveness of solid pseudopapillary neoplasm of the pancreas: A literature review and meta-analysis. Medicine (Baltimore). 2018;97(49):e13147.
34. Eidt S, Jergas M, Schmidt R, Siedek M. Metastasis to the pancreas—an indication for pancreatic resection? Langenbecks Arch Surg. 2007;392(5):539-42.
35. Koomalsingh KJ, Fazylov R, Chorost MI, Horovitz J. Cystic teratoma of the pancreas: presentation, evaluation and management. JOP. 2006;7(6):643-6.
36. Seki M, Ninomiya E, Aruga A, Yamada K, Koga R, Saiura A, et al. Image-diagnostic features of mature cystic teratomas of the pancreas: report on two cases difficult to diagnose preoperatively. J Hepatobiliary Pancreat Surg. 2005;12(4): 336-40.
37. Kim H, Koh Y. Mature Cystic Teratoma of the Pancreas: A Rare Cystic Neoplasm. Open Med (Wars). 2019;14:872-4.
38. Matsushita D, Kurahara H, Mataki Y, Maemura K, Higashi M, Iino S, et al. Pancreatic hamartoma: a case report and literature review. BMC Gastroenterol. 2016;16:3.
39. Zhang J, Wang H, Tang X, Jiang Q, Wang C. Pancreatic hamartoma, a rare benign disease of the pancreas: A case report. Oncol Lett. 2016;11(6):3925-8.
40. Cui H, Lian Y, Chen F. Imaging findings for pancreatic Hamartoma: two case reports and a review of the literature. BMC Gastroenterol. 2020;20(1):37.
41. Eriksson B, Oberg K. Neuroendocrine tumours of the pancreas. Br J Surg. 2000;87(2):129-31.
42. Lewis RB, Lattin GE Jr, Paal E. Pancreatic endocrine tumors: radiologic-clinicopathologic correlation. Radiographics. 2010;30(6):1445-64.
43. Metz DC, Jensen RT. Gastrointestinal neuroendocrine tumors: pancreatic endocrine tumors. Gastroenterology. 2008;135(5):1469-92.
44. Guilmette JM, Nosé V. Neoplasms of the Neuroendocrine Pancreas: An Update in the Classification, Definition, and Molecular Genetic Advances. Adv Anat Pathol. 2019;26(1): 13-30.
45. Lu L, Shang Y, Mullins CS, Zhang X, Linnebacher M. Epidemiologic trends and prognostic risk factors of patients with pancreatic neuroendocrine neoplasms in the US: an updated population-based study. Future Oncol. 2021;17(5):549-63.
46. Hruban RH, Pitman MB, Klimstra DS, American Registry of Pathology, Armed Forces Institute of Pathology (U.S.). Tumors of the Pancreas. American Registry of Pathology in collaboration with the Armed Forces Institute of Pathology; 2007.
47. Rindi G, Klimstra DS, Abedi-Ardekani B, Asa SL, Bosman FT, Brambilla E, et al. A common classification framework for neuroendocrine neoplasms: an International Agency for Research on Cancer (IARC) and World Health Organization (WHO) expert consensus proposal. Mod Pathol. 2018;31(12):1770-86.
48. Galgano SJ, Morani AC, Gopireddy DR, Sharbidre K, Bates DDB, Goenka AH, et al. Pancreatic neuroendocrine neoplasms: a 2022 update for radiologists. Abdom Radiol (NY). 2022;47(12):3962-70.
49. Khanna L, Prasad SR, Sunnapwar A, Kondapaneni S, Dasyam A, Tammisetti VS, et al. Pancreatic Neuroendocrine Neoplasms: 2020 Update on Pathologic and Imaging Findings and Classification. Radiographics. 2020;40(5):1240-62.
50. Zhu JK, Wu D, Xu JW, Huang X, Jiang YY, Edil BH, et al. Cystic pancreatic neuroendocrine tumors: A distinctive subgroup with indolent biological behavior? A systematic review and meta-analysis. Pancreatology. 2019;19(5):738-50.
51. Kartalis N, Mucelli RM, Sundin A. Recent developments in imaging of pancreatic neuroendocrine tumors. Ann Gastroenterol. 2015;28(2):193-202.
52. Fidler JL, Fletcher JG, Reading CC, Andrews JC, Thompson GB, Grant CS, et al. Reoperative detection of pancreatic insulinomas on multiphasic helical CT. AJR Am J Roentgenol. 2003;181(3):775-80.
53. Gouya H, Vignaux O, Augui J, Dousset B, Palazzo L, Louvel A, et al. CT, endoscopic sonography, and a combined protocol for preoperative evaluation of pancreatic insulinomas. AJR Am J Roentgenol. 2003;181(4):987-92.
54. Thoeni RF, Mueller-Lisse UG, Chan R, Do NK, Shyn PB. Detection of small, functional islet cell tumors in the pancreas: selection of MR imaging sequences for optimal sensitivity. Radiology. 2000;214(2):483-90.
55. Zimmer T, Scherübl H, Faiss S, Stölzel U, Riecken EO, Wiedenmann B. Endoscopic ultrasonography of neuro-endocrine tumours. Digestion. 2000;62(Suppl 1):45-50.
56. Matsumoto T, Okabe H, Yamashita YI, Yusa T, Itoyama R, Nakao Y, et al. Clinical role of fludeoxyglucose (18F) positron emission tomography/computed tomography (18F-FDG PET/CT) in patients with pancreatic neuroendocrine tumors. Surg Today. 2019;49(1):21-6.
57. Howe JR, Merchant NB, Conrad C, Keutgen XM, Hallet J, Drebin JA, et al. The North American Neuroendocrine Tumor Society Consensus Paper on the Surgical Management of Pancreatic Neuroendocrine Tumors. Pancreas. 2020;49(1):1-33.
58. Falconi M, Bartsch DK, Eriksson B, Klöppel G, Lopes JM, O'Connor JM, et al. ENETS Consensus Guidelines for the

management of patients with digestive neuroendocrine neoplasms of the digestive system: well-differentiated pancreatic non-functioning tumors. Neuroendocrinology. 2012;95(2):120-34.

59. Singh RR, Gopakumar H, Sharma NR. Diagnosis and Management of Pancreatic Cysts: A Comprehensive Review of the Literature. Diagnostics (Basel). 2023;13(3):550.
60. Mansour JC, Chen H. Pancreatic endocrine tumors. J Surg Res. 2004;120(1):139-61.
61. Whipple AO, Frantz VK. Adenoma of islet cells with hyperinsulinism: a review. Ann Surg. 1935;101(6):1299-335.
62. Choi TW, Kim JH, Yu MH, Park SJ, Han JK. Pancreatic neuroendocrine tumor: prediction of the tumor grade using CT findings and computerized texture analysis. Acta Radiol. 2018;59(4):383-92.
63. Canellas R, Burk KS, Parakh A, Sahani DV. Prediction of Pancreatic Neuroendocrine Tumor Grade Based on CT Features and Texture Analysis. AJR Am J Roentgenol. 2018;210(2):341-6.

SECTION

5

Miscellaneous

CHAPTER 22

Madhurima Sharma, Mandeep Kang, Anindita Sinha, Uma Debi

Nontraumatic Acute Abdomen

INTRODUCTION

The term "acute abdomen" includes a spectrum of medical and surgical conditions ranging from benign self-limiting to life-threatening conditions in a patient presenting with severe abdominal pain, developing over a period of hours.[1] Acute abdominal pain comprises of 4–5% of all admissions to the emergency department.[2] Acute abdomen may be due to a variety of diseases which may involve the gastrointestinal (GI) system, biliary tree, solid viscera, or genitourinary system. Acute appendicitis is the most common cause of an acute abdomen, particularly in young adults. In a review of 10,682 patients presenting with an acute abdomen, acute appendicitis accounted for 28% of cases, followed by acute cholecystitis (9.7%), small bowel obstruction (4.1%), gynecologic disorders (4%), acute pancreatitis (2.9%), renal colic (2.9%), peptic ulcer disease (2.5%), cancer (1.5%), diverticular disease (1.5%), and a variety of less common conditions (9%).[3] In about one-third of cases, the cause of the abdominal pain remains indeterminate or nonspecific. Early identification of patients who require surgical management allows for timely management thereby reducing associated morbidity and mortality. However, on account of the considerable overlap of symptoms and signs in an acute abdomen, the clinical accuracy for the specific diagnosis is low, ranging from 50 to 65%.[4] This limitation emphasizes the importance of imaging in the diagnostic workup of the acute abdomen.

Various imaging modalities available for investigating the acute abdomen include conventional radiography, contrast studies, ultrasound, computed tomography (CT), and magnetic resonance imaging (MRI). The choice of the initial modality to be used should be guided by the disease suspected on clinical grounds, e.g., plain radiographs continue to be the initial imaging modality in cases of intestinal obstruction and perforation.[5] Contrast examinations have a limited role in evaluation of acute abdomen. US is the ideal screening modality for suspected hepatobiliary disease or for suspected pelvic pathology such as ectopic gestation or acute pelvic inflammatory disease (PID).

The introduction of multidetector computed tomography (MDCT) has impacted imaging of all organs of the body, especially the abdomen.[6] Because of the greater speed of *Z*-axis coverage and thinner sections with 3D reconstruction, MDCT has become the imaging modality of choice for evaluation of the acute abdomen. It provides a comprehensive view of all the intra-abdominal solid and hollow viscera, as well as the peritoneum, mesentery, lymph nodes, and retroperitoneum. Data can be acquired in different phases making MDCT an ideal modality for evaluation of suspected mesenteric ischemia or vascular disorders like abdominal aortic aneurysms. Low dose unenhanced CT has replaced excretory urography as the screening method of choice for the evaluation of renal colic in most centers.[6] Recent improvements in resolution and development of faster breath-hold sequences have drastically increased the utility of MRI in evaluation of the gut. However, MRI is still not routinely used for evaluation of an acute abdomen except in situations where iodinated contrast cannot be administered or in pregnant patients.

According to American College of Radiology (ACR) appropriateness criteria, contrast enhanced CT of the abdomen and pelvis is considered the imaging modality of choice for initial evaluation of acute nonlocalized abdominal pain and fever.[7] US is considered as the initial imaging modality of choice in patients with right upper quadrant pain with suspected biliary disease. For initial imaging evaluation of patients with right lower quadrant pain (including suspected appendicitis) ACR recommends contrast enhanced CT of the abdomen and pelvis.[8] However, in pregnant patients with right lower quadrant pain and suspected appendicitis, ACR recommends US and MRI as the initial imaging modalities of choice.[9]

PLAIN RADIOGRAPHS IN EVALUATION OF THE ACUTE ABDOMEN

Conventional radiography has limited diagnostic accuracy in workup of the patients with acute abdominal pain. One study has reported accuracy of 56% in the diagnosis of acute abdomen.[10] In another study, only 4% of patients had a change in the treatment based upon conventional radiography.[11] In a retrospective study of 871 patients, Ahn et al., reported best sensitivity of plain radiographs for detection of foreign bodies (90%) and bowel perforation (47%), while the sensitivity of plain radiographs was 0% in detection of acute appendicitis, pyelonephritis, diverticulitis, and pancreatitis.[12] However, plain radiographs still remain an important initial investigation in the evaluation of a patient with acute abdomen. Conventional radiography is widely available, can be easily performed, and can be used to exclude intestinal obstruction and hollow viscus perforation in the emergency department. Interpretation of these radiographs represents a formidable challenge to the radiologist, as the findings may be nonspecific, confusing, or even misleading at times.[5]

Perforation

In the past, a minimum three film radiographic series was recommended for evaluation of an acute abdomen. These included a supine film of the abdomen and erect radiographs of the abdomen and chest **(Figs. 1A to C)**. More recently, it has been demonstrated that the erect film of the abdomen can be eliminated from the initial series without significant loss of the diagnostic information.[13] The upright chest film is ideal for demonstrating free air as the X-ray beam strikes the hemidiaphragms tangentially at their highest point and at an optimal exposure. Classical studies have shown that as little as 1 mL of free air can be detected below the right hemidiaphragm, provided the patient has been in an erect position for at least 10–15 minutes prior to obtaining the radiograph.[14,15] The chest radiograph may also reveal chest diseases such as pneumonia, pulmonary or myocardial infarction which may mimic an acute abdomen. If the patient cannot sit or stand up a left lateral decubitus film will demonstrate air between the opacity of the liver and the abdominal wall. If the patient is too ill to roll over, a cross-table lateral view of the abdomen is obtained **(Fig. 2)**.

Various signs of pneumoperitoneum can be seen even on supine films if carefully searched for. The signs include "Rigler's" or "double wall" sign describing visualization of both the mucosal and serosal aspect of the bowel wall due to presence of intra- and extraluminal air **(Fig. 3)**. The falciform ligament may be outlined by air in the epigastrium just to the right of the midline. The "football" sign is due to presence of large quantity of air which fills the peritoneal cavity. The lateral umbilical ligaments may be visualized in the lower abdomen known as the "inverted V" sign. Free air in Morrison's pouch may be seen as an oval radiolucency in the subhepatic region. The right upper quadrant may appear radiolucent due to air collecting between the anterior surface of liver and the abdominal wall. The under surface of the central part of the diaphragm may be visualized—the "cupola" sign.[16] Retroperitoneal perforation of a duodenal ulcer results in air outlining the renal or psoas shadows **(Fig. 4)**. Large bowel may also perforate into the retroperitoneal space resulting in mottled extraluminal air lucencies. Plain films are inferior to CT for the detection of free intraperitoneal air. Supine abdominal films may detect free air in only about 60% of the cases, whereas CT can reliably detect even small amounts of free air which is usually seen just beneath the anterior abdominal wall or in the peritoneal recesses. Viewing the scan at wide window settings (lung window) increases the sensitivity of CT for the detection of free air.[14]

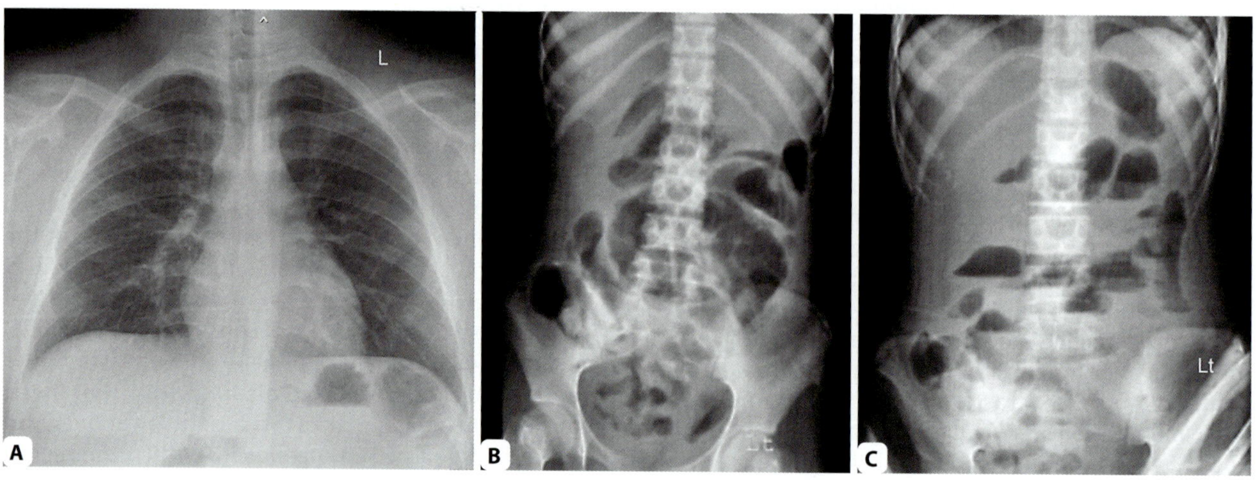

FIGS. 1A TO C: Abdominal series (Three views of the abdomen): (A) Chest X-ray reveals absence of free air under the domes of diaphragm; (B) Supine film shows dilated jejunal and ileal loops with no air in the large bowel; (C) Erect film demonstrates multiple air-fluid levels in a case of distal small bowel obstruction.

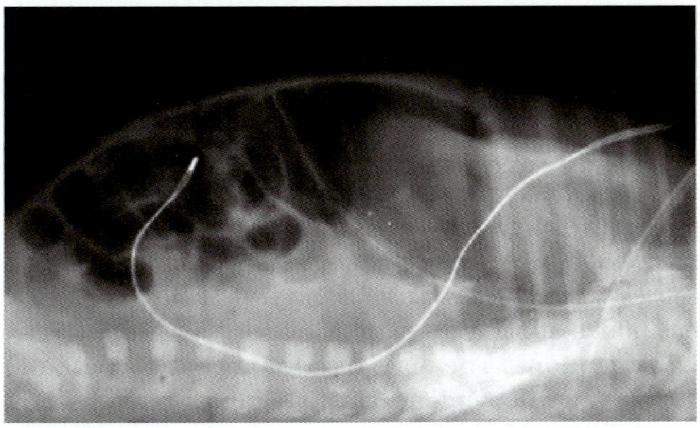

FIG. 2: Cross-table lateral view of a premature neonate reveals free intraperitoneal air in a case of necrotizing enterocolitis.

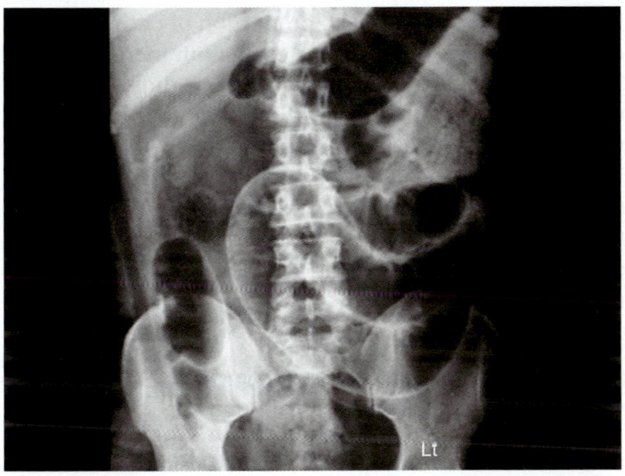

FIG. 3: X-ray abdomen, supine film. Both the inner and outer walls of the small bowel loop are visualized due to the presence of free intraperitoneal air. Air is also seen in the subhepatic region (Morrison's pouch).

Intestinal Obstruction

The diagnosis of intestinal obstruction may be correctly suggested on the basis of plain films alone in nearly 80% of the cases. Additional imaging with US and CT is required in equivocal cases and also to determine the level and cause of obstruction. In mechanical obstruction, plain films reveal dilated, gas-filled bowel loops with air-fluid levels proximal to the obstruction with collapsed loops with absence of air distal to the obstruction **(Figs. 1A to C)**. Dilatation of both small and large bowel loops from stomach to rectum indicates a diagnosis of paralytic ileus. It may not always be possible to differentiate between mechanical obstruction and paralytic ileus. A lateral view to look for air in the rectum may aid in the differentiation, however CT or contrast studies may be required in equivocal cases.[5,14]

Distinction between small and large bowel loops on plain films is based on the central position of the small bowel, presence of valvulae conniventes in the jejunum, and tubular featureless appearance of the ileum. The dilated loops measure between 3 and 5 cm. The valvulae conniventes form thin, 1–2 mm complete rings at intervals of 1 mm. In contrast, the large bowel loops are located peripherally, usually measure >5 cm in diameter and display haustral markings that are incomplete, 2–3 mm wide and occurring at intervals of 1 cm.[17] The erect film in a normal person usually displays 2–3 fluid levels in the small bowel which do not exceed 3 cm in caliber. Dilated fluid-filled loops of small bowel may be identified as oval or round soft tissue densities.[5] At times, the bowel loops proximal to the site of obstruction may get completely filled with fluid resulting in a gasless abdomen. When a tiny amount of gas accompanies a large amount of intraluminal fluid, small gas bubbles get trapped between the valvulae conniventes resulting in the "string-of-beads" sign **(Fig. 5)**.[2] This appearance is virtually diagnostic of mechanical obstruction as it is never seen with paralytic ileus.

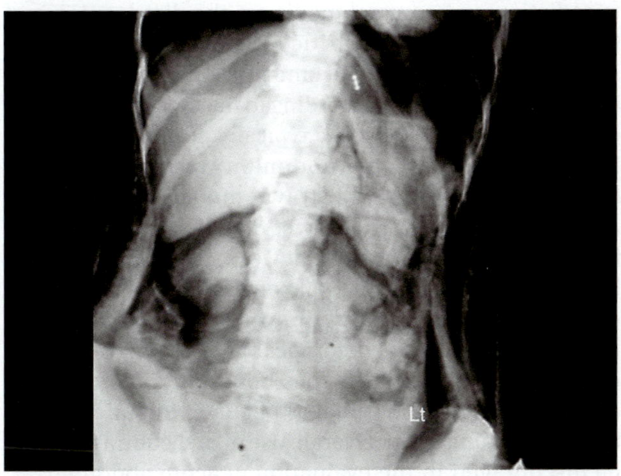

FIG. 4: Plain radiograph abdomen, erect film shows large amount of free air in the upper abdomen. In addition, air is also seen outlining the right kidney suggestive of pneumoperitoneum in a case of perforated duodenal ulcer.

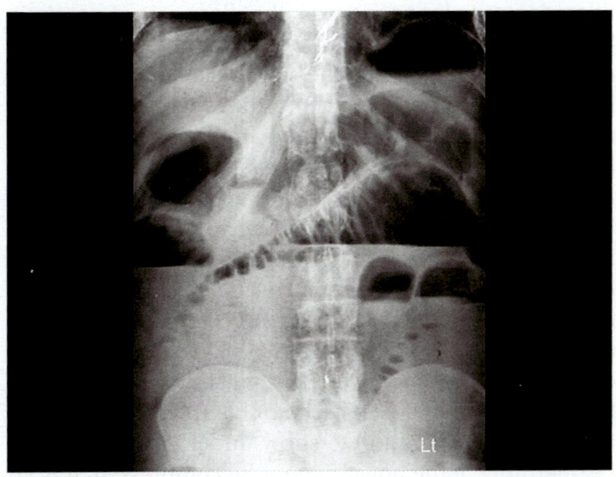

FIG. 5: X-ray abdomen, erect view shows multiple air-fluid levels in the proximal jejunal loops with "string of beads" sign.

Miscellaneous Conditions

Apart from perforation and intestinal obstruction, plain films may sometimes reveal important findings which may clinch the diagnosis or indirectly suggest the possible diagnosis such as:

- Presence of intramural and intraluminal gas in the gallbladder in patients with emphysematous cholecystitis.
- Presence of air in the biliary tree with small gut obstruction due to gallstone ileus caused by erosion of the gallstone into the duodenum.
- Presence of localized duodenal ileus (sentinel loop), dilated transverse colon with "colon cut-off" in case of acute pancreatitis.
- Presence of extraluminal mottled gas in patients with abdominal abscess.
- Presence of soft tissue mass with obliteration of properitoneal fat line in the right lower quadrant and scoliosis with convexity to the left in patients of acute appendicular abscess.
- Presence of gas in the perinephric region in cases of emphysematous pyelonephritis.
- Presence of intestinal pneumatosis or portomesenteric air in mesenteric ischemia.

ULTRASONOGRAPHY

Ultrasonography (US) is another imaging modality commonly used in the diagnostic workup of patients with acute abdominal pain. Wide availability, low cost, and absence of radiation exposure are few of the advantages of US. US is a real-time dynamic examination that can reveal the presence or absence of peristalsis and depict blood flow. Thus, US can be beneficial in cases of suspected intestinal obstruction when it is difficult to differentiate between mechanical obstruction and paralytic ileus on plain radiographs. It demonstrates increased peristalsis in cases of mechanical obstruction, whereas presence of dilated, atonic loops suggests the diagnosis of paralytic ileus. US is also helpful in localizing intra-abdominal abscesses, particularly in the solid viscera. Furthermore, it is possible to correlate US findings with the point of maximal tenderness. Dynamic examination is also useful in the evaluation of bowel hernias through the Valsalva maneuver. This maneuver may reveal an intermittent hernia and may show the contiguity of a mass with the intraperitoneal space thereby allowing better depiction of the hernial sac or abdominal wall defect, and showing reducibility.[18] The most common US technique used to examine patients with acute abdominal pain is the graded-compression procedure.[19] With this technique, interposing fat and bowel can be displaced or compressed by means of gradual compression to show underlying structures. Furthermore, if the bowel cannot be compressed, it is an indication of inflammation.

Color and power Doppler imaging supplement the information provided by gray-scale imaging. Increased vascularity is visualized in a number of inflammatory, infectious, or neoplastic diseases. For example, hyperemia, both of the bowel wall and adjacent mesentery, is a marker of disease activity in inflammatory bowel disease while diminished vascularity is a sign of ischemia. US may be as effective as radiography at diagnosing pneumoperitoneum. Transvaginal imaging could be very useful in the evaluation of acute abdominal pain from gynecologic causes. It could also be useful for the evaluation of deeply positioned appendixes, terminal ileitis, sigmoid, or rectal inflammation.[20] The main disadvantages of ultrasound are operator dependence, including high interobserver variability, and lack of tissue penetration in obese patients. In one study, US reportedly provided useful information for 56% of the patients with acute abdominal pain,[21] and in another study, it either yielded unique diagnostic information or confirmed one of the differential diagnoses in 65% of the patients.[22] The proportion of patients with a correct diagnosis after clinical evaluation increased from 70 to 83% after evaluation with US in a study conducted on 496 patients presenting with acute abdominal pain in the emergency department.[23] In a study by Lameris et al., US was used as the primary imaging modality, followed by CT only in cases of negative or indeterminate sonographic findings, resulted in the highest sensitivity for acute abdominal and pelvic conditions while reducing exposure to ionizing radiation.[24]

COMPUTED TOMOGRAPHY

The utility of CT in the diagnosis and management of acute abdominal emergencies is well established. CT is easily available, has short acquisition time, and provides multiplanar reconstructions. CT provides greater accuracy than US or plain radiography for the evaluation of acute abdomen. It has high sensitivity and specificity for evaluating most common emergent pathologies such as acute appendicitis and diverticulitis. However, exposure to radiation and contrast media are the disadvantages of CT.[1] The technique used for acquisition of the image data set is of paramount importance for accurate diagnosis and should be tailored according to the most likely clinical diagnosis. Traditionally, the typically described protocol for evaluating an acute abdomen was to administer both positive oral and intravenous contrast media. Although rectal or oral contrast material may be helpful in differentiating fluid-filled bowel loops from abscesses in some cases, the use of oral contrast material can slow down patient throughput and negatively impacts the management in cases of surgical abdomen. The lack of enteral contrast medium does not seem to hamper the accurate reading of CT images obtained in patients with acute abdominal pain. Overall, use of oral contrast should be discouraged in the evaluation of acute abdomen.[25,26] Intravenous nonionic iodinated contrast helps in better depiction of inflammatory as well as neoplastic pathology, enables differentiation of lymph nodes from vessels and detection of vascular complications. 100–120 mL of contrast is injected at a rate of 2.8–3.5 mL/s and images routinely obtained in the portal venous phase at a delay of 70 seconds. Arterial phase imaging or dual energy scanning can be added, depending on the most likely clinical diagnosis. Scanning should be performed from the domes of the diaphragm to the pubic symphysis using a slice thickness of 5–10 mm which can be retrospectively reconstructed to thinner sections for various 3D reconstructions.

Prospective studies have shown that CT findings have a significant effect on diagnoses in cases of acute abdomen. In one study, the accuracy of the clinical diagnosis made before performing CT improved from 71 to 93% after CT was performed.[27] Another study revealed a significant increase in the level of confidence of the diagnosis made with CT: The treatment management for 60% of patients was changed.[28] In a cohort study comparing US and CT in 1,021 consecutive patients, CT was significantly more sensitive than ultrasound (89% vs. 70%, $p < 0.001$).[24]

In recent years, dual energy CT has emerged as a promising tool in the evaluation of various acute abdominal pathologies. Because of its ability to characterize materials based upon their differential attenuation, dual energy CT can selectively identify iodine, thereby allowing for identification of hyperenhancement (in inflammatory conditions) or hypoenhancement (in ischemic conditions) of an organ. Dual energy CT can also determine composition of stone in urolithiasis and can accurately distinguish between uric acid and nonuric acid calculi. Virtual noncontrast images can be reconstructed in cases of GI hemorrhage or acute aortic syndromes, obviating the need for true noncontrast scan. Active contrast extravasation can be more visible on dual energy CT due to increased conspicuity of iodine.[29]

MAGNETIC RESONANCE IMAGING

The MRI is potentially an attractive alternative to CT for evaluation of acute abdominal pain. Although MRI currently plays only a limited role in the assessment of acute abdominal pain, its utility in the pregnant and pediatric population has already been demonstrated. Lack of exposure to ionizing radiation and high intrinsic soft tissue contrast are the major advantages of MRI. MRI also allows for additional opportunities such as diffusion-weighted imaging (DWI), which are not available with CT, which may prove valuable in the assessment of the acute abdomen.[30] However, availability, cost, and long acquisition time of MRI with multiple breath-hold sequences remain the limiting factors for its utilization in the emergency department. Recent technical advances have led to development of faster imaging sequences particularly suited to the emergency department. Currently MRI is indicated for evaluation of pregnant patients with suspected appendicitis and has shown high sensitivity and specificity.[30] MRI also can be used to evaluate hepatobiliary pathologies, particularly magnetic resonance cholangiopancreatography (MRCP) for choledocholithiasis.

ROLE OF CROSS-SECTIONAL IMAGING IN SPECIFIC DISEASE ENTITIES

Acute Appendicitis

Acute appendicitis is one of the most common causes of acute abdominal pain. Clinical diagnosis of appendicitis can be difficult due to nonspecific clinical features overlapping with other diseases. In about one-third of patients, presentation of acute appendicitis is atypical, resulting in a negative laparotomy rate of 20%, which rises to 35–45% in young women of reproductive age, in whom distinction from acute PID and other gynecological conditions such as torsion of ovarian cyst is difficult on clinical grounds alone.[31] Thus, imaging plays an important role in the diagnostic workup of patients with suspected acute appendicitis, thereby minimizing the rates of negative laparotomy. Plain radiography and contrast studies have a limited role in the diagnosis of acute appendicitis. On plain radiography, although the presence of an appendicolith suggests appendicitis, it is visualized on properly exposed radiographs in only 14% of all patients with appendicoliths.[13] At barium enema, lack of appendiceal visualization and presence of a cecal mass impression are nonspecific findings and not definitely diagnostic of appendicitis. Filling of the appendix up to its bulbous tip virtually excludes appendicitis, however, the appendix may not fill completely in up to one-third of normal individuals.[32] US is the screening modality of choice for initial evaluation in suspected appendicitis, followed by CT in selected cases. Graded compression sonography using high frequency linear transducers is a highly accurate technique with a sensitivity of 80–93%, specificity of 94–100% and an accuracy of 95–97% for the diagnosis of acute appendicitis.[33] Another technique for improving visualization of retrocecal appendix in obese or muscular patients is posterior manual compression of right lower quadrant in anterior or anteromedial direction using the left hand with simultaneous anterior graded compression by transducer. Turning the patient from supine position to left oblique lateral decubitus position also displaces cecum, terminal ileum, and appendix medially onto the psoas muscle, and reduces the depth of the lateral portion of the retrocecal area, thereby improving visualization of retrocecal appendix.[34]

The US criteria for a normal appendix are presence of a compressible, tubular, blind-ending structure filled with fluid, gas or feces, originating from the base of the cecum having a wall thickness of 2 mm or less and diameter of 6 mm or less. The sonographic diagnosis of acute appendicitis is based on one or more of the following: direct visualization of a concentrically layered, aperistaltic, noncompressible appendix with an anteroposterior diameter >6 mm, or echogenic incompressible periappendicular inflamed fat with or without an appendicolith **(Fig. 6)**. On color Doppler, increased flow signals in the appendiceal wall or periappendicular space allow confirmation of the diagnosis. Perforation should be suspected if there is loss of symmetry of the concentric layers of the wall or a right lower quadrant fluid collection without visualization of the inflamed appendix. However, inconclusive US studies may be seen in a right lower quadrant phlegmon or abscess without a visible appendix, retrocecal inflamed appendix, cecal edema or terminal ileum thickening, distal or tip appendicitis with a normal proximal appendix, obesity, and if there is pain limiting compression. A false-positive sonogram may be seen in Crohn's disease, cecal diverticulitis, and salpingitis.

Helical CT using thin sections (4–5 mm) has a higher reported sensitivity of 90–100%, specificity of 91–99%, and accuracy of 94–98% compared to US.[35] One of the CT hallmarks of acute appendicitis is appendiceal dilatation. Most authors have defined appendiceal thickening on CT as outer-wall-to-outer-wall transverse diameter greater than 6 mm (as mentioned in ultrasound literature). However, sonographic data of appendiceal diameter are based on graded compression technique, which may alter appendiceal diameter. Thus, sonographic criteria of appendiceal thickening may not be valid on CT. Brown et al.[36] reported that in 42% of asymptomatic patients, the normal appendix measures greater than 6 mm; they defined the upper limit of normal as 10 mm. Because of overlap between normal and abnormal appendix, the appendiceal diameter should be interpreted in conjunction with other clinical and CT findings.[37] Other CT signs of appendicitis include thickened and enhancing walls, an appendicolith, and periappendicular inflammatory changes in the form of fat stranding, phlegmon, fluid, abscess, or adenopathy **(Figs. 7A and B)**. Inflammatory changes can be seen in

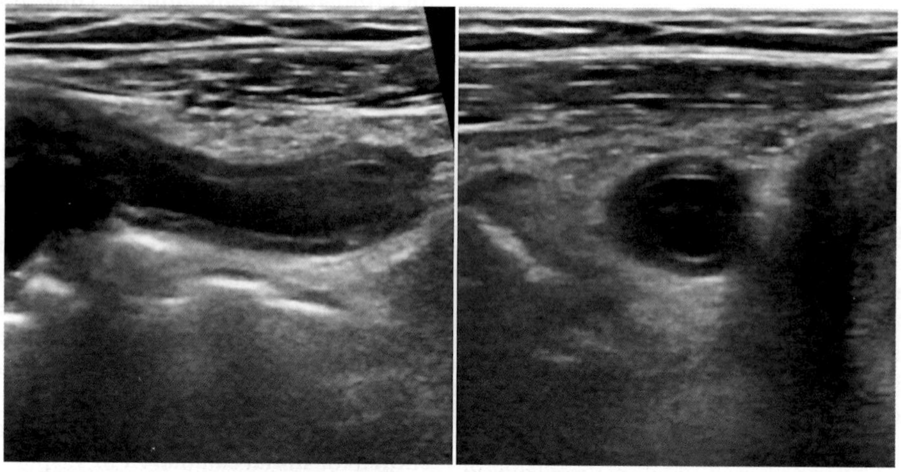

FIG. 6: Acute appendicitis: Longitudinal and transverse sonogram images showing the classical target lesion in the right iliac fossa due to inflamed, incompressible appendix with thickened walls.

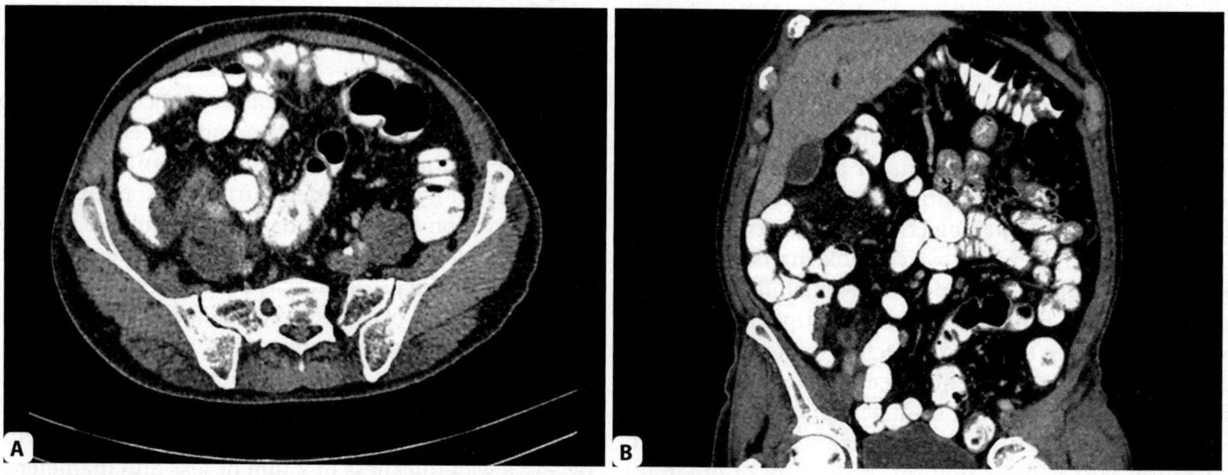

FIGS. 7A AND B: Acute appendicitis: Contrast-enhanced computed tomography (CECT) abdomen, (A) Axial; and (B) Coronal images show fluid filled dilated appendix with mural thickening and adjacent fat stranding in a case of acute appendicitis. Also note the soft tissue thickening at base of appendix separating it from cecum suggestive of cecal bar sign.

adjacent cecum like circumferential mural thickening, cecal apical thickening, or the "arrowhead" sign which results due to funneling of contrast medium on both sides of the inflamed cecal apex coming to a point at the occluded orifice of the appendix. As the "arrowhead" sign highlights extension of inflammation to the upper portion of cecum, it may identify patients who require more than standard ligation appendectomy. The "cecal bar" sign refers to inflammatory soft tissue at the base of the appendix that separates the appendix from the contrast-filled cecum. CT can also demonstrate various complications of appendicitis like perforation **(Fig. 8)**, periappendiceal abscess, gangrenous appendicitis, peritonitis, and bowel obstruction. In addition, CT is also of special value in suggesting an alternative diagnosis in patients who do not have appendicitis. MRI is a good imaging modality in pregnant patients and pediatric population, in whom ionizing radiation is of high concern. MRI has demonstrated high specificity and sensitivity for appendicitis in pediatric and pregnant patients.[30]

Acute Cholecystitis

Acute cholecystitis is a potentially life-threatening emergency requiring prompt diagnosis and treatment. Sonography is the primary imaging modality of choice for evaluating acute inflammatory conditions of the gallbladder (GB). Acute cholecystitis is associated with gallstones in 90–96% of patients with a calculus causing cystic duct obstruction being the most common cause. Sensitive sonographic features are positive Murphy's sign (in 96% of patients with acute cholecystitis), calculi (in 95%), and a thickened GB wall (in 73%).[38] However, these signs are not specific and may occur in other conditions such as chronic cholecystitis, pancreatitis, cirrhosis, or hepatitis. Other sonographic signs include distension of the GB, edematous wall, mucosal irregularity, intramural gas, and/or pericholecystic collection **(Fig. 9)**. Doppler sonography improves diagnostic confidence in acute cholecystitis by revealing mural hypervascularity. Acalculous cholecystitis accounts for minority of acute cholecystitis cases but carries high mortality and morbidity. Increased intraluminal pressure in GB due to decreased motility and bile stasis in critically-ill patients is the cause of acalculous cholecystitis.[39] Imaging findings are similar to calculous cholecystitis except for presence of GB stones. Sonographic Murphy's sign is difficult to elicit in these patients due to altered mental status and sedation.

The CT scan may be used as an adjunct to US if sonography is inconclusive, especially in acalculous cholecystitis or when complications such as perforation or emphysematous cholecystitis are suspected.[40] CT findings of acute cholecystitis include wall thickening, pericholecystic stranding, GB distension, pericholecystic fluid, subserosal edema, high attenuation bile and sloughed membranes, gas, or septations within the GB.[41] MRI can be a valuable complement to US and CT in demonstrating impacted calculi in the GB neck or cystic duct which are often difficult to detect on US. Also, conditions causing acalculous cholecystitis such as adenomyomatosis, GB polyp, malignant neoplasm, or other cancers can be depicted on magnetic resonance (MR).[42]

Complications of acute cholecystitis include the following:

- *Empyema*: It occurs when pus fills the distended and inflamed GB, typically in diabetic patients. On US and CT, pus resembles sludge. Heavily T2-weighted image (T2WI) is sensitive in demonstrating purulent bile as a dependent hypointense layer relative to normal bile.
- *Gangrenous cholecystitis*: Gangrenous cholecystitis is an advanced, severe form of acute cholecystitis, seen more commonly in elderly men. It results from marked distension of the GB with resultant increase in tension in the wall. Associated inflammation leads to

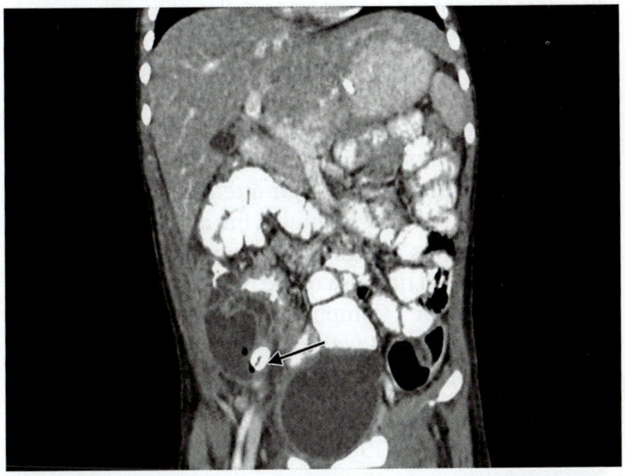

FIG. 8: Acute appendicitis with perforation: Coronal oblique reformatted computed tomography (CT) image demonstrating fluid filled inflamed appendix with appendicolith at its base (arrow) with adjacent air containing loculated collection in right iliac fossa.

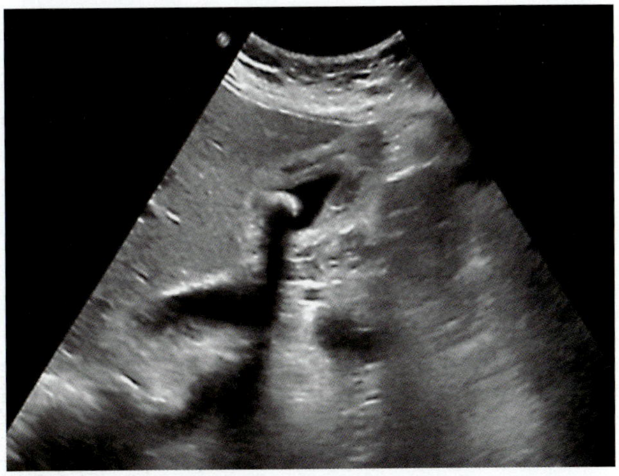

FIG. 9: Acute cholecystitis: Ultrasound image showing calculus in gallbladder (GB) lumen with diffusely thickened walls. Sonographic Murphy's sign was positive.

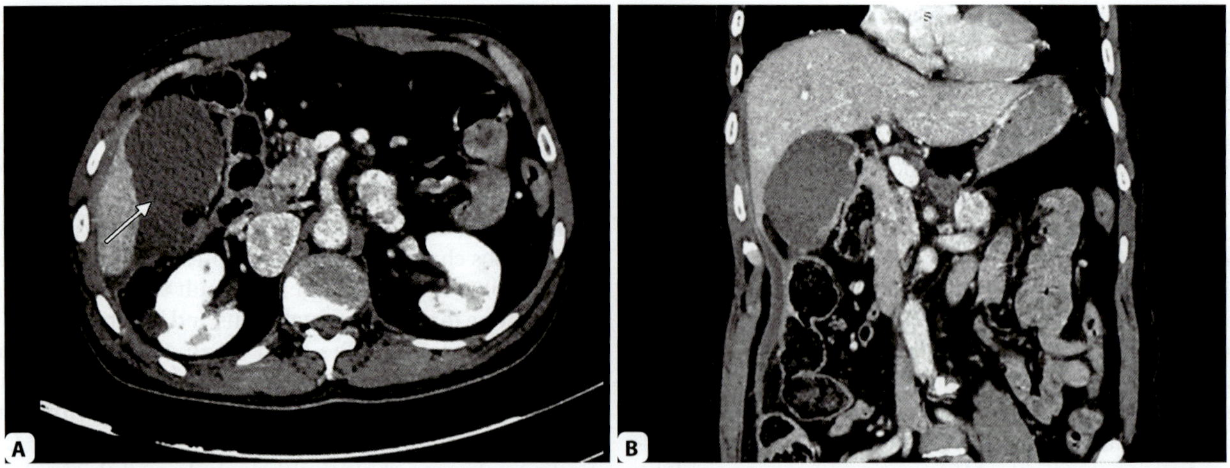

FIGS. 10A AND B: Gangrenous cholecystitis: (A) Axial; and (B) Coronal computed tomography (CT) images showing absent mural enhancement of gallbladder at places with indistinct wall and pericholecystic collection (arrow).

ischemic necrosis. US reveals heterogeneous or striated thickening of GB wall or intraluminal membranes representing desquamated mucosa. US findings typical of uncomplicated acute cholecystitis may be absent in this subset of patients. GB wall thickness may be <3 mm or Murphy's sign may be absent due to denervation of the GB wall.[43] CT features consist of intraluminal membranes, irregular wall, pericholecystic fluid/abscess, and lack of mural enhancement **(Figs. 10A and B)**.

- *Gallbladder perforation*: Gallbladder perforation is most often a complication of acute gangrenous cholecystitis. As blood supply is poor in the region of fundus, this is the most common site of perforation. Perforation can be classified into three types:
  1. Acute free perforation into peritoneal cavity,
  2. Subacute perforation with pericholecystic abscess, and
  3. Chronic perforation with a cholecystoenteric fistula.[44] Subacute perforations are the most common. Following perforation, US, CT, and MR show complex pericholecystic fluid collections and the wall of GB can appear focally disrupted **(Figs. 11 and 12)**.
- *Emphysematous cholecystitis*: Emphysematous cholecystitis is a rare form of acute cholecystitis seen in patients with diabetes and peripheral atherosclerotic disease. The majority of patients are between 50 and 70 years. US demonstrates intraluminal and intramural gas as highly echogenic foci. CT is the most sensitive and specific imaging modality to identify gas in the lumen or wall **(Fig. 13)**.[45]
- *Hemorrhagic cholecystitis*: It can complicate acute calculous or acalculous cholecystitis, and the patient presents with acute biliary colic, jaundice, melena, and hematemesis.[45] It needs to be differentiated from other causes of GB hemorrhage, which include trauma, tumors, and coagulopathy states. US shows echogenic or heterogeneous material within the GB lumen or wall, which are seen as high-attenuation contents on CT. MRI can be quite helpful in the diagnosis. Subacute blood products are generally hyperintense on both T1WI and T2WI because of the presence of extracellular methemoglobin.[45] Complications of hemorrhagic cholecystitis include GB wall perforation and associated potentially life-threatening hemoperitoneum.[46]

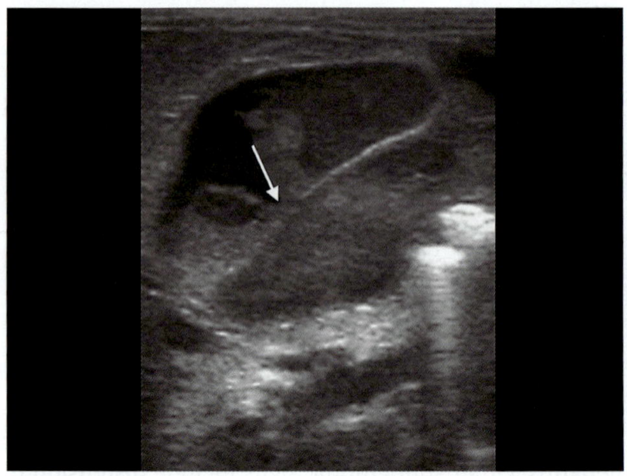

FIG. 11: Gallbladder perforation: Ultrasound image showing a rent in the gallbladder wall (arrow) with a large collection adjacent to the rent in a case of acute cholecystitis with gallbladder perforation.

Acute Pancreatitis

Acute pancreatitis is an acute inflammatory process of the pancreas which may range in severity from a mild parenchymal edema to severe necrotizing pancreatitis with variable involvement of other regional tissues or remote

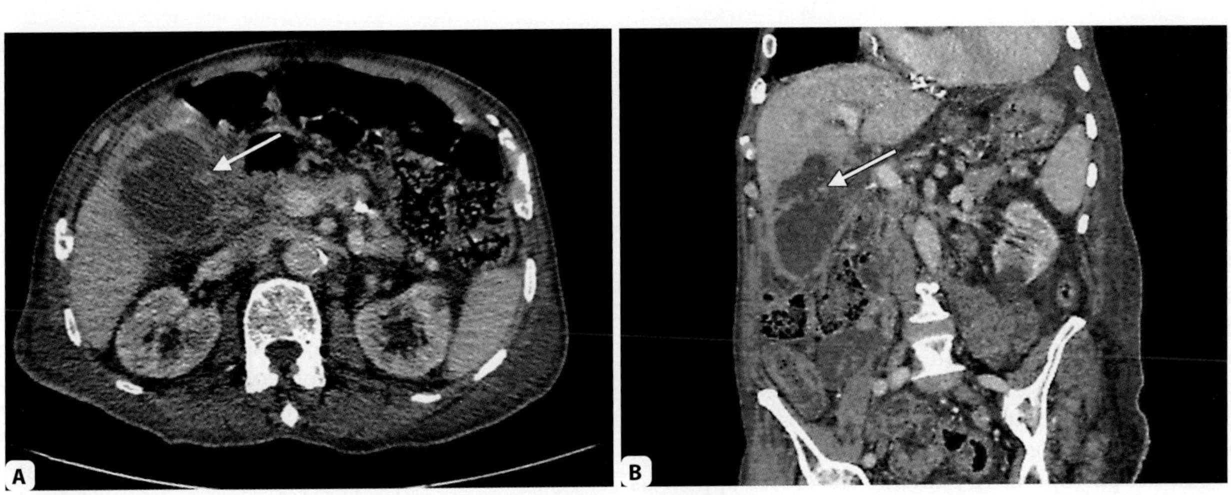

FIGS. 12A AND B: Gallbladder perforation: (A) Axial; and (B) Coronal computed tomography (CT) images showing thickened gallbladder wall with a rent (arrow) and adjacent intrahepatic collection in a case of acute cholecystitis with gallbladder perforation.

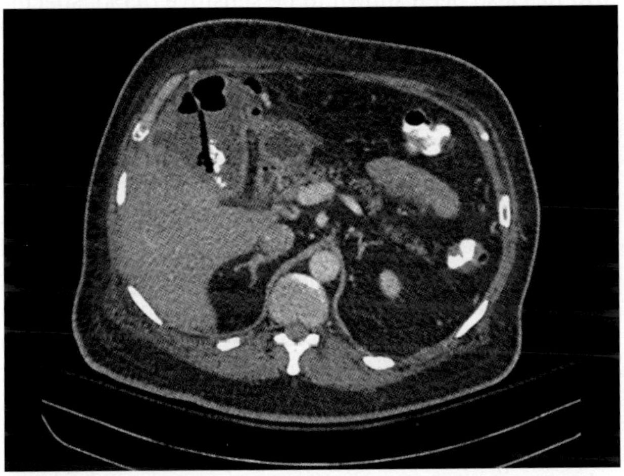

FIG. 13: Emphysematous cholecystitis: Axial CT image showing cholelithiasis with irregularity of gallbladder wall with multiple intraluminal air foci.

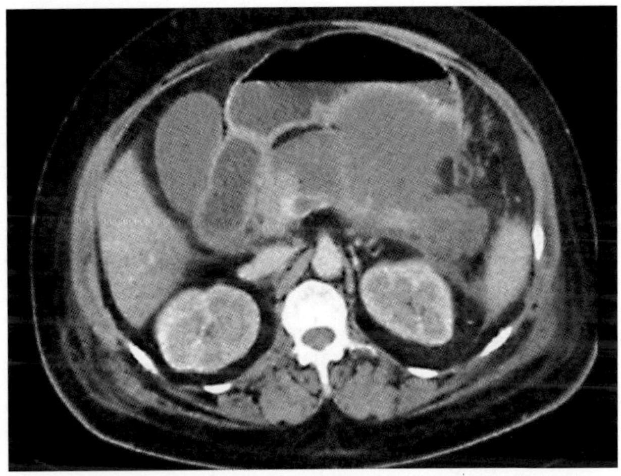

FIG. 14: Acute necrotizing pancreatitis: Axial CT Image shows the body and tail of the pancreas are hypodense with only a small amount of normally enhancing parenchyma seen in the head of pancreas. There are extrapancreatic collections with a hypodense filling defect in the portal vein due to thrombosis [modified computed tomography severity index (CTSI)-10].

organ systems. Most of the patients with the mild form of the disease have an uneventful recovery, however, the cases with severe pancreatitis show significant mortality and morbidity with development of failure of various organ systems and require aggressive management. The diagnosis of acute pancreatitis is usually made on clinical grounds supported by laboratory data. The role of imaging is to confirm the diagnosis in inconclusive cases, stage the severity of disease, and detect complications such as infection, pseudocyst formation, or vascular involvement. US may reveal an enlarged, hypoechoic pancreas in the early stages with presence of peripancreatic fluid. It may also detect the presence of cholelithiasis or choledocholithiasis which is a major etiological factor for acute pancreatitis. It can also be used in the follow-up of acute fluid collections or pseudocysts particularly after percutaneous catheter drainage.

Contrast-enhanced CT is the modality of choice not only to confirm the diagnosis or detect extra-pancreatic intra-abdominal disease, but also to stage the severity of disease which is required for prognostication.[47] It is also highly accurate for the detection of necrosis and complications **(Fig. 14)**. The various grading systems, complications related to pancreatitis as well as pancreatic interventions have already been discussed in detail in Chapter 18 of this book: Acute Pancreatitis: Imaging and Interventions.

The MRI has also been reported to have similar accuracy to MDCT for the diagnosis of acute pancreatitis and assigning a severity index. MRI is useful in patients with deranged renal functions, allergy to iodinated contrast, and pregnant patients. MRI is more sensitive than CT for detection of hemorrhagic pancreatitis and for demonstrating ductal communication of the collection. Associated choledocholithiasis is also better depicted on MRI. MRI with DWI is equivalent to contrast enhanced CT for diagnosis of acute pancreatitis.[48]

Intra-abdominal Abscess

A localized collection of pus can occur anywhere in the abdomen including the parenchyma of solid organs, in the peritoneal or extraperitoneal spaces. Early detection, accurate localization, and prompt drainage are the mainstay of successful management. US is an excellent modality for the detection of visceral abscesses and is also useful for screening for intraperitoneal abscesses, like in the postoperative patient.[49] Abscesses appear as a rounded, complex fluid collection with irregular walls, posterior acoustic enhancement, low level internal echoes, septations, or debris **(Fig. 15A)**. A fluid-fluid level may be seen. At times, the abscess may have a solid appearance. Color Doppler demonstrates peripheral hypervascularity. CT has a high sensitivity and specificity with an overall accuracy of 95% for the detection of intra-abdominal abscesses.[50] CT will show a low attenuation fluid collection with mass effect and peripheral rim enhancement with or without gas bubbles or an air-fluid level. MDCT allows accurate delineation of the complex anatomy which may exist in intra-abdominal collections and thus enables proper planning of a safe approach route for percutaneous catheter drainage **(Fig. 15 B)**.

Intestinal Obstruction

Intestinal obstruction accounts for approximately 20% cases of acute surgical emergencies of the abdomen. The role of imaging is to confirm the diagnosis of intestinal obstruction, determine the cause, level, and severity of obstruction, and to look for associated complications such as strangulation, ischemia, and perforation.[51] Plain radiography is the initial imaging investigation performed in patients with suspected bowel obstruction. Radiographic findings of bowel obstruction have already been described in detail earlier in this chapter. CT is the imaging modality of choice for evaluation of bowel obstruction and has overall accuracy of 90–95% for the diagnosis of high-grade obstruction.[52] CT is useful for detecting an obstruction not visualized on plain films, e.g., closed loop obstruction. More importantly, CT can detect complications like strangulation which require emergent surgery. Intraluminal fluid and gas already present within the obstructed bowel serve as excellent contrast agents, thereby obviating the need for positive oral contrast. CT enterography with neutral oral contrast is also helpful in cases of partial small bowel obstruction demonstrating the exact site and the cause of obstruction. It helps in improved visualization of mucosal lesions as compared with conventional CT.[53] Fast MRI has also been shown to be sensitive (95%), specific (100%), and accurate (96%) in the setting of small bowel obstruction.[54]

The CT diagnosis of bowel obstruction is based on the presence of dilated loops (small bowel >2.5 cm, large bowel >5 cm) with air-fluid levels proximal to a transition zone with collapsed distal bowel. The "small bowel feces" sign refers to the presence of gas bubbles mixed with particulate matter in dilated loops proximal to the site of obstruction. This is a less common but reliable indicator of mechanical obstruction. Strangulating obstruction is a mechanical obstruction caused when two limbs of a loop are incarcerated within a hernia so as to cause vascular compromise by compression of the mesenteric vessels. Presence of thumb-printing due to submucosal edema or hemorrhage should suggest ischemia in the loops. If left untreated, the ischemia may progress causing breach of

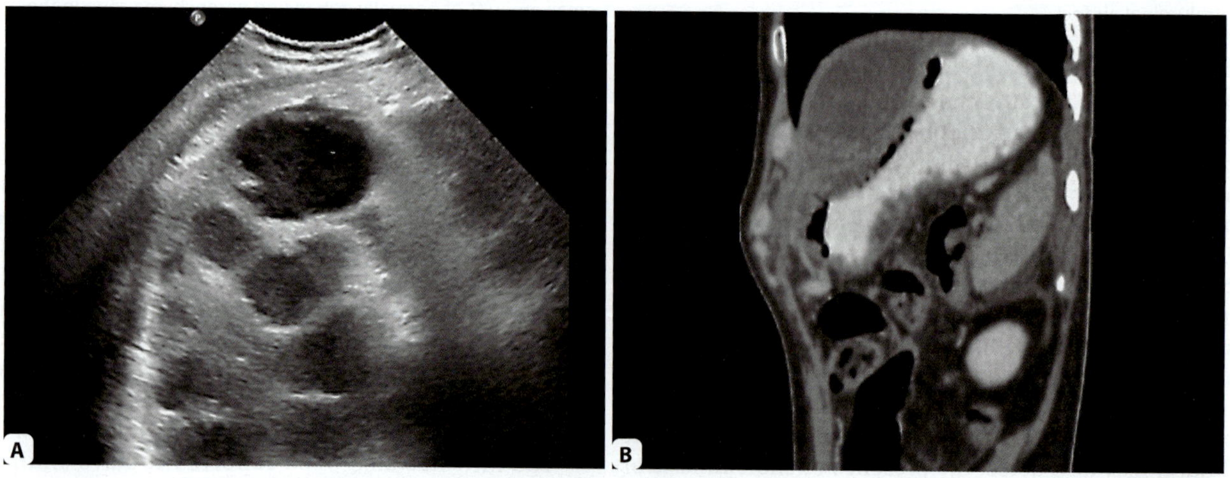

FIGS. 15A AND B: Intra-abdominal abscess: (A) Ultrasound of abdomen shows multiple intrahepatic fluid collections with internal echoes, debris, and irregular walls in a case of pyogenic liver abscess; (B) Coronal multiplanar reconstruction (MPR) image in another case shows a large, left subphrenic, low-attenuation fluid collection elevating the left hemidiaphragm. The transpleural approach had to be employed for percutaneous drainage of this abscess.

the mucosa, intramural air, air in the mesenteric and portal veins, and frank perforation which are all ominous signs. Intramural air in the form of parallel streaks of gas along the bowel wall or as rings may also be seen in infants with necrotizing enterocolitis. This appearance should not be confused with the bubbly appearance of pneumatosis coli which is a benign condition affecting the colon in adults.

The causes of intestinal obstruction vary with the age of the patient. In neonates and infants, the usual causes of obstruction are congenital conditions such as hypertrophic pyloric stenosis, duodenal stenosis or atresia, ileal atresia, etc. Duodenal atresia shows the typical "double-bubble" sign. In young children, intussusception or Ladd's bands are common causes of obstruction. Intussusception may be seen as a mass-like soft tissue shadow with a crescent of gas surrounding the leading edge. A barium examination will reveal the coil-spring appearance of the intussuscipiens with the "claw" sign. Adhesions are the most common cause of small bowel obstruction comprising of two-thirds cases.[51] Diagnosis of adhesions on imaging is a diagnosis of exclusion. CT findings include abrupt transition from dilated bowel loops to collapsed bowel loops without an apparent cause with beaking at the transition point. Minimal mural thickening with enhancement may at times be seen at the transition zone in cases of adhesions **(Fig. 16)**.[55] External hernias occur at sites of abdominal wall weakness, while internal hernias occur at sites of mesenteric and omental weakness or in the postoperative abdomen. Gas filled loops, mesenteric vessels and fat may be seen in the inguinal canal or other sites of external hernias. CT may reveal tapering of the bowel loops entering and exiting the hernial sac **(Figs. 17A and B)**. Dilatation of the small bowel proximal to the hernia indicates obstruction at the entry site, while dilatation of loops within the hernia and proximal to it suggests obstruction at the exit site.[51] Circumferential mural thickening of the dilated bowel loops with increased attenuation in the mesentery or bowel wall denotes the presence of strangulation. An internal hernia can be diagnosed if a cluster of dilated small bowel loops which appears to be enclosed in a sac is seen in an ectopic location (e.g., lesser sac or anterior to transverse colon) with crowding and twisting of the mesenteric vessels. A markedly dilated, fluid-filled bowel segment with abrupt tapering ends denotes a closed loop obstruction **(Figs. 18A and B)**. These show relatively little dilatation of the proximal bowel and are at greater risk for strangulation. Adhesive bands, internal and external hernias are the cause of closed loop obstruction. Fixed radial distribution of several dilated small bowel loops with stretched and prominent mesenteric vessels converging toward the point of torsion (whirl sign) with mesenteric edema

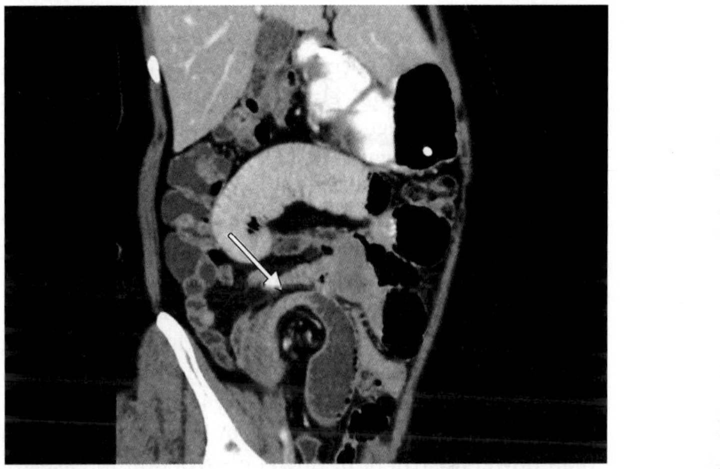

FIG. 16: Adhesion: Oblique multiplanar reconstruction (MPR) computed tomography (CT) image showing abrupt angulation of an ileal loop with minimal mural thickening (arrow) at the site of postoperative adhesion in a case of small bowel obstruction.

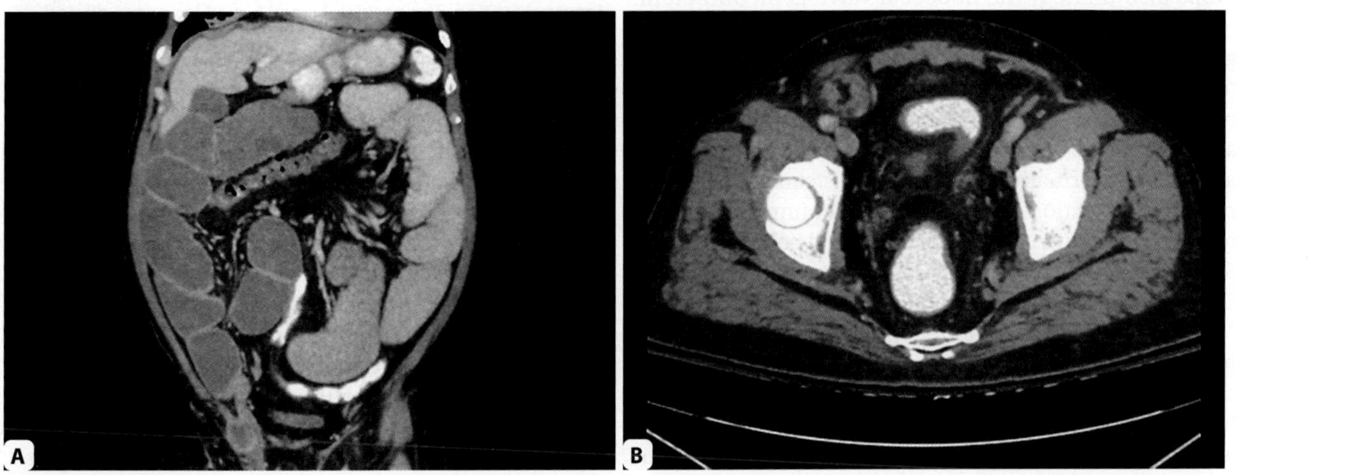

FIGS. 17A AND B: Obstructed right inguinal hernia: (A) Coronal; and (B) Axial contrast-enhanced computed tomography (CECT) images showing dilated small bowel loops with transition point at the level of inguinal hernia.

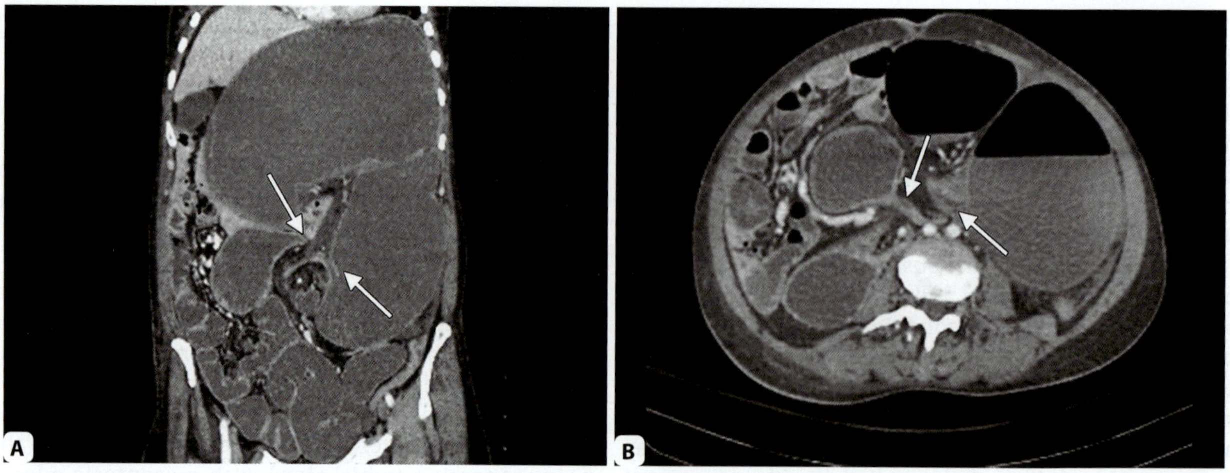

FIGS. 18A AND B: Closed loop obstruction: (A) Coronal; and (B) Axial contrast-enhanced computed tomography (CECT) images showing dilated small bowel loops with abrupt tapering at proximal and distal ends (arrows).

indicates a small bowel volvulus. A target appearance on cross section with a bowel-within-bowel appearance on longitudinal scans suggests a diagnosis of intussusception. Mesenteric fat and vessels can be identified within the mass and the lead point if present **(Fig. 19)**. Enteroenteric intussusceptions without proximal dilatation that are <3.5 cm in length are probably not significant in adults. Intussusceptions involving the colon that are 4 cm in length or longer have proximal dilatation or mural thickening which should be carefully evaluated for an underlying neoplasm. Foreign bodies, gallstones, and bezoars can all cause obstruction and can be readily identified on CT. In India, tuberculosis also remains an important cause of small bowel obstruction. Bowel obstruction in cases of tuberculosis can be caused by strictures **(Figs. 20A and B)**, ileocecal mass or adhesions.

Large bowel obstruction is 4–5 times less common than small bowel obstruction and differs in etiology. In mechanical large bowel obstruction, the small bowel loops also dilate if the ileocecal valve is incompetent. However, if the ileocecal valve is competent, it can result in gross gaseous distension of the cecum with the attendant dangers of ischemia and perforation. Neoplasm is the most common cause of large bowel obstruction accounting for approximately 55% cases **(Fig. 21)**. Pericolic inflammation and abscess formation in diverticulitis can cause partial colonic obstruction. Volvulus is also an important cause of obstruction and can affect the sigmoid colon or cecum. Sigmoid volvulus is generally seen in the older age group. The distended ahaustral sigmoid loop assumes an inverted "U" shape with its apex under either dome. The opposed inner walls of the loops appear as a single line giving the "coffee bean" appearance **(Fig. 22)**. "Whirl" sign has been described on CT in volvulus constituted by the afferent and efferent limbs of the volvulus. Cecal volvulus generally occurs in younger individuals. The cecum twists and inverts so that its pole and appendix lie in the left upper quadrant.

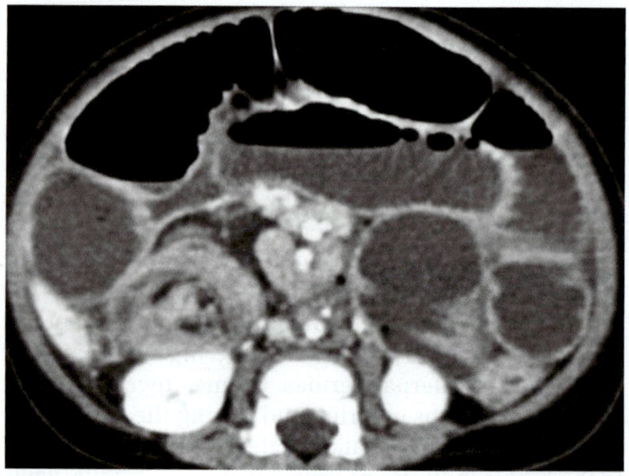

FIG. 19: Intussusception: Axial contrast-enhanced computed tomography (CECT) image demonstrates a heterogeneous mass in the right lumbar region showing a target appearance with mesenteric fat and vessels within the lesion suggestive of intussusception. The proximal small bowel loops are dilated.

Bowel Perforation

Gastrointestinal tract perforation can be caused by peptic ulcer disease, foreign body, appendicitis, bacterial enteritis, Crohn's disease, diverticulitis, bowel ischemia, and obstruction or malignant neoplasms. Some studies have reported US to be a more sensitive modality than plain radiography for the diagnosis of pneumoperitoneum.[56] Sonographic findings of perforated hollow viscus include demonstration of free air as echogenic spots or lines with posterior ring-down artifacts that shift with change in patient position, enhancement of the peritoneal stripe, echogenic free peritoneal fluid, and decreased peristalsis.[57] When patient is in supine position, the reverberations are seen between anterior surface of left lobe of liver and anterior abdominal wall **(Fig. 23)**. Shifting phenomenon

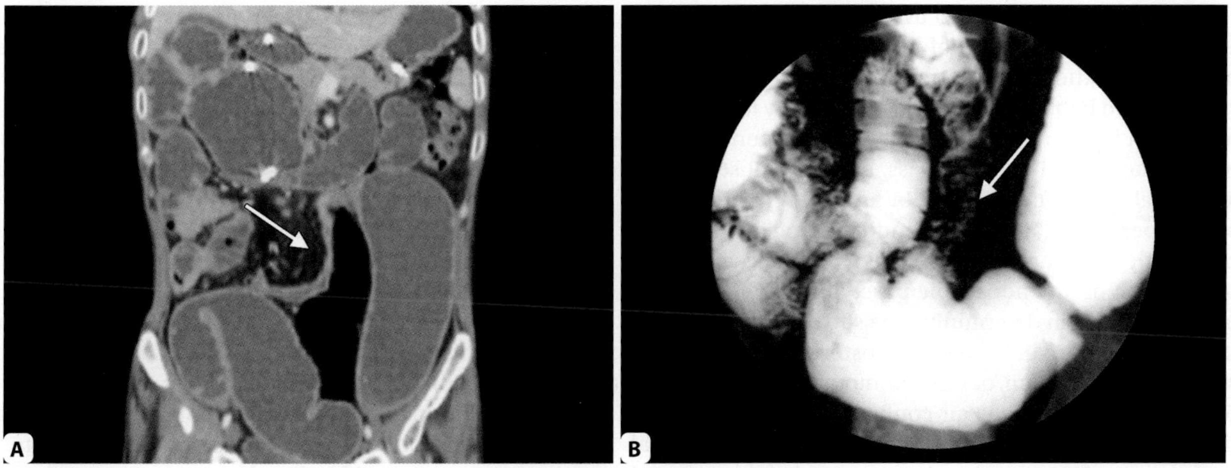

FIGS. 20A AND B: Stricture: (A) Computed tomography (CT) enterography coronal multiplanar reconstruction (MPR) image showing a long segment distal ileal stricture (arrow) causing obstruction with dilatation of the proximal small bowel loops. (B) Barium enteroclysis done subsequently confirms the stricture (arrow) in a case of tuberculosis.

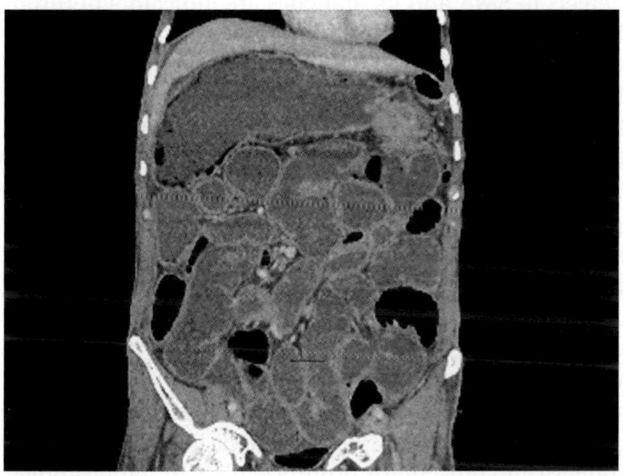

FIG. 21: Large bowel obstruction: Coronal reformatted computed tomography (CT) image showing irregular nodular thickening at splenic flexure causing large bowel obstruction in a case of colon cancer.

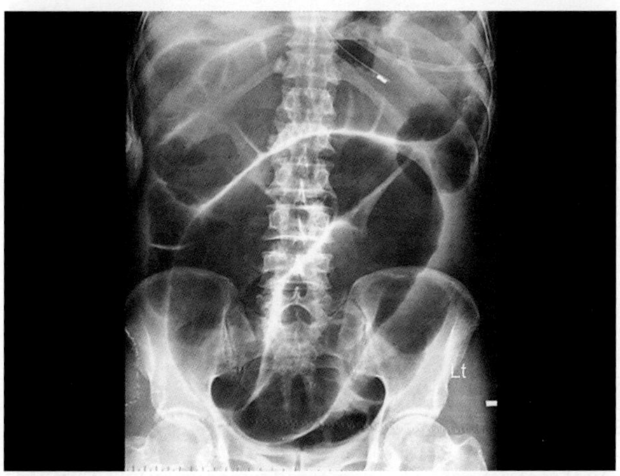

FIG. 22: Sigmoid volvulus: X-ray abdomen, supine view shows a hugely dilated ahaustral loop arising from the pelvis with the "coffee-bean" sign in a case of sigmoid volvulus.

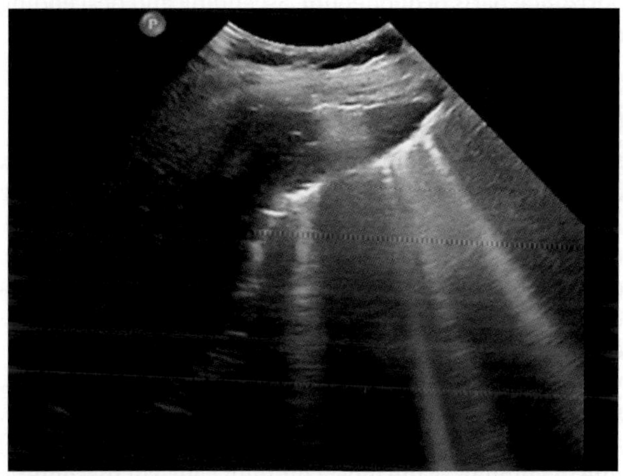

FIG. 23: Pneumoperitoneum on ultrasonography (US): US image shows echogenic foci with reverberation artefact anterior to left lobe of liver suggestive of pneumoperitoneum.

is seen on rolling the patient to left lateral position as free air rises to the highest portion of the right hypochondrium. Enhancement of peritoneal stripe refers to increased echogenicity and thickening of the peritoneal stripe due to free intraperitoneal air with associated dirty shadowing.

The CT is superior to both plain films and US for the detection of presence, cause, and site of perforation. Preoperative localization of the site of perforation is beneficial for the surgeon, with the laparoscopic approach currently being used for most surgical procedures instead of open surgery. Extraluminal contrast extravasation, when seen, is pathognomonic. Other direct signs are the presence of extraluminal air or discontinuity of the bowel wall. Inflammatory changes may also be seen at the site of perforation. CT images should be assessed in wide window settings to distinguish free air from fat density. Careful analysis of anterior peritoneal surfaces of liver and mid-abdomen as well as of peritoneal folds should be done, so as not to overlook a small amount of extraluminal air. The site of bowel perforation may be predicted by the site of extraluminal contrast leakage, concentrated bubbles of air in close proximity to the bowel wall, focal interruption of bowel wall, segmental bowel wall thickening, ill-defined mass, adjacent fat stranding, and extraluminal fluid **(Figs. 24A and B)**. A large amount of intraperitoneal air usually indicates gastroduodenal perforation, except for bowel perforation caused by obstruction or an endoscopic procedure.[58] The location of air also helps in determining the site of perforation. Air in the lesser sac can be seen in posterior perforation of stomach or duodenum, or less commonly, from perforation of transverse colon. Free air confined to the intrahepatic ligamentum teres is commonly due to gastroduodenal perforations. Air trapped in the mesenteric folds is found in colon and small bowel perforation, but seldom in gastric perforation. Retroperitoneal air is caused by perforation of extraperitoneal sites of GI tract, viz. descending and horizontal parts of duodenum, ascending and descending colon, sigmoid colon, and rectum.

Mesenteric Ischemia

Bowel ischemia or infarction is a common but complex disorder with a plethora of primary causes and a wide range of clinical and pathological manifestations. Acute mesenteric ischemia is therefore a diagnostic challenge, particularly in view of its high mortality rate, which ranges from 50 to 90% depending upon the cause and degree of bowel wall damage. Acute mesenteric ischemia can result from arterial occlusion (thrombotic or embolic), mesenteric venous thrombosis, or nonocclusive cause. Acute occlusion of the superior mesenteric artery (SMA) due to embolus is the most common cause of mesenteric ischemia accounting for nearly 50% of cases.[59] High flow rate in SMA and its narrow angle of branching from abdominal aorta make it susceptible for embolism. The manifestation may range from a self-limiting superficial ischemia involving the watershed zones to a diffuse ischemic injury to the entire bowel "shock bowel" which requires immediate surgical intervention.[60] Plain films reveal the characteristic thick-walled dilated loops with thumb-printing in only 20–30% of cases.[61] Intramural air or portomesenteric air is also rarely visualized on the plain radiograph.

The CT angiography is the modality of choice for the evaluation of bowel ischemia with a sensitivity approaching that of angiography. Reduction or cessation of arterial blood supply in arterial thromboembolic disease leads to reduced or absent bowel wall enhancement. Restoration of intestinal perfusion may cause mural thickening, hyperenhancement, and stratification. However, progression of ischemia with transmural infarction results in intramural nerve destruction, loss of muscle tone and tissue volume, with resultant "paper thin" appearance. Hypodense filling defects in SMA and its branches are indicators of thromboembolism.[62] Luminal dilatation with air-fluid levels can be seen in 56–91% of cases of mesenteric ischemia. Pneumatosis and portomesenteric gas are less common but more specific findings of ischemia, being present in 6–28% and 3–14% of cases, respectively **(Figs. 25A and B)**.[59,60] The presence of pneumoperitoneum or focal peritonitis signifies perforation. Synchronous infarcts in solid abdominal organs (particularly kidneys) point toward the diagnosis of arterial ischemia.[62]

Mesenteric venous ischemia is due to venous outflow obstruction leading to vascular engorgement and bowel wall edema. Continued arterial inflow with impaired venous drainage leads to increased intramural hydrostatic pressure leading to submucosal edema between enhancing mucosa and muscularis propria leading to "target appearance". Adjacent mesenteric stranding and edema is also commonly seen resulting from extravasation of fluid

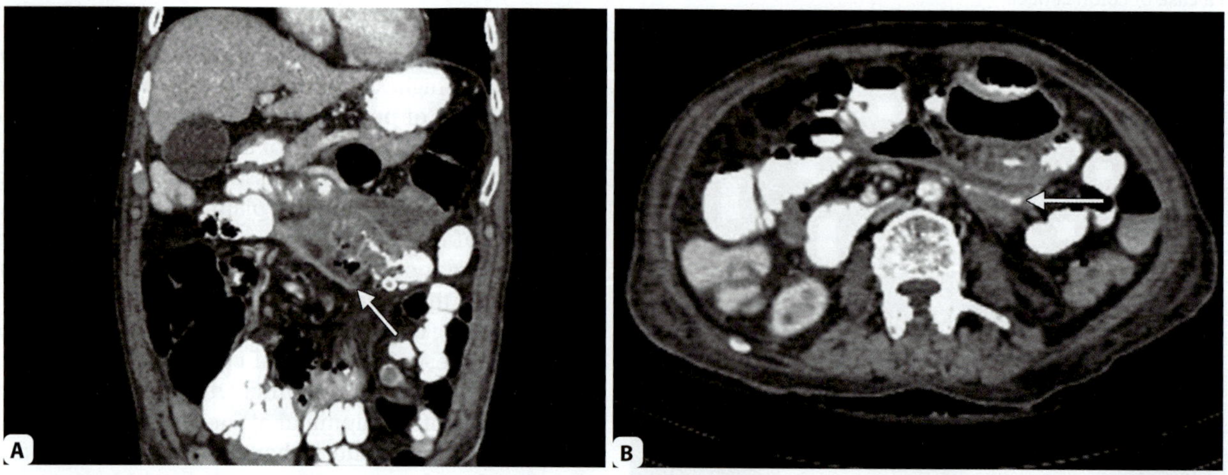

FIGS. 24A AND B: Perforated jejunal diverticula: (A) Coronal; and (B) Axial contrast-enhanced computed tomography (CECT) images showing jejunal diverticula with concentric mural thickening of jejunum and adjacent collection showing air foci (arrow in A) with pooling of oral contrast (arrow in B) suggestive of perforation.

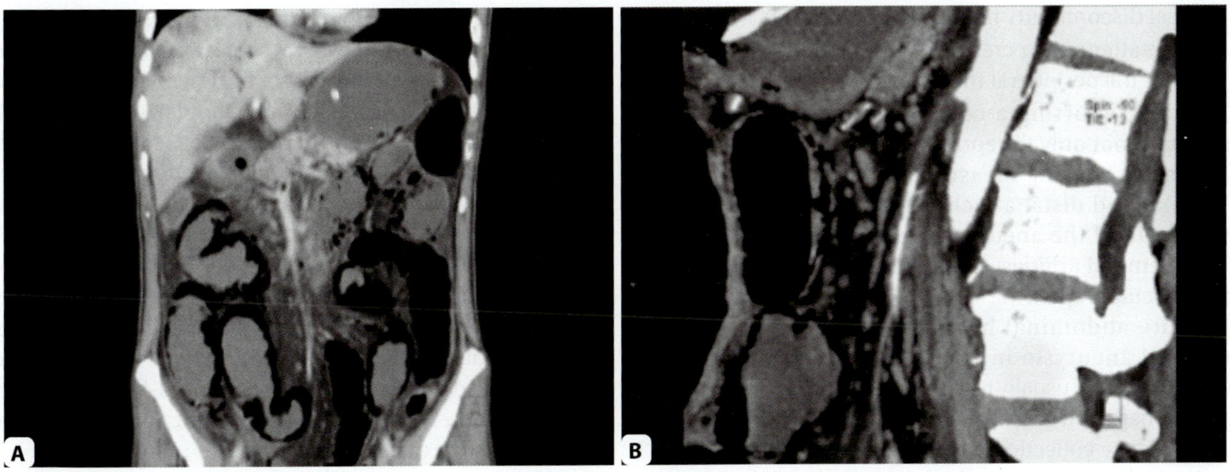

FIGS. 25A AND B: Mesenteric ischemia, computed tomography (CT) angiography. (A) The small bowel loops are dilated with thinned-out walls and gross pneumatosis. Air is also seen in the mesenteric veins and the portal radicles in the liver. Note the irregular, nonenhancing hypodense areas in the periphery of the liver due to infarcts. (B) Sagittal maximum intensity projection (MIP) image demonstrates the occlusion of the proximal superior mesenteric artery.

into the mesentery. Filling defect is seen in mesenteric veins with engorgement of collateral venous pathways. Concurrent thrombosis of portal and splenic vein can also be seen. Nonocclusive mesenteric ischemia is poorly understood and challenging to diagnose on imaging. Reduced caliber of mesenteric arteries is seen with features of CT hypoperfusion complex (hyperenhancement of kidneys, adrenals, and bowel wall). Bowel findings are often discontinuous and segmental.[62]

Vascular Causes

Vascular conditions that may present as acute abdomen include rupture of an aortic aneurysm, spontaneous aortic occlusion, aortic dissection, penetrating atherosclerotic ulcer, intramural hematoma, acute hemorrhage, and hepatic or splenic vascular occlusion. Aneurysmal dilatation of the abdominal aorta is rare before the age of 50 with average age at the time of diagnosis being 65–70 years. Most abdominal aortic aneurysms are true aneurysms and occur below the level of renal arteries. An abdominal aortic aneurysm is defined as an aortic diameter of 3 cm (measured perpendicular to the long axis of lumen) or more while a diameter of 5.5 cm or more warrants urgent intervention.[63] Presence of a pulsatile mass and sudden hypotension in the clinical setting of acute pain abdomen suggests the diagnosis of a ruptured aortic aneurysm. Although US may detect the aneurysm as well as the associated thrombus and hematoma, frequently the entire aorta cannot be evaluated due to overlying bowel gas or body habitus. Multidetector CT is the modality of choice for evaluation of acute aortic syndrome. The most common finding of rupture of aortic aneurysm is a retroperitoneal hematoma adjacent to the aneurysm **(Fig. 26)**. Other CT features may include active extravasation of contrast, extension of periaortic blood into perirenal or pararenal spaces or the psoas muscle or peritoneal cavity. Signs predictive of impending rupture are:

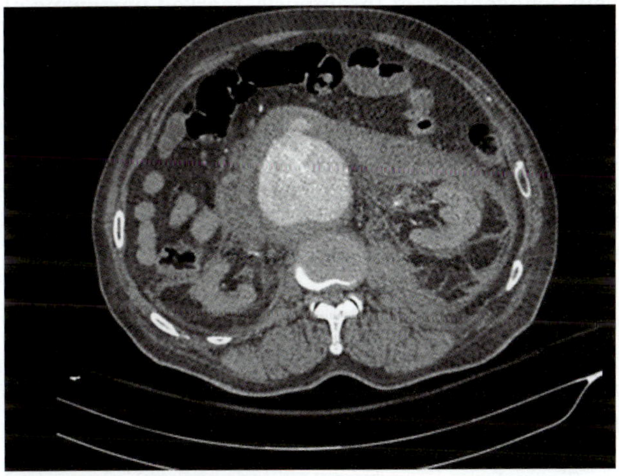

FIG. 26: Ruptured aortic aneurysm: Axial contrast-enhanced computed tomography (CECT) image shows abdominal aortic aneurysm with extravasation of intravenous contrast and retroperitoneal hematoma suggestive of rupture.

- *Draped aorta sign*: It is seen with contained leak. The posterior wall of aorta cannot be defined due to close application and lateral "draping" of the aneurysm around the adjacent vertebral bodies.[64]
- *Increase in aneurysm size*: A patient with a very large aneurysm (>7 cm diameter) who presents with acute aortic syndrome has a high likelihood of aneurysmal rupture. Also, a rate of enlargement of >10 mm/year warrants surgical repair.
- *Thrombus-to-lumen ratio*: This ratio decreases with increasing aneurysm size. A thick circumferential thrombus is protective against rupture.

- Focal discontinuity in intimal calcification.
- Hyperattenuating crescent sign due to hemorrhage in either the peripheral thrombus or aneurysm wall.

While reporting a case of aortic aneurysm, it is important not only to report the aneurysmal dimensions but also to provide measurements of the aorta at the proximal and distal attachment sites, the morphology and length of the aneurysm neck, and the diameter of the iliofemoral arteries, all of which have implications for endovascular repair.[65]

Acute abdominal hemorrhage may result due to ruptured aneurysm in a case of polyarteritis nodosa, ruptured tumor (usually renal cell carcinoma) or in a patient on anticoagulant therapy. Noncontrast CT demonstrates a hyperdense collection at the site of hemorrhage. MDCT angiography can accurately delineate the site and cause of hemorrhage. Rare vascular causes of acute abdomen include hepatic vein thrombosis (acute Budd-Chiari syndrome) and portal vein thrombosis. US in the acute phase may show liver enlargement, partial or complete inability to visualize hepatic veins, intraluminal hepatic vein echogenicity or thrombosis, marked narrowing of intrahepatic inferior vena cava (IVC) and ascites. Color Doppler is the technique of choice for initial evaluation. Absence of flow or flow in an abnormal direction in all or part of the hepatic veins may be seen. CT and MR are complimentary techniques for definitive diagnosis which provide a more complete evaluation of the hepatic parenchyma, hepatic veins, and IVC.

Pelvic Disease

The various entities that have to be additionally thought of while evaluating a young female in the reproductive age group presenting with acute abdomen are ruptured ectopic pregnancy, PID, twisted ovarian cyst, and complications of early pregnancy, etc.

- Signs of a ruptured ectopic pregnancy on ultrasound include an inhomogeneous adnexal mass, pelvic fluid or hematoma, and decidual reaction without intrauterine gestation sac, in the presence of a positive pregnancy test. Visualization of an echogenic adnexal ring separate from the ovary that has prominent peripheral flow on color Doppler is highly suggestive of ectopic gestation. Corpus luteum is a useful guide while looking for an ectopic pregnancy and is usually seen in the ipsilateral ovary in 70–85% cases.[66] Using transvaginal ultrasound, the live embryo can be detected in up to 17% of all ectopic pregnancies.
- Fibroids may present with acute pain if there is torsion or degeneration of a submucosal or subserosal fibroid. On imaging, uterine enlargement with a focal mass or contour deformity are seen. Degenerated fibroids may have a cystic appearance.
- Ovarian torsion usually occurs in children and is attributed to excessive mobility of the ovary. In adults, a cyst or mass, frequently a cystic teratoma, is present in the ovary undergoing torsion. Sonographic findings include an enlarged ovary with peripherally distributed follicles, an associated cyst or mass, with diminished or absent central venous flow on Doppler. On CT or MRI, deviation of the uterus to the twisted side, obliteration of fat planes, and an enlarged ovary displaced from its adnexal location is seen **(Fig. 27)**. Contrast enhanced CT may show surrounding enhancing blood vessels due to congestion.[67]
- Hemorrhage into a corpus luteal or follicular cyst may manifest with abrupt onset of pelvic pain. On imaging, hemorrhagic ovarian cysts can mimic a variety of solid and mixed solid-cystic masses. A fluid-fluid level may be present. On CT, high attenuation components are usually seen due to hemorrhage.
- PID is among the common causes of acute pain in young women. In the early stage of PID, US may demonstrate a small amount of fluid in the cul-de-sac or endometrial canal. On CT, there may be stranding in the parapelvic fat, thickening of the uterosacral ligament, and ovarian enlargement with oophoritis.[67] In advanced stages, there is development of pyosalpinx or tubo-ovarian abscess.
- Ovarian vein thrombosis (OVT) should be suspected as a cause of abdominal pain in the postpartum period, in women with PID, recent abdominal surgery, malignancy, or known hypercoagulable state. Pregnancy increases the risk for venous thrombosis due to stasis, alteration in coagulation factors, and by nearly tripling the diameter of the ovarian veins. In 90% of cases, the right ovarian vein is involved due to dextrotorsion of the uterus. OVT may be diagnosed by US, CT, or MRI; however, CT is the modality of choice and demonstrates a low attenuation thrombus in lumen of ovarian vein.

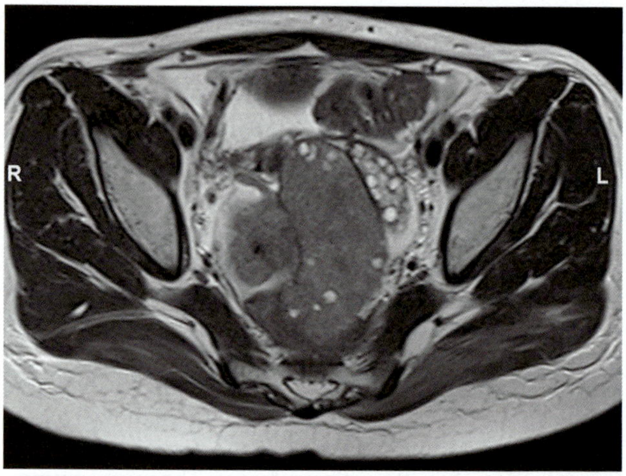

FIG. 27: Ovarian torsion: Axial magnetic resonance (MR) T2-weighted image (T2WI) shows an enlarged right ovary with peripheral follicles displaced into the midline. Note the adjacent normal left ovary.

MISCELLANEOUS

Diverticulitis

The tetrad of left lower quadrant pain and tenderness, fever, and leukocytosis is the classic presentation of diverticulitis. Diverticular disease of the colon affects 65% of the Western population by the age of 65 years, and diverticulitis eventually develops in up to 25% of individuals with diverticulosis.[68] Findings on barium enema include diverticula, muscular wall hypertrophy, intramural or extramural mass effect on the barium column, colonic obstruction or peritoneal extravasation of contrast material, such as with fistula or sinus tract formation. The full extent of peritoneal involvement cannot be estimated on barium examination, hence it has largely been replaced by CT for imaging of suspected diverticulitis. Findings on CT include diverticula, muscular wall hypertrophy, symmetrical mural thickening >3 mm, pericolonic fat stranding **(Fig. 28)**, phlegmon, extraluminal gas bubbles, extravasation of contrast in case of perforation, and paracolic abscess formation. Oral and rectal contrast is not necessary in acute setting, however can be given in chronic setting to detect fistulae. The differential diagnosis includes carcinoma: presence of enlarged lymph nodes, mural thickening >1.5 cm, and an abrupt change from normal to abnormal colon favors carcinoma over diverticulitis.[69]

Toxic Megacolon

Toxic megacolon is an acute transmural fulminant colitis which can occur as a complication of any colitis but is most commonly seen with ulcerative colitis (1.6–13% of cases). Plain radiographs show marked colonic dilatation (>8 cm) particularly of the transverse colon as this is the least dependent part of the large bowel in the supine position. The wall has a shaggy appearance with mucosal islands or pseudopolyps with absence of haustra due to profound inflammation and ulceration. There may be air-fluid levels and small bowel dilatation. CT shows the distended colon filled with air, fluid, and blood with a distorted or absent haustral pattern and irregular, nodular wall.[70] There may be presence of intramural air or blood. The prognosis is poor in the presence of perforation and complications.

Acute Pyelonephritis

Acute pyelonephritis is the bacterial or fungal infection of the renal parenchyma and collecting system. Presenting features include flank pain, dysuria, and high grade fever with rigors. On US, renal enlargement, decreased visualization of sinus fat secondary to compression, loss of corticomedullary differentiation, and focal poorly marginated hypoechoic areas representing interstitial edema or complications like abscesses may be seen. Harmonic imaging and contrast-enhanced ultrasound can increase the conspicuity of renal parenchymal abnormalities in acute pyelonephritis.[71] CT scan is the imaging modality of choice and can reveal calculi, obstruction, renal enlargement, striated nephrogram, ill-defined, wedge-shaped areas of decreased attenuation radiating from the papillae to the cortical surface, abscess, thickening of Gerotas' fascia, and perinephric stranding **(Fig. 29)**. Emphysematous pyelonephritis usually occurs in patients with poorly controlled diabetes with the most common infecting organism being *Escherichia coli*. Presence of air in the renal parenchyma is pathognomonic of this condition.

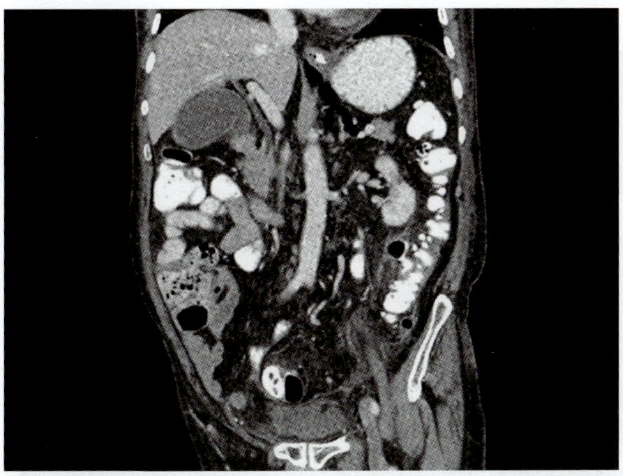

FIG. 28: Acute diverticulitis: Coronal reformatted contrast-enhanced computed tomography (CECT) image shows multiple diverticula in descending colon with inflammatory fat stranding around one of the diverticula suggestive of diverticulitis.

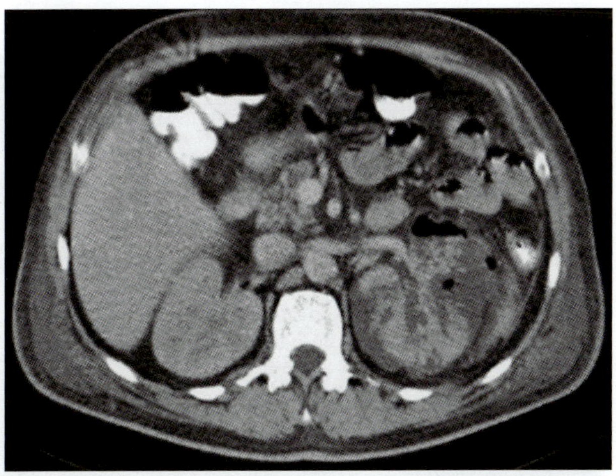

FIG. 29: Acute pyelonephritis: Axial computed tomography (CT) image shows multiple, irregular, linear, hypodense areas in the left kidney due to pyelonephritis. A hypodense area with an air-fluid level is seen in anterior cortex suggestive of renal abscess. In addition, perinephric collection with air is also visualized.

Acute Urinary Colic

Impacted ureteric stone is the most common cause of acute postrenal obstruction. US is useful for the detection of small/radiolucent calculi missed on plain films. Secondly, direct visualization of the effects of these calculi on the urinary tract is also possible. However, because pelvicaliectasis may be mild to negligible in acute obstruction, US may miss up to one-third of acute obstructions. Color Doppler US helps demonstrate absence of the normal urinary jet on the obstructed side. Unenhanced helical CT has emerged as an attractive modality in the diagnostic workup of urinary tract disease. NCCT KUB is performed rapidly, without patient preparation and without risk of contrast reaction. It can provide information about size, localization, and chemical composition of the stone. In addition to direct stone visualization, secondary CT signs of urinary obstruction, including ureteral dilatation, perinephric or periureteric fat stranding, and blurring of renal sinus fat and ureteral wall edema, are usually present to confirm the diagnosis even after recent stone passage.[72]

Acute Epiploic Appendagitis, Omental Infarction

Epiploic appendages are fat-containing peritoneal outpouchings that arise from cecum to rectosigmoid junction, along the serosal surface of the colon. These are 0.5–5.0 cm long and contain fat and small vessels. Epiploic appendagitis occurs due to torsion of an epiploic appendage leading to venous occlusion and ischemia. It is usually associated with obesity, hernia, and unaccustomed exercise. The condition manifests as acute left lower quadrant pain, predominantly in males in the fourth to fifth decades of life. On US, a hyperechoic, incompressible mass delineated by a hypoechoic ring is seen at the point of maximum tenderness **(Fig. 30A)**. The lesions are hyperechoic due to their fat content or hemorrhagic necrosis. CT features include an oval, fat attenuation lesion <5 cm in diameter that abuts the anterior or anterolateral serosal aspect of the colonic wall, surrounded by inflammatory changes **(Fig. 30B)**.[73] A hyperattenuating rim corresponding to the hypoechoic ring on US is seen on CT due to swollen serosa covered by fibrinoleukocyte exudate.

Omental infarction commonly involves the inferior aspect of right side of omentum. It is characteristically situated between the anterior abdominal wall and the transverse or ascending colon, corresponding in location to the greater omentum. Predisposing factors include obesity, strenuous activity, congestive heart failure, digitalis administration, recent abdominal surgery, and abdominal trauma. Pain is localized to the right lower or upper quadrant and the presumptive diagnosis is usually appendicitis. Both US and CT show an ovoid, soft tissue mass just beneath the anterior abdominal wall. The infarcted omental fat is hyperechoic on ultrasound and appears heterogeneous with no enhancement on CT. Although omental infarction may resemble acute epiploic appendagitis on CT, it lacks the hyperattenuating ring seen in the latter. Moreover, omental infarction is larger than epiploic appendagitis which is often <5 cm. Omental infarction is commonly located next to the cecum and ascending colon whereas acute epiloic appendagitis is usually located adjacent to sigmoid colon.[73]

Acute Abdomen in Neutropenic Patients

Neutropenic enterocolitis and acute graft versus host disease are common causes of acute abdominal pain in immunocompromised patients and patients with

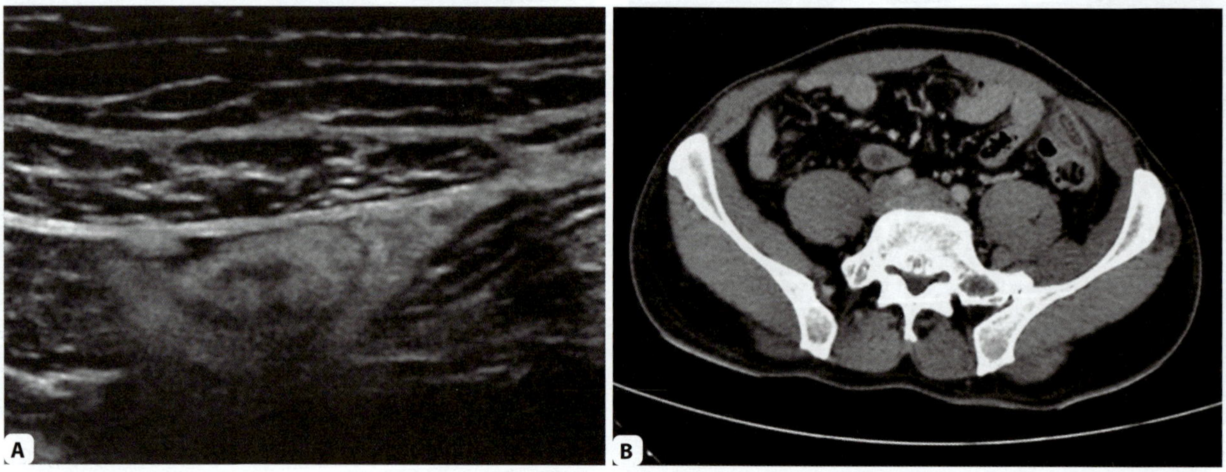

FIGS. 30A AND B: Acute epiploic appendagitis: (A) Ultrasound image showing oval hyperechoic noncompressible mass with hypoechoic rim in left iliac fossa; (B) Axial contrast-enhanced computed tomography (CECT) image of the same patient demonstrates fat attenuation lesion with hyperdense rim along anterior wall of descending colon with adjacent inflammatory changes.

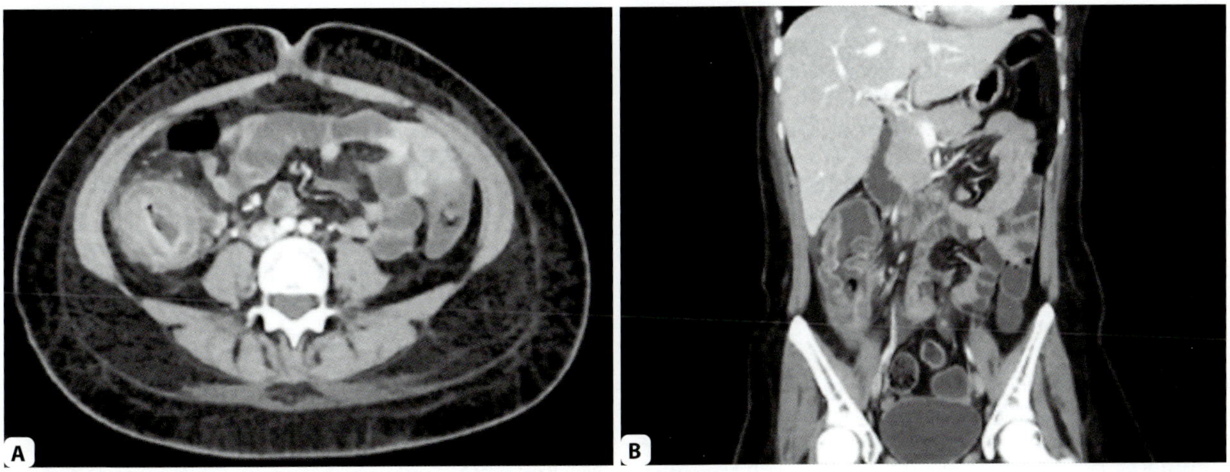

FIGS. 31A AND B: Neutropenic colitis: (A) Axial; and (B) Coronal images demonstrate the gross mural thickening in the cecum and ascending colon.

allogeneic bone marrow transplants. Cecal wall thickening and involvement of the right side of the colon is the most common finding in neutropenic colitis **(Figs. 31A and B)**.[74] In acute graft versus host disease, bowel wall thickening and abnormal mucosal enhancement are common, with small bowel being most commonly affected.[75]

CONCLUSION

The presentation of an acute abdomen maybe due to a heterogeneous variety of conditions. Helical CT is the imaging modality of choice to evaluate these patients, with plain radiographs, US, and MRI having contributory roles.

REFERENCES

1. Gangadhar K, Kielar A, Dighe MK, O'Malley R, Wang C, Gross JA, et al. Multimodality approach for imaging of non-traumatic acute abdominal emergencies. Abdom Radiol (NY). 2016;41(1):136-48.
2. Stoker J, van Randen A, Laméris W, Boermeester MA. Imaging patients with acute abdominal pain. Radiology. 2009;253(1):31-46.
3. de Bombal FT. Introduction. In: de Bombal FT (Ed). Diagnosis of acute abdominal pain, 2nd edition. Churchill Livingstone: Edinburgh; 1991. pp. 1-10.
4. Balthazar EJ, Chako AC. Computerized tomography in acute gastrointestinal disorders. Am J Gastroenterol. 1990;85(11):1445-52.
5. Field S, Morrisom I. The acute abdomen. In: Sutton D (Ed). Textbook of radiology and imaging, 7th edition. Edinburgh: Churchill Livingstone; 2003. pp. 663-90.
6. Kundra V, Silverman P. Impact of mutlislice CT on imaging of acute abdominal disease. Radiol Clin N Am. 2003;41(6):1083-93.
7. Expert Panel on Gastrointestinal Imaging:; Scheirey CD, Fowler KJ, Therrien JA, Kim DH, Al-Refaie WB, Camacho MA, et al. ACR Appropriateness Criteria® acute nonlocalized abdominal pain. J Am Coll Radiol. 2018;15(11S):S217-31.
8. Expert Panel on Gastrointestinal Imaging:; Peterson CM, McNamara MM, Kamel IR, Al-Refaie WB, Arif-Tiwari H, Cash BD, et al. ACR appropriateness criteria® right upper quadrant pain. J Am Coll Radiol. 2019;16(5S):S235-43.
9. Expert Panel on Gastrointestinal Imaging; Russo GK, Zaheer A, Kamel IR, Porter KK, Archer-Arroyo K, Bashir MR, et al. ACR Appropriateness Criteria® right upper quadrant pain: 2022 update. J Am Coll Radiol. 2023;20(5S):S211-23.
10. MacKersie AB, Lane MJ, Gerhardt RT, Claypool HA, Keenan S, Katz DS, et al. Nontraumatic acute abdominal pain: unenhanced helical CT compared with three view acute abdominal series. Radiology. 2005;237(1):114-22.
11. Kellow ZS, MacInnes M, Kurzencwyg D, Rawal S, Jaffer R, Kovacina B, et al. The role of abdominal radiography in the evaluation of the nontrauma emergency patient. Radiology. 2008;248(3):887-93.
12. Ahn SH, Mayo-Smith WW, Murphy BL, Reinert SE, Cronan JJ. Acute non-traumatic abdominal pain in adult patients: abdominal radiography compared with CT evaluation. Radiology. 2002;225(1)159-64.
13. Mirvis SE, Young JWR, Keramati B, McCrea ES, Tarr R. Plain film evaluation of patients with abdominal pain: Are three radiographs necessary? AJR Am J Roentgenol. 1986;147(3):501-3.
14. Morrison ID, McLaughlin P, Maher MM. Current status of imaging of the gastrointestinal tract: Imaging techniques and radiation issues. In: Adam A, Dixon AK, Gillard JH, Schaefer-Prokop CM (Eds). Grainger and Allison's diagnostic Radiology, 6th edition. Edinburgh: Churchill Livingstone; 2015. pp. 593-609.
15. Miller RE, Nelson SW. The roentgenological demonstration of tiny amounts of free intra-peritoneal gas: experimental and clinical studies. Am J Roentgenol Radium Ther Nucl Med. 1971;112(3):574-85.
16. Rubesin SE, Levine MS. Radiologic diagnosis of gastrointestinal perforation. Radiol Clin N Am. 2003;41(6):1095-115.

17. Messmer JM, Levine MS. Gas and soft tissue abnormalities. In: Gore RM, Levine MS (Eds). Textbook of gastrointestinal radiology, 4th edition. Philadelphia: WB Saunders company; 2015. pp. 178-96.
18. Jamadar DA, Jacobson JA, Morag Y, Girish G, Dong Q, Al-Hawary M, et al. Characteristic locations of inguinal region and anterior abdominal wall hernias: sonographic appearances and identification of clinical pitfalls. Am J Roentgenol. 2007;188(5):1356-64.
19. Puylaert JB, Rutgers PH, Lalisang RI, de Vries BC, van der Werf SD, Dörr JP, et al. A prospective study of ultrasonography in the diagnosis of appendicitis. N Engl J Med. 1987; 317(11):666-9.
20. Mazzei MA, Guerrini S, Cioffi Squitieri N, Cagini L, Macarini L, Coppolino F, et al. The role of US examination in the management of acute abdomen. Crit Ultrasound J. 2013;5(Supp 1):S6.
21. Walsh PF, Crawford D, Crossling FT, Sutherland GR, Negrette JJ, Shand J, et al. The value of immediate ultrasound in acute abdominal conditions: a critical appraisal. Clin Radiol. 1990; 42(1):47-9.
22. McGrath FP, Keeling F. The role of early sonography in the management of the acute abdomen. Clin Radiol. 1991;44(3): 172-4.
23. Allemann F, Cassina P, Rothlin M, Largiadèr F. Ultrasound scans done by surgeons for patients with acute abdominal pain: a prospective study. Eur J Surg. 1999;165:966-70.
24. Lameris W, van Randen A, van Es HW, van Heesewijk JP, van Ramshorst B, Bouma WH, et al. Imaging strategies for detection of urgent conditions in patients with acute abdominal pain: diagnostic accuracy study. BMJ. 2009;338:b2431.
25. Uyeda JW, Yu H, Ramalingam V, Devalapalli AP, Soto JA, Anderson SW, et al. Evaluation of acute abdominal pain in the emergency setting using computed tomography without oral contrast in patients with body mass index greater than 25. J Comp Assist Tomogr. 2015;39(5):681-6.
26. Alabousi A, Patlas MN, Sne N, Katz DS. Is oral contrast necessary for multidetector computed tomography imaging of patients with acute abdominal pain? Can Assoc Radiol J. 2015;66(4):318-22.
27. Tsushima Y, Yamada S, Aoki J, Motojima T, Endo K. Effect of contrast-enhanced computed tomography on diagnosis and management of acute abdomen in adults. Clin Radiol. 2002;57(6):507-13.
28. Rosen MP, Sands DZ, Longmaid HE 3rd, Reynolds KF, Wagner M, Raptopoulos V. Impact of abdominal CT on the management of patients presenting to the emergency department with acute abdominal pain. AJR Am J Roentgenol. 2000;174(5):1391-6.
29. Murray N, Darras KE, Walstra FE, Mohammed MF, McLaughlin PD, Nicolaou S. Dual-energy CT in evaluation of the acute abdomen. Radiographics. 2019;39(1):264-86.
30. Bannas P, Pickhardt PJ. MR evaluation of the nontraumatic acute abdomen with CT correlation. Radiol Clin North Am. 2015;53(6):1327-39.
31. Bongard F, Landers DV, Lewis F. Differential diagnosis of appendicitis and pelvic inflammatory disease. Am J Surg. 1985;150(1):90-6.
32. Rao PM, Rhea JT, Novelline RA, McCabe CJ, Lawrason JN, Berger DL, et al. Helical CT technique for the diagnosis of appendicitis: Prospective evaluation of a focused appendix CT examination. Radiology. 1997;202(1):139-44.
33. Gaitini D, Beck-Razi N, Mor-Yosef D, Fischer D, Itzhak OB, Krausz MM, et al. Diagnosing acute appendicitis in adults: accuracy of color Doppler sonography and MDCT compared with surgery and clinical follow-up. AJR Am J Roentgenol. 2008;190(5):1300-6.
34. Lee JH, Jeong YK, Park KB, Park JK, Jeong AK, Hwang JC. Operator dependent techniques for graded compression sonography to detect the appendix and diagnose acute appendicitis. AJR Am J Roentgenol. 2005;184(1):91-7.
35. Poortman P, Lahle PNM, Schoemaker CMC, Oostvogel HJ, Teepen HJ, Zwinderman KA, et al. Comparison of CT and sonography in the diagnosis of acute appendicitis: A blinded prospective study. AJR Am J Roentgenol. 2003; 181(5):1355-9.
36. Brown MA, Tamburrini S, Furtado CD, Nanigan D, Sirlin CB, Casola G. Prospective evaluation of normal appendiceal diameter on CT. AJR Am J Roentgenol. 2003;180(American Roentgen Ray Society 103rd Annual Meeting Abstract Book suppl):2s.
37. Pinto Leite N, Pereira JM, Cunha R, Pinto P, Sirlin C. CT evaluation of appendicitis and its complications: imaging techniques and key diagnostic findings. AJR Am J Roentgenol. 2005;185(2):406-17.
38. Uggowitzer M, Kugler C, Schramayer G, Kammerhuber F, Gröll R, Hausegger KA, et al. Sonography of acute cholecystitis: comparison of color and power Doppler sonography in detecting a hypervascularized gallbladder wall. AJR Am J Roentgenol. 1997;168(3):707-12.
39. Maddu K, Phadke S, Hoff C. Complications of cholecystitis: a comprehensive contemporary imaging review. Emerg Radiol. 2021;28(5):1011-27.
40. Blankenberg F, Wirth R, Jeffry BR Jr, Mindelzun R, Francis I. Computed tomography as an adjunct to ultrasound in the diagnosis of acute a calculous cholecystitis. Gastrointestinal Radiol. 1991;16(2):149-53.
41. Fidler J, Paulson EK, Layfield L. CT evaluation of acute cholecystitis: Findings and usefulness in diagnosis. AJR Am J Roentgenol. 1996;166(5):1085-8.
42. Watanabe Y, Nagayama M, Okumura A, Amoh Y, Katsube T, Suga T, et al. MR imaging of acute biliary disorders. Radiographics. 2007;27(2):477-95.
43. Bennett GL, Rusinek H, Lisi V, Israel GM, Krinsky GA, Slywotzky CM, et al. CT findings in acute gangrenous cholecystitis. AJR Am J Roentgenol. 2002;178(2):275-81.
44. Morris BS, Balpande PR, Morani AC, Chaudhary RK, Maheshwari M, Raut AA. The CT appearances of gall bladder perforation. BJR. 2007;80(959):898-901.
45. Gore RM, Yaghmai V, Newmark GM, Berlin JW, Miller FH. Imaging benign and malignant disease of the gallbladder. Radiol Clin North Am. 2002;40(6):1307-23.
46. Smith EA, Dillman JR, Elsayes KM, Menias CO, Bude RO. Cross-sectional imaging of acute and chronic gallbladder inflammatory disease. AJR Am J Roentgenol. 2009;192(1): 188-96.
47. Balthazar EJ, Ranson JHC, Naidich DP, Megibow AJ, Caccavale R, Cooper MM. Acute pancreatitis: prognostic value of CT. Radiology. 1985;156(3):767-72.

48. Barral M, Taouli B, Guiu B, Koh DM, Luciani A, Manfredi R, et al. Diffusion-weighted MR imaging of the pancreas: current status and recommendations. Radiology. 2015;274(1):45-63.
49. Joseph AEA, MacVicar D. Ultrasound in the diagnosis of abdominal abscess. Clin Radiol. 1990;42(3):154-6.
50. Go HI, Baarslaq HJ, Vermeulen H, Laméris JS, Legemate DA. A comparative study to validate the use of ultrasonography and computed tomography in patients with post-operative intra-abdominal sepsis. Eur J Radiol. 2005;54(3):383-7.
51. Gore RM, Silvers RI, Thakrar KH, Wenzke DR, Mehta UK, Newmark GM, et al. Bowel obstruction. Radiol Clin North Am. 2015;53(6):1225-40.
52. Canon CL. Gastrointestinal Tract. In: Lee JKT, Sagel SS, Stanley RJ, Heiken JP (Eds). Computed body tomography with MRI correlation, 4th edition. Philadelphia PA: Lippincott Williams and Wilkins; 2005.
53. Ilangovan R, Burling D, George A, Gupta A, Marshall M, Taylor SA. CT enterography: review of technique and practical tips. Br J Radiol. 2012;85(1015):876-86.
54. Beall DP, Fortman BJ, Lawler BC, Regan F. Imaging bowel obstruction: a comparison between fast magnetic resonance imaging and helical computed tomography. Clin Radiol. 2002;57(8):719-24.
55. Federle MP, Anne VS. Small bowel obstruction. In: Federle MP (Ed). Diagnostic imaging - Abdomen, 1st edition. Utah: Amirsys Inc; 2004.
56. Chen SC, Wang HP, Chen WJ, Lin FY, Hsu CY, Chang KJ, et al. Selective use of ultrasonography for the detection of pneumoperitoneum. Acad Emerg Med. 2002;9(6):643-5.
57. Jones R. Recognition of pneumo-peritoneum using bedside ultrasound in critically ill patients presenting with acute abdominal pain. Am J Emerg Med. 2007;25(7):838-41.
58. Furukawa A, Sakoda M, Yamasaki M, Kono N, Tanaka T, Nitta N, et al. Gastrointestinal tract perforation: CT diagnosis of presence, site, and cause. Abdom Imaging. 2005;30(5): 524-34.
59. Rha SE, Ha HK, Lee S, Kim JH, Kim JK, Kim JH, et al. CT and MR imaging findings of bowel ischemia from various primary causes. Radiographics. 2000;20(1):29-42.
60. Wiesner W, Khurana B, Ji H, Ros PR. CT of acute bowel ischemia. Radiology. 2003;226(3):635-50.
61. Ha HK, Rha SE, Kim AY, Auh YH. CT and MR diagnosis of intestinal ischemia. Semin Ultrasound CT MR. 2000;21(1):40-55.
62. Olson MC, Bach CR, Wells ML, Andrews JC, Khandelwal A, Welle CL, et al. Imaging of bowel ischemia: an update, from the AJR special series on emergency radiology. AJR Am J Roentgenol. 2023;220(2):173-85.
63. Scott RA, Ashton HA, Kay DN. Abdominal aortic aneurysm in 4,237 screened patients: prevalence, development and management over 6 years. Br J Surg. 1991;78(9):1122-5.
64. Rakita D, Newatia A, Hines JJ, Siegel DN, Friedman B. Spectrum of CT findings in rupture and impending rupture of abdominal aortic aneurysms. Radiographics. 2007;27(2): 497-507.
65. Mellnick VM, Heiken JP. The acute abdominal aorta. Radiol Clin North Am. 2015;53(6):1209-24.
66. Condous G, Okaro E, Khalid A, Lu C, Van Huffel S, Timmerman D, et al. The accuracy of transvaginal ultrasonography for the diagnosis of ectopic pregnancy prior to surgery. Hum Reprod. 2005;20(5):1404-9.
67. Donaldson CK. Acute Gynecologic Disorders. Radiol Clin North Am. 2015;53(6):1293-307.
68. Rao PM, Rhea JT, Novelline RA, Dobbins JM, Lawrason JN, Sacknoff R, et al. Helical CT with only colonic contrast material for diagnosing diverticulitis: Prospective evaluation of 150 patients. AJR Am J Roentgenol. 1998;170(6):1445-9.
69. Chintapalli KN, Esola CC, Chopra S, Ghiatas AA, Dodd GD 3rd. Pericolic mesenteric lymph nodes: An aid in distinguishing diverticulitis from cancer of the colon. AJR AJR Am J Roentgenol. 1997;169(5):1253-5.
70. Imbriaco M, Balthazar EJ. Toxic megacolon: role of CT in evaluation and detection of complications. Clin Imaging. 2001;25(5):349-54.
71. Kim B, Lim HK, Choi MH, Woo JY, Ryu J, Kim S, et al. Detection of parenchymal abnormalities in acute pyelonephritis by pulse inversion harmonic imaging with or without microbubble ultrasonographic contrast agent: Correlation with computed tomography. J Ultrasound Med. 2001;20(1):5-14.
72. Sourtzis S, Thibeau JF, Damry N, Raslan A, Vandendris M, Bellemans M. Radiologic investigation of renal colic: unenhanced helical CT compared with excretory urography. AJR Am J Roentgenol. 1999;172(6):1491-4.
73. Singh AK, Gervais DA, Halin PF, Sagar P, Mueller PR, Novelline RA, et al. Acute epiploic appendagitis and its mimics. Radiographics. 2005;25(6):1521-34.
74. Iain D, Kirkpatrick C, Greenberg HM. Gastrointestinal complications in the neutropenic patient: Characterization and differentiation with abdominal CT. Radiology. 2003;226(3): 668-74.
75. Kalantari BN, Mortelé KJ, Cantisani V, Ondategui S, Glickman JN, Gogate A, et al. CT features with pathologic correlation of acute gastrointestinal graft-versus-host disease after bone marrow transplantation in adults. AJR Am J Roentgenol. 2003;181(6):1621-5.

CHAPTER 23

Atin Kumar, Shivanand Gamanagatti, Chandrashekhara SH

Imaging in Abdominal Trauma

INTRODUCTION

Blunt abdominal trauma in isolation accounts for 5% of trauma mortality and further contributes 15% to mortality as part of polytrauma.[1] Excessive bleeding accounts for 80–90% of acute deaths from abdominal injury. In recent years, advances in cross-sectional imaging coupled with image-guided interventional therapy have made significant contributions in enabling nonsurgical management of blunt abdominal trauma in hemodynamically stable patients.

A radiologist must have a detailed understanding of the patterns of injury, imaging appearance of traumatic injuries, assessment of hemodynamic status, and common image artifacts. The imaging evaluation must take place within the context of systematic and orderly resuscitation of the patient.

Abdominal trauma can be blunt or penetrating. Blunt trauma accounts for approximately two-thirds of abdominal injury patients. Motor vehicle accidents account for up to 80% of blunt trauma with the remainder being caused by falls, assault, and industrial accidents. Penetrating injuries commonly result due to gunshot injuries and stab wounds.

The spleen, liver, and kidneys are the most frequently injured organs in order of frequency followed by small bowel/mesentery, bladder, colon, diaphragm, pancreas, and major vessels. Multiple organs are involved in many patients.[2]

Up to two-thirds of the patients with abdominal trauma have a significant injury to other systems as well and these injuries may take precedence for both diagnosis and treatment.

Radiology plays an important role in the diagnosis and management of patients with abdominal trauma. This has become even more relevant in the last two decades because there is an increasing trend toward conservative management of most solid abdominal organ trauma. The emergence of imaging as a strong marker for extent of injury has made the surgeons more comfortable with a trial of nonoperative management of these patients and has improved the outcome.

The various imaging modalities are used, and their current role is discussed below.

PLAIN RADIOGRAPHY

Plain radiography of the abdomen is not routinely recommended in an abdominal trauma patient. It is insensitive for the detection of hemoperitoneum as intraperitoneal volume of >800 cc is usually necessary for the demonstration of classic plain radiographic signs, e.g., "dog ear" or "bladder ear" sign when there is accumulation of intraperitoneal blood in the pouch of Douglas. According to Advanced Trauma Life Support (ATLS) guidelines, chest radiograph and pelvic radiographs are recommended as an adjunct to primary survey and resuscitation of an abdominal trauma patient. The chest radiograph, besides being required for detecting chest injuries, can also detect pneumoperitoneum. It is possible with optimal radiographic technique to demonstrate as little as 1 cc of free air on an upright chest radiograph. However, in this setting, it is often not feasible to obtain an upright radiograph. The supine chest radiograph which is usually done is not that sensitive for detecting pneumoperitoneum. The pelvic radiographs are done to detect pelvic fractures in suspected pelvic injuries.

ULTRASONOGRAPHY

Sonography is commonly used for the initial assessment of abdominal trauma. Abdominal ultrasound in cases of major trauma is usually performed with a FAST (Focused

Assessment with Sonography in Trauma) examination. It provides a fast overview of the abdomen to detect free fluid which indicates hemoperitoneum and visceral organ injury in this setting. The FAST scan should be completed within a few minutes with an aim to primarily search for free intraperitoneal fluid. While parenchymal organ injuries may be detected, search for such injuries should not delay the examination especially in the setting of hemorrhage. Following standard views are recommended:

- Transverse view of epigastrium to detect pericardial fluid.
- Longitudinal view of right upper quadrant for Morison's pouch and perihepatic free fluid. This may be extended along the right flank to look for free fluid in the right paracolic gutter.
- Longitudinal view of left upper quadrant for perisplenic free fluid. This may be extended along the left flank to look for free fluid in the left paracolic gutter.
- Longitudinal views of bilateral flanks
- Transverse and longitudinal views of suprapubic region for free fluid in pelvis and pouch of Douglas.

The FAST examination is often extended to include chest to look for hemothorax which is referred to as Extended FAST (eFAST). The pleural cavities are also screened for presence of pneumothorax, which is referred to as pneumoscan. This can be done by extending the ultrasound probe cranially while examining the right and left upper quadrant planes. The eFAST technique for detection of pneumothorax is covered in the chapter on chest trauma in a different book in this series.

The reported sensitivity of FAST for detection of free intraperitoneal fluid ranges from 64 to 98% and specificity from 86 to 100%.[3] The false negative rate of FAST is about 15% for free-fluid detection. Negative FAST should be interpreted as indicative of the absence of hemoperitoneum, not the absence of intra-abdominal injury. However, it should be remembered that the sensitivity of FAST for free fluid is less than that of CT. A negative FAST should be viewed with suspicion if the finding is not commensurate with the patient's clinical presentation. On the other hand, a positive FAST does not necessarily mandate laparotomy. Hemodynamically stable patients with positive FAST should have their injuries staged with CT, giving them the benefit of nonoperative management whenever possible. FAST is not reliable for assessment of the retroperitoneum.

The sensitivity of ultrasound for detection of liver injury ranges from 0.15 to 0.883 and it misses an average of 15% injuries to the liver. The sensitivity for splenic injuries is reported to be between 37 and 85% with an average false negative rate of >50%. Sensitivity for renal and pancreatic injuries is less than of liver and spleen and even lesser for bowel and mesenteric injuries. The sensitivity for pericardial effusion is high (97–100%).[3] Hence, ultrasound as a modality to detect abdominal injuries is not recommended.

In a technically successful examination, hemoperitoneum **(Fig. 1)** is visualized as a lenticular collection in the subphrenic space, triangular in Morison's pouch and ovoid in the pelvis.

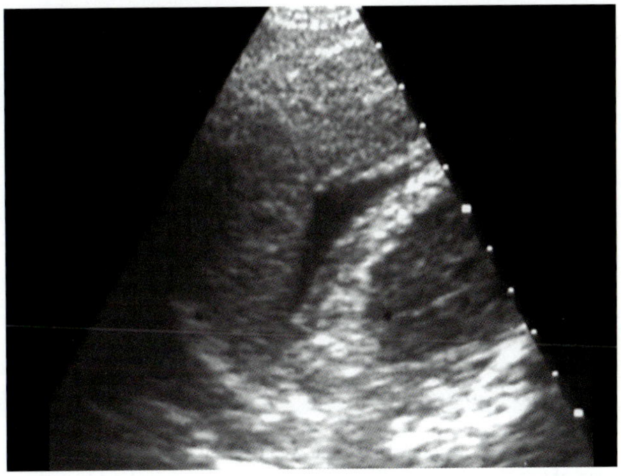

FIG. 1: Axial ultrasound image shows free fluid in hepatorenal pouch.

Recently contrast-enhanced ultrasound (CEUS) has been used for improving the detection of solid abdominal organ injuries. It has been shown to detect hepatic, splenic, and renal injuries including vascular injuries **(Figs. 2A to C)**. However, the assessment of bowel, mesentery, and retroperitoneum is not possible. Hence, it can be used as an alternative to contrast-enhanced computed tomography (CECT) for use in low energy localized trauma in patients with contraindication to CT contrast. It may also be useful in follow-up of patients to monitor the organ injury especially in pediatric patients where radiation dose is a concern.[4]

Ultrasound has certain limitations as the technique is operator dependent and may be limited by excessive bowel gas (especially in posttraumatic paralytic ileus). It may also be limited by open wounds, surgical dressings, and by subcutaneous emphysema.

COMPUTED TOMOGRAPHY

Computed tomography (CT) is now firmly established as the principal imaging modality for diagnostic evaluation of abdominal trauma. It is useful in detecting otherwise occult injuries to both intra-abdominal and retroperitoneal structures and grading the severity of specific parenchymal injury. Associated injuries of head and chest, etc. can also be evaluated. According to the American College of Radiology (ACR) guidelines, if the initial CT abdomen of a stable patient is negative, then the patient can be safely discharged from the emergency department without a period of observation.[5]

Computed Tomography Technique

Meticulous attention to scanning technique is essential. Scans should be done expeditiously, and care should be taken to avoid artifacts and repeat scanning. Current

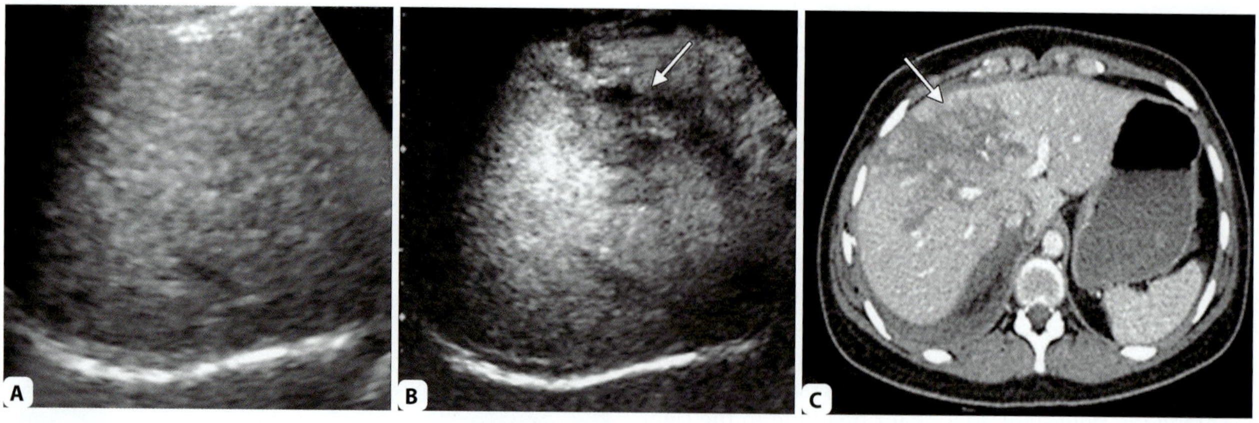

FIGS. 2A TO C: Contrast-enhanced ultrasound of right hypochondrium (B) shows the hypoechoic linear lacerations within the right lobe of the liver (arrow). These were not well appreciated on the gray scale ultrasound (A). Contrast-enhanced computed tomography (CECT) axial scan (C) also clearly shows multiple lacerations (arrow).

multidetector computed tomography (MDCT) scanners have significantly reduced the scan time with less motion artifacts besides providing excellent quality reconstructions in coronal and sagittal planes. Administration of intravenous iodinated contrast material is mandatory as it makes detection and location of parenchymal contusions and hematoma more conspicuous, identifies great vessels and provides information regarding integrity of organs or extent of the injury. MDCT protocols vary from institution to institution but typically involve a venous phase imaging at sub-millimeter slice thickness, 60–70 seconds after initiating an injection of 100–120 mL of 300 mg/dL low osmolar intravenous contrast medium at 2.5–3.0 mL/second. This phase is best for parenchymal injury detection. A lot of trauma centers in the world now do a dual phase CT in which an arterial phase is also acquired.[6] This phase is best suitable for detection of vascular injuries which may sometimes be evident only on the arterial phase. This is most useful in the spleen. Characterization of the vascular injuries often requires two phases. If the venous phase is the first acquired phase, and there is evidence of a contained vascular injury (pseudoaneurysm or fistula) or active contrast extravasation, a localized repeat phase is taken immediately to confirm the same. If the scan shows renal injury, then a delayed scan after 5–10 minutes during urographic phase is essential to detect collecting system injuries.[7] Some centers include an arterial phase (25–30 seconds after start of contrast injection) to better delineate vascular injuries. Routine use of dual phase (arterial and venous) has a concern of increased radiation exposure. At the authors institution, a dual-phase CT is done in all patients who are FAST positive as these have a high index of suspicion for a significant abdominal injury. We do a complete torso scan including chest and abdomen together as associated injuries are often present. The arterial phase covers the chest and abdomen whereas the venous phase is done only for the abdomen. In all other sets of patients who are FAST negative but in which an abdominal CT is indicated as per the clinical evaluation or history like dangerous mechanism of injury, we do a single-phase CT in the venous phase as the suspicion for a significant abdominal injury is less. There is no role for a noncontrast scan or a precontrast phase as it is not shown to be useful except to detect pneumoperitoneum.

Computed tomography cystography may be done in specific situations like hematuria with no renal injury seen on CT or hematuria along with pelvic fracture.[2] It is done by instillation of approximately 300–400 mL of diluted (1:10) iodinated contrast into bladder via Foley's catheter or suprapubic catheter. A delayed phase with passive filling of urinary bladder by renal contrast excretion is not a substitute for the same.

Oral contrast is not administered in the setting of acute trauma in most trauma centers across the world.[2,5] It has a potential use for detecting bowel injuries by showing extravasated oral contrast. But, the presence of pneumoperitoneum or pneumoretroperitoneum is an indirect marker for the same. Also, usually there is not enough time available at hand to administer oral contrast. Rectal contrast is used occasionally in specific situations to detect colorectal injuries in patients with perineal lacerations and penetrating flank or back wounds.[5]

At the authors' institution, kidney function test is not required before administering IV contrast as it may delay the scan where time is of essence. The contrast is a concern only in patients who are known patients of chronic renal disease.

Viewing on the bone window for detecting subtle fractures and upper sections with lung windows for unsuspected pneumothorax, lung contusion or free peritoneal gas should be done.

MAGNETIC RESONANCE IMAGING

Currently, magnetic resonance imaging (MRI) does not play much role in the initial evaluation of the acutely injured patient. Magnetic resonance cholangiopancreatography (MRCP) may be useful in detecting biliary transection. MRI is useful only for niche indications in hemodynamically stable patients. It has been shown to be useful in detection of pancreatic injuries. The pancreatic parenchymal lacerations and contusions are sometimes better demonstrated on MRI than CT in the acute setting. However, CT remains the first modality for evaluation. If there are equivocal findings on CT pertaining to pancreatic parenchymal injury, then MRI can subsequently be done to aid in the diagnosis. Moreover, involvement of main pancreatic duct is also better characterized on MRI (and MRCP) which is important for deciding management.[8]

DIGITAL SUBTRACTION ANGIOGRAPHY

With the recent trend toward nonoperative management of abdominal trauma patients, digital subtraction angiography (DSA) with embolization has been increasingly used in the management of posttraumatic hemorrhage. Angiographic embolization is indicated when CT shows evidence of vascular injury (pseudoaneurysm and arteriovenous fistula) and in active contrast extravasation as an alternative to surgery. It has also been used in controlling bleeding in patients with high grade (IV and V) liver and spleen injuries especially in hemodynamically stable patients with falling hematocrit.

IMAGING AND MANAGEMENT PROTOCOLS

When a patient of suspected abdominal trauma presents to the emergency department, the initial evaluation and assessment is done as per the Advanced Trauma Life Support (ATLS) guidelines. Chest and pelvic radiograph along with FAST ultrasound are considered as an adjunct of this primary survey and resuscitation. The subsequent management and further role of imaging is dependent upon the hemodynamic stability of the patient. As per the ACR guidelines/appropriateness criteria (first published in 1996 and subsequently updated in 2012 and 2019),[5] the trauma patients are divided into following categories:

- *Category A:* Patients who remain hemodynamically unstable after initial evaluation and resuscitation. The further management and imaging protocol in this group is outlined in **Flowchart 1**.
- *Category B:* Patients who are hemodynamically stable either at presentation or get stabilized after resuscitation. The imaging and management protocol in this group is outlined in **Flowchart 2**.
- *Category C:* Patients of abdominal trauma who have hematuria. This group requires some modification of imaging workup which is outlined in **Flowchart 3**.

DIAGNOSTIC IMAGING

CT Signs in Blunt Abdominal Trauma

- *Hemoperitoneum:* Blood collects in the peritoneum following injury to the liver, spleen, bowel, or mesentery. CT is sensitive in detecting intra-abdominal or pelvic hemorrhage. Nonclotted blood typically has an attenuation value of 30–45 HU whereas clotted blood has attenuation values between 45 and 70 HU. However, a quarter of patients may have HU value <20 HU. Therefore, hemoperitoneum may not be distinguishable from ascites, extravasated small intestinal fluid from bowel perforation or from intraperitoneal urine from ruptured urinary bladder. Detection of fluid within the abdomen in a suspected patient of abdominal trauma is considered as hemoperitoneum unless proven otherwise. It should, however, be remembered that in women of child-bearing age small amounts of intraperitoneal fluid may be a normal finding. Detection

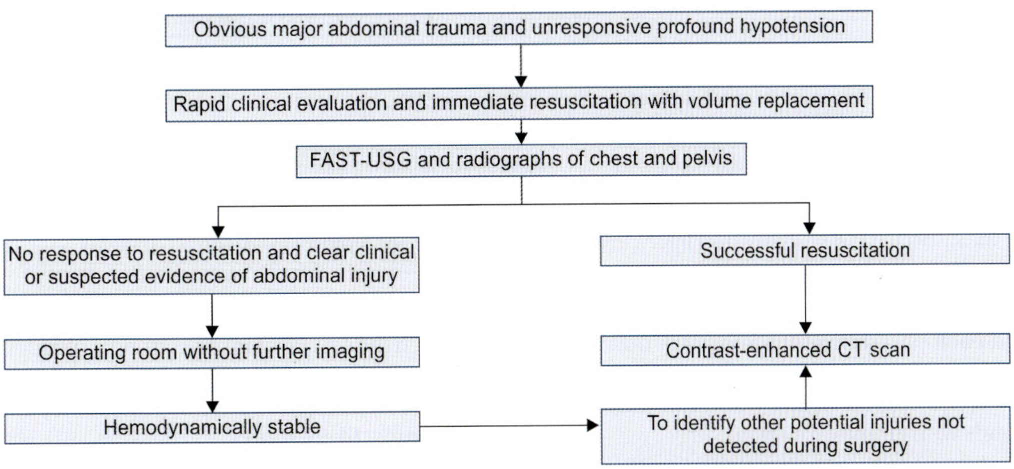

FLOWCHART 1: Hemodynamically unstable patient. Imaging and management protocol in Category A patients.
(FAST-USG: focused assessment with sonography for trauma)

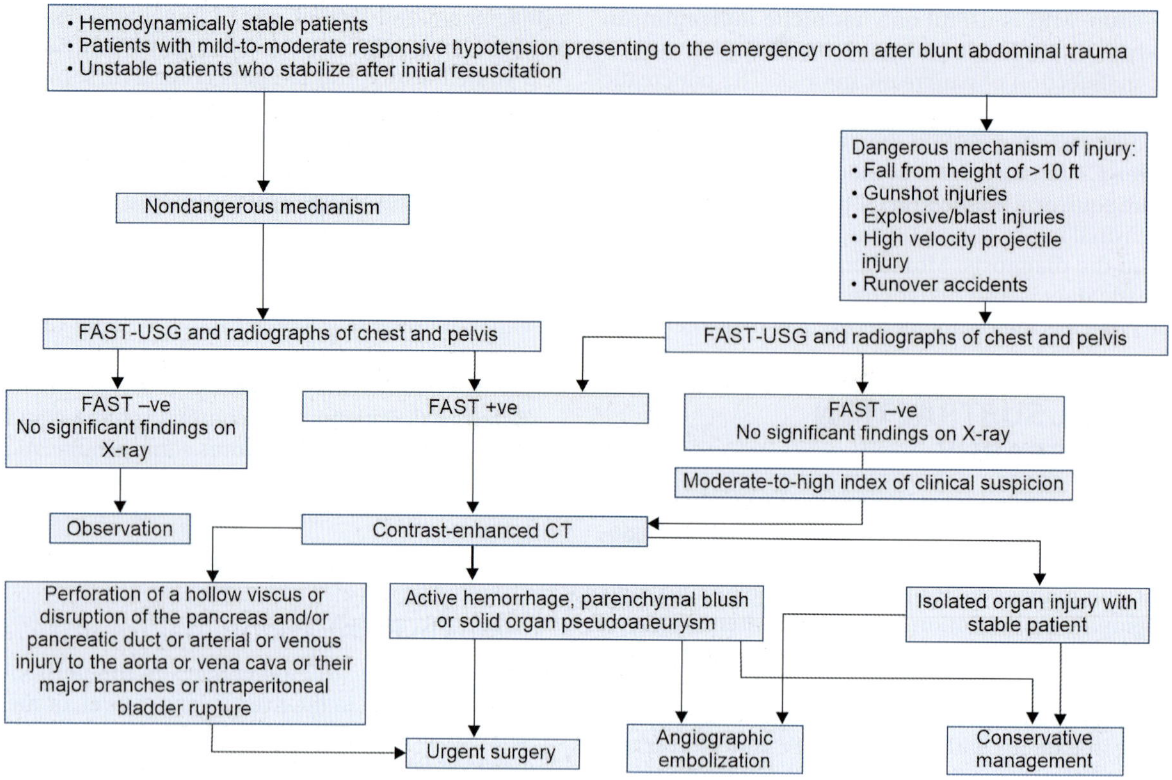

FLOWCHART 2: Hemodynamically stable patient. Imaging and management protocol in Category B patients.

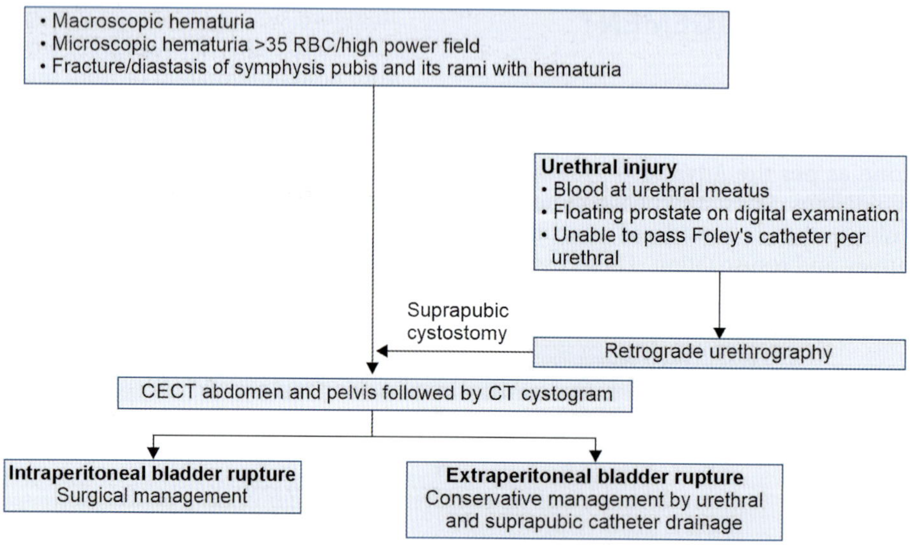

FLOWCHART 3: Suspected lower urinary tract injury. Imaging and management protocol in Category C patients.
(CECT: contrast-enhanced computed tomography)

of fluid in each paracolic gutter indicates that at least 200 mL of blood must be present in each gutter. CT visualization of blood in the abdomen and pelvis corresponds with amounts >500 mL.

- *Sentinel clot sign:* Clotted blood adjacent to the site of injury is of higher attenuation (45–70 HU) than unclotted blood which flows away **(Figs. 3A and B)**. When the source of intraperitoneal bleed is not evident or in the situation of multiple organ injuries, the location of highest attenuating blood clot is a clue to the most likely source.
- *Interloop fluid:* Triangular fluid collection(s) between the leaves of mesentery are important indicators of bowel or mesenteric injury. Hemoperitoneum from

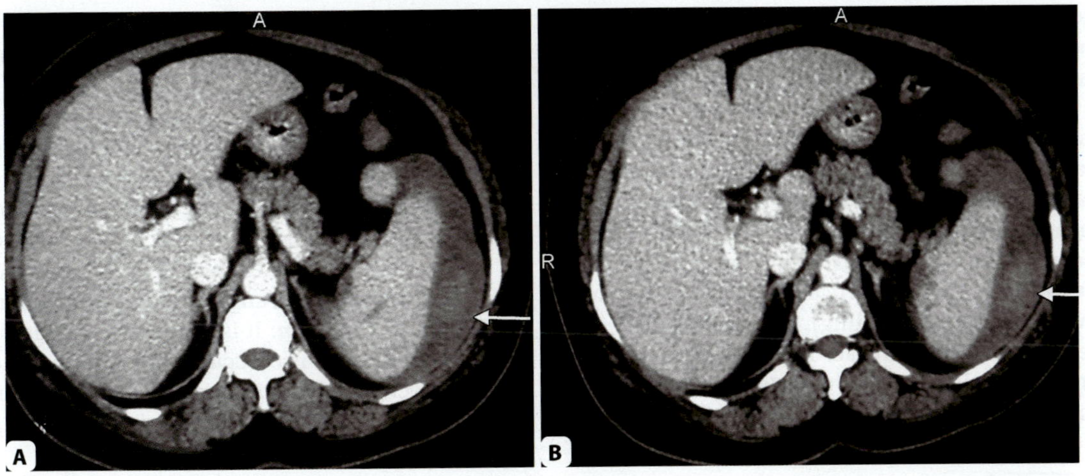

FIGS. 3A AND B: Axial contrast-enhanced computed tomography (CECT) scans show hemoperitoneum in perisplenic region. Note the presence of higher density clotted blood adjacent to the spleen (arrows)—the "sentinel clot sign".

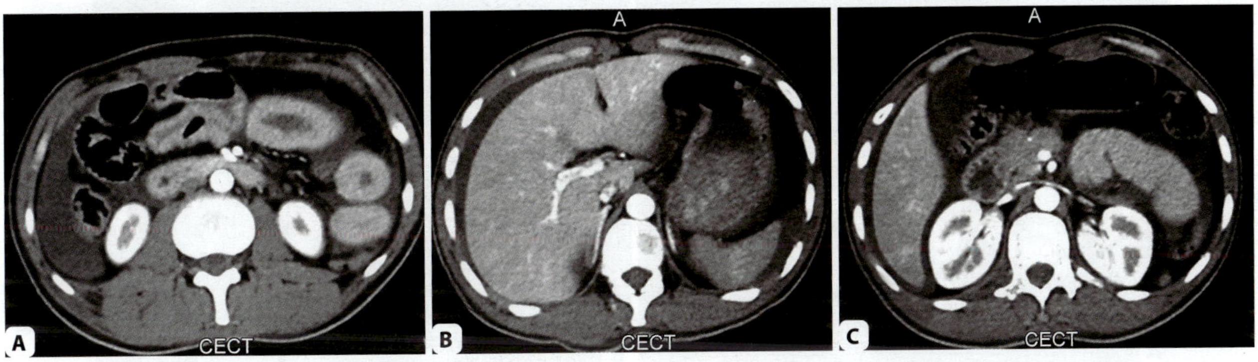

FIGS. 4A TO C: Hypoperfusion complex. Axial contrast-enhanced computed tomography (CECT) scan through mid-abdomen (A) shows diffuse thickening and hyperenhancement of jejunal loops (shock bowel). Note the presence of hemoperitoneum. Axial scan through adrenals (B) show hyperenhancing bilateral adrenal glands. Axial scan through kidneys (C) show flat inferior vena cava (IVC).

TABLE 1: Computed tomography (CT) signs for hypoperfusion complex.

Vascular signs	Visceral signs
Diminished caliber of inferior vena cava (IVC): Anteroposterior (AP) diameter <9 mm on three slices of intrahepatic IVC, at and 2 cm below renal veins	*Hollow visceral abnormalities*: • Increased bowel wall mucosal • Enhancement and gastric dilatation
Diminished caliber of aorta: AP diameter < 1.3 cm, 2 cm above, at and below renal arteries	*Solid visceral abnormalities*: • Intense adrenal gland enhancement (greater than IVC) • Renal cortical enhancement (greater than that of aorta) • Hypoenhancing spleen • Only pancreatic parenchymal enhancement

liver or spleen injury typically does not form such collections, but instead tracks from the upper abdomen along the paracolic gutters into the pelvis. When interloop fluid is of low attenuation (<15 HU), bowel injury is suspected and when it is of high attenuation (>30 HU), mesenteric hematoma is likely.

- *Hemodynamic status:* There are a combination of CT findings which give valuable morphological information that correlates with the intravascular volume and cardiac output. Hypoperfusion complex is a gamut of visceral and vascular manifestations which signify the presence of clinical shock in the patient **(Figs. 4A to C)**. They are outlined in **Table 1**.[9]
- *Vascular injuries:* Vascular injuries are classified as free/uncontained and contained vascular injuries. The uncontained vascular injury is seen as active arterial

contrast extravasation which is defined as leakage of intravascular contrast from vessel into surrounding extravascular tissues. The active contrast leak appears as a poorly marginated high attenuation contrast density (85–350 HU) seen outside the confines of a vessel **(Figs. 5A and B)**. It may be lobulated or may be spreading. It is usually surrounded by a hematoma. The extravasation appears more hyperdense than clotted blood which has HU values in the range of 45–70. On a repeat delayed scan, the active contrast leak can show change in shape (spreading). The attenuation may either increase or decrease. The contained vascular injuries (pseudoaneurysm or arteriovenous fistula) are seen as contrast outpouching which is usually rounded and well-marginated **(Figs. 6A and B)**. It is typically of the same attenuation as the adjacent major artery or aorta.

In the delayed phase, it does not change in shape and the attenuation parallels the attenuation of the adjacent artery or aorta. The vascular injuries must be actively looked for as they (especially uncontained) signify active arterial bleeding in the patient at the time of CT scanning. Detection of these injuries is often an indicator for surgical/angiographic intervention.

- *Pneumoperitoneum:* It is a sign of perforated hollow viscus, but may also occur following pneumothorax and mechanical ventilation. The small amount of air is easily detectable under the right hemidiaphragm

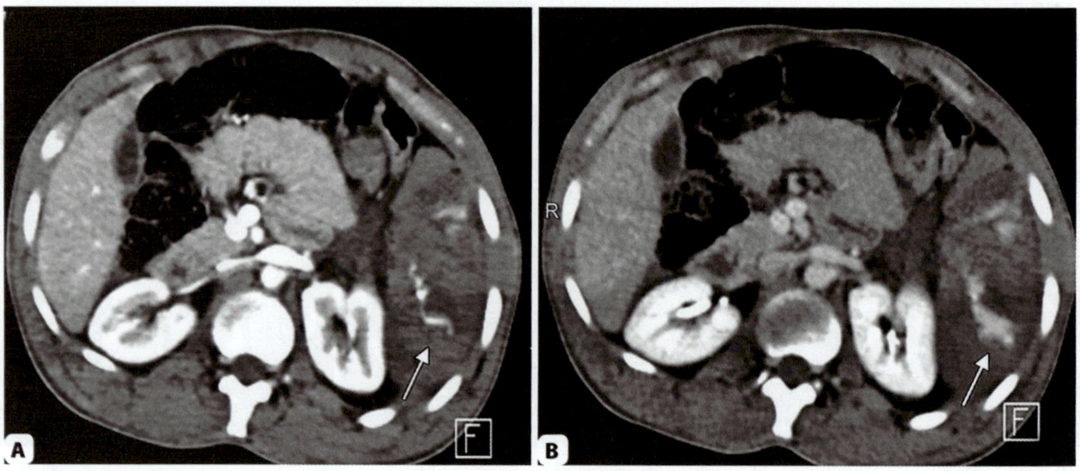

FIGS. 5A AND B: Contrast-enhanced computed tomography (CECT) abdomen axial image through the level of spleen (A) shows an irregular contrast density (arrow) in the region of splenic bed. The spleen is showing a large hematoma. The delayed image (B) acquired immediately after the first scan shows the contrast density to be spreading and changing in shape (arrow) confirming active contrast extravasation.

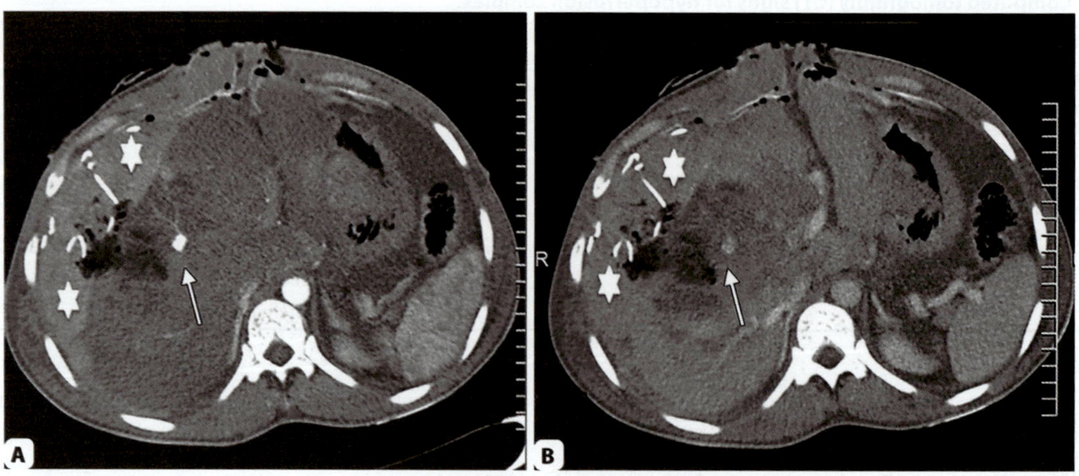

FIGS. 6A AND B: Contrast-enhanced computed tomography (CECT) abdomen axial image through the level of liver in a patient who underwent an urgent damage control surgery with perihepatic packing (A) shows a well-marginated, rounded-contrast density lesion (arrow) in the liver which is of same density as the aorta. On the delayed image (B) acquired immediately after the first scan, the lesion (arrow) maintains the same shape but shows decrease in attenuation paralleling the attenuation of the aorta. Note the presence of a large perihepatic hematoma (stars in A and B) with surgical packs.

on erect chest radiograph. CT is the most sensitive investigation for detection for free peritoneal air. In order not to miss small amounts of free air, the images should be viewed on lung window settings. It may be detected on CT over the liver and anteriorly in the mid abdomen **(Fig. 7)**. Bubbles of free air may be trapped between the leaves of the mesentery or in the peritoneal recesses.

- *Contusion/hematoma*: The contusion/hematoma within the parenchyma of solid abdominal organs appears as focal, poorly marginated areas of low attenuation representing edema, hemorrhage, and necrotic tissue **(Fig. 8)**. Subcapsular hematomas are characterized by their lenticular configuration and flattening of the adjacent parenchyma. The compression of underlying parenchyma helps to differentiate subcapsular location of hematoma from free intraperitoneal fluid or blood. Acute hematomas show increased density (40–60 HU) relative to the adjacent normal liver parenchyma at unenhanced CT.
- *Laceration:* Lacerations are seen as nonenhancing linear or branching areas usually at the periphery of the parenchyma **(Fig. 9)**. They are commonly multiple and may involve different areas including different segments. Lacerations decrease in size and number with time. When delayed phase images are taken, the lacerations appear to 'fill-in' from the periphery and become less visible.
- *Infarction/devascularization:* Infarct appears as a well-demarcated wedge-shaped area of low attenuation which remains unchanged on delayed images. It may decrease in size or remain unchanged on follow-up scans. Devascularization occurs secondary to vascular pedicle injury. The entire organ or a large segment does not show enhancement **(Fig. 10)**. Often the occluded major artery is also seen.

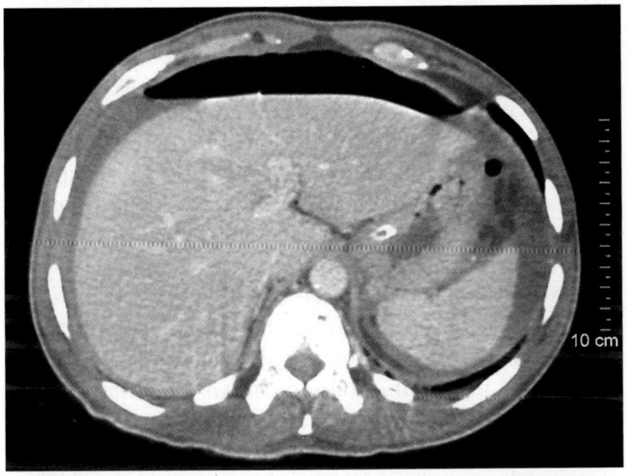

FIG. 7: Axial contrast-enhanced computed tomography (CECT) scan through upper abdomen in lung window settings shows pneumoperitoneum anterior to liver.

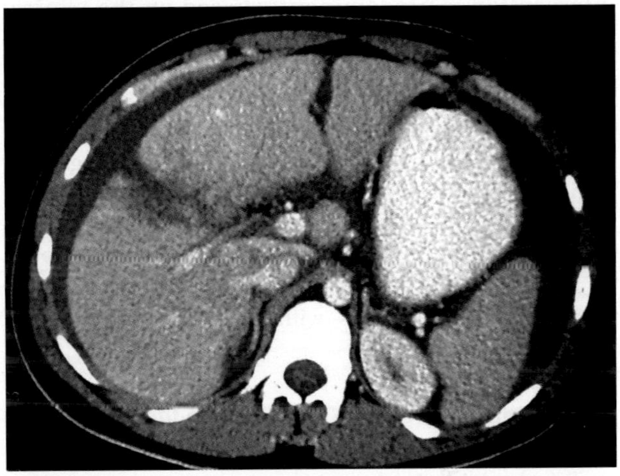

FIG. 9: Axial contrast-enhanced computed tomography (CECT) scan shows a linear liver laceration.

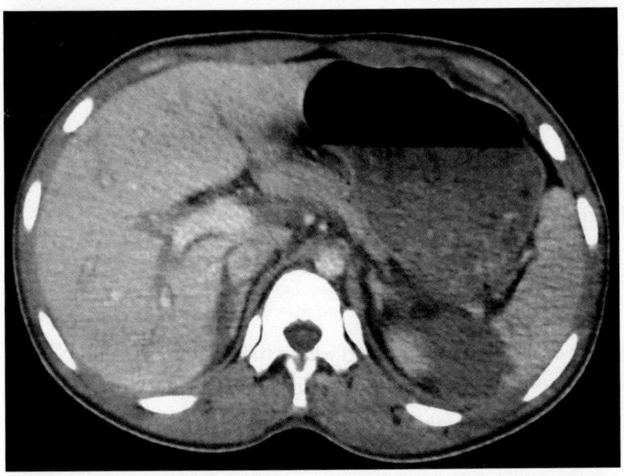

FIG. 8: Axial contrast-enhanced computed tomography (CECT) scan through upper abdomen shows a splenic parenchymal hematoma.

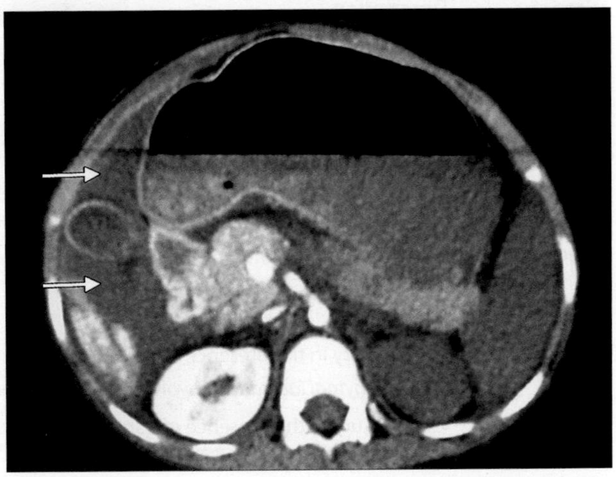

FIG. 10: Axial contrast-enhanced computed tomography (CECT) scan shows nonenhancing left kidney and spleen (devascularized) (arrows).

Computed Tomography Staging of Abdominal Injuries

Most of the organs in the abdomen are staged according to the American Association for Staging in Trauma (AAST) grading system. It is a surgical grading but can be very well correlated with CT. All organ injuries should be staged accordingly as it is an important marker for extent of injury and deciding further course of management. Majority of the injuries to the liver, spleen, and kidneys can be managed nonoperatively.

However, the higher-grade injuries require a close observation and often surgical intervention.

Computed Tomography Signs for Operative/Angiographic Intervention

As already discussed, most abdominal injuries are currently treated by nonoperative management. The surgical intervention is predominantly based on the clinical condition of the patient. The CT grading aids the trauma surgeon to monitor the patient. The higher-grade injury *per se* is not an indication for surgical intervention but is more likely to be associated with an unstable hemodynamic condition of the patient which may require surgery or angiography. However, there are a few CT findings which when seen may warrant a surgical repair. These are:

- Pneumoperitoneum—signifies full thickness bowel injury (exclude other causes as described later)
- Pancreatic transection—with involvement of pancreatic duct
- Diaphragmatic injury
- Intraperitoneal rupture of urinary bladder
- Mesenteric hematoma/vascular injury
- Renal pelvic injury.

The following CT features when seen are relative indications for either a surgical or angiographic intervention:

- Grade 4/5 liver injuries
- Grade 4/5 splenic injuries
- Vascular injuries—uncontained (active contrast extravasation) or contained (pseudoaneurysm or arterio-venous fistula).

SPLEEN

Spleen is the most commonly injured organ following blunt abdominal trauma. It is the most vascular organ of the body containing approximately 500–600 mL of blood. Although it may occur as an isolated injury, most patients with splenic trauma have associated intra-abdominal injuries.[10] The AAST splenic injury grading scale (2018 revised version) is depicted in **Table 2**.[11]

The earlier versions of AAST injury grading score did not take into account vascular injuries and active hemorrhage. Marmery et al.[12] had proposed a modified splenic injury grading system taking into account the findings of active splenic hemorrhage and vascular injuries on CT. They found it to be a better predictor for surgical or angiographic intervention in patients of splenic trauma (grade IV patients). Subsequently the 2018 revised version of AAST organ injury scale has now included the vascular injuries in the grading.[11] It has now been well established that the presence of active hemorrhage and vascular injuries is predictive of the need for splenic artery transcatheter embolization or splenic surgery.

- Arterial phase, if obtained, shows vascular injuries better and they may sometimes be difficult to detect on venous phase alone.[6] However, it is important to evaluate spleen on portal venous phase of CT as

TABLE 2: AAST organ injury scale for spleen.

Grade*	Description
Grade I	• *Hematoma:* Subcapsular, <10% surface area • *Laceration:* <1 cm in parenchymal depth • *Capsular tear*
Grade II	• *Subcapsular hematoma*: 10–50% surface area • *Intraparenchymal hematoma*: <5 cm in diameter • *Parenchymal laceration:* 1–3 cm in parenchymal depth
Grade III	• *Subcapsular hematoma*: >50% surface area or expanding; ruptured subcapsular or intraparenchymal hematoma > 5 cm • *Parenchymal laceration:* >3 cm in depth
Grade IV	• Any injury in the presence of a *splenic vascular injury or active bleeding* confined within the splenic capsule • *Parenchymal laceration:* Involving segmental or hilar vessels producing major devascularization (>25% of spleen)
Grade V	• Any injury in the presence of a *splenic vascular injury with active bleeding extending beyond the spleen* into the peritoneum • *Shattered spleen*

*Advance one grade for multiple injuries up to grade III.
(AAST: American Association for the Surgery of Trauma)

heterogenous enhancement in the arterial phase can simulate injury. If the arterial phase has not been obtained and the venous phase shows suspicion of a vascular injury then, as already stated above, another immediate delayed phase should be obtained. This will help to confirm vascular injury and also differentiate between contained and uncontained injury.

- Delayed phase may also be useful in differentiating a laceration from a splenic cleft.[10,13] When delayed phase images are taken, the lacerations appear to "fill-in" from the periphery and become less visible. In contrast, splenic clefts remain unchanged in appearance on delayed phase images besides having smooth or rounded margins.

A common pitfall in interpretation of vascular injuries of spleen is the red pulp injury.[14] It appears as focal rounded areas of hyperdensity on the arterial phase which gets isodense on the venous phase. It has been labeled as unidentified bright objects (UBO) and does not have a correlation on the DSA. On arterial phase CT, it is seen as a hyperdense string of beads appearance adjacent to a laceration with normal parenchyma on one side and gets inconspicuous on the portal venous phase. It can be differentiated from the pseudoaneurysm which is usually single, is surrounded by a laceration rather than being on the edge, and follows the attenuation of the artery on the portal venous phase.

Splenic artery embolization (SAE) has now been established as an effective tool to aid in the nonsurgical management of splenic injuries.[13,15] Currently, SAE is considered in all patients showing vascular injuries (active leak or pseudoaneurysms) **(Figs. 11A and B)**. It may also be done in patients with other grade 4 and 5 injuries without vascular injury depending upon the clinical status of the patient **(Figs. 12)**. Selected cases of grade 3 with large hemoperitoneum who may be transiently responding to resuscitative efforts can also benefit by SAE. The embolization aims to reduce the perfusion pressure to the spleen by blocking the arterial supply. However, development of collaterals from pancreatic and gastric circulation prevents clinically significant infarction thereby preserving splenic function. SAE has been shown to have beneficial effect on hematocrit drop and fluid requirements of the patient besides decreasing the length of hospital stay.[13,15]

LIVER AND BILIARY TRACT

The liver is the second most frequently injured solid abdominal organ after spleen.[2] The right lobe is injured more frequently and severely than the left and posterior segments are more frequently injured than anterior. As with spleen, CT is currently the diagnostic modality of choice for the evaluation of blunt liver trauma in

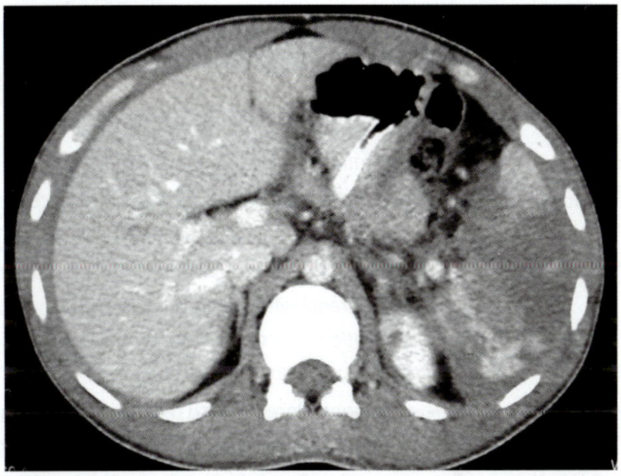

FIG. 12: Axial contrast-enhanced computed tomography (CECT) scan through the spleen shows a shattered splenic parenchyma consistent with grade V injury.

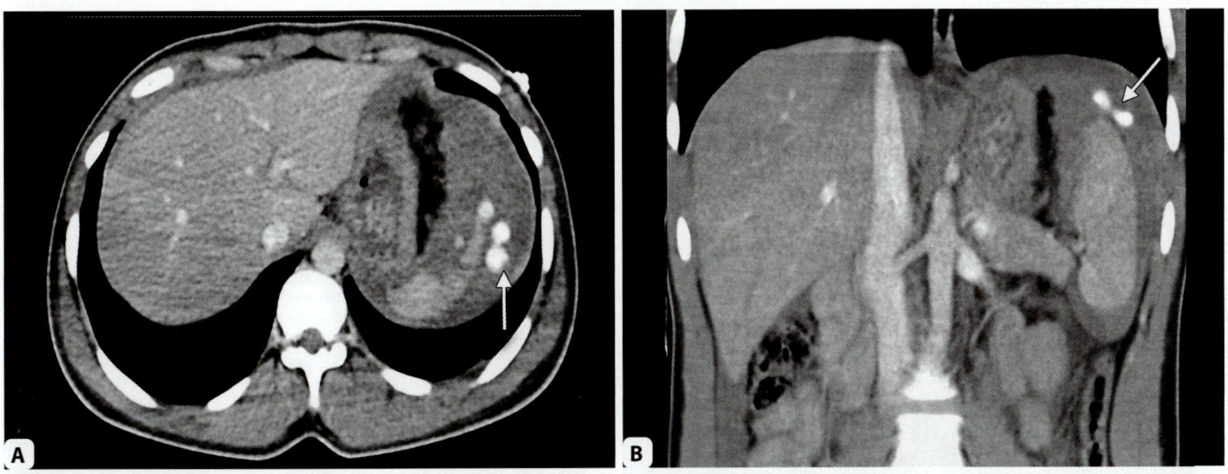

FIGS. 11A AND B: Contrast-enhanced computed tomography (CECT) axial (A) and coronal reformatted (B) images shows active contrast extravasation (arrows) from the spleen into peritoneum. The upper pole of the spleen shows a laceration. There is hemoperitoneum in perisplenic region.

hemodynamically stable patients. The AAST liver injury grading system is depicted in **Table 3**.[11]

- Majority (80%) of liver injuries cause hemoperitoneum. The finding of integrity of the liver capsule is important because it correlates with the amount of blood loss. Few specific features of liver injuries are discussed below. The subcapsular hematomas are located most commonly in the anterolateral aspect of the right lobe of liver **(Figs. 13A and B)**.
- Laceration is the most common type of liver injury. They frequently course along the vascular planes (portal vein branches and hepatic veins) and fissures (ligamentum teres and venosum), which are anatomic weak zones. They can be classified as superficial (≤3 cm in depth) or deep (>3 cm).
- Periportal tracking is seen as low-density areas along the portal vein branches. When accompanied by an adjacent parenchymal laceration, it indicates blood tracking along the periportal connective tissue **(Fig. 14)**.[14] It may also be secondary to distention of periportal lymphatic vessels due to increased central venous pressure of any cause most commonly following vigorous intravenous fluid replacement.
- The contained (pseudoaneurysm and arteriovenous fistula) and uncontained (active contrast extravasation) vascular injuries are similar to as described in spleen. Like in spleen, the revised 2018 version of AAST has included these in the grading.
- Major hepatic venous injury should be suspected if CT shows lacerations or hematomas extending into one or more major hepatic veins or IVC. These are classified as juxtahepatic venous injury and may be an indicator for surgical treatment.
- Uncommonly intrahepatic or subcapsular air may be seen up to 2 days after the injury, and it is attributed to necrosis rather than infection.

TABLE 3: AAST organ injury scale for liver (2018).

Grade*	Description
Grade I	• *Subcapsular hematoma:* <10% surface area • *Laceration:* <1 cm in parenchymal depth
Grade II	• *Hematoma:* Subcapsular, 10–50% surface area; intraparenchymal, <10 cm in diameter • *Laceration:* 1–3 cm in parenchymal depth, <10 cm in length
Grade III	• *Subcapsular hematoma:* >50% surface area; ruptured subcapsular or parenchymal hematoma; • *Intraparenchymal hematoma*: >10 cm • *Laceration:* >3 cm in parenchymal depth • Any injury in the presence of a liver *vascular injury or active bleeding contained within liver parenchyma*
Grade IV	• *Laceration:* Parenchymal disruption involving 25–75% hepatic lobe • *Active bleeding extending beyond the liver parenchyma into the peritoneum*
Grade V	• *Laceration:* Parenchymal disruption involving >75% hepatic lobe • *Vascular:* Juxtahepatic venous injuries (i.e., central major hepatic veins or retrohepatic vena cava)

*Advance one grade for multiple injuries up to grade III.
(AAST: American Association for the Surgery of Trauma)

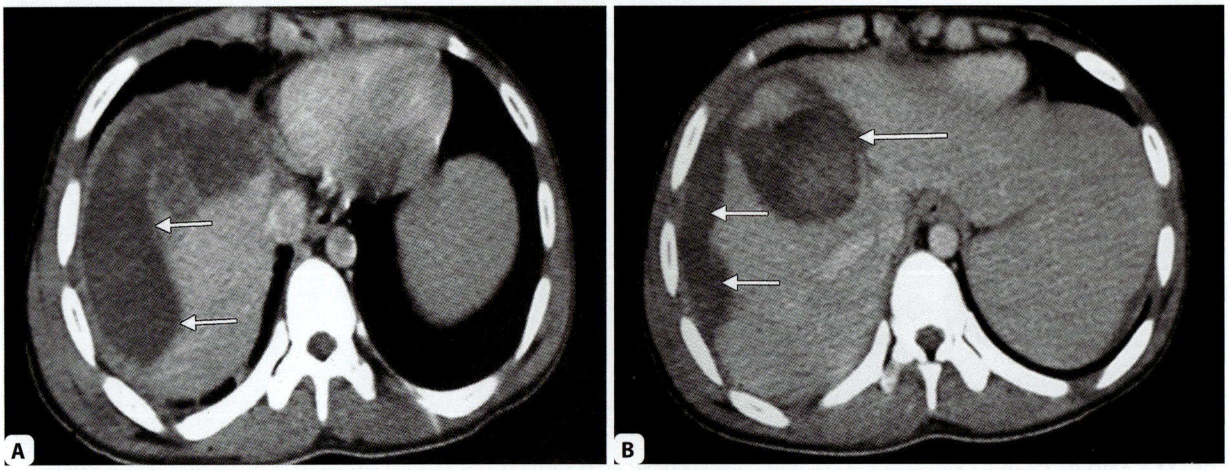

FIGS. 13A AND B: Axial contrast-enhanced computed tomography (CECT) scans show a large subcapsular liver hematoma (small arrows in A and B) caused due to rupture of a parenchymal hematoma (long arrow in B).

- Hemobilia is seen as high-attenuating material in the gallbladder or biliary channels **(Figs. 15A and B)**. It is caused when persistent arterial hemorrhage elevates intrahepatic pressure leading to parenchymal necrosis and blood spilling into the biliary tree and gut.
- Intraperitoneal bile leak and peritonitis can occur secondary to disruption of biliary system by trauma. Bile leaks are seen as relatively low-attenuation fluid collections as compared to hemoperitoneum. These may be intrahepatic or extrahepatic, diffuse, focal or encapsulated (biloma).[16]

With the current concept of nonsurgical conservative management being employed in the majority of patients of liver injury including those with severe grades, there is an increased frequency of delayed complications visualized on follow-up CT. These include:[16]

- *Delayed hemorrhage:* Secondary to rupture of pseudoaneurysm formed by a biloma or secondary to an initially minimal but expanding injury.

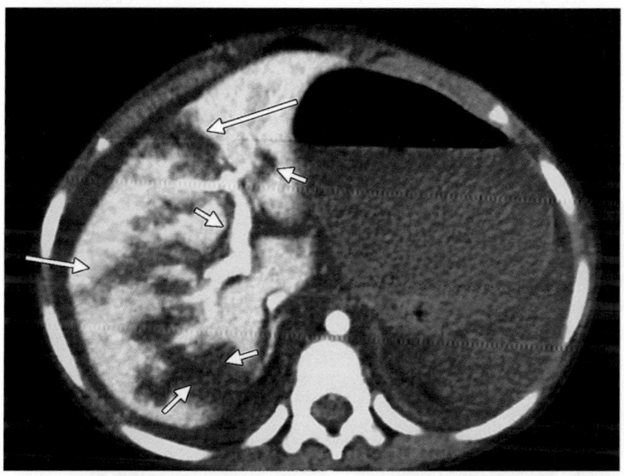

FIG. 14: Axial contrast-enhanced computed tomography (CECT) scan though liver shows periportal fluid tracking (small arrows). The liver shows multiple lacerations (long arrows) and contusion.

- *Hepatic artery pseudoaneurysm and hemobilia:* A pseudoaneurysm is formed when the arterial continuity is disrupted and blood extravasates into a parenchymal hematoma with formation of a fibrous tissue capsule. They appear as focal rounded enhancing lesions paralleling the attenuation of arterial blood in all phases. When the pseudoaneurysm ruptures into the biliary system it leads to hemobilia and subsequent drainage into duodenum can lead to hematemesis or melena. These pseudoaneurysms should be treated early and angiographic embolization is the modality of choice.
- *Abscess:* Usually seen in follow-up of high-grade liver injuries. It is visualized as fluid containing a focal lesion with air bubbles or air-fluid levels. The treatment of choice is percutaneous catheter drainage.
- *Biliary complications:* Biliary leaks are usually self-limiting with no definitive treatment required. Hepatic scintigraphy and MRCP may be helpful in detecting bile leaks. Bile leak into a hematoma may cause necrosis of surrounding liver tissue leading to formation of biloma which on CT appears as low-attenuating well-circumscribed collection. Enlarging or symptomatic bilomas can be treated with percutaneous catheter drainage with or without endoscopic retrograde cholangiopancreatography (ERCP)-guided endobiliary stent placement. Bile leak into the peritoneal cavity leads to biliary peritonitis which may be suspected on CT if peritoneal thickening and enhancement is seen with increasing amount of low-attenuation fluid.

Follow-up CT is usually not required in low-grade injuries unless the patient's clinical status demands so. However, in high-grade injuries (grades IV or V), due to increased incidence of delayed complications a follow-up ultrasound is usually required and should be done between 7 days and 10 days after injury.[17] CEUS, if available, can improve the diagnostic accuracy. CT scan may be required in selected complicated cases.

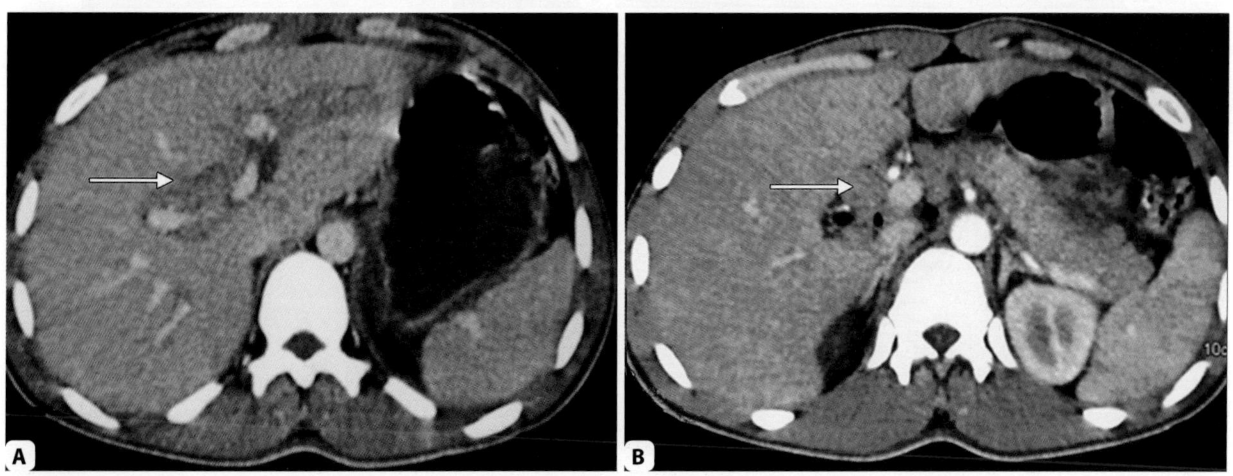

FIGS. 15A AND B: Axial contrast-enhanced computed tomography (CECT) scans through upper abdomen show hyperdensity within intrahepatic bile ducts (arrow in A) and within the common bile duct (CBD) (arrow in B) suggesting hemobilia.

Hepatic artery embolization (HAE) has also been increasingly used in the management of liver injuries.[17] It is indicated when CT shows presence of a vascular injury in the form of active contrast extravasation or pseudoaneurysm **(Figs. 16A to D)**. It can also be done prophylactically for grades 4 and 5 injuries and has been shown to decrease morbidity and mortality. The dual blood supply to the liver from hepatic artery and portal venous system helps in this regard wherein the hepatic artery or its branches can be sacrificed without much risk of infarction.

Gallbladder injuries are unusual. CT findings of ill-defined contour of gallbladder, wall thickening, intraluminal hemorrhage, or collapsed lumen, especially in the presence of pericholecystic fluid suggests primary gallbladder injury in patients with abdominal trauma. Injuries to the extrahepatic bile ducts are uncommon and occur at the points of fixation, i.e., where the hepatic ducts enter the liver and where common bile duct enters the pancreas. The diagnosis is most often made at surgery.

PANCREAS

The pancreas is the least commonly injured solid organ, accounting for 3–12% of all abdominal injuries.[18] This injury occurs after a sudden force that compresses the pancreatic neck against lumbar spine, e.g., in motor vehicle accidents in adults and bicycle accidents in children. Pancreatic injuries are difficult to diagnose. The presence of abdominal pain, leukocytosis, and hyperamylasemia is nonspecific and frequently not present.

CT has sensitivity and specificity of about 85% for the detection of pancreatic injuries. The routine venous phase which is acquired for the rest of the abdomen is often sufficient to diagnose pancreatic injuries. The injuries are classified according to the AAST grading for pancreatic injuries **(Table 4)**.[19] The following points are most relevant for clinical management:

- The presence of a laceration involving the pancreatic duct. However, the pancreatic duct may not often be seen. When a central laceration is seen extending for >50% of anteroposterior or craniocaudal width of the pancreatic parenchyma, then it is presumed to involve the main pancreatic duct. Hence, it is required to quantitate the depth of laceration as a percentage of parenchymal width.[8,18,20] This is best delineated on the CT workstation by visualizing the pancreas in multiplanar reformation or reconstruction (MPR) in all planes. Curved reformatted images in the plane of pancreas are useful in this setting.

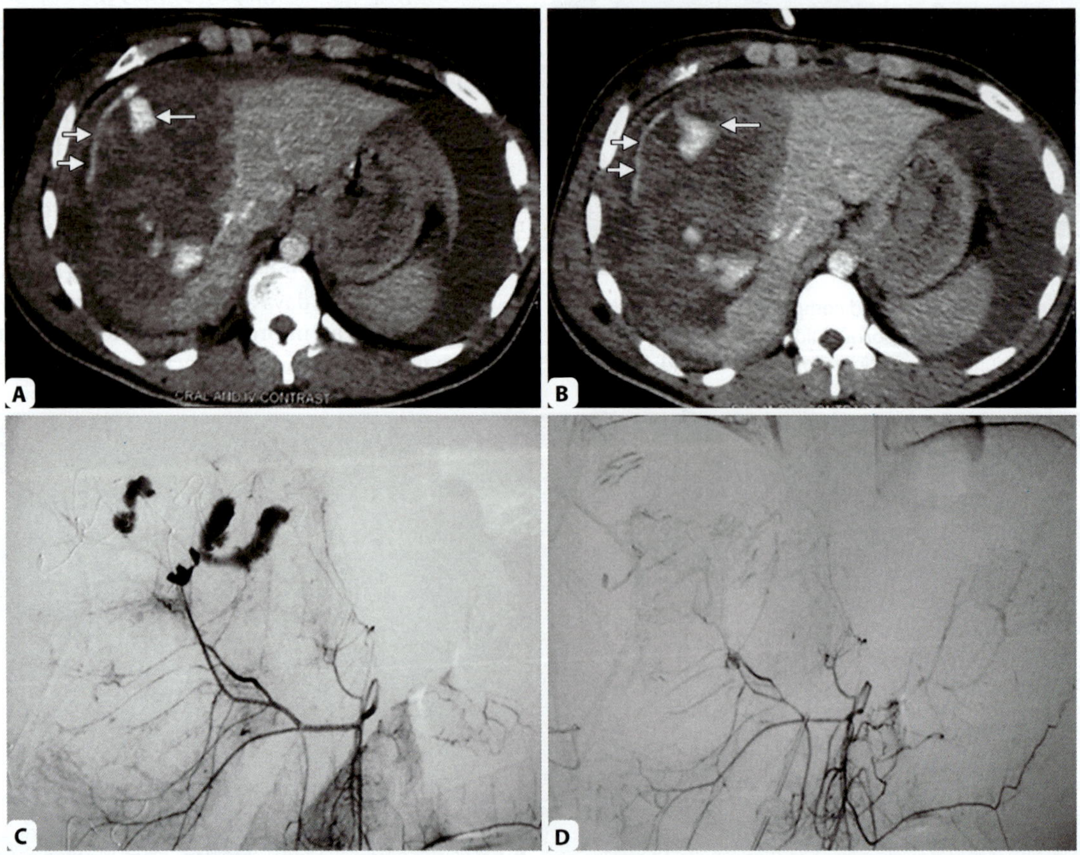

FIGS. 16A TO D: Axial contrast-enhanced computed tomography (CECT) scans (A and B) show active contrast extravasation within liver parenchyma (arrows) extending into peritoneal space (small arrows). digital subtraction angiography (DSA) image (C) of selective hepatic artery injection shows active contrast extravasation. Post coil embolization (D) the extravasation has stopped.

TABLE 4: AAST organ injury scale for pancreas.

Grade*	Description of injury
Grade I	• Minor contusion without duct injury • Superficial laceration without duct injury
Grade II	• Major contusion without duct injury or tissue loss • Major laceration without duct injury or tissue loss
Grade III	Distal transection or parenchymal injury with duct injury
Grade IV	Proximal transection or parenchymal injury involving ampulla
Grade V	Massive disruption of pancreatic head

*Advance one grade for multiple injuries up to grade III.
(AAST: American Association for the Surgery of Trauma)

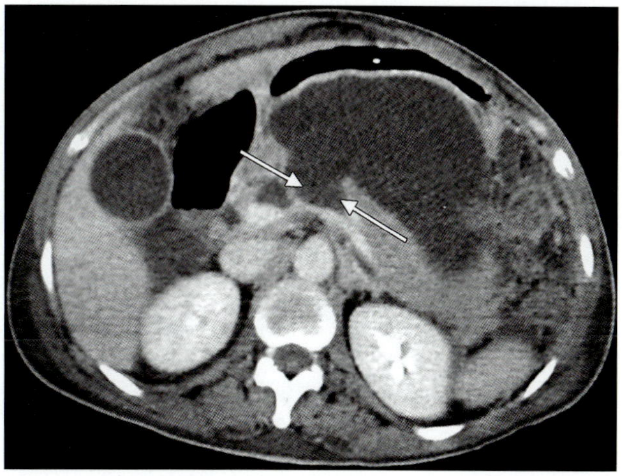

FIG. 17: Axial contrast-enhanced computed tomography (CECT) scan through pancreas shows a laceration/transection involving neck/proximal body of pancreas (arrows) with a large collection seen anterior to pancreas.

- *Location of the laceration:* It most commonly involves the region of pancreatic neck **(Fig. 17)**. Within the neck region, it is important to describe whether it is to the right or left of superior mesenteric vein and splenic vein confluence. If the laceration (>50%) or transection is seen to the right of the confluence, then it is managed either conservatively or may require Whipple's surgery. If it lies to the left of the confluence, then a distal pancreatectomy is done.[20] Similarly, large lacerations and hematomas in the head of pancreas may require Whipple's surgery **(Fig. 18)**. However, there is an increasing trend in conservative management of these patients.
- Often the direct evidence of injury to pancreas is not visualized on CT especially when done within 24–48 hours of injury. Indirect CT signs of pancreatic injury include focal or diffuse enlargement of the gland, fluid in the peripancreatic fat, around the superior mesenteric artery (SMA), in the transverse mesocolon and lesser peritoneal sac, fluid separating pancreas from the splenic vein, and thickening of left anterior renal fascia. The pancreatic injuries are shown to evolve over time. In a patient with suspected pancreatic injury in whom the initial CT scan shows a normal pancreas, a follow-up thin section CT scan within 24–48 hours of injury may show an injury not evident initially.

Recent studies have shown an increasing role of MRI with MRCP in the diagnosis of pancreatic injuries. MRI has been shown to increase the diagnostic confidence for detection of parenchymal contusions and lacerations especially the involvement of the main pancreatic duct which is essential for planning treatment **(Figs. 19A and B)**.[8] At the authors' institution, MRI with MRCP is done in all patients who have a doubtful contusion or laceration on the initial CT and the patient is stable. The patients showing a definite laceration in which involvement or sparing of pancreatic duct is clear on CT are not subjected to MRI.

The role of ERCP is mainly limited to pancreatic ductal stenting for treatment of ductal injury.

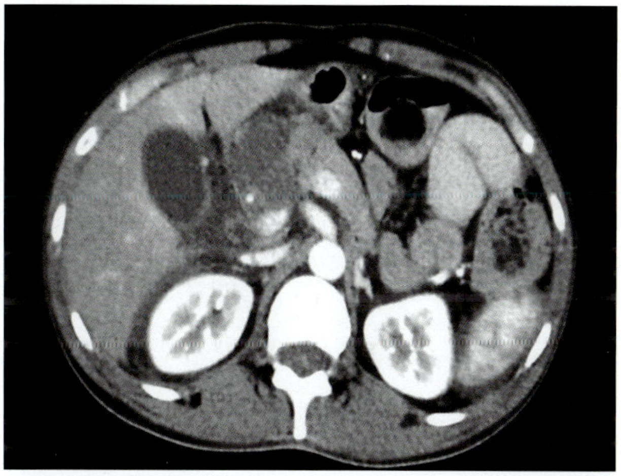

FIG. 18: Axial contrast-enhanced computed tomography (CECT) scans show a contusion involving the head of pancreas.

Major complications can result following pancreatic trauma, e.g., pancreatic fistula, intra-abdominal abscess, pseudocyst formation **(Fig. 20)**, hemorrhage, pseudo-aneurysm formation, acute recurrent pancreatitis, etc.

URINARY TRACT

Urinary tract injuries are outside the purview of this book and will be described in detail in a forthcoming book of this series on "Urogenital Imaging".

ADRENAL

With the increasing use of CT, adrenal injuries are now recognized as the most common retroperitoneal injury.[21] It is usually associated with injury to other organs especially liver and kidneys. Adrenal hemorrhage due

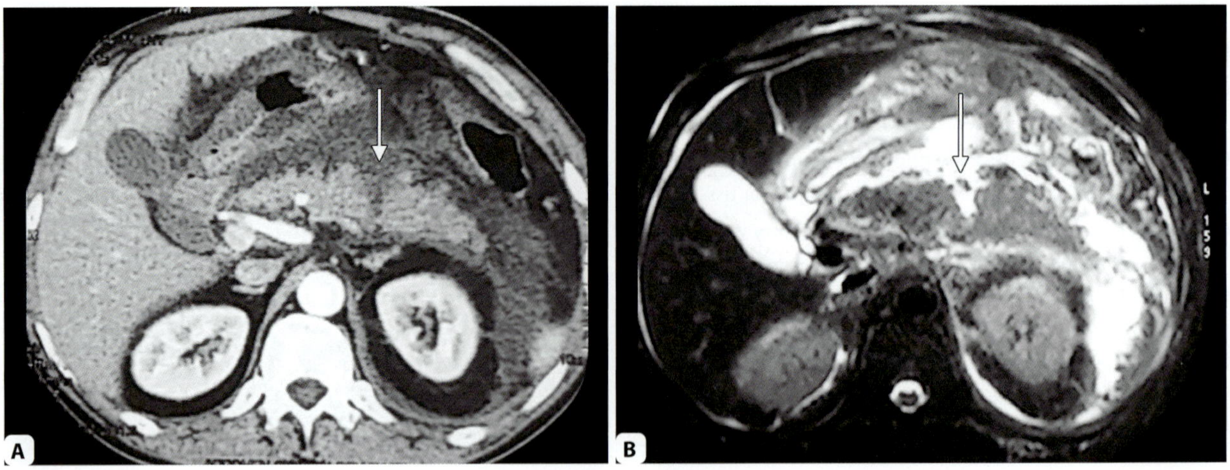

FIGS. 19A AND B: Contrast-enhanced computed tomography (CECT) axial scan (A) at level of pancreas shows a laceration (arrow) involving the distal body of the pancreas. The laceration extends to >50% of parenchymal depth, hence it is likely involving the main pancreatic duct. Note the surrounding inflammatory changes of pancreatitis. HASTE (Half fourier Single-shot Turbo spin-Echo) axial MRI (magnetic resonance imaging) image (B) at same level clearly shows the pancreatic laceration (arrow) with surrounding inflammatory changes.

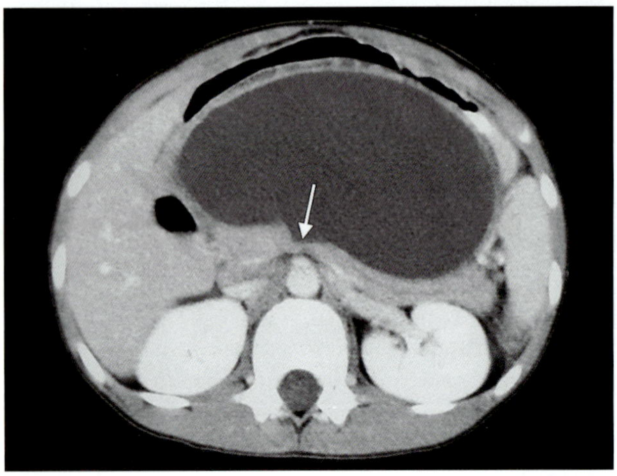

FIG. 20: Axial contrast-enhanced computed tomography (CECT) scan at the level of pancreas shows a large pseudocyst anterior to pancreas with a beak-shape extension (arrow) in the neck of pancreas representing partial transection of pancreas.

to trauma is unilateral in >90% of cases and usually the right adrenal gland is involved. The mechanism of injury may be compression of the adrenal gland between the liver and spine. On CT, adrenal hematoma appears as a round to oval homogeneous density mass (40–75 HU) that replaces all or a portion of the normal adrenal gland **(Figs. 21A and B)**. In addition, there may be stranding of the periadrenal fat that extends to the upper pole of the kidney and apparent thickening of the ipsilateral diaphragmatic crus due to adjacent hemorrhage.[21] A posttraumatic cyst or calcification may be seen as a sequel on long-term follow-up. Adrenal hemorrhage is of little clinical significance, particularly when it is unilateral.[22] Rarely, bilateral adrenal hemorrhage has been shown to precipitate adrenal insufficiency.[23]

HOLLOW VISCUS, OMENTAL, AND MESENTERIC INJURY

The diagnosis of intestinal injury is one of the most difficult and controversial aspects of trauma care. The symptoms may be delayed for many hours. If not surgically repaired, it may lead to bleeding and leakage of gastrointestinal contents into the peritoneal cavity or retroperitoneum, leading to peritonitis or sepsis. The plain radiographs of the abdomen are relatively insensitive in detecting bowel injury. Rupture of a hollow viscus may produce free air either in the peritoneal cavity or retroperitoneum. Additional findings of free intraperitoneal fluid may be seen. MDCT is the diagnostic modality of choice for detection of bowel and mesenteric injuries and has been shown to be more sensitive and specific than clinical examination, diagnostic peritoneal lavage, and abdominal ultrasound.[24] The signs of bowel injury are frequently subtle. The most specific signs of bowel injury are:[24-26]

- Pneumoperitoneum or pneumoretroperitoneum
- Extravasation of oral contrast material (if administered)
- Low-attenuating fluid between loops
- Bowel wall discontinuity **(Figs. 22A to C)**

Retroperitoneal air tends to localize near the site of injury, often accompanied by fluid, either blood or intestinal. The presence of these signs usually mandates urgent laparotomy. All the above signs, though highly specific, are not as sensitive.[26] Also care must be taken to exclude other causes of extraluminal contrast (bladder injury) and extraluminal air (mechanical ventilation, pneumothorax, chest injury, peritoneal lavage prior to CT, Foley's catheter in an intraperitoneal bladder rupture). Another important consideration is "pseudopneumoperitoneum" which leads to false positive diagnosis. It refers to trapped air between the parietal peritoneum and the abdominal wall. So, it is actually extraperitoneal, but can be confused

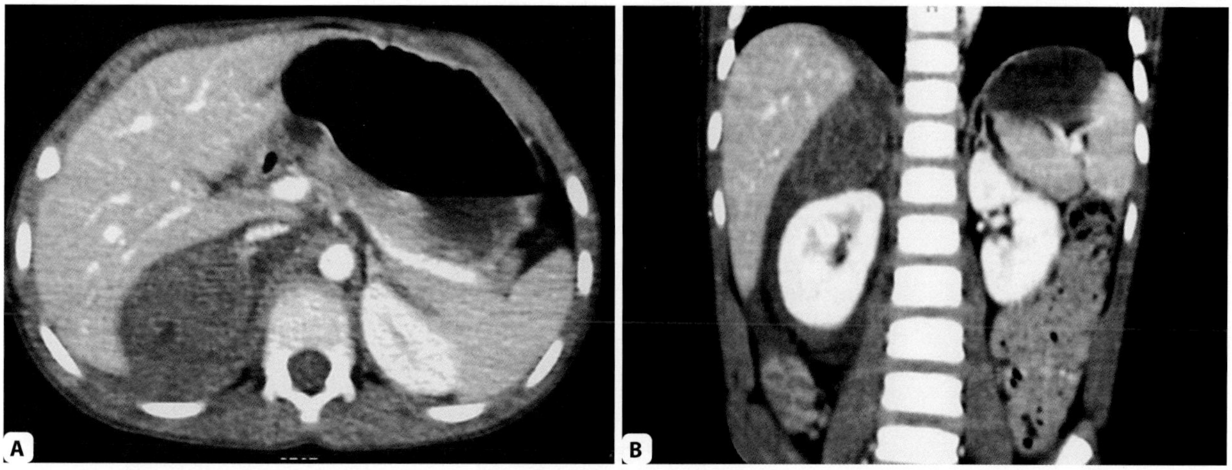

FIGS. 21A AND B: Axial (A) and coronal reformat (B) contrast-enhanced computed tomography (CECT) scans show a right adrenal hematoma.

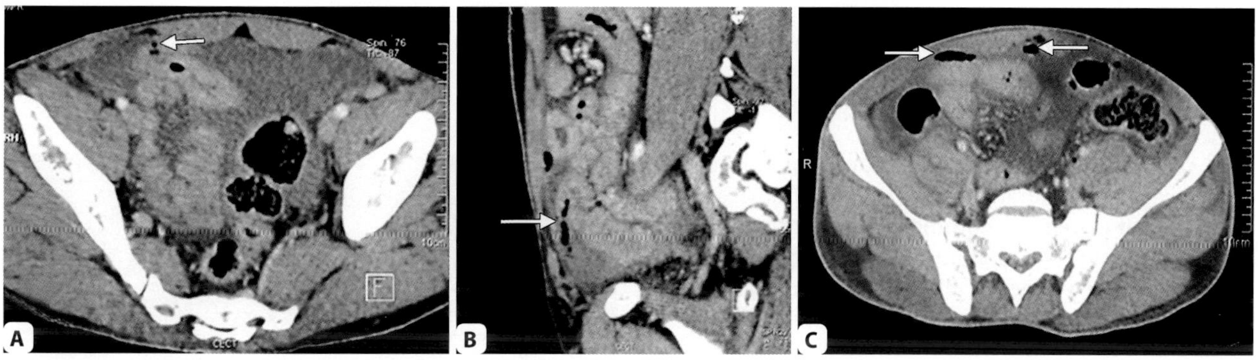

FIGS. 22A TO C: Axial (A) and sagittal reformat (B) images of contrast-enhanced computed tomography (CECT) shows a focal defect in wall of ileum (arrows) with air extending outside bowel lumen. An axial section at a different level with changed window settings shows the presence of pneumoperitoneum (arrows).

as intraperitoneal on images. It is seen in patients with pneumothorax and pneumomediastinum especially on positive pressure ventilation where the air dissects and extends caudally beneath the abdominal wall. Careful evaluation of the CT images especially with coronal and sagittal reconstructions often helps in localizing this air to be extraperitoneal.

It should also be remembered that absence of pneumoperitoneum does not rule out bowel perforation. This can occur due to multiple causes like very early imaging posttrauma, spontaneous healing of perforation, paralytic ileus causing failure of gas to escape from intestine, or reabsorption of small quantity of gas through the peritoneal lining. Hence, other suggestive signs should also be looked for. Often the clinical signs on abdominal examination alone can warrant exploratory laparotomy.

Less specific signs of bowel injury include:[24-26]

- Peritoneal fluid without a known cause
- Focal bowel wall thickening > 3 mm
- Mesenteric infiltration, thickening or hematoma
- Abnormal bowel wall enhancement **(Figs. 23A and B)**.

Patients manifesting these signs may have bowel perforation requiring surgery, a less severe bowel contusion, or hematoma that may be managed without surgery or no bowel injury at all. It must be remembered that diffuse bowel wall thickening may also be noted in fluid overload or in hypoperfusion state (shock bowel) wherein it would have other accompanying features of hypoperfusion complex as detailed earlier in this chapter. There can be various abnormal patterns of bowel wall enhancement secondary to trauma:

- Increased enhancement as in hypoperfusion state (due to increased vascular permeability with interstitial leakage of contrast)
- Patchy and irregular enhancement due to wall injury
- Decreased or absent enhancement due to ischemia

Blunt injuries to the stomach are uncommon. The second and third parts of duodenum are the most frequently injured portion of small bowel as they are fixed.[24] Duodenal hematoma has a characteristic appearance on CT scan. In the absence of duodenal perforation, focal thickening or high-attenuating mass in the duodenal

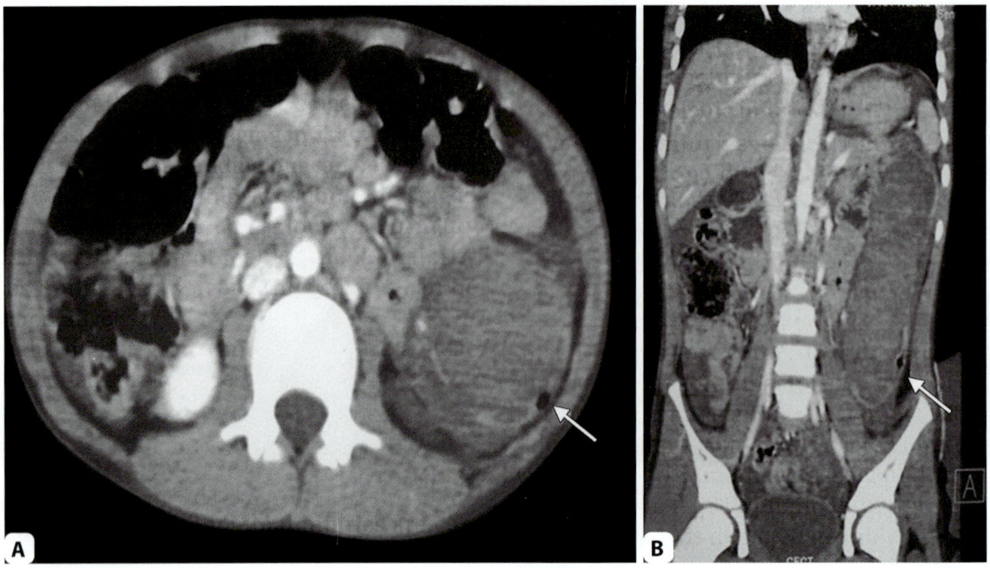

FIGS. 23A AND B: Axial (A) and coronal reformat (B) contrast-enhanced computed tomography (CECT) scans of abdomen show entire descending colon distended with hyperdense contents representing hematoma with thinned out abnormally enhancing walls and air within the wall (arrow in A and B) suggesting colonic injury.

wall, possibly associated with retroperitoneal fluid, is suggestive of intramural hematoma. Blunt injuries of the small intestine are most commonly seen at the points of fixation (ligament of Treitz and terminal ileum) but may occur anywhere along the length of the small intestine. Blunt colonic injuries are rare.

The mesentery and omentum are most often associated with injuries elsewhere in the abdomen and pelvis. Avulsion of the SMA and vein occurs most commonly near their origin, because of shearing effect. Massive hemorrhage can result from rupture or tear of these vessels. Vascular thrombosis and occlusion by an intimal flap may also result from trauma. CT scan can be used to determine the extent and location of mesenteric injury.

Mesenteric injury has certain specific and nonspecific features on MDCT.[24,25] The specific CT features of mesenteric vascular injury are:

- Active contrast extravasation within mesentery
- Beaded appearance of mesenteric vessels
- Abrupt termination of mesenteric vessels

The relatively nonspecific findings include:

- Mesenteric hematoma **(Fig. 24)**
- Mesenteric infiltration
- Bowel wall thickening
- Abnormal wall enhancement secondary to ischemia
- Increased fluid within the bowel lumen
- Pneumatosis intestinalis

It must be remembered that some of these signs may also be seen in bowel injury alone without concomitant mesenteric injury.

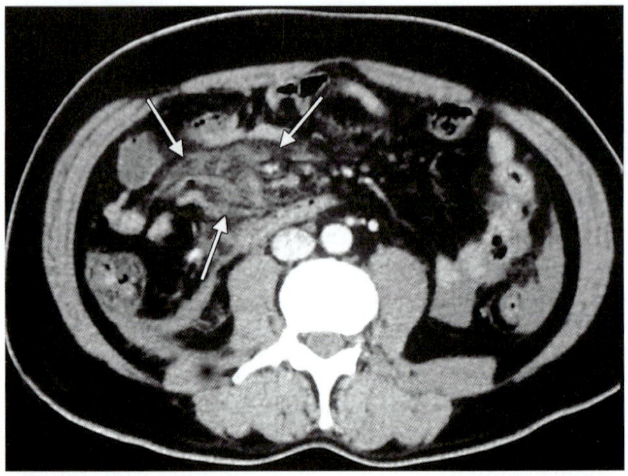

FIG. 24: Axial contrast-enhanced computed tomography (CECT) scan through lower abdomen shows infiltration and hematoma (arrows) in mesenteric root representing mesenteric injury.

DIAPHRAGM

Diaphragmatic rupture and subsequent herniation of abdominal contents into thorax is nine times more common on left side than right due to the protective effect of the liver.[1] On the right side, most injuries to the diaphragm go unrecognized during the acute phase. In the interval phase, the abdominal viscus may not have herniated, or the patient may have acclimatized to the presence of abdominal contents in the thorax. In the later phase, obstruction or strangulation presents with severe abdominal or chest pain. The injury may also be evident at a later stage in those patients who were earlier on positive pressure ventilation and extubated later.

Chest radiograph may diagnose diaphragmatic rupture if the following specific signs are visualized:

- Visualization of bowel loops or solid masses above the diaphragm
- Loss of the normal diaphragmatic contour
- Detection of a nasogastric tube above the left hemidiaphragm

The diagnosis may also be suspected on chest radiograph if a combination of following nonspecific signs is visualized:

- Indistinct or elevated hemidiaphragm **(Fig. 25A)**
- Pleural effusion
- Atelectasis with shift of the mediastinum to the contralateral side
- Hemothorax
- Pneumothorax
- Lower rib fractures

Contrast studies (barium meal or enema) can be used to clearly delineate the herniation.

The advent of MDCT with multiplanar reconstructions has significantly improved the sensitivity of CT in detecting diaphragmatic injuries.[27] The various CT signs which are seen in diaphragmatic rupture are:

- Focal diaphragmatic discontinuity or elevation
- Focal diaphragmatic thickening (retraction)
- Herniated abdominal contents into thorax
- "Collar" sign—narrowed waist of a herniated intra-abdominal organ due to compression at the neck (diaphragm tear)
- "Dependent viscera" sign—herniated intra-abdominal contents abutting the posterior thoracic wall without intervening diaphragmatic slip **(Figs. 25A and B)**.

Among the above features the "dependent viscera" sign and the "collar" signs are reported to be 100% specific.[1] MRI also has been reported to be highly sensitive in detecting diaphragmatic rupture.[28]

RETROPERITONEUM

The most frequently injured retroperitoneal structures include the adrenals, pancreas, great vessels, gastrointestinal tract, genitourinary tract, and musculoskeletal system.[1,2] Inability to account for blood loss either in the chest or abdomen in a patient with ongoing transfusion requirements should dictate angiographic investigation. The potential for simultaneous angiographic embolization of actively bleeding vessels is well documented and may be lifesaving since opening the retroperitoneum to control bleeding is associated with high mortality.

ABDOMINAL WALL INJURY

Abdominal wall injuries are easily overlooked if not specifically looked for. Most common are bruises, which appear on CT as skin thickening and soft-tissue infiltration of subcutaneous fat. Intramuscular hematomas may be seen **(Fig. 26)**. Tearing of lateral abdominal wall or rectus abdominis is an unusual occurrence that results in subcutaneous hematoma and occasionally bowel herniation. Morel Lavallee lesion representing internal degloving injury is seen on CT as separation of skin from the subcutaneous with intervening fluid collection.

PENETRATING ABDOMINAL TRAUMA

Traditionally, almost all stab and gunshot wounds to the abdomen used to undergo surgical exploration. With

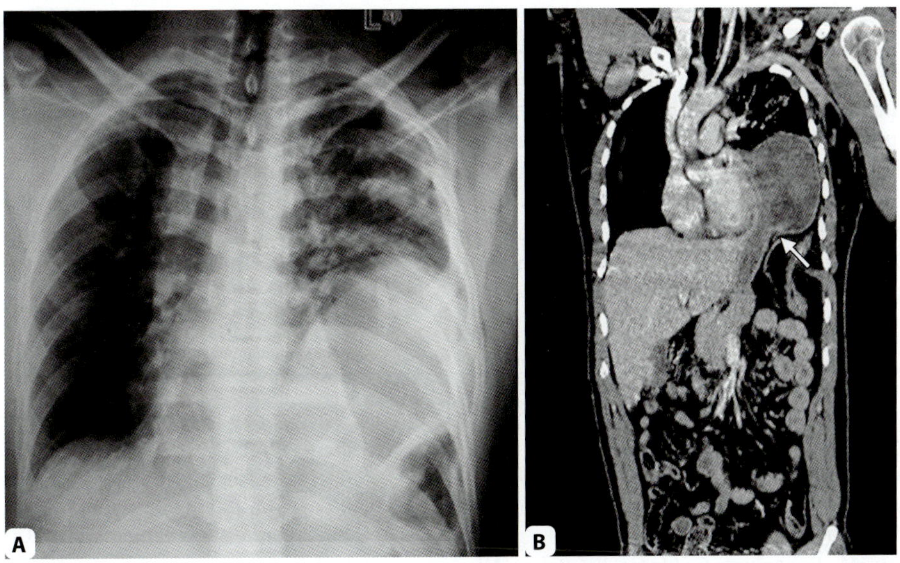

FIGS. 25A AND B: Chest radiograph posteroanterior (PA) view (A) shows opacity in left lower zone with smooth convex upper margin and air lucencies within. Coronal reformatted contrast-enhanced computed tomography (CECT) image (B) shows clearly the diaphragmatic defect (arrow) with stomach herniating through it into the thorax.

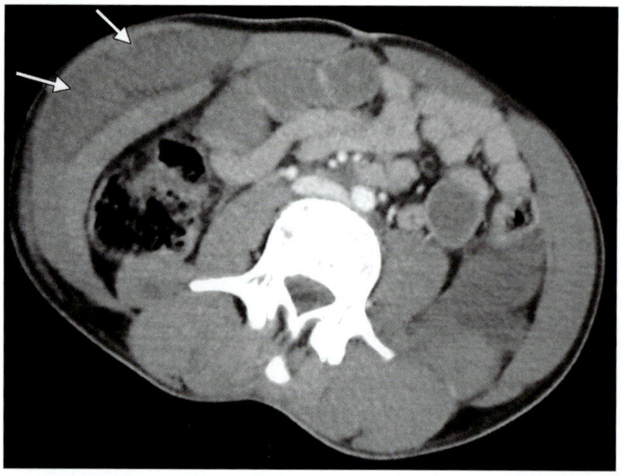

FIG. 26: Axial contrast-enhanced computed tomography (CECT) scan through mid-abdomen shows a large abdominal wall hematoma (arrows).

increasing interest in nonoperative management of penetrating injuries, CT has become important in evaluating extent of injury in selected hemodynamically stable patients. The most important information required by the surgeon is whether or not there is a breach of the peritoneum by the penetrating wound. If the wound is deep then it is important to look for solid organ laceration, bowel perforation, retroperitoneal hematoma, and hemoperitoneum. It is often difficult to detect small perforations of the bowel that result in only small amounts of peritoneal fluid on CT. In contrast to stab wounds, gunshot wounds are potentially complex injuries and depend upon the type of weapon, distance between the weapon and victim among others. CT is directly able to demonstrate the path of the bullet.

CONCLUSION

Diagnostic imaging technology has evolved considerably during the past decade and CT, in particular, has increased the sensitivity and specificity of imaging in abdominal trauma. Currently, CT is universally accepted as a valuable tool for evaluating hemodynamically stable patients. The value of CT in diagnosis of abdominal injuries can be optimized by using state of art MDCT scanners, maintaining adequate patient physiologic support and monitoring devices within the CT suite, using appropriate intravenous contrast, paying careful attention to CT technique and timely interpretation of CT images. However, CT must be considered as an adjunct to the clinical evaluation of the patient, which remains the most important criteria for guiding management of the patient with abdominal trauma. Increasing role of angioembolization in the management of hepatic, splenic, and pelvic injuries has widened the role of radiologist in successful nonsurgical management of these patients.

TAKE HOME KEY POINTS

- Chest and pelvic radiographs along with FAST ultrasound are done as initial investigations in all patients of suspected abdominal trauma.
- Multidetector computed tomography is done in patients for further evaluation depending upon the hemodynamic stability, mechanism of injury and findings of the initial radiological investigations.
- Role of radiologist is to detect and characterize the solid and visceral organ injuries and to grade them as per American Association for the Surgery of Trauma (AAST) grades.
- Most of the abdominal injuries are managed conservatively if the patient's condition remains hemodynamically stable.
- The few surgical indications which can be detected on CT should be carefully looked for and communicated to the surgeon. These include full thickness bowel injury, pancreatic transection, intraperitoneal rupture of urinary bladder, diaphragmatic tear, mesenteric hematoma/vascular injury, and renal pelvic injury.
- Other CT findings which require close monitoring of patients and would often require a surgical or angiographic intervention which also needs to be specifically looked for. These include uncontained vascular injury (depicted by active arterial contrast extravasation), contained vascular injury (pseudoaneurysm of arteriovenous fistula), and high grade (4/5) liver and splenic injuries.
- Angiographic embolization procedures are frequently used to aid the nonoperative management of patients with vascular injuries and high-grade liver and spleen injuries.

REFERENCES

1. Stanescu AL, Gross JA, Bittle M, Mann FA. Imaging of blunt abdominal trauma. Semin Roentgen. 2006;41(3):196-204.
2. Soto JA, Anderson SW. Multidetector CT of blunt abdominal trauma. Radiology. 2012;265(3):678-93.
3. Korner M, Krotz M, Degenhart C, Pfeifer KJ, Reiser MF, Linsenmaier U. Current role of emergency US in patients with major trauma. Radiographics. 2008;28:225-44.
4. Cokkinos D, Antypa E, Stefanidis K, Tserotas P, Kostaras V, Parlamenti A, et al. Contrast-enhanced ultrasound for imaging blunt abdominal trauma—indications, description of the technique and imaging review. Ultraschall Med. 2012; 33(1):60-7.
5. American College of Radiology. (2019). ACR Appropriateness Criteria®: Major Blunt Trauma. [online] Available from https://

acsearch.acr.org/docs/3102405/Narrative/ [Last accessed July, 2024].

6. Hemachandran N, Gamanagatti S, Sharma R, Shanmuganathan K, Kumar A, Gupta A, et al. Revised AAST scale for splenic injury (2018): does addition of arterial phase on CT have an impact on the grade? Emerg Radiol. 2021;28(1):47-54.
7. Stuhlfaut JW, Lucey BC, Varghese JC, Soto JA. Blunt abdominal trauma: utility of 5-minute delayed CT with a reduced radiation dose. Radiology. 2006;238(2):473-9.
8. Panda A, Kumar A, Gamanagatti S, Bhalla AS, Sharma R, Kumar S, et al. Evaluation of diagnostic utility of multidetector computed tomography and magnetic resonance imaging in blunt pancreatic trauma: a prospective study. Acta Radiol. 2015;56(4):387-96.
9. Prasad KR, Kumar A, Gamanagatti S, Chandrashekhara SH. CT in post-traumatic hypoperfusion complex-a pictorial review. Emerg Radiol. 2011;18(2):139-43.
10. Boscak A, Shanmuganathan K. Splenic Trauma: What is New? Radiol Clin North Am. 2012;50(1):105-22.
11. Kozar RA, Crandall M, Shanmuganathan K, Zarzaur BL, Coburn M, Cribari C, et al.; AAST Patient Assessment Committee. Organ injury scaling 2018 update: Spleen, liver, and kidney. J Trauma Acute Care Surg. 2018;85(6):1119-22.
12. Marmery H, Shanmuganathan K, Alexander M, Mirvis S. Optimisation of selection for nonoperative management of blunt splenic injury: Comparison of MDCT grading systems. AJR. 2007;189:1421-7.
13. Gamanagatti S, Rangarajan K, Kumar A, Jineesh. Blunt abdominal trauma: imaging and intervention. Curr Probl Diagn Radiol. 2015;44(4):321-36.
14. Hemachandran N, Gamanagatti S, Sharma R, Kumar A, Gupta A, Kumar S. Unidentified bright objects of spleen on arterial phase CT: mimicker of splenic vascular injury in blunt abdominal trauma. Diagn Interv Radiol. 2021;27(4): 497-503.
15. Parihar ML, Kumar A, Gamanagatti S, Bhalla AS, Mishra B, Kumar S, et al. Role of splenic artery embolization in management of traumatic splenic injuries: a prospective study. Indian J Surg. 2013;75(5):361-7.
16. Yoon W, Jeong YY, Kim JK, Seo JJ, Lim HS, Shin SS, et al. CT in blunt liver trauma. Radiographics. 2005;25:87-104.
17. Kumar R, Kumar A, Baliyan V, Bhalla AS, Sharma R, Gupta A, et al. Correlating MDCT liver injury grade and clinical outcome in patients without significant extrahepatic injury. Indian J Surg. 2016;78:275.
18. Melamud K, LeBedis CA, Soto JA. Imaging of pancreatic and duodenal trauma. Radiol Clin North Am. 2015;53(4):757-71.
19. Moore EE, Cogbill TH, Malangoni MA, Jurkovich GJ, Champion HR, Gennarelli TA, et al. Organ injury scaling II: Pancreas, duodenum, small bowel, colon and rectum. J Trauma. 1990;30:1427-9.
20. Kumar A, Panda A, Gamanagatti S. Blunt pancreatic trauma: A persistent diagnostic conundrum? World J Radiol. 2016; 8(2):159-73.
21. To'o KJ, Duddalwar VA. Imaging of traumatic adrenal injury. Emerg Radiol. 2012;19:499-503.
22. Panda A, Kumar A, Gamanagatti S, Bhalla AS, Sharma R, Kumar S, et al. Are traumatic bilateral adrenal injuries associated with higher morbidity and mortality?-A prospective observational study. J Trauma Manag Outcomes. 2015;9:6.
23. Francque SM, Schwagten VM, Ysebaert DK, Van Marck EA, Beaucourt LA. Bilateral adrenal hemorrhage and acute adrenal insufficiency in a blunt abdominal trauma: a case-report and literature review. Eur J Emerg Med. 2004;11:164-7.
24. Brofman N, Atri M, Epid D, Hanson JM, Grinblat L, Chughtai T, et al. Evaluation of bowel and mesenteric blunt trauma with multidetector CT. Radiographics. 2006;26:1119-26.
25. Iaselli F, Mazzei MA, Firetto C, D'Elia D, Squitieri NC, Biondetti PR, et al. Bowel and mesenteric injuries from blunt abdominal trauma: a review. Radiol Med. 2015;120:21.
26. Panda A, Kumar A, Gamanagatti S, Das R, Paliwal S, Gupta A, et al. Can multidetector computed tomography detect the site of gastrointestinal tract injury in trauma? – A retrospective study. Diagn Interv Radiol. 2017;23(1):29-36.
27. Panda A, Kumar A, Gamanagatti S, Patil A, Kumar S, Gupta A. Traumatic diaphragmatic injury: a review of CT signs and the difference between blunt and penetrating injury. Diagn Interv Radiol. 2014;20(2):121-8.
28. Barbiera F, Nicastro N, Finazzo M, Lo Casto A, Runza G, Bartolotta TV, et al. The role of MRI in traumatic rupture of the diaphragm. Our experience in three cases and review of the literature. Radiol Med. 2003;105(3):188-94.

CHAPTER 24

Anju Garg, Anjali Prakash, Alpana Manchanda

Imaging of Peritoneum and Mesentery

INTRODUCTION

The peritoneum is a thin, translucent, serous membrane made up of a single layer of mesothelial cells. It is supported by submesothelial connective tissue containing lymphatics, blood vessels, inflammatory cells such as lymphocytes and plasma cells and a variable amount of fat. Just like the pleura, the peritoneum also has two layers—the *parietal peritoneum* lines the anterior, lateral, and posterior walls of the peritoneal cavity and the *visceral peritoneum* which envelops the hollow and solid abdominal organs. Between these two layers lies the *peritoneal cavity*—a potential space containing a small amount of fluid which acts as a lubricant. The peritoneal cavity is a closed continuous space in males, but in females, it communicates with the extraperitoneal compartment of the pelvis through the ostia of the fallopian tubes.[1]

IMAGING MODALITIES

Conventional Radiographs

The role of plain radiography in peritoneal imaging is very limited. However, it serves as a valuable tool for preliminary assessment of patients presenting with abdominal distension or abdominal pain to exclude pneumoperitoneum or peritoneal calcification and to monitor postoperative patients.

Ultrasonography

Ultrasonography (US) plays only a minor role in the evaluation of peritoneal disease. As it is a readily available and noninvasive imaging modality, it is often the first modality used to evaluate any abdominal pathology. It offers real-time imaging and dynamic assessment, making it particularly useful in identification of ascites with or without peritoneal/omental nodules and masses within the peritoneal cavity. When evaluating peritoneal disease, high-frequency linear transducers (7–15 MHz) are typically employed to achieve detailed visualization of superficial structures and detect subtle peritoneal abnormalities. Ultrasound also plays a useful role in the assessment of abdominal collections, postoperative complications, and guiding intervention.

Doppler sonography aids in assessing vascularity within peritoneal lesions, with increased vascularity suggestive of malignancy. Contrast-enhanced ultrasound (CEUS) can provide further characterization of enhancing peritoneal lesions, offering insights into their vascular supply and perfusion dynamics.

Computed Tomography

Multidetector computed tomography (MDCT) is the primary modality of choice in the radiological evaluation of peritoneal disease, owing to its wide availability, superior spatial resolution, rapid acquisition times, and multiplanar reconstruction capability. It is generally performed with both oral and intravenous contrast. The use of a negative contrast medium or a water density contrast is recommended for optimal visualization of the bowel wall, serosa, and peritoneum. Contrast-enhanced computed tomography (CECT) is particularly valuable for detecting and characterizing peritoneal implants, peritoneal thickening, nodularity, and omental caking.

Multiplanar reformations and three-dimensional reconstructions aid in accurately delineating the extent of disease spread, assessing for associated complications such as bowel obstruction or perforation and guiding percutaneous interventions such as biopsy or drain placement. Furthermore, advancements in CT technology, such as dual-energy CT and CT perfusion imaging, offer additional functional information that may aid in distinguishing between benign and malignant peritoneal lesions. Dual-energy CT techniques provide quantitative information regarding tissue composition and iodine uptake, potentially aiding in the characterization of peritoneal lesions.

Magnetic Resonance Imaging

Magnetic resonance imaging (MRI) provides excellent soft tissue contrast resolution without ionizing radiation, and is particularly valuable in cases where detailed anatomical and functional assessment is required. T1-weighted (T1W), T2-weighted (T2W), and fat-suppressed sequences allow for comprehensive characterization of peritoneal lesions based on their signal intensity (SI) and morphological features. MRI with intravenous contrast administration enables detailed assessment of vascular involvement and visceral organ invasion by peritoneal implants. The use of fat suppression, delayed postcontrast enhancement, and water soluble enteric contrast have allowed detection sensitivities over CT. Diffusion-weighted imaging (DWI) allows evaluation of tissue cellularity and diffusion characteristics, aiding in the differentiation between benign and malignant peritoneal processes and to differentiate postoperative scar tissue from residual/recurrent disease. Dynamic contrast-enhanced MRI (DCE-MRI) provides information on lesion vascularity and enhancement patterns, facilitating the assessment of tumor aggressiveness and treatment response. Additionally, magnetic resonance (MR) spectroscopy can offer metabolic insights into peritoneal lesions, potentially aiding in their characterization and prognostication.

Positron Emission Tomography-Computed Tomography

Whole body positron emission tomography-computed tomography (PET-CT) imaging plays a valuable role in the staging and evaluation of primary peritoneal malignancies and distant metastases. It combines anatomical imaging (CT) with functional imaging (PET) with 18F-2-deoxy-2-fluoro-D-glucose (FDG), being the most commonly used radiotracer.

It can detect occult peritoneal metastases and assess treatment response following chemotherapy or radiation therapy. Quantitative analysis of FDG uptake, the standardized uptake value (SUV), provides valuable information regarding tumor aggressiveness and treatment response. Integration of PET imaging with CT allows for precise anatomical localization of metabolic abnormalities within the peritoneal cavity, enhancing diagnostic accuracy and treatment planning.

RADIOMICS

Radiomics plays a significant role in peritoneal imaging by extracting quantitative data from medical images, such as CT scans or MRI, and translating it into clinically relevant insights for diagnosis, prognosis, and treatment planning. Radiomics enables the detection of subtle changes in peritoneal tissues that may indicate the presence of diseases such as peritoneal carcinomatosis (PC) or peritoneal mesothelioma, as well as can predict PC and its response to treatment.[2]

EMBRYOLOGY

Knowledge of the developmental anatomy of the peritoneum, helps to understand the peritoneal ligaments, spaces, and their relationship with the abdominal organs. The majority of the ligaments in the abdomen are formed from remnants of the ventral and dorsal mesenteries which suspend the primitive gut. The liver and its ligaments arise in the *ventral mesentery*. The anterior part of the ventral mesentery becomes the falciform, coronary, and triangular ligaments and the posterior part of the ventral mesentery becomes the lesser omentum. The stomach, spleen, and pancreatic tail and their ligaments develop in the *dorsal mesentery* of the foregut. At the level of spleen, the anterior part of the dorsal mesentery becomes the gastrosplenic ligament, and the posterior part of the dorsal mesentery becomes the splenorenal ligament **(Figs. 1A to C)**. Above the level of spleen the dorsal mesentery gives rise to gastrophrenic ligament and below the level of spleen it gives rise to the greater omentum (gastrocolic ligament).[3]

Below the level of the transverse colon, the ventral mesentery regresses while the dorsal mesentery forms the transverse mesocolon, small bowel mesentery, and sigmoid mesocolon. During development, the duodenum, ascending and descending colon lose their mesenteries and become retroperitoneal.

ANATOMY OF THE PERITONEUM[4-7]

The peritoneum forms double layered folds, or ligaments, that interconnect the organs and viscera within the peritoneal cavity. The *peritoneal ligaments* are named according to the two major structures connected by them, e.g., splenorenal ligament or gastrohepatic ligament (GHL), etc. *Omentum* is a specialized ligament that attaches the stomach to other structures whereas *mesentery* is the ligament attaching the bowel to the posterior abdominal wall. These ligaments divide the peritoneal cavity into a number of compartments and recesses **(Figs. 2A and B)**.

The peritoneal ligaments carry vessels, nerves, and lymphatics from the extraperitoneal spaces to the intraperitoneal organs. They act as boundaries for spread of pathological processes within the abdomen, but may also become conduits for spread of disease. They are not directly visible on cross-sectional imaging but can be identified either by their typical position, organ relationships, or by the anatomical landmarks provided by their constituent vessels. They may become directly visible when they get thickened by edema, inflammation or neoplastic infiltration, or when

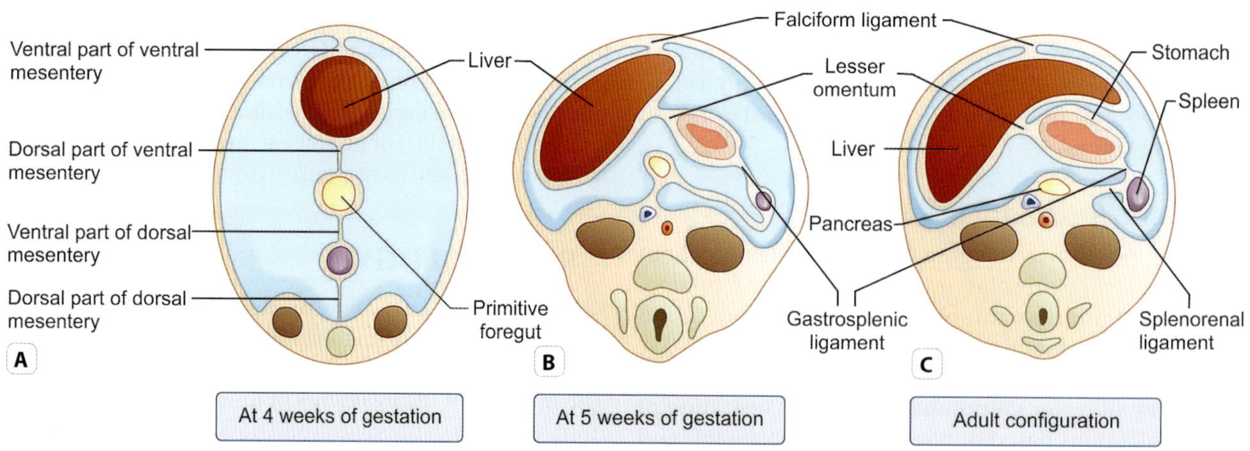

FIGS. 1A TO C: Embryologic development and rotation of the peritoneal structures to the eventual adult position. The ventral part of the ventral mesentery becomes the falciform ligament, the dorsal part of the ventral mesentery becomes the lesser omentum, the ventral part of the dorsal mesentery becomes the gastrosplenic ligament, and the dorsal part of the dorsal mesentery becomes the splenorenal ligament. The liver arises in the ventral mesentery, whereas the stomach, spleen, and pancreatic tail develop in the dorsal mesentery. The liver fills and moves to the right side of the peritoneal cavity as it grows. The spleen moves to the left.

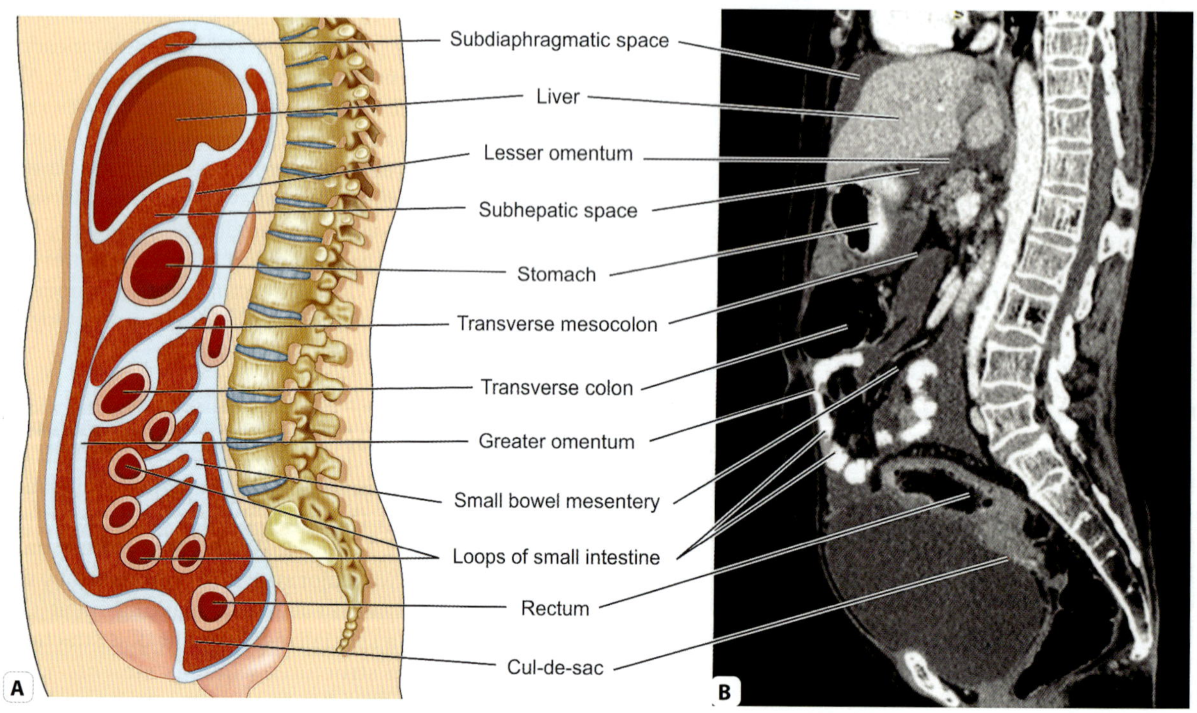

FIGS. 2A AND B: Sagittal illustration and corresponding sagittal computed tomography (CT) scan in a patient with ascites, showing the peritoneal ligaments in the midline sagittal section.

they are outlined by air or fluid in the peritoneal cavity. They can be grouped into the following:

- Ligaments of the stomach
- Ligaments of the liver and spleen
- Ligaments attached to the small bowel
- Ligaments attached to the large bowel
- Ligaments of the pelvis.

Ligaments of Stomach (Figs. 2 and 3)

The peritoneal ligaments of the stomach include two main groups: Ligaments attached to the lesser curvature, i.e., the lesser omentum, and ligaments attached to the greater curvature which include gastrophrenic, gastrosplenic ligaments, and the greater omentum.

Lesser omentum: The lesser omentum is formed by the gastrohepatic and hepatoduodenal ligaments (HDLs) **(Fig. 2)**. *The GHL* is attached to the lesser curve of the stomach and the visceral surface of the liver and contains the coronary vein and left gastric artery **(Figs. 3A and D)**. The GHL can be involved by pancreatitis or metastatic disease from esophageal, gastric, and biliary tumors. It is also the site for coronary varices. The *HDL* attaches the first part of the duodenum to the liver and contains the portal vein, hepatic artery, common hepatic ducts, and part of the cystic duct **(Fig. 3D)**. It is a common site for spread of biliary and gallbladder neoplasms.

Greater omentum: It is also known as the *gastrocolic ligament* **(Figs. 2 and 3)**. It attaches to the greater curvature of the stomach and proximal part of duodenum. Its descending and ascending portion fuse to form a four layer vascular fatty apron which hangs down covering the small bowel. It has mostly fatty tissue with few gastroepiploic vessels. On CT, it is seen as a band of fatty tissue, just beneath the anterior abdominal wall and anterior to the stomach, transverse colon, and small bowel. It is a mobile structure and has an important role in limiting spread of infections and confining injuries to the bowel. However, it is a common site of spread of metastatic peritoneal disease and is also commonly involved in tubercular peritonitis.

Gastrosplenic ligament: It attaches the greater curvature of the stomach to the spleen and contains the short gastric and left gastroepiploic vessels and lymphatics **(Figs. 3A and D)**. It is a leftward continuation of the greater omentum and is also in continuity with the splenorenal and phrenicocolic ligaments. The gastrosplenic ligament is a frequent route for spread of pancreatitis-related fluid and its vessels form a collateral route of venous flow in cases of splenic vein thrombosis.

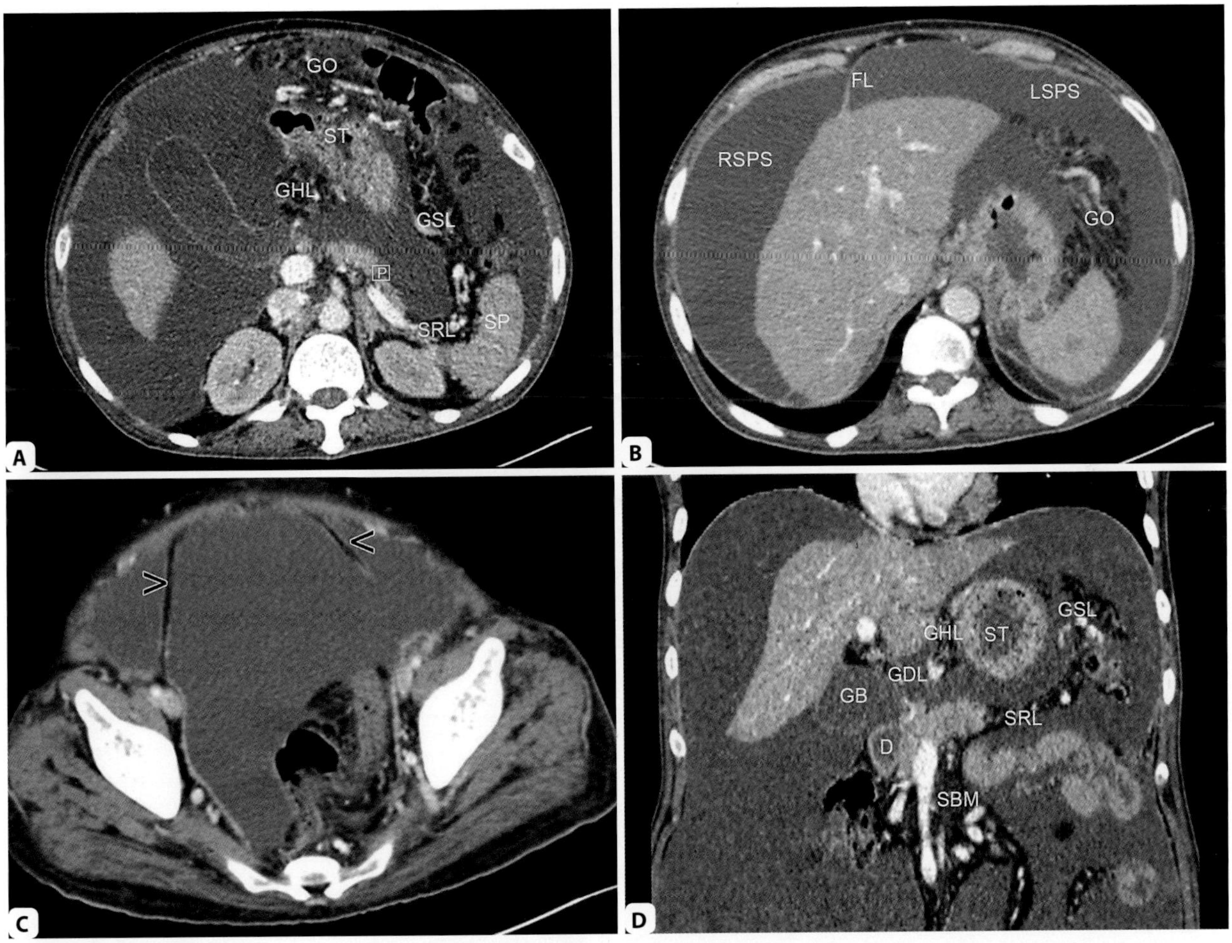

FIGS. 3A TO D: (A to C) Axial; and (D) Coronal contrast-enhanced computed tomography (CECT) scans showing the peritoneal ligaments in a 61-year-old man with peritoneal carcinomatosis with ascites, thickened enhancing peritoneum, and omental nodularity.

[FL: falciform ligament; GO: greater omentum; GHL: gastrohepatic ligament; GDL: gastroduodenal ligament; GSL: gastrosplenic ligament; SRL: splenorenal ligament; SBM: small bowel mesentery; ST: stomach; SP: spleen; D: duodenum; RSPS: right subphrenic space; LSPS: left subphrenic space; and medial umbilical ligaments (arrowheads)]

Gastrophrenic ligament is attached to the posterior surface of the stomach. The attachment of the gastrophrenic ligament lies in apposition with the diaphragm, and frequently with the upper portion of the left suprarenal gland.

Ligaments of the Liver and Spleen

The peritoneal ligaments of the liver include the suspensory ligaments of the liver and lesser omentum. The suspensory ligaments of the liver include the falciform, coronary and triangular ligaments. The peritoneal ligaments of spleen include gastrosplenic and lienorenal ligaments.

Triangular and coronary ligaments: These are peritoneal attachments between the liver and the parietal peritoneum. The triangular ligaments are formed by fusion of the coronary ligaments and outline the bare area of the liver. The right triangular ligament is long and separates the right subphrenic space from the right subhepatic space while the left triangular ligament is short and does not compartmentalize the left subphrenic space.

Falciform ligament: It attaches the ventral surface of the liver to the anterior abdominal wall and contains the ligamentum teres, i.e., obliterated umbilical vein **(Fig. 3B)**. The recanalized paraumbilical vein is also found in the falciform ligament. It is an important site of peritoneal seeding of metastatic tumors which may be mistaken for hepatic metastases.

Splenorenal ligament: It is the connecting peritoneal reflection between the spleen and the left kidney. It contains the tail of the pancreas, splenic vessels, and small vessels to the retroperitoneum. Tumor spread and systemic portal collaterals can develop in this space.

Ligaments Attached to Small Bowel

Small bowel mesentery: It is a broad fan-shaped peritoneal fold that attaches the jejunum and ileum to the retroperitoneum and contains branches of the superior mesenteric vessels, lymph nodes, nerves, and varying amounts of fat **(Figs. 2 and 4)**. The root of the mesentery extends from the ligament of Trietz to the ileocecal valve, a length of approximately 15 cm, whereas the intestinal border is 6–8 m long, and so the mesentery is thrown into a number of folds **(Figs. 4A and B)**.

The small bowel mesentery is commonly involved by metastatic disease and infectious processes of the peritoneum. Inflammation and tumor from the pancreatic body or jejunum can involve the small bowel mesentery directly or by way of neurovascular plexus or lymphatics. Rotational and fusion anomalies may lead to volvulus or internal hernias.

Ligaments Attached to Large Bowel

Transverse mesocolon: It is a peritoneal fold that attaches the transverse colon to the anterior surface of the pancreas **(Figs. 2 and 5)**. It contains the middle colic vessels and lymph nodes. Local extension of pancreatic head cancers occurs along the transverse mesocolon.

Sigmoid mesocolon: It is the peritoneal attachment of the sigmoid colon to the posterior pelvic wall **(Fig. 5C)**. It contains the hemorrhoidal and sigmoid vessels. It serves as a medial and caudal boundary for the spread of material from the left paracolic space. Acute diverticulitis, Crohn's disease, and tumors of the sigmoid colon can involve the sigmoid mesocolon.

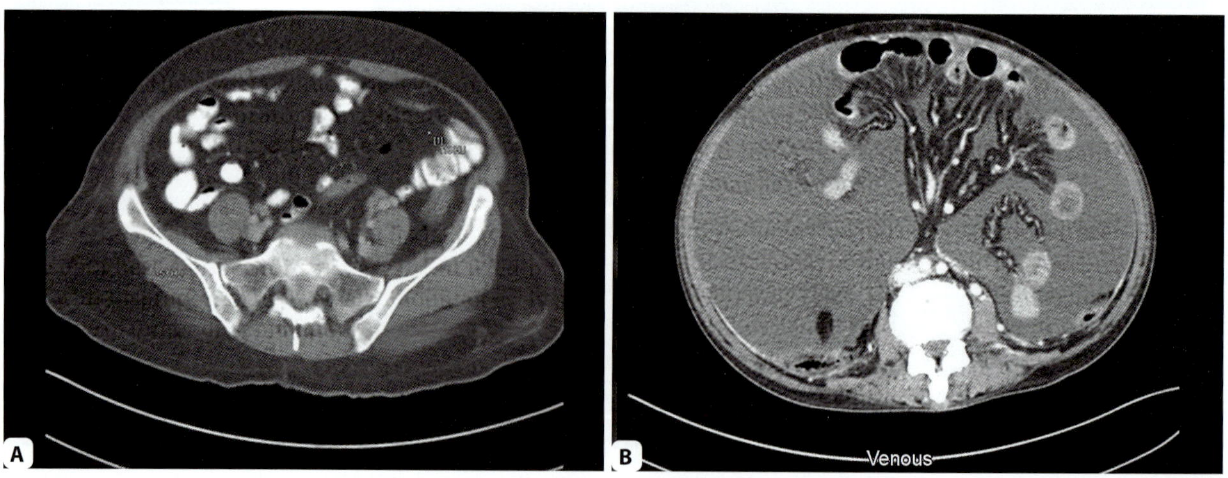

FIGS. 4A AND B: Axial contrast-enhanced computed tomography (CECT) scans through abdomen in two different patients showing normal mesentery. (A) Mesentery is seen as diffuse fat density structure with mesenteric vessels within. The leaves of the mesentery cannot be made out separately. (B) In a patient with ascites, the leaves of the mesentery are separated by the ascitic fluid.

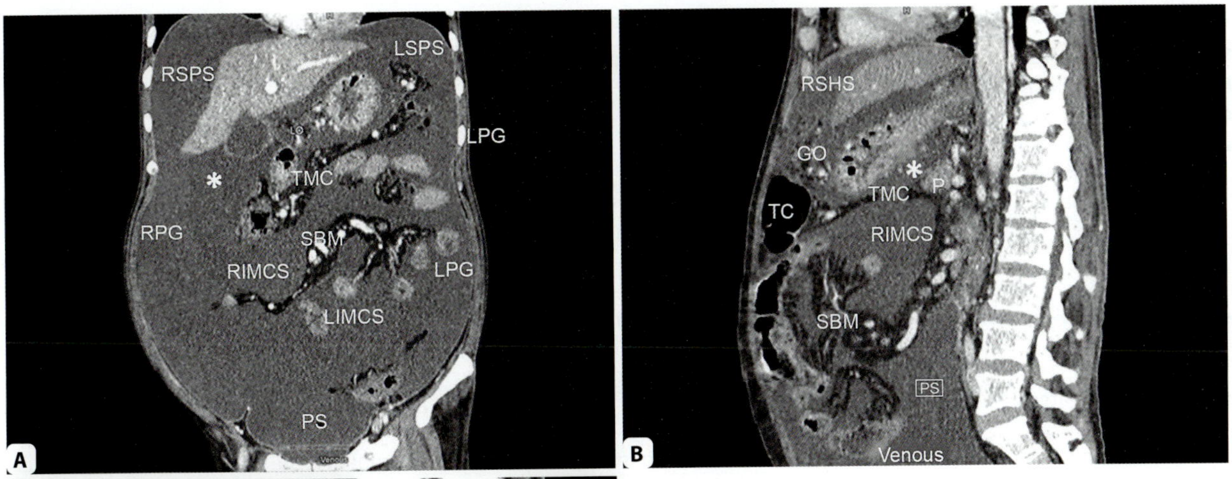

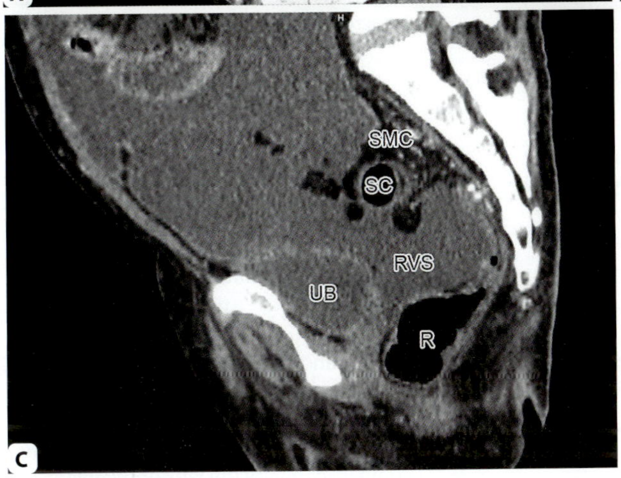

FIGS. 5A TO C: (A) Coronal; and (B and C) sagittal reformats in the same patient as in Figure 3, showing the peritoneal spaces. (RSPS: right subphrenic space; LSPS: left subphrenic space; RSPS: right subhepatic space (asterisk in A), lesser sac (asterisk in B); RPG: right paracolic gutter; LPG: left paracolic gutter; RIMCS: right inframesocolic space; LIMCS: left inframesocolic space; PS: pelvic space; TMC: transverse mesocolon; GO: greater omentum; TC: transverse colon; p: pancreas; SC: sigmoid colon; RVS: rectovesical space; R: rectum; SBM: small bowel mesentery; SMC: sigmoid mesocolon; UB: urinary bladder)

Phrenicocolic ligament: It attaches the proximal descending colon to the left hemidiaphragm. It separates the supramesocolic compartment from the left paracolic gutter. Pancreatic disease can spread via this ligament to involve the splenic flexure of the colon.

Table 1 lists the peritoneal ligaments, their attachments, contents, and the major pathological processes involving these ligaments.

Ligaments of the Pelvis

The *broad ligaments* extend from the uterus to the pelvic sidewalls and envelop the parametria, fallopian tubes, ovaries, uterine vessels, and ureters. These ligaments can be involved by inflammatory and neoplastic processes affecting the uterus, ovaries, and fallopian tubes.

Round ligaments are the anterior suspensory ligaments of the uterus. They run lateral to the deep inferior epigastric vessels, enter the inguinal canal, and insert on the labia majora. They contain lymphatic channels.

There are two paired *lateral and medial umbilical ligaments* and *one median umbilical ligament* in the midline. The lateral folds are formed by reflection of the peritoneum over the deep inferior epigastric vessels, the medial folds are peritoneal reflections over the obliterated umbilical arteries and the median fold lies over the obliterated urachus **(Fig. 3C)**.

PERITONEAL SPACES[4,5,7]

The peritoneal ligaments divide the peritoneal space into multiple compartments and recesses. On imaging these spaces are visualized only when they are distended with fluid or air. The transverse mesocolon divides the peritoneal cavity into the supramesocolic and the inframesocolic compartments.

Supramesocolic space: It extends from the diaphragm to the transverse mesocolon. It includes the perihepatic spaces and the lesser sac. The perihepatic spaces consist of the subphrenic and subhepatic spaces which are right, left, anterior, and posterior.

The *subphrenic space* lies adjacent to the lateral and superior portion of the liver, between the diaphragm and the abdominal wall. The right subphrenic space is limited medially by the falciform ligament, which separates it from the left subphrenic space **(Figs. 5A to C)**. Inferiorly it is continuous with the right subhepatic space and the right paracolic space. The left subphrenic space is located below and around the left lobe of liver and stomach. It is limited inferiorly by the phrenicocolic ligament.

The *right subhepatic space*, also known as the Morrison's pouch or hepatorenal space, lies adjacent to the gallbladder and duodenum, and extends posteriorly to the anterior surface of the right kidney **(Figs. 2 and 5)**. It is an important

TABLE 1: Peritoneal ligaments, attachments, contents, and major pathological processes which involve these ligaments.

Peritoneal ligaments	Attachments	Contents	Other relevant information
Ligaments of stomach and duodenum:			
• Attached to lesser curvature: – Lesser omentum: ▪ Gastrohepatic ligament	Lesser curvature of the stomach and the visceral surface of liver	Coronary vein and left gastric artery	• Can be involved by pancreatitis or metastatic disease from esophageal, gastric, and biliary tumors • Can be a site for coronary varices
• Hepatoduodenal ligament	First part of duodenum and liver	Portal vein, hepatic artery, common hepatic ducts, and part of the cystic duct	• Common site for spread of biliary and gallbladder neoplasms
• Attached to greater curvature: – Gastrosplenic ligament	• Greater curvature of the stomach and spleen	Short gastric vessels	• Frequent route for subperitoneal spread of pancreatitis-related fluid
– Gastrophrenic ligament	• Posterior surface of the stomach and diaphragm	Left inferior phrenic artery	
– Greater omentum	• Greater curvature of the stomach and proximal part of duodenum	Fatty tissue with few gastroepiploic vessels	• Common site of spread of metastatic peritoneal disease • Commonly involved in tubercular peritonitis • Important role in limiting spread of infections and confining injuries to bowel
Ligaments of liver and spleen:			
• Triangular and coronary ligaments	Liver and the diaphragm	No vessels	• Right triangular ligament separates the right subphrenic space from the right subhepatic space • Left triangular ligament does not compartmentalize the left subphrenic space
• Falciform ligament	Ventral surface of the liver and the anterior abdominal wall	Ligamentum teres (obliterated umbilical vein) and recanalized paraumbilical vein	• Important site of peritoneal seeding of metastatic tumors
• Lesser omentum	As above		
• Ligaments of spleen: – Splenorenal ligament – Gastrosplenic ligament	Spleen and left kidney As above	Tail of the pancreas, splenic vessels, and small vessels to the retroperitoneum	• Systemic portal collaterals can develop in this space • Renal and splenic neoplasm can spread
Ligaments attached to small bowel:			
• Small bowel mesentery	Jejunum and ileum and the retroperitoneum (root of mesentery extends from the ligament of Trietz to ileocecal valve)	Branches of superior mesenteric vessels, lymph nodes, nerves and varying amounts of fat	• Commonly involved by metastatic disease and infectious processes of peritoneum • Rotational and fusion anomalies may lead to volvulus or internal hernias
Ligaments attached to large bowel:			
• Transverse mesocolon	Transverse colon and the anterior surface of the pancreas	Middle colic vessels and lymph nodes	Local extension of pancreatic head cancer
• Sigmoid mesocolon	Sigmoid colon and the posterior pelvic wall	Hemorrhoidal and sigmoid vessels	Serves as medial and caudal boundary for spread of material from left paracolic space. Can be involved by acute diverticulitis, Crohn's disease, and tumor of the sigmoid colon
• Phrenicocolic ligament	Proximal descending colon and the left hemidiaphragm		Separates the supramesocolic compartment from left paracolic gutter

site of fluid collection as it is the most gravity dependent space. Medially, it extends into the lesser sac through the foramen of Winslow. The *left subhepatic space* lies between the lateral segment of the left lobe of liver and the stomach.

The *lesser sac* also known as the *omental bursa*, lies behind the stomach, anterior to the pancreas **(Fig. 5)**. It is further subdivided by the reflection over the left gastric artery into two recesses—a smaller superior recess and a larger inferior recess. The *superior recess* surrounds the caudate lobe of the liver. It communicates with the subhepatic space through the foramen of Winslow that is located posterior to the free edge of the HDL. The larger *inferior recess* lies between the stomach and the anterior surface of the spleen and pancreas. Abnormalities of the pancreas, posterior wall of stomach, duodenum, caudate lobe, and transverse colon may all extend into the lesser sac.

Inframesocolic space: The right and left inframesocolic spaces are separated by the root of the mesentery. The *left inframesocolic space* is larger and communicates freely with the pelvic spaces. The *right inframesocolic space* is limited inferiorly by the attachment of the small bowel mesentery to the cecum and does not communicate with the pelvis **(Figs. 5A and B)**.

Paracolic spaces: They lie lateral to the peritoneal reflections of the left and right side of the colon. The right space is larger and deeper than the left. It communicates freely with the right perihepatic space, whereas the left is partially limited by the phrenicocolic ligament. Both paracolic spaces communicate freely with the pelvic spaces **(Fig. 5A)**.

Pelvic Peritoneal Spaces

The pelvic cavity can be divided into the anterior and posterior paravesical spaces. The anterior paravesical space is divided by the medial umbilical folds, into lateral and medial compartments. On each side, the inferior epigastric artery divides the lateral pelvic compartments into lateral and medial inguinal fossae, the sites of direct and indirect inguinal hernias, respectively.

In males, the posterior paravesical space is subdivided into the *rectovesical* and *pararectal space* by the peritoneal coverings of the rectum and bladder. In females, peritoneal coverings of the uterus divide the rectovesical space into the *vesicouterine* and *rectouterine space* (cul-de-sac or pouch of Douglas). The rectouterine space is the most dependent portion of the pelvis in women while the rectovesical space is the most dependent portion of pelvis in men and these spaces are a common location for fluid, drop metastases, and abscesses in women and men, respectively **(Fig. 5)**.[4]

PERITONEAL FLUID DYNAMICS

The peritoneal cavity contains a small amount of fluid—approximately 50–100 mL.[8] This fluid has a natural tendency to move inferiorly toward the pelvis due to gravity. However, due to the respiratory motion of the diaphragm, gravitational pull of the liver and peristalsis of bowel, there is an active flow of the peritoneal fluid laterally and upwards toward the diaphragm. It predominantly flows up the right paracolic gutter which is deeper and wider than the left to the subphrenic space where majority (about 90%) of the peritoneal fluid is cleared by the submesothelial lymphatics. These lymphatics are connected with lymphatics on the other side of the diaphragm. Thus, metabolic, infectious, and neoplastic processes in the peritoneal cavity may pass through the diaphragm to the subdiaphragmatic lymph nodes.[9] Ascites and tumor cells may also pass through the lymphatics and produce an ipsilateral pleural effusion. As these lymphatics have unidirectional valves, pleural effusion cannot pass into the peritoneal cavity. There are some areas of fluid stasis in the peritoneal cavity namely ileocolic region, root of sigmoid mesentery, and pouch of Douglas, which become important in harboring disease.

ASCITES

Ascites is the pathological accumulation of fluid in the peritoneal cavity. It can occur due to a large number of causes. Common causes are listed in **Box 1**. Ascitic fluid is traditionally characterized as either *transudate*—thin, with a low protein count and low specific gravity, and *exudate*—high protein count and specific gravity. It has been seen that the serum-ascites albumin gradient is more accurate in classification of the causes of ascites.[10]

The imaging appearance of ascites depends on the amount of fluid, its contents, and whether it is free flowing

BOX 1 Causes of ascites.

- Hepatic:
  - Cirrhosis, portal hypertension, Budd–Chiari syndrome, alcoholic hepatitis, fulminant hepatic failure
- Cardiac:
  - Congestive heart failure, constrictive pericarditis, cardiac tamponade
- Renal:
  - Nephrotic syndrome, renal failure
- Hypoalbuminemia
- Infective peritonitis:
  - Bacterial, tuberculosis, viral, fungal
- Neoplasms:
  - Primary neoplasms of abdominal organs—colon, pancreas, ovary, liver, etc.
  - Primary peritoneal malignancy
  - Metastatic peritoneal disease
- Trauma
- Blunt, penetrating or iatrogenic trauma to abdominal organs can lead to collection of blood, bile, chyle, urine, etc., depending on the organ involved

or loculated. In uncomplicated *transudative* ascites which is usually free flowing, the fluid tends to collect in dependent areas such as pelvic cul-de-sac, Morrison's pouch, and paracolic gutters in early stages. Due to the suction effect of the diaphragm, fluid also accumulates in the subphrenic spaces. Larger amounts of fluid will fill the entire peritoneal cavity and displace the small bowel loops centrally. The fluid collection is shaped by the surrounding structures, forms acute angles where fluid borders organs and does not deform the normal shape of adjacent organs. Complicated ascites, i.e., exudative or loculated ascites is associated with adhesions, malignancy, or infection. Loculated ascites is noncompressible and has rounded margins with mass effect and frequently displaces adjacent structures.

Ultrasound is a sensitive modality for detection, quantification, localization, and characterization of ascitic fluid. As little as 0.8 mm of fluid has been detected in the pouch of Douglas by transvaginal scanning.[11] US can also be very helpful in differentiating transudative from exudative ascites. In patients with transudative ascites, the US appearances are predominantly those of anechoic, mobile fluid. Features associated with exudative ascites due to inflammatory or malignant causes include loculated fluid collections, particulate ascites, septa, and matted bowel loops with interposed fluid. US can also help determine whether identified fluid is free or loculated, as free ascites moves when the patient changes position.

The CT is most sensitive to small amounts of fluid in the peritoneum which collects preferentially in the dependent regions. The CT density of intraperitoneal fluid can give a clue to the underlying etiology, transudative ascites density is approximately that of water (–10 to +10 HU), whereas exudative ascites density is greater than 15 HU and increases with increasing protein content, hemoperitoneum density is higher still (~45 HU) and chylous fluid density is <0 HU. Enhancement of the peritoneum may be seen on CECT in infective and neoplastic ascites. As CT provides a more complete evaluation of the abdomen and pelvis than sonography, other intra- or extra-abdominal CT features may give further evidence to the origin of the ascites (e.g., features of heart failure, features of cirrhosis, peritoneal catheter in situ, etc.).

It is often difficult to characterize the nature and underlying cause of peritoneal fluid collections on basis of imaging alone and a diagnostic paracentesis may be required to sample the fluid. US can be used to guide aspiration for diagnostic or therapeutic purpose.

PNEUMOPERITONEUM

Normally, there is no free air within the peritoneal cavity. The most common cause of a pneumoperitoneum is due to rupture of an abdominal viscus. Other causes are postoperative status, patient on peritoneal dialysis, rupture of a cyst in pneumatosis intestinalis, etc. It is important to be able to recognize the signs of a pneumoperitoneum on various imaging modalities and to be able to differentiate a true pneumoperitoneum from a pseudopneumoperitoneum. This has been discussed in detail elsewhere in the book.

INTERNAL HERNIAS

Internal hernia is the protrusion of a viscus through a normal or abnormal aperture in the peritoneum or mesentery, within the confines of the peritoneal cavity. This aperture can be congenital or acquired, such as postsurgical, post-traumatic, or even postinflammatory. Congenital hernias may occur through a normal aperture, e.g., foramen of Winslow, or abnormal defects which arise from anomalies of internal rotation and peritoneal attachment.

Based on the location, Meyers traditionally classified these hernias as paraduodenal (53%), pericecal (13%), foramen of Winslow (8%), transmesenteric and transmesocolic (8%), intersigmoid (6%), retroanastomotic (5%), and paravesical (7%—not a true internal hernia).[12] The most common internal hernias have been the paraduodenal hernias which are congenital hernias, however, with the increase in surgical procedures being performed these days, the incidence of the acquired postoperative hernias is increasing.[13]

Clinically, internal hernias can have a variable presentation ranging from asymptomatic to mild colicky abdominal pain to acute intestinal obstruction. Imaging plays an important role in diagnosis as they are difficult to identify clinically. Imaging features on barium studies and CT include cluster of dilated/nondilated bowel loops in an abnormal location **(Figs. 6A and B)**, crowding of loops in a hernia sac and/or features of obstruction. CT may additionally show mesenteric vessel abnormalities as engorgement, twisting, or stretching of the vessels. **Table 2** lists the various hernias with their characteristic clinical and imaging findings.

PERITONEAL INFECTIONS AND INFLAMMATION

Peritonitis

Peritonitis is defined as a diffuse inflammation of the parietal and visceral peritoneum. It is most often caused by introduction of an infection into the otherwise sterile peritoneal environment through perforation of an abdominal viscus, but it may also result from other irritants, such as foreign bodies (talc or barium), bile from a perforated gallbladder or a lacerated liver, or gastric acid from a perforated ulcer. Gynecologic disease processes such as salpingitis may also cause peritonitis. Uncommonly, primary bacterial peritonitis may occur due to hematogenous spread of organisms in association with chronic liver or renal disease.

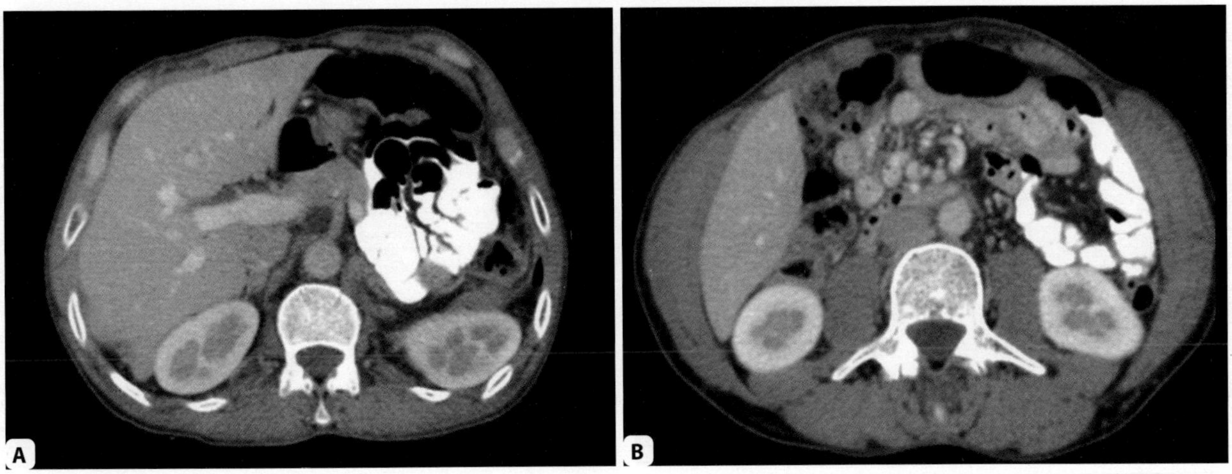

FIGS. 6A AND B: Left paraduodenal hernia in a 45-year-old man with chronic postprandial abdominal pain. (A) Axial contrast-enhanced computed tomography (CECT) image shows a sac like mass of jejunal loops between stomach and pancreatic body. (B) Section obtained at lower level shows crowded and dilated mesenteric vessels.

TABLE 2: **Internal hernias: Clinical and imaging features.**[13]

Type of hernia	Congenital/acquired site	Findings on plain radiographs and barium studies	Computed tomography findings
Left paraduodenal	Congenital Through Landzert's fossa behind the fourth part of the duodenum	Cluster of jejunal loops in left hypochondrium, lateral to the fourth part of duodenum; may have mass effect indenting posterior wall of stomach or displacing transverse colon inferiorly	• Encapsulated cluster of dilated small-bowel loops between stomach and pancreas, behind pancreas itself, or between transverse colon and left adrenal gland • Inferior mesenteric vein displaced superoanteriorly in neck of hernia sac
Right paraduodenal	Congenital Through Waldeyer's fossa (representing a defect in the first part of the jejunal mesentery)	Clustered loops lateral and inferior to the second part of duodenum; associated with nonrotation of small bowel	• Encapsulated cluster of loops lateral and inferior to the second part of duodenum; associated with small-bowel nonrotation • Superior mesenteric artery displaced anteriorly
Pericecal	Congenital/acquired Through a defect in the cecal mesentery and extending into the right paracolic gutter	Clustered small-bowel loops (usually distal ileal) posterior and lateral to the cecum in right paracolic gutter	Clustered small-bowel loops (usually distal ileum) posterior and lateral to the cecum in right paracolic gutter
Foramen of Winslow	Congenital Through Foramen of Winslow	Circumscribed loops medial and posterior to the stomach	Loops in the lesser sac between liver and inferior vena cava
Intersigmoid	Congenital/acquired Fossae/defects in and around sigmoid mesocolon	U- or C-shaped cluster of small bowel posterior and lateral to the sigmoid colon	U- or C-shaped cluster of small bowel posterior and lateral to the sigmoid colon
Transmesenteric	• Congenital in children through defect in small bowel mesentery • Acquired in adults associated with abdominal surgery	Variable, air within gastric remnant in postoperative cases; may simulate a left paraduodenal hernia	Small bowel lateral to colon; displaced omental fat with small bowel directly abutting abdominal wall
Retroanastomotic	Acquired Through a defect related to a surgical anastomosis	Variable	Variable

Source: Adapted from Martin LC, Merkle EM, Thompson WM. Review of internal hernias: radiographic and clinical findings. AJR Am J Roentgenol. 2006;186(3):703-17.

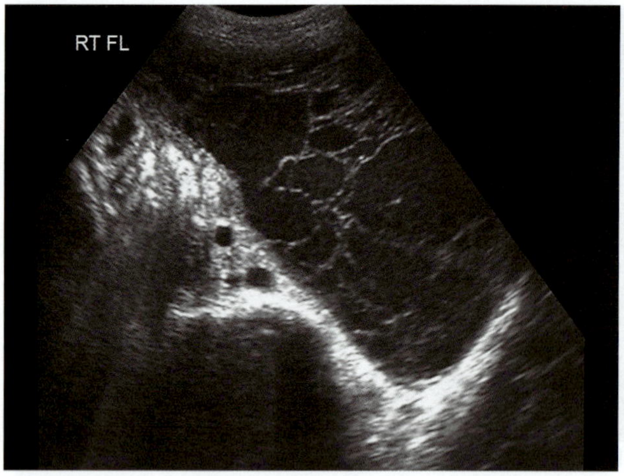

FIG. 7: Purulent peritonitis. Transverse ultrasonography (US) image through right flank shows ascites with peritoneal thickening and ascitic fluid. The fluid shows internal echoes characteristic of exudative nature and multiple septa within.

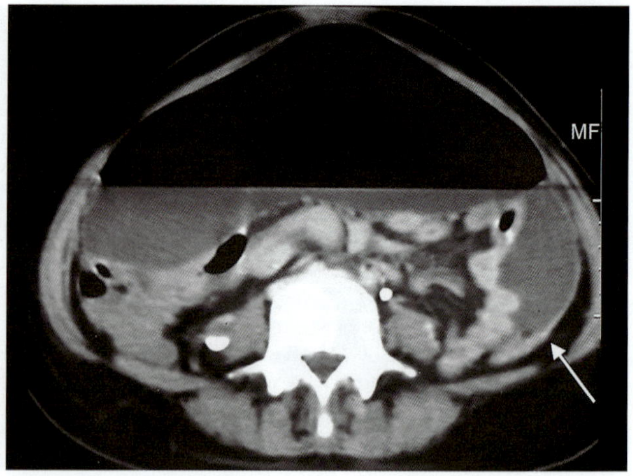

FIG. 8: Perforation peritonitis: Contrast-enhanced computed tomography (CECT) axial section through the abdomen, shows fluid in the peritoneal cavity with a large air fluid level. Smooth, enhancing, thickening of the peritoneal lining is seen (arrow).

Clinically, patients may present with an acute or insidious onset of symptoms, limited and mild disease, or systemic and severe disease with septic shock. On imaging, there is presence of ascites which may be loculated or show presence of debris, septa, or gas **(Fig. 7)**. US is superior to CT in demonstrating the nature of the ascitic fluid.[14] In association with ascites there is peritoneal and mesenteric thickening. The thickened peritoneum is seen to enhance on contrast administration, and is often smooth **(Fig. 8)**. In some cases, evidence of the underlying primary pathology can be seen such as diverticulitis, appendiceal perforation, bowel ischemia, etc.

Peritoneal abscess is an infected fluid collection encapsulated by fibrinous exudate, omentum, and/or adjacent visceral organs. The majority of abscesses occur secondary to spread of infection from an adjacent infected organ or viscus, e.g., inflamed appendix, pancreatitis, diverticulitis, Crohn's disease, liver abscess, etc. Abscess formation may also occur as a complication of abdominal or pelvic surgery or penetrating trauma. The risk of abscess increases in cases of preoperative perforation of the hollow viscus, significant fecal contamination of the peritoneal cavity, bowel ischemia, as well as in the setting of immunosuppression.

Clinically, patients present with fever, tachycardia, and symptoms localized to area of abscess, e.g., with a subphrenic collection, there may be shoulder tip pain, hiccups, and unexplained pulmonary symptoms (pleural effusion, basal atelectasis). Sometimes, clinical features may be minimal, especially in immunocompromised patients.

The CT appearance of an abscess varies depending on its age. In early stages, it may appear as a mass with soft tissue attenuation values. As the liquefaction progresses, a central hypodense, nonenhancing area with a definable, enhancing wall is seen. Gas may be seen within the abscess cavity as multiple small bubbles or as an air fluid level **(Figs. 9 and 16B)**. Occasionally, septations may be seen. There is thickening and obliteration of adjacent fat planes, and mass effect on surrounding structures. Features of the predisposing cause of the abscess, e.g., acute appendicitis, Crohn's disease, or diverticulitis, etc., may be seen.

On US, an abscess is seen as a round or oval fluid collection with a well-defined irregular wall, with occasional internal septa or debris. Small pockets of air within the abscess cavity can be seen as echogenic foci with posterior reverberation artefact.[15] However, US detection of abscess is hampered by bowel gas, intra-abdominal fat, gas within the abscess cavity, and in postoperative cases, there is limited availability of scanning surface. Thus, US has a low sensitivity in abscess detection. CT is the preferred modality and can confidently rule out intra-abdominal abscess if the CT examination is negative.

On MRI, abscesses are seen as well-defined fluid collection with low SI on T1W and high SI on T2W images. Adjacent inflammation can be seen as diffusely increased SI on T2W images.

Percutaneous aspiration is frequently required to confirm the presence of pus in a suspected abscess. Percutaneous drainage has become the widely accepted treatment for abdominal abscesses and can be done under US or CT guidance. US can be used for the follow-up evaluation of abscess under treatment.[7]

Tuberculous Peritonitis

The peritoneum and its reflections can also be commonly involved by tuberculosis (TB). Isolated involvement is rare, mostly occurring in association with other sites of involvement. The mode of transmission may be hematogenous or lymphatic, reactivation of latent tuberculous foci in the peritoneum or peritoneal spill from tubercular salpingitis. Discharge of caseous material

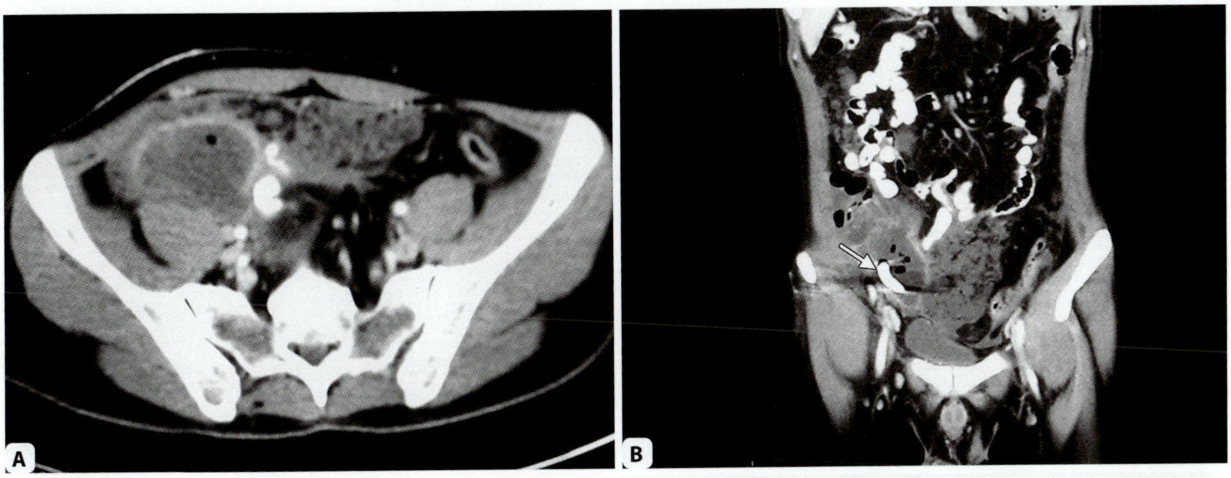

FIGS. 9A AND B: Appendicular abscess: (A) Contrast-enhanced computed tomography (CECT) axial and coronal scans; (B) show a well-defined hypodense collection with a thin peripheral enhancing rim in the right iliac fossa. Small gas bubbles are seen within the abscess. There is evidence of associated inflammatory changes in the adjacent fat. A drain can be seen in the abscess in (B) (arrow).

from diseased lymph nodes may also lead to tubercular peritonitis.

Classically, three forms of tuberculous peritonitis have been described:[16-18]

1. *Wet ascitic type*: Seen in 90% cases characterized by large amount of free or loculated ascitic fluid. This may be accompanied by diffuse and smooth peritoneal thickening.
2. *Fibrotic fixed type*: Characterized by mesenteric and omental thickening and matted bowel loops resembling masses, with formation of cocoon in some cases.
3. *Dry or plastic type*: Predominant peritoneal and mesenteric thickening with caseous nodules, lymph node enlargement, and dense adhesions.

Imaging features: Tubercular infection diffusely involves the peritoneum, mesentery, and omentum. Free or loculated ascites is seen in 30–100% cases and is demonstrated by both ultrasound and CT.[19-21]

Ultrasound may show fine, multiple, complete, or incomplete mobile strands of fibrin and debris in the ascites **(Fig. 10A)**. Peritoneal thickening and tiny nodules are better visualized in presence of ascites on US. On CT, usually high density (25–45 HU) ascitic fluid due to high fibrin content and cellular debris is characteristic of TB.[17] However, ascites may be near water density, representing an earlier transudative stage of immune reaction. Fat fluid level, a feature of chylous ascites with supportive evidence of mesenteric adenopathy has been described in TB.[22] CT fails to show the multiple, thin interlacing septa in most patients **(Figs. 11A to C)**. Smooth, slight peritoneal thickening, and/or pronounced enhancement are seen in presence of ascites on CT in almost all cases. Enhancement of peritoneal lining is seen on delayed contrast-enhanced MRI.

Mesenteric involvement is seen as linear striations, vascular engorgement, nodular lesions, increased density at the root of mesentery, mesenteric thickening, and loss of normal mesenteric configuration. On US, the mesentery becomes echogenic as a result of increased fat deposition due to lymphatic obstruction. Presence of enlarged lymph nodes adds to the diagnosis of early TB **(Figs. 10A to C)**. Mesenteric nodular lesions may present as micro (<5 mm) or macro (>5 mm) nodules. Mesenteric abscess may form as result of extension of caseous material from diseased lymph nodes. Fixed loops of bowel and mesentery standing out as spokes radiating out from the mesenteric root are described as ultrasound "stellate" sign. CT demonstrates the thickened mesentery by its increased vascularity and thickened strands and tethering of bowel loops forming an abdominal mass **(Figs. 11 and 12)**. "Club sandwich sign" or the "sliced bread" appearance is due to localized or focal ascites between radially oriented bowel due to local exudation from inflamed bowel or ruptured lymph nodes.

Omental thickening is a feature of both TB and PC and many different appearances "nodular", "smudged", or "caked" have been described. The thickened omentum shows heterogeneous iso- to hyperintense signal on T2W sequences on MRI.[23] A marked degree of enhancement is seen on enhanced CT and MRI **(Figs. 13 and 14)**. Sclerosing encapsulating peritonitis (SEP) (abdominal cocoon) formation has also been described in tubercular involvement of peritoneum **(Figs. 17A to D)**.

Associated features of intra-abdominal TB may also be present, such as thickening of the bowel wall, particularly the terminal ileum, focal abnormalities in the liver or spleen due to granulomas, and occasionally adrenal pathology. Notably, the chest radiograph is abnormal in only 50% of patients with tuberculous peritonitis.[24]

The *differential diagnosis* of tubercular peritonitis constitutes PC, mesothelioma, peritonitis, and rarely lymphoma. A marked overlap exists between the imaging appearances of tubercular peritonitis and PC. Features favoring carcinomatosis are nodular implants with

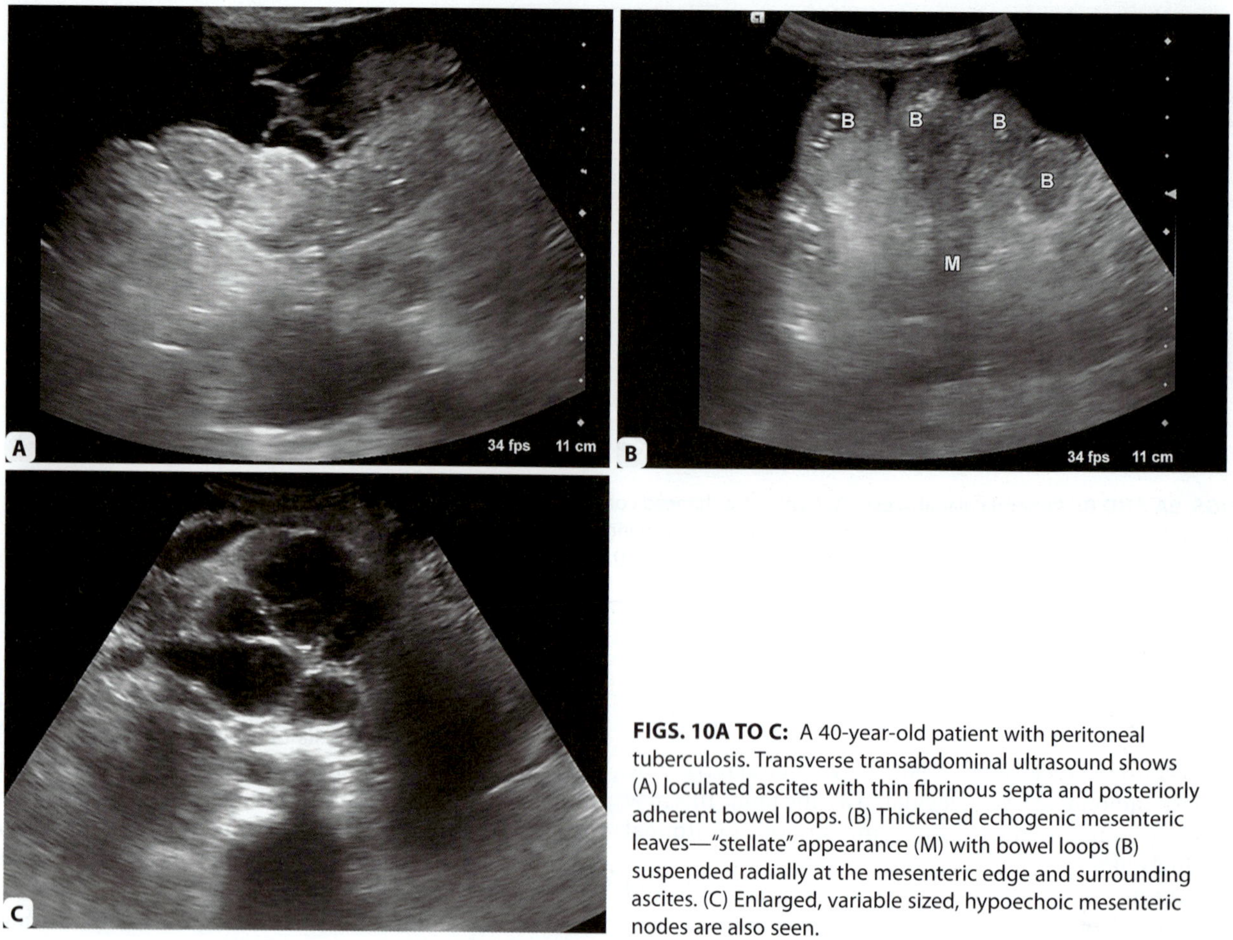

FIGS. 10A TO C: A 40-year-old patient with peritoneal tuberculosis. Transverse transabdominal ultrasound shows (A) loculated ascites with thin fibrinous septa and posteriorly adherent bowel loops. (B) Thickened echogenic mesenteric leaves—"stellate" appearance (M) with bowel loops (B) suspended radially at the mesenteric edge and surrounding ascites. (C) Enlarged, variable sized, hypoechoic mesenteric nodes are also seen.

irregular thickening. Irregularly thickened outer contour of the infiltrated peritoneum favors malignancy, whereas a thin omental line, suggestive of a fibrous wall covering the infiltrated omentum is more common in tubercular peritonitis.[25,26] However, a clinical background of malignancy along with laboratory investigations are often required to differentiate between them. Peritoneal mesothelioma shows multifocal peritoneal thickening of either sheet or nodular type which can be up to 3 cm in thickness, omental or mesenteric soft tissue masses, thick rigid septa between peritoneal leaves, and fixed bowel loops with disproportionately small amount of ascites to the degree of tumor dissemination.

Peritoneal Hydatidosis

Peritoneal hydatidosis is an uncommon manifestation of hydatid disease and is almost always secondary to hepatic disease. It occurs as a result of traumatic or surgical rupture of a hepatic or splenic hydatid cyst. However, spontaneous, asymptomatic microruptures of hepatic cysts into the peritoneal cavity are not uncommon leading to peritoneal seeding. Primary hydatidosis is a rare entity accounting for just 2% of all intra-abdominal hydatid disease.[27]

Clinical picture: Most patients remain asymptomatic for years. Symptoms such as nonspecific pain, abdominal fullness, dyspepsia, anorexia, and vomiting arise due to enlarging abdominal cysts. Rupture of the cyst into the peritoneum may present as acute abdominal pain. Antigenic fluid released into the peritoneal cavity and absorbed into the circulation may present with acute allergic manifestations.[28]

Imaging features: Hydatid cysts can be well seen on US, CT, and MRI. Cysts may be multiple and located anywhere in the peritoneal cavity **(Figs. 15A to C)**. The imaging appearances of hydatid cysts are similar to those in hepatic disease. Sometimes, peritoneal hydatid disease occupies the entire peritoneal cavity, simulating a multiloculated mass which is known as encysted peritoneal hydatidosis.[27]

Secondary Inflammatory Processes

Inflammation of any part of the abdominal viscera may be accompanied by inflammatory change of the regional fatty tissue. This may progress to phlegmon formation, abscess, or even generalized peritonitis. Appendicitis, diverticulitis, pancreatitis, inflammatory bowel disease,

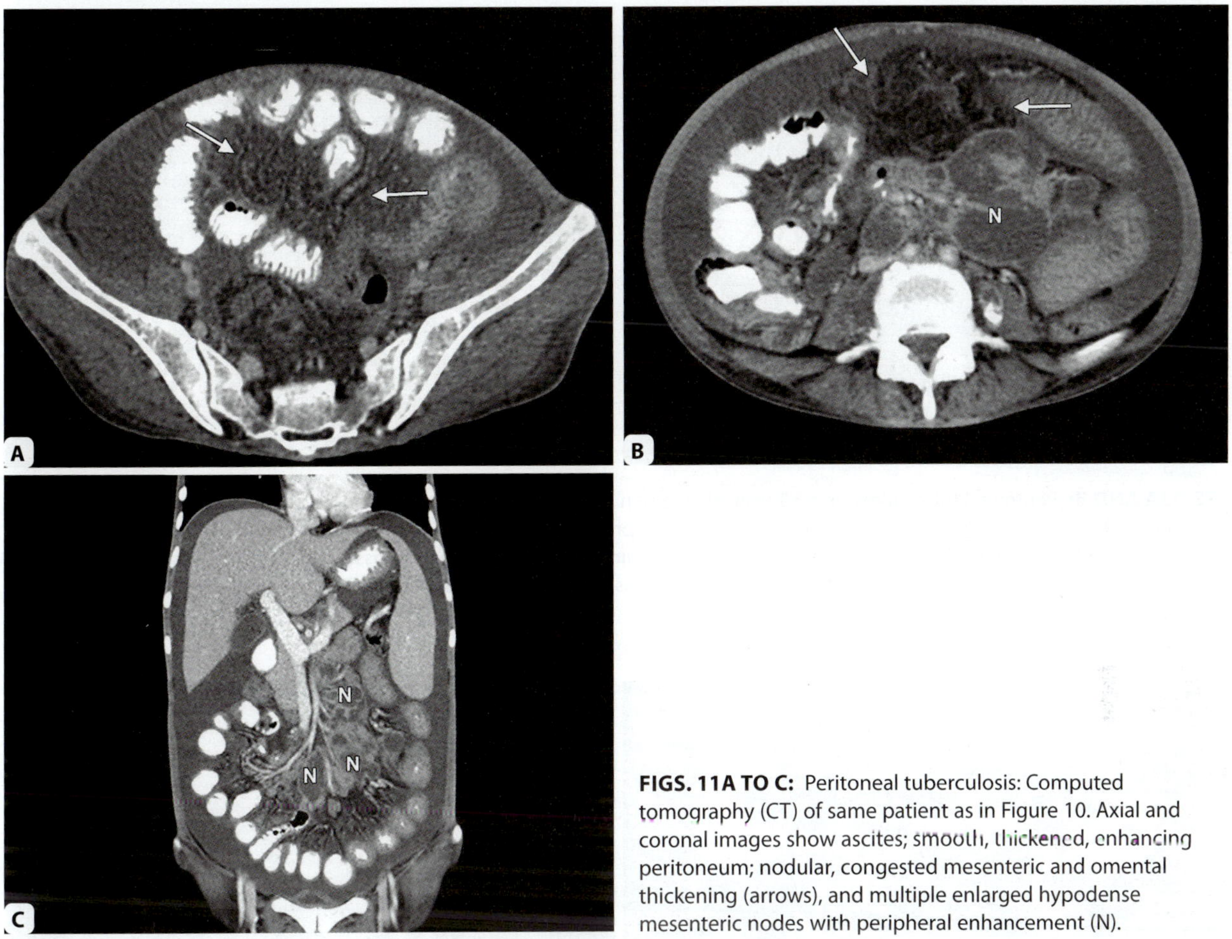

FIGS. 11A TO C: Peritoneal tuberculosis: Computed tomography (CT) of same patient as in Figure 10. Axial and coronal images show ascites; smooth, thickened, enhancing peritoneum; nodular, congested mesenteric and omental thickening (arrows), and multiple enlarged hypodense mesenteric nodes with peripheral enhancement (N).

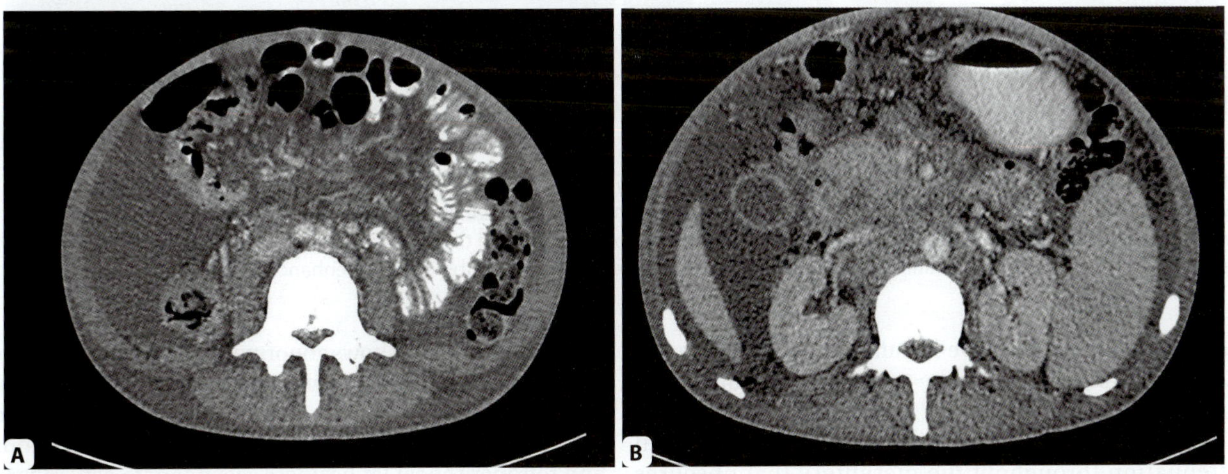

FIGS. 12A AND B: Tubercular peritonitis—wet ascitic type. Contrast-enhanced computed tomography (CECT) axial scans show (A) the presence of ascites with small nodules and haziness in the mesentery and omentum. (B) At a more cranial level, conglomerate caseous lymphadenopathy is seen in mesenteric and retroperitoneal regions.

cholecystitis, etc., are conditions which commonly give rise to these localized inflammatory changes. They are best visualized on CT as soft tissue stranding of adjacent fat, fluid, phlegmon or abscess formation, sinus tracts, and fistulas **(Figs. 16A and B)**.

Besides the above inflammatory changes, Crohn's disease may show other mesenteric abnormalities in the form of hypertrophied mesenteric fat (fibrofatty proliferation), engorged vasa recta (the comb's sign), and small mesenteric nodes. The presence of engorged

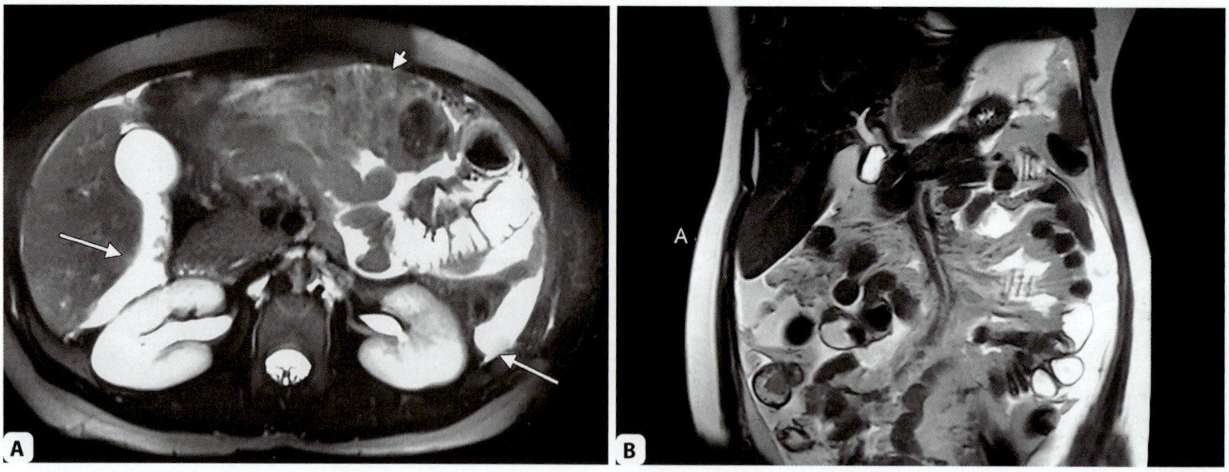

FIGS. 13A AND B: Peritoneal tuberculosis in a 35-year-old woman with loss of weight and abdominal fullness for 1 month. (A) Axial T2-weighted (T2W) haste magnetic resonance (MR) image shows presence of ascitic fluid in Morrison's pouch, left paracolic gutter (arrows) and in interloop regions. The omentum is thickened showing a heterogeneous soft tissue signal (arrowhead). (B) Coronal T2W haste MR image shows diffuse infiltration of the mesenteric fat by isointense soft tissue. Ascites is seen in the paracolic gutters and subhepatic space.

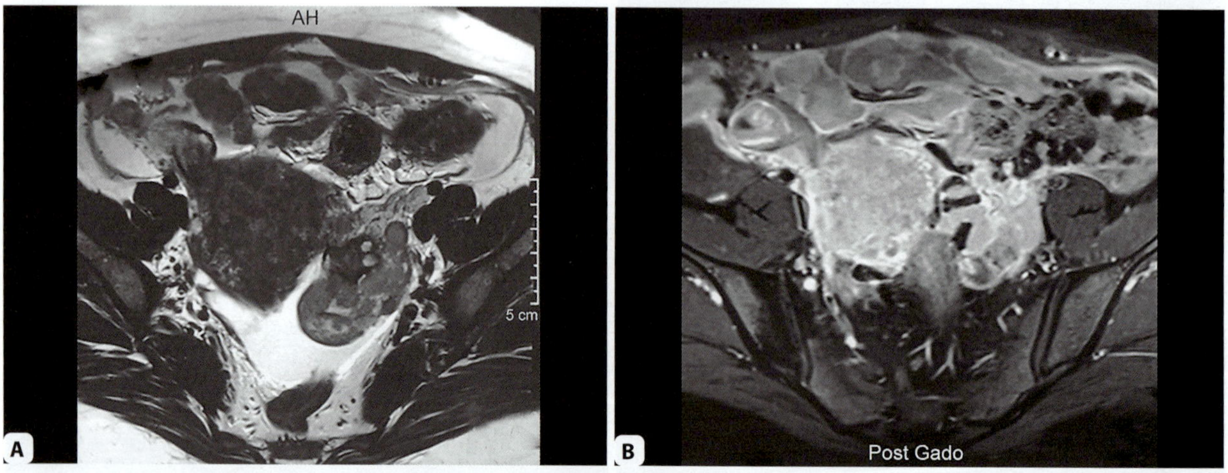

FIGS. 14A AND B: Peritoneal tuberculosis—same patient as in Figure 13, axial T2W haste (A) and postcontrast (B) magnetic resonance (MR) images show presence of ascites, clumped bowel loops, with thickened and enhancing serosa. Left tubo-ovarian mass was seen which also enhanced on the postcontrast scan. On laprotomy the bowel serosa and the adnexal mass were studded with multiple small granulomas, which were not identifiable individually on the MR images, but caused the intensely enhancing peritoneal lining.

vasa recta indicates active inflammation, whereas the fibrofatty proliferation can be seen even with quiescent disease.

Mesenteric edema is defined as diffuse increase in attenuation throughout the mesentery that obscures visualization of the blood vessels as they course through the mesentery, also termed as "misty mesentery". It may be secondary to various causes, including hypoalbuminemia, cirrhosis, nephrosis, heart failure, tricuspid disease, constrictive pericarditis, portal hypertension, portal vein thrombosis, mesenteric ischemia, vasculitis, or trauma. On CT, mesenteric edema increases the density of the mesenteric fat from –100 to –160 HU, which is similar to the density of subcutaneous fat, to values of –40 to –60 HU.[29] On MRI, the mesentery shows abnormal signal. The mesenteric arteries and veins lose their sharp definition and are not clearly visualized as they course to the bowel. Associated ascites may be present and generalized subcutaneous and retroperitoneal fat haziness secondary to generalized edema can be seen. The extent and site of involvement gives a clue to the differential diagnosis.

Sclerosing Encapsulating Peritonitis/ Abdominal Cocoon

Sclerosing encapsulating peritonitis (SEP) is a rare chronic inflammatory process of the peritoneum which is characterized by total or partial encasement of the small bowel

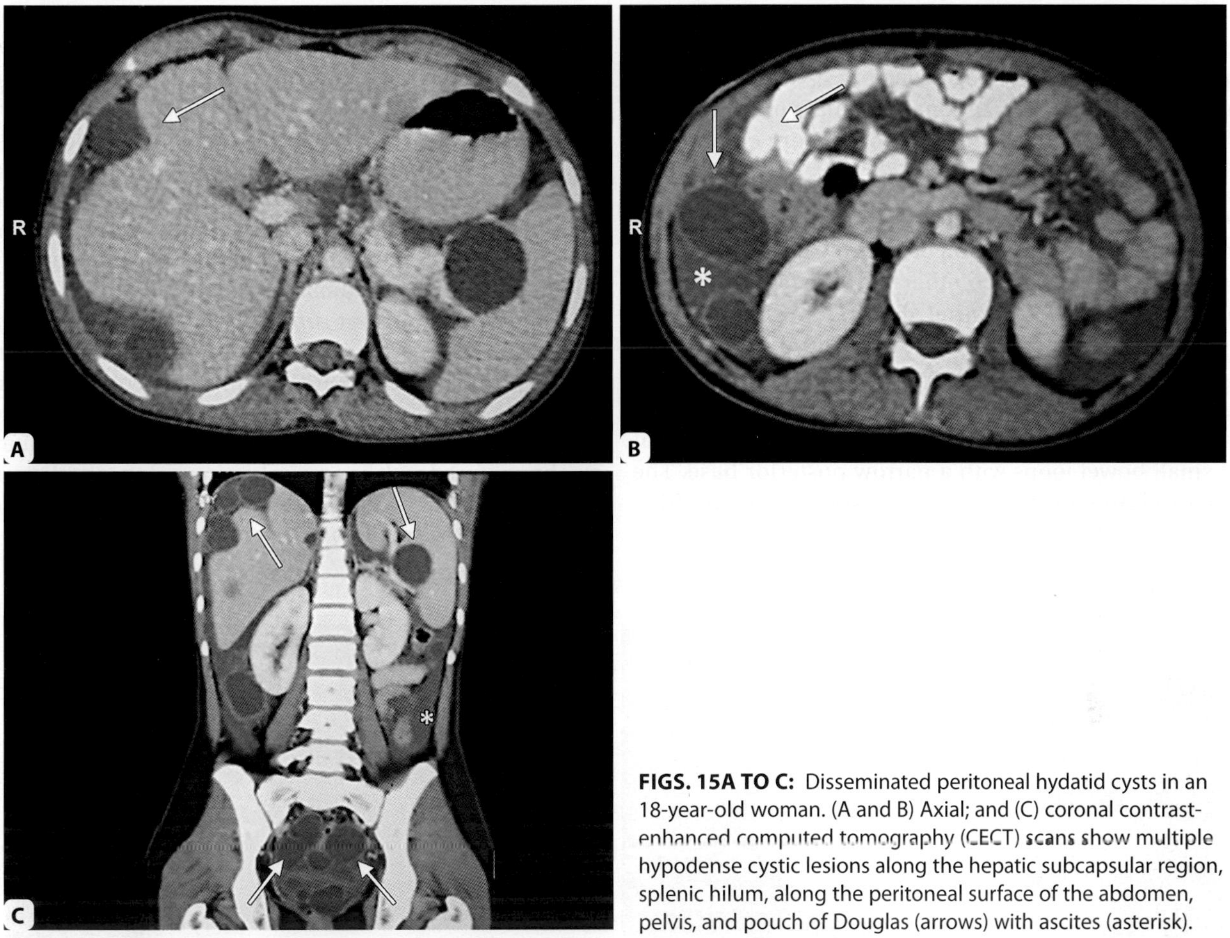

FIGS. 15A TO C: Disseminated peritoneal hydatid cysts in an 18-year-old woman. (A and B) Axial; and (C) coronal contrast-enhanced computed tomography (CECT) scans show multiple hypodense cystic lesions along the hepatic subcapsular region, splenic hilum, along the peritoneal surface of the abdomen, pelvis, and pouch of Douglas (arrows) with ascites (asterisk).

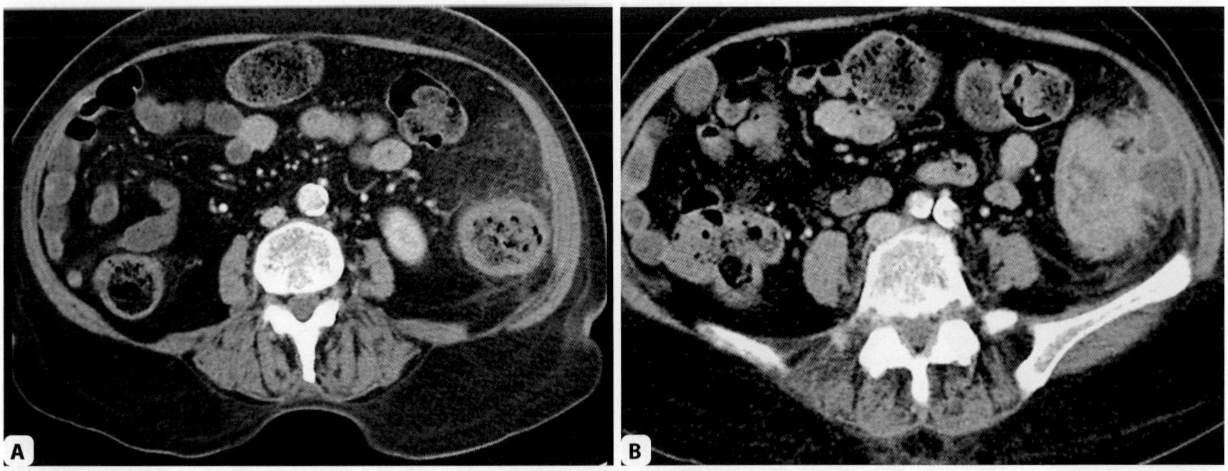

FIGS. 16A AND B: Acute diverticulitis showing local extension of inflammation. Contrast-enhanced computed tomography (CECT) axial scans (A) inflammatory fat stranding seen around the thickened segment of descending colon. (B) In another patient, there is formation of abscesses seen as rim enhancing hypodense masses in the left pericolonic region.

within a thick fibrocollagenous membrane. SEP is most commonly associated with abdominal TB in our country. It can occur as a complication in patients who undergo continuous peritoneal dialysis. It has also been described in association with long-term β-blocker treatment, sarcoidosis, systemic lupus erythematosus (SLE), indwelling abdominal catheter, etc.[30] These conditions predispose patients to peritoneal irritation and inflammation which can lead to peritoneal fibroneogenesis. Sometimes, no predisposing condition may be found.

Clinically, patients may be asymptomatic or have abdominal distension, pain, and vomiting that resolve spontaneously suggesting recurrent episodes of small bowel obstruction. A soft nontender mass may be felt on abdominal palpation. It is seen to be more common in young adolescent girls.

Imaging features: A barium meal follow-through study may show a conglomeration of multiple bowel loops that appear to adhere to each other with or without delayed passage of contrast material **(Fig. 17A)**. Characteristic sonographic findings include altered peristalsis, adherence of the bowel to the anterior abdominal wall, and a membranous sac seen to encase the small bowel loops **(Fig. 17B)**. There is a concertina-like arrangement of small bowel loops with a narrow posterior base. The encapsulating membrane may be identified with high frequency linear probes.[31]

The CECT shows conglomeration of small bowel loops in the central abdomen with a thick enhancing membrane surrounding the bowel, forming a saclike structure or a cocoon **(Figs. 17C and D)**. Small amount of fluid may be seen within the cocoon. Bowel loops may be of normal caliber or dilated. The fibrous membrane surrounding the bowel loops is best visualized on CT. CT also gives more accurate information on the degree of obstruction and the types of bowel loops involved. Multiple foci of linear calcification may develop or there can be diffuse peritoneal calcification.[32,33]

The most important *differential diagnosis* of SEP is an internal hernia that also causes localized collection of small bowel loops with symptoms of obstruction. However, there is no membrane-like sac around the clustered small bowel loops in internal hernias. SEP may also be confused with congenital peritoneal encapsulation, which is characterized by a thin accessory peritoneal sac surrounding the small bowel.

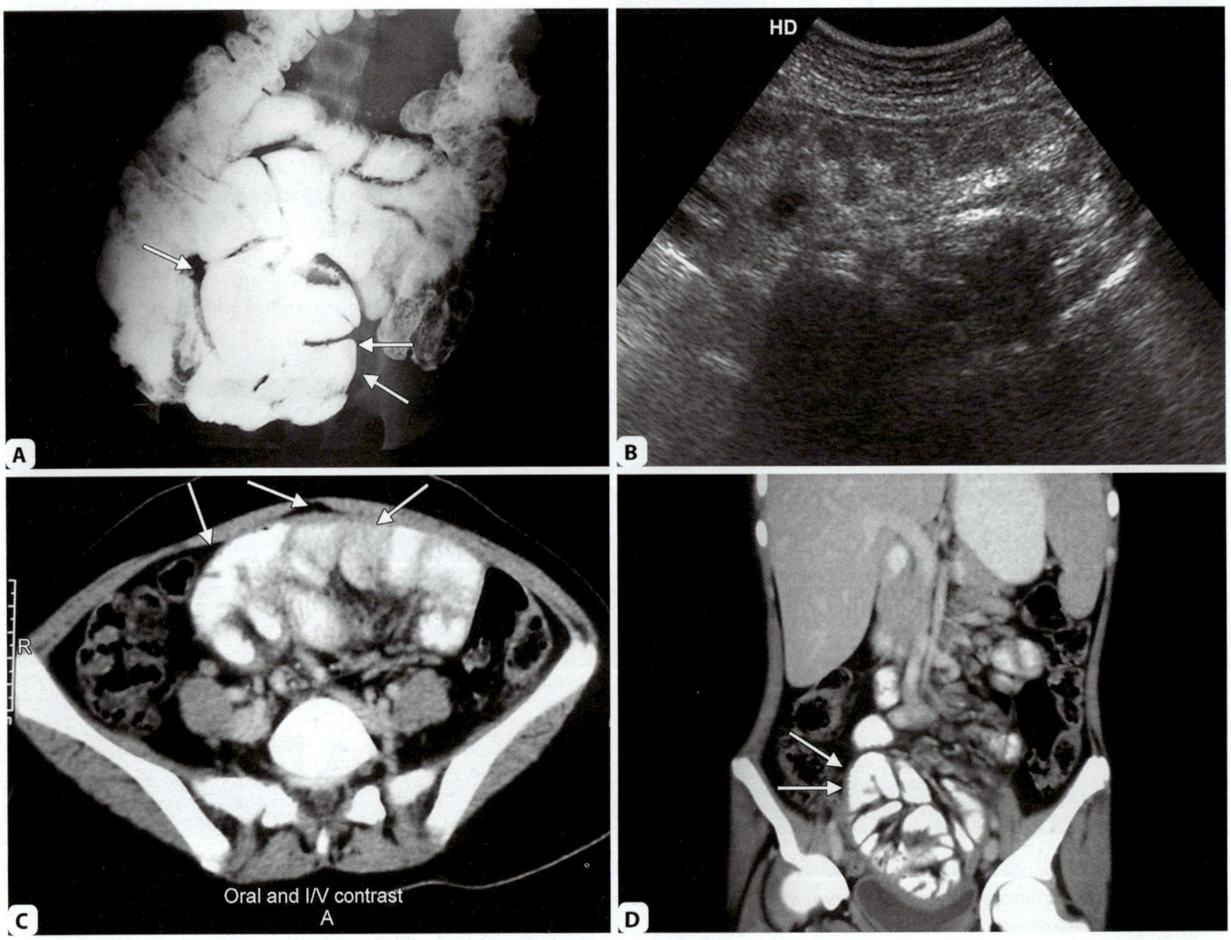

FIGS. 17A TO D: Sclerosing peritonitis: A 14-year-old girl with recurrent episodes of intestinal obstruction. (A) Barium meal follow through study shows clustered bowel loops in pelvis and lower abdomen (arrows). (B) Transverse ultrasonography (US) through lower abdomen show clumped bowel loops adherent to the anterior abdominal wall. An increased peristalsis was noted in the loops on real-time. (C) Axial; and (D) coronal contrast-enhanced computed tomography (CECT) scans show clumped small bowel loops in the lower abdomen with a thin surrounding membrane (arrows). Small mesenteric nodes are also seen.

Sclerosing Mesenteritis/Mesenteric Panniculitis/Mesenteric Lipodystrophy

Sclerosing mesenteritis is a rare, slowly progressive disorder characterized by nonspecific inflammation of the mesenteric fat. It usually involves the root of the small bowel mesentery, but may affect the transverse mesocolon, peripancreatic region, omentum, retroperitoneum, or pelvis.[34]

Histologically, it has varying amounts of fibrosis, chronic inflammation, and fat necrosis. Depending on the predominant component it has been categorized into three subgroups:

1. Sclerosing/retractile mesenteritis, when the fibrous component is dominant.
2. Mesenteric panniculitis, when chronic inflammation predominates.
3. Mesenteric lipodystrophy, when fat necrosis is the predominant component.[35]

These three subgroups have been considered to be different stages of the same disease or could represent different entities. Although their exact cause remains unknown, various underlying possibilities have been suggested such as prior surgery or trauma, ischemia, an autoimmune process [can be immunoglobulin G4 (IgG4)-related], or malignancy. An association with other idiopathic inflammatory disorders such as retroperitoneal fibrosis, Reidel's thyroiditis, orbital pseudotumors, and sclerosing cholangitis has been noted.

Clinical picture: They occur more commonly in males and the average age of presentation is around 60 years. Patients present with abdominal pain, fever, mass, weight loss, obstructive symptoms, or diarrhea, or may even be completely asymptomatic.

Imaging features: The imaging findings reflect the underlying histology of the lesion. CT is the most useful imaging modality for the evaluation, with US showing nonspecific increase in mesenteric echogenicity, with small lymph nodes. When the fibrous component is dominant, i.e., sclerosing type of mesenteritis, an infiltrative soft tissue mass with variable degree of enhancement is seen on CT. Central calcification or necrosis, radiating strands of soft tissue (desmoplastic reaction), and small lymph nodes in the adjacent fat may all be seen **(Figs. 18A and B)**. There may be preservation of fat around the mesenteric vessels and the lymph nodes, a phenomenon that is referred to as the *"fat ring or halo sign"*.[36] On MRI, the SI pattern is consistent with fibrosis, showing low SI on both T1W and T2W images. Sometimes, a high signal on T2W image may be seen which corresponds to myxomatous change or hypervascularity accompanying active proliferation of fibrosis. Secondary changes may be seen in the adjacent bowel as angulations by the fibrotic process in the mesentery, or edematous thickening due to obstruction of lymphatics and veins.[35]

The classical CT signs of mesenteric panniculitis (when the inflammatory component is dominant) are presence of an inhomogeneous increase in attenuation of mesenteric fat, more than adjacent retroperitoneal or mesocolonic fat, with a well-defined "mass effect" on neighboring structures and presence of small lymph nodes **(Figs. 19A and B)**. Presence of the "fat ring sign" may be seen.[37] A tumoral pseudocapsule, i.e., a thin, usually <3 mm, band of soft tissue attenuation on CT, appearing hypointense on T2W MR images, may be seen around the mass, which together with the fat rim sign are considered as radiologic hallmarks of the disease.

On FDG PET-CT these lesions are non-FDG avid, and this helps in differentiating between sclerosing mesenteritis and malignant mesenteric involvement.

Differential diagnosis: Several conditions can mimic the CT appearance of sclerosing mesenteritis, including lymphoma, carcinoid tumor, carcinomatosis, primary

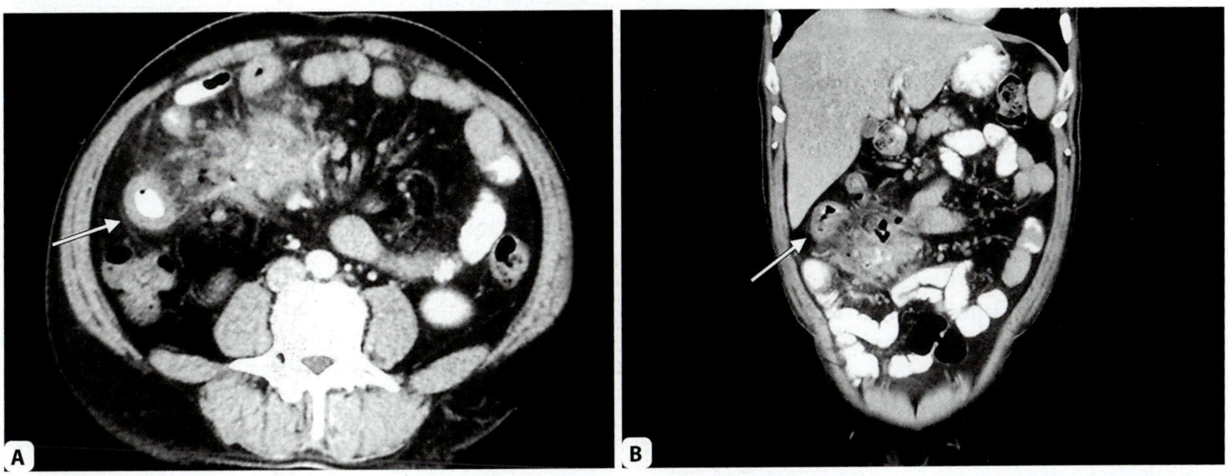

FIGS. 18A AND B: Sclerosing mesenteritis. (A) Enhanced axial; and (B) coronal computed tomography (CT) scans show an ill-defined soft tissue mesenteric mass with irregular, spiculated margins and thickening of adjacent jejunal loops (arrow). Small mesenteric lymph nodes are seen.

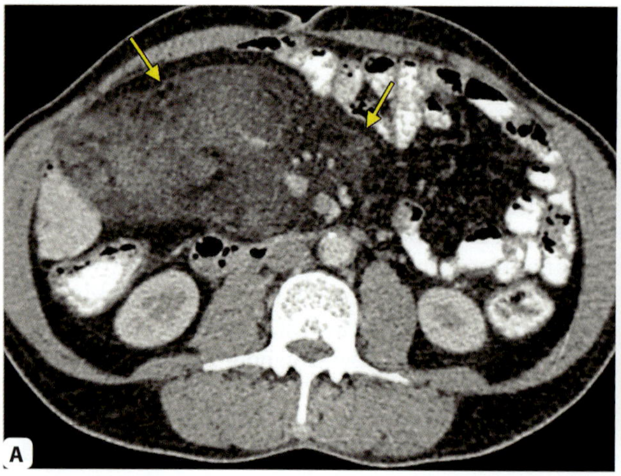

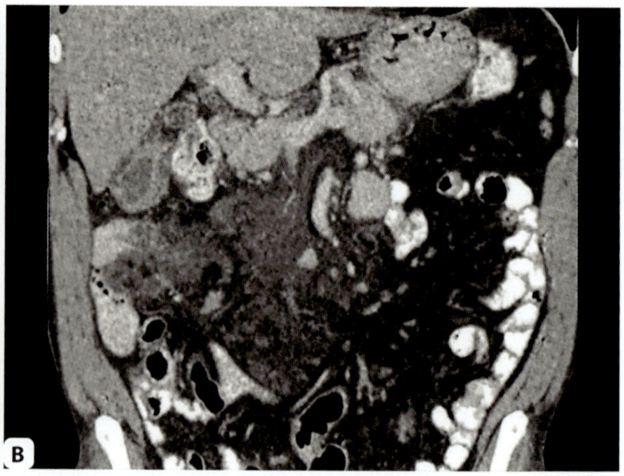

FIGS. 19A AND B: Mesenteric panniculitis. (A) Enhanced axial; and (B) coronal computed tomography (CT) scans show a large mesenteric mass with a pseudocapsule (yellow arrows), with small lymph nodes and vessels inside the mass displacing the adjacent bowel. The fat around vessels and lymph nodes within the mass has the same density as the normal fat "the fat ring sign".

mesenteric mesothelioma, and mesenteric edema.[38] Except for primary mesenteric mesothelioma, these conditions are considerably more common than sclerosing mesenteritis. Mesenteric panniculitis can be mimicked by mesenteric edema resulting from various conditions such as cirrhosis, hypoalbuminemia, heart failure, portal or mesenteric vein thrombosis, and vasculitis. Trauma can also result in edema and hemorrhage in the mesentery. Mesenteric edema secondary to systemic disease is often diffuse and coexists with generalized subcutaneous edema and ascites, which will not be present in patients with sclerosing mesenteritis. Also, the clinical history will often be the clue to the correct diagnosis. A biopsy is often necessary for diagnosis and although results of the biopsy may suggest the diagnosis, surgical excisional biopsy is often required for complete histologic analysis.

Mesenteric panniculitis is typically self-limiting, whereas sclerosing mesenteritis is more aggressive. Management is mainly supportive with anti-inflammatory drugs and corticosteroids. Immunomodulating drugs can be given in cases which do not respond to steroids.[39]

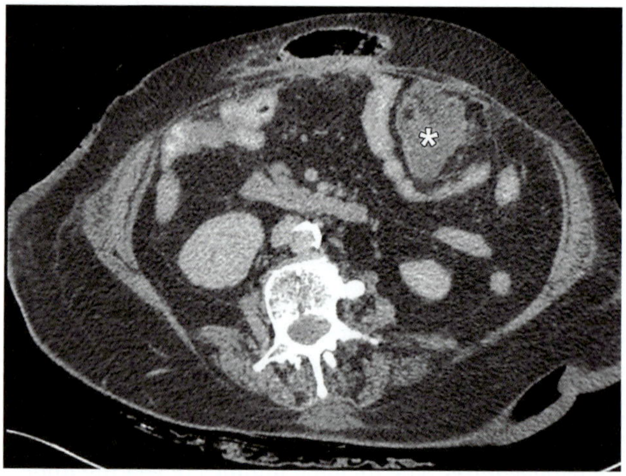

FIG. 20: Omental infarction. A 60-year-old patient with complaint of pain in abdomen 6 days after undergoing abdominal surgery. Contrast-enhanced computed tomography (CECT) axial scan shows a hypodense, heterogeneous soft tissue mass with focal fatty areas within and adjacent fat stranding between the anterior abdominal wall and the transverse colon (asterisk). A pocket of air is seen in the subcutaneous tissue due to dehiscence of the distal sutures.

Omental Infarction

Omental infarction (OI) occurs due to vascular compromise, torsion or venous thrombosis, of the greater omentum. It can be primary or secondary. Primary OI is generally right-sided and is related to the tenuous blood supply to the right edge of the greater omentum. Secondary OI occurs due to vascular insult after trauma, surgery or inflammation of the greater omentum, and it is located near the site of the initial insult. Unaccustomed exercise, straining, or coughing can precipitate this condition.

Clinical findings: Primary OI is more common in children. Obesity is an important risk factor. Patients present with subacute onset of pain most often localized in the right upper or lower quadrant without any other gastrointestinal (GI) symptoms. There can be mild leucocytosis. Establishing a preoperative diagnosis of OI is difficult as it often mimics acute appendicitis or cholecystitis. The management is conservative.

Imaging features: On CT, it appears as a fatty, large (>5 cm) encapsulated mass, with soft-tissue stranding adjacent to the ascending colon. Early or mild infarction may manifest as ill-defined, mild haziness. It is classically located between the anterior abdominal wall and the ascending or transverse colon **(Fig. 20)**. Swirling of vessels may be seen in omental torsion. At US, OI may appear as a focal area of echogenic, noncompressible fat that corresponds to the site of focal tenderness.

MESENTERIC LYMPHADENOPATHY

The mesentery contains multiple small lymph nodes which may get enlarged in a number of disease processes notably infective, inflammatory, and neoplastic **(Box 2)**. Normal mesenteric lymph nodes can be routinely identified at the mesenteric root and throughout the mesentery on US, CT, and MRI, and are generally <5 mm in short axis diameter. The size of the nodes alone does not always reflect disease, the number and distribution of lymph nodes is also important. Lymph nodes greater than 6 mm in short axis diameter or a group of three or more clustered together in one anatomic location are taken as abnormal.[40,41]

Tuberculous Lymphadenitis

Lymphadenopathy in abdominal TB usually occurs in mesenteric, peripancreatic, periportal, and para-aortic groups of lymph nodes. It can occur through lymphatic spread, hematogenous route, or direct spread from adjacent infected organs. The nodes may vary from increased number of normal-sized nodes to massive conglomerates with matting, the latter resulting from adhesions due to periadenitis. Pathologically, tuberculous infection of a lymph node follows a spectrum from early exudative to caseous to late fibro-calcification phases.

On sonography, the lymph nodes are seen either as discrete or conglomerate masses. Enlarged nodes show central hypoechoic areas with a mixed heterogeneous echotexture **(Fig. 10C)** in contrast to homogeneously hypoechoic nodes seen in lymphoma. Heterogeneity of echo pattern in nodes of a single anatomic subgroup, prior to treatment is strongly suggestive of TB, rather than lymphoma. Larger areas of caseation may coalesce with adjacent nodes, resulting in larger collections. Lymph nodes may be adherent to intra-abdominal vasculature and a fibrous reaction surrounding clusters of nodes may be seen as increase in background echogenicity.[42,43]

On CT, the multicompartmental localization of nodes with relative sparing of the retroperitoneal compartment is the most characteristic feature of TB. On unenhanced scans, the nodes may display low attenuation values <30 HU or soft tissue attenuation values similar to muscle. Four different patterns of nodal enhancement have been described by Pombo et al.[44]

- Peripheral enhancement, the most frequent pattern, is characterized by peripheral rim enhancement, with or without low attenuation center. This pattern is seen in younger patients and reflects significant central liquefactive or caseous necrosis and a highly vascular perinodal inflammatory reaction which is relatively diagnostic for TB, although not pathognomic **(Fig. 11)**.
- Inhomogeneous enhancement is also a frequent manifestation of tubercular adenitis, due to intranodal granulomas and relatively less necrosis than in nodes that show peripheral enhancement **(Fig. 12B)**.
- Homogeneous contrast enhancement represents a less frequent manifestation. These are indistinguishable from untreated lymphomatous nodes and are seen in patients with infection with mycobacterium avium intracellulare and acquired immunodeficiency syndrome (AIDS).
- Nonenhancing nodes

MRI shows majority of nodes to be hypointense on T1W and hyperintense on T2W images when compared to abdominal muscle, with a few demonstrating a rim which is hypointense on T1W and hyperintense on T2W images. Minority of nodes are hypo- to isointense on both T1W and T2W images. The varying SI on T2W images is explained on the stage of evolution of the disease—the central T2 hyperintensity reflects caseous necrosis while central T2 hypointensity denotes presence of paramagnetic free radicals secreted from phagocytic cells. On contrast-enhanced images, different enhancement patterns, including peripheral, heterogeneous, and less frequently homogeneous enhancement may be seen, similar to CT.[45,46]

With the institution of appropriate treatment, nodal masses tend to show a transient increase in size for 3–4 weeks followed by a gradual reduction in overall dimensions. Focal calcification may occur in nodal and omental masses and collections, which may be clustered along the periphery or may be central in location. Tubercular adenitis may be confused with nodes of lymphoma and metastatic disease, and clinical and radiological differentiation may be difficult. Lymphoma nodes have a different anatomical distribution and near homogeneous enhancement pattern prior to treatment. Caseation and calcification are highly suggestive of tubercular etiology.[47]

BOX 2 Causes of mesenteric lymphadenopathy.

Infective processes:
- Tuberculosis
- Mesenteric adenitis syndrome
- Celiac disease
- Intestinal infection—*Yersinia*
- *Mycobacterium avium* intracellulare (MAC) infection
- Human immunodeficiency virus (HIV)
- Whipple's disease

Inflammatory lesions:
- Local inflammatory processes such as acute appendicitis, diverticulitis, pancreatitis, etc.
- Crohn's disease
- Mesenteric panniculitis/sclerosing mesenteritis
- Connective tissue disorders—rheumatoid arthritis, scleroderma, systemic lupus erythematosus (SLE), etc.
- Others

Neoplastic processes:
- Lymphoma
- Metastatic disease
- Kaposi's sarcoma

Miscellaneous:
- Castleman's disease
- Sarcoidosis
- Amyloidosis, etc.

Differential diagnosis: Lymph nodes with hypodense centers are also seen in metastatic nodes, lymphoma after treatment, inflammatory conditions (such as Crohn's disease), pyogenic infection, and Whipple's disease, however, other imaging findings and clinical features are helpful in diagnosis. Lymphatic involvement is also a common feature in patients with AIDS. The nodes in these are usually located in mesenteric and retroperitoneal region. Nonenhancing low attenuation nodes may be seen in AIDS.

Primary Mesenteric Adenitis

Primary mesenteric adenitis consists of right-sided mesenteric adenopathy without any associated identifiable inflammatory process. Although it has been termed as primary, it is thought that the enlarged nodes arise from an infective process (e.g., *Yersinia sp*) causing a terminal ileitis that may or may not be seen on imaging.

Clinically, patients present with nonspecific abdominal pain which may be acute or chronic, often mimicking appendicitis. US and CT will show clustered, discrete, and moderately enlarged nodes in the right lower quadrant with a short axis diameter of generally <10 mm. Occasionally, thickening of the terminal ileum may also be seen **(Figs. 21A and B)**.[48]

This is a self-limiting condition, which resolves on conservative treatment. The most important differential diagnosis is acute appendicitis, as enlarged reactive nodes may often be seen in the right lower quadrant in appendicitis. The identification of a normal appendix on imaging favors primary mesenteric adenitis.[49]

Neoplastic Lymphadenopathy

Lymphoma is the most common cause of neoplastic mesenteric lymph node enlargement. Non-Hodgkin's lymphoma (NHL) involves the mesenteric nodes along with the retroperitoneal para-aortic nodes. Approximately, 30–50% cases of NHL spread to the mesenteric nodes, commonly from the retroperitoneal nodes.[50] The enlarged nodes can show three patterns of involvement—in the mesenteric root, scattered throughout the peripheral mesentery, or a mixed root-peripheral pattern **(Figs. 22A and B)**. In early cases, the lymph nodes may be small and discrete, but they progressively increase in size to form coalescent conglomerate masses. As they are soft tumors, they tend to grow around the vessels and the bowel without causing pressure effect. On CECT images, lymphomatous nodes are seen as multiple round, mildly enhancing, and homogeneous masses that often surround mesenteric arteries and veins. Pretreatment calcification is rare. Associated peritoneal and mesenteric involvement can be seen.[34]

Metastatic involvement of mesenteric nodes can occur from GI malignancies, however is rare from tumors of genitourinary or extra-abdominal malignancies.

Kaposi's sarcoma is a low grade mesenchymal tumor seen in patients of AIDS involving the blood and lymphatic vessels. Mesenteric lymphadenopathy is seen as homogeneously enhancing, large nodes, measuring 3–5 cm in short axis diameter. They may coalesce to form large masses. Associated lymphadenopathy may be seen in the porta hepatis, retroperitoneum, and pelvis. Bowel, spleen, and liver involvement may occur.[34]

NEOPLASTIC DISEASE OF PERITONEUM

The peritoneum can be involved by both primary and secondary neoplastic disease, with secondary involvement being much more common than primary tumors. **Table 3** lists the more common neoplastic diseases that arise from or involve the peritoneum.

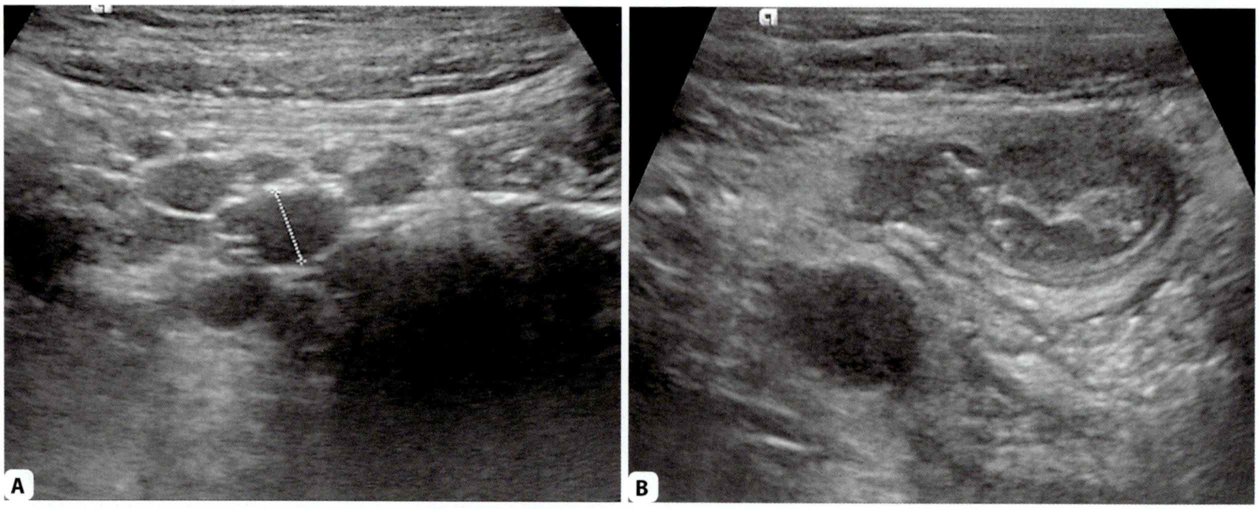

FIGS. 21A AND B: Mesenteric adenitis in a 10-year-old boy presenting with pain in right iliac fossa. (A) Ultrasonography (US) shows multiple small nodes in the right iliac fossa. (B) A more caudal scan shows a thickened distal ileal loop.

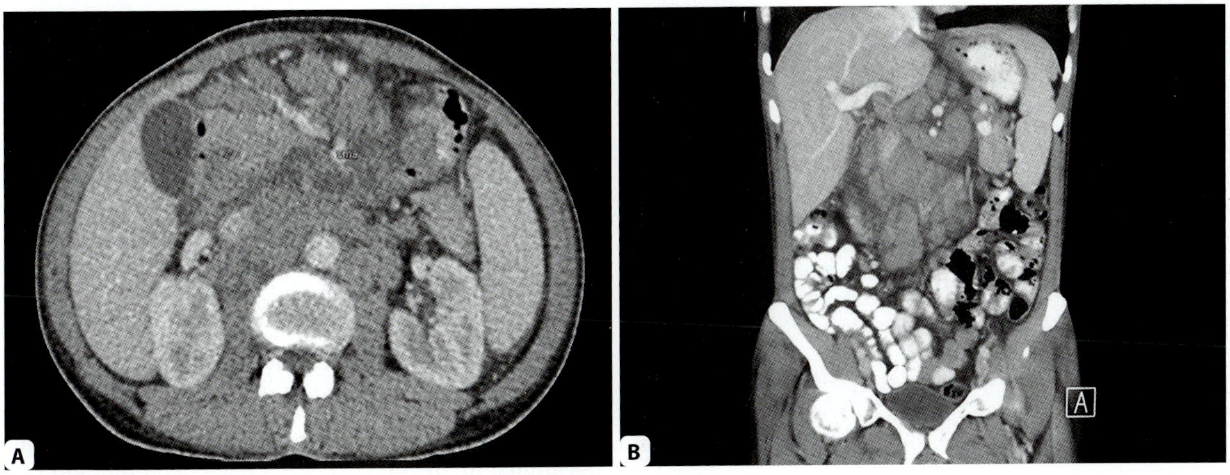

FIGS. 22A AND B: Lymphoma: Contrast-enhanced computed tomography (CECT) (A) Axial; and (B) coronal scans show multiple homogeneously enhancing mesenteric and retroperitoneal lymph nodes in a 45-year-old man with non-Hodgkin's lymphoma.

TABLE 3: List of peritoneal neoplastic diseases.

Primary tumors of the peritoneum	
Mesothelial tumors	Peritoneal malignant mesothelioma
	Well-differentiated papillary mesothelioma
	Multicystic mesothelioma
	Adenomatoid tumors
	Primary peritoneal serous borderline tumor
Smooth muscle tumor	Leiomyomatosis peritonealis disseminata
Tumors of uncertain origin	Desmoplastic small round cell tumor
	Solitary fibrous tumor
Connective tissue tumors	Desmoid tumor, lipoma, liposarcoma, leiomyosarcoma, GIST, nerve sheath tumors, synovial sarcoma, etc.
Vascular/lymphatic tumors	Primary peritoneal lymphoma
	Hemangioma, angiosarcoma, etc.
Secondary tumors of the peritoneum	
Metastatic neoplasms	Carcinomatosis
	Pseudomyxoma peritonei
	Lymphomatosis
	Sarcomatosis
	Neuroendocrine tumor/carcinoid

Primary peritoneal tumors are defined as tumors both benign and malignant, with primary manifestation in the peritoneum in the absence of a visceral site of origin.[51] They are uncommon lesions which arise from the mesothelial cells, submesothelial cells, and uncommitted stem cells. As they share a common anatomic site of origin, they have similar clinical manifestations. Patients frequently present with abdominal discomfort and distension, GI complaints, and, less commonly, pelvic pain or a palpable mass.

Malignant Peritoneal Mesothelioma

Malignant peritoneal mesothelioma (MPM) is an aggressive tumor arising from serous membranes of pleura, peritoneum, pericardium, and tunica vaginalis. Peritoneal mesotheliomas are the second most common site of involvement after pleural mesotheliomas and account for 10–15% of all mesotheliomas.[52] Histologically, three main subtypes have been described—*epithelioid* (most common with best prognosis), *sarcomatoid* (least common with worst prognosis), and the *biphasic* type which contains both epithelioid and sarcomatoid components.

Clinical picture: Similar to pleural mesotheliomas, peritoneal malignant mesotheliomas are also associated with asbestos exposure, but in lesser proportion than pleural mesotheliomas and usually develop in individuals exposed to higher levels of asbestos. The majority of malignant mesotheliomas occur in men, with a median age at presentation of 60 years, whereas in women, the mean age is 50 years.[53] Patients present with abdominal pain, abdominal distension, nausea, anorexia, and weight loss. Intestinal obstruction may occur with advanced disease.

Imaging features: The features will depend on the histological subtype. Epithelioid mesothelioma has a "wet appearance" similar to that of PC. There is diffuse involvement, with sheet-like thickening of the peritoneum, leading to an irregular and nodular peritoneum. There is associated moderate amount of ascites and omental caking **(Fig. 23)**. Sarcomatoid mesothelioma shows a "dry appearance" with heterogeneous, solid intraperitoneal masses. The margins are often irregular. The ascites is small in amount and may be loculated. The biphasic type shows a combination of these appearances. Local invasion can be seen into the abdominal wall, mesentery, liver, and other organs in both forms. Rarely calcification may occur. Mesenteric involvement can be seen as "pleated" or "stellate" appearance and sheet-like thickening can be seen to encase the small bowel loops in some cases. Generally, lymph node enlargement does not

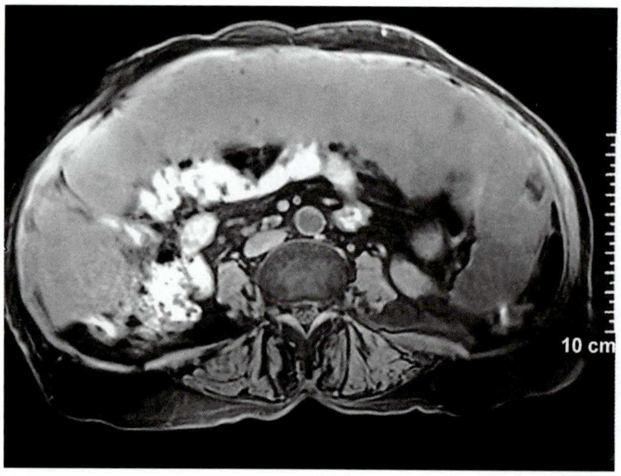

FIG. 23: Peritoneal mesothelioma. A 57-year-old woman presenting with abdominal discomfort and distension. T2-weighted (T2W) magnetic resonance (MR) image shows a thick characteristic "omental cake" appearance.

occur which is differentiating point from lymphomatosis and tubercular peritoneal involvement. Calcified pleural plaques and other asbestos-related changes such as pleural thickening and masses may be present within the chest.[54] CT findings of large tumor burden with significant bowel distortion or the presence of a small bowel obstruction is predictive of incomplete resectability. MRI imaging may quantify the extent of disease more accurately. On MRI, the nodules are seen as low T1 and intermediate to high T2 SI. The role of PET scan is not well-defined and may have some limited use in the detection of recurrent disease.[55]

Biopsy is required to establish a diagnosis and can be performed under imaging guidance or surgically. Ascitic fluid cytology has a variable sensitivity of 32–76% with the major limitation being difficulty in distinguishing benign from malignant lesions.[56] On immunohistochemistry (IHC), positive staining for mesothelial markers such as calretinin, CK 5/6, WT-1, and D2-40 is characteristic for mesotheliomas. Loss of expression of BAP1 (*BRCA*-associated protein 1) has been shown to have high specificity for differentiating peritoneal mesothelioma from benign mesothelial proliferation.

Differential diagnosis: The presence of peritoneal masses with or without ascites in the abdominal cavity is most suggestive of PC in the majority of patients. However, when a sheet like thickening is seen, the diagnosis of a primary mesothelioma must be kept in mind. IHC staining has proved to be of great benefit in differentiating MPMs from secondary tumors affecting the peritoneum. Current recommendation is to use two mesothelioma markers and two carcinoma markers. MPM will stain positive for mesothelioma markers but negative for carcinoma markers. Other differentials to be considered are tuberculous peritonitis—shows a smooth peritoneum with mild thickening and marked enhancement; lymphomatous peritonitis—which shows marked mesenteric and retroperitoneal lymphadenopathy; and sarcomatous peritonitis—which is characterized by heterogeneous, bulky, hypervascular masses with a variable amount of ascites.

The overall prognosis is poor. Cytoreductive surgery (CRS) with hyperthermic intraperitoneal chemotherapy (HIPEC) have become the most widely adopted methods of treatment for peritoneal mesothelioma, however, are associated with significant morbidity. Studies using novel molecular targets are under process to develop targeted therapies.[57]

Multicystic Peritoneal Mesothelioma/ Peritoneal Inclusion Cyst

Over the years, multicystic peritoneal mesothelioma and peritoneal inclusion cyst (PIC) have been thought of as the same condition. However, more recently the term *multicystic mesothelioma* is being used to describe a true neoplasm, a benign, multilocular cystic tumor that most commonly arises from the pelvic surface of the peritoneum. Although it has a benign, indolent course in most patients, it is known to recur and can also undergo malignant transformation. It typically comprises of grape like clusters of cysts which on histological examination are lined by a single layer of flat to cuboidal mesothelial cells separated by fibrous tissue components.

The term *peritoneal inclusion cyst (PIC)* is used to describe non-neoplastic cysts which are formed secondary to intra-abdominal inflammation. The development of a PIC depends on the presence of a functioning ovary and peritoneal adhesions. The normal peritoneum absorbs fluid easily but this absorptive capacity is reduced in the presence of injury, inflammation, and peritoneal adhesions. PICs occur almost exclusively in premenopausal women with a history of previous abdominal or pelvic surgery, trauma, pelvic inflammatory disease, or endometriosis. Pathologically, the cysts are lined by non-neoplastic, reactive cuboidal, or flattened mesothelial cells and can vary in size from few centimeters to large masses.[58,59]

Clinical features: Patients often present with nonspecific symptoms—chronic or intermittent lower abdominal or pelvic pain, abdominal distension, tenderness, mass, and rarely pressure symptoms such as dyspareunia, urinary hesitancy, or constipation. Sometimes, these cysts are discovered incidentally.

Imaging features: Both of these entities show similar features on imaging. Ultrasound is often the first modality in detection of these lesions. They are seen as large, multiseptated, cystic structures commonly seen in the pelvis and lower abdomen. They are frequently anechoic, but sometimes may show internal echoes due to debris or hemorrhage. Septations may be complete, incomplete, of varying thickness, and may be nodular or polypoid. Unilocular, multifocal cysts may also be seen. In men, multicystic mesothelioma typically arises from the peritoneal surface along the superior margin of the bladder or in the retrovesical space.[54]

In PICs the ovary is often completely surrounded by the cystic mass/es. The characteristic "spider in web" sign describes when a morphologically normal ovary can be seen within a web of adhesions. As PICs occur due to loculated fluid collection, they may show irregular shape with sleeves of fluid extending between adjacent structures **(Figs. 24A to C)**.

CT and MRI are useful in defining the exact extent of the lesion and for identifying presence of multiple cysts. Large mutiseptated cyst with fluid attenuation can be seen on CT, while MR shows homogeneous fluid SI that is hypointense on T1W and hyperintense on T2W images. The septations enhance with contrast administration.

Differential diagnosis: Lymphangioma, complex loculated ascites, paraovarian cysts, hydrosalpinx, pseudomyxoma peritonei (PMP) in the early stages, and cystic ovarian neoplasms can all be considered in the differential diagnosis of multicystic mesothelioma and PICs.

Management: As multicystic mesotheliomas can undergo malignant transformation, they need to be removed surgically. However, they tend to recur and so a complete surgical cytoreduction with HIPEC is recommended.[60] PICs also tend to recur after surgical resection, however, they do not have a malignant potential. Conservative symptomatic treatment is recommended for PICs along with suppression of ovulation.

Primary Peritoneal Serous Carcinoma

Primary peritoneal serous carcinoma (PPSC) is an epithelial tumor of the peritoneum, arising from the extraovarian mesothelium with Mullerian potential. This tumor occurs in postmenopausal women and an association with *BRCA1* gene has been demonstrated.[61] Serum CA-125 may be elevated in a majority of cases. On immunohistochemical studies, PPSC is generally positive for BerEP4, CLDN, and PAX8.[62] The clinical and histological features closely resemble advanced epithelial ovarian carcinoma.

Imaging features: Ascites, peritoneal nodules and thickening, and omental nodules and masses are the most common cross-sectional imaging features of PPSC. A minority of patients have either no ascites or only a small amount at initial presentation. Calcifications within peritoneal and omental nodules representing psammoma bodies may be seen in 30% cases **(Fig. 25)**.[54]

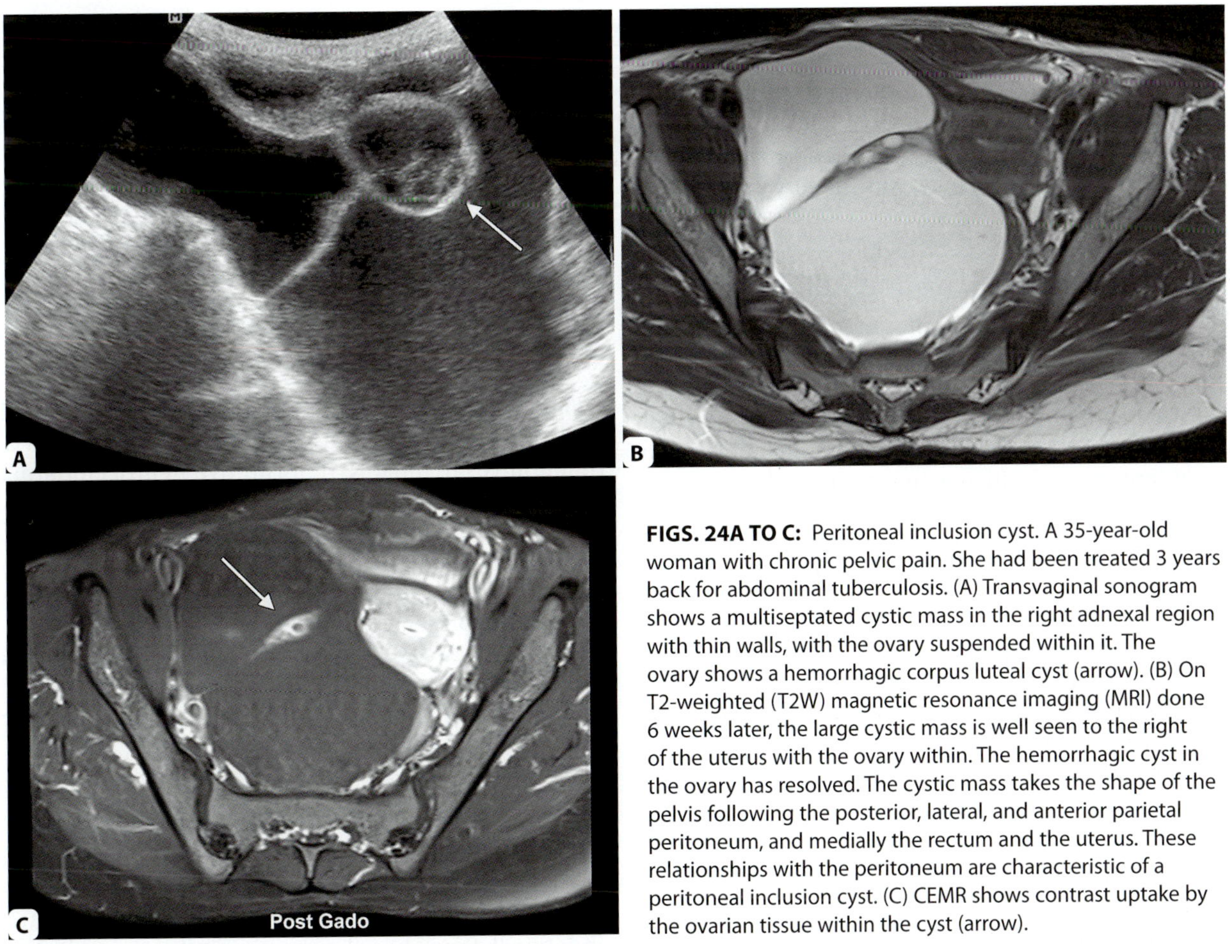

FIGS. 24A TO C: Peritoneal inclusion cyst. A 35-year-old woman with chronic pelvic pain. She had been treated 3 years back for abdominal tuberculosis. (A) Transvaginal sonogram shows a multiseptated cystic mass in the right adnexal region with thin walls, with the ovary suspended within it. The ovary shows a hemorrhagic corpus luteal cyst (arrow). (B) On T2-weighted (T2W) magnetic resonance imaging (MRI) done 6 weeks later, the large cystic mass is well seen to the right of the uterus with the ovary within. The hemorrhagic cyst in the ovary has resolved. The cystic mass takes the shape of the pelvis following the posterior, lateral, and anterior parietal peritoneum, and medially the rectum and the uterus. These relationships with the peritoneum are characteristic of a peritoneal inclusion cyst. (C) CEMR shows contrast uptake by the ovarian tissue within the cyst (arrow).

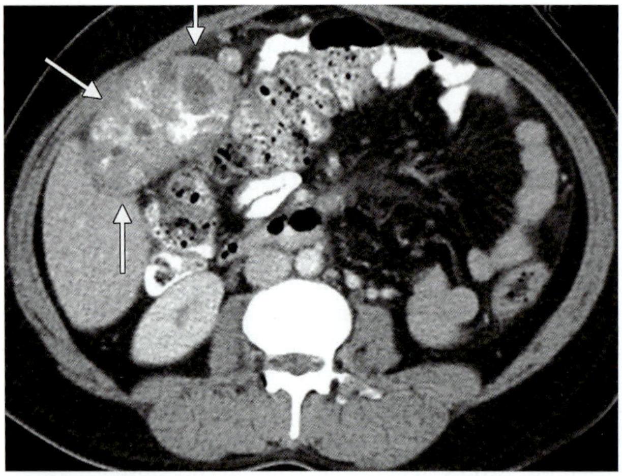

FIG. 25: Papillary serous carcinoma. A large well defined, enhancing, peritoneal mass is seen in the subhepatic region (arrows) with psammomatous calcification and few nonenhancing necrotic areas within.

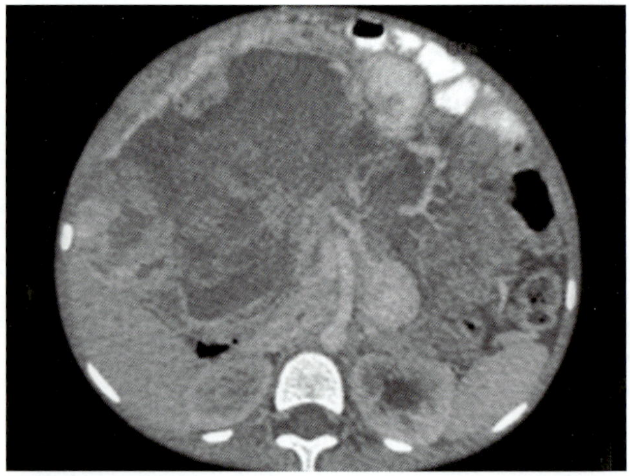

FIG. 26: Desmoplastic round cell tumor in a 15-year-old boy. Axial contrast-enhanced computed tomography (CECT) shows a large necrotic mass in the mesentery.

Histological confirmation is required to differentiate from metastatic ovarian disease and make a correct diagnosis. The criteria for diagnosing PPSC are:

- Both ovaries should be normal.
- Involvement of extraovarian sites should be greater than involvement of ovarian surface.
- Ovarian involvement should only be limited to surface epithelium.

The therapeutic approach is also similar to advanced epithelial ovarian malignancy, with surgery and chemotherapy.

Desmoplastic Small Round Cell Tumor

Desmoplastic small round cell tumor (DSRCT) is a rare aggressive malignancy occurring in adolescents and young adults. Histologically, it is composed of small, round, blue cells, belonging to the family of "small round blue cell tumors" a group that includes Wilms tumor, neuroblastoma, Ewing sarcoma, primitive neuroectodermal tumor, and rhabdomyosarcoma. DSRCT most often develops as a primary tumor of the peritoneal cavity but can also arise in other sites including pleura, bone, testes, or salivary glands.[63]

Clinical features: The mean age of presentation of DSRCT is 22 years (range 5–30 years) with a marked male preponderance. The most common signs at presentation are an intra-abdominal mass, abdominal pain, and increased abdominal girth.[63]

Imaging features: It is characterized by bulky, peritoneal masses in the omentum or paravesical region, which are heterogeneous, or have central low-attenuation areas on CT, suggestive of intratumoral necrosis, hemorrhage, or fibrous components. The masses can vary in size from 3 to 22 cm **(Fig. 26)**. When multiple masses are present, nearly all patients have a single dominant mass (>10 cm), usually in the retrovesical or retrouterine space. They may show small, punctate calcifications. Ascites is frequently present. At MR imaging, the tumors are typically heterogeneous in SI but predominantly hypointense on T1W sequences and hyperintense on T2W sequences. Postcontrast CT/MRI shows heterogeneous enhancement. DWI can increase the conspicuity of peritoneal/visceral lesions, thus, helping to detect subtle lesions. Lymph nodal metastases and hematogenous metastasis to the liver, lung, and bone may occur.[64]

DSRCT is intensely FDG-avid with a mean SUV of 11.1 (range, 3.7–15.0). FDG PET/CT has also been shown to detect occult lesions that may not be seen on CT or MRI. PET-CT plays a useful role in the initial staging of the disease and also in assessment of treatment response.[65]

Differential diagnosis: Other malignant conditions with multiple peritoneal and mesenteric masses such as rhabdomyosarcoma, NHL, primitive neuroectodermal tumor (PNET), neuroblastoma, mesothelioma, PC or sarcomatosis, etc., can be kept in the differential diagnosis of DSRCT. Factors which favor DSRCT are male adolescent status, no definite organ of origin with extensive peritoneal masses, and presence of calcifications.

DSRCT has a very aggressive clinical course with a 5-year survival rate of <15% despite the use of aggressive multimodality treatment such as debulking surgery, chemotherapy, and radiotherapy.

Desmoid Tumor/Mesenteric Fibromatosis

Desmoids are locally aggressive fibrous tumors with a tendency to recur, but no metastatic potential. They can be intra-abdominal, in the abdominal wall, or extra-abdominal. Small bowel mesentery is the most common site of involvement. Most cases are sporadic and are characterized by a mutation in the *CTNNB1* gene, while few show a hereditary pattern associated with *APC* gene mutation.[66] Approximately 10–15% occur in patients with familial adenomatous polyposis (FAP), particularly those with Gardener's syndrome. More than 80% of patients with FAP have a history of previous abdominal surgery, whereas only 10% of patients with sporadic mesenteric fibromatosis have had abdominal surgery.[34]

Clinical features: Desmoids may occur at any age but have a peak incidence in the third decade with a predilection for the female sex. Clinically, they may be asymptomatic or may present with abdominal pain or intestinal obstruction due to mass effect on the small or large bowel.

Imaging features: They are commonly seen as focal, solid masses with well-defined or infiltrative margins within the mesentery **(Figs. 27A to C)**. The internal features depend on the relative content of collagen and myxoid stroma within the tumor mass. A striated or whorled appearance may be seen due to the presence of alternate areas of myxoid stroma which are hyperdense on CT, hyperintense on MR, and areas of collagen—isodense/hyperdense on CT, hypointense on MR, within the masses. Contrast enhancement is also variable as the myxoid component does not enhance. Some lesions that do not enhance on CT may show enhancement on MRI.[67] Desmoids show low to moderate FDG uptake on FDG PET-CT scans which can help in differentiating from malignant lesions.

Differential diagnosis: On the basis of imaging findings, desmoid tumors are difficult to differentiate from GI stromal tumor and other malignant neoplasms of the mesentery, such as lymphoma, metastatic disease, and soft-tissue sarcoma. GISTs more commonly have areas of hemorrhage and necrosis, which are seen as focal areas of hypoattenuation. Immunohistochemical profile can help in differentiating from GIST as desmoids are c-KIT negative. They may closely resemble lymphoma whenever the lesions manifest with well-defined margins, homogeneous attenuation, and involvement of adjacent small bowel segments.

Due to the close association with vital structures, resection of the tumor may not be possible. Also, desmoid tumors have a tendency to recur, even after complete surgical resection. Therefore, conservative management has been recommended whenever possible, using analgesia and minimally invasive therapy as needed. Radiotherapy and chemotherapy have also been used in the management of desmoid tumors.[68]

Inflammatory Myofibroblastic Tumor/ Inflammatory Pseudotumor

Inflammatory myofibroblastic tumors (IMFT) are rare solid tumors of mesenchymal origin, which may originate in virtually any anatomic site but are most often found in the lung, mesentery, and omentum. They have a low metastatic potential with a high recurrence rate after excision. Histologically, IMFTs contain proliferating neoplastic, fibroblastic, and myofibroblastic cells along with chronic inflammatory infiltrates. More than half of the cases (40–100%) are associated with anaplastic lymphoma

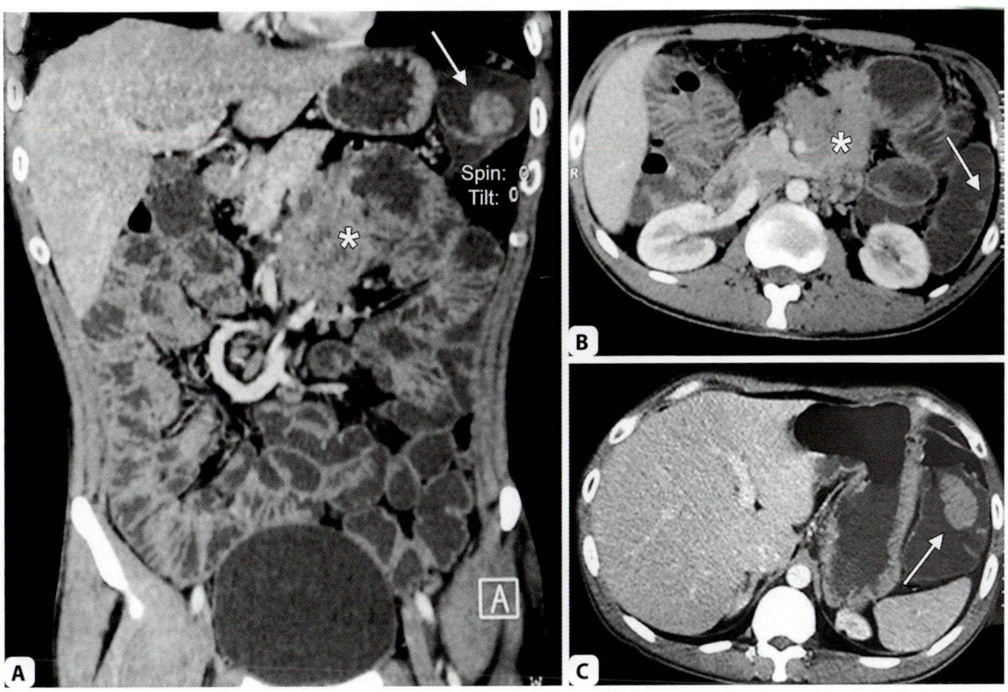

FIGS. 27A TO C: Desmoid tumor in a 31-year-old man with familial adenomatous polyposis. Contrast-enhanced computed tomography (CECT) (A) coronal; and (B and C) axial scans show an irregular, heterogenous mass with infiltrative margins in the mesentery (asterisk). Multiple polypoid lesions can be seen in the large bowel (arrows).

kinase (*ALK*) gene mutations and its expression suggesting the neoplastic origin of the lesion. IMFTs have also been associated with IgG4-related disease.

Inflammatory pseudotumors (IPT), on the other hand, are a broad category of rare inflammatory conditions which present as a mass, either infective or autoimmune in etiology. Histologically, they consist of fibroblasts, and/or myofibroblasts together with lymphocytes, plasma cells, histiocytes, and eosinophils. Previously, the terms IMFT and IPT were used interchangeably, however, IMFT is now regarded as a neoplastic lesion whereas IPT as a mass-forming inflammatory lesion. [69]

Clinical features: IMFT is most commonly seen to affect children and young adults, with a slight tendency to occur more frequently in girls. The clinical symptoms are nonspecific and depend on the site of origin. The most common presenting symptom is abdominal pain due to mass effect. A minority of patients present with systemic signs and symptoms suggestive of infection.[70]

Imaging features: A variable appearance is seen on imaging depending on the amount of fibrotic tissue present within the lesion. At CT, these tumors typically manifest as bulky, well-demarcated, homogeneous or heterogeneous, spherical or multilobulated mass lesions **(Figs. 28A and B)**. A few cases may show central calcifications. Large tumors may demonstrate hypoattenuating, nonenhancing areas that represent central necrosis. These tumors rarely show aggressive growth patterns such as circumferential growth around vessels and extension into the bowel with mural infiltration and ulceration.[70,71] On MR imaging, IMFTs appear hypointense on T1W images and hyperintense on T2W images, although tumors with a great deal of fibrotic stroma may be dark on both T1W and T2W images. Contrast enhancement is variable and includes early peripheral enhancement due to vascular tissue and delayed central enhancement of fibrotic components.[72] FDG-PET shows nonspecific increased uptake of radiotracer, similar to other malignancies. On IHC, B and T cell markers such as CD34, CD117, S-100, and c-Kit can be used to differentiate from other soft tissue lesions.[73]

As IMFTs are locally aggressive with potential for local recurrence, therefore, complete surgical excision is associated with the best outcomes. However, adjuvant therapy including anti-inflammatory agents, chemotherapy, and radiotherapy have been tried on a case-by-case basis with some success. For the subset of IMT patients who show *ALK* positivity, ALK tyrosine kinase inhibitors are being tried for targeted neoadjuvant or adjuvant therapy.

Leiomyomatosis Peritonealis Disseminata

Leiomyomatosis peritonealis disseminata (LPD) also known as diffuse peritoneal leiomyomatosis, is a rare, benign disorder characterized by innumerable smooth muscle nodules throughout the peritoneal cavity. These nodules are derived from metaplasia of the submesothelial cells.

Clinical features: LPD is almost always seen in women. It may be associated with high estrogen states, caused by pregnancy and oral contraceptive use, but rarely may occur in postmenopausal women, and even sometimes in men.[74] It is often discovered incidentally during surgery or imaging examinations of women who have uterine leiomyomas. The clinical course is often benign, with spontaneous regression of the leiomyomas or regression can occur after withdrawal of hormonal stimulus. In rare cases, sarcomatous degeneration of the tumor nodules, may occur.[75]

Imaging features: CT and MRI show numerous well-circumscribed, variable-sized solid masses in the peritoneal cavity with no ascites, lymphadenopathy, or visceral metastases. Heterogeneous attenuation is seen on CT.

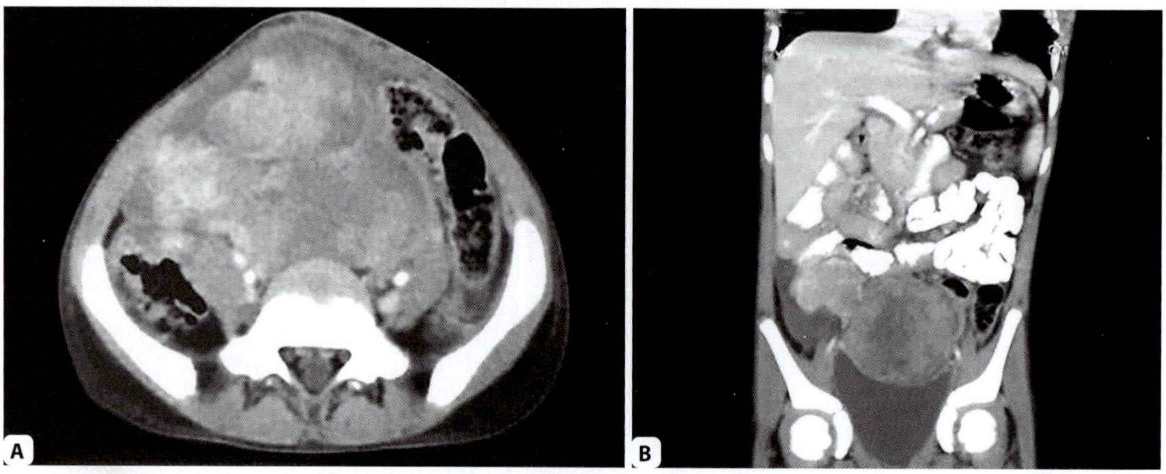

FIGS. 28A AND B: Inflammatory myofibroblastic tumor in a 7-year-old girl. Contrast-enhanced computed tomography (CECT) (A) axial; and (B) coronal images show a large well circumscribed, multilobulated, heterogeneously enhancing mass in the lower abdomen displacing the bowel loops superiorly and laterally. Associated ascites is present.

On MR imaging, the masses are isointense relative to muscle on T1W sequences with low SI on T2W sequences. The masses enhance similarly to uterine leiomyomas.[54]

The main *differential diagnoses* are PC, disseminated leiomyosarcomatosis, and endometriosis. Treatment decision depends on patient's age, hormonal and reproductive status, and clinical symptoms. Asymptomatic disseminated peritoneal leiomyomatosis does not require treatment, but if the patient is symptomatic then surgical excision is recommended with hormone suppressive therapy reserved as an alternative.

Miscellaneous Primary Peritoneal Tumors

Well-differentiated papillary mesothelioma, adenomatoid tumor, primary peritoneal serous borderline tumor, and solitary fibrous tumor are uncommon primary tumors of the peritoneum. Connective tissue tumors include benign entities such as leiomyoma, lipoma, neurofibroma and their malignant counterparts such as leiomyosarcoma, liposarcoma, fibrosarcoma, and hemangiopericytoma, etc. Imaging findings are nonspecific. Benign tumors are usually well circumscribed and localized whereas malignant tumors have indistinct or infiltrative margins with invasion into surrounding structures. Lipomas and liposarcomas are more distinctive due to their characteristic features of fat containing masses.

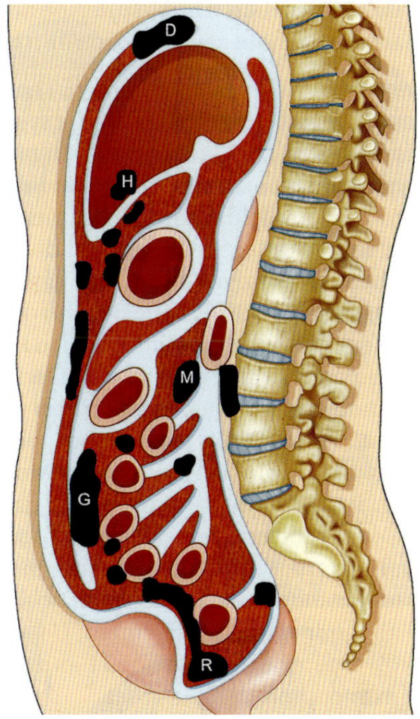

FIG. 29: Sagittal schematic illustration of the abdomen and pelvis showing common locations of peritoneal deposits. Commonly involved sites include greater omentum (G), rectouterine pouch (R), subdiaphragmatic region (D), subhepatic region (H), and small bowel mesentery (M).

SECONDARY PERITONEAL NEOPLASMS

Secondary neoplasms are the most common malignancies involving the peritoneum. The dissemination of tumor cells within the peritoneal cavity can occur by several mechanisms:

(1) Intraperitoneal seeding, (2) Direct invasion, (3) Embolic hematogenous dissemination, and (4) Lymphatic permeation.

Intraperitoneal seeding occurs most commonly from GI and ovarian tumors due to intramural tumor growth and invasion through bowel wall or extension through the peritoneal lining of organs such as ovary, pancreas, or liver. Seeding can also occur due to iatrogenic spillage of tumor cells into the peritoneal cavity during biopsy or surgery. These tumor cells are carried by the peritoneal fluid and disseminated throughout the peritoneal cavity. They get preferentially deposited in the areas of fluid stasis, i.e., pouch of Douglas in women, rectovesical space in men, distal small bowel mesentery near the ileocecal junction, sigmoid mesocolon, right paracolic gutter, Morrison's pouch, and the right subdiaphragmatic space **(Fig. 29)**, and these areas should be carefully examined in all cases when evaluating for metastatic disease. Two unusual sites of PC are the umbilicus and the ovaries; such metastases are respectively called Sister Mary Joseph's nodule and Krukenberg tumors. Ovarian carcinoma is the most common tumor to spread by this mechanism. Gastric, pancreatic, colonic, biliary, and endometrial tumors also spread through intraperitoneal seeding.

Direct invasion: Intra-abdominal primary malignancies can directly invade into the leaves of mesentery along the mesenteric vessels or through ligamentous attachments to involve adjacent organs. Pancreatic, gastric, biliary, colonic, small bowel, hepatic, splenic, and ovarian tumors may spread in this way. Small bowel carcinoid tumor commonly invades the mesentery. Lymphoma and tumors arising from retroperitoneal structures may spread directly to the root of the small bowel mesentery along its retroperitoneal attachment.

Hematogenous spread: Tumor emboli from extra-abdominal tumors such as malignant melanoma, lung or breast carcinoma, and sarcomas may spread to the mesentery by hematogenous spread. These tumors usually involve the antimesenteric margins of the small bowel producing soft issue nodules that may cause bowel obstruction and/or intussusception.

Lymphatic extension: Lymphatic dissemination plays a minor role in spread of GI malignancies to the peritoneum, but it is the main pathway for spread of lymphomas to mesenteric lymph nodes. Chronic lymphocytic leukemia may also spread through the lymphatics and produce large mesenteric nodal masses which encase the branches of abdominal aorta-celiac trunk, superior and inferior mesenteric arteries without causing vascular compression.

Quantification of peritoneal tumor burden: The peritoneal cancer index (PCI) is a preoperative scoring system, which was initially developed by Jacquet and Sugarbaker[76] to assess the volume and extent of peritoneal disease, but later adapted to quantify peritoneal disease on imaging as well. It combines the intra-abdominal distribution of lesions with their size, to give a semiquantitative indicator for determining the extent of peritoneal tumor deposits. The method for calculating the PCI is illustrated in **Figures 30A to D**. The radiological PCI correlates well with surgical PCI and facilitates communication between radiologists and surgeons. If the CT-PCI is 20 or greater, the likelihood of complete cytoreduction is minimized.[77] More recently the acronym "PAUSE" has been proposed as a method for communicating the radiological extent of a peritoneal malignancy. The term "PAUSE" incorporates the following: P—primary tumor and peritoneal carcinomatosis index; A—ascites and abdominal wall involvement; U—unfavorable sites of involvement; S—small bowel and mesenteric disease; E—extraperitoneal metastases.[78]

Peritoneal Carcinomatosis

Peritoneal carcinomatosis is the malignant tumor seeding of the peritoneum with the most common primaries being the ovarian, gastric, and colorectal malignancies. Other less common primary sites include pancreas, uterus, kidney, bladder, and melanoma.

Patients with PC may be asymptomatic at the onset, but may progress to abdominal distension from ascites, or nausea, vomiting, and abdominal pain from bowel obstruction.

Imaging features: The classic feature of PC is *tumor nodules* studding the peritoneal surfaces. A fibrotic response can occur as the tumor grows along the peritoneal surface or invades into the subperitoneal tissues, replacing the omental fat with tumor and fibrosis which produces the gross appearance of *omental caking*. PC can also exhibit a *sheet-like growth* pattern encircling and encasing intraperitoneal viscera producing an appearance similar to malignant mesothelioma. A variable amount of ascites may accompany the peritoneal seeding, but is not always present. Adenocarcinoma with abundant mucin and signet ring cell morphology is the most frequent tumor type seen on histopathology.

On US, the ascitic fluid seen in patients with PC may be anechoic or may contain echogenic particulate matter, which reflects proteinaceous exudate. Tumor nodules on peritoneal surfaces appear as hypoechoic nodules or sheet like masses **(Figs. 31A and B)**.[79] The omentum with tumor infiltration appears as an echogenic, plaque like structure either floating in the ascitic fluid or it may be adherent to the anterior abdominal wall or serosal surface of the bowel.

The MDCT is the optimal technique for detecting the presence, location, and extent of PC with reported overall diagnostic accuracy of 94%, specificity of 92%, and sensitivities between 75 and 81%. However, CT sensitivities for detection of smaller nodules, <1 cm, is much lower.[80] The parietal peritoneum shows smooth, nodular, or plaque like thickening which enhances on postcontrast scans. Omental fat stranding, nodularity, or caking may be seen. As the

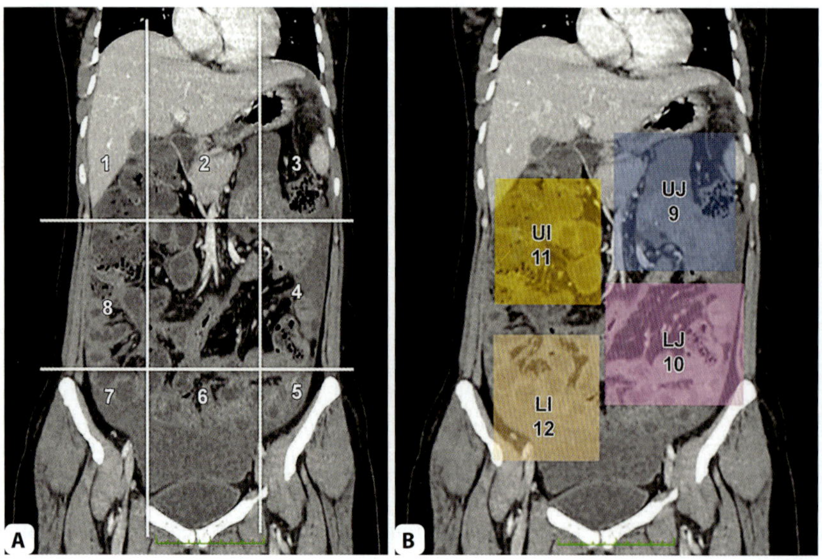

C

Lesion size score
LS 0—no tumor seen
LS 1—tumor up to 0.5 cm
LS 2—tumor up to 5 cm
LS 3—tumor >5 cm or confluence

D

Regions	Lesion size
Central	
Right upper	
Epigastrium	
Left upper	
Left flank	
Left lower	
Pelvis	
Right lower	
Right flank	
Upper jejunum	
Lower jejunum	
Upper ileum	
Lower ileum	
PCI score:	

FIGS. 30A TO D: Sugarbaker's peritoneal cancer index (PCI): The peritoneal cavity is divided into nine regions (0–8) as shown in (A) by 2 transverse planes (upper plane at lowest aspect of costal margin and lower plane at level of anterior superior iliac spines) and two sagittal planes which divide the abdomen into three equal parts. Further, the small bowel is divided into upper jejunum (UJ 9), lower jejunum (LJ10), upper ileum (UI11), and lower ileum (LI12) as shown in (B). The lesions are scored from 0–3, according to the size of the largest lesion in a region, (C and D). The final PCI is the sum total of the scores in each region, with a minimum score of 0 and a maximum score of 39.

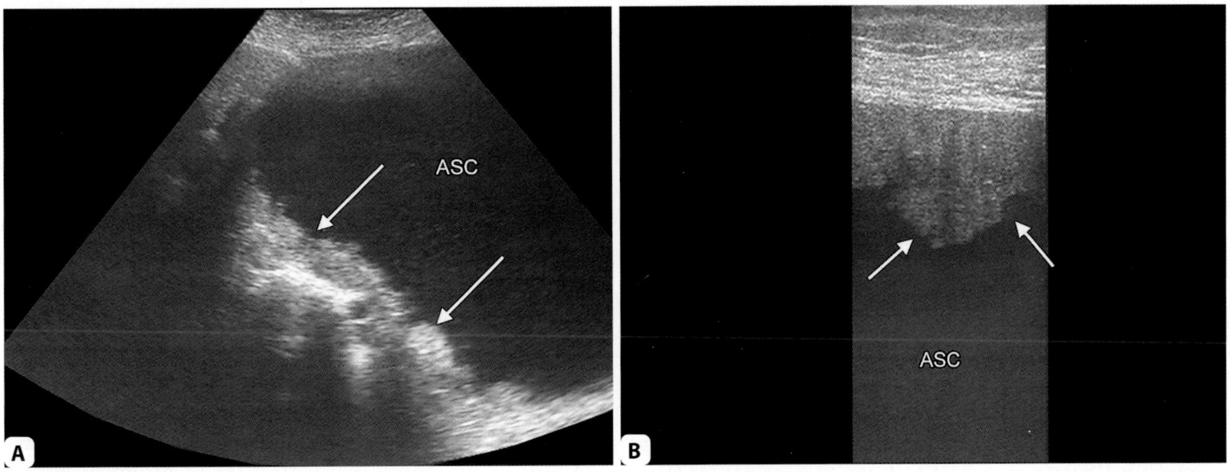

FIGS. 31A AND B: Peritoneal carcinomatosis with metastatic peritoneal deposits. (A) Transverse ultrasonography (US) image of right flank shows a large amount of ascites with fine internal echoes and multiple small peritoneal implants along the right paracolic gutter. (B) High frequency US image in a different patient shows an irregular solid hypoechoic mass projecting within the ascitic fluid (ASC) from the anterior peritoneal margin (arrows).

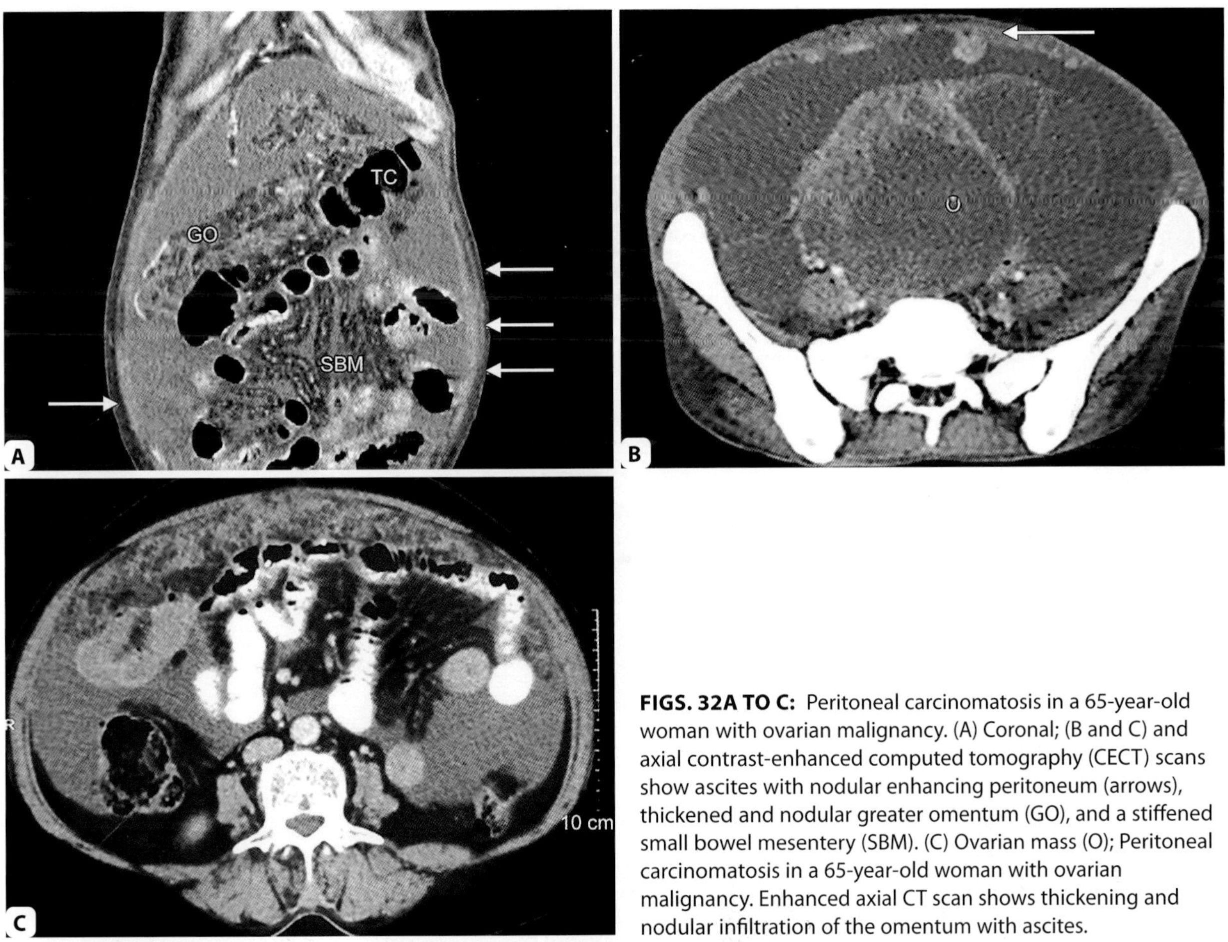

FIGS. 32A TO C: Peritoneal carcinomatosis in a 65-year-old woman with ovarian malignancy. (A) Coronal; (B and C) and axial contrast-enhanced computed tomography (CECT) scans show ascites with nodular enhancing peritoneum (arrows), thickened and nodular greater omentum (GO), and a stiffened small bowel mesentery (SBM). (C) Ovarian mass (O); Peritoneal carcinomatosis in a 65-year-old woman with ovarian malignancy. Enhanced axial CT scan shows thickening and nodular infiltration of the omentum with ascites.

tumor infiltrates the small bowel mesentery, it becomes stiff and loses its normal undulations. There is a characteristic straightening of the mesenteric vasculature producing a "pleated" appearance on CT images. A "stellate" pattern of mesenteric involvement may occur when the tumor infiltrates the perivascular spaces, causing the vessels within the mesentery to appear denser than the surrounding fat and appears like stars in the sky on axial CT scans **(Figs. 32A to C)**. Nodular or diffuse thickening can occur along the serosal surface of the bowel, leading to small bowel obstruction.[37]

Calcification can be seen in the peritoneal deposits from serous papillary ovarian carcinoma **(Figs. 33A to C)**, rarely gastric carcinomas, or in metastases after chemotherapy.

Magnetic resonance imaging can improve the detection of small peritoneal implants. These are best seen on contrast-enhanced T1W images with fat suppression, as the peritoneum enhances slowly after intravenous administration of gadolinium, and images should be obtained 5–10 minutes after injection. The normal peritoneum has an enhancement similar to that of liver. An abnormal enhancement should be suspected when peritoneum enhances more than liver or shows associated thickening, nodularity, or mass. Typically, omental and mesenteric masses are of low T1W and mixed T2W SI compared with surrounding soft tissues which show restricted diffusion on DWI. A combination of DWI and conventional sequences improves the accuracy for detection[81] **(Figs. 34A to D)**.

The FDG PET/CT is another promising modality for evaluation of peritoneal implants. Metastatic foci appear as round, oval, globular, or conglomerate areas of increased activity on FDG-PET.[82] **(Figs. 35A and B)**. One of the primary limitations of FDG PET/CT is that benign infectious or inflammatory peritoneal conditions may be FDG avid and therefore may mimic malignant peritoneal disease. Other sources of false-positive FDG PET/CT findings in the peritoneal cavity include physiologic bowel activity, motion artefact at the diaphragm, and urinary excretion of FDG.[83]

Differential diagnosis: There are several non-neoplastic and neoplastic conditions that may mimic PC on imaging. The most important differential is the involvement of the peritoneum by TB, which is very common in our country. The differentiating points have been discussed earlier. Other differentials include lymphomas, sarcomatous involvement of the peritoneum **(Table 4)**, and primary peritoneal malignancies such as mesothelioma. Primary peritoneal mesothelioma may be indistinguishable from carcinomatosis when the predominant imaging findings are multifocal peritoneal nodules and omental involvement ranging from finely infiltrated fat to omental caking. A history of asbestos exposure favors mesothelioma.

The treatment and prognosis of PC is variable and depends on multiple factors—histology of the primary tumor, presence/absence of extraperitoneal disease, the extent of peritoneal spread (PCI score), and involvement of unfavorable sites which could preclude surgery. CRS and HIPEC/PIPAC (pressurized intraperitoneal aerosolized chemotherapy) are the treatment of choice and it is essential to have an extremely accurate preoperative

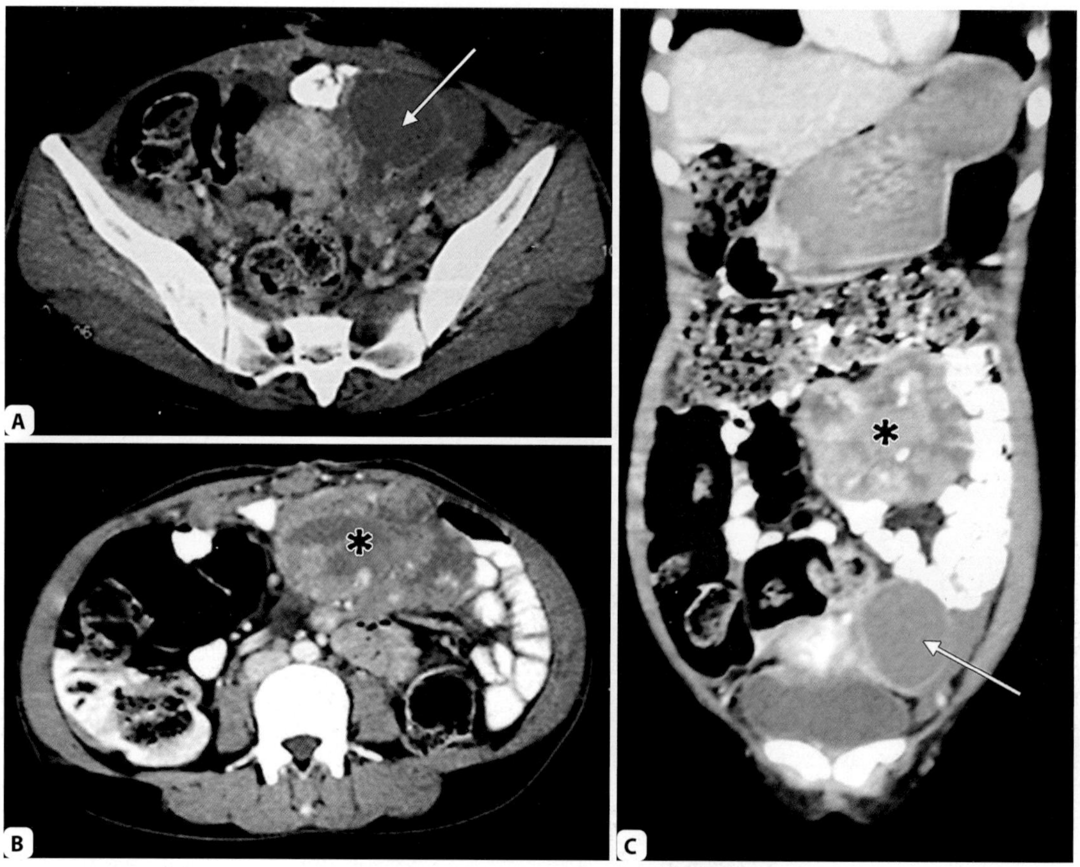

FIGS. 33A TO C: Peritoneal carcinomatosis from ovarian mucinous adenocarcinoma in a 45-year-old woman. (A and B) Axial; (C) coronal contrast-enhanced computed tomography (CECT) scan shows a solid-cystic mass lesion in the left adnexa (arrow). There is an associated large heterogeneously enhancing solid mass lesion (asterisk) in the mesentery with foci of calcification within.

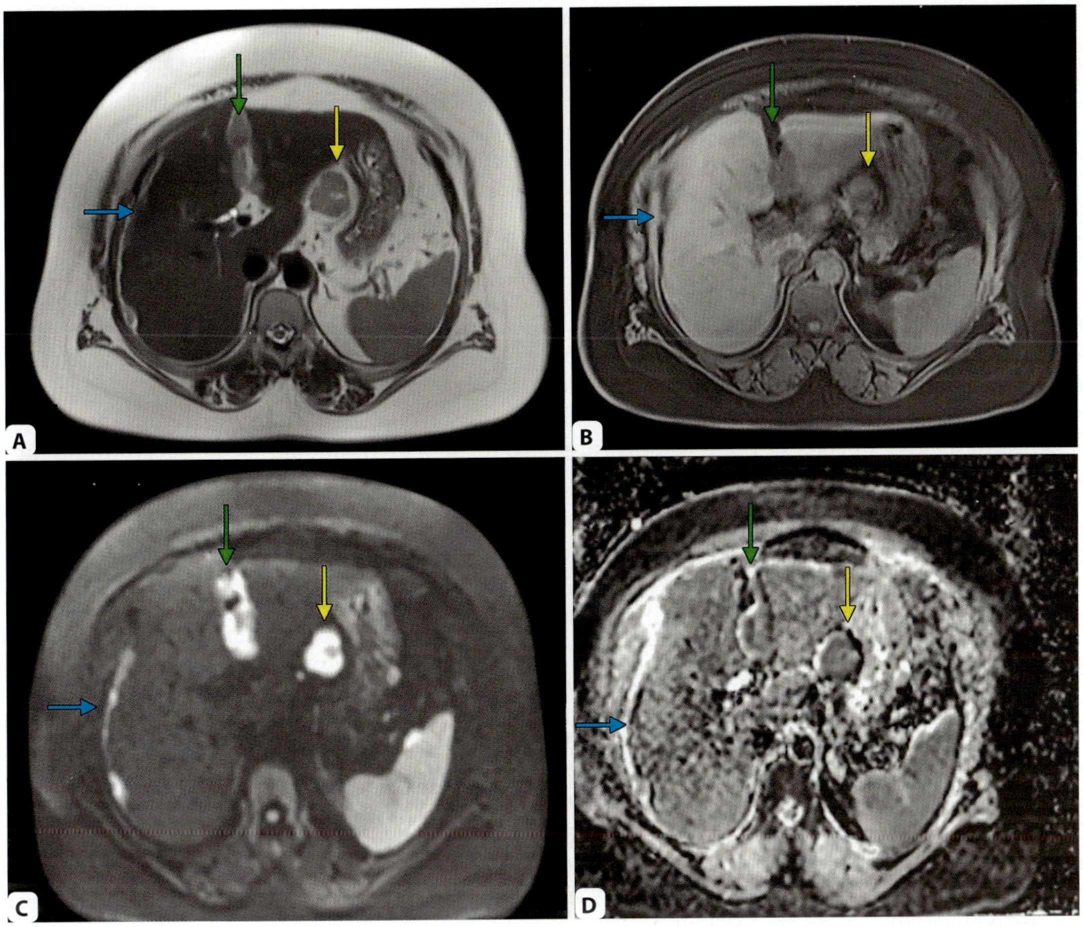

FIGS. 34A TO D: Peritoneal carcinomatosis in a 47-year woman with history of surgically excised ovarian carcinoma presenting with abdominal pain. (A) Axial magnetic resonance (MR) T2-weighted image (T2WI); (B) T1 weighted image (T1WI); (C) Diffusion-weighted imaging (DWI) at b 800; and (D) apparent diffusion coefficient (ADC) map. Images show T2 intermediate intensity, T1 isointense soft tissue nodular masses scattered in peritoneum along ligamentum teres (green arrow), gastrohepatic ligament (yellow arrow), and capsular surface of liver (blue arrow), showing high signal on DWI and low signal on ADC map, suggestive of restricted diffusion with an average ADC value of 0.6×10^{-3} mm^2/s. In comparison to T1WI and T2WI, deposits along capsular surface of liver are more conspicuous on DWI and ADC map images.

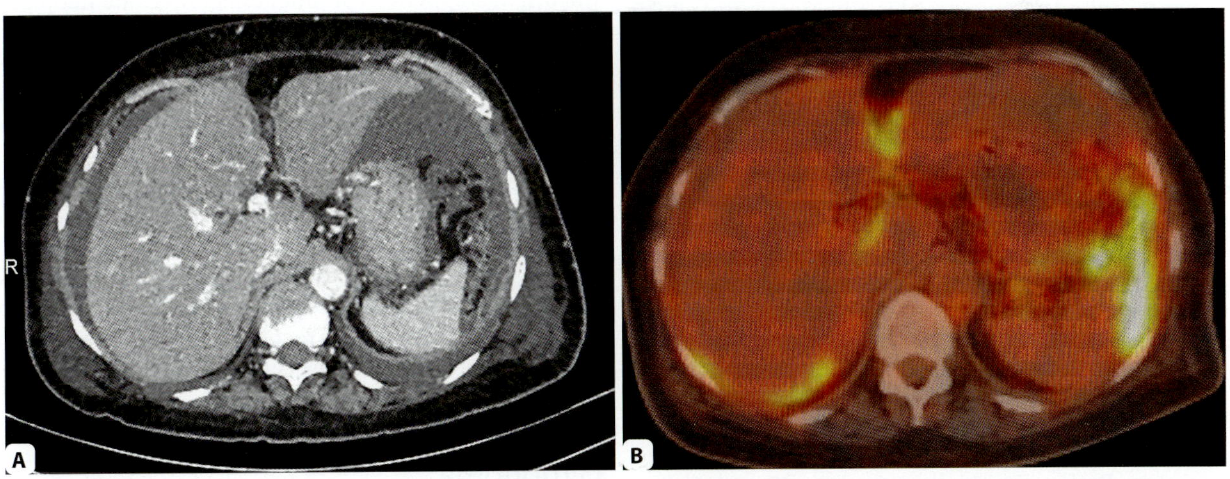

FIGS. 35A AND B: Positron emission tomography (PET)-CT in a 55-year-old man with colon carcinoma. (A) Axial contrast-enhanced computed tomography (CECT); and (B) corresponding axial fused PET-CT image, show metabolically active lesions along the posterior serosal surface of liver, falciform ligament, gastrosplenic ligament, and greater omentum with associated ascites.

TABLE 4: Main differentiating features between peritoneal carcinomatosis, lymphomatosis and sarcomatosis.[85]

	Peritoneal carcinomatosis	Peritoneal lymphomatosis	Peritoneal sarcomatosis
Peritoneal lesions	Multiple small nodules	Bulky homogeneous masses	Bulky heterogeneous masses
Lymphadenopathy	Lymph nodes around primary mass	Diffuse enlarged lymph nodes	None
Ascites	++	+	+/–

Source: Cabral FC, Krajewski KM, Kim KW, Ramaiya NH, Jagannathan JP. Peritoneal lymphomatosis: CT and PET/CT findings and how to differentiate between carcinomatosis and sarcomatosis. Cancer Imaging. 2013;13(2):162-70.

assessment of the overall disease burden, and the exact sites of involvement in specific areas of the peritoneum. Analysis of imaging findings need to be done on a site to site basis, and presence, type, and size of the deposits reported, so as to be able decide on the feasibility and extent of surgery.[84]

Pseudomyxoma Peritonei

Pseudomyxoma peritonei or "jelly belly" is a clinical or radiological description and not a pathological diagnosis resulting in large amount of thick, mucinous, or gelatinous material in the peritoneal cavity. It is most commonly seen with rupture of a benign or malignant mucin producing tumor of the appendix or ovary and occasionally pancreas, stomach, colon, or urachus. The relationship between appendiceal and ovarian mucinous tumors has long been observed, and a controversy exists as to whether in patients with PMP and synchronous manifestation of ovarian and appendiceal tumors, the ovarian tumors are primary or secondary, as the ovarian tumors are frequently seen to occur on the right side or are bilateral. Results of several clinical, histopathological and immunohistochemical studies strongly suggest that in these patients ovarian tumor deposits are almost always metastases of an appendiceal primary.[86]

The Peritoneal Surface Oncology Group have classified PMP into three basic groups:[87]

1. *PMP with low grade histological features (disseminated peritoneal adenomucinosis)* is a benign entity which spreads along the peritoneal surfaces, and does not invade the stroma. It is seen in association with low-grade mucinous carcinomas of appendix that penetrate or rupture into the peritoneal cavity. It has 5-year survival rate of around 90–100%.
2. *PMP with high grade histological features (peritoneal mucinous carcinomatosis)* which occurs from high grade mucinous carcinomas of the GI tract, gallbladder, pancreas, or ovary, and has a 5-year survival rate of around 40–60%.
3. *PMP with signet ring cells* which is similar to high grade PMP but with signet ring cells, more aggressive in behavior, and has a 5-year survival rate of around 20%.

Clinical features: PMP occurs more commonly in women than men. Patients typically complain of progressive abdominal pain, increasing abdominal girth, and weight loss. Small bowel obstruction can occur in later stages.

Imaging features: On sonography, PMP is seen as echogenic ascites, with nonmobile echoes in the ascitic fluid, in contrast to mobile echoes seen with other exudative ascites. Echogenic septations representing the margins of the mucinous nodules can be seen within the ascites.[88] Scalloping of the visceral surfaces of the abdominal organs, specially liver and spleen, is an important hallmark of PMP. This scalloping represents indentations of the margins of organs due to extrinsic pressure of the intraperitoneal mucinous implants.[88]

On CT, the mucinous nodules are seen as hypodense areas filling the peritoneal cavity. Soft-tissue attenuation masses may be seen representing solid tumor elements, fibrosis, or compression of the mesentery and mucin. There may be curvilinear or amorphous calcifications. Peritoneal and omental nodules and even omental caking can be seen. Scalloping of margins of liver and spleen is well visualized on CT **(Figs. 36A and B)**. On MRI, the mucinous masses can be seen as T1-hypointense and T2-hyperintense but the SI may vary with the mucin concentration. On DWI, mucinous lesions show hyperintensity on intermediate b-values (400–500 s/mm^2) with high apparent diffusion coefficient (ADC) values.[89]

PET-CT is not recommended as mucinous neoplasms generally have low metabolic activity.

The regions of the appendix and ovaries should be closely evaluated in all newly diagnosed cases of PMP. However, in many cases, it may be impossible to identify the original appendiceal mucinous low-grade neoplasm or cystadenocarcinoma. It may be difficult to differentiate PMP from mucinous PC as they have overlapping findings. Carcinomatosis tends to involve thorax more commonly. Pleural effusions, pleural masses, enlarged mesenteric or retroperitoneal lymph nodes, omental caking, and invasion into parenchymal organs are characteristically seen. In contrast, PMP does not invade visceral organs or spread by lymphatic or hematogenous routes.

Surgical debulking of the tumor and surgery combined with HIPEC with or without chemotherapy in the immediate postoperative period, is the recommended management of PMP in majority of specialist centers.[90]

Peritoneal Lymphomatosis/Peritoneal Lymphoma

Peritoneal lymphomatosis is defined as the intraperitoneal spread of lymphoma. Lymphomatous involvement of

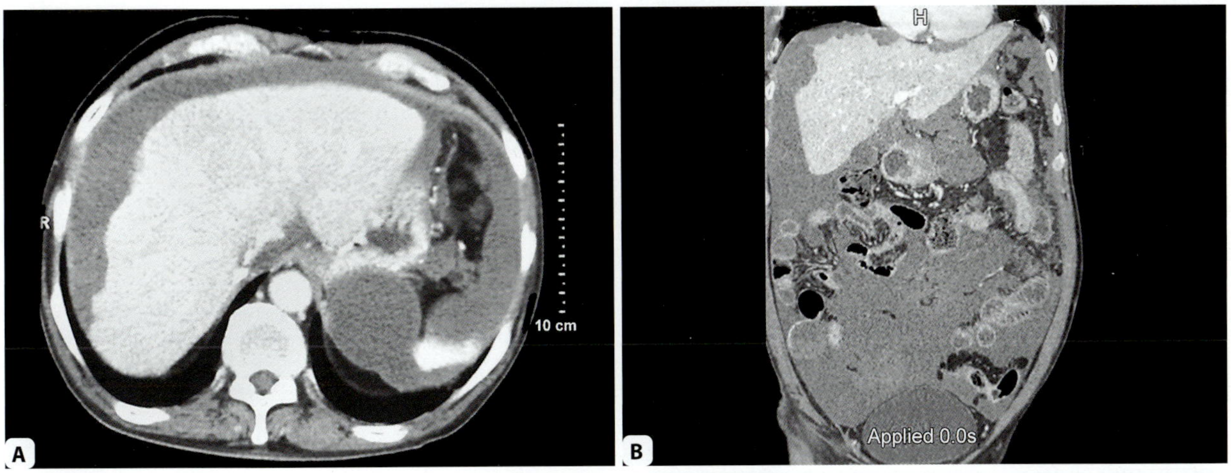

FIGS. 36A AND B: Pseudomyxoma peritonei from mucinous adenocarcinoma of appendix manifesting as increasing abdominal girth. (A) Axial; and (B) coronal contrast-enhanced computed tomography (CECT) images show large locules of high density intraperitoneal fluid. Scalloping of the liver margins by the mucin locules can be very well seen.

the peritoneum may be a primary or secondary process. *Secondary* involvement is more common, and can occur from nodal or extranodal NHLs, such as small B-cell lymphoma, diffuse large B-cell lymphoma, or Burkitt lymphoma. *Primary lymphomas* of the peritoneum, also called body cavity-based lymphomas or primary effusion lymphomas, are uncommon and nearly exclusively found in immunocompromised patients, most of whom are infected with the HIV.[91]

Imaging features: Diffuse thickening of peritoneal surfaces with multifocal nodules and masses that mimic PC can be seen. There can be associated ascites, peritoneal enhancement and thickening, omental caking, infiltration of the small bowel mesentery, and fine nodularity in the mesentery.[92] Enlarged lymph nodes, especially in the retrocrural, retroperitoneal region and in the small bowel mesentery are commonly seen in association with the mesenteric disease and are a clue to the diagnosis. Associated GI involvement, hepatosplenomegaly and hepatic/splenic nodules may also be seen in some cases.

In primary effusion lymphoma, the most common imaging manifestation is ascites without associated lymphadenopathy, organomegaly, or masses. In later stages, lymph node enlargement and nodular peritoneal thickening may occur, however, ascites remains the most predominant manifestation.[91,93]

The FDG-PET/CT has been shown to improve staging, evaluation of therapy response, and earlier detection of recurrent disease in peritoneal lymphomatosis. FDG-PET/CT shows two patterns of glucose metabolism in peritoneal lymphomatosis—a nodular and a diffuse metabolic pattern. The FDG avidity in lymphoma is variable with aggressive and highly aggressive NHL and Hodgkin lymphomas showing high FDG avidity and indolent lymphomas showing an overall low-grade or no FDG uptake because of low metabolic activity. FDG-PET/CT not only has greater sensitivity than CT for depicting peritoneal involvement in subtle cases but it also has greater accuracy in identifying extranodal sites other than the peritoneum, even in the absence of CT findings. Due to its improved usefulness in distinguishing residual active lymphoma and benign fibrosis, FDG-PET/CT has been found valuable in assessment of treatment response.[85]

Sporadic Burkitt lymphoma is the most common form of NHL diagnosed in children younger than 15 years, accounting for 30–50% of cases.[94] It is a very aggressive B-cell lymphoma with a doubling time of only 24 hours, and thus needs to be diagnosed urgently. Burkitt lymphoma involving the peritoneum may appear as a large solitary mass or multiple abdominal masses **(Figs. 37A to C)**. Encasement of mesenteric vessels is a characteristic feature. Large tumors may show central necrosis. Associated peritoneal thickening or nodularity along the liver capsule and peritoneal reflections may be noted. Omental caking is not a feature of Burkitt lymphoma. Intrinsic involvement of the GI tract is common, which is seen as bowel wall thickening or mural masses. Other solid organs such as liver, spleen, kidneys, and pancreas may be involved either intrinsically or by direct invasion by the peritoneal masses. Malignant ascites is found in 25% of cases of abdominal Burkitt lymphoma. Enlarged abdominal lymph nodes may be seen.[69]

Peritoneal lymphomatosis is treated nonsurgically, and often shows dramatic improvement with chemotherapy, and therefore its early and precise diagnosis is of utmost importance.

Peritoneal Sarcomatosis

Peritoneal sarcomatosis or the disseminated intraperitoneal spread of sarcoma occurs most frequently from intra-abdominal sarcomas such as malignant gastrointestinal stromal tumors (GIST), leiomyosarcomas, or liposarcomas,

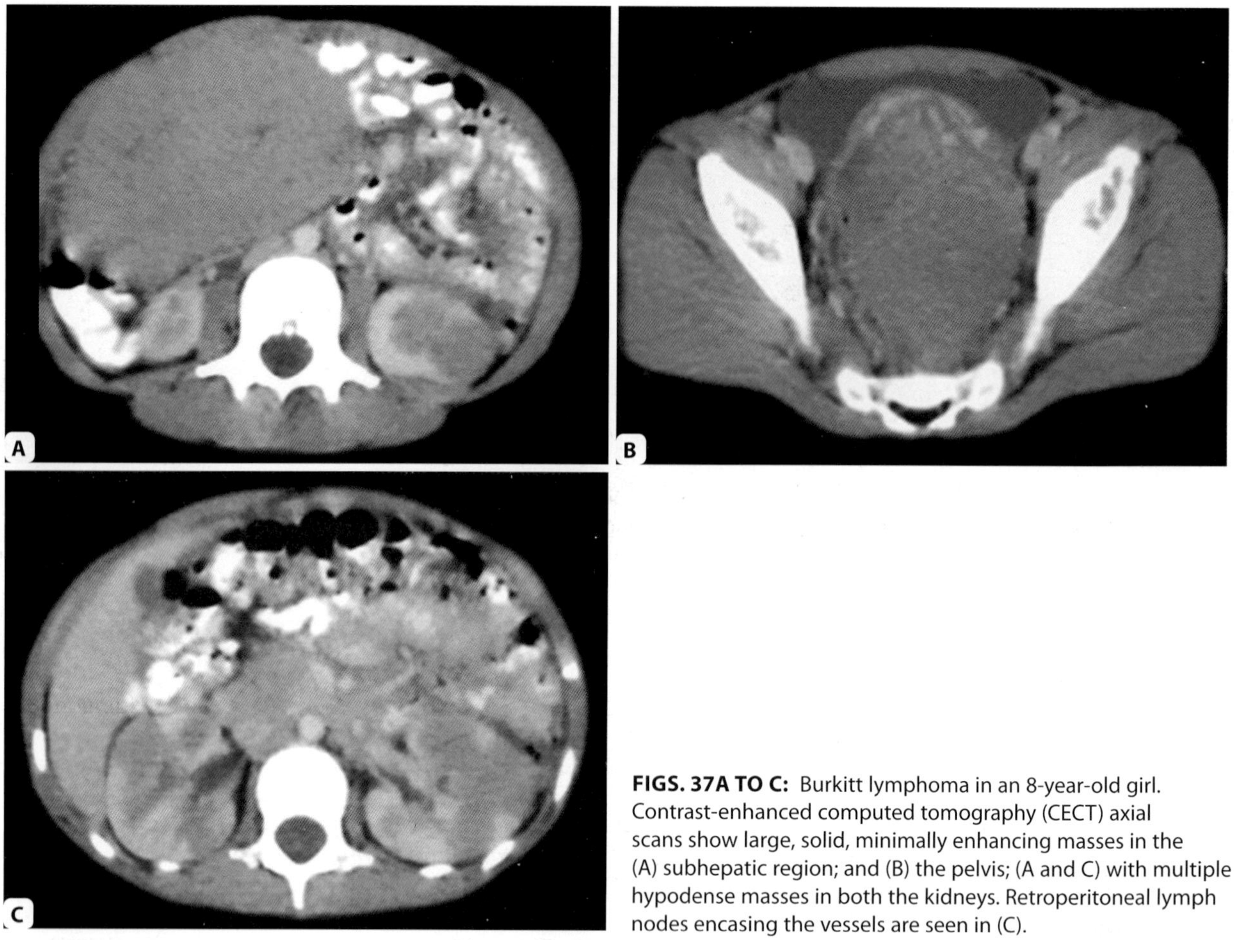

FIGS. 37A TO C: Burkitt lymphoma in an 8-year-old girl. Contrast-enhanced computed tomography (CECT) axial scans show large, solid, minimally enhancing masses in the (A) subhepatic region; and (B) the pelvis; (A and C) with multiple hypodense masses in both the kidneys. Retroperitoneal lymph nodes encasing the vessels are seen in (C).

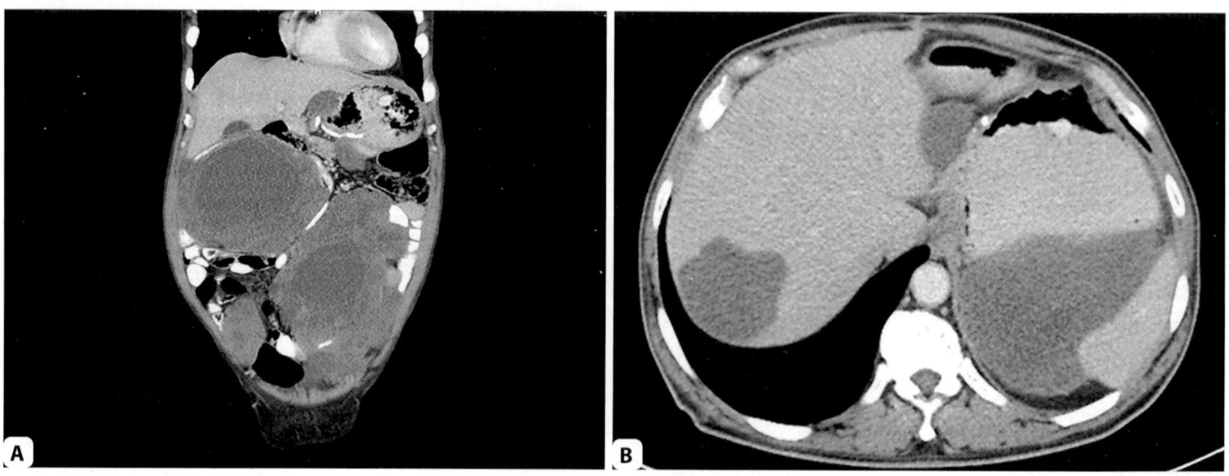

FIGS. 38A AND B: A 60-year-old man with gastrointestinal stromal tumor. (A) Coronal; and (B) axial contrast-enhanced computed tomography (CECT) images show bulky, heterogeneous peritoneal masses. Metastatic lesion seen in the liver on the axial scan (B). There is no evidence of ascites.

by direct seeding of the peritoneal cavity. Metastases to peritoneum from extremity sarcomas are unusual and presumed to occur through the hematogenous route.

On imaging, peritoneal sarcomatosis may show focal, large soft-tissue masses, nodular infiltration, or confluent areas of increased attenuation within the mesentery and omentum **(Figs. 38A and B)**. Visceral deposits can occur and are seen as soft-tissue masses on serosal surfaces of the liver and spleen. Ascites is generally minimal and occurs late in the course of disease. GIST is the most common soft tissue sarcoma metastasizing to the peritoneum, seen in 21–45% of cases of GISTs.[95,96]

The peritoneal deposits in GIST are seen as large, discrete, often spherical masses with necrosis with heterogeneous enhancement. Less commonly, diffuse hypervascular peritoneal involvement may occur with omental "cake" formation. The hypervascular nature of the metastases may lead to GI bleeding and hemoperitoneum.[94]

Differential diagnosis: The appearance of peritoneal sarcomatosis may show overlap with carcinomatosis and lymphomatosis, although bulky heterogeneous masses, hypervascularity, minimal ascites, and hemoperitoneum are more characteristic of sarcomatosis. **Table 4** lists the main differentiating features between PC, lymphomatosis, and sarcomatosis.

Mesenteric Neuroendocrine Tumor (Carcinoid)

The small intestine is the most common location for GI neuroendocrine tumors (NET). Independent of site of origin, aggressive NET typically spread to the mesentery, mesenteric lymph nodes, liver, ovaries, and spleen.

Approximately 40–80% of GI NETs spread to the mesentery, either by direct extension or through the local lymphatics.[97] The primary intestinal mass is often small and difficult to detect, the mesenteric tumor is usually discovered first. Secondary involvement of the mesentery leads to a desmoplastic reaction incited by local release of serotonin and other vasoactive substances.

Imaging features: CT/MR enterography is an appropriate imaging modality for evaluating patients suspected of having a NET as it may show both the components of carcinoid tumor, the primary mural nodule and the secondary mesenteric mass.

NET incites a strong desmoplastic reaction thought to be due to the effect of serotonin and other vasoactive peptides produced by the tumor. It is usually seen as an enhancing soft-tissue mass with linear bands radiating in the mesenteric fat **(Figs. 39A to C)**. Segmental thickening of adjacent bowel loops resulting from chronic ischemia or tumor infiltration as well as angulation can be seen. Dystrophic calcification may be seen in up to 40% of carcinoids on CT.[98] On MRI, the lesions exhibit low T1 SI, high T2 SI, and moderately intense gadolinium

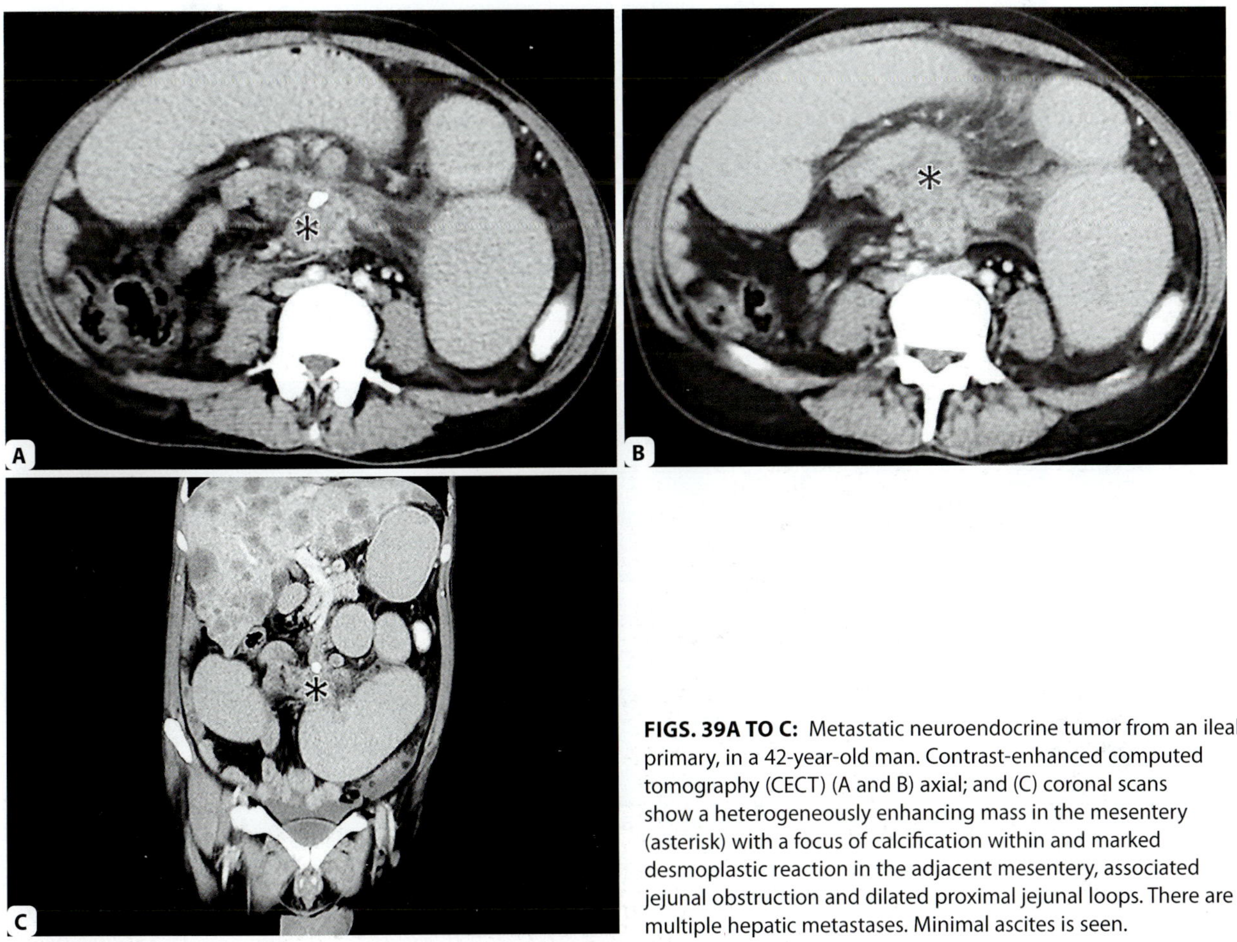

FIGS. 39A TO C: Metastatic neuroendocrine tumor from an ileal primary, in a 42-year-old man. Contrast-enhanced computed tomography (CECT) (A and B) axial; and (C) coronal scans show a heterogeneously enhancing mass in the mesentery (asterisk) with a focus of calcification within and marked desmoplastic reaction in the adjacent mesentery, associated jejunal obstruction and dilated proximal jejunal loops. There are multiple hepatic metastases. Minimal ascites is seen.

enhancement.[99] Functional imaging such as octreotide scintigraphy and G-68 DOTANOC PET/CT play an important role in the diagnosis and management of these lesions.

MISCELLANEOUS LESIONS OF THE PERITONEUM

Lymphatic Malformations/Lymphangioma

Lymphatic malformations (LMs) are rare nonmalignant masses consisting of fluid-filled channels or spaces thought to be caused by the abnormal development of the lymphatic system. Abdominal LMs occur most commonly in the mesentery, followed by the omentum, mesocolon, retroperitoneum, and abdominal viscera.[100,101]

Clinical features: Although LMs can occur at any age, they are seen more commonly in infants and young children.[101] Abdominal pain and distension are the common presenting features. Rarely, patients may present with acute abdominal pain due to complications such as torsion, infarction, or intestinal obstruction.

Imaging features: LMs are thin-walled unilocular or multilocular cystic masses containing serous or chylous fluid. On US, these LMs are seen as cystic, unilocular or multilocular masses with echogenicity varying from anechoic to hypoechoic depending on the internal content **(Figs. 40 and 41)**. CT shows enhancing cyst wall and internal septa with homogeneous, low attenuation fluid content. The attenuation of the fluid may have negative values in the presence of chyle. MRI also shows similar

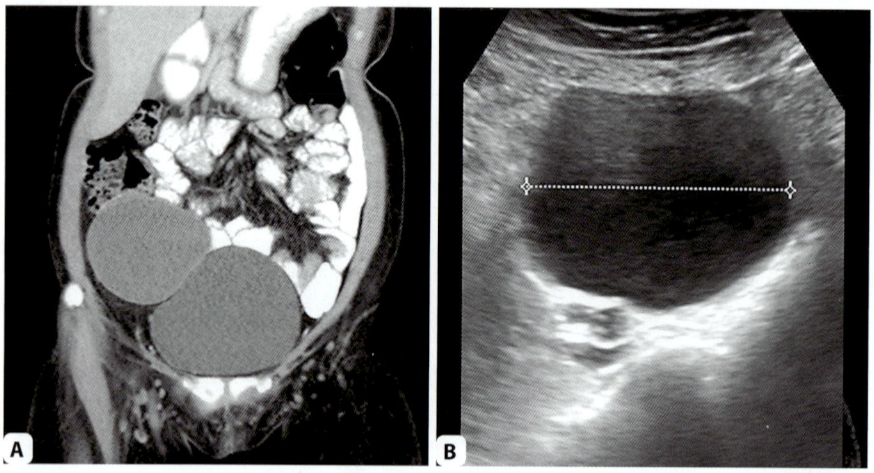

FIGS. 40A AND B: Mesenteric cyst in a 34-year-old woman with chronic pain in right iliac fossa. (A) Coronal computed tomography (CT) image; and (B) Ultrasonography (US) scan show an anechoic, unilocular thin-walled cyst in the peritoneal fat.

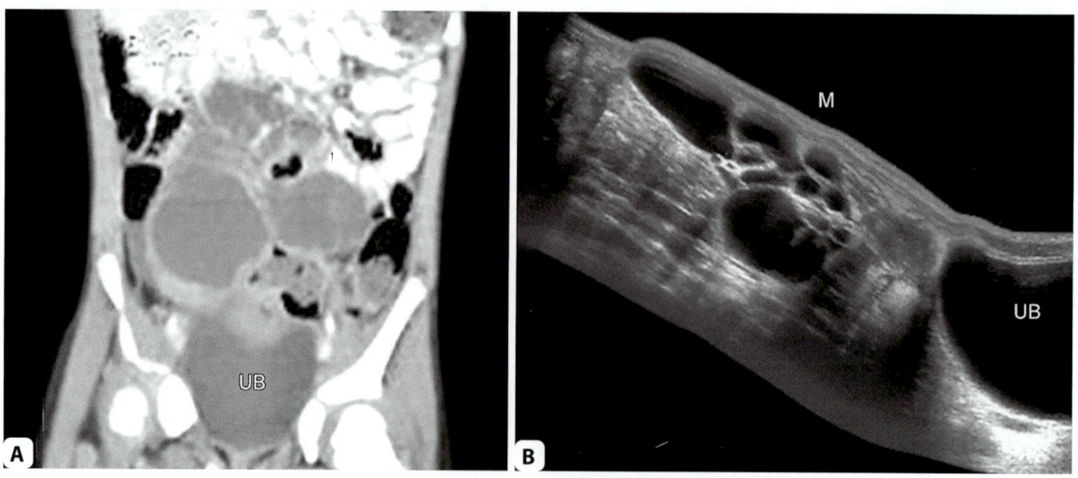

FIGS. 41A AND B: Mesenteric lymphangioma (A) Contrast-enhanced computed tomography (CECT) coronal image shows a multiloculated cystic mass in the mesentery with enhancing septa. (B) Longitudinal section US, panoramic image, shows the whole extent of the mesenteric lymphangioma as a multiloculated cystic mass (M) with varying sized cysts.

(UB: urinary bladder)

findings with low SI on T1W and high on T2W images. The presence of hemorrhage or infection in the cysts may change the CT attenuation or MR signal pattern. Calcification is uncommon.[100]

Differential diagnosis: Large mesenteric lymphangiomas need to be differentiated from ascites. The presence of septa, compression of the adjacent intestinal loops, and lack of fluid in the dependent peritoneal recesses help to establish a diagnosis of lymphangioma. Other differentials to be considered are benign ovarian neoplasms and PICs. Duplication cyst or mesothelial cyst are uncommon.

Gliomatosis Peritonei

In gliomatosis peritonei (GP) multiple nodules of benign, mature glial tissue occur throughout the peritoneum. This condition is seen almost exclusively in association with immature ovarian teratomas, but has rarely been reported to occur in patients with ventriculoperitoneal shunts.

Two theories have been put forward as to the etiology of GP. The first theory is that it occurs due to a rupture of the ovarian teratoma capsule or by angiolymphatic spread from the tumor.[102] The second theory suggests that foci of peritoneal glial tissue arise autonomously from pluripotent stem cells of Mullerian origin and is not related to primary ovarian teratoma.[103]

On CT, it is seen as multiple soft-tissue peritoneal nodules varying in size from 0.3 to 1.2 cm in diameter, along with omental caking, and ascites. These nodules show a high signal on T2W MR image, are generally homogeneous, may be multilobulated and do not have any fat or calcific content. A pelvic mass suggestive of a teratoma is generally seen in these patients, which is more often an immature teratoma, but in some cases can even be a mature teratoma. The imaging findings can be indistinguishable from tuberculous peritonitis or PC. GP can only be confirmed on histopathology, where GP nodules show presence of mature glial tissue.[91]

Endometriosis

Endometriosis is a common condition affecting almost 10% of women in the reproductive age group. It commonly involves the ovaries forming endometriomas, but may also involve peritoneal surfaces in two forms—superficially and as part of deep infiltrating endometriosis where the endometriotic lesions infiltrate peritoneum to a depth of at least 5 mm. Majority of the endometriotic lesions are confined to the pelvis but extrapelvic endometriosis occurs in approximately 1% of patients generally involving the serosal surfaces of bowel segments closest to the pelvis and rarely forming fibrotic nodules in the upper abdominal peritoneal surfaces.

The MR imaging is the modality of choice in imaging of extrapelvic peritoneal endometriotic implants which are seen as nodular or fibrotic retractile masses with low SI on T1W and T2W images. Hyperintense foci may be seen within these masses on T1W images representing hemorrhagic foci, and on T2W images representing dilated endometrial glands. Associated features of pelvic endometriosis can be well visualized on both US and MRI.

Splenosis

Splenosis is defined as the presence of nodules of splenic tissue throughout the abdomen due to a traumatic or iatrogenic splenic rupture. These nodules may mimic malignant peritoneal implants. Patients are often asymptomatic, with an incidental detection of nodules. On imaging, they show features identical to the spleen with CT showing a heterogeneous contrast uptake in arterial phase, becoming homogeneous in the portal phase, and on MRI they show the same signal as normal spleen on all sequences. Technetium-99 m-labelled red blood cells scintigraphy can be used to confirm the splenic nature of the nodules in case of doubt.

CONCLUSION

Diseases of the peritoneum are common, but there is a considerable overlap in their imaging appearances. This often results in misinterpretation of the findings, and thus peritoneal diseases present a diagnostic challenge. With the appropriate clinical setting, CT and MRI substantially aid in the identification of peritoneal disease. Radiologists must be familiar with the anatomy of the peritoneal ligaments and spaces, and a knowledge of the various diseases that can involve the peritoneum, to provide an accurate interpretation of findings.

REFERENCES

1. Standring S. Gray's anatomy: the anatomical basis of clinical practice, Peritoneum and peritoneal cavity, 39th edition. London: Churchill Livingstone; 2004.
2. Song XL, Ren JL, Yao TY, Zhao D, Niu J. Radiomics based on multisequence magnetic resonance imaging for the preoperative prediction of peritoneal metastasis in ovarian cancer. Eur Radiol. 2021;31(11):8438-46.
3. Le O. Patterns of peritoneal spread of tumor in the abdomen and pelvis. World J Radiol. 2013;5(3):106-12.
4. DeMeo JH, Fulcher AS, Austin RF. Anatomic CT demonstration of the peritoneal spaces, ligaments, and mesenteries: normal and pathologic processes. Radiographics. 1995;15(4):755-70.
5. Tirkes T, Sandrasegaran K, Patel AA, Hollar MA, Tejada JG, Tann M, et al. Peritoneal and retroperitoneal anatomy and its relevance for cross-sectional imaging. Radiographics. 2012;32(2):437-51.
6. Sharma M, Rai P, Rameshbabu CS, Senadhipan B. Imaging of peritoneal ligaments by endoscopic ultrasound. Endosc Ultrasound. 2015;4(1):15-27.

7. Haaga JR, Pickhardt PJ. Peritoneum. In: Haaga JR, Dogra VS, Frosting M, Gilkeson RC, Ha HK, Sundaram M (Eds). CT and NRI of the whole body, 5th edition. Philadelphia, PA: Mosby; 2009. pp. 1675-730.
8. Turnage RH, Li BD, McDonald JC. Abdominal wall, umbilicus, peritoneum, mesenteries, omentum and retroperitoneum. In: Townsend CM, Beauchamp RD, Evers BM, Mattox KI (Eds). Sabiston Textbook of Surgery, 17th edition. Philadelphia, PA: Saunders; 2004. pp. 1181-2.
9. Feldman GB, Knapp RC. Lymphatic drainage of the peritoneal cavity and its significance in ovarian cancer. Am J Obstet Gynecol. 1974;119(7):991-4.
10. Runyon BA, Montano AA, Akriviadis EA, Antillon MR, Irving MA, McHutchison JG. The serum-ascites albumin gradient is superior to the exudate-transudate concept in the differential diagnosis of ascites. Ann Intern Med. 1992;117(3):215-20.
11. Nicholas JE, Steinkampf MP. Detection of free peritoneal fluid by transvaginal sonography. J Clin Ultrasound. 1993;21(3):171-4.
12. Meyers MA. Dynamic radiology of the abdomen: normal and pathologic anatomy, 4th edition. New York, NY: Springer-Verlag; 1994.
13. Martin LC, Merkle EM, Thompson WM. Review of internal hernias: radiographic and clinical findings. AJR Am J Roentgenol. 2006;186(3):703-17.
14. Edell SL, Gefter WB. Ultrasonic differentiation of types of ascitic fluid. AJR Am J Roentgenol. 1979;133(1):111-4.
15. Gazelle GS, Mueller PR. Abdominal abscess: imaging and intervention. Radiol Clin North Am. 1994;32(5):913-32.
16. Batra A, Gulati MS, Sarma D, Paul SB. Sonographic appearances in abdominal tuberculosis. J Clin Ultrasound. 2000;28(5):233-45.
17. Leder RA, Low VHS. Tuberculosis of the abdomen. Radiol Clin North Am. 1995;33(4):691-705.
18. Burill J, Williams CJ, Bain G, Conder G, Oren C, Williams B. Tuberculosis: A radiological review. Radiographics. 2007;27(5):1255-73.
19. Hulnick DH, Megibow AJ, Nadiach DP, Hilton S, Cho KC, Balthazar EJ. Abdominal tuberculosis: CT evaluation. Radiology. 1985;157(1):199-204.
20. Lundstedt C, Nymon R, Brimsar J, Hugosson C, Kagevi I. Imaging of abdominal tuberculosis. Abdominal manifestations in 112 patients. Acta Radiol. 1996;37(4):489-95.
21. Malik A, Saxena NC. Ultrasound in abdominal tuberculosis. Abdom Imaging. 2003;28(4):574-9.
22. Anbarasu A, Upadhyaya A, Merchant SA, Amonkar P, Devarbhavi H, Bhatnagar M. Tuberculous chylous ascites: pathognomic CT findings. Abdom Imaging. 1997;22(1):50-1.
23. Joshi AR, Basantani AS, Patel TC. Role of CT and MRI in abdominal tuberculosis. Current Radiology Reports. 2014;2:66.
24. Healy JC, Reznek RH. The peritoneum, mesenteries and omenta: normal anatomy and pathological processes. Eur Radiol. 1998;8(6):886-900.
25. Ha HK, Jung JM, Lee MS, Choi BG, Lee MG, Kim YH, et al. CT differentiation of tuberculous peritonitis and peritoneal carcinomatosis. AJR Am J Roentgenol. 1996;167(3):743-48.
26. Rodriquez E, Pombo F. Peritotneal tuberculosis versus peritoneal carcinomatosis: Distinction based on CT findings. J Comput Asst Tomogr. 1996;20(2):269-72.
27. Pedrosa I, Saíz A, Arrazola J, Ferreirós J, Pedrosa CS. Hydatid disease: radiologic and pathologic features and complications. Radiographics. 2000;20(3):3795-817.
28. Acharya AN, Gupta S. Peritoneal hydatidosis: a review of seven cases. Tropical Gastroenterology. 2009;30(1):32-4.
29. Mindelzun RE, Brooke Jeffrey R, Lane MJ, Silverman PM. The misty mesentery on CT: differential diagnosis. AJR Am J Roentgenol. 1996;167(1):61-5.
30. Demir MK, Akinci O, Onur E, Koksal N. Case 108: sclerosing encapsulating peritonitis. Radiology. 2007;242(3):937-9.
31. Vijayaraghavan SB, Palanivelu C, Sendhilkumar K, Parthasarathi R. Abdominal cocoon: sonographic features. J Ultrasound Med. 2003;22:719-21.
32. Hur J, Kim KW, Park MS, Yu JS. Abdominal cocoon: preoperative diagnostic clues from radiologic imaging with pathologic correlation. AJR Am J Roentgenol. 2004;182:639-41.
33. Gupta S, Shirahatti RG, Anand J. CT findings of an abdominal cocoon. AJR Am J Roentgenol. 2004;183(6):1658-60.
34. Auh YH, Kung S, Shih G. Mesentery. In: Haaga JR, Dogra VS, Frosting M, Gilkeson RC, Ha HK, Sundaram M (Eds). CT and MRI of the whole body, 5th edition. Philadelphia, PA: Mosby; 2009. pp.1731-70.
35. Horton KM, Lawler LP, Fishman ER. CT Findings in Sclerosing Mesenteritis (Panniculitis): Spectrum of Disease. Radiographics. 2003;23(6):1561-7.
36. Valls C. Fat-Ring Sign in Sclerosing Mesenteritis. AJR Am J Roentgenol. 2000;174(1):259-60.
37. Coulier B. Mesenteric panniculitis. Part 1: MDCT--pictorial review. JBR-BTR. 2011;94(5):229-40.
38. Hamrick-Turner J, Chiechi M, Abbitt P, Ros P. Neoplastic and inflammatory processes of the peritoneum, omentum and mesentery: diagnosis with CT. Radiographics. 1992;12(6):1051-68.
39. Nyberg L, Björk J, Björkdahl P, Ekberg O, Sjöberg K, Vigren L. Sclerosing mesenteritis and mesenteric panniculitis – clinical experience and radiological features. BMC gastroenterol. 2017;17(1):75.
40. Lucey BC, Stuhlfaut JW, Soto JA. Mesenteric lymph nodes: Detection and significance on MDCT. AJR Am J Roentgenol. 2005;184(1):41-4.
41. Lucey BC, Stuhlfaut JW, Soto JA. Mesenteric lymph nodes seen at imaging—causes and significance. Radiographics. 2005;25(2):351-65.
42. Jain R, Sawhney S, Bhargava DK, Berry M. Diagnosis of abdominal tuberculosis: Sonographic findings in patients with early disease. AJR Am J Roentgenol. 1995;165(6):1391-5.
43. Kedar RP, Shah PP, Shirde RS, Malde HM. Sonographic findings in gastrointestinal and peritoneal tuberculosis. Clin Radiol. 1994;49(1):24-9.
44. Pombo F, Rodriquez E, Mato J, Pérez-Fontán J, Rivera E, Valvuena L. Patterns of contrast enhancement of tuberculous lymph nodes demonstrated by CT. Clin Radiol. 1992;46(1):13-7.
45. De Backer AI, Mortele KJ, Deeren D, Vanschoubroeck IJ, De Keulenaer BL. Abdominal tuberculous lymphadenopathy: MRI features. Eur Radiol. 2005;15(10):2104-9.
46. Rocha ELD, Pedrassa BC, Bormann RL, Kierszenbaum ML, Torres LR, D'Ippolito G. Abdominal tuberculosis: a radiological review with emphasis on CT and MRI findings. Radiol Bras. 2015;48(3):181-91.

47. Yang ZG, Min P, Sone S, He ZY, Liao ZY, Zhou XP, et al. Tuberculosis versus lymphoma in the abdominal lymph nodes. Evaluation with contrast-enhanced CT. AJR Am J Roentgenol. 1999;172(3):619-23.
48. Macari M, Hines J, Balthazar E, Megibow A. Mesenteric adenitis: CT diagnosis of primary versus secondary causes, incidence, and clinical significance in pediatric and adult patients. AJR Am J Roentgenol. 2002;178(4):853-8.
49. Rao PM, Rhea JT, Novelline RA. CT diagnosis of mesenteric adenitis. Radiology. 1997;201(1):145-9.
50. Yenarkam P, Theni RF, Hanks D. Lymphoma of the mesentery. Radiology. 2007;242(2):628-31.
51. Mok SC, Schorge JO, Welch WR, Hendrickson MR, Kempson RL. Peritoneal tumors. In: Tavassoli FA, Devilee P (Eds). Pathology and genetics of tumours of the breast and female genital organs, 3rd edition. Lyon, France: IARC; 2003. pp. 197-202.
52. Boffetta P. Epidemiology of peritoneal mesothelioma: a review. Ann Oncol. 2007;18(6):985-90.
53. Churg A, Cagle PT, Roggli VL. Tumors of the serosal membranes, 4th edition. Silver Spring, Maryland: ARP Press; 2006.
54. Levy AD, Arnáiz J, Shaw JC, Sobin LH. From the archives of the AFIP: primary peritoneal tumors—imaging features with pathologic correlation. Radiographics. 2008;28(2):583-607.
55. Cao Q, Lu M, Heath J, Hausner PF, Alexander HR, Dilsizian V, et al. 18F-FDG PET/CT in a recurrent diffuse malignant peritoneal mesothelioma. Clin Nucl Med. 2012;37(5):492-4.
56. Turner KM, Varghese S, Alexander HR. Surgery for peritoneal mesothelioma. Curr Treat Options Oncol. 2011;12:189-200.
57. Raza A, Huang WC, Takabe K. Advances in the management of peritoneal mesothelioma. World J Gastroenterol. 2014;20(33):11700-12.
58. Rapisarda AMC, Cianci A, Caruso S, Vitale SG, Valenti G, Piombino E, et al. Benign multicystic mesothelioma and peritoneal inclusion cysts: are they the same clinical and histopathological entities? A systematic review to find an evidence-based management. Arch Gynecol Obstet. 2018;297(6):1353-75.
59. Ross MJ, Welch WR, Scully RE. Multilocular peritoneal inclusion cysts (so-called cystic mesotheliomas). Cancer. 1989;64(6):1336-46.
60. Noiret B, Renaud F, Piessen G, Eveno C. Multicystic peritoneal mesothelioma: a systematic review of the literature. Pleura Peritoneum. 2019;4(3):20190024.
61. McLaughlin P, Flippone A, Maher MM. Neoplastic diseases of Peritoneum and Mesentery. AJR Am J Roentgenol. 2013;200(5):W420-30.
62. Kawai T, Tominaga S, Hiroi S, Ogata S, Nakanishi K, Kawahara K, et al. Peritoneal malignant mesothelioma (PMM), and primary peritoneal serous carcinoma (PPSC) and reactive mesothelial hyperplasia (RMH) of the peritoneum. Immunohistochemical and fluorescence in situ hybridisation (FISH) analyses. J Clin Pathol. 2016;69(8):706-12.
63. Zhang J, Xu H, Ren F, Yang Y, Chen B, Zhang F. Analysis of clinicopathological features and prognostic factors of desmoplastic small round cell tumor. Pathol Oncol Res. 2014;20(1):161-8.
64. Arora VC, Price AP, Fleming S, Sohn MJ, Magnan H, LaQuaglia MP, et al. Characteristic imaging features of desmoplastic small round cell tumor. Pediatr Radiol. 2013;43(1):93-102.
65. Morani AC, Bathala TK, Surabhi VR, Yedururi S, Jensen CT, Huh WW, et al. Desmoplastic small round cell tumor: imaging pattern of disease at presentation. AJR Am J Roentgenol. 2019;212(3):W45-54.
66. Garci-Ortega DY, Martin-Tellez KS, Cuellar-Hubbe M, Martínez-Said H, Álvarez-Cano A, Brener-Chaoul M, et al. Desmoid type fibromatosis. Cancers (Basel). 2020;12(7):1851.
67. Azizi I, Bali M, Belkacem A, Lewin M, Tubiana JM, Arrivé L. MRI Features of mesenteric desmoids tumors in familial adenomatous polyposis. AJR Am J Roentgenol. 2005;184(4): 1128-35.
68. Shinagare AB, Ramaiya NH, Jagannathan JP, Krajewski KM, Giardino AA, Butrynski JE, et al. A to Z of desmoids tumours. AJR Am J Roentgenol. 2011;197(6):W1008-14.
69. Rodríguez CR, Fontán GEM, Ramos BM, Magdalena Benavides LJ, Otero Lozano D, Moldes Rodriguez M, et al. Inflammatory pseudotumor and myofibroblastic inflammatory tumor. Diagnostic criteria and prognostic differences. Cir Esp (Engl Ed). 2022;100(6):329-35.
70. Aptel S, Gervaise A, Fairise A, Henrot P, Leroux A, Guillemin F, et al. Abdominal inflammatory myofibroblastic tumour. Diagn Interv Imaging. 2012;93(5):410-2.
71. Narla LD, Newman B, Spottswood SS, Narla S, Kolli R. Inflammatory pseudotumor. Radiographics. 2003;23(3): 719-29.
72. Sedlic T, Scali EP, Lee WK, Verma S, Chang SD. Inflammatory pseudotumors in the abdomen and pelvis: a pictorial essay. Can Assoc Radiol J. 2014;65(1):52-9.
73. Cantera JE, Alfaro MP, Rafart DC, Zalazar R, Muruzabal MM, Barquín PG, et al. Inflammatory myofibroblastic tumours: a pictorial review. Insights Imaging. 2015;6(1):85-96.
74. Lausen I, Jensen OJ, Andersen E, Lindahl F. Disseminated peritoneal leiomyomatosis with malignant change in a male. Virchows Arch A Pathol Anat Histopathol. 1990;417(2): 173-5.
75. Xu S, Qian J. Leiomyomatosis Peritonealis disseminata with sarcomatous transformation: a rare case report and literature review. Case Rep Obstet Gynecol. 2019;2019:1-4.
76. Jacquet P, Sugarbaker PH. Clinical research methodologies in diagnosis and staging of patients with peritoneal carcinomatosis. Cancer Treat Res. 1996;82:359-74.
77. Bhatt A, Rousset P, Benzerdjeb N, Kammar P, Mehta S, Parikh L, et al. Prospective correlation of the radiological, surgical and pathological findings in patients undergoing cytoreductive surgery for colorectal peritoneal metastases: implications for the preoperative estimation of the peritoneal cancer index. Colorectal Dis. 2020;22(12):2123-32.
78. Chandramohan A, Thrower A, Smith SA, Shah N, Moran B. "PAUSE": a method for communicating radiological extent of peritoneal malignancy. Clin Radiol. 2017;72(11):972-80.
79. Hanbridge AE, Lynch D, Wilson SR. US of the peritoneum. Radiographics. 2003;23(3):663-83.
80. Marin D, Catalano C, Baski M, Di Martino M, Geiger D, Di Giorgio A, et al. 64-section multidetector row CT in the preoperative diagnosis of peritoneal carcinomatosis: Correlation with histopathological findings. Abdom Imaging. 2010;35(6):694-700.
81. Iafrate F, Ciolina M, Sammartino P, Baldassari P, Rengo M, Lucchesi P, et al. Peritoneal carcinomatosis: Imaging with 64-MDCT and 3T MRI with diffusion-weighted imaging. Abdom Imaging. 2012;37(4):616-27.

82. Soussan M, Des Guetz G, Barrau V, Aflalo-Hazan V, Pop G, Mehanna Z, et al. Comparison of FDG-PET/CT and MR with diffusion-weighted imaging for assessing peritoneal carcinomatosis from gastrointestinal malignancy. Eur Radiol. 2012;22(7):1479-87.
83. Anthony MP, Khong PL, Zhang J. Spectrum of 18F-FDG PET/CT appearances in peritoneal disease. AJR Am J Roentgenol. 2009;193(6):1646.
84. Tentes KA, Courcoutsakis N, Prasopoulos P. Combined cytoreductive surgery and perioperative intraperitoneal chemotherapy for the treatment of advanced ovarian cancer—clinical and therapeutic perspectives. In: Samir F (Ed). Ovarian Cancer—Clinical and Therapeutic Perspectives. New York: InTech; 2012. pp. 143-67.
85. Cabral FC, Krajewski KM, Kim KW, Ramaiya NH, Jagannathan JP. Peritoneal lymphomatosis: CT and PET/CT findings and how to differentiate between carcinomatosis and sarcomatosis. Cancer Imaging. 2013;13(2):162-70.
86. Seidman JD, Elsayed AM, Sobin LH, Tavassoli FA. Association of mucinous tumors of the ovary and appendix: a clinicopathologic study of 25 cases. Am J Surg Pathol. 1993;17(1):22-34.
87. Carr NJ, Cecil TD, Mohamed F, Sugarbaker PH, González-Moreno S, Taflampas P, et al. A consensus for classification and pathologic reporting of pseudomyxoma peritonei and associated appendiceal neoplasia: the results of the Peritoneal Surface Oncology Group International (PSOGI) modified Delphi process. Am J Surg Pathol. 2016;40(1):14-26.
88. Seshul MB, Coulam CM. Pseudomyxoma peritonei: Computed tomography and sonography. AJR Am J Roentgenol. 1981;136(4):803-6.
89. Mahmoud BE, Abdelzaher AA, Mohamed AA, Metwally LIA. The role of diffusion-weighted MR imaging in assessment of peritoneal lesions: radiologic-pathologic correlation. Egypt J Radiol Nucl Med. 2020;51:149.
90. Campos NMF, Almeida V, Curvo Semedo L. Peritoneal disease: key imaging findings that help in the differential diagnosis. Br J Radiol. 2022;95(1130):20210346.
91. Levy AD, Shaw JC, Sobin LH. Secondary tumors and tumor like lesions of the peritoneal cavity: imaging features with pathologic correlation. Radiographics. 2009;29(2):347-73.
92. KimY, Cho O, Song S, Lee H, Rhim H, Koh B. Peritoneal lymphomatosis: CT findings. Abdom Imaging. 1998;23(1):87-90.
93. Ferrozzi F, Tognini G, Mulonzia NW, Bova D, Pavone P. Primary effusion lymphomas in AIDS: CT findings in two cases. Eur Radiol. 2001;11(4):623-5.
94. International Agency for Research on Cancer, World Health Organization. In: Swerdlow SH, Campo E, Harris NL, Jaffe ES, Pileri SA, Stein H, et al. (Eds). WHO classification of tumors of hematopoietic and lymphoid tissues, 4th edition. Lyon, France: International Agency for Research on Cancer; 2008.
95. Katz SC, DeMatteo RP. Gastrointestinal stromal tumors and leiomyosarcoma. J Surg Oncol. 2008;97(4):350-9.
96. Burkill GJ, Badran M, Thomas JM, Meirion Thomas J, Judson IR, Fisher C, et al. Malignant gastrointestinal stromal tumor: distribution, imaging features, and pattern of metastatic spread. Radiology. 2003;226(2):527-32.
97. Sheth S, Horton KM, Garland MR, Fishman EK. Mesenteric neoplasms: CT appearances of primary and secondary tumors and differential diagnosis. Radiographics. 2003;23(2):457-73.
98. Levy AD, Sobin LH. From the archives of the AFIP: Gastrointestinal carcinoids: Imaging features with clinicopathologic comparison. Radiographics. 2007;27:237-57.
99. Elsayes KM, Staveteig PT, Narra VR, Leyendecker JR, Lewis JS Jr, Brown JJ. MRI of the peritoneum: spectrum of abnormalities. Am J Roentgenol. 2006;186:1368-79.
100. Levy AD, Cantisani V, Miettinen M. Abdominal lymphangiomas: imaging features with pathologic correlation. AJR Am J Roentgenol. 2004;182(6):1485-91.
101. Merrot T, Chaumoitre K, Simeoni-Alias J, Alessandrini P, Guys JM, Panuel M. Abdominal cystic lymphangiomas in children. Clinical, diagnostic and therapeutic aspects: apropos of 21 cases. Ann Chir. 1999;53(6):494-9.
102. Robboy SJ, Scully RE. Ovarian teratoma with glial implants on the peritoneum: an analysis of 12 cases. Hum Pathol. 1970;1(4):643-53.
103. Dallenbach-Hellweg G. Critical commentary to "Gliomatosis peritonei combined with mature ovarian teratoma" Pathol Res Pract. 1995;191(10):1037.

CHAPTER 25

Mukesh Kumar Yadav, Priyanka Naranje, Ekta Dhamija

Imaging of Spleen

INTRODUCTION AND ANATOMY

The spleen is an encapsulated organ located intraperitoneally in the left subdiaphragmatic region of the abdomen. Multiple ligaments support the spleen in its normal position. The important ones are gastrosplenic ligament and lienorenal ligament. Others are phrenicosplenic, splenocolic, pancreaticosplenic, phrenocolic, and pancreaticocolic ligaments. The capsule is penetrated at the hilus located anteromedially, by the splenic artery, splenic vein, lymphatics, and nerves **(Figs. 1A and B)**. Within the spleen, the branches of arteries, veins, nerves, and lymphatics form a trabecular network.

The splenic parenchyma has a unique arrangement of white pulp (25%) and red pulp (75%).[1] Splenic cords and vascular sinuses containing predominantly erythrocytes constitute the red pulp, whereas lymphatic tissue, macrophages and lymphocytes compose the white pulp area of spleen. Some of the normal variations in enhancement pattern of spleen seen on contrast-enhanced computed tomography (CECT) as well as gadolinium enhanced magnetic resonance imaging (MRI) are attributed to this unique anatomy of the spleen.

The spleen arises from aggregations of mesenchymal tissue between the layers of the dorsal mesogastrium during the 5th gestational week giving a lobulated pattern of the fetal spleen. The principal function of the embryonic spleen is erythropoiesis, which increases from the first to mid-second trimester and subsequently reduces. In later life, the spleen filters the damaged or aged red blood cells, bacteria, antigen-coated cells and foreign particles. The spleen comprises the largest functional mass of lymphoid

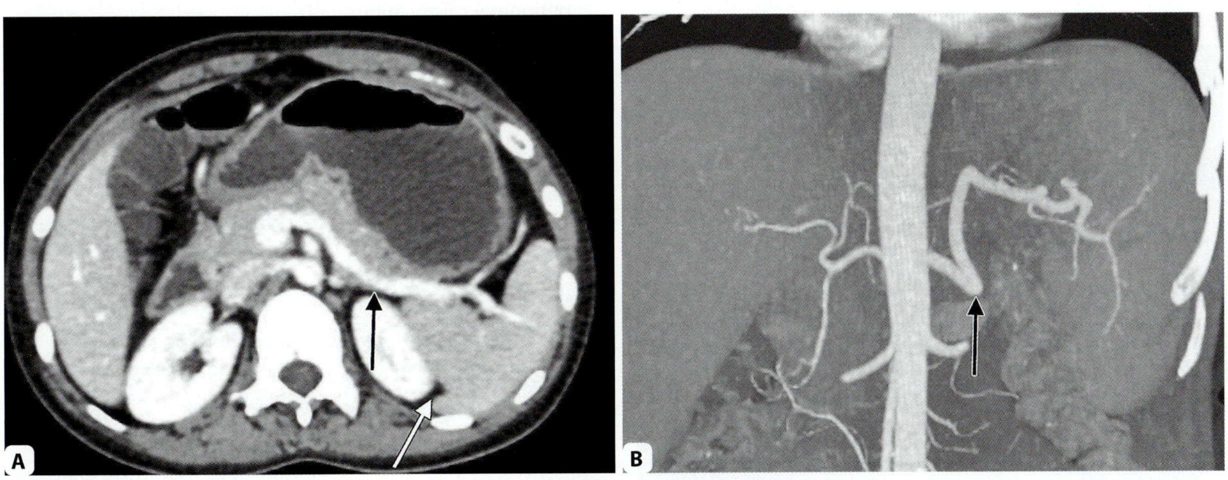

FIGS. 1A AND B: Normal spleen anatomy. (A) Axial contrast-enhanced computed tomography (CECT) image shows the retropancreatic location of the splenic vein (black arrow), coursing from splenic hilum to confluence with superior mesenteric vein (SMV). White arrow depicts the normal splenic notch. (B) Splenic artery arising from the celiac axis shows a more tortuous course (arrow) superior to pancreas and enters the splenic hilum to supply splenic parenchyma as a functional end artery.

tissue in the body. It consumes the circulating platelets when there is splenomegaly and also functions as reservoir for platelets, releasing them in response to epinephrine.[1]

IMAGING MODALITIES

Plain Abdominal Radiograph

A plain radiograph of the abdomen normally shows the spleen below the left hemidiaphragm in the upper quadrant, lateral to the gastric bubble and superior to the colon. Enlarged spleen is seen as a soft-tissue opacity displacing the stomach medially and colonic gas inferiorly **(Fig. 2)**. Plain radiograph helps in identifying splenic calcifications, which may be curvilinear, coarse, or punctate in appearance **(Table 1)**.

Ultrasonography

Sonography is a nonionizing, radiation free, noninvasive, and inexpensive modality for evaluating the spleen. It is frequently the initial imaging tool used for suspected splenic pathology **(Table 2)**.

Sonography is used for evaluating splenic size, shape, location, and multiplicity, especially in children **(Figs. 3A to E)**. Characterization of focal splenic lesions, splenic size evaluation in portal hypertension, and cases of extrahepatic portal venous obstruction (EHPVO) along with assessment of perisplenic collaterals, splenic vein assessment in cases of pancreatitis, identification of splenic arterial aneurysms, preoperative work-up and postoperative follow-up of cases requiring splenectomy and as a guidance tool for various interventions such as fine-needle aspiration cytology (FNAC), biopsies, or drainages are other common indications for using ultrasound for spleen. Sonography is ideally suited to study the internal architecture of a focal mass within the spleen, and distinguish a solid from a cystic lesion. Diffuse splenic involvement in infections such as tuberculosis, fungal infections or in sarcoidosis or in cases of lymphoma, ultrasound may reveal the abnormality better than computed tomography **(Figs. 3A and B)**. Some lesions are known to have characteristic sonographic morphology and this modality helps to narrow the differential diagnosis and triage patients for further imaging work-up. The major drawback of this technique is that it is highly operator dependent. The details of sonographic features of different pathologies will be discussed subsequently. USG plays a vital role in the follow-up of patients with splenic trauma, who have undergone nonoperative management, to look for vascular complications like pseudoaneurysm and arteriovenous fistula, which is covered in detail in the chapter on abdominal trauma.

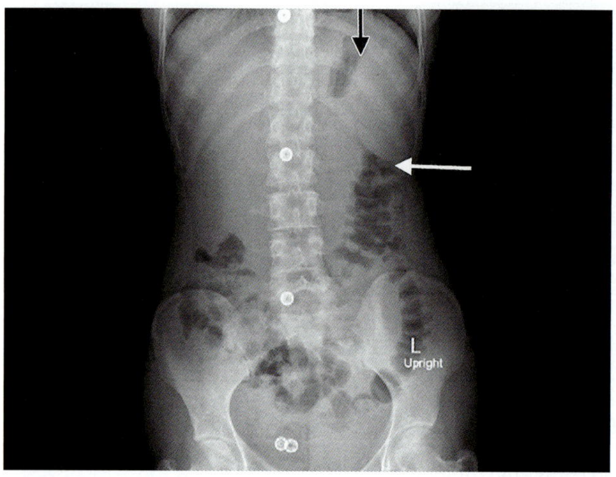

FIG. 2: Plain radiograph of abdomen shows indentation of splenic flexure (inferiorly) and greater curvature of stomach by soft tissue in left upper abdomen due to splenomegaly.

Technique

The spleen is usually scanned in the supine or right decubitus position with a 3.5–5 MHz convex array transducer in the sagittal and oblique planes as well as transversely, usually from an intercostal approach in suspended deep inspiration and end expiration. Sometimes due to deep inspiration, the lateral margin of the left lung obscures the visualization of spleen **(Fig. 3D)**. In such a situation, either scanning in expiration **(Fig. 3E)** or scanning with a small footprint probe in intercostal space may be helpful. An attempt is made to localize the splenic hilum, which represents the mid portion of the spleen, and the scanning is done taking a swipe posterior and anterior to the visualized hilum. Color Doppler is useful to assess the splenic vein and artery at the hilum.

TABLE 1: Patterns of calcified splenic lesions.

Mass with wall calcifications:	
• Thin peripheral calcifications • Thick curvilinear peripheral calcifications	True epithelial cyst; epidermoid cyst; pseudocyst; splenic artery aneurysm; and *Echinococcus*
Mass with both wall and internal calcifications:	
Complete calcification with central clearing	*Pneumocystis carinii* infection
Mass with internal calcifications:	
• Coarse calcifications	• Myelofibrosis; epithelioid hemangioendothelioma; peritoneal metastasis of nonsplenic neoplasm; and lymphoma
• Punctate calcifications	• Pleomorphic sarcoma; hemangioma; angiosarcoma
Diffuse calcifications without associated mass:	
• Coalescent calcifications	• Autosplenectomy, thorium dioxide (Thorotrast) exposure-related fibrosis
• Scattered punctate calcifications	• Gamna–Gandy bodies; tuberculosis; *Histoplasma capsulatum* infection

TABLE 2: Role of ultrasonography (USG) in splenic evaluation.

Clinical setting	Role of USG
Splenomegaly	Accurate size assessment, e.g., in portal hypertension, EHPVO
Focal splenic lesions	• To characterize the internal architecture of a focal mass • Solid versus cystic mass assessment
Diffuse splenic lesions	• Infections—e.g., tuberculosis and fungal infections • Sarcoidosis • Lymphoma *Note*: USG may reveal the abnormality better than computed tomography
Trauma	Evaluation of extent of injury and monitoring of complications
Infection	Assessment of abscess formation and its complications such as rupture
Neoplasms	Detection of both benign and malignant masses
Pancreatitis	• Splenic vein assessment • Assessment of pseudocyst formation in spleen/perisplenic regions • Splenic arterial aneurysms detection
EHPVO, portal hypertension	Splenic size, assessment of perisplenic collaterals
Splenic infarction	Detecting wedge-shaped hypoechoic areas with relative avascularity
Splenic cysts	Assessment of epithelial cysts versus hydatid cysts versus pseudocysts
Preoperative assessment	Prior to splenectomy assessment of size, shape, any anomalies, and splenunculi detection
Postoperative follow-up	Detection of collection, infection, and bleed
Fine-needle aspiration cytology (FNAC), biopsies or drainage of focal splenic lesions	USG provides real-time guidance for these interventions
• Wandering spleen • Asplenia • Polysplenia evaluation	• Helps in determining the location • Multiplicity of spleen • Useful especially in children

(EHPVO: extrahepatic portal venous obstruction)

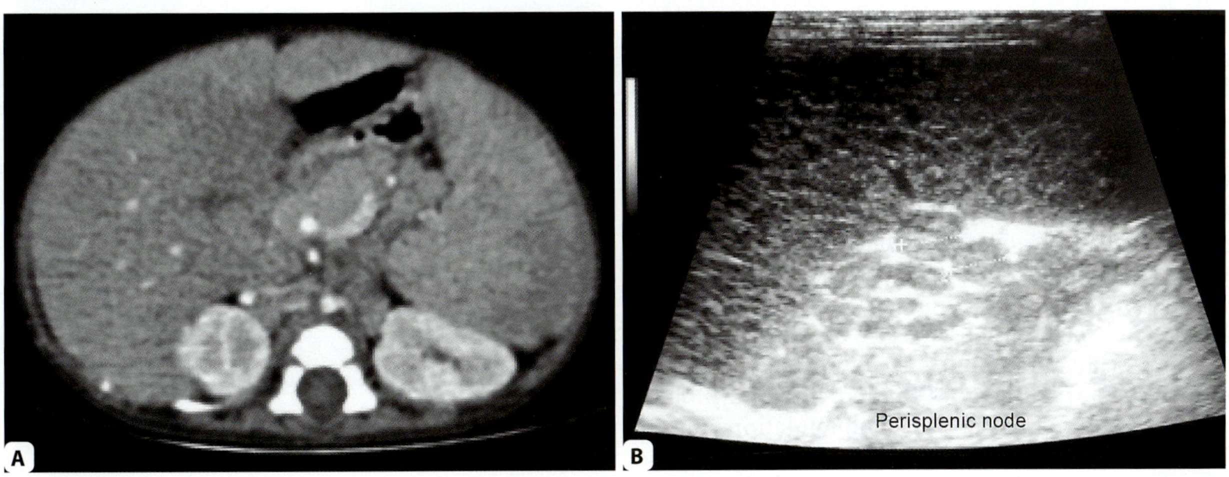

FIGS. 3A TO E: *Continued*

Continued

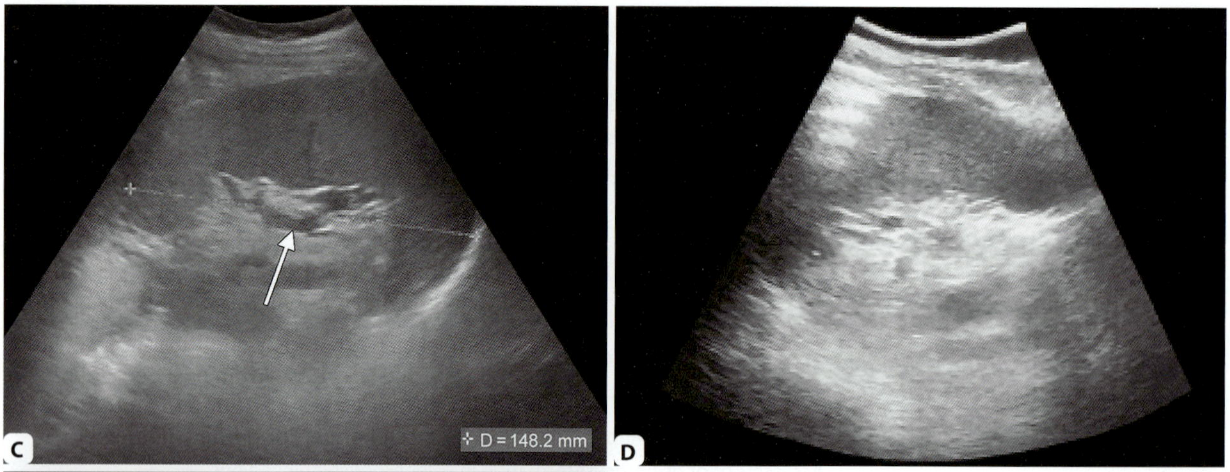

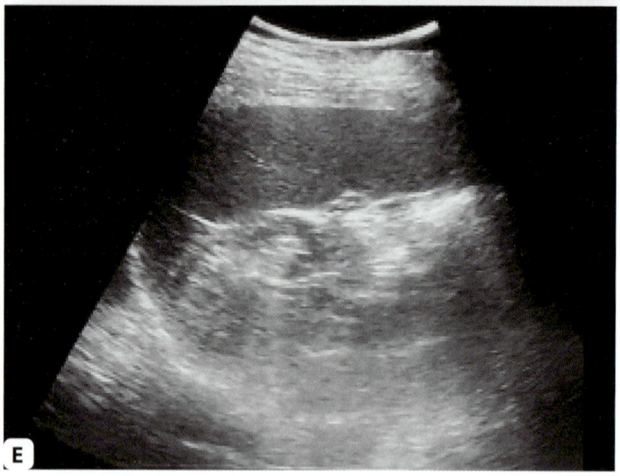

FIGS. 3A TO E: Contrast-enhanced computed tomography (CECT) image (A) in a known case of non-Hodgkin's lymphoma (NHL) showing multiple retroperitoneal, perisplenic lymph nodes, and heterogeneous attenuation of spleen without obvious discernible lesions. USG image (B) for the same patient revealed multiple hypoechoic lesions in the spleen which were not identified on CT. USG image of normal spleen (C) at the level of splenic hilum showing homogeneous echotexture of spleen. Anechoic tubular splenic vessels noted at the splenic hilum (arrow); (D and E) USG images in inspiration and expiration show obscuration of upper aspect of spleen in inspiration which is overcome in expiration.

On ultrasonography, normal spleen shows a homogeneous echotexture **(Fig. 3C)**. Its echogenicity is a little more than that of the kidneys **(Fig. 4)** and is isoechoic to slightly hyperechoic compared to the liver. Tubular anechoic tortuous structures on gray-scale at the hilum of the spleen are the splenic vessels **(Fig. 3C)** and intrasplenic vessels are visualized on color Doppler imaging.

Elasticity of the spleen can be measured with the real-time elastography, which measures the stiffness of parenchyma and it can be utilized as a marker for portal hypertension in patients with chronic liver disease.[2]

Contrast-enhanced ultrasound (CEUS) of spleen enhances the diagnostic confidence of the radiologist in interpretation of the lesions detected on two-dimensional (2D) gray-scale ultrasound.[3-5] The European Federation of Societies for Ultrasound in Medicine and Biology (EFSUMB) Guidelines and Recommendations on the Clinical Practice of CEUS, updated in 2011, recommend several indications where CEUS may be utilized in the spleen and they include:[6]

- To characterize inhomogeneity of splenic parenchyma or to characterize suspected lesions on conventional US.
- To characterize accessory spleens or splenosis.
- To confirm suspected splenic infarction.

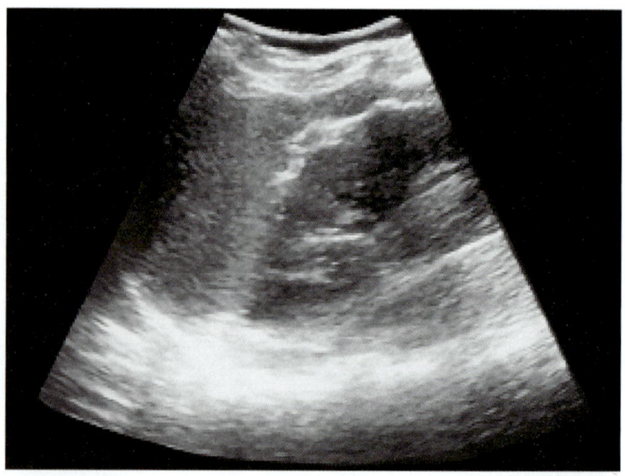

FIG. 4: Ultrasonography (USG) image showing normal splenic echotexture as slightly more than the adjacent left kidney.

- To detect malignant splenic lesions in oncologic patients when CT and/or MRI and positron emission tomography (PET) are contraindicated or inconclusive.
- To evaluate the spleen in selected patients following trauma.

Computed Tomography

On a noncontrast CT (NCCT), a normal spleen shows a homogeneous attenuation which is higher than the liver by 1–18 Hounsfield Unit (HU).[7] Normal HU of spleen is 40–60 HU. Splenic artery follows a tortuous course normally and splenic vein shows a straighter course and is usually located posterior to pancreatic body and tail.

In routine clinical practice for identification and characterization of any focal lesion in the spleen and also in trauma setting, CECT is frequently required.

Most often transient inhomogeneous splenic attenuation patterns are identified during the 1st minute of CECT, particularly with rapid intravenous injection of iodinated contrast media.[8] This is a normal flow phenomenon and must not be misinterpreted as an indication of focal abnormality. It is thought to be due to different blood flow rates through the cords of red pulp[9] and white pulp. As the internal architecture of the spleen develops, this phenomenon gets more evident in children older than 1 year. Frequently described heterogeneity patterns include: (1) Archiform pattern, consisting of ring-like or zebra-stripe bands of alternating low- and high-attenuation (the most common pattern) **(Figs. 5A and B)**; (2) Diffuse, mottled areas of heterogeneity; and (3) Focal areas of low density.[8] More homogeneous splenic enhancement is seen about 70 seconds after commencement of the contrast injection. This heterogeneous splenic enhancement pattern can obscure pathologic lesions. With increasing age, the heterogeneous pattern is less often seen and in adults, several other factors may be responsible for the heterogeneous splenic enhancement, such as the liver disease, portal vein thrombosis, and congestive heart failure.[10] CT angiography is performed for the detection of splenic artery aneurysms. Multiplanar reformation (MPR), maximum intensity projections (MIP), and volume rendered (VR) imaging help in the complete morphological assessment of these aneurysms.

Magnetic Resonance Imaging

Magnetic resonance imaging offers major advantages due to its high-contrast resolution, lack of ionizing radiation and multiplanar capability. Technical advances in MR hardware and software have allowed the introduction of faster pulse sequences with significantly reduced motion artifacts that previously posed limitations to abdominal MRI. Indications for performing MRI for splenic pathology are mainly as a problem-solving technique for focal splenic lesions or tumors, proliferative lymphatic diseases, or in iron deposition conditions.

Normal Appearance of Spleen

On MRI, normal adult spleen is T2 hyperintense relative to the liver **(Figs. 6A to D)**. On T1-weighted images (T1WI), the normal spleen shows lower signal intensity (SI) than that of liver and slightly greater SI than that of muscle. Such a signal intensity of spleen is attributed to large fractional heme content, which results in long T1 and T2 relaxation times.[11] However, in a neonate, due to the immaturity of the white pulp, the spleen is T1 as well as T2 hypo- to isointense compared to the liver **(Figs. 7A and B)**. After 8 months of age as white pulp matures, the spleen becomes hyperintense on T2-weighted image (T2WI) relative to the liver and it maintains this appearance through adulthood.[12] On diffusion-weighted imaging, the spleen shows physiologically restricted diffusion **(Figs. 6A to D)**.[13]

Dynamic gadolinium-enhanced MRI has potential advantages over conventional MRI of the spleen because it can potentially provide differential contrast enhancement between splenic lesions and normal splenic tissue with better contrast resolution compared with CT. Heterogeneous enhancement patterns of the normal spleen, seen commonly on early phase CECT scans, are also seen on dynamic contrast-enhanced MRI **(Figs. 8A to C)**.

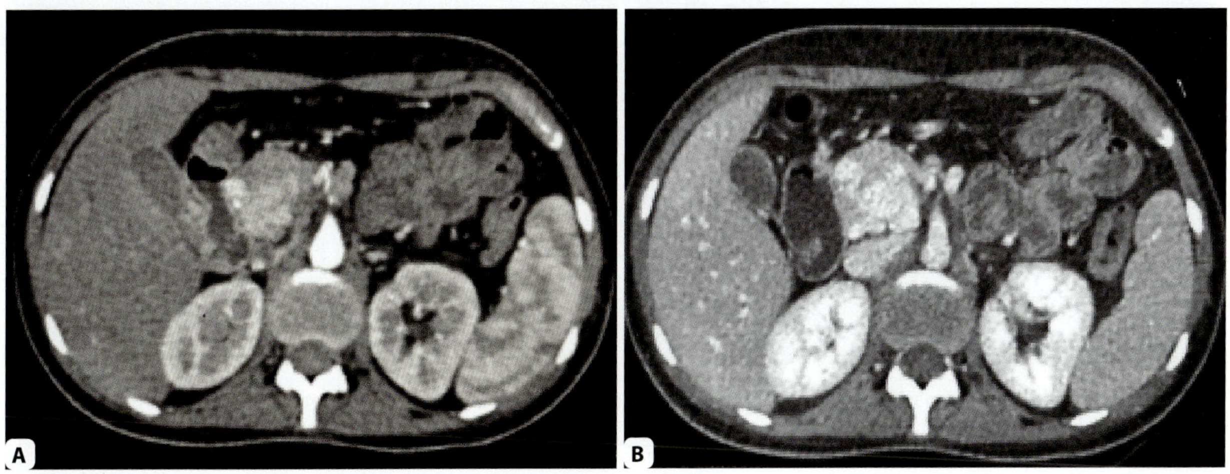

FIGS. 5A AND B: Contrast-enhanced CT images in arterial phase (A) showing normal Zebra-stripe/archiform enhancement pattern and venous phase (B) showing homogeneous enhancement.

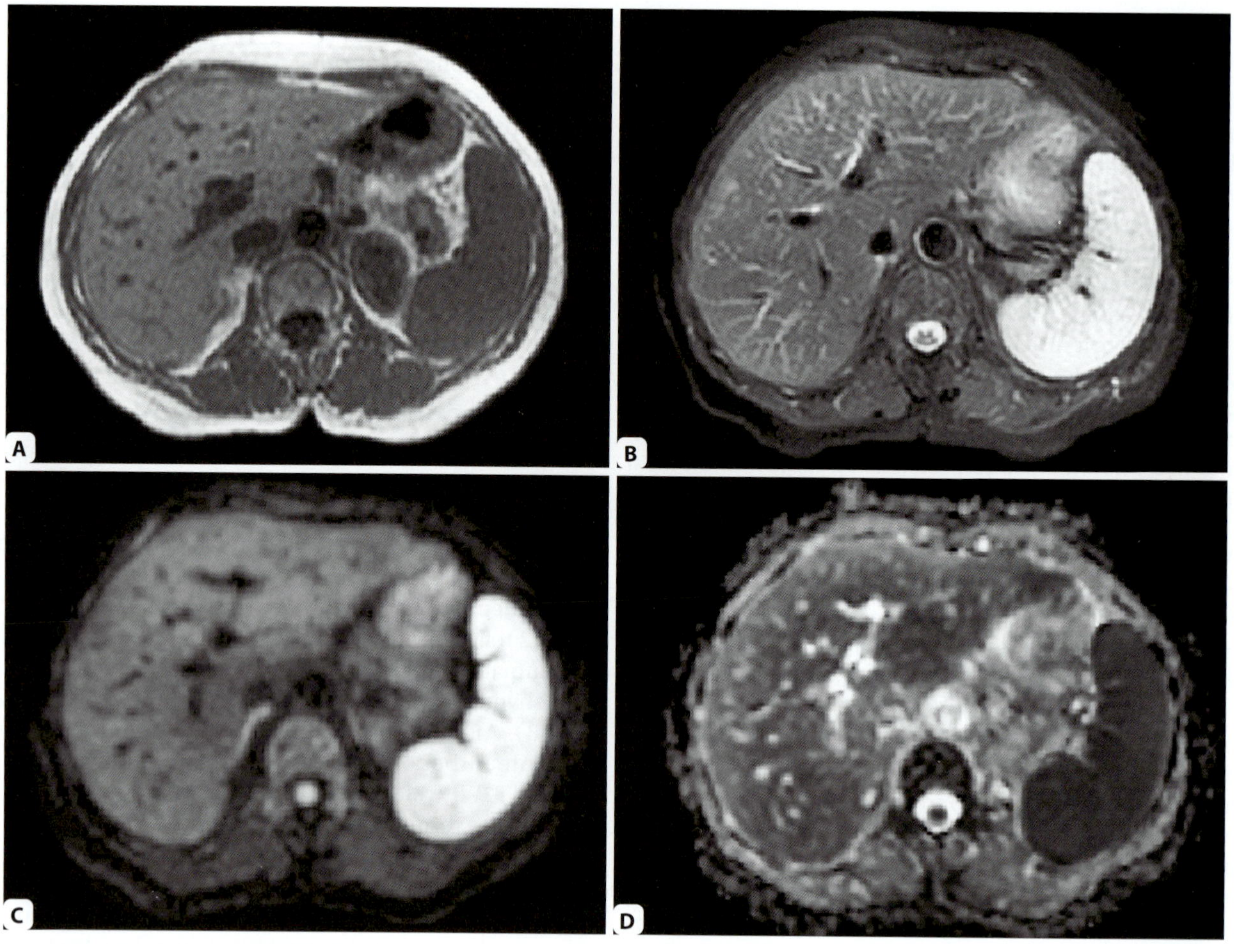

FIGS. 6A TO D: Axial T1-weighted imaging (T1WI) (A), T2-weighted imaging (T2WI) (B), diffusion-weighted imaging (DWI)-b 1,000 (C), and apparent diffusion coefficient (ADC) map (D) showing T1 hypointensity, T2 hyperintensity, and restricted diffusion on DWI and ADC maps of normal spleen.

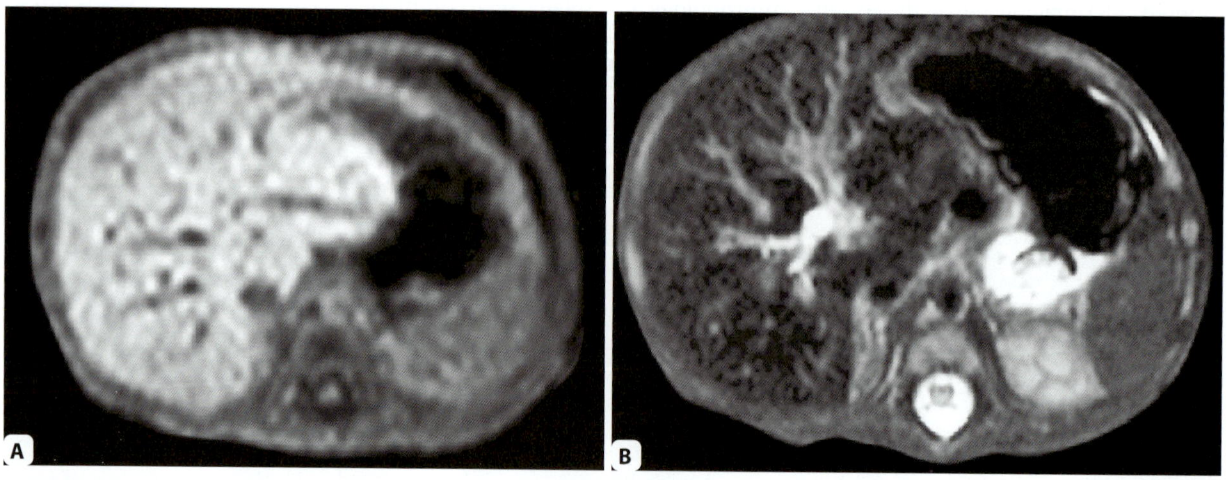

FIGS. 7A AND B: Magnetic resonance imaging (MRI) T1-weighted imaging (T1WI) (A) and T2-weighted imaging (T2WI) (B) images showing normal hypointense spleen in a neonate.

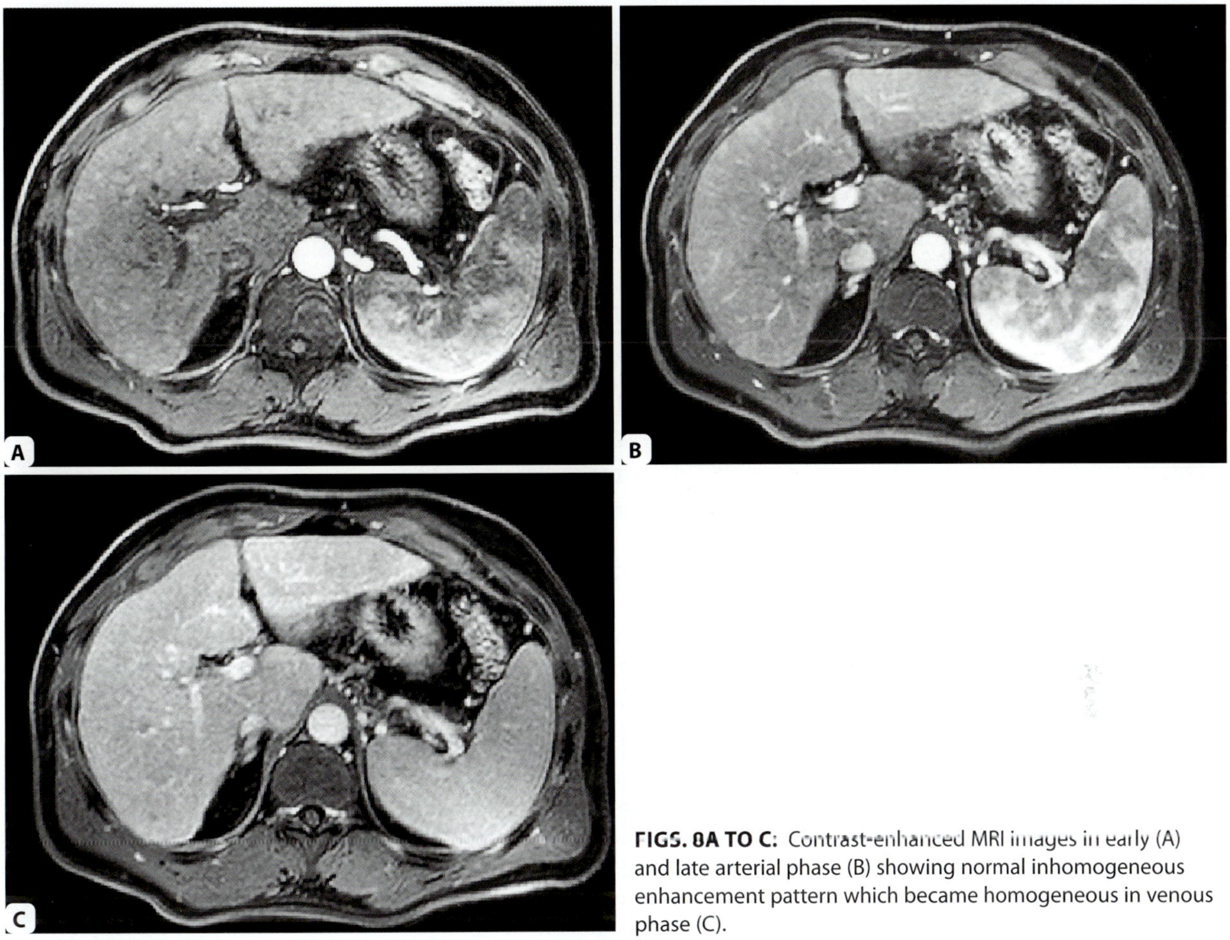

FIGS. 8A TO C: Contrast-enhanced MRI images in early (A) and late arterial phase (B) showing normal inhomogeneous enhancement pattern which became homogeneous in venous phase (C).

Scintigraphy

Scintigraphic splenic imaging involves the use of technetium-99m–labeled sulfur colloid. The tracer is taken up by the reticuloendothelial system and hence is helpful for the assessment of splenic congenital anomalies, e.g., splenic ectopia, accessory spleen, splenic hamartoma, etc.

Positron Emission Tomography/Computed Tomography

It plays a role in evaluation of staging for lymphoma. Involvement of the spleen can be more accurately assessed using ^{18}F-fluorodeoxyglucose positron-emission tomography (FDG-PET) or fused PET/CT.[14]

Angiography

The high quality of images provided by cross-sectional imaging techniques has led to a dramatic change in the indications for splenic artery angiography. This technique is now seldom used for diagnostic purpose; however, it is widely used for vascular interventions for the management of splenic artery aneurysms and traumatic splenic injuries. CT angiography and MR angiography offer excellent visualization of the spleen and its vessels for diagnostic purposes.

SPLENIC SIZE

On USG, the measurement of splenic length is done by measuring maximum distance on a longitudinal coronal view obtained at the level of splenic hilum, between the most inferolateral and the most superomedial points **(Fig. 3C)**. CT and MRI also readily allow for more standardized and reproducible measurement. Splenic volume can be readily measured with CT or MRI.

Normal splenic size in children and adolescents varies according to age and the upper limit of normal at various age range are given in **Table 3**. In a normal adult, the spleen measures approximately 12 cm in length, 4 cm in thickness, and 7 cm in anteroposterior (AP) diameter. However, due to high variability in the shape of the spleen, these measurements are not very useful in evaluating splenic size. A more precise approach for the estimation of splenic volume is the splenic index, a product of length, width, and thickness of the spleen, expressed in centimeters **(Figs. 9A to C)**. Length is determined by summing the number of contiguous sections on which the

TABLE 3: Spleen length in children and adolescents.*[16]

Group	No.	10th percentile	Median	90th percentile	Upper limit
0–3 months	28	3.3	4.5	5.8	6.0
3–6 months	13	4.9	5.3	6.4	6.5
6–12 months	17	5.2	6.2	6.8	7.0
1–2 years	12	5.4	6.9	7.5	8.0
2–4 years	24	6.4	7.4	8.6	9.0
4–6 years	39	6.9	7.8	8.8	9.5
6–8 years	21	7.0	8.2	9.6	10.0
8–10 years	16	7.9	9.2	10.5	11.0
10–12 years	17	8.6	9.9	10.9	11.5
12–15 years	26	8.7	10.1	11.4	12.0
15–20 years (male)	5	9.0	10.0	11.7	12.0
15–20 years (female)	12	10.1	11.2	12.6	13.0

*All measurements are in centimeters.

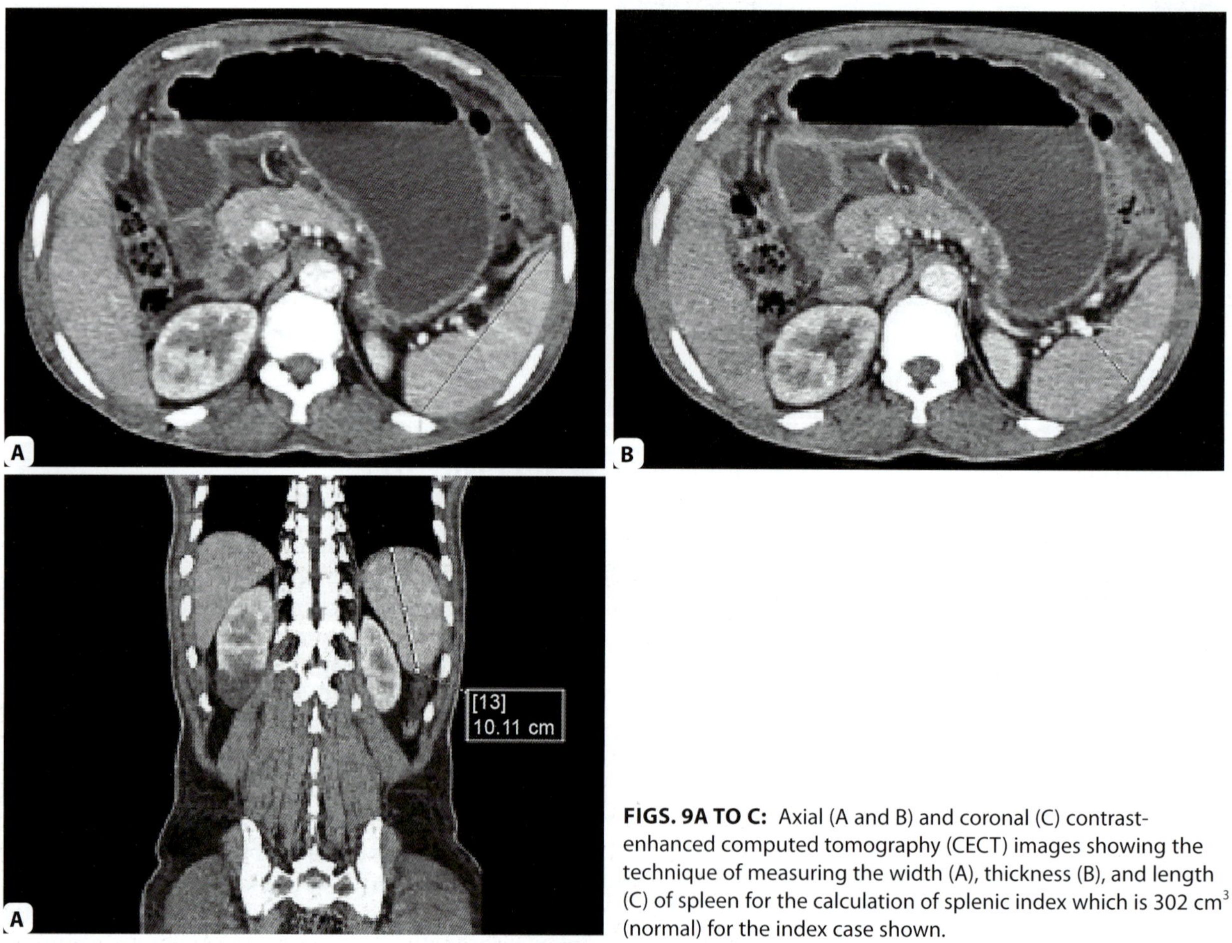

FIGS. 9A TO C: Axial (A and B) and coronal (C) contrast-enhanced computed tomography (CECT) images showing the technique of measuring the width (A), thickness (B), and length (C) of spleen for the calculation of splenic index which is 302 cm^3 (normal) for the index case shown.

spleen is visible or simpler is to measure the craniocaudal length in coronal reconstruction. Width is the longest AP splenic diameter in an axial image. Thickness is measured between the inner and outer borders of the spleen, at the level of the splenic hilum (normal splenic index is 120–480 cm^3).[15]

NORMAL VARIANTS/ DEVELOPMENTAL ANOMALIES

Various developmental anomalies are seen resulting from deficient fusion of separate splenic masses of the dorsal mesogastrium during embryogenesis. These include complete agenesis, persistent lobulations **(Fig. 10)**, clefts **(Figs. 11A and B)**, notches, and isolated small splenunculi and polysplenia.

Splenunculus/Accessory Spleen

Accessory spleen is the most frequent congenital abnormality of the spleen. They can be found virtually anywhere in the abdomen **(Figs. 12A and B)**, but the most common sites are hilus and vascular pedicle of the spleen, around tail of the pancreas, along the greater curvature of the stomach, greater omentum, mesentery, near left ovary or left testicle and in the pouch of Douglas.[17] Splenunculi are found in 10–44% of autopsies.[18] They are usually found incidentally on imaging done for unrelated reasons and generally require no treatment. The clinical significance of accessory spleen is that after splenectomy, the accessory spleen may dramatically enlarge and cause recurrence of symptoms if splenectomy was done for some hematologic or other disorders. Intrapancreatic location of accessory splenic tissue is also described, which may, if missed at surgery, be a cause of recurrence of the symptoms **(Figs. 12C and D)**. It enhances markedly in the arterial phase and is a rare differential diagnosis for neuroendocrine tumor of the pancreas. Splenunculi are usually six or fewer in number and they have histological features same as primary organ and blood supply is from a branch of the splenic artery.[17] They rarely exceed 2 cm in diameter and can be confused with splenic hilar or peripancreatic lymph nodes. Splenunculi can be identified on imaging modalities such as ultrasound, CT, or MRI, as of same attenuation or signal intensity as that of normal spleen **(Figs. 12E and F)** both before as well as after intravenous administration of contrast material but when there is doubt ^{99m}Tc sulfur colloid liver-spleen scan is definitive. Ectopic splenic tissue can also be found due to acquired causes such as trauma (splenosis).

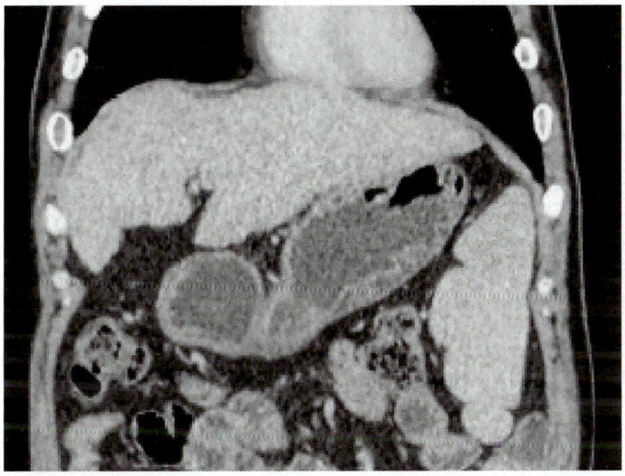

FIG. 10: Contrast-enhanced CT images (coronal reformat) showing prominent lobules of splenic tissue on medial and inferior aspect of spleen (suggesting persistence of fetal lobulations).

Wandering Spleen

Spleen changing its position within the abdomen due to ligamentous laxity, traumatic injury, and maldevelopment of suspensory ligaments is referred to as wandering spleen. It may present as mobile unexplained mass in the abdomen or may present with acute pain in the abdomen, if torsion occurs.

It is thought to result from congenital abnormal fusion of the posterior mesogastrium.[19] Incidence of wandering

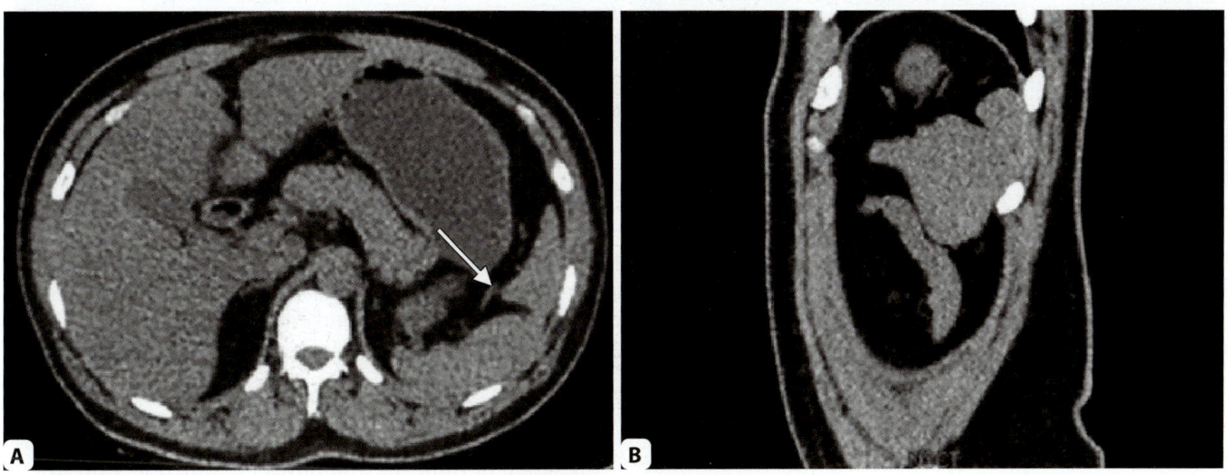

FIGS. 11A AND B: Noncontrast CT images [axial (A) and sagittal (B) reformat] showing splenic cleft (arrow). This may be confused with laceration in case of history of trauma.

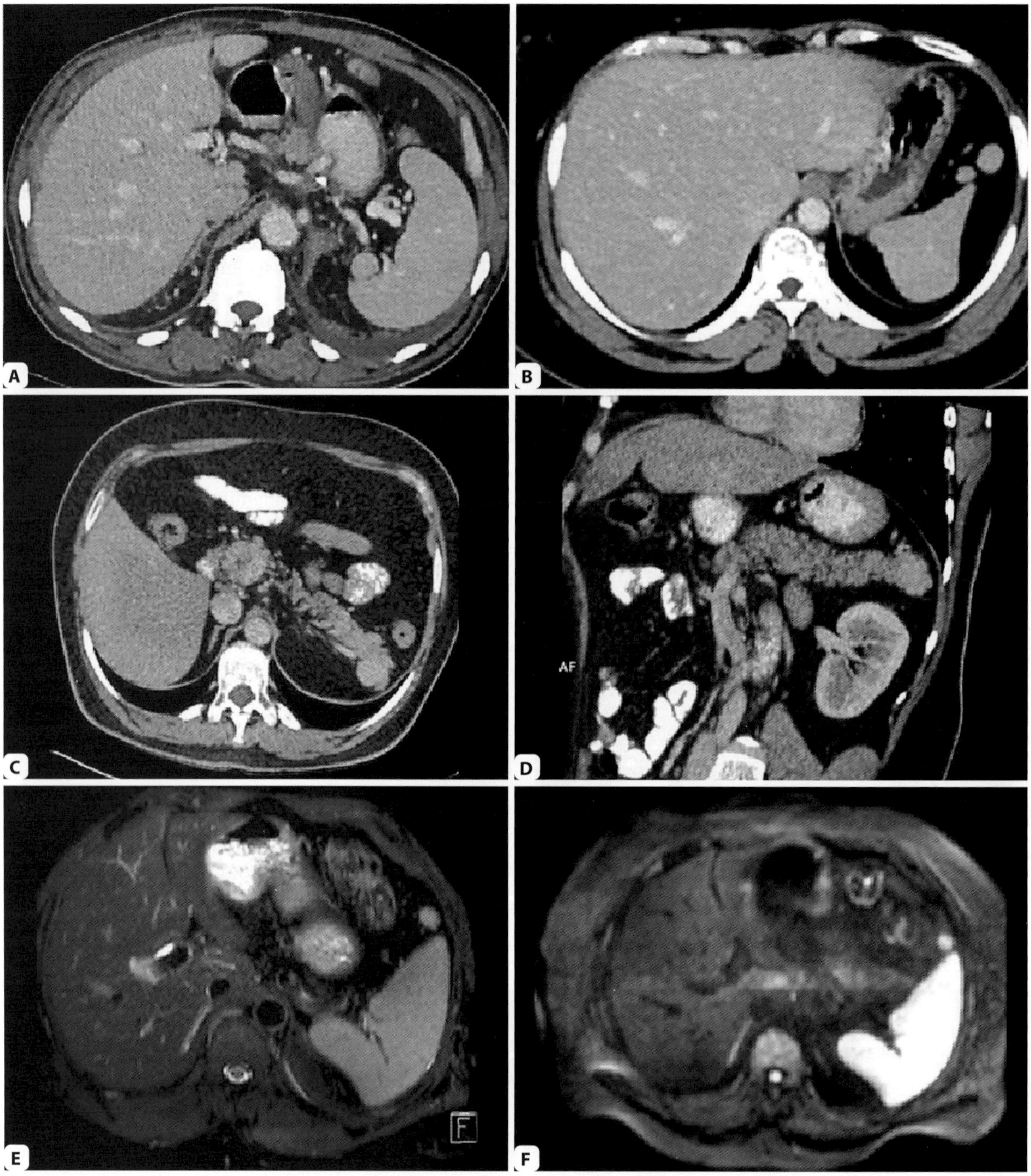

FIGS. 12A TO F: Axial contrast-enhanced CT images showing small rounded nodular well-defined structures having same enhancement as spleen at hilum (A), near pole (B), and within pancreatic parenchyma (C and D). Axial T2-weighted image (T2WI) MRI image (E) and b-1,000 diffusion-weighted image (F) reveal splenunculus showing similar T2 hyperintensity and restricted diffusion respectively as an adjacent normal spleen.

spleen is higher in multiparous women. On imaging, the changing position of the spleen can be determined on USG. CT **(Figs. 13A and B)** also can depict the same and in case of torsion may show a "whorled appearance" of splenic pedicle. Splenic infarcts, ascites, and pancreatic tail necrosis can also be identified.

Polysplenia

Presence of multiple splenules is known as polysplenia. It is seen in association with left-sided atrial isomerism syndrome and is more common in females than males. Patients with polysplenia may be asymptomatic or

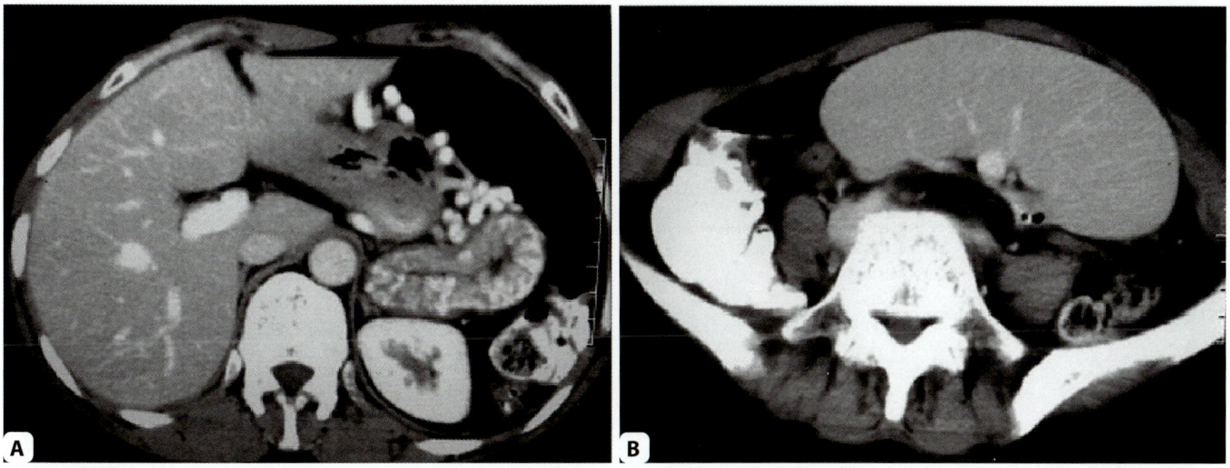

FIGS. 13A AND B: Axial contrast-enhanced CT showing absence of spleen in left upper abdomen (A) with centrally and inferiorly located spleen in lower abdomen (B).

symptoms may occur due to congenital heart disease, biliary atresia, or intestinal malrotation. On imaging, numerous small splenic masses are seen in the left **(Fig. 14)** or right hypochondrium.

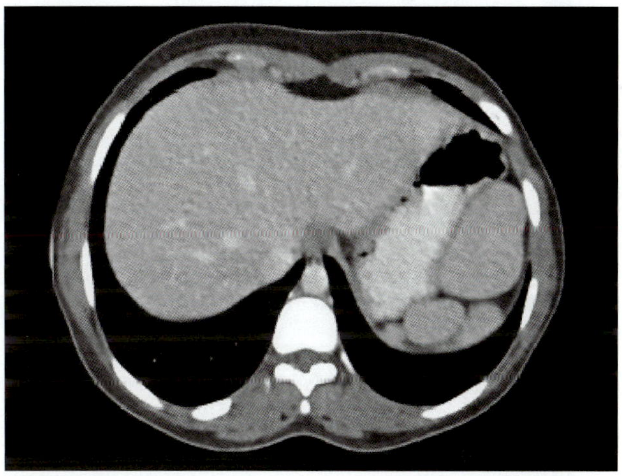

FIG. 14: Axial contrast-enhanced CT showing multiple small splenic masses in left subphrenic region suggestive of polysplenia.

Asplenia

Congenital absence of spleen is termed "asplenia" and it is seen in association with situs ambiguous. The condition is more common in males and association with congenital heart diseases is seen in 99–100% of the patients.[20]

CYSTIC LESIONS OF SPLEEN

The cystic lesions of the spleen can be primary (true) or secondary (pseudocyst) cysts, depending on whether there is cellular or fibrous lining respectively.[21]

Primary cysts are divided into parasitic and nonparasitic. Primary nonparasitic cysts may be of epithelial origin (congenital cysts), such as epidermoid, dermoid, or transitional cell cysts, or of endothelial origin, such as lymphatic malformations and hemangiomas. Primary parasitic cysts include echinococcal cysts. Secondary/false or pseudocysts may form secondary to trauma, hematoma, infarction-degeneration or inflammation.

Congenital Cysts

Congenital or epithelial splenic cysts such as epidermoid, dermoid, or transitional cell cysts, account for about 25% of primary cysts of the spleen.[21] They are usually solitary, but can be multiple, and are commonly seen in pediatric population and young adults. The exact etiopathogenesis of congenital splenic cysts is unknown. In general, these cysts are asymptomatic. Symptoms develop due to increase in size, trauma, hemorrhage, rupture, or infection of the cyst.

When symptomatic, surgery in the form of partial or total splenectomy is the treatment of choice.

On USG, these cysts are generally anechoic, or may show fine internal echoes. CT shows splenic cysts as being characteristically spherical and well-defined lesions **(Figs. 15A to C)**. Attenuation value of near water and a thin or imperceptible nonenhancing wall are other features of a congenital cyst.[22] Internal debris, hemorrhage, and peripheral calcifications of the cyst wall may give a more complex picture.

Epidermoid cyst **(Figs. 15D to G)** has a complex imaging appearance due to epithelial peripheral trabeculations causing thickening and irregularity of the posterior wall and due to presence of internal blood clots.

False Cyst (Pseudocyst)

False cysts/pseudocysts are lined by dense fibrous tissue which is often calcified and have no epithelial lining, and account for approximately 75% of the cysts of the spleen.[21]

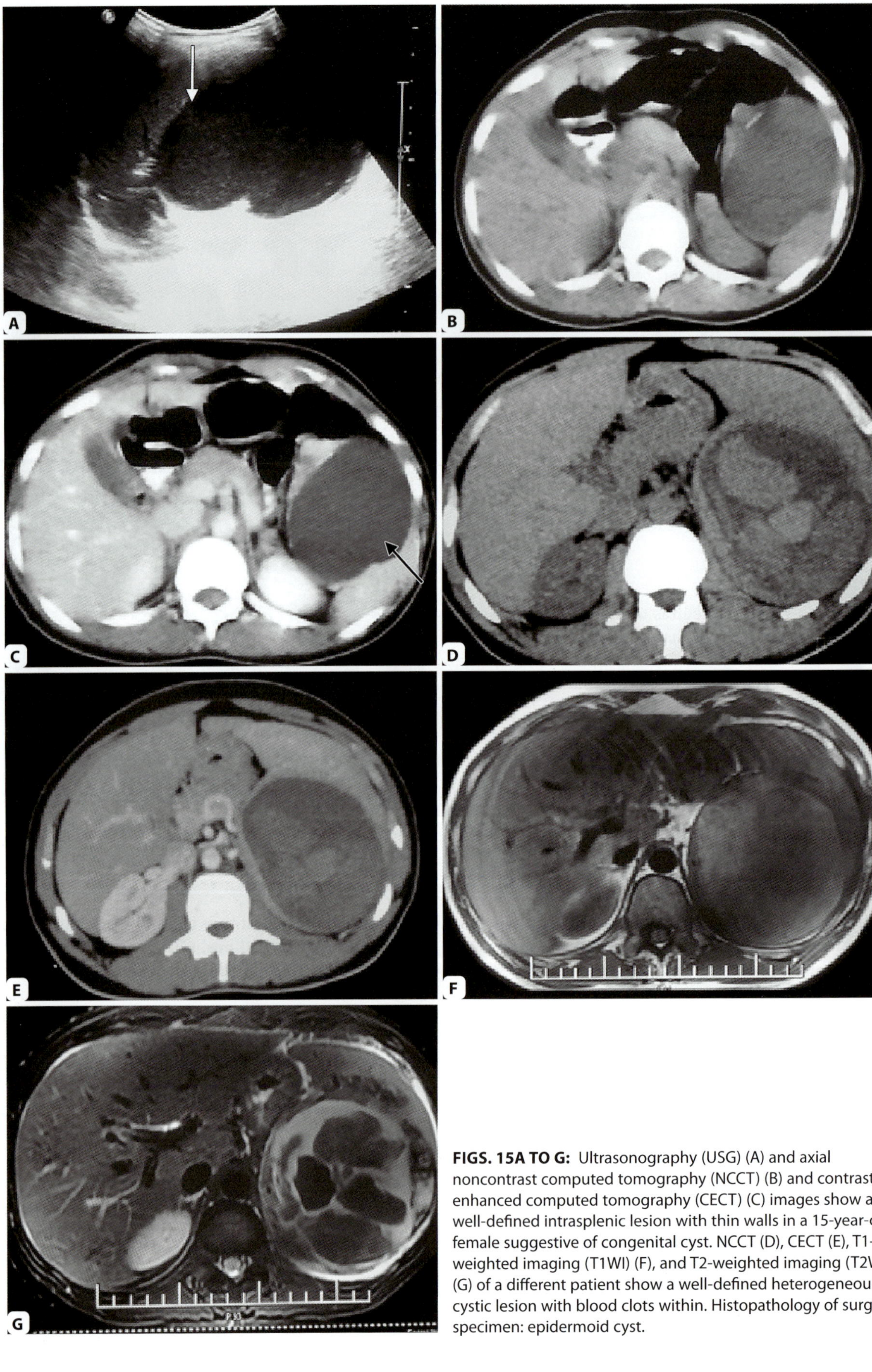

FIGS. 15A TO G: Ultrasonography (USG) (A) and axial noncontrast computed tomography (NCCT) (B) and contrast-enhanced computed tomography (CECT) (C) images show a well-defined intrasplenic lesion with thin walls in a 15-year-old female suggestive of congenital cyst. NCCT (D), CECT (E), T1-weighted imaging (T1WI) (F), and T2-weighted imaging (T2WI) (G) of a different patient show a well-defined heterogeneous cystic lesion with blood clots within. Histopathology of surgical specimen: epidermoid cyst.

Trauma, infarction, or infection are common causes. The most apparent etiologic factor is trauma. The majority of these cysts are solitary and asymptomatic. Cyst contains mostly blood and necrotic debris. It is often not possible to differentiate between primary and secondary cysts based on radiological appearance alone **(Figs. 16A and B)**. Patient's history and clinical presentation may sometimes help to narrow the differential diagnosis.

Echinococcal Cyst

Splenic involvement by hydatid disease is uncommon. It can be seen in endemic areas. Clinical findings are nonspecific and patients may present with abdominal pain, fever, and splenomegaly.

Ultrasonography demonstrates a cystic lesion which is either anechoic or with internal debris, membranes, daughter cysts or calcification depending upon the stage of cyst growth.

The three layers of hydatid cyst consist of the following:
1. The outer pericyst, composed of modified host cells that form a dense and fibrous protective zone.
2. Middle laminated layer, which is also referred to as ectocyst, allows passage of nutrients.
3. Inner germinal layer, where the scolices (the larval stage of the parasite) and the laminated membrane are produced. The true wall of the cyst is formed by this innermost germinal layer.

Daughter cysts are small spherical vesicles formed from the rest of the germinal layer and contain the protoscolices. Cyst fluid secreted by the germinal layer is antigenic and may also contain scolices. When vesicles rupture within the cyst, scolices are mixed with cyst fluid and form white sediment known as "hydatid sand".

Imaging features on USG, CT, or MRI depend on the stage of growth of the cyst, i.e., whether it is unilocular, have daughter vesicles, partially calcified or completely calcified signifying a dead parasite.

The ultrasonographic appearance of hydatid cysts are:
- A well-defined anechoic cyst **(see Fig. 17C)**.
- A well-defined anechoic cyst with hydatid sand.
- Detachment of the endocyst from pericyst resulting in "floating membranes" within the cavity.
- The honeycomb pattern due to the presence of daughter cysts.
- Calcification of either cyst wall or internal matrix. Partial calcification of the cyst does not always indicate the death of the parasite, nevertheless, densely calcified cysts may be assumed to be inactive.

Infected hydatid may give an appearance of abscess with thick irregular walls and internal debris and lose its characteristic sonographic appearance.

The CT scans show the cyst as a well-defined, round, or oval cystic mass of near water density **(Figs. 17A to E)**. A multilocular appearance may be seen with the presence of multiple low-attenuating daughter cysts. Detached membranes can be seen as curvilinear increased attenuation areas within the cyst. Homogeneous higher attenuation within the lesion is frequently encountered and may occur secondary to the formation of daughter cysts or as a result of the collection of dense debris (hydatid sand) within the cyst. Enhancement of internal septations may be seen with contrast administration. Calcification of cyst wall or internal septa is easily detected at CT.

Splenic hydatid cysts are T1-hypointense and T2-hyperintense on MRI. Collagen makes the pericyst to appear T1 and T2 hypointense and this low-signal intensity rim on T2WI has been proposed as a characteristic sign of hydatid cyst. MR also demonstrates daughter cysts as hypo- to isointense on T1WI and isointense on T2WI relative to hyperintense hydatid fluid of the mother cyst. The floating membranes appear as low-intensity structures within the degenerating cyst. Intraparenchymal rupture of the cyst appears as a defect in the low intensity rim. Thick calcifications may produce a signal void on MRI, however, are better demonstrated by CT.

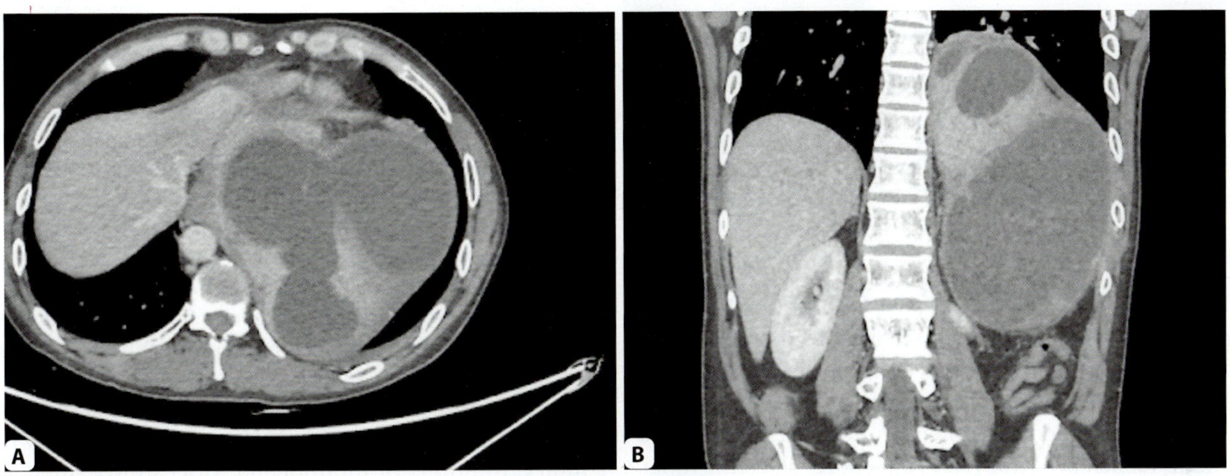

FIGS. 16A AND B: Splenic pseudocyst. Axial (A) and coronal (B) contrast-enhanced computed tomography (CECT) abdomen shows thin-walled, multiloculated, intrasplenic cystic lesion with internal fluid density involving predominantly the lower pole of the spleen. No calcifications or solid enhancing components are seen within the lesion.

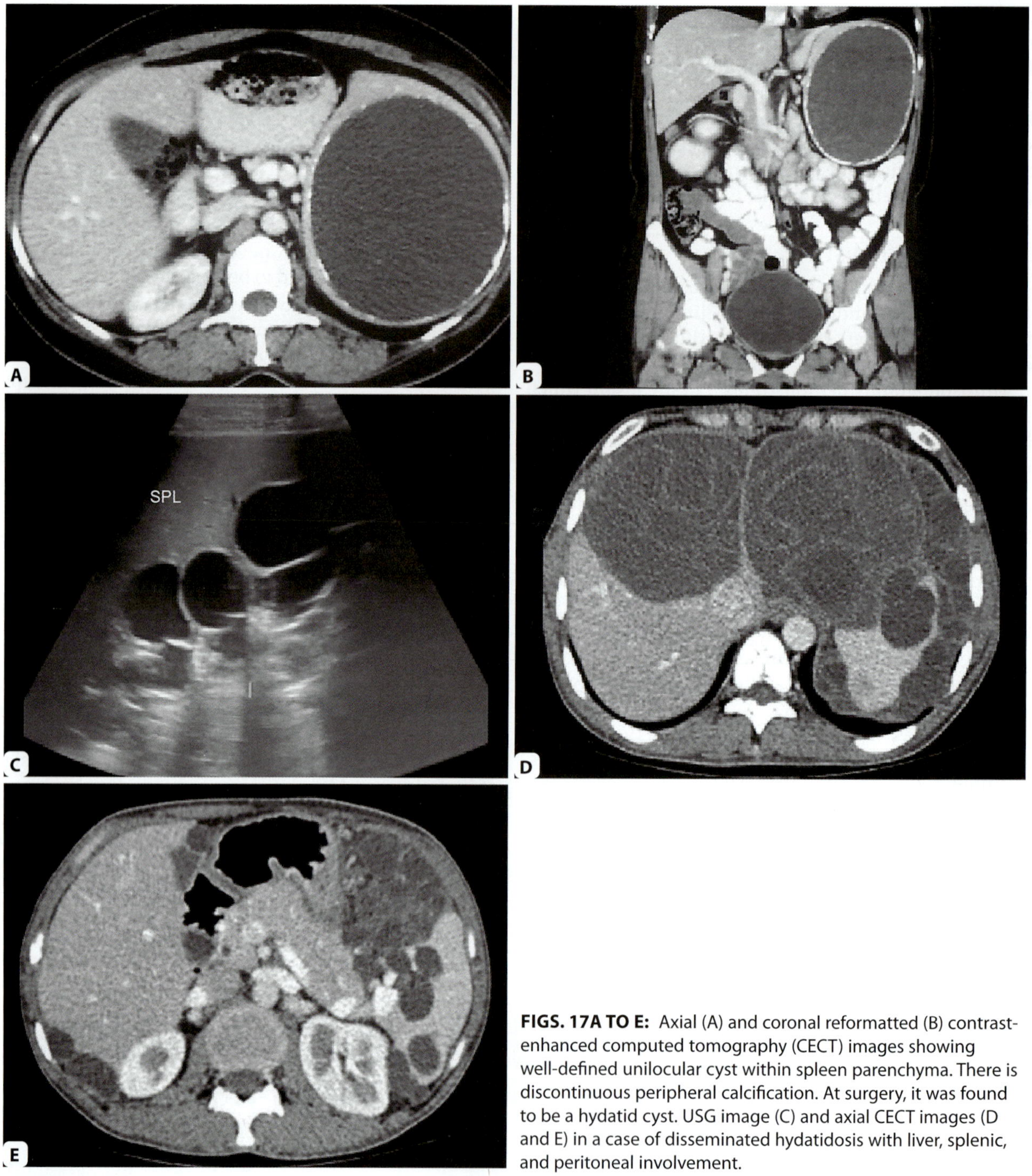

FIGS. 17A TO E: Axial (A) and coronal reformatted (B) contrast-enhanced computed tomography (CECT) images showing well-defined unilocular cyst within spleen parenchyma. There is discontinuous peripheral calcification. At surgery, it was found to be a hydatid cyst. USG image (C) and axial CECT images (D and E) in a case of disseminated hydatidosis with liver, splenic, and peritoneal involvement.

INFECTIOUS DISEASES OF SPLEEN

Involvement of the spleen in systemic infectious processes is commonly seen in immunocompromised patients, and the prevalence has increased as a result of the increased use of steroids and chemotherapeutic agents and human immunodeficiency virus (HIV) infection.[11] Bacteria, fungi, and *Mycobacterium tuberculosis* are frequent agents. Splenic involvement can also occur in immunocompetent hosts with cat scratch disease, granulomatous diseases such as histoplasmosis, parasitic diseases such as hydatid cyst, and viral infections. Nonspecific splenomegaly can be seen in viral infections and enteric fever.

Splenic abscesses are localized collections of pus and they are found in 0.14–0.7% of autopsy cases.[23] It may be solitary, multiple, or multilocular. USG shows single or multiple hypoechoic to frankly anechoic lesions. Larger lesions may show internal echoes or septations. On CT and

MRI, the abscess appears as a lesion of fluid attenuation or signal intensity respectively and shows peripheral enhancement on contrast administration when the capsule develops **(Figs. 18A and B)**.

Bacterial causes of splenic abscess include infection with aerobic organisms, commonly *Staphylococcus, Streptococcus, Escherichia coli,* and *Salmonella*. The route of infection is mainly hematogenous (75%), penetrating trauma (15%), and prior splenic infarction (10%).[21] The factors leading to involvement of the spleen are metastatic infection (bacterial endocarditis and sepsis), contiguous infection (pancreatitis and periphrenic abscess), embolic noninfectious events causing ischemia and superadded infection, trauma, and immunodeficiency.[24]

On CT and MRI, the lesion shows thick, irregular, and dense peripheral enhancing rim with internal nonenhancing area. Sometimes, air foci may also be seen within the bacterial abscesses. Peripheral enhancement of the wall of the abscess on a venous phase CT is less often seen than in liver abscesses. Postgadolinium MRI is more sensitive to depict the rim enhancement.

Fungal abscesses are mainly seen in immunocompromised patients including postsolid organ transplantation, patients on chemotherapy for malignancy or leukemia and children with immunodeficiency, such as chronic granulomatous disease. *Candida albicans, Aspergillus fumigatus,* and *Cryptococcus neoformans* are the commonly encountered fungi. Fungal infections of the spleen are mostly due to hematogenous spread and form microabscesses in the splenic parenchyma which may not be detectable on imaging at times even in the presence of disseminated infection and may only present with diffuse splenomegaly. When visible on CT, fungal abscesses are seen as multiple well-defined small hypoattenuating lesions and vary from a few millimeters to 2 cm in size. Rim enhancement is usually not seen. Occasionally, CT may demonstrate a wheel within a wheel pattern/bulls-eye (e.g., Candidial infection) or a central focus of higher attenuation corresponding to ultrasound findings (echoic lesion with central hypoechoic nidus due to necrosis containing fungal elements). Histoplasmosis of the spleen demonstrates multiple scattered hypointense lesions on both T1WI and T2WI on MRI **(Figs. 19A to D)**. Old granulomas can be calcified.

Tuberculosis

Splenic involvement is seen in 80–100% of autopsies of disseminated tuberculosis since it has a rich network of reticuloendothelial cells.[25] Three forms of splenic involvement include splenomegaly, micronodular/miliary, and macronodular form. USG may show normal spleen or mild heterogeneous echotexture whereas CT may demonstrate multiple low-density intrasplenic foci with nodules that range from 0.5 to 2.0 mm in diameter in the micronodular form of disease **(Figs. 20A to D)**. Macronodular form manifests as solitary or multifocal 1–3 cm sized lesions which are hypodense on CT **(Figs. 21A to F)**, and sometimes show peripheral rim of enhancement and may demonstrate calcification. MRI features vary depending on the stage of evolution of tuberculomas. A tuberculoma with central caseous necrosis appears as a centrally nonenhancing lesion with peripheral enhancement and this is one of their typical features. Such caseous necrosis might show hypointensity or hyperintensity on T2WI. The reason for the variable signal on T2WI is not clearly understood; however, internal hypointensity could suggest more solid caseation **(Fig. 21C)**.[26] Lesions with no central caseous necrosis may demonstrate gradual peripheral enhancement with complete fill-in of the lesions. Other imaging findings may be abdominal lymphadenopathy with low central attenuation, high-attenuation ascites with nodular peritoneal thickening, hepatomegaly, and pleural effusion.

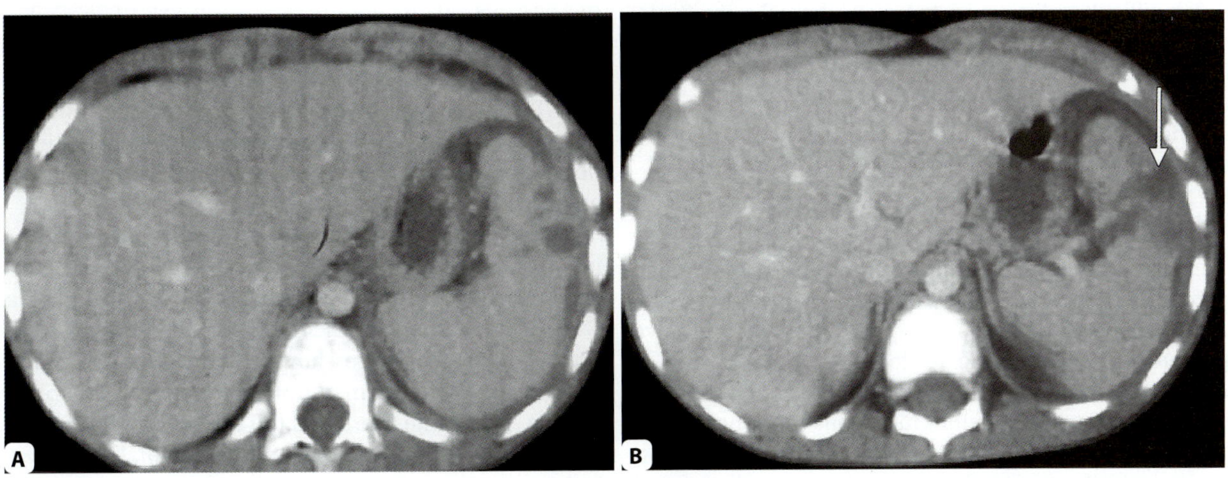

FIGS. 18A AND B: Axial contrast-enhanced computed tomography (CECT) images (A and B) showing multiple small peripherally enhancing lesions in the spleen suggestive of abscesses. Presence of perisplenic fluid (arrow) indicates rupture.

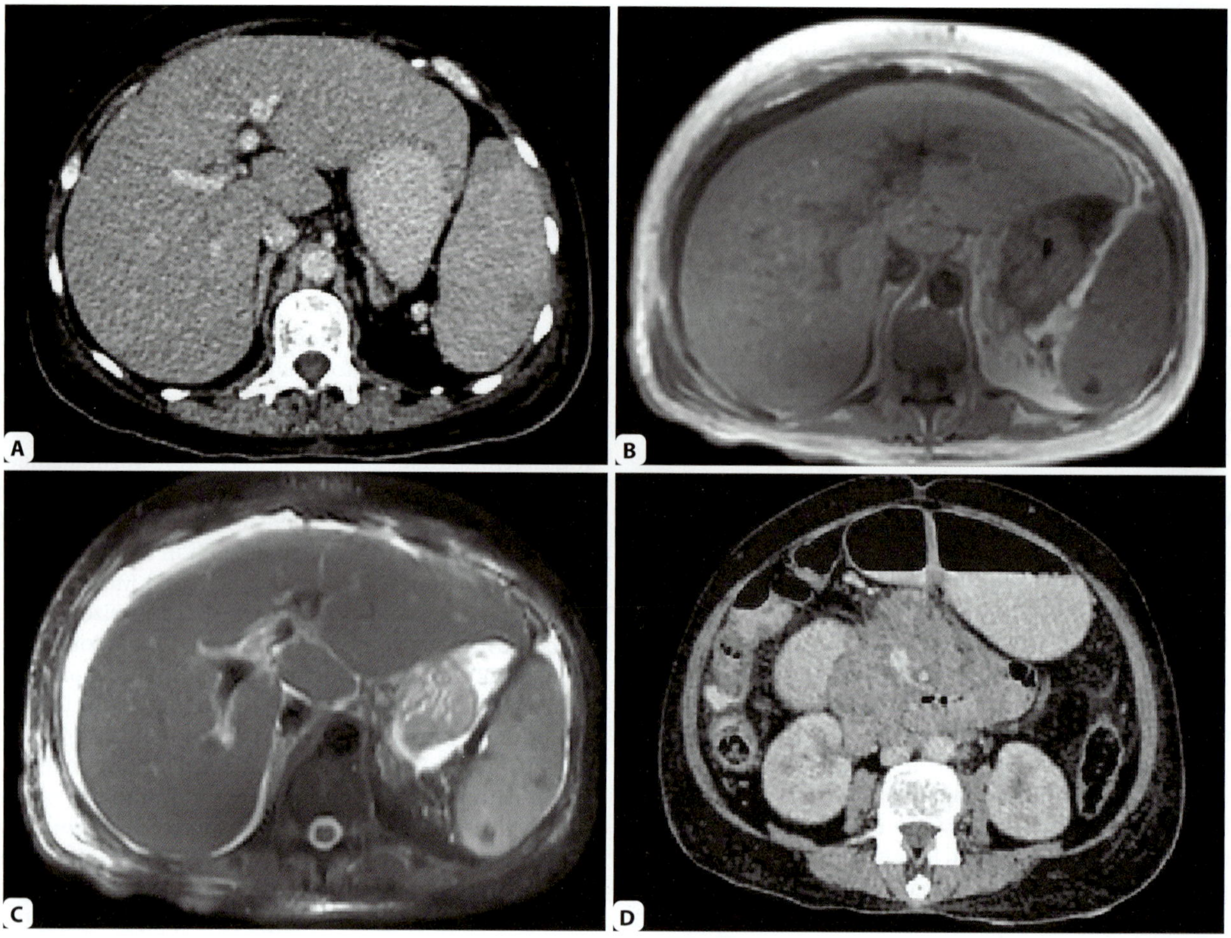

FIGS. 19A TO D: Axial contrast-enhanced computed tomography (CECT) image (A) showing ill-defined focal lesions in spleen. Axial T1-weighted image (T1WI) (B) and T2-weighted image (T2WI) (C) shows hypointense lesions on both sequences. Axial CECT image (D) showing multiple lymph nodes with necrosis—Biopsy proven histoplasmosis.

Other organ involvement or presence of necrotic lymph nodes makes a diagnosis of tuberculosis more certain.

It is difficult to distinguish between tubercular, pyogenic, and disseminated fungal infections as well as leukemic and lymphomatous infiltration. FNAC from splenic focal lesions is required to reach a definitive diagnosis if there is no other focus of tuberculosis or in case of nonresponders to treatment.

Splenic Infarcts

Splenic infarcts are a relatively common entity. It is usually secondary to arterial occlusion. The various recognized causes of splenic infarct are arterial embolism, massive splenomegaly secondary to myeloproliferative disorders or hematological malignancies, storage disorders, lymphoma, portal hypertension, torsion, infectious mononucleosis, etc. Imaging findings of splenic infarct depend upon the "age of infarct". On USG, it is seen as an ill-defined hypoechoic area in acute phase which progressively becomes more well-defined. In later stage, secondary to fibrosis and calcification it may appear as a hyperechoic area also. Splenic rupture and superimposed infection are complications seen in the areas of infarction.[9]

CT is the imaging investigation of choice for evaluation of splenic infarcts. Imaging should be performed in the portal venous phase, which better depicts the infarcted areas.

On CT, various imaging findings are described for infarcts. There are multiple, heterogeneous areas of patchy enhancement in the acute phase. Typical peripheral, wedge-shaped nonenhancing or hypoenhancing area is seen with further progression with time **(Fig. 22A)**. Entire splenic parenchyma may not enhance, e.g., in splenic torsion. With time, the infarcted area may decrease and sometimes may vanish entirely or may remain as a cystic lesion (pseudocyst).

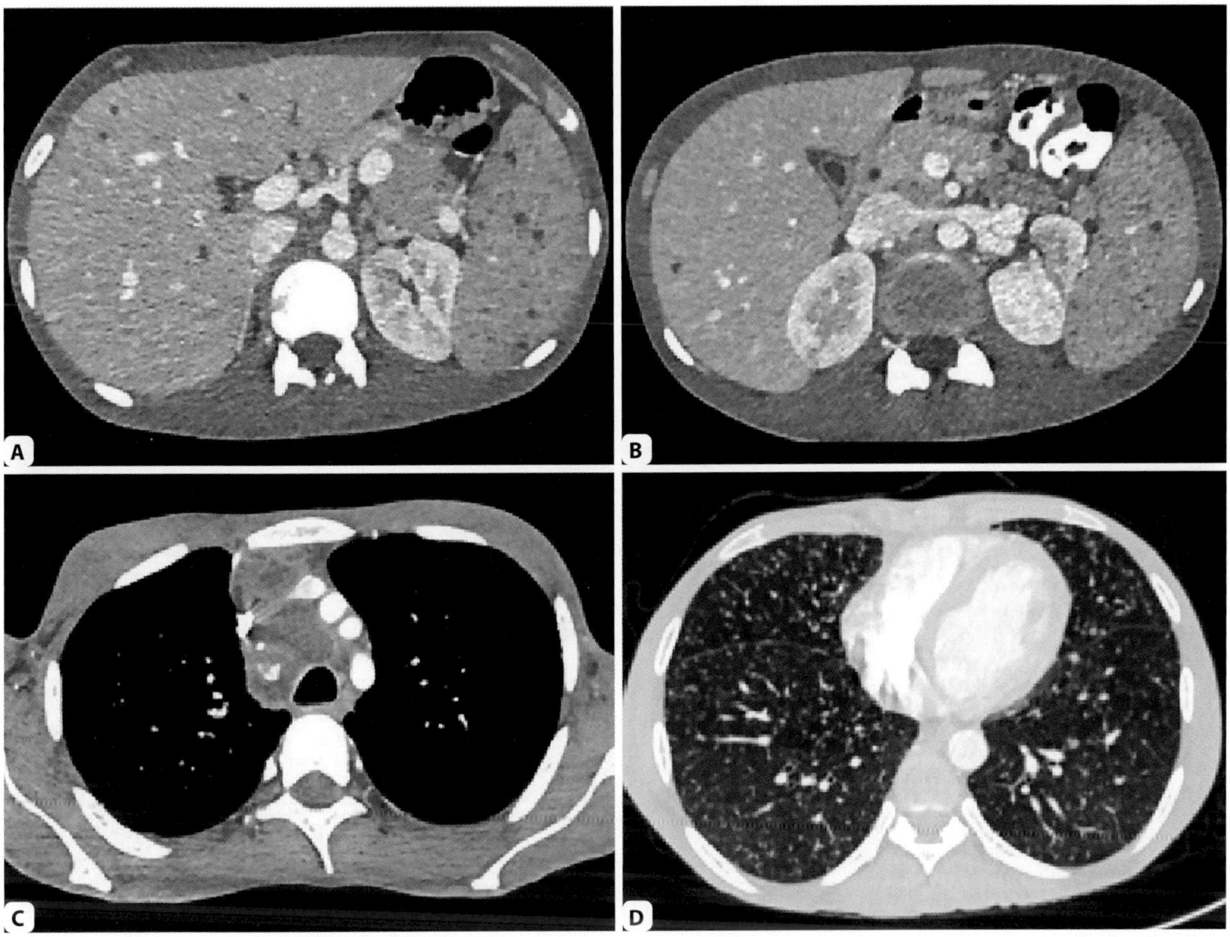

FIGS. 20A TO D: Axial contrast-enhanced computed tomography (CECT) images (A and B) of 20-year-male patient with disseminated tuberculosis showing multiple diffusely scattered tiny hypodense lesions in spleen (arrow). Similar lesions are also noted in liver and pancreas. Mediastinal (C) and lung window images (D) showing necrotic lymph nodes and miliary nodules, respectively.

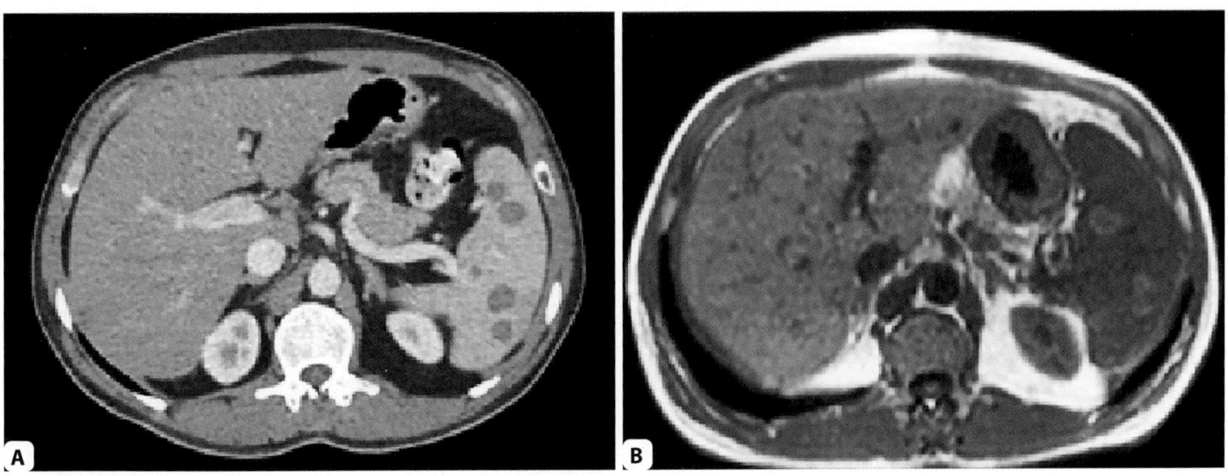

FIGS. 21A TO F: *Continued*

Continued

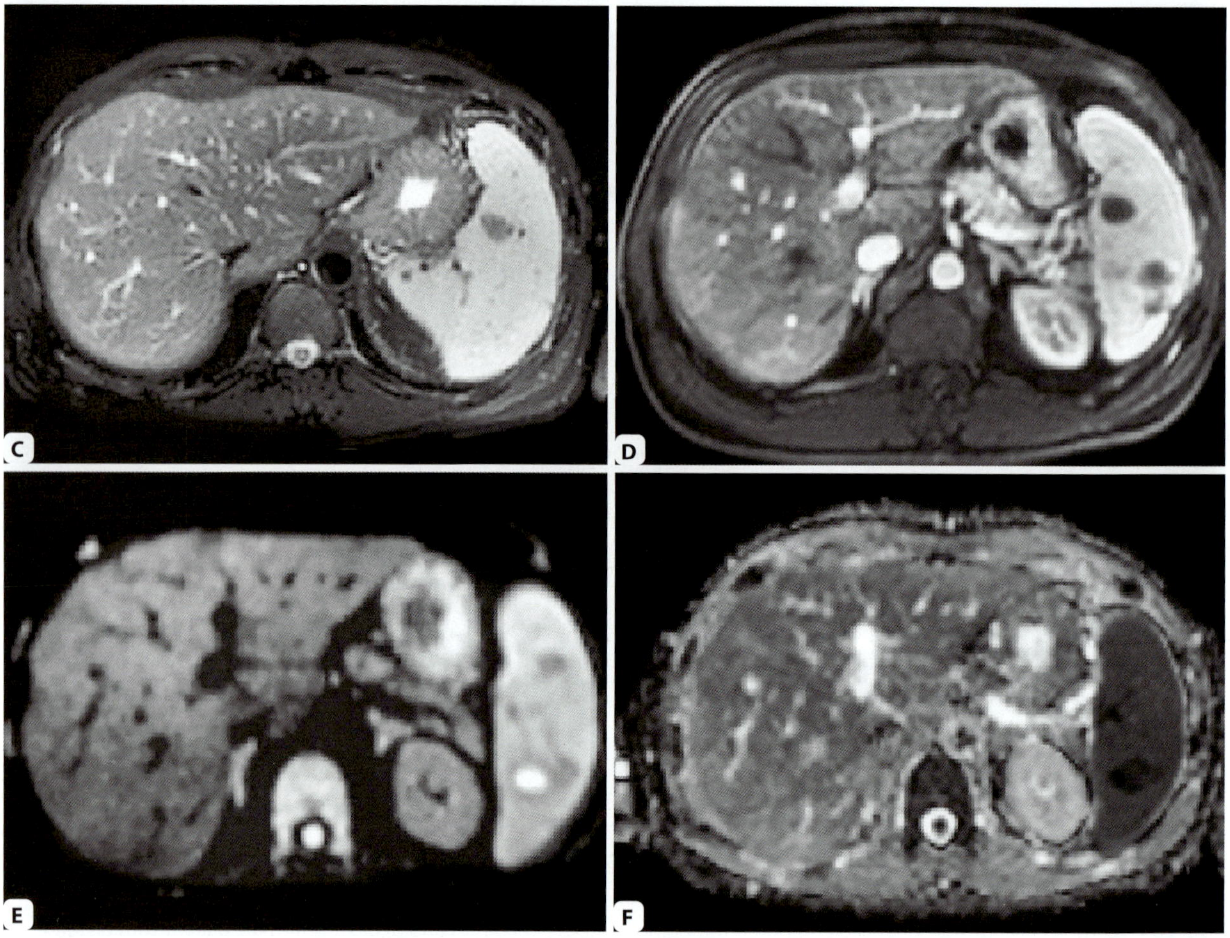

FIGS. 21A TO F: Axial contrast-enhanced computed tomography (CECT) (A) image showing multiple large hypodense lesions in the spleen. Axial MRI images of the same patient, lesions are T1 hyperintense (B), T2 hypointense (C), showing peripheral rim enhancement (D), with diffusion restriction on diffusion-weighted imaging (DWI) (E and F) consistent with macronodular form of tuberculosis (FNAC proven).

MRI shows various signal intensities in splenic infarct based on its chronicity and composition. If infarct is hemorrhagic, it may appear as hyperintense on T1WI as well as T2WI. Chronic infarcts will be relatively well-defined; wedge-shaped and usually have hypointense signal on T1WI and hyperintense signal on T2WI **(Figs. 22A to H)**.[27]

Trauma

Please refer to the chapter on Abdominal Trauma for full discussion of splenic trauma.

Splenic Rupture

Splenic rupture most commonly occurs secondary to significant trauma. However, there are many uncommon causes of splenic rupture other than trauma.[28] This condition of atraumatic splenic rupture has been variously described as "spontaneous", "pathological", or "occult" splenic rupture. Practically, it refers to rupture of spleen in the absence of any perceivable significant injury to spleen. Various causes of atraumatic splenic rupture are malaria, leukemia, lymphomas, secondary to pancreatitis, congestive splenomegaly, amyloidosis, infectious mononucleosis or splenic abscess, etc.

Exact pathogenesis of truly idiopathic splenic rupture (with unknown causes) is still not clear. Majority of these patients have associated splenomegaly. Imaging findings associated with splenic rupture are commonly similar to cases of post-traumatic splenic rupture, however, the incidence of splenomegaly is more common in these atraumatic patients. On USG, fluid with internal echoes is seen in the perisplenic area and peritoneal cavity. Other findings may be subcapsular hematoma and hypoechoic splenic laceration **(Figs. 23A to C)**. CECT will depict similar findings **(Figs. 23B and D)**. On arterial phase CT images, sometimes areas of active extravasation may be seen which signifies ongoing active bleed. MRI may be helpful in deciding the "age" of hematoma. Majority of these patients are treated by surgery.

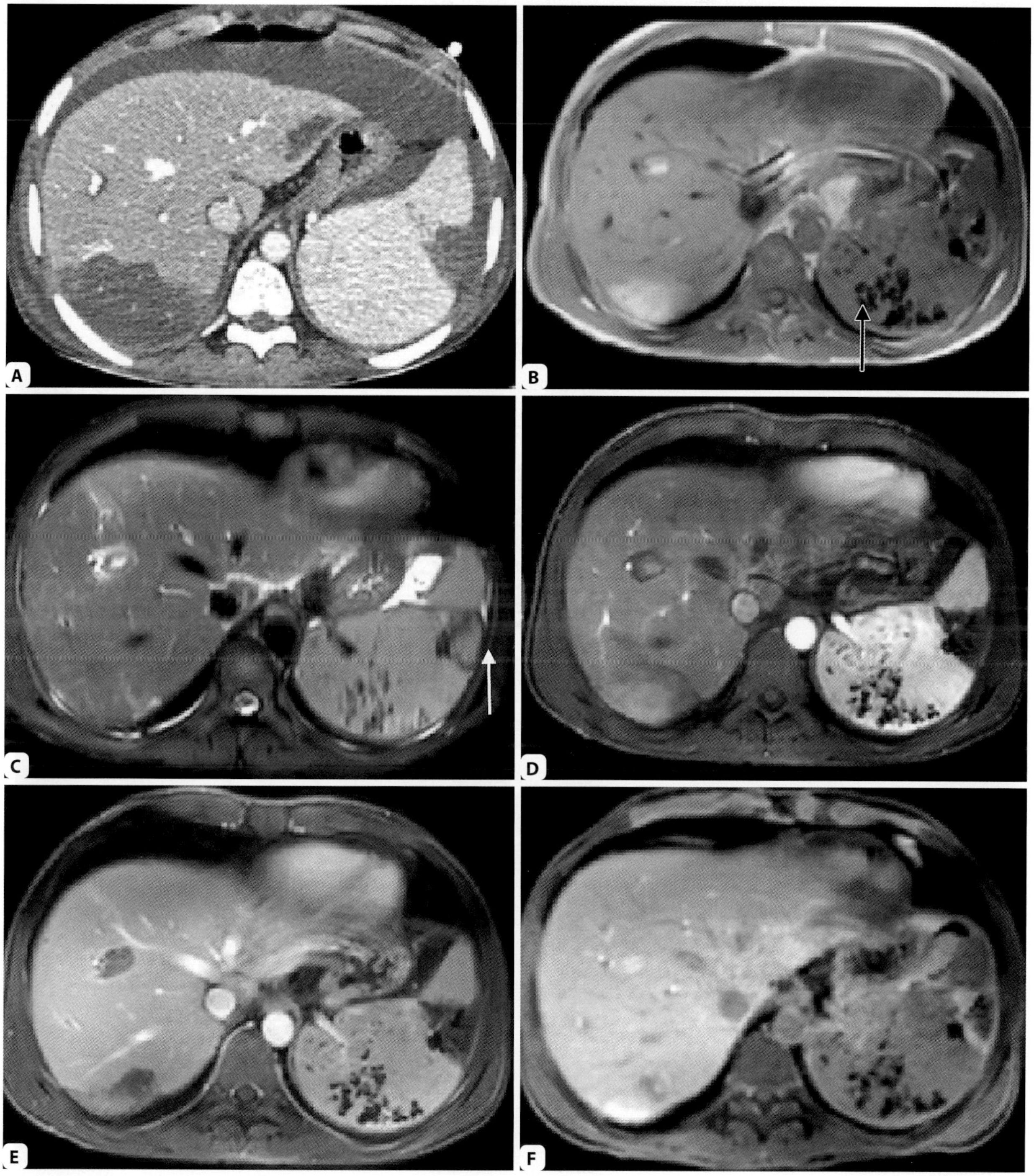

FIGS. 22A TO H: *Continued*

Continued

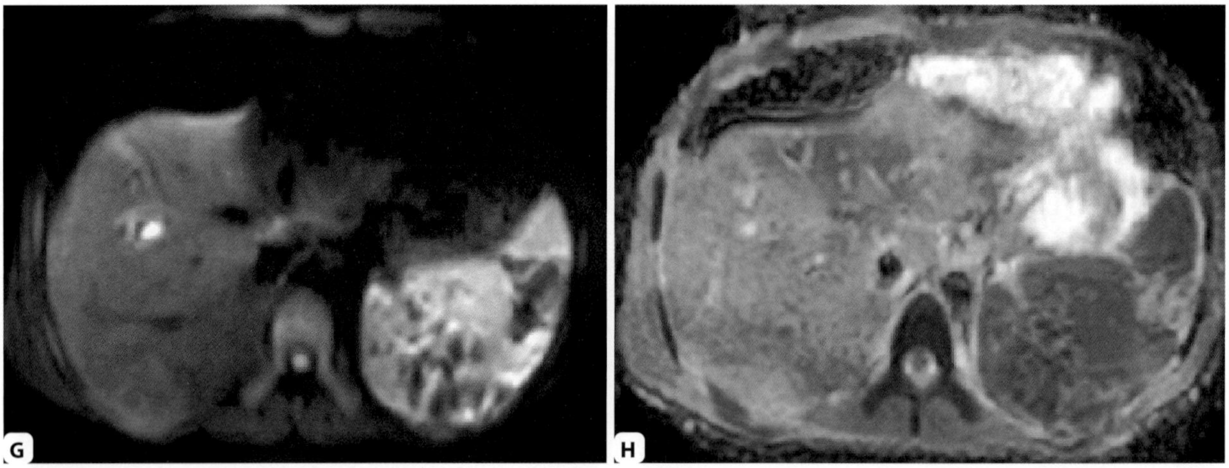

FIGS. 22A TO H: Contrast-enhanced CT scan (A) showing peripheral wedge-shaped hypodensity in spleen suggestive of infarct. Incidentally, liver infarct is also seen. T1-weighted imaging (T1WI) (hyperintense) (B) and T2-weighted imaging (T2WI) (C) (hyperintense with hypointense rim) respectively showing peripheral wedge-shaped altered signal intensity (white arrow). Multiple T1 and T2 hypointense Gamna–Gandy bodies are also noted (black arrow). Arterial (D) venous (E) and delayed (F) MR images showing nonenhancing area with peripheral enhancement on delayed phase. Diffusion-weighted imaging (DWI) (G) and ADC map (H) showing no restriction (suggestive of chronic infarct—3 months).

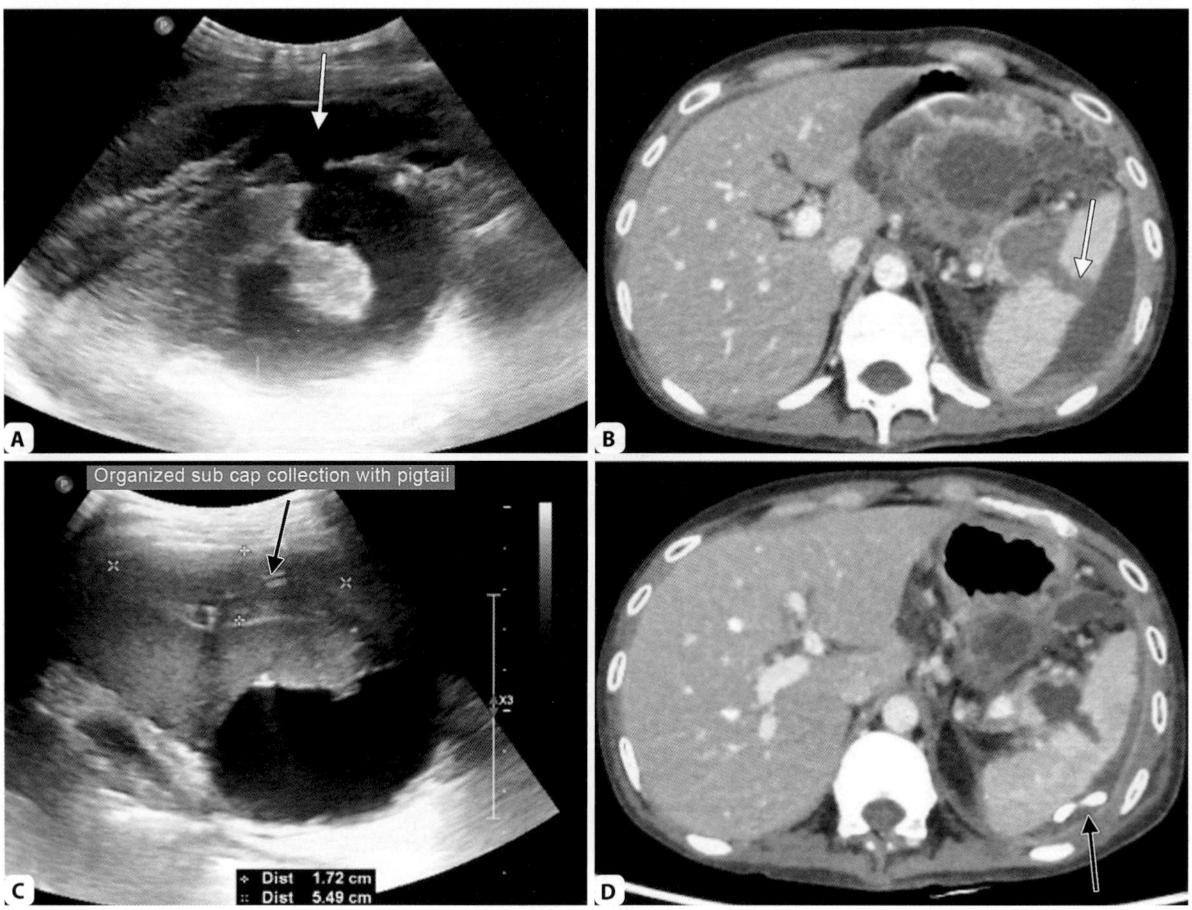

FIGS. 23A TO D: Ruptured splenic abscess drainage. (A) USG shows anechoic fluid collection with few septations in perisplenic region (arrow); (B) Corresponding CT showed hypodense region in splenic parenchyma (arrow) communicating with the perisplenic collection suggestive of ruptured splenic abscess. (C and D) USG and CT images after pigtail catheter drainage (arrows) shows reduction in the volume of collection with residual mild organized collection.

SPLENIC NEOPLASMS

Splenic neoplasms can be divided into benign and malignant neoplasms. Among the benign lesions, hemangioma, lymphangioma, hamartoma, littoral cell angioma, peliosis, and inflammatory pseudotumors are common. Among the malignant lesions, metastasis, lymphoma, and angiosarcoma are common entities **(Table 4)**.

TABLE 4: Splenic neoplasms.

Benign splenic neoplasms:	*Malignant splenic neoplasms*:
• Hemangioma	• Metastases
• Lymphangioma	• Lymphoma
• Hamartoma	• Angiosarcoma
• Angioma	*Miscellaneous*:
• Peliosis	• Sarcoidosis
• Pseudotumor	• Gaucher's disease
• Hemangioendothelioma	• Hemochromatosis
• Fibroma	• Amyloidosis
• Lipoma	• Gamma–Gandy bodies
• Angiofibromas	

Benign Neoplasms

Hemangioma

Hemangioma is the most common benign primary neoplasm of spleen with prevalence ranging from 0.3 to 14%.[29] Most hemangiomas are small in size and detected incidentally on imaging. When large, it may present with pain in the left hypochondrium with presence of palpable nontender mass. Splenic hemangiomatosis **(Fig. 24)** may occur in cases with generalized angiomatosis, like Klippel–Trenaunay syndrome.[30] Spontaneous rupture may occur in 25% of the patients having large hemangiomas.[31]

On USG, they are seen as echogenic solid or cystic lesions which are iso- to hypodense on unenhanced CT. Hemangioma can be capillary and cavernous on histology. The cavernous hemangiomas have solid isodense components which show enhancement on contrast administration while the cystic component remains hypodense **(Fig. 25)**. Peripheral punctate calcification may be seen on CT. On MRI, the lesions are hyperintense relative to spleen on T2WI and hypo- to isointense on T1WI. After

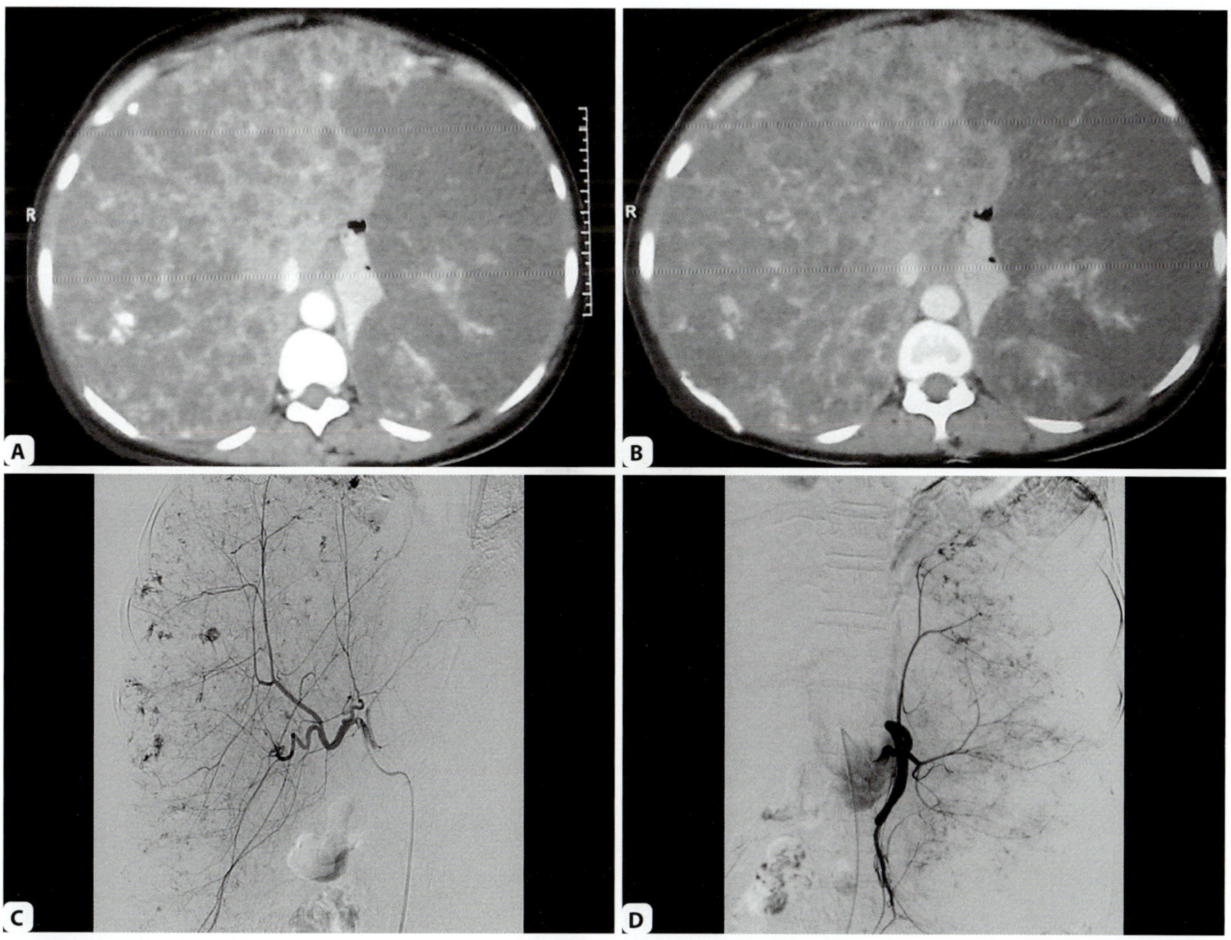

FIGS. 24A TO D: *Hemangiomatosis:* Contrast-enhanced computed tomography (CECT) images (A and B) reveal presence of multiple hypodense lesions involving the liver as well as spleen; few showing central enhancement. Subsequent angiography of hepatic artery (C) and splenic artery (D) corroborates with CT findings by illustrating multiple foci of contrast blush.

injection of gadolinium, three patterns of enhancement have been described:
1. Immediate homogeneous enhancement which persists
2. Early peripheral enhancement with delayed uniform enhancement, and
3. Peripheral enhancement which progresses centripetally with presence of enhancing central fibrous scar.[32]

Lymphangioma

Lymphangioma is a congenital malformation of lymphatic system that occurs most commonly in neck, mediastinum, and retroperitoneum; rarely affecting the spleen.[33] Splenic lymphangiomas are asymptomatic in the majority of patients and are detected incidentally. Spleen may be normal in size or enlarged and shows presence of predominantly cystic masses. These lesions are seen as anechoic to hypoechoic well-defined intrasplenic cysts on USG and hypodense lesions on CT; with few showing fine internal septations **(Figs. 26A and B)** or echogenic debris within. Thin calcification may be seen along the periphery.[34] The signal intensity on MRI corresponds to simple fluid; however, the cysts containing hemorrhage and proteinaceous material demonstrate high signal intensity on T1WI.[35]

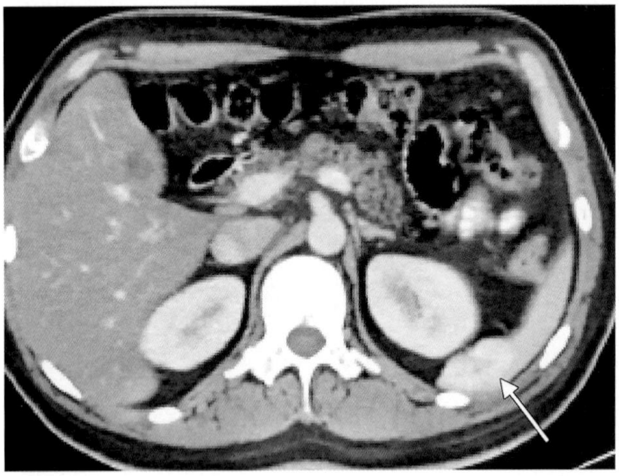

FIG. 25: Axial contrast-enhanced computed tomography (CECT) showing an enhancing lesion in lower pole of spleen suggestive of hemangioma (Incidental lesion). A metastatic lesion in segment 5 of liver is noted in a known case of malignancy.

Hamartoma

Splenic hamartoma is a rare benign neoplasm, which is composed of malformed red pulp elements without organized lymphoid follicles. Incidence in autopsy series is estimated to be 0.024–0.13%.[36] Most patients have no symptoms and the lesion is detected incidentally.

On USG, it is depicted as a solid mass with homogeneous or heterogeneous echo pattern showing intense vascularity on color Doppler owing to presence of red pulp within it. CT scan reveals homogeneous or heterogeneous low density or isodense masses causing contour deformity with or without presence of calcification and fatty component within. Persistent enhancement in delayed images has also been documented due to stagnation of contrast within the sinusoids of red pulp.[37] The lesion shows variable signal intensity on MRI depending upon the amount of fibrous content within it. The nonfibrous hamartoma is isointense on T1WI and hyperintense on T2WI and fibrous hamartoma shows iso- to hyperintense signal on T1 and hypointense signal on T2WI. However, both variants show mild early enhancement after IV contrast and uniform enhancement on delayed phase.[38]

Littoral Cell Angioma

Littoral cell angioma (LCA) is a very rare neoplasm arising from cells lining the sinuses of splenic red pulp, the Littoral

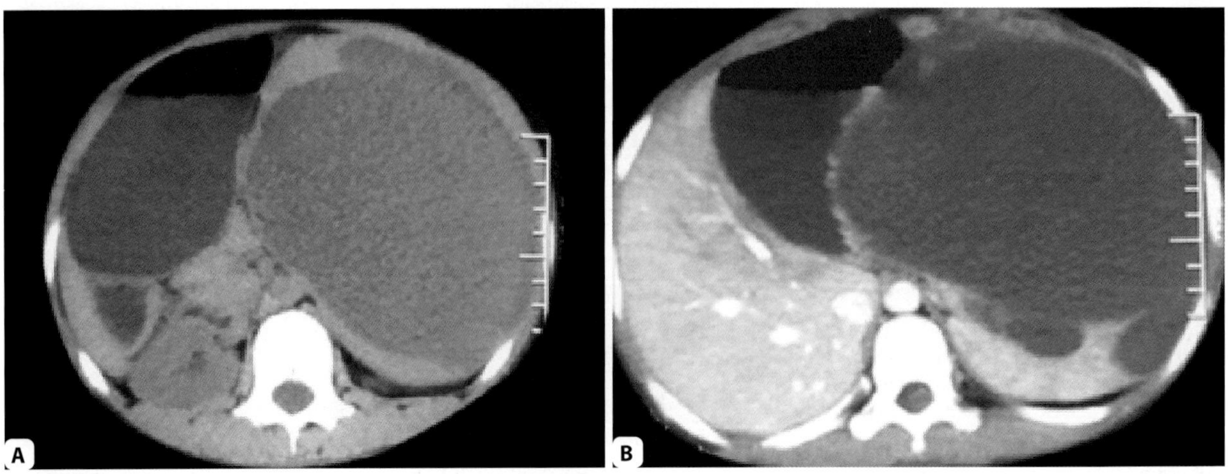

FIGS. 26A AND B: Axial noncontrast computed tomography (NCCT) (A) and CECT (B) images showing intrasplenic hypodense lesion with septations in a case of lymphangioma.

cells. It may be asymptomatic or may present with anemia or splenomegaly. Sonography reveals splenomegaly with heterogeneous echotexture and presence of multiple masses which are of low or iso-attenuation on noncontrast CT and demonstrate minimal delayed enhancement on postcontrast CT.[39] MRI depicts markedly hypointense signal on T1WI and T2WI due to presence of hemosiderin within the lesions.[32]

Peliosis

Peliosis is an uncommon condition, which is characterized by presence of blood-filled spaces within the splenic parenchyma. It may occur in isolation or along with peliosis hepatis. Usually asymptomatic; rupture of the hemorrhagic cyst leading to intraperitoneal hemorrhage has been described. It may appear as echogenic or heteroechoic mass lesion in the left upper quadrant on USG which shows rapid enhancement on contrast-enhanced USG without any centripetal enhancement.[40] Noncontrast CT demonstrates hypodense lesions with fine internal septations which enhance significantly on contrast administration. Variable signal intensity is seen on MRI owing to blood products at different stages. Fluid-fluid level may be visualized within these cysts due to hematocrit effect.[41] Based on these imaging features, the differential diagnosis would include hemangiomatosis, angiosarcoma, and lymphangioma.

Inflammatory Pseudotumor

Inflammatory pseudotumors, also known as inflammatory myofibroblastic tumor, are basically myofibroblastic neoplasms which result from an unusual inflammatory response to any injury or infection. They may present with features of mass effect on surrounding structures or may remain asymptomatic. Imaging features include well-circumscribed mass on USG with hetero- or homogeneous enhancement on CT and there may be calcification within or a central scar which does not show enhancement. Diagnosis solely based on imaging is difficult and is mostly established after surgery.[35,39]

The other tumors like hemangioendothelioma, fibroma, lipoma, and angiofibromas are extremely rare.

Malignant Neoplasms

Lymphoma

Spleen is affected in many hematological malignancies such as lymphoma, leukemia, plasma cell malignancies; most common being diffuse large B-cell lymphoma (DLBCL) type of non-Hodgkin's lymphoma (NHL).[42] Hodgkin's lymphoma (HD) also involves the spleen in one third of patients when it is considered as nodal disease in contrast to NHL in which its infiltration is considered to be extranodal.[43] The lymphomatous involvement of spleen may be primary or secondary. The diagnostic criteria of primary splenic lymphoma include involvement of only spleen with or without hilar lymph nodes; and no lesion in any other site at the time and within 6 months of detection of splenic disease. Primary splenic lymphoma is rare, constituting approximately 1–2% of all lymphomas and is usually DLBCL variant.[44] Secondary splenic involvement is more commonly seen in patients with lymphomas having enlarged lymph nodes at multiple other sites in abdomen.

On imaging, four patterns have been described:
1. Homogeneous splenomegaly without any focal lesion
2. Diffuse infiltration with miliary lesions (<5 mm)
3. Multiple focal nodular lesions (1–10 cm); and
4. Large solitary mass. Li M et al. documented single large mass as the most common pattern.[44] Diffuse involvement may occur in normal sized spleen **(Figs. 27A and B)** and mild-to-moderate enlargement may

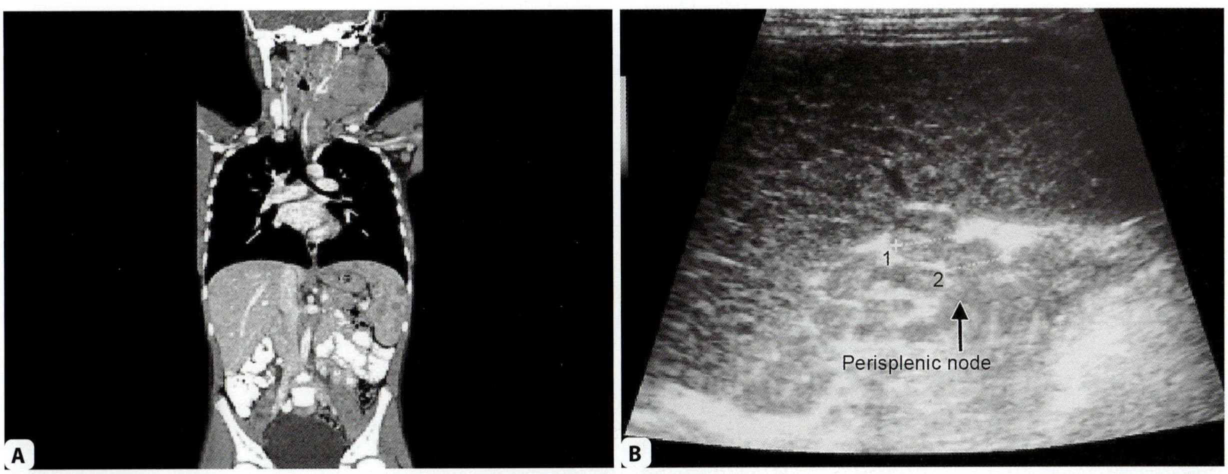

FIGS. 27A AND B: Coronal reformatted contrast-enhanced computed tomography (CECT) image (A) showing bulky cervical lymphadenopathy and multiple lesions seen in the spleen in a case of Hodgkin's lymphoma. USG image (B) in a different patient of NHL showing multiple small hypoechoic nodular lesions diffusely distributed in the splenic parenchyma. Note is made of multiple homogeneous, nonnecrotic perisplenic lymph nodes (arrow).

represent reactive splenomegaly in 30% of cases.[45] However, marked splenomegaly almost always suggests infiltration.[46] Diffuse involvement of spleen is commonly seen in Hodgkin's disease due to predominant involvement of periarteriolar lymphoid sheath.[42,47] The nodules appear hypoechoic on ultrasound and hypoenhancing on contrast-enhanced CT.[48] On MRI, the lesions are hyperintense on T2WI, iso- to hypointense on T1WI and show reduced enhancement on contrast administration.[11]

^{18}F-fluorodeoxyglucose positron-emission tomography/computed tomography is considered superior to CT in staging and restaging of lymphoma by virtue of detecting FDG avid normal sized nodes and detection of extranodal sites like liver, spleen **(Figs. 28A and B)** and bone marrow.[43] Sensitivity and specificity of CT, PET, and PET/CT have been reported to be 91% and 96%, 75% and 99%, and 100% and 95%, respectively in a series of 111 patients.[49] Hence, for the staging of patients with FDG-avid, potentially curable lymphomas (e.g., DLBCL and Hodgkin disease), PET is recommended routinely to delineate the disease extent more accurately and monitor response to therapy.[43] In lymphoma patients, the posttherapy inflammatory changes may persist for up to 2 weeks after chemotherapy alone and for up to 2–3 months or longer after radiation therapy or chemoradiotherapy. Thus, to avoid false positive results, PET scans should not be performed for at least 3 weeks, and preferably 6–8 weeks, after completion of therapy.[50,51]

Angiosarcoma

Splenic angiosarcoma is a rare and aggressive neoplasm, which arises from the splenic vascular endothelium and the mesothelial cells of the sinusoids.[52] It is considered to be the most common primary nonlymphoid neoplasm of spleen with an estimated annual incidence of 0.14–0.25 cases per million persons.[53] The exact etiopathogenesis is unknown; although, it has been postulated that the benign splenic tumors like hemangioma and lymphangioma may act as precursors. It presents with upper abdominal pain in 80% of patients and anemia in 75–81%.[52] Angiosarcoma of spleen is a fatal neoplasm and may present as splenic rupture in 13–32% of cases.[53] It is associated with high rate of metastases at the time of presentation (69–100%); liver being the most common site followed by lungs, lymph nodes, and bone.[54] Early diagnosis and splenectomy are the treatment of choice with less defined role of chemoradiotherapy. Despite prompt measures, it has a dismal prognosis.

There is limited literature available on the imaging features of angiosarcoma in the form of anecdotal case reports and a few case series. Splenomegaly with heterogeneous mass is seen in 60% cases on all imaging modalities.[55] On ultrasound, it appears as solid-cystic mass in an enlarged spleen with mixed echogenicity. CT demonstrates single or multiple masses, which show mixed attenuation and ill-defined margins. Nonenhancing areas represent necrosis and active contrast blush is seen in the areas of active bleeding. Areas of active hemorrhage appear hyperdense on noncontrast CT and the lesions may show peripheral enhancement after contrast administration **(Figs. 29A and B)**.[55] On MRI, the nodules are hypointense on T1WI and T2WI relative to splenic parenchyma; however, hyperintense signal may be seen due to presence of hemorrhage or necrosis within. Chronic hemorrhage leading to hemosiderin deposition causes reduction in signal intensity. The pattern of contrast enhancement includes peripheral nodular enhancement with nonenhancing areas due to necrosis or hemorrhage.[55]

Metastases

Splenic metastases occur mostly in the setting of multisystem metastatic disease. The prevalence ranges from 1.3 to 7.1%, reported in autopsy series.[56] It has been postulated that the relative lower incidence of splenic metastases is due

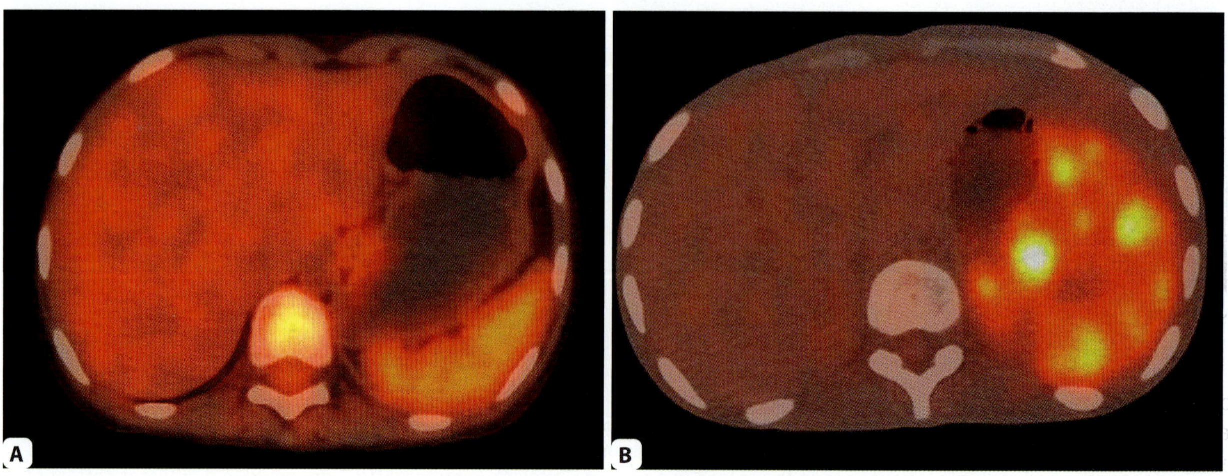

FIGS. 28A AND B: ^{18}F-fluorodeoxyglucose positron-emission tomography-computed tomography (^{18}F-FDG-PET-CT) image showing diffuse involvement (A) and focal nodules (B) in patient of non-Hodgkin's lymphoma (NHL) as areas of avid uptake of FDG.

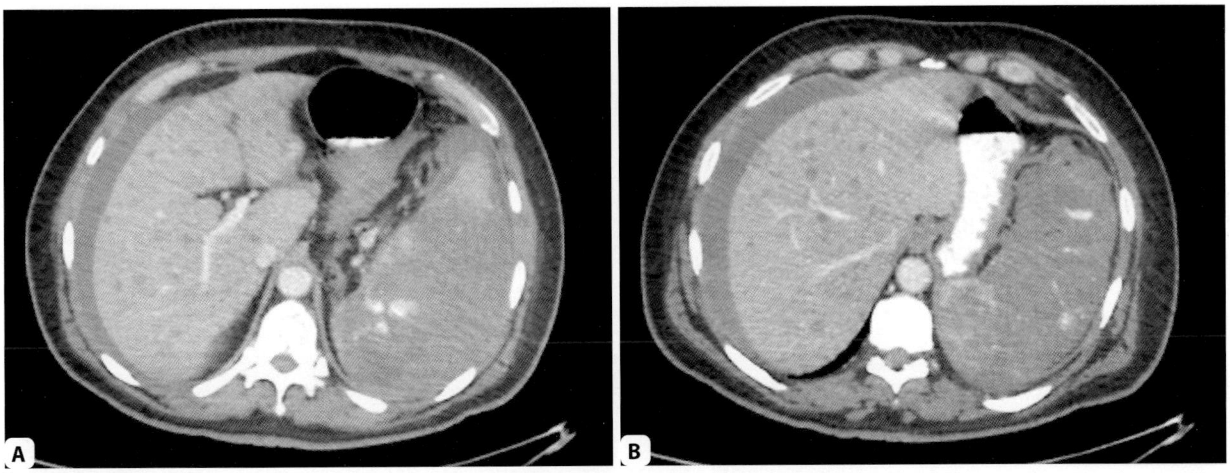

FIGS. 29A AND B: Angiosarcoma—axial contrast-enhanced computed tomography (CECT) sections of upper abdomen reveal a diffusely hypodense lesion involving almost the entire spleen with internal hyperdense areas representing active hemorrhage.

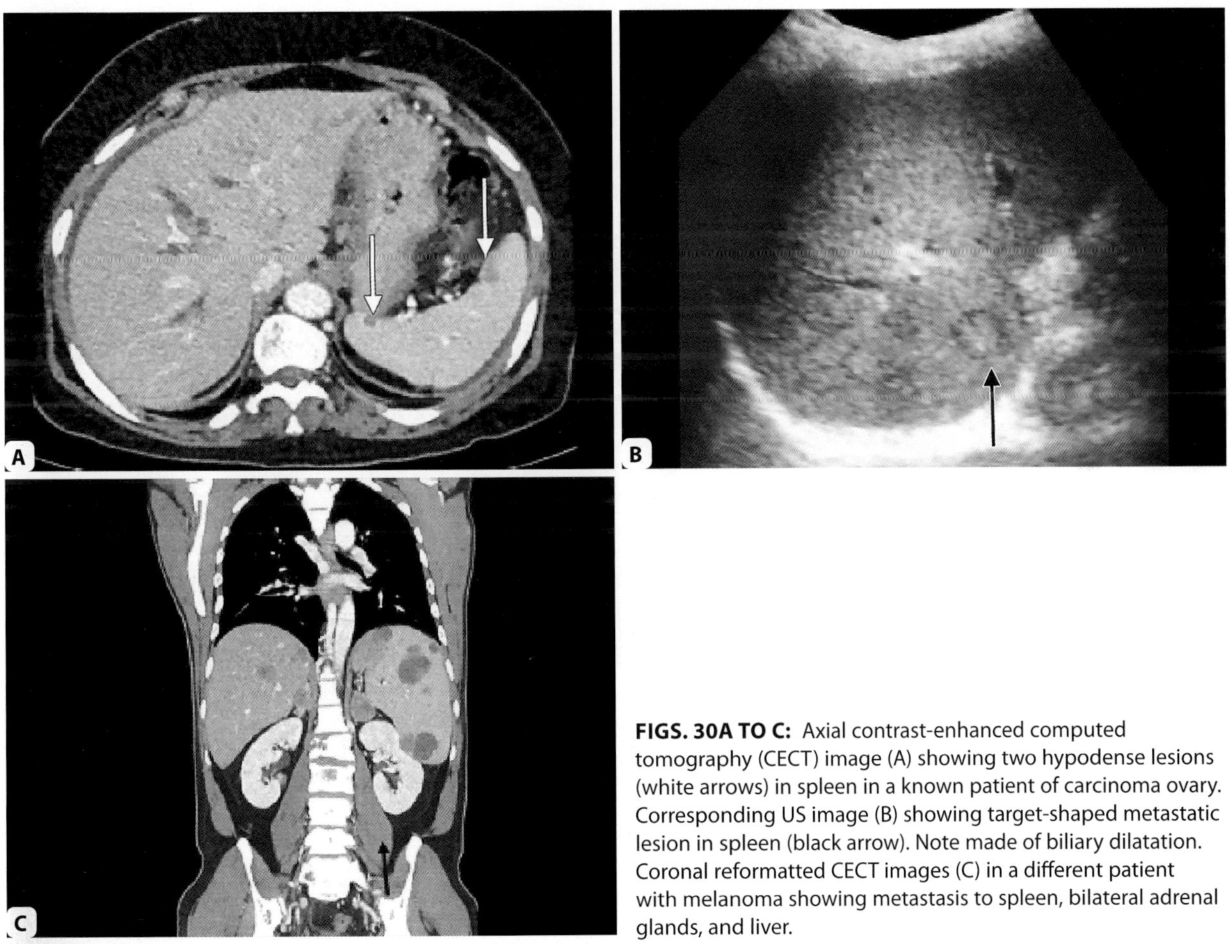

FIGS. 30A TO C: Axial contrast-enhanced computed tomography (CECT) image (A) showing two hypodense lesions (white arrows) in spleen in a known patient of carcinoma ovary. Corresponding US image (B) showing target-shaped metastatic lesion in spleen (black arrow). Note made of biliary dilatation. Coronal reformatted CECT images (C) in a different patient with melanoma showing metastasis to spleen, bilateral adrenal glands, and liver.

to innate hostile environment for malignant invasion, the reticuloendothelial system inhibiting tumor cell seeding and lack of afferent lymphatics.[57] Gynecological malignancy is the most common primary neoplasm followed by colorectal, lung, and gastric cancer to be associated with splenic metastases.[58] The lesions are hypodense on imaging with majority being lobulated, well-defined, nonenhancing nodules on CT **(Figs. 30A to C)**.[59] On MRI, the lesions typically appear as hyperintense on T2WI and hypo- to isointense on T1WI.[11]

Miscellaneous Conditions

Sarcoidosis

Splenic involvement in sarcoidosis is much less common than lungs, mediastinum, and eyes. However, when involved it may be seen on CT as multiple hypodense nodules in the spleen, which may vary in shape and size. If the nodules increase with time these may also look like confluent masses. These nodules and masses are hypodense and show less enhancement as compared to splenic parenchyma.[60] On MRI, these show hypointense signal on T1WI and T2WI as compared to background parenchyma with hypoenhancement on early arterial phase.[61] These nodules may show enhancement on delayed phase images **(Figs. 31A to E)**.

Gamna–Gandy Bodies

Histologically, these are small siderotic nodules which contain hemosiderin, calcium, and fibrosis. These are

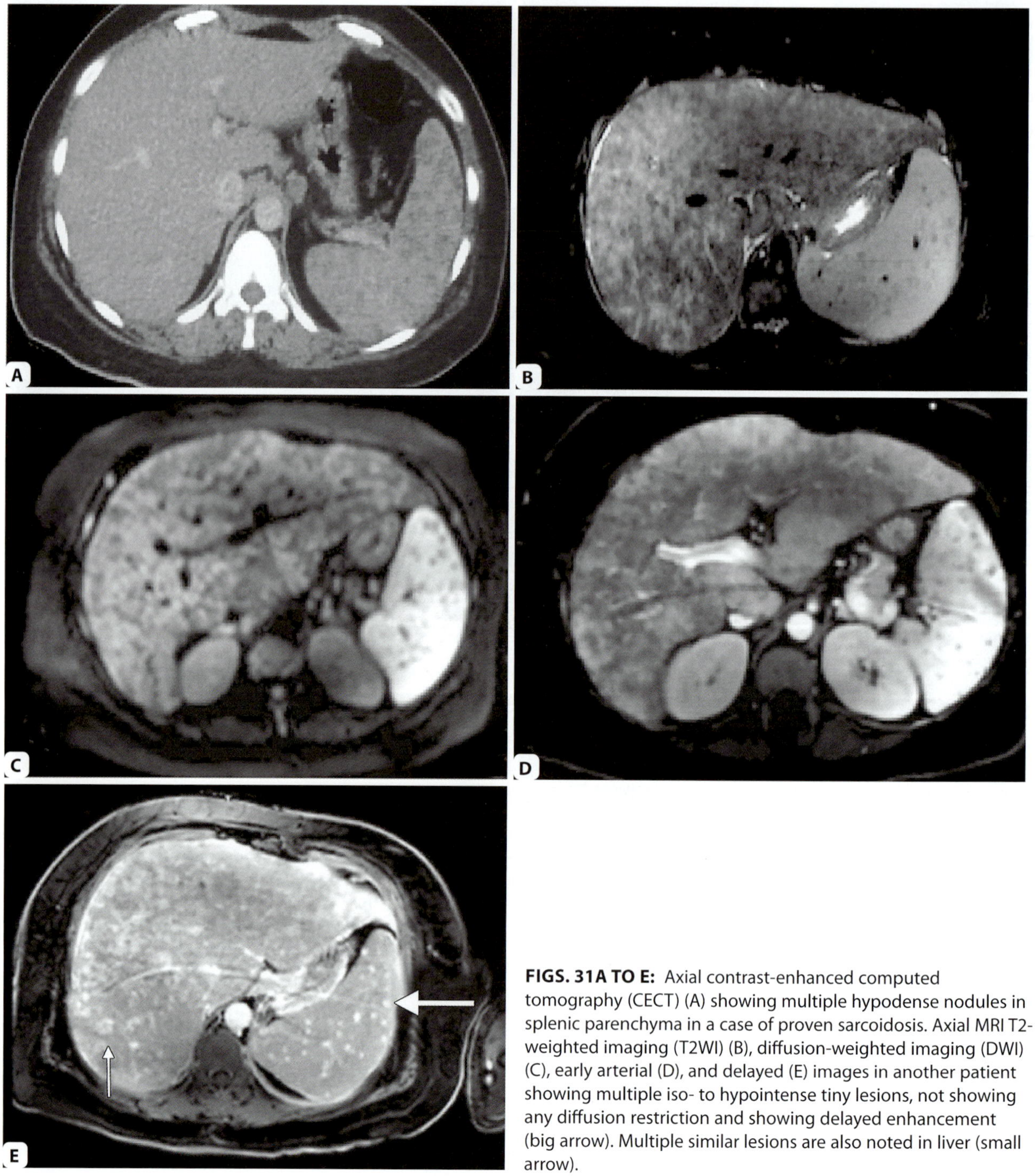

FIGS. 31A TO E: Axial contrast-enhanced computed tomography (CECT) (A) showing multiple hypodense nodules in splenic parenchyma in a case of proven sarcoidosis. Axial MRI T2-weighted imaging (T2WI) (B), diffusion-weighted imaging (DWI) (C), early arterial (D), and delayed (E) images in another patient showing multiple iso- to hypointense tiny lesions, not showing any diffusion restriction and showing delayed enhancement (big arrow). Multiple similar lesions are also noted in liver (small arrow).

commonly seen in the clinical setting of portal hypertension.[62] Other conditions in which these are seen include portal vein or splenic vein thrombosis and hemolytic anemias. They are best seen on MRI as hypointense foci in all sequences **(Figs. 32A to D)**.[63] Their usual size is from few millimeters to up to a centimeter.

Gaucher's Disease

Gaucher's disease occurs due to deficiency of lysosomal enzyme glucocerebrosidase. This disease affects the skeleton, spleen, and liver most dominantly. The majority of times the patient is already diagnosed before they reach the radiology department. Skeletal involvement is in the form of osteopenia, osteoporosis, and fractures. Spleen may be massively enlarged with frequent findings of focal lesions and infarcts. On CT, these focal lesions are hypodense and enhance less as compared to splenic parenchyma. On MRI, most of these lesions are hyperintense on T2WI although occasionally they may be hypointense on T2WI also. These are hypointense on T1WI with hypoenhancement as compared to splenic parenchyma.[64] Liver enlargement is less striking as compared to splenic enlargement.

Hemochromatosis

Hemochromatosis may be primary [due to increased absorption from gastrointestinal tract (GIT)] or secondary (due to increased extravascular hemolysis or repeated transfusions). In primary form, liver involvement is much more as compared to spleen and in secondary form, the spleen is predominantly involved. The usual imaging feature on CT is presence of increased attenuation involving these organs. On MRI, these involved organs show decreased signal on T2WI due to susceptibility artifacts because of presence of iron in visceral organs.[65,66] Spleen is also hypointense on T2WI; however, the involvement of liver is much more in primary forms **(Fig. 33)**. Conversely, spleen is more profoundly hypointense than liver if the etiology is secondary hemochromatosis. MR using gradient echo sequences is also used to quantify liver iron load in an attempt to avoid the need of repeated biopsies. Iron

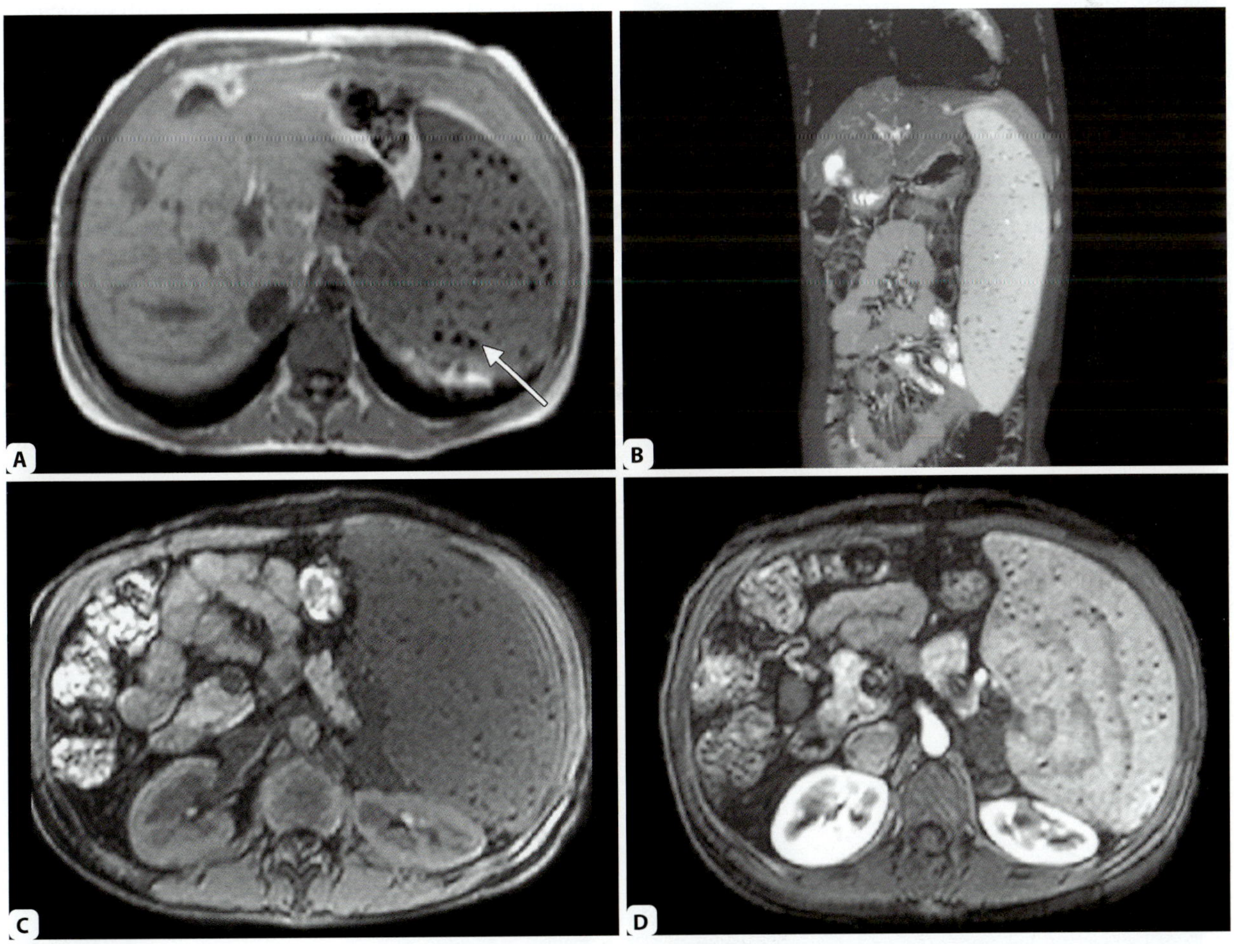

FIGS. 32A TO D: Axial T1-weighted imaging (T1WI) (A), coronal T2-weighted imaging (T2WI) (B), T1 weighted fat-saturated image (T1FS) noncontrast (C), and postcontrast (D) MRI showing numerous hypointense tiny focal lesions (arrow) in enlarged spleen on all sequences with no enhancement on postcontrast images suggestive of Gamna–Gandy bodies in a patient with portal hypertension.

overload causes loss of signal on the in-phase image of the in- and opposed-phase sequence.

Amyloidosis

Pathologically, in amyloidosis, there is abnormal accumulation of some fibrillar material in the extracellular matrix in a wide variety of tissues in the body. Based on the biochemical property of this fibrillar material, it can be divided into primary (type AL, monoclonal proliferation) and secondary type (AA type, secondary to chronic inflammatory diseases). Both of these types can involve the spleen which may be diffuse (more commonly) or focal. Splenomegaly is quite uncommon.[67] Various imaging features are focal tumor such as lesions,[68] diffuse low attenuation,[69] and decreased enhancement. Occasionally, extensive focal splenic calcification has also been described in splenic involvement of amyloidosis.[69] On MRI, decreased signal on T2WI has been described.[70]

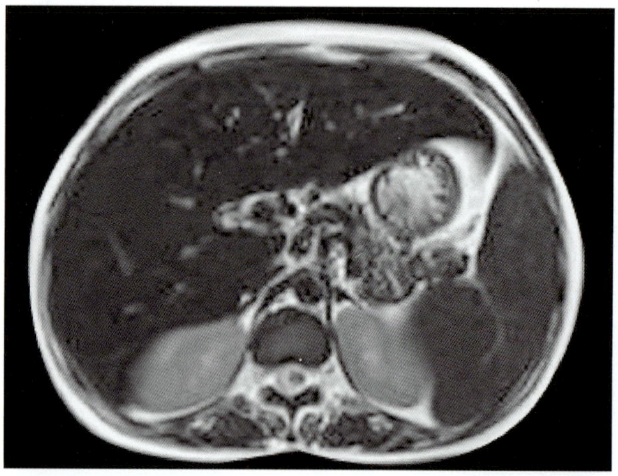

FIG. 33: Axial T2-weighted imaging (T2WI) showing diffuse hypointense signal in spleen in a case of hemolytic anemia.

SPLENIC INTERVENTIONS FINE-NEEDLE ASPIRATION CYTOLOGY AND BIOPSY OF SPLEEN

Fine-needle aspiration cytology of the spleen is a relatively safe procedure. Common indications of performing FNAC in the spleen are infectious diseases, sarcoidosis, and neoplastic conditions like metastases. Uncommonly, FNAC is also performed to rule out storage disorders, amyloidosis, hemophagocytic syndrome and primary splenic benign and malignant diseases. In India, because of the very high prevalence of tuberculosis, focal splenic lesions even in patients of a known malignancy may be infectious in nature. This is a relatively common clinical scenario for performing FNAC to differentiate these two possibilities.

There is a reluctance to do guided interventions in spleen because of potential risk of hemorrhage that may necessitate urgent splenectomy. However, with the use of thinner gauge biopsy needles for splenic biopsy, the risk of complication is similar to the risk associated with other large organ biopsies.[71]

Most common indication for splenic biopsy is to sample a focal lesion in spleen found on imaging with suspicion of lymphoma or metastasis.[72,73]

A significant percentage of patients of lymphomas (HD as well as NHL) has involvement of the spleen.[72] Another important consideration is that splenic involvement in lymphoma has got prognostic importance and overall treatment of the patient changes according to whether spleen is involved or not.

It is important to consider the fact that if metastasis is also present at some other site in addition to spleen, then it is advisable to obtain biopsy from these accessible sites.[74]

Whenever chances of bleeding are high, e.g., in presence of coagulopathy, it is advisable to obtain FNAC rather than core biopsy. FNAC is normally performed with 20–23G Chiba needle **(Figs. 34A and B)**, which

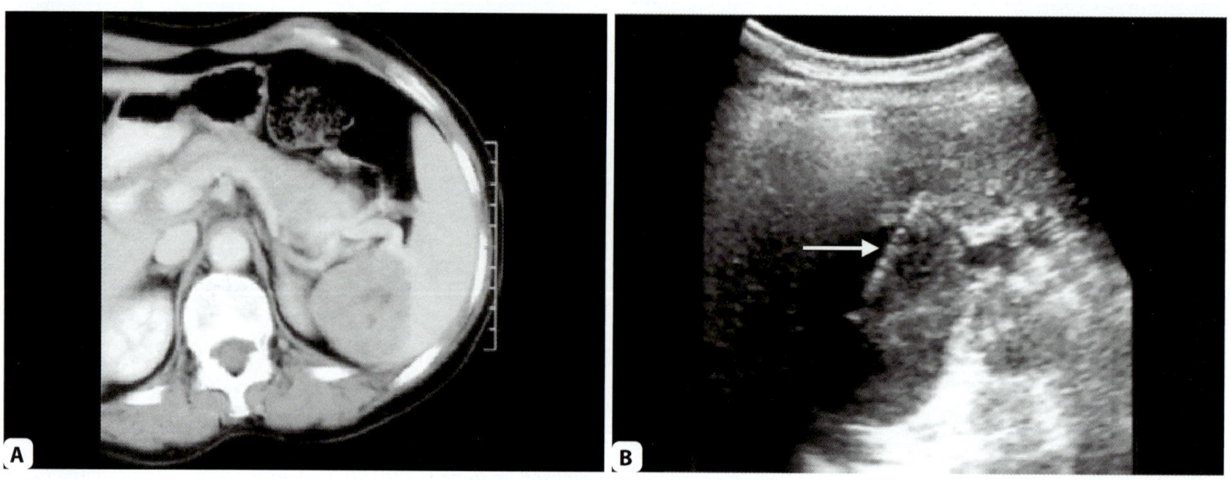

FIGS. 34A AND B: Axial contrast-enhanced computed tomography (CECT) image (A) showing focal hypodense mass lesion in spleen. USG-guided fine-needle aspiration cytology (FNAC) procedure (B) showing echogenic needle in situ (arrow). FNAC was reported as non-Hodgkin's lymphoma (NHL).

has a safer profile compared to core biopsy which is done with 14–18G needles. However, it is important to note that FNAC is not useful in evaluation of lymphoma because the obtained sample is usually insufficient to further subtype lymphomas. With the advent of specific targeted chemotherapeutic agents of different subtypes of lymphoma, it is essential to provide larger tissues to the pathologist for subtyping, which results in better selection of chemotherapeutic regimen. Additional samples are taken for flow cytometry if lymphoma is one of the clinical possibilities.

Contraindications for splenic biopsy or drainage are uncorrectable coagulopathy, lack of safe access route, and uncooperative patient. For biopsy, a minimal caliber needle should be chosen which can give sufficient diagnostic yield so as to decrease chances of postprocedural bleeding. It is advisable to traverse some normal splenic tissue before obtaining access to the target lesion in the spleen to help to decrease bleeding by way of tamponade effect. Biopsy tract can be embolized either with gelfoam slurry or glue if there is risk of bleeding. Frequent hemodynamic monitoring and placing the patient in left lateral decubitus is advisable.

Drainage

Drainage of splenic abscess is done uncommonly for tubercular, fungal, or bacterial abscesses which are more common in patient with altered immune status.[75]

The success rate of percutaneous drainage for splenic abscess is >80%[74,76,77] with reduced success in presence of loculations and multiple internal septations. Usually, collections <3 cm^3 can be managed by single-time needle aspiration only.[78] If lesion is bigger than 3 cm^3, then drainage is usually considered. Seldinger's techniques and tandem trocar techniques are both feasible for splenic drainage. Normally, 8–10 F pigtail catheters are selected, however, if on initial aspiration thick pus is aspirated it should be drained with a bigger pigtail catheter (e.g., 12–14 F). Intermittent (every 8 hours) flushing of the catheter with 10 mL of saline helps in improving the patency of catheters. If the drainage from the catheter drops to <10 mL/24 hours, white blood cell (WBC) counts return to normal and fever subsides, then catheter removal should be planned. Repeat USG screening is useful before removing the catheter to rule out significant residual collection.

Ultrasonography guidance is better than CT for evaluating internal architecture of fluid collection/abscess in spleen as the thin internal septations are better seen on USG.

Splenic Artery Aneurysm and Intervention

In abdomen, only aorta and iliac artery aneurysms are more common sites of aneurysm than splenic artery.[79] With more frequent use of USG and CT, incidental splenic artery aneurysms are also seen more commonly.[80] The difference between true aneurysm and pseudoaneurysm is with respect to the adventitial layer of the wall; which is present in true aneurysm but absent in pseudoaneurysm. The exact etiopathogenesis of true aneurysm is not yet completely elucidated. The clinical settings in which it is seen include atherosclerosis, pregnancy, portal hypertension, cirrhosis, and post liver transplantation.[81-83] Inflammatory and infectious conditions, collagen vascular diseases, and arterial fibrodysplasia are other conditions, which are associated with it. In pancreatitis, release of proteolytic enzymes may cause weakening of the wall of splenic artery with consequent pseudoaneurysm formation. Other causes of pseudoaneurysms are iatrogenic or accidental trauma and postoperative causes.[84]

A large majority of unruptured splenic artery true aneurysms are clinically silent.[81] In contrast, ruptured splenic artery aneurysms are almost always symptomatic with pain abdomen, gastrointestinal hemorrhage, and hemodynamic instability as presenting features. Rupture rate has been described as approximately 2–3%.[85,86] Liver transplantation, pregnancy, and portal hypertension are associated with increased frequency of rupture.[87] CECT scan is the most commonly used modality for diagnosing splenic artery aneurysms and pseudoaneurysms, however, the gold standard for diagnosing these conditions still remains direct catheter angiography. If CECT is utilized, a meticulous evaluation of arterial phase images is vital which reveals a well-defined rounded intensely enhancing outpouching from the splenic artery **(Figs. 35A and B)** or its branch. Other findings which may be seen are presence of calcification in its wall, mural thrombosis in the peripheral part of the aneurysm or extravasation of contrast in its vicinity or within the lumen of adjacent bowel loops. If aneurysm is large, it may be seen on USG or color Doppler **(Fig. 35C)**, however, small aneurysms may be missed on USG/Doppler as frequently there is poor sonographic window in presence of pancreatitis and postoperative changes.

The treatment strategies for splenic artery aneurysm and pseudoaneurysms are quite different. All the splenic pseudoaneurysms irrespective of size should be treated due to increased risk of rupture. However, treatment of true aneurysms needs to be assessed on a case-to-case basis. If a patient is symptomatic, then splenic artery true aneurysm should be treated.[81] For asymptomatic patients, treatment should be contemplated for certain high-risk factors such as pregnant women, size > 2 cm, hypertension, and liver transplantation.[88] Treatment is also recommended for asymptomatic aneurysms larger than 2 cm in those patients with life expectancy > 2 years and having reasonable operative risk.[79-81]

The modality of treatment depends on many factors such as clinical condition of the patient, location of aneurysm, and operative risks associated in a given scenario. Elective surgery is associated with >0.5% mortality rate; hence, patient selection and treatment modality selection are of paramount importance.[87] Previously, surgical treatment for proximal and middle splenic artery used to be simple

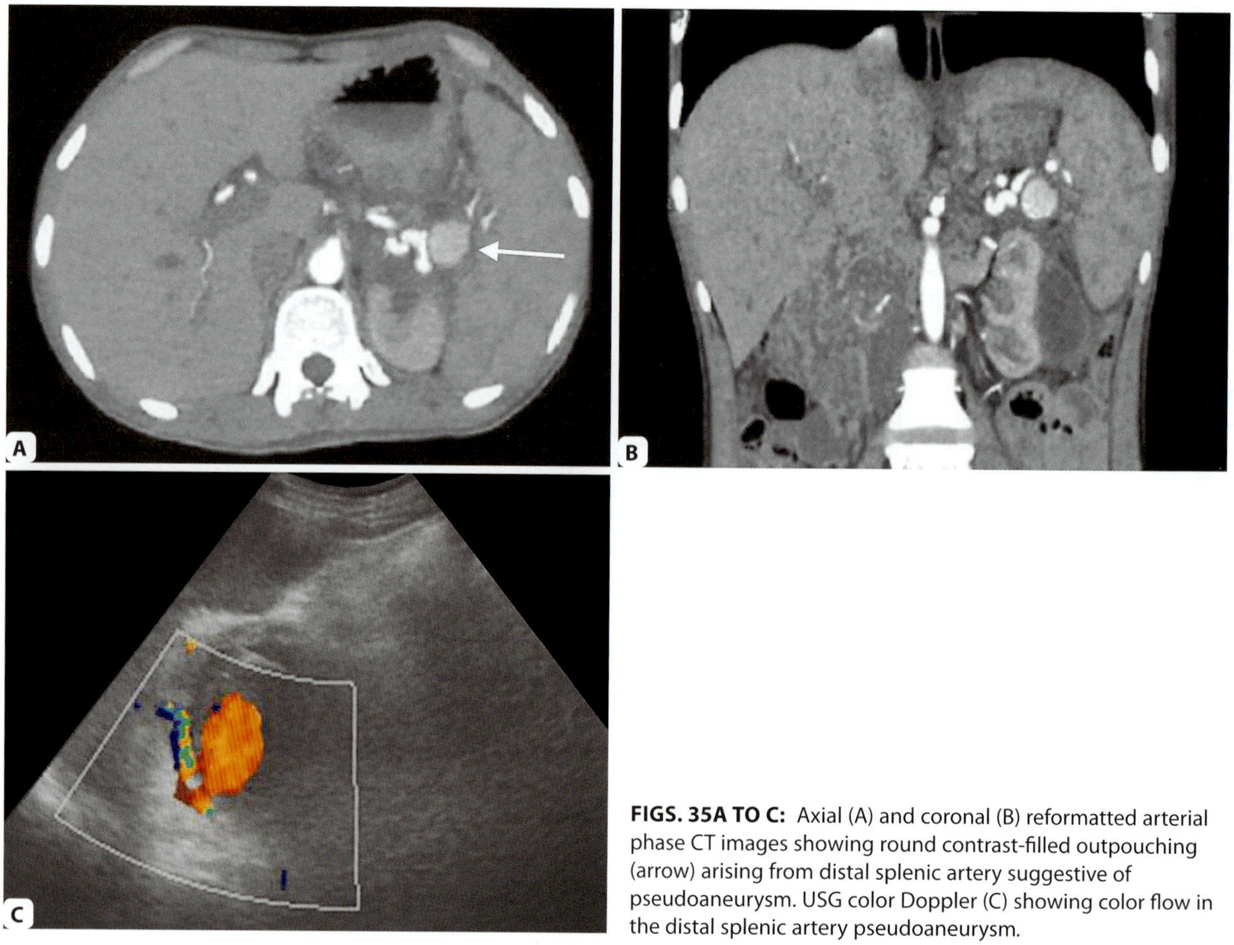

FIGS. 35A TO C: Axial (A) and coronal (B) reformatted arterial phase CT images showing round contrast-filled outpouching (arrow) arising from distal splenic artery suggestive of pseudoaneurysm. USG color Doppler (C) showing color flow in the distal splenic artery pseudoaneurysm.

excision with ligation of proximal and distal stumps; in which case short gastric arteries may help to preserve splenic supply through collateralization. Surgical treatment for distally located aneurysms is splenectomy.[88]

Endovascular repair of splenic artery aneurysm is more efficacious than open surgical treatment in short-term follow-up with lesser perioperative mortality. However, late complications and reintervention rate are more with endovascular repair as compared to open surgical repair.[89] Endovascular repair has also been found to be more cost effective for treatment of splenic artery true aneurysms.[90]

The technique of pseudoaneurysm embolization is described in detail under Chapters of Acute Pancreatitis and GI Hemorrhage.

Acceptable success rates have been achieved with endovascular techniques using embolization with coils **(Figs. 36A and B)** and gel foam.[91]

Partial splenic artery embolization has also been used successfully for treatment of hypersplenism.[92]

Occasionally, use of percutaneous thrombin has been shown to be successful if the patients are not good candidates for endovascular treatment.[93,94]

Transsplenic vascular interventions: In addition to the above-described vascular interventions in spleen, occasionally transsplenic puncture has also been employed.

Direct splenoportography is an old obsolete technique used for performing diagnostic angiography for the splenoportal axis.

Transsplenic vascular access has also been employed to perform gastric variceal obliteration **(Figs. 37A to C)**, and for performing portal vein embolization in cases where transhepatic route is difficult due to acute angulation of right-sided portal vein branches.

CONCLUSION

The spleen is affected by a wide variety of disorders ranging from developmental abnormalities to storage disorders, infective, vascular, and neoplastic pathologies. A thorough knowledge of available imaging modalities and judicious utilization of these is necessary for optimal patient care. USG and CT are the most commonly used imaging modalities for evaluation of splenic disorders. MRI can be used as a problem-solving tool. FNAC, biopsy, and splenic artery embolization are major interventions performed, which need meticulous planning using these imaging modalities. FNAC with or without cell block is a safe and useful procedure for diagnosis of focal splenic lesions, especially granulomatous diseases such as tuberculosis.

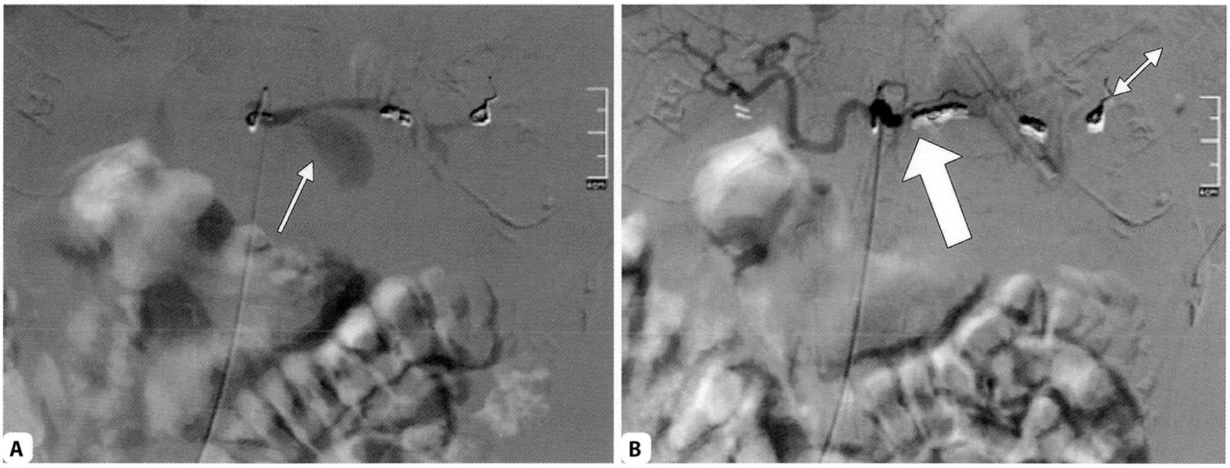

FIGS. 36A AND B: Angiogram (A) showing aneurysm in proximal part of splenic artery (arrow). Coils have been placed distal to splenic artery aneurysm. Incidentally, a coil is seen migrated in the distal most part of splenic artery (double-headed arrow). Coils have been placed proximal to aneurysm (thick arrow) also to "trap" the aneurysm (B).

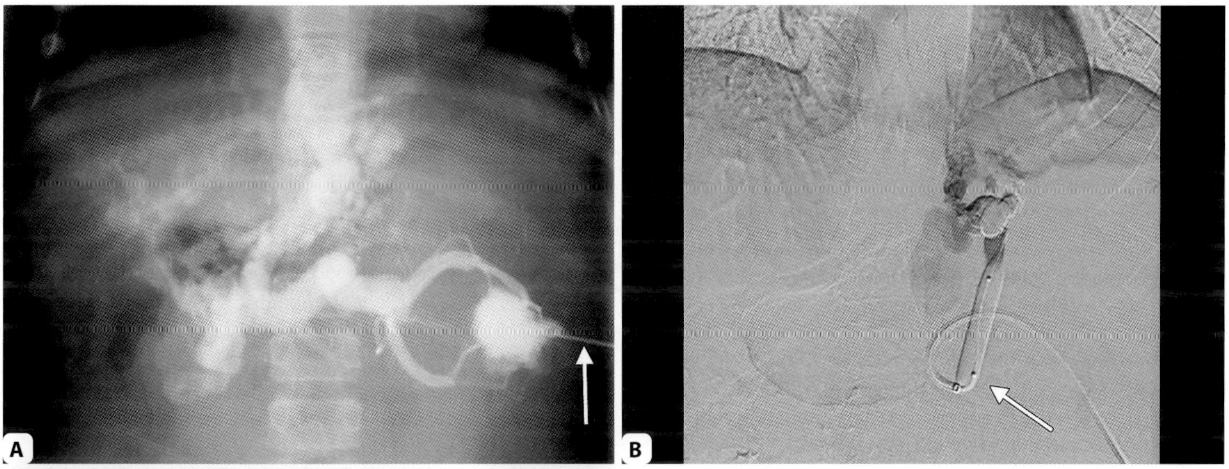

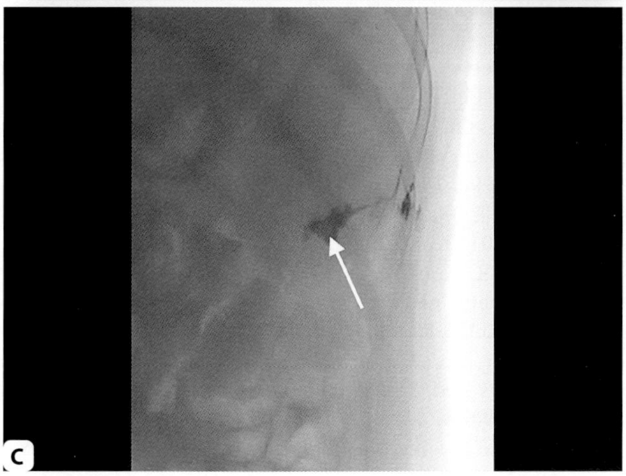

FIGS. 37A TO C: Radiographic spot image. (A) Showing the technique of direct splenoportography which is performed by using large bore needle (arrow) to puncture the splenic parenchyma blindly followed by injecting iodinated contrast medium into the splenic parenchyma and multiple spot images were taken. Spot image is showing dilated splenoportal axis with dilated left gastric vein and esophageal varices in a patient with portal hypertension. (B) Spot image is showing technique of transsplenic fundal variceal obliteration; glue was injected into the fundal varices after accessing the splenic vein under combined ultrasound fluoroscopic guidance followed by placing vascular sheath into the short gastric vein. *Note:* forward flow through short gastric vein was reduced using balloon catheter (arrow). (C) Spot image is showing the technique of access tract embolization following vascular transsplenic intervention. The access tract was embolized using glue (arrow) to prevent intraperitoneal bleeding.

REFERENCES

1. Chadburn A. The spleen: anatomy and anatomical function. Semin Hematol. 2000;37(1 Suppl 1):13-21.
2. Hirooka M, Ochi H, Koizumi Y, Kisaka Y, Abe M, Ikeda Y, et al. Splenic elasticity measured with real-time tissue elastography is a marker of portal hypertension. Radiology. 2011;261(3):960-8.
3. Grzelak P, Augsburg L, Majos A, Stefanczyk L, Gorski P, Piotrowski W, et al. Diagnostic potential of contrast-enhanced ultrasound (CEUS) in the assessment of spleen and liver granulomas in the course of sarcoidosis. Pneumonol Alergol Pol. 2013;81(5):424-8.
4. Omar A, Freeman S. Contrast-enhanced ultrasound of the spleen. Ultrasound. 2016;24(1):41-9.
5. Miele V, Piccolo CL, Galluzzo M, Ianniello S, Sessa B, Trinci M. Contrast-enhanced ultrasound (CEUS) in blunt abdominal trauma. Br J Radiol. 2016;89(1061):20150823.
6. Piscaglia F, Nolsoe C, Dietrich CF, Cosgrove DO, Gilja OH, Bachmann Nielsen M, et al. The EFSUMB Guidelines and Recommendations on the Clinical Practice of Contrast Enhanced Ultrasound (CEUS): update 2011 on non-hepatic applications. Ultraschall Med. 2012;33(1):33-59.
7. Park YS, Park SH, Lee SS, Kim DY, Shin YM, Lee W, et al. Biopsy-proven nonsteatotic liver in adults: estimation of reference range for difference in attenuation between the liver and the spleen at nonenhanced CT. Radiology. 2011;258(3):760-6.
8. Donnelly LF, Foss JN, Frush DP, Bisset GS 3rd. Heterogeneous splenic enhancement patterns on spiral CT images in children: minimizing misinterpretation. Radiology. 1999;210(2):493-7.
9. Rabushka LS, Kawashima A, Fishman EK. Imaging of the spleen: CT with supplemental MR examination. Radiographics. 1994;14(2):307-32.
10. Urban BA, Fishman EK. Helical CT of the spleen. AJR Am J Roentgenol. 1998;170(4):997-1003.
11. Elsayes KM, Narra VR, Mukundan G, Lewis JS Jr, Menias CO, Heiken JP. MR imaging of the spleen: spectrum of abnormalities. Radiographics. 2005;25(4):967-82.
12. Donnelly LF, Emery KH, Bove KE, Bissett GS 3rd. Normal changes in the MR appearance of the spleen during early childhood. AJR Am J Roentgenol. 1996;166(3):635-9.
13. Yoshikawa T, Kawamitsu H, Mitchell DG, Ohno Y, Ku Y, Seo Y, et al. ADC measurement of abdominal organs and lesions using parallel imaging technique. AJR Am J Roentgenol. 2006;187(6):1521-30.
14. Rini JN, Leonidas JC, Tomas MB, Palestro CJ. 18F-FDG PET versus CT for evaluating the spleen during initial staging of lymphoma. J Nucl Med. 2003;44(7):1072-4.
15. Lee JKT. Spleen. In: Lee JKT, Sagel SS, Stanley RJ, Heiken JP (eds). Computed Body Tomography with MRI Correlation, 4th edition. Philadelphia: Lippincott Williams and Wilkins; 2006.
16. Rosenberg HK, Markowitz RI, Kolberg H, Park C, Hubbard A, Bellah RD. Normal splenic size in infants and children: sonographic measurements. AJR Am J Roentgenol. 1991;157(1):119-21.
17. Radu CC, Mutiu G, Pop O. Accessory spleen. Rom J Morphol Embryol. 2014;55(3 Suppl):1243-6.
18. al-Ahmadi M, Brundage S, Brody F, Jacobs L, Sackier JM. Splenosis of the mesoappendix: case report and review of the literature. J R Coll Surg Edinb. 1998;43(3):200-2.
19. Costello P, Kane RA, Oster J, Clouse ME. Focal splenic disease demonstrated by ultrasound and computed tomography. J Can Assoc Radiol. 1985;36(1):22-8.
20. Fulcher AS, Turner MA. Abdominal manifestations of situs anomalies in adults. Radiographics. 2002;22(6):1439-56.
21. Zech CJ, Bartolozzi C, Baron R, Reiser MF (eds). Multislice-CT of the Abdomen. Berlin, Heidelberg: Springer-Verlag; 2012.
22. Dachman AH, Ros PR, Murari PJ, Olmsted WW, Lichtenstein JE. Nonparasitic splenic cysts: a report of 52 cases with radiologic-pathologic correlation. AJR Am J Roentgenol. 1986;147(3):537-42.
23. Al-Hajjar N, Graur F, Hassan AB, Molnar G. Splenic abscesses. Rom J Gastroenterol. 2002;11(1):57-9.
24. Ooi LL, Leong SS. Splenic abscesses from 1987 to 1995. Am J Surg. 1997;174(1):87-93.
25. Tirumani SH, Ojili V, Gunabushanam G, Shanbhogue AK, Nagar A, Fasih N, et al. Imaging of tuberculosis of the abdominal viscera: beyond the intestines. J Clin Imaging Sci. 2013;3:17.
26. Murata Y, Yamada I, Sumiya Y, Shichijo Y, Suzuki Y. Abdominal macronodular tuberculomas: MR findings. J Comput Assist Tomogr. 1996;20(4):643-6.
27. Ito K, Mitchell DG, Honjo K, Fujita T, Uchisako H, Matsumoto T, et al. MR imaging of acquired abnormalities of the spleen. AJR Am J Roentgenol. 1997;168(3):697-702.
28. Renzulli P, Hostettler A, Schoepfer AM, Gloor B, Candinas D. Systematic review of atraumatic splenic rupture. Br J Surg. 2009;96(10):1114-21.
29. Husni EA. The clinical course of splenic hemangioma with emphasis on spontaneous rupture. Arch Surg. 1961;83:681-8.
30. Louis TH, Sanders JM, Stephenson JS, Harbour LN, Ford KL 3rd. Splenic hemangiomatosis. Proc (Bayl Univ Med Cent). 2011;24(4):356-8.
31. Shinde J, Pandit S, Kolte S, Singh SP. Laparoscopic splenectomy for haemangioma of the spleen. J Minim Access Surg. 2014;10(1):42-4.
32. Abbott RM, Levy AD, Aguilera NS, Gorospe L, Thompson WM. From the archives of the AFIP: primary vascular neoplasms of the spleen: radiologic-pathologic correlation. Radiographics. 2004;24(4):1137-63.
33. Yang F, Chen WX. Splenic lymphangioma that manifested as a solid-cystic mass: a case report. World J Gastroenterol. 2013;19(5):781-3.
34. Ioannidis I, Kahn AG. Splenic lymphangioma. Arch Pathol Lab Med. 2015;139(2):278-82.
35. Kaza RK, Azar S, Al-Hawary MM, Francis IR. Primary and secondary neoplasms of the spleen. Cancer Imaging. 2010;10:173-82.
36. Lam KY, Yip KH, Peh WC. Splenic vascular lesions: unusual features and a review of the literature. Aust N Z J Surg. 1999;69(6):422-5.
37. Ohtomo K, Fukuda H, Mori K, Minami M, Itai Y, Inoue Y. CT and MR appearances of splenic hamartoma. J Comput Assist Tomogr. 1992;16(3):425-8.
38. Yu RS, Zhang SZ, Hua JM. Imaging findings of splenic hamartoma. World J Gastroenterol. 2004;10(17):2613-5.
39. Giovagnoni A, Giorgi C, Goteri G. Tumours of the spleen. Cancer Imaging. 2005;5:73-7.

40. Davidson J, Tung K. Splenic peliosis: an unusual entity. Br J Radiol. 2010;83(990):e126-8.
41. Maves CK, Caron KH, Bisset GS 3rd, Agarwal R. Splenic and hepatic peliosis: MR findings. AJR Am J Roentgenol. 1992;158(1):75-6.
42. Saboo SS, Krajewski KM, O'Regan KN, Giardino A, Brown JR, Ramaiya N, et al. Spleen in haematological malignancies: spectrum of imaging findings. Br J Radiol. 2012;85(1009):81-92.
43. Paes FM, Kalkanis DG, Sideras PA, Serafini AN. FDG PET/CT of extranodal involvement in non-Hodgkin lymphoma and Hodgkin disease. Radiographics. 2010;30(1):269-91.
44. Li M, Zhang L, Wu N, Huang W, Lv N. Imaging findings of primary splenic lymphoma: a review of 17 cases in which diagnosis was made at splenectomy. PLoS One. 2013;8(11):e80264.
45. Fishman EK, Kuhlman JE, Jones RJ. CT of lymphoma: spectrum of disease. Radiographics. 1991;11(4):647-69.
46. Guermazi A, Brice P, de Kerviler EE, Ferme C, Hennequin C, Meignin V, et al. Extranodal Hodgkin disease: spectrum of disease. Radiographics. 2001;21(1):161-79.
47. Bhatia K, Sahdev A, Reznek RH. Lymphoma of the spleen. Semin Ultrasound CT MR. 2007;28(1):12-20.
48. Manzella A, Borba-Filho P, D'Ippolito G, Farias M. Abdominal manifestations of lymphoma: spectrum of imaging features. ISRN Radiol. 2013;2013:483069.
49. de Jong PA, van Ufford HM, Baarslag HJ, de Haas MJ, Wittebol SH, Quekel LG, et al. CT and 18F-FDG PET for noninvasive detection of splenic involvement in patients with malignant lymphoma. AJR Am J Roentgenol. 2009;192(3):745-53.
50. Cheson BD, Pfistner B, Juweid ME, Gascoyne RD, Specht L, Horning SJ, et al. Revised response criteria for malignant lymphoma. J Clin Oncol. 2007;25(5):579-86.
51. Juweid ME, Stroobants S, Hoekstra OS, Mottaghy FM, Dietlein M, Guermazi A, et al. Use of positron emission tomography for response assessment of lymphoma: consensus of the Imaging Subcommittee of International Harmonization Project in Lymphoma. J Clin Oncol. 2007;25(5):571-8.
52. Hamid KS, Rodriguez JA, Lairmore TC. Primary splenic angiosarcoma. JSLS. 2010;14(3):431-5.
53. Badiani R, Schaller G, Jain K, Swamy R, Gupta S. Angiosarcoma of the spleen presenting as spontaneous splenic rupture: A rare case report and review of the literature. Int J Surg Case Rep. 2013;4(9):765-7.
54. Manouras A, Giannopoulos P, Toufektzian L, Markogiannakis H, Lagoudianakis EE, Papadima A, et al. Splenic rupture as the presenting manifestation of primary splenic angiosarcoma in a teenage woman: a case report. J Med Case Rep. 2008;2:133.
55. Thompson WM, Levy AD, Aguilera NS, Gorospe L, Abbott RM. Angiosarcoma of the spleen: imaging characteristics in 12 patients. Radiology. 2005;235(1):106-15.
56. Comperat E, Bardier-Dupas A, Camparo P, Capron F, Charlotte F. Splenic metastases: clinicopathologic presentation, differential diagnosis, and pathogenesis. Arch Pathol Lab Med. 2007;131(6):965-9.
57. Showalter SL, Hager E, Yeo CJ. Metastatic disease to the pancreas and spleen. Semin Oncol. 2008;35(2):160-71.
58. Agha-Mohammadi S, Calne RY. Solitary splenic metastasis: case report and review of the literature. Am J Clin Oncol. 2001;24(3):306-10.
59. Senturk S, Karcaaltincaba M, Akata D. CT diagnosis of intrasplenic metastasis from ovarian carcinoma. Eur J Radiol. 2012;81(6):1094-9.
60. Hoeffel C, Bokemeyer C, Hoeffel JC, Gaucher H, Galanski M, Fornes P. CT hepatic and splenic appearances with sarcoidosis. Eur J Radiol. 1996;23(2):94-6.
61. Torres GM, Terry NL, Mergo PJ, Ros PR. MR imaging of the spleen. Magn Reson Imaging Clin North Am. 1995;3(1):39-50.
62. Minami M, Itai Y, Ohtomo K, Ohnishi S, Niki T, Kokubo T, et al. Siderotic nodules in the spleen: MR imaging of portal hypertension. Radiology. 1989;172(3):681-4.
63. Sagoh T, Itoh K, Togashi K, Shibata T, Nishimura K, Minami S, et al. Gamna-Gandy bodies of the spleen: evaluation with MR imaging. Radiology. 1989;172(3):685-7.
64. Hill SC, Damaska BM, Ling A, Patterson K, Di Bisceglie AM, Brady RO, et al. Gaucher disease: abdominal MR imaging findings in 46 patients. Radiology. 1992;184(2):561-6.
65. Housman JF, Chezmar JL, Nelson RC. Magnetic resonance imaging in hemochromatosis: extrahepatic iron deposition. Gastrointest Radiol. 1989;14(1):59-60.
66. Long JA Jr, Doppman JL, Nienhus AW, Mills SR. Computed tomographic analysis of beta-thalassemic syndromes with hemochromatosis: pathologic findings with clinical and laboratory correlations. J Comput Assist Tomogr. 1980;4(2):159-65.
67. Kim SH, Han JK, Lee KH, Won HJ, Kim KW, Kim JS, et al. Abdominal amyloidosis: spectrum of radiological findings. Clin Radiol. 2003;58(8):610-20.
68. Liu TY, Chen SC, Wang LY, Chuang WL, Chang WY, Liu CS. Systemic amyloidosis presenting as splenic tumor. Gastrointest Radiol. 1991;16(2):137-8.
69. Kennan NM, Evans C. Case report: hepatic and splenic calcification due to amyloid. Clin Radiol. 1991;44(1):60-1.
70. Monzawa S, Tsukamoto T, Omata K, Hosoda K, Araki T, Sugimura K. A case with primary amyloidosis of the liver and spleen: radiologic findings. Eur J Radiol. 2002;41(3):237-41.
71. McInnes MD, Kielar AZ, Macdonald DB. Percutaneous image-guided biopsy of the spleen: systematic review and meta-analysis of the complication rate and diagnostic accuracy. Radiology. 2011;260(3):699-708.
72. Tam A, Krishnamurthy S, Pillsbury EP, Ensor JE, Gupta S, Murthy R, et al. Percutaneous image-guided splenic biopsy in the oncology patient: an audit of 156 consecutive cases. J Vasc Interv Radiol. 2008;19(1):80-7.
73. Lucey BC, Boland GW, Maher MM, Hahn PF, Gervais DA, Mueller PR. Percutaneous nonvascular splenic intervention: a 10-year review. AJR Am J Roentgenol. 2002;179(6):1591-6.
74. Kang M, Kalra N, Gulati M, Lal A, Kochhar R, Rajwanshi A. Image guided percutaneous splenic interventions. Eur J Radiol. 2007;64(1):140-6.
75. Kamaya A, Weinstein S, Desser TS. Multiple lesions of the spleen: differential diagnosis of cystic and solid lesions. Semin Ultrasound CT MR. 2006;27(5):389-403.
76. Thanos L, Dailiana T, Papaioannou G, Nikita A, Koutrouvelis H, Kelekis DA. Percutaneous CT-guided drainage of splenic abscess. AJR Am J Roentgenol. 2002;179(3):629-32.
77. Singh AK, Shankar S, Gervais DA, Hahn PF, Mueller PR. Image-guided percutaneous splenic interventions. Radiographics. 2012;32(2):523-34.

78. Sammon J, Twomey M, Crush L, Maher MM, O'Connor OJ. Image-guided percutaneous splenic biopsy and drainage. Semin Intervent Radiol. 2012;29(4):301-10.
79. Trastek VF, Pairolero PC, Joyce JW, Hollier LH, Bernatz PE. Splenic artery aneurysms. Surgery. 1982;91(6):694-9.
80. Rokke O, Sondenaa K, Amundsen S, Bjerke-Larssen T, Jensen D. The diagnosis and management of splanchnic artery aneurysms. Scand J Gastroenterol. 1996;31(8):737-43.
81. Abbas MA, Stone WM, Fowl RJ, Gloviczki P, Oldenburg WA, Pairolero PC, et al. Splenic artery aneurysms: two decades experience at Mayo clinic. Ann Vasc Surg. 2002;16(4):442-9.
82. Lee PC, Rhee RY, Gordon RY, Fung JJ, Webster MW. Management of splenic artery aneurysms: the significance of portal and essential hypertension. J Am Coll Surg. 1999;189(5):483-90.
83. Selo-Ojeme DO, Welch CC. Review: spontaneous rupture of splenic artery aneurysm in pregnancy. Eur J Obstet Gynecol Reprod Biol. 2003;109(2):124-7.
84. Tessier DJ, Stone WM, Fowl RJ, Abbas MA, Andrews JC, Bower TC, et al. Clinical features and management of splenic artery pseudoaneurysm: case series and cumulative review of literature. J Vasc Surg. 2003;38(5):969-74.
85. Stanley JC, Wakefield TW, Graham LM, Whitehouse WM Jr, Zelenock GB, Lindenauer SM. Clinical importance and management of splanchnic artery aneurysms. J Vasc Surg. 1986;3(5):836-40.
86. Trastek VF, Pairolero PC, Bernatz PE. Splenic artery aneurysms. World J Surg. 1985;9(3):378-83.
87. Mattar SG, Lumsden AB. The management of splenic artery aneurysms: experience with 23 cases. Am J Surg. 1995;169(6): 580-4.
88. de Perrot M, Buhler L, Schneider PA, Mentha G, Morel P. Do aneurysms and pseudoaneurysms of the splenic artery require different surgical strategy? Hepatogastroenterology. 1999;46(27):2028-32.
89. Hogendoorn W, Lavida A, Hunink MG, Moll FL, Geroulakos G, Muhs BE, et al. Open repair, endovascular repair, and conservative management of true splenic artery aneurysms. J Vasc Surg. 2014;60(6):1667-76, e1.
90. Hogendoorn W, Lavida A, Hunink MG, Moll FL, Geroulakos G, Muhs BE, et al. Cost-effectiveness of endovascular repair, open repair, and conservative management of splenic artery aneurysms. J Vasc Surg. 2015;61(6):1432-40.
91. Guillon R, Garcier JM, Abergel A, Mofid R, Garcia V, Chahid T, et al. Management of splenic artery aneurysms and false aneurysms with endovascular treatment in 12 patients. Cardiovasc Intervent Radiol. 2003;26(3):256-60.
92. Gu JJ, He XH, Li WT, Ji J, Peng WJ, Li GD, et al. Safety and efficacy of splenic artery coil embolization for hypersplenism in liver cirrhosis. Acta Radiol. 2012;53(8):862-7.
93. Puri S, Nicholson AA, Breen DJ. Percutaneous thrombin injection for the treatment of a post-pancreatitis pseudoaneurysm. Eur Radiol. 2003;13(Suppl 4):L79-82.
94. Krueger K, Zaehringer M, Lackner K. Percutaneous treatment of a splenic artery pseudoaneurysm by thrombin injection. J Vasc Interv Radiol. 2005;16(7):1023-5.

CHAPTER 26

Harish Bhujade, Mandeep Kang, Nidhi Prabhakar, Anmol Bhatia

Imaging of the Postoperative Abdomen

INTRODUCTION

Recent advances in the understanding of the pathophysiology of disease processes have led to improved medical as well as surgical management. There have been substantial advances in the technique and type of surgical procedures being performed with an increasing trend toward minimally invasive techniques. This, in turn, has led to an increasing number of requests for radiological investigations for the evaluation of postoperative patients. These include the detection of complications both in the early (<4 weeks) and late phases (>4 weeks) as well as disease recurrence. To be able to recognize these complications, the radiologist needs to be familiar with the normal postoperative appearances of the surgery that has been performed as well as the complications that can occur after the procedure. It becomes critical here to be able to differentiate between what are the expected postoperative changes (relative to the temporal profile) and what findings constitute pathology, which in turn can alter patient management.

In this chapter, we will address the basics of imaging of the postoperative abdomen, the general complications which may occur, the normal postoperative anatomy as well as specific complications which are peculiar to certain commonly performed surgical procedures.

IMAGING MODALITIES

Plain X-rays of the abdomen are commonly performed in the immediate postoperative period and are useful for the detection of pneumoperitoneum, ileus, or intestinal obstruction. Ultrasonography (US) is often asked for to detect fluid collections or abscess or to look for biliary radicle dilatation after biliary procedures. The presence of surgical dressings on the abdominal wall and pneumoperitoneum or ileus in the immediate postoperative period limit its usefulness.[1] However, its portability as well as the use of nonionizing radiation is of advantage, particularly when children or young women have to undergo repeated imaging.

Helical CT is now the modality of choice for the radiological evaluation of the postoperative patient. Rapid acquisition is of advantage when critically sick patients need to be imaged. The ability to reconstruct multiplanar images is useful when complex postoperative anatomy has to be evaluated.

CT PROTOCOL

Before proceeding for CT, the radiologist must be familiar with the type of surgery done, intraoperative details and specific clinical question which demands CT. Positive water-soluble iodinated oral contrast should be used in most postoperative examinations, particularly when anastomotic leakage has to be ruled out. It is also most useful for differentiating distended bowel loops from extra-luminal fluid collections. Sick patients may not be able to tolerate larger volumes, administering between 500 and 1,000 mL of oral contrast should be enough to achieve an optimal diagnostic study. If plain radiographs of the abdomen reveal evidence of bowel obstruction, oral contrast can be avoided as the fluid in the dilated bowel loops provides a natural contrast. If there is suspected bowel ischemia or acute gastrointestinal bleeding, one should perform a biphasic contrast-enhanced computed tomography (CECT) with negative or neutral oral contrast. In both these clinical scenarios, performing dual energy CT (DECT) has the benefit of reducing the patient's radiation dose as well as improving the diagnostic accuracy. By using DECT and generating virtual nonenhanced images, one can omit the precontrast acquisition which is generally performed to detect presence of hyperattenuation, signifying bleed in the bowel lumen.[2] Subtle differences in the enhancement of ischemic bowel loops become more conspicuous with the use of iodine maps or quantitative measurements of the iodine content in the wall of the bowel.[3] Rectal contrast should be used, particularly following colorectal surgery.

Intravenous iodinated contrast should be used in all patients unless there is a specific contraindication such as deranged renal parameters or history of allergy to contrast. Besides the clinical scenarios mentioned previously where one should acquire a biphasic CECT, a single portal venous phase acquisition is adequate. The anatomical coverage should be from the domes of the diaphragm to the public symphysis, even if the surgery has been performed in the upper abdomen or pelvis. This is because both the compartments are interconnected and fluid may track along anatomical pathways from one to the other.[4] Secondly, many new pathways come into existence because of defects in the mesentery created due to the surgical procedure and so fluid may track to a location remote from the surgical bed.

NORMAL RADIOLOGICAL FINDINGS IN THE POSTOPERATIVE ABDOMEN

Some amount of changes will occur following surgery which do not represent complications but are due to the procedure itself. Soft-tissue stranding or patchy increased density will be seen in the subcutaneous fat around the incision site and in the intra-abdominal fat around the operative site. When the surgical procedure has involved significant handling of the bowel loops, these can show mural thickening or ileus **(Fig. 1)**. Subcutaneous emphysema may be seen in the anterior abdominal wall which may be extensive following laparoscopic procedures.[5]

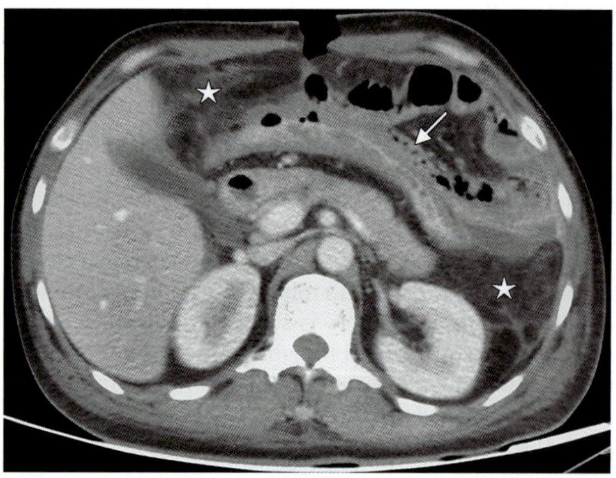

FIG. 1: A 42-year-old male underwent right hemicolectomy for carcinoma ascending colon. An axial contrast-enhanced CT image on postoperative day 4 shows diffuse mural thickening of the small bowel loops (arrow) due to edema and increased density of intra-abdominal fat (star).

The presence of free intraperitoneal air can pose a diagnostic dilemma to the radiologist as it can be due to the procedure itself or represent a complication such as an anastomotic leak or development of infection. Detection of pneumoperitoneum on plain radiographs formed the basis of initial literature. CT shows a much higher sensitivity for the detection of free intraperitoneal air in comparison to plain radiographs (87% on day 3 on CT vs. 53% on X-ray).[6] Pneumoperitoneum is reported to be present in up to 44% of CT scans performed on the third postoperative day, decreasing with time to 30% of cases between days 14 and 18 following surgery. The volume does not usually exceed 10 mL but larger volumes up to 40 mL may be seen in some patients.[7]

Laparoscopic surgery involves insufflation of carbon dioxide to create an artificial pneumoperitoneum. Carbon dioxide is more rapidly absorbed than nitrogen which is the main component of room air. Therefore, the amount of postoperative free intraperitoneal air is less with laparoscopic surgeries in comparison to open surgeries and is expected to be completely resorbed by 48 hours. It may, however, be seen up to the 9th postoperative day on plain X-rays[8] and up to 2 weeks on CT.[5] Presence of pneumoperitoneum >7–10 days following open surgery and >2 days after laparoscopic surgery is a cause for concern. Individual cases normally require clinic-radiological correlation. If there is still a doubt, one can consider follow-up radiological evaluation as any increase in the volume of pneumoperitoneum over time is definitely due to a complication.[9] One must also remember that surgical drains or percutaneous catheter in situ also lead to free intraperitoneal air and their presence must be kept in mind while interpreting the significance of the pneumoperitoneum.

Imaging features of generalized fluid retention may be seen in the postoperative period as a result of hypoproteinemia, fluid retention, and fluid overload. This is more commonly seen in patients with comorbidities, particularly, renal, or cardiac problems. This may result in a "Wet" patient with combinations of pleural effusion, mild ascites and mesenteric or subcutaneous fat edema **(Fig. 2)**.[9] Due to the surgical procedure, there is some accumulation of blood, lymph, and intraperitoneal fluid in the operative bed. These appear radiologically as unencapsulated, crescentic collections which do not anatomically displace any surrounding structures. These are generally absorbed spontaneously.[10] There may be mild peritoneal enhancement **(Fig. 3)**. Due to the decreased diaphragmatic excursion secondary to the pain associated with movement of the abdominal wall, some degree of bilateral basal passive atelectasis of the lungs is also expected in the immediate postoperative period.

Hemostatic compounds may be used by the surgeons to control intraoperative bleeding. The most commonly used is "Surgicel", made of oxidized regenerated cellulose, which may be left behind in the abdomen as it is bioabsorbable. On CT, it appears hypodense with a bubbly appearance,

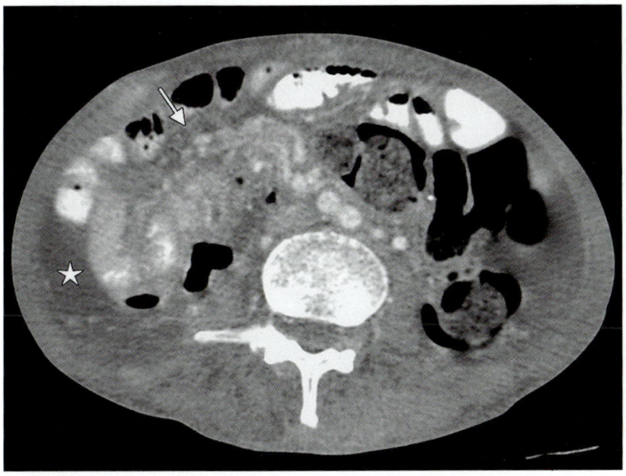

FIG. 2: A 53-year-old male underwent palliative distal gastrectomy with feeding jejunostomy for carcinoma distal stomach. An axial contrast-enhanced CT image on day 8 shows ascites (star) with diffuse increased density of the mesentery (arrow) with generalized edema of the subcutaneous fat.

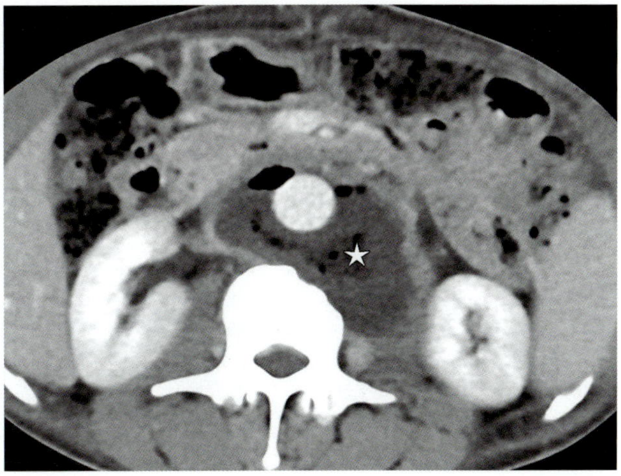

FIG. 4: A 70-year-old male underwent aortic aneurysm repair with graft placement. Contrast-enhanced computed tomography (CECT) axial image on postoperative day 3 shows Surgicel (star) as a hypodense area with a bubbly appearance surrounding the graft with air foci.

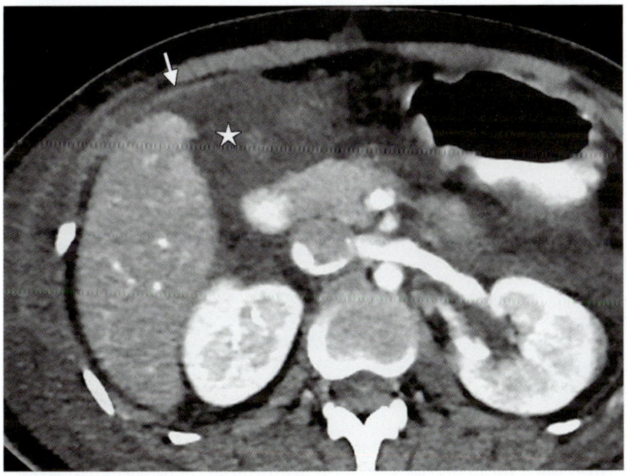

FIG. 3: A 28-year-old female postlaparoscopic cholecystectomy. Contrast-enhanced computed tomography (CECT) on day 4 following surgery shows mild peritoneal enhancement (arrow) with fluid (star) in the gallbladder fossa.

containing multiple gas foci which may be peripheral, located in the operative bed **(Fig. 4)**. This may be mistaken for an abscess, however, "Surgicel" will not show any enhancement following contrast.[11]

POSTOPERATIVE COMPLICATIONS

Postsurgical complications are common as they are part of the inherent risk of the procedure. In the immediate postoperative period, they are commonly related to infections or the surgical technique. Later complications may occur due to the altered anatomy, or recurrence of the primary disease process.

Anastomotic Leak

Anastomotic leaks are common to all reconstructive gastrointestinal surgeries and have an incidence of 1–5% after upper gastrointestinal surgeries and of 5–10% following colon resections.[12] They are associated with a high mortality (up to 50%) and morbidity and therefore require prompt recognition and early treatment.[10] Leaks occur at the anastomotic margins due to devascularization leading to necrosis, and therefore usually manifest clinically within the first fortnight following the surgery. Clinical symptoms are usually of sudden onset and consist of fever, which may show spikes, intense abdominal pain with guarding and rebound tenderness, tachycardia, and rising leukocyte counts. Fluoroscopic gastrointestinal studies using water soluble iodinated contrast have been shown to be useful for the detection and localization of leaks,[4,10] however, helical CT with its multiplanar reformation (MPR) capability is a better modality. It has been reported to confirm clinically suspected leaks in 48–100% of cases.[13] The hallmark of an anastomotic leak is extraluminal extravasation of oral or rectal contrast with air in the operative bed **(Fig. 5)**. At times oral contrast may not have had time to reach the anastomotic site due to the associated ileus. In this case, presence of loculated fluid with excess of extraluminal air in the surgical bed should raise the possibility of leak **(Figs. 6A and B)**.[14] At times, one can also see disruption of the staple line at the anastomotic site.

Postoperative Abscess

Postoperative intra-abdominal abscesses are a serious complication associated with increased morbidity and mortality rates of 10–40%.[10] They usually occur due to anastomotic leaks, in association with wound infections or operative contamination. Enteric pathogens such as

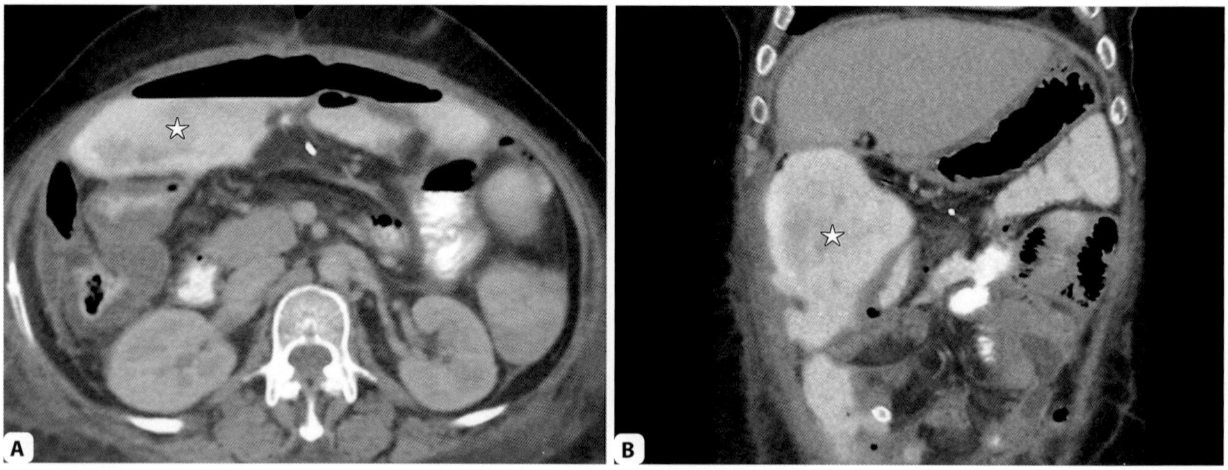

FIGS. 5A AND B: A 58-year-old female underwent transverse colon resection for colonic perforation. Following surgery on day 8, patient presented with fecal discharge from main wound and drain. Axial (A) and coronal multiplanar reformation or reconstruction (MPR) (B) demonstrates extraluminal oral contrast (star) due to anastomotic leak.

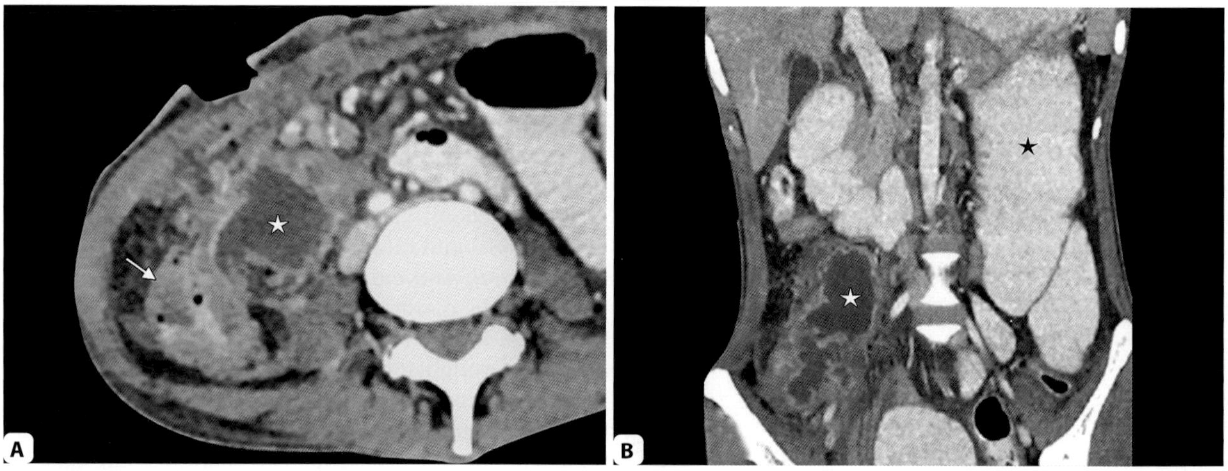

FIGS. 6A AND B: A 26-year-old female underwent ileal resection for bowel gangrene with end jejunostomy. Post-restoration of bowel continuity with jejunocolic anastomosis on day 4, patient presented with high-grade fever and abdominal distension. (A) Axial contrast-enhanced CT image shows a multiloculated collection (white star) with surrounding stranding fat strandings adjacent to the anastomotic site. The ascending colon shows diffuse mural thickening (arrow). (B) Coronal reconstructed CT image shows grossly dilated proximal jejunal loops (black star) and multiloculated collection (white star).

Klebsiella, *Escherichia coli*, and *Proteus* are the usual causative organisms. Helical CT is reported to have a high accuracy of >90% for the detection of intra-abdominal abscesses.[10,15,16] On CT, these appear as a low-attenuating fluid collection, spherical or elliptical in shape, which is usually well-defined. They usually show a peripheral enhancing rim. Air foci, air-fluid levels, or septations may be seen at times. There may be mass effect with displacement or distortion of adjacent structures. The abscess may be located in the surgical bed or at a remote location due to spread of inflammation along anatomical pathways in the peritoneal cavity or along the surgically created nonanatomic pathways and spaces.[4,10] As an example, the gastrosplenic and gastrocolic ligaments are transected during gastrectomy while the gastrohepatic ligament is partially transected. This creates a communication between the lesser sac, left subphrenic, gastrosplenic, and gastrohepatic spaces. Hence, an anastomotic leak may cause a fluid collection or abscess in this newly created compartment with spread to the left subphrenic space **(Figs. 7A and B)**. Abscesses in the left subphrenic space usually have associated left pleural effusion and basal consolidation.[17] Inter-loop abscesses may be accompanied by paralytic ileus.[10]

Image-guided percutaneous catheter drainage is the preferred management option, and therefore, the initial CT report should mention the suitability for safe drainage of the abscess, especially regarding the location and access route. The true internal character of the abscess may not be evident on CT. US and MR are better at determining the

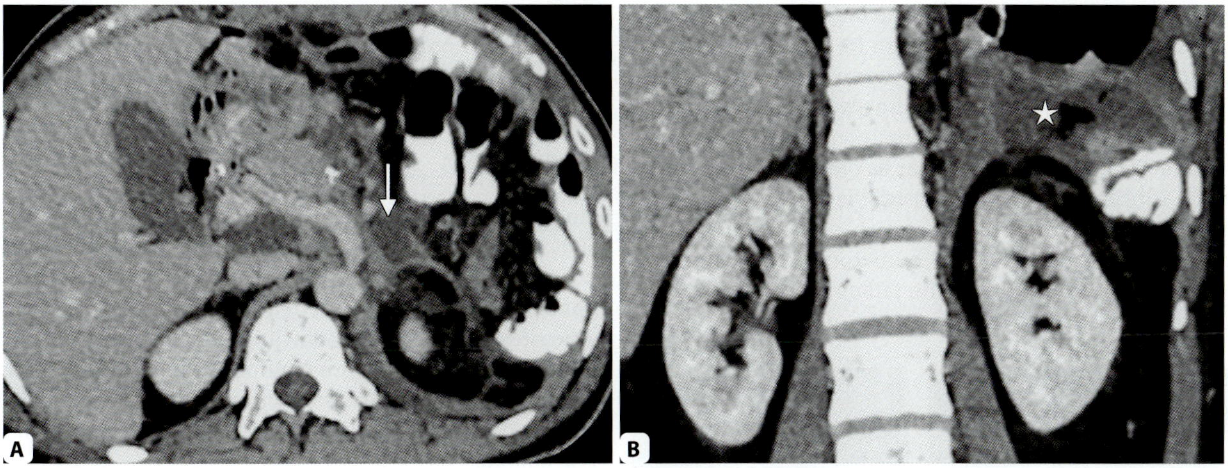

FIGS. 7A AND B: A 47-year-old male with gastrointestinal stromal tumor (GIST) underwent a total gastrectomy, distal pancreatectomy, and splenectomy. Patient developed spiking fever on seventh postoperative day. (A) Axial contrast-enhanced computed tomography (CECT) image shows small amount of fluid (arrow) and fat stranding in the operative bed; (B) Coronal multiplanar reformation (MPR) CT image demonstrates a fluid collection (star) with specks of air and thick-enhancing rim in the left subphrenic space.

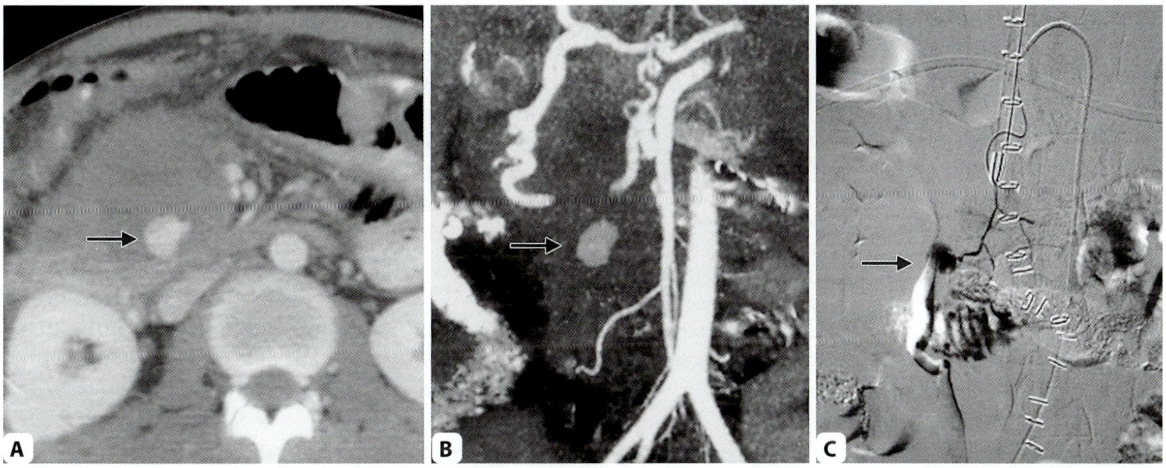

FIGS. 8A TO C: A 36-year-old male underwent laparotomy for ascending colon perforation. Presented with hematemesis on day 3. CT angiography axial (A) and coronal maximum intensity projection (MIP) (B) image shows a pseudoaneurysm (arrow) arising from a branch of the superior mesenteric artery (SMA) with surrounding hematoma. Digital subtraction angiography (C) shows contrast-filled outpouching suggestive of pseudoaneurysm (arrow) from SMA branch.

degree of liquefaction and presence of septations which in turn help to predict whether this particular abscess will respond to percutaneous catheter drainage alone or will surgical intervention be required.[9,18] Percutaneous catheter drainage is also less likely to succeed, if the abscess is due to an anastomotic leak, or if there is a fistulous communication with the bowel.[9,10]

Postoperative Bleeding

Hemorrhage is a serious complication of abdominal surgery which may be due to inadvertent vessel or organ injury, inadequate hemostasis, or vascular ligation. In addition, in patients with obstructive jaundice or hepatic dysfunction, deficiency of vitamin K, or coagulation factor may cause a hemorrhagic diathesis. Clinically, the patients present with signs of hypovolemia with falling hematocrit, tachycardia, and hypotension. The surgical drains (if placed) may reveal bloody fluid output or there may be oozing of blood through the incision site.[4,10,17] As mentioned previously, a biphasic CT scan should be done with negative/neutral oral contrast as intraluminal high attenuation can be masked by the positive oral contrast. A bleeding vessel may at times be seen on the CT scan showing active extravasation of the intravenous contrast **(Figs. 8 and 9)**. These patients may be managed by endovascular embolization. Acute hematomas are hyperdense on CT with attenuation values between 20 and 60 HU with a layered appearance, with gradual decrease in density over time as hemoglobin is removed from the clot **(Figs. 10A and B)**. Chronic hematomas have fluid attenuation and may be indistinguishable from other fluid collections. There can be mass effect on the adjacent structures depending upon their location and size. Postoperative hematomas involving the solid organs (spleen, liver, or kidneys) are usually confined by the organ capsule. Therefore, they appear as crescentic collections in the subcapsular space with variable compression of the underlying parenchyma.

Anterior abdominal wall hematomas can occur due to injury to perforators in the subcutaneous fat during the placement of trocars in laparoscopic surgery. High-attenuation collections in the subcutaneous fat with thickening of the abdominal wall muscles which appear hyperdense will be visualized on CT **(Fig. 11)**.[5]

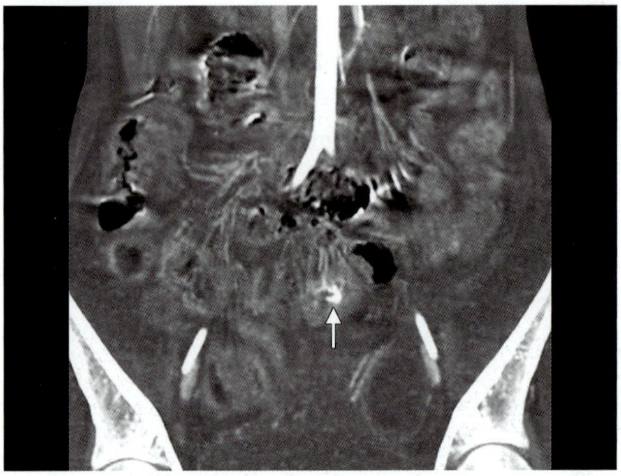

FIG. 9: A 32-year-old female who had undergone a right hemicolectomy for abdominal tuberculosis developed an enterocutaneous fistula. Presented with history of bleeding from site of fistula. CT angiography maximum intensity projection (MIP) image demonstrates high attenuation in the bowel lumen due to active extravasation of contrast (arrow) from a branch of the superior mesenteric artery.

Anastomotic Strictures

Hold-up in the passage of contrast across the anastomotic sites on fluoroscopic examinations done in the immediate postsurgical period is generally due to edema and resolves spontaneously over time. Nevertheless, anastomotic strictures may develop following surgical procedures due to ischemia and are more common when there has been an anastomotic leak. Anastomotic strictures can usually be managed with balloon dilatation, if an endoscopic approach is available.[19]

Postoperative Bowel Obstruction

Postoperative ileus is commonly seen in the early phase following abdominal surgery and may be due to excessive handling of the bowel loops during the procedure. It may later be a manifestation of inter-loop abscesses. Plain radiographs show mild dilatation of the small bowel loops. On CT, the small bowel is distended with fluid and air with no obvious transition point.[10] At times, there may be accompanying dilatation of the ascending and transverse colon extending till the splenic flexure with collapse of the distal colon. This is said to be due to the increase in the intra-abdominal pressure resulting in collapse of the left colon which lies in a dependent position posteriorly **(Fig. 12)**.[20] Small bowel mechanical obstruction can occur in the postoperative period due to the formation of adhesions, internal hernias or incisional or port site hernias, volvulus, strictures or tumor recurrence. Adhesions

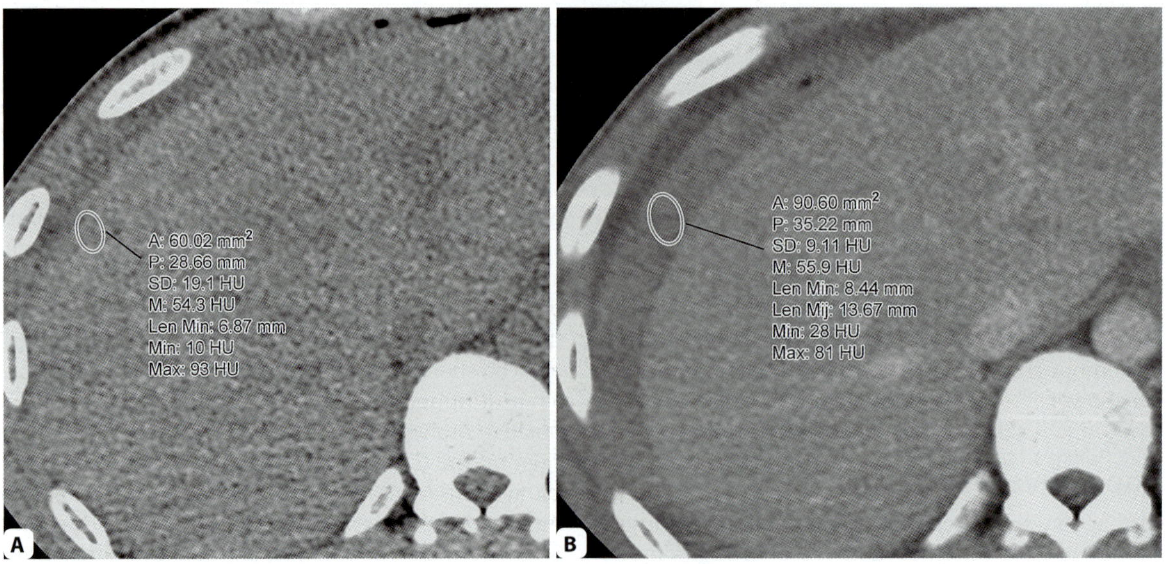

FIGS. 10A AND B: A 45-year-old male underwent cholecystectomy. An axial noncontrast image (A) and axial contrast-enhanced CT image on postoperative day 1 show a large hyperdense collection (circle) in the right perihepatic region with a layered appearance consistent with acute hematoma. Note is made of high HU value (54 HU) seen on noncontrast image. An axial contrast-enhanced venous phase image (B) is better delineating the the perihepatic hematoma.

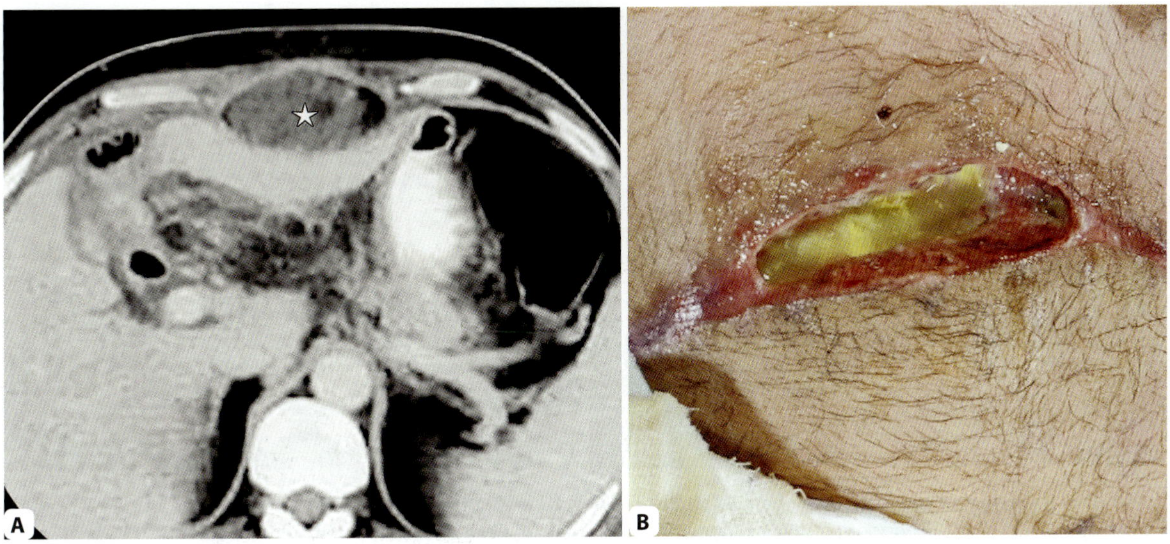

FIGS. 11A AND B: A 53-year-old male underwent a whipple's procedure with development of postoperative sepsis with pus discharge from the wound. Axial contrast-enhanced computed tomography (CECT) image (A) on day 15 demonstrates a large hypodense collection (star) just beneath abdominal wall. (B) Clinical picture of infected wound showing pus at the incision site.

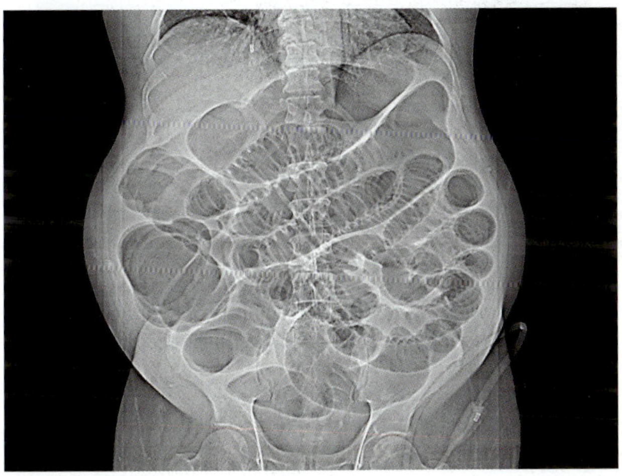

FIG. 12: A 46-year-old female developed abdominal distention on the second postoperative day following open cholecystectomy. Scout film prior to CT shows moderately dilated small bowel loops with dilatation of the small and large bowel due to ileus.

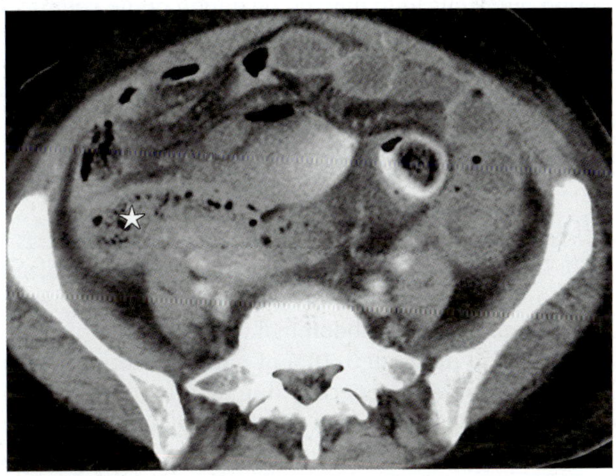

FIG. 13: A 58-year-male underwent a low anterior resection for carcinoma rectum. Presented with pain in abdomen and vomiting on day 9 of surgery. contrast-enhanced computed tomography (CECT) axial image shows dilatation of a small bowel loop with mottled air lucencies—the "small bowel feces" sign (star).

can occur in >90% of patients who have undergone major abdominal surgery.[21] Internal hernias can occur when the surgical procedure has involved creating defects in the mesentery or mesocolon, for example, following Roux-en-Y gastrojejunostomy (GJ). Typical radiological features include dilated proximal small loops with collapsed loops distal to the transition point. There may be particulate feculent matter seen in the small bowel loop just proximal to the point of obstruction known as the "small bowel feces" sign **(Fig. 13)**.[22] An abrupt transition with no identifiable cause is likely due to adhesions **(Fig. 14)**. A cluster of dilated loops may be seen in cases of internal hernias or volvulus. The mesenteric vessels may be engorged and demonstrate the "swirl" sign as the mesentery is pulled into an abnormal location.

One must carefully look for signs of ischemia in the obstructed loop as the management of the patient may be radically altered, if present. In brief, these include mural thickening which can give a stratified appearance, abnormal enhancement of the involved segment of bowel and soft-tissue stranding or fluid in the subtending mesentery. The presence of pneumatosis in the wall of the involved segment of bowel or gas in the portal venous radicles are signs of irreversible ischemia.[23]

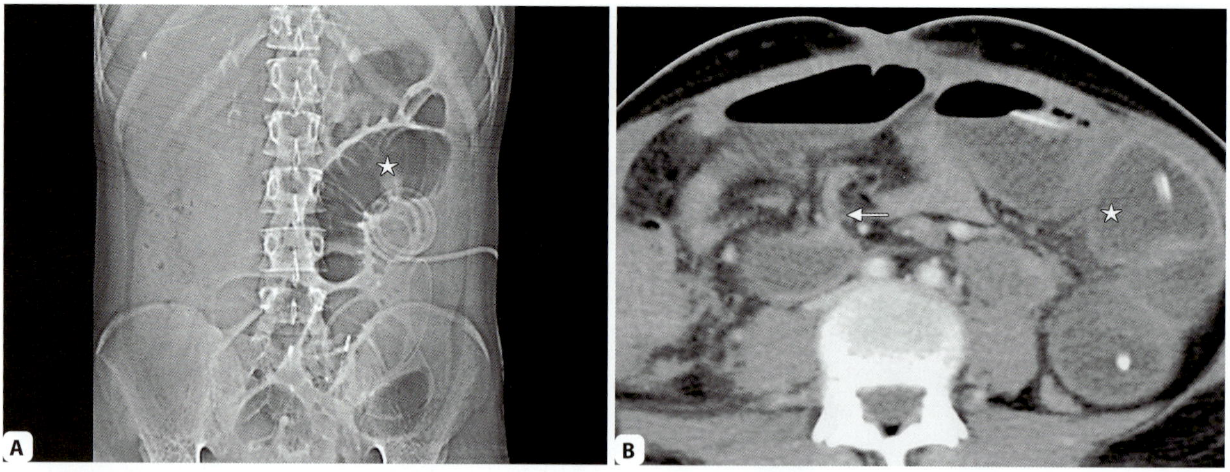

FIGS. 14A AND B: A 40-year-old male underwent Whipple's repair with feeding jejunostomy. Presented with episodes of vomiting and no passage of flatus. (A) CT Topogram shows dilated proximal small bowel loops (star) in left side of abdomen. (B) Axial contrast-enhanced CT image shows the dilated fluid-filled proximal small bowel loops (star) with an abrupt transition point (arrow) beyond which the loops are collapsed. The cause of obstruction is most likely due to adhesions.

Colonic obstruction is less common in the postoperative period but can lead to marked dilatation of the colon. As the cecum is the most distensible segment of the large bowel, it bears the brunt of the dilatation. In the presence of a competent ileocecal valve, thereby preventing decompression into the small bowel, there is a grave risk of cecal ischemia or perforation.[9]

Wound Complications

On CT, the surgical incision site can be easily recognized as an area of increased attenuation in the subcutaneous fat and muscles of the abdominal wall.[24] Wound infection may develop in about 5–10% of patients who undergo abdominal surgery generally due to contamination by anaerobic organisms.[10] The resultant inflammation can lead to necrosis and pus accumulation at the incision site, with the potential adverse sequelae of wound dehiscence, necrotizing fasciitis, incisional hernia formation, peritonitis, and systemic sepsis. Various risk factors associated with increased incidence of wound infections include elderly patients, obesity, tobacco, drugs or alcohol abuse, and presence of comorbidities. The risk also depends upon the kind of surgery performed with abdominoperineal resections having a higher incidence.[25,26]

Computed tomography scan can detect the presence of wound infection even before it becomes clinically apparent as small collections of fluid and air in the subcutaneous fat and muscles of the abdominal wall at and around the incision site **(Fig. 15)**.[4,10] Unless this condition is recognized early and treated promptly, it can lead on to frank abscess formation and ultimately separation of the fascia at the incision and wound dehiscence. On CT, one needs to meticulously evaluate all the layers of the abdominal wall around the incision site, including the anterior and posterior fascial sheaths for evidence of any separation which portends dehiscence.[27]

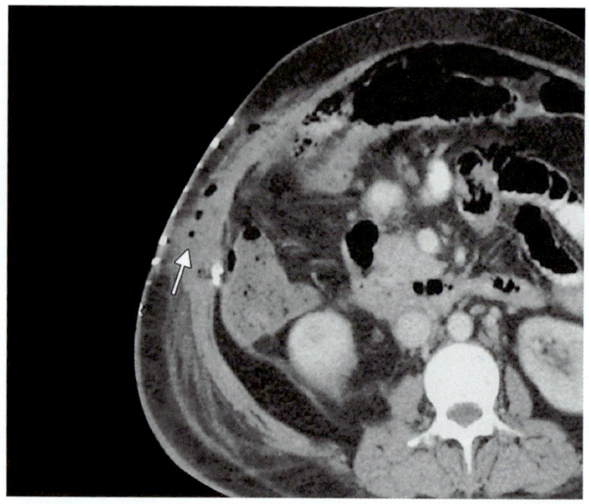

FIG. 15: A 41-year-old female underwent extended cholecystectomy for carcinoma gallbladder. Postoperative day 14 contrast-enhanced computed tomography (CECT) shows thickening of the layers of the anterior abdominal wall at the incision site with multiple foci of air suggestive of wound infection (arrow).

Incisional Hernia

Despite improvements in surgical techniques, incisional hernias may develop in about 3–30% of cases[24,28] with the incidence rising in the presence of wound infection.[29] It is also more common when median or paramedian vertical incisions are used in comparison to horizontal incisions as vertical incisions transect the muscular fibers rather than dissect along them. These transected muscles are rendered more prone to disruption in the presence of increased abdominal pressure.[10,30] Most incisional hernias develop within the first year following surgery but may manifest clinically much later. Clinical examination usually suffices to reach the diagnosis, however, in the presence of obesity or a thick keloid, the abdominal wall defect may not be palpable. Secondly, the omentum is usually the initial content of the hernia and may not be palpable, if the sac has dissected between the layers of the abdominal wall. In this clinical setting, a CT may be asked for in order to find a cause for the patient's symptoms and will establish the correct diagnosis.[24-26] Once bowel loops also herniate into the sac, they can get incarcerated and obstructed.

Computed tomography scans will show a defect in the layers of the abdominal wall with protrusion of omentum, a loop of small bowel or mesentery through it into the subcutaneous fat. Presence of stranding in the fat, small fluid collections or mural thickening of the herniated bowel loop are early changes that suggest strangulation.[25] Herniation may also occur at port sites following laparoscopy with a reported incidence of 0.5% with a higher risk associated with the use of trocars over 12 mm and large diameter ports.[5] Parastomal herniation may also occur along ileostomy or colostomy sites **(Figs. 16A and B)**.[10]

Retained Surgical Foreign Material

Unintended retention of a surgical material in a patient poses a serious risk of complications for the patient and lays the surgical team open for a malpractice suit. Usual operating theater procedures include repeated counts of all surgical material being used in order to prevent this complication, but it still occurs though the exact incidence is not known. Reports reveal that surgical sponges are the most often retained foreign object (RFO) followed by instruments.[31] Septic or aseptic complications result due to the RFO. If the RFO remains sterile, fibrosis occurs due to a foreign body response leading to adhesions or fistula formation. Retained surgical swabs are referred to as gossypibomas or textilomas and appear on CT as well-defined soft-tissue masses with a whorled texture and multiple internal foci of air **(Figs. 17A and B)**. Enhancement of the rim is seen following intravenous contrast. It is helpful to identify the wavy radiopaque markers which are now incorporated into most surgical sponges[9,32] which may be better appreciated on the scout image rather than the axial images. In the setting of infection, there is abscess formation with a loculated fluid collection often showing a thick enhancing rim. On magnetic resonance imaging (MRI), retained sponges show an intermediate signal intensity on T1-weighted images similar to skeletal muscle. Internal high-signal intensity fluid may be seen on T2-weighted images with low-signal intensity structures having a whorled appearance.[31]

NORMAL POSTOPERATIVE ANATOMY AND COMPLICATIONS SPECIFIC TO PROCEDURE

It is beyond the scope of this chapter to discuss the normal postoperative anatomy of the myriad surgical procedures performed in the abdomen. This chapter will limit itself to discuss some of the most commonly performed surgical procedures.

Esophageal Surgeries

Esophageal resections are commonly performed for malignancy but may also be performed for benign strictures refractory to balloon dilatation. The Ivor Lewis esophagectomy involves resection of the diseased part of the mid and distal esophagus, and mobilization of the stomach which is then placed vertically inside the mediastinum after fashioning it into a tubular structure by resection of

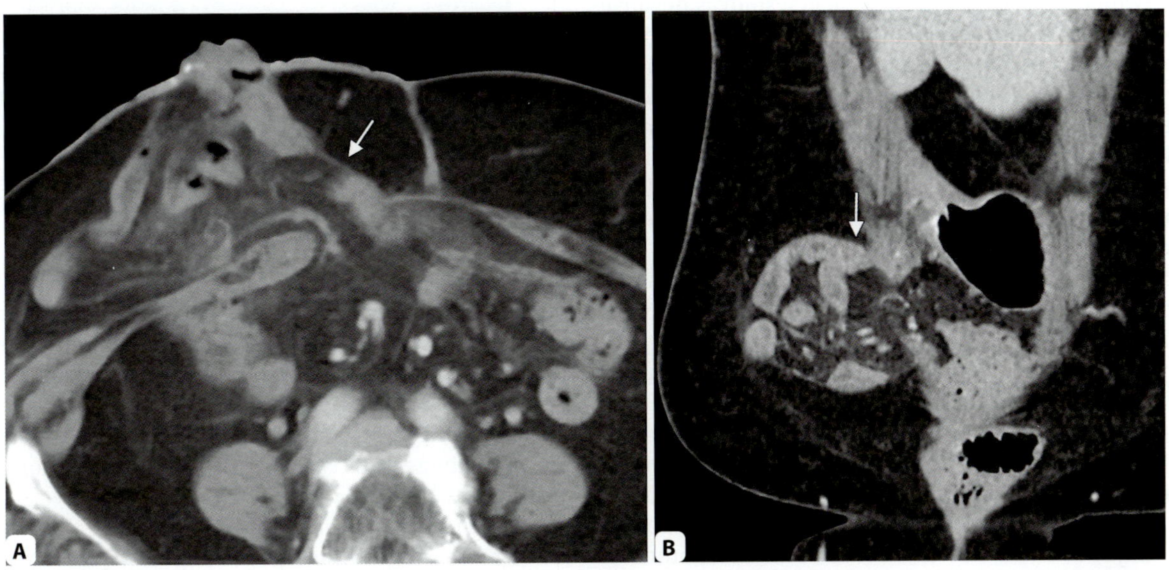

FIGS. 16A AND B: (A) Axial and (B) coronal contrast-enhanced computed tomography (CECT) images of a 65-year-old male showing a large parastomal hernia containing mainly bowel loops along with omental fat and vessels (arrow).

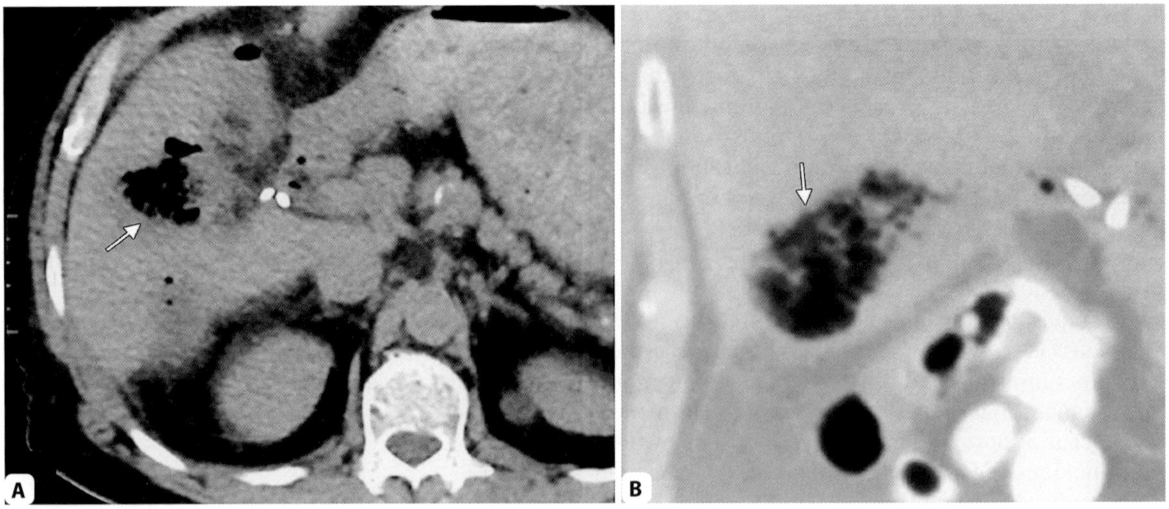

FIGS. 17A AND B: A 28-year-old female complained of intermittent right hypochondrial pain following a laparoscopic cholecystectomy. (A) contrast-enhanced computed tomography (CECT) axial image shows an ill-defined hypodense area with multiple air foci adjacent to the surgical clips consistent with gossypiboma (arrow); (B) The internal whorled appearance (arrow) is better appreciated on viewing at lung window settings.

the greater curvature. This is then anastomosed with the esophagus in an end-to-end or end-to-side manner. In case of disease involving the upper esophagus, a neck dissection is also done and the esophagogastric anastomosis is created in the neck. These are usually accompanied with a pyloroplasty to drain the stomach as the vagus nerve is sacrificed during the procedure.[33]

Upper gastrointestinal contrast studies are routinely performed between 5 and 10 days postoperatively to look for any anastomotic leak before the patient is allowed oral intake. Water-soluble nonionic contrast is preferred as it does not carry the risk of chemical pneumonia in case of aspiration.[34] Many authors advocate the use of repeating the study with dilute barium in case the first study is negative in order to increase the sensitivity.[35,36] A plain radiograph should be obtained prior to administering contrast so that any subtle difference in density in pleural effusions can be detected which denote leak. It also aids in differentiating between a small leak and a surgical clip. CT may be done, if the contrast study is negative but the patient is unwell and improves the sensitivity for the detection of anastomotic leaks.[36]

Major complications occur in about 20% of patients which can be grouped into general complications of a thoracotomy such as pneumonia, atelectasis, and respiratory failure or specific to the esophageal surgery. There can be vascular injury leading to a hemothorax or injury to the thoracic duct leading to a chylothorax, but the most common complication is an anastomotic leak which carries significant morbidity and mortality. The leak usually occurs early in the postoperative period (2–3 days) due to technical failure of the anastomoses. Leaks occurring later at around 3–7 days are usually due to ischemia of the anastomotic margins. The leak may occur from the esophagogastric anastomoses, from the margins of the stomach where the greater curvature has been resected or from the pyloroplasty, hence all these sites need to be carefully examined. A leak can lead to formation of an esophago-bronchial or esophago-pleural fistula, mediastinitis and sepsis **(Fig. 18)**. These patients are also at increased risk for the subsequent development of strictures.[37]

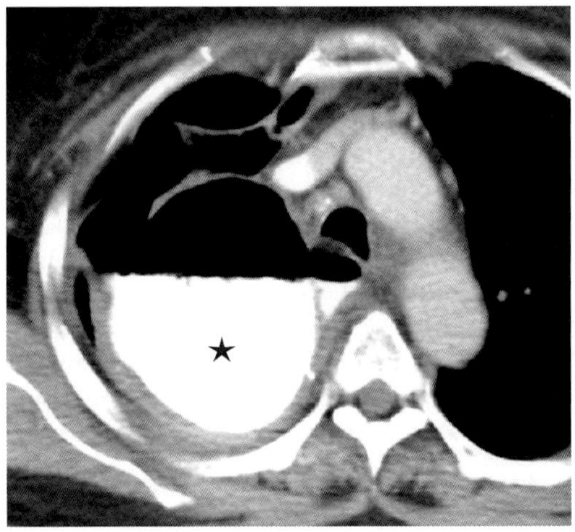

FIG. 18: A 42-year-old male underwent thoracoscopic assisted esophagectomy for carcinoma. He presented with complaints of chest pain, dyspnea, and had tachycardia. contrast-enhanced computed tomography (CECT) axial image demonstrates a leak (star) from the esophagogastric anastomotic site with formation of an esophagopleural fistula.

Imaging has a similar role to look for anastomotic leaks following bypass procedures where colonic, jejunal, or myocutaneous flaps are used. A more dreaded complication is ischemia of the conduit which is diagnosed endoscopically.

Surgeries of the Stomach and Duodenum

Gastric resections are commonly performed surgical procedures for malignancies involving the stomach or complicated peptic ulcer disease. In the Billroth I partial gastrectomy, the distal stomach is resected and an anastomosis created between the duodenum and proximal stomach. The Billroth II/Polya partial gastrectomy involves resection of the distal stomach, closure of the duodenal stump and creation of a GJ in an antecolic or retrocolic position. In a Roux-en-Y procedure, the bowel continuity after distal gastrectomy is restored through construction of a Roux loop. Direct anastomoses of the distal esophagus with a jejunal Roux loop are performed following total gastrectomy. A contrast fluoroscopic study is usually performed using water soluble contrast media in the immediate postoperative period to rule out leakage. However, the study can detect subclinical leaks in 7% of cases which do not require any further surgical intervention. The study may also return false negative results with leaks identified on subsequent endoscopy.[38] Hence, some surgeons reserve the contrast study to cases where there is a clinical suspicion of leak. The afferent limb may not opacify with oral contrast, hence a CT examination should be done in case of clinical suspicion of duodenal stump blow-out. It may show complex, air/fluid collections in the region of the duodenal stump which can be identified by the surgical staples line **(Figs. 19A and B)**. Collections may also be seen in the subhepatic or peripancreatic spaces.[17]

The afferent loop may get obstructed due to adhesion or twisting of the bowel at the gastroenterostomy site. Acute obstruction can cause duodenal stump blow-out and is an emergent situation. CT can demonstrate the dilated, fluid-filled loop passing posterior to the superior mesenteric vessels to the left side. Obstruction to the outflow of bile usually results in associated dilatation of the biliary tree.[39]

Tumor recurrence becomes a more common cause for obstructive symptoms developing later in the time course after the surgery. CT is the imaging modality of choice in this situation and should be carefully evaluated for recurrence in the surgical bed or anastomotic site and any evidence of spread of disease to the lymph nodes, liver, or peritoneum.[40] If the initial malignancy was a gastrointestinal stromal tumor, addition of an arterial phase to the imaging protocol is of benefit as these tumors are typically hypervascular.

Bariatric Surgery

Morbid obesity has shown an alarming increasing trend in its prevalence even in India over the last few years, and has now reached epidemic proportions. A body mass index (BMI) over 25 kg/m^2 is considered overweight internationally. However, updated guidelines released by the Indian Council of Medical Research and the Ministry of Health and Family Welfare in 2012 consider the BMI over 23 kg/m^2 as overweight. This is due to a genetic tendency of Indians toward abdominal obesity with its attendant risk of lifestyle diseases. Despite the morbidly obese forming a high-risk group, surgery for weight loss is offered to these patients as it reduces the long-term associated morbidity and improves life expectancy.[41]

Two kinds of procedures are used—malabsorptive procedures wherein the length of the absorptive surface is reduced by bypassing a segment of the small bowel. These are seldom used in isolation these days due to significant associated complications. Restrictive procedures aim to reduce the capacity of the stomach in order to induce early satiety. These include sleeve gastrectomy, vertical

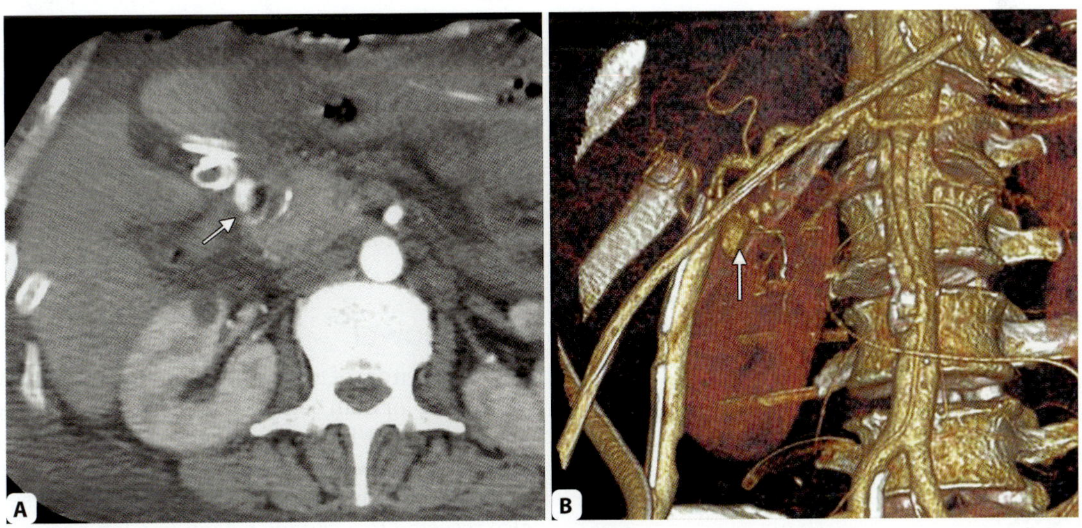

FIGS. 19A AND B: A 57-year-old male with gastric carcinoma, status postgastrectomy and Billroth II gastrojejunostomy. He had duodenal stump blow-out which was being managed conservatively with placement of a subhepatic drain. Now presented with bloody discharge from the drain. CT angiography (A) axial image shows active extravasation of intravenous contrast (arrow) with pooling in the duodenum (arrow) adjacent to the surgical drain; (B) Coronal volume-rendered image shows pseudoaneurysms (arrow) arising from the gastroduodenal artery, probably due to leak of the pancreatic enzymes from the duodenal stump.

gastroplasty, and laparoscopic adjustable gastric banding (LAGB). The Roux-en-Y gastric bypass (RYGB) and biliopancreatic diversion are combination procedures with both restrictive and malabsorptive components. Sleeve gastrectomy involves creating a narrow gastric tube along the lesser curvature by resecting 70–85% of the stomach along the greater curvature. In LAGB, an inflatable band is placed just below the gastroesophageal junction, thereby creating a small gastric pouch. The band is connected to a port in the anterior abdominal wall through which the volume of the band can be adjusted and therefore the degree of restriction. In the RYGB, a small gastric pouch is created in its proximal part and anastomosed to a Roux loop. The rest of the stomach and duodenum forms the biliopancreatic limb which is also anastomosed to the Roux loop. The length of the Roux loop determines the degree of malabsorption with more distal loops having more malabsorptive effect.[42]

Early in the postoperative period, a contrast fluoroscopic examination is usually performed to rule out anastomotic leaks. Following sleeve gastrectomy, most of the leaks occur from the proximal end, close to the gastroesophageal junction. CT is required for evaluation of the biliopancreatic limb in RYGB procedures. It is also the best modality for investigating a patient with suspected efferent loop obstruction, which may be due to adhesions, strictures, internal hernias, or incisional hernias. Three types of internal hernias can occur following RYGB procedures:

1. Through the defect created in the transverse mesocolon when a retrocolic anastomosis has been created. Multiple and dilated small bowel loops will be seen superior to the transverse mesocolon, rather than the single anastomotic Roux loop on CT.
2. Through the defect created in the small bowel mesentery due to the jejunojejunostomy. In this case, a cluster of loops will be seen located beneath the anterior abdominal wall with absence of any intervening omental fat. The colon may be centrally displaced.
3. Through the defect in the mesentery posterior to the Roux loop (Peterson type).[43] Characteristically, there will be a cluster of small bowel loops in the left upper abdomen with shift of the superior mesenteric vessels to the left.

The gastric band placed in LAGB may migrate away from the gastroesophageal junction. The usual orientation of the balloon is at 45°, with migration it takes up a more vertical or horizontal position ("O" sign), which will be evident on plain radiographs.[44] A contrast swallow will confirm dilated stomach above the band. If the migration remains unrecognized or untreated, it may lead to gastric necrosis.

Small Bowel

Surgeries on the small bowel are commonly performed for resection of diseased segments or resections of segments which are required to be used as a conduit elsewhere. As mentioned earlier, the most common immediate postoperative complication is an anastomotic leak which is best evaluated by a CT with oral and intravenous contrast. Delayed complications such as intestinal obstruction or recurrence of disease are usually evaluated with a combination of fluoroscopic contrast studies and cross-sectional imaging such as CT or MR enteroclysis or enterography.

Blind Pouch Syndrome

Side-to-side small bowel anastomoses or incorrectly performed end-to-side anastomoses can result in the formation of a blind pouch which is an enlarged, blind-ended, aperistaltic small bowel loop. These usually manifest late after surgery with features of malabsorption or due to complications such as perforation or bleeding. A dynamic investigation such as fluoroscopic enteroclysis will demonstrate the preferential filling of the blind pouch with dilatation of the loop. CT will demonstrate a saccular structure filled with oral contrast in close relation to surgical clips/staples.

Ileal Pouch-anal Anastomoses

A total proctocolectomy is the definitive treatment for patients with ulcerative colitis or familiar adenomatous polyposis (FAP). This is followed by the creation of an ileal pouch which is anastomosed to the anal canal, thus maintaining continence by preserving the anal sphincter. The ileal reservoir is created from the terminal ileum in a J, S, or W manner of which the J-shape is the most commonly performed.[45] The pouch is usually allowed to heal by performing a proximal temporary ileostomy with restoration of the bowel continuity after 8–12 weeks. Routine fluoroscopic contrast studies are performed before closure of the ileostomy to rule out any leaks. CT may be done, if there is clinical suspicion of an abscess or obstruction.

Pouchitis is a nonspecific inflammation of the pouch with uncertain etiology which can affect up to half the patients. The usual clinical presentation is with diarrhea, bleeding, and tenesmus. The radiologic features are nonspecific with dilatation of the pouch, mural thickening, mucosal enhancement, and stranding in the surrounding fat.[46]

Large Bowel

Various kinds of resections of the large bowel are performed for both benign and malignant diseases. A right hemicolectomy involves resection of the right colon and terminal ileum with an ileotransverse colon anastomosis. In extended right hemicolectomy, the transverse colon is also resected to a varying extent. In a left hemicolectomy, the left colon including the splenic flexure and proximal sigmoid colon are resected. A Hartmann's procedure involves closing off of the rectum and sigmoid colon after a diverting colostomy when a primary anastomosis is not considered safe. This rectal stump can later be reattached to the distal colon. At times, instead of closing off the stump, a distal mucous fistula is created by bringing the stump up to the anterior abdominal wall. Anterior resection consists of resecting the sigmoid colon and varying part of the rectum with a colorectal anastomosis. When the upper rectum is resected above the peritoneal reflection, it is termed a "high anterior resection" while in the low or extended low anterior resection, the middle or distal rectum are also resected. Abdominoperineal excision of the rectum involves resection of the anal canal as well. Restorative proctocolectomy involves resection of the entire colon and rectum with formation of an ileal pouch.

Some surgeons routinely ask for fluoroscopic contrast studies to rule out anastomotic leaks. These are most often posterior in location after procedures involving the rectum and may cause anterior displacement of the rectum (3–5 cm from the anterior sacral margin). The patient must be fluoroscoped again after being asked to void as some leaks may become evident only after emptying the rectum.[25]

Computed tomography may be asked for in the early postoperative period, if there is clinical suspicion of an anastomotic leak, abscess, fistula, or bowel obstruction. Rectal contrast should always be administered prior to the scan. The "double rectum" sign has been described in rectal anastomotic leaks. This is due to the anteriorly displaced rectum with a fluid collection in the presacral space due to the leak **(Figs. 20A to C)**.[25,47] Other signs of leaks are frank extravasation of the rectal contrast, air within or outside the bowel wall, fluid collections, disruption of the staple line and pneumoperitoneum.

Diversion Colitis

Once the temporary colostomy has to be taken down with restoration of bowel continuity, a fluoroscopic contrast study is normally asked for by the surgeon prior to closure. The unused segment often appears nondistensible with diffuse mucosal nodularity or even punctuate ulcerations. The exact etiology is unclear, however, the colon returns to normal once the bowel continuity is restored with resumption of the fecal stream through it.[25]

HEPATOBILIARY SURGERIES

Curative liver surgeries are performed for many benign and malignant liver diseases. The type of surgery depends on the nature and location of the disease and expertise of the surgeon.[48] Most common indications for liver resections are malignancies such as colorectal metastasis, hepatocellular carcinoma (without underlying cirrhosis), neuroendocrine metastasis, cholangiocarcinoma, benign diseases such as hepatic adenomas, symptomatic cysts, intrahepatic biliary calculi, and traumatic hepatic lacerations.[49]

Surgical Procedures

Liver resections can be anatomical or nonanatomical resections. The former includes removing contiguous hepatic segments whereas latter is a wedge resection which is usually small and peripheral. A standardized nomenclature for anatomical resections has been suggested by the Brisbane 2000 Terminology of Hepatic Anatomy and Resection.[50] Right hepatectomy includes removal of segments 5, 6, 7, and 8, i.e., resecting the entire liver parenchyma to the right of the middle hepatic vein. Extended right hepatectomy includes additional removal of segment 4 in addition to right lobe. Left hepatectomy involves removal of segments 2, 3, and 4, i.e., resection of liver parenchyma to the left of the middle hepatic vein. Extended left hepatectomy includes additional resection of segments 5 and 8. Monosegmentectomy is resection of a single segment, whereas bisegmentectomy involves resection of two contiguous segments. Nonanatomical resections are suitable for small peripheral lesions.[48]

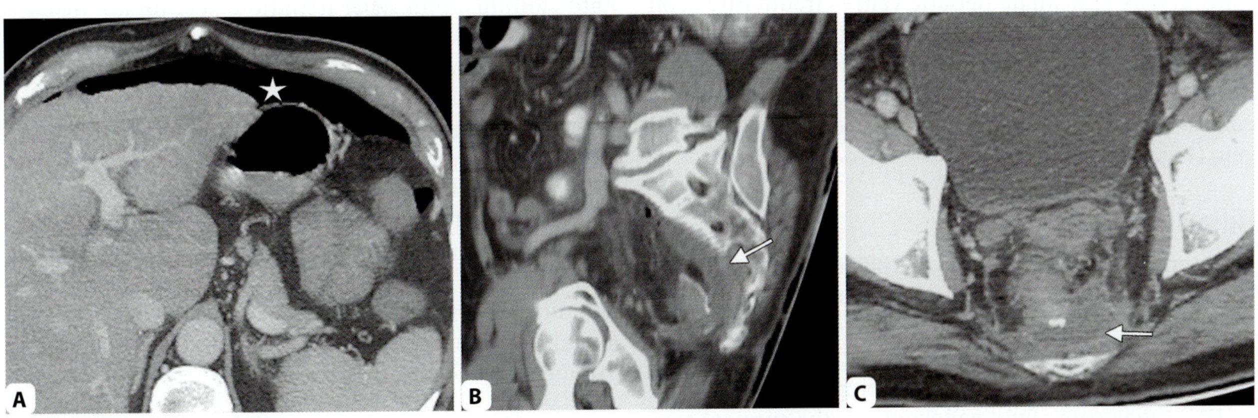

FIGS. 20A TO C: A 68-year-old male post-extended low anterior resection for carcinoma rectum had fever with abdominal distention. (A) Contrast-enhanced CT axial image shows a large pneumoperitoneum (star) beneath the anterior abdominal wall; (B) Oblique multiplanar reformation (MPR) and (C) Axial images reveal a displaced staple with a collection showing specks of air posterior to the rectum due to an anastomotic leak—the double-barrel sign (arrow in B and C).

Normal Postoperative Imaging Features

Small fluid collections, hematomas, or bilomas can be routinely observed in the early postoperative period and generally regress over a period of few weeks. In addition, metallic surgical clips, extra-luminal gas accumulation, and pleural effusions are also routine findings on imaging. Portal branch stump thrombosis may also be seen in the early postoperative period. In addition, a linear band of low-attenuating area may be observed adjacent to the resection margins. This finding is transient and is possibly due to accumulated bile or blood, or devascularized parenchyma.[48]

Late Postoperative Period

The volume of the remnant liver rapidly reaches up to 100% during 6 months to 1 year, with up to 60% in the first 7 days following the surgery.[51,52] After right hepatectomy, the left and caudate lobes hypertrophy and shift to the right. There is upward displacement of the right kidney, hepatic flexure, and small bowel loops with posterior displacement of the inferior vena cava (IVC). After left hepatectomy, there is hypertrophy of right and caudate lobes, right kidney is usually displaced caudally and stomach or colon occupy the left hepatic fossa. Transient splenic enlargement during initial 6 months after liver resection may be observed.[53]

EARLY POSTOPERATIVE COMPLICATIONS

The most common early postoperative complications are fluid collections, vascular thrombosis, and biliary injuries. Fluid collections are usually adjacent to surgical margins, and correspond to seromas or hematomas (50%), bilomas (25%), or infected collections (25%).[48]

Vascular Thrombosis

Thrombosis of a single hepatic vein is frequently seen after liver resections and is usually partial and seen close to the resection margins. Portal vein and hepatic artery thrombosis are rare, with segmental portal thrombosis more commonly observed than thrombosis of the main portal vein **(Fig. 21)**.[48]

Biliary Injuries

Biliary injuries can be bile leaks and biliary obstruction. Bile leak after hepatobiliary surgery may arise from the biliary-enteric anastomosis site, or may be related to the withdrawal of an external drainage tube, or to intraprocedural bile duct injury.[54] US and multidetector computed tomography (MDCT) may show fluid collections at the surgical site. Magnetic resonance cholangiopancreatography (MRCP) may be used to identify the location and the nature of the leak.[54]

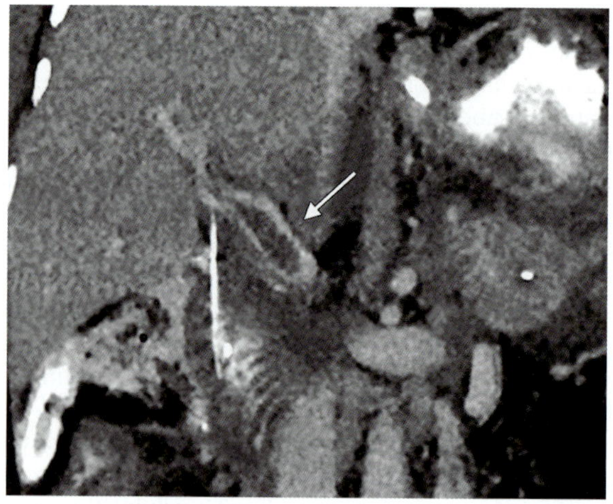

FIG. 21: A 61-year-old male underwent a left hepatectomy. contrast-enhanced computed tomography (CECT) coronal multiplanar reformation (MPR) reveals a thrombus as a hypodense filling defect in the main portal vein (arrow).

Biliary obstruction results from postoperative fibrosis at the bile duct stump or inadvertent bile duct ligation. It is most frequently seen after biliary-enteric anastomosis, with obstruction of the Roux-en-Y loop.[55] MDCT will show dilated biliary tree with dilated fluid-filled Roux-en-Y loop.[48]

Intraoperative Diaphragmatic Injury

Diaphragmatic injuries are very rare and mostly seen after right hepatectomy. Right pleural effusion with increased pleural enhancement may be seen on MDCT. They may present with early small bowel obstruction, if the bowel herniates through the diaphragmatic defect.[48]

LATE POSTOPERATIVE COMPLICATIONS

Late complications after hepatic resection are disease recurrence and ischemic cholangitis. Follow-up MDCT or MR are performed depending on the nature of the resected hepatic neoplasm for the detection of tumor recurrence. Presence of segmental or subsegmental biliary dilatation although not specific may suggest disease recurrence, even without visible focal lesion.[48]

Ischemic cholangitis may occur after hepatic resection within a few months to several years in cases of arterial injury during surgery. The clinical presentation is nonspecific with jaundice and fever. MRCP is the imaging modality of choice and may show irregular and multiple bile duct stenoses with intrahepatic bile duct dilatations.[48]

Laparoscopic Cholecystectomy

Laparoscopic cholecystectomy is the preferred procedure in patients with symptomatic gallstones. However, complications after laparoscopic cholecystectomy, especially bile duct injuries, have been described more commonly in comparison to open surgery.[56] US, CT, endoscopic retrograde cholangiopancreatography (ERCP), MRCP, and radionuclide imaging play an important role in evaluating the postoperative patient.[57-59] These imaging modalities are complementary and the primary imaging technique to be used will depend on the clinical scenario and availability.

Normal Appearances after Laparoscopic Cholecystectomy

- A small amount of fluid in the operative bed is a common finding during the first week. These fluid collections have no distinct or well-defined margins on CT.[60]
- Increased density in the abdominal wall fat at the site of the laparoscopic ports and small amounts of free pelvic fluid may also be seen.[61]
- The diameter of the common bile duct (CBD) may increase postcholecystectomy, with a maximal caliber of 13 mm identified.[62] When biliary dilatation is seen on postoperative imaging, correlation with preoperative imaging and current clinical features and biochemistry is required.

Complications

Major complications after cholecystectomy can be divided into biliary, vascular, and laparoscopic complications. Biliary complications include bile duct injury, biliary obstruction, and dropped stones.

Biliary Injury

Bile leak secondary to bile duct injury is the most common complication of laparoscopic cholecystectomy.[63] Most leakages occur from the cystic duct stump. A few common mechanisms for the leak are dislodgment of clips from the cystic duct stump, laceration, transection, or thermal injuries of the duct.[64] The initial assessment in these patients is usually with US or MDCT which may show perihepatic fluid. Hepatobiliary scintigraphy is a less frequently used method of assessing the patients with suspected bile duct injury, however, it has been claimed to be more sensitive and specific than US or CT in detecting bile leaks.[65] Although it is an invasive procedure, ERCP is useful as it can detect the exact site of leak and can successfully treat the leak using internal stents. ERCP is more likely to be successful, if the injury to the duct is <5 mm, the injury is extrahepatic, and there is no associated abscess or biloma.[66] Open surgery may be required, if the leak persists. MRCP is a noninvasive way of evaluating the anatomy of bile ducts. The use of mangafodipir trisodium, a contrast agent that has primary biliary excretion, helps to both diagnose a bile leak and identify the source of the leak.[67]

Biliary Obstruction

Retained gallstones, misplaced surgical clips, fibrosis due to inflammation from adjacent clips, and thermal injury from cautery devices are causes of biliary obstruction **(Fig. 22)**.[66] Patients present with progressive postoperative obstructive jaundice. US and MRCP detect duct dilatation and exclude CBD stones. ERCP is useful in confirming the diagnosis and may be therapeutic.

Stone Retention

Stone retention is an important complication of laparoscopic cholecystectomy with an incidence of 1.1–7%.[68] Factors which predispose to retained stones are a long cystic duct pedicle and partial excision of gallbladder due to adhesions. Similarly, since the CBD is not explored during laparoscopic cholecystectomy, a gallbladder stone can migrate into the CBD in patients with patulous cystic duct when the gallbladder is pulled in a cephalad direction during cholecystectomy, causing biliary obstruction. In patients with suspected stone retention, MRCP is helpful in depicting these stones, while ERCP is both diagnostic and therapeutic.[64]

Dropped Gallstones

Spillage of gallstones occurs due to inadvertent entry into the gallbladder during dissection or at the time of gallbladder extraction through the port site. The majority of "dropped" gallstones are found in the right upper quadrant, but they may migrate to dependent areas (right paracolic gutter or pelvis).[69] Most remain asymptomatic, however,

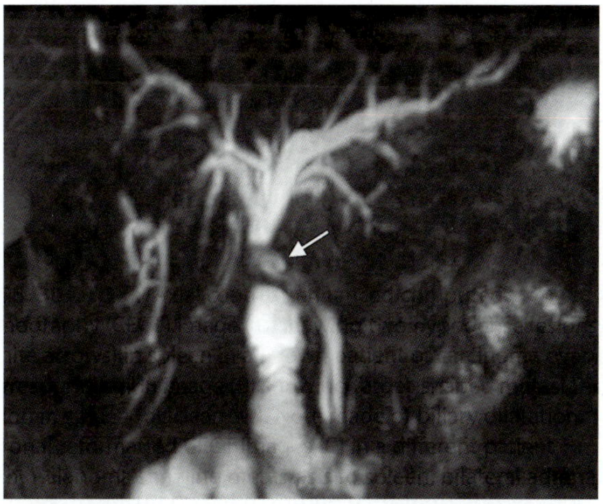

FIG. 22: A 25-year-old female underwent a laparoscopic cholecystectomy for gallstone disease. She presented with obstructive jaundice 6 months later. Magnetic resonance cholangiopancreatography (MRCP) maximum intensity projection (MIP) image shows a stricture (arrow) in the proximal common bile duct (CBD).

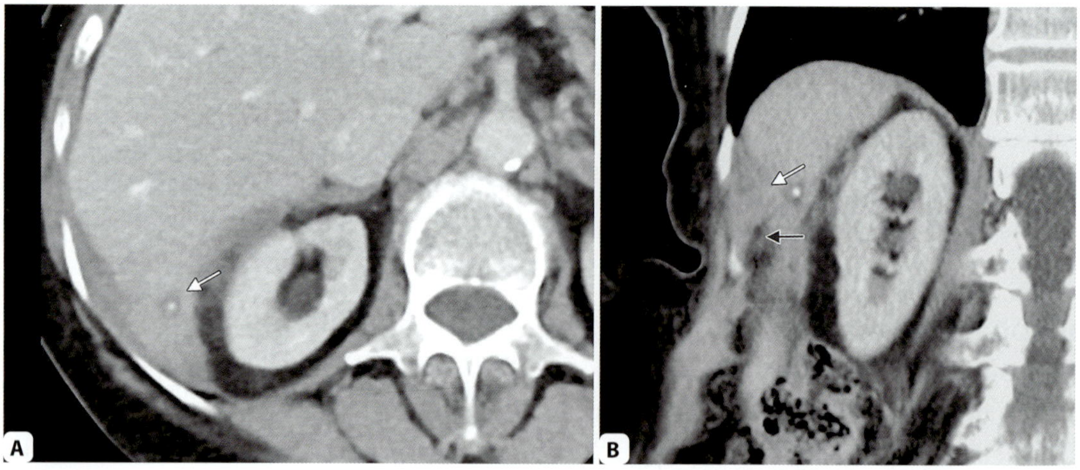

FIGS. 23A AND B: A 42-year-old female with history of laparoscopic cholecystectomy 6 months back, presented with pain in right upper quadrant of abdomen. Axial (A) and (B) coronal contrast-enhanced computed tomography (CECT) image show hyperdense focus with halo (black arrow) with surrounding inflammatory changes (white arrows) consistent with dropped stone.

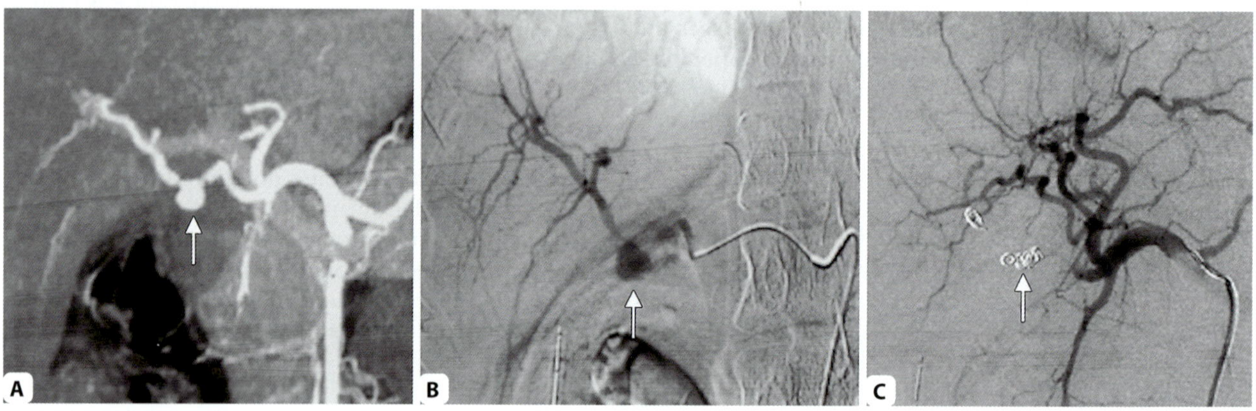

FIGS. 24A TO C: A 32-year-old female had a laparoscopic cholecystectomy following which she developed hemobilia and malena. (A) CT angiography coronal maximum intensity projection (MIP) image shows a large pseudoaneurysm (arrow) arising from the right hepatic artery; (B) Selective right hepatic artery angiogram confirms the presence of pseudoaneurysm (arrow); (C) Check angiogram post successful endovascular coiling (arrow) demonstrates no filling of the aneurysm.

significant complications can occur since they cause a local foreign body reaction.[70] Abscess formation is the most common complication resulting from "dropped" stones and may develop months later following cholecystectomy (**Fig. 23** dropped calculus).[69]

Vascular Injury

Injury to blood vessels during trocar insertion is responsible for peri- or postoperative hemorrhage.[71] During dissection of Calot's triangle, the right hepatic artery is the most common vessel to be injured followed by the portal vein **(Figs. 24A to C)**.[70] Hepatic artery ligation may lead to the development of a delayed ischemic cholangiopathy. MRCP may show irregular ductal dilatation and stenosis.

PANCREATIC SURGERIES

Pancreatic resection surgeries for tumors and chronic pancreatitis include Whipples' and Beger's procedures as well as central and distal pancreatectomy, while drainage procedures include Puestow and Frey's operations.[72,73] Information regarding the type of surgery the patient has undergone as well as the interval between surgery and imaging is important for interpretation of postoperative scans.

Whipples' procedure: This procedure involves resection of pancreatic head, jejunum, gastric antrum, and duodenum, followed by hepaticojejunostomy (HJ), pancreaticojejunostomy (PJ), and duodenojejunostomy

(DJ), or GJ. The normal postoperative findings include the presence of these different anastomoses.[72,73] Following pancreatic head resection, the splenomesenteric venous junction and superior mesenteric vein (SMV) will be seen to the right of the residual pancreatic parenchyma and in close proximity to the IVC posteriorly.

Beger's procedure: It includes resection of the pancreatic head with preservation of duodenum. PJ is done at two locations of the Roux-en-Y limb following pancreatic head removal. A sleeve of the pancreatic parenchyma is left behind along with duodenum ensuring the preservation of blood supply of the duodenum.[72,73]

Puestow procedure: It consists of side-to-side longitudinal PJ with dilated pancreatic duct draining directly into a loop of jejunum. The Roux-en-Y loop following this surgery lies immediately anterior to pancreatic body or tail.[72,73]

Frey's procedure: It includes partial resection of pancreatic head and a longitudinal PJ, with an intact biliary duct.[72,73]

Central pancreatectomy: Part of the pancreatic body or neck is resected, followed by a Roux-en-Y PJ to the remaining pancreatic tissue in the distal part. The distal end of the pancreas may, however, be anastomosed to the stomach. The proximal cut end is sutured, and the Roux-en-Y bowel is seen at the level of the splenoportal confluence, separating the pancreatic head from its body and tail.[73]

Distal pancreatectomy: The pancreatic parenchyma lying to the left of SMV is resected, and the cut end is sutured to prevent pancreatic juice leakage. The pancreas thereby ends abruptly, and the surgical bed will not have any bowel related to the pancreas, stomach, or duodenum, as against in the above-described surgeries. As the blood supply to the tail of pancreas comes mostly from splenic artery branches, splenectomy becomes necessary at times along with distal pancreatectomy.[73]

Normal Postoperative Findings

Several normal postoperative CT and MRI findings may be misdiagnosed as the disease process, hence, knowledge of normal postoperative appearances is highly essential.

- Pneumobilia (tends to persist) and periportal hepatic edema (usually resolves within a month) are universally seen. Air may be seen in the MPD also as a normal finding. However, pneumobilia should not be seen following surgeries in which there are no biliary anastomoses.[72,73]
- The afferent loop of bowel following Frey procedure which drains the biliary ducts and pancreas may be thick and edematous for the first 3 weeks following surgery, and should not be misdiagnosed as hemorrhage or ischemia.[72,73]
- Roux loop following the Puestow procedure lies between the body of the pancreas and stomach in the lesser sac, and may be falsely diagnosed to be a pancreatic mass or internal hernia.[72] The use of positive oral contrast for distending the bowel and changing the patient from a supine to a lateral decubitus position during CT, characteristic location as well as course of the Roux loop, and the presence of valvulae conniventes help in preventing a misdiagnosis.[73,74]
- Transient fluid collections in the surgical bed are common in the first month following surgery. The presence of air foci within these collections does not necessarily indicate infection but should raise the suspicion of a pancreatic fistula.[75-77]
- Reactive lymphadenopathy (nodes up to 1.5 cm in the short axis diameter) is seen up to 2 months after the surgery and regresses on follow-up imaging.[78]
- Perivascular cuffing around the celiac artery and its branches, and superior mesenteric artery (SMA) is seen for up to 6 weeks following Whipples' and Beger's procedures. This cuffing is inflammatory in nature in patients having negative surgical margins and should not be wrongly diagnosed as tumor recurrence. Follow-up imaging becomes necessary to distinguish between the perivascular cuffing and disease recurrence.[73]
- Mild pancreatic duct dilation (1–2 mm in comparison to preoperative imaging) is an expected postoperative appearance, and does not correlate with subsequent pancreatitis.[72,73]
- There may be a cavity detected in the head of the pancreas after Frey's procedure, which may be falsely diagnosed as a pancreatic pseudocyst or cystic neoplasm.[72,73] This cavity usually decreases with time.

Complications

Minor complications are relatively more frequent (seen in 28–29% patients), as against major complications that may require surgical intervention or vascular embolization (seen in 11% patients).[72]

- *Delayed gastric emptying:* Seen in up to 50% of patients during the early postoperative course following pylorus preserving pancreatoduodenectomy.[79,80] Gastric outlet obstruction may also be seen due to narrowing of the gastric outlet.
- *Arterial complications:* Splenic artery and common hepatic artery pseudoaneurysms are known to occur after pancreatic surgery. Stenosis in the celiac artery can also be seen following pancreatic surgery, but is treated only when there are symptoms attributable to it, as isolated vessel stenosis is usually asymptomatic due to presence of rich collaterals between the celiac and SMA.[73]

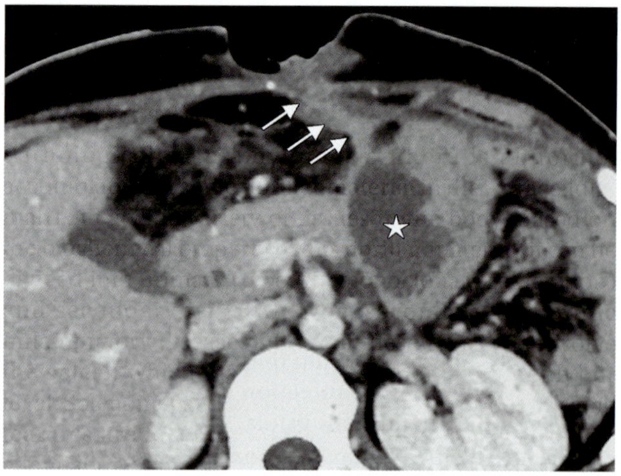

FIG. 25: A 38-year-old male underwent a distal pancreatectomy, gastrectomy, and splenectomy for a desmoid tumor of the tail of pancreas. Presented with history of watery discharge from incision site. An axial contrast-enhanced CT image shows an irregular collection (star) with thick enhancing wall in the region of the tail of pancreas with a fistulous track (arrows) seen extending anteriorly to the anterior abdominal wall.

- *Thrombosis of portal vein and splenic infarction:* Due to postoperative pancreatitis or as a result of iatrogenic injury.[73]
- *Pancreatic fistula and postoperative pancreatitis:* Detection of amylase-rich fluid after the 10th post-operative day in the drainage tube kept in the surgical bed raises the suspicion of a PJ fistula **(Fig. 25)**.[72,73]
- Extrahepatic CBD dilatation of >10 mm is abnormal and is likely due to ischemia of the distal CBD.[72,73]

CONCLUSION

Knowledge of the normal postoperative appearance following abdominal surgery is essential for the accurate interpretation of postoperative imaging. A two-way communication between the radiologist and clinical colleagues is required so that the radiologist is aware of the exact nature of the procedure the patient has undergone. Helical CT with its multiplanar capability is the modality of choice for the detection and characterization of postoperative complications.

REFERENCES

1. Bader FG, SchrÖder M, Kujath P, Muhl E, Bruch HP, Eckmann C. Diffuse post-operative peritonitis: value of diagnostic parameters and impact of early indication for relaparotomy. Eur J Med Res. 2009;14(11):491-6.
2. Okamura-Kawasaki M, Uesugi Y, Yabusaki S. Dual-energy CT for gastrointestinal bleeding. BJR Open. 2023;5(1):20220054.
3. Trabzonlu TA, Mozaffary A, Kim D, Yaghmai V. Dual-energy CT evaluation of gastrointestinal bleeding. Abdom Radiol (NY). 2020;45(1):1-14.
4. Pannu HK, Oliphant M. The subperitoneal space and peritoneal cavity: basic concepts. Abdom Imaging. 2015;40(7):2710-22.
5. Hindman NM, Kang S, Parikh MS. Common post-operative findings unique to laparoscopic surgery. Radiographics. 2014;34:119-38.
6. Earls JP, Dachman AH, Colon E, Garrett MG, Molloy M. Prevalence and duration of postoperative pneumoperitoneum: sensitivity of CT vs left lateral decubitus radiography. AJR Am J Roentgenol.1993;161(4):781-5.
7. Gayer G, Jonas T, Apter S, Amitai M, Shabtai M, Hertz M. Postoperative pneumo-peritoneum as detected by CT: prevalence, duration, and relevant factors affecting its possible significance. Abdom Imaging. 2000;25(3):301-5.
8. Hope WW, Herriford BT, Norton HJ, Lincourt AE, Teigland CM, Kercher KW. Duration and clinical significance of radiographically detected "free air" after laparoscopic nephrectomy. Surg Laparosc Endosc Percut Tech. 2009;19(5):415-8.
9. Chalmers AG, Macafee D, Tolan DJM, Brittenden J. Introduction to the postsurgical abdomen. In: Brittenden J, Tolan DJM (Eds). Radiology of the postsurgical abdomen. London: Springer-Verlag. 2012. pp.1-40.
10. Gore RM, Berlin JW, Yaghmai V, Mehta U, Newmark GM, Ghahremani GG. CT diagnosis of post-operative complications. Semin Ultrasound CT MR. 2004;25(3):207-21.
11. Roshkovan L, Singhal S, Katz SI, Galperin-Aizenberg M. Multimodality imaging of Surgicel®, an important mimic of post-operative complication in the thorax. BJR Open. 2021;3(1):20210031.
12. Bertelsen CA, Andreasen AH, Jørgensen T, Harling H. Danish Colorectal Cancer Group. Anastomotic leakage after anterior resection for rectal cancer: risk factors. Colorectal Dis. 2010;12(1):37-43.
13. Nicksa GA, Dring RV, Johnson KH, Sardella WV, Vignati PV, Cohen JL. Anastomotic leaks: what is the best diagnostic imaging study? Dis Colon Rectum. 2007;50(2):197-203.
14. Pouli S, Kozana A, Papakitsou I, Daskalogiannaki M, Raissaki M. Gastrointestinal perforation: clinical and MDCT clues for identification of aetiology. Insights Imaging. 2020;11(1):31.
15. Burke C, Maura M, Molina PL. Interventional computed tomography. In: Lee J, Sagel SS, Stanley RJ (Eds). Computed Body Tomography. Philadelphia: Lippincott Williams & Wilkins; 2006. pp. 95-144.
16. Kambadakone A, Mueller PR. Abdominal abscesses. In: Gore RM, Levine MS (Eds). Textbook of Gastrointestinal Radiology, 4th edition. Philadelphia: Elsevier-Saunders; 2015. pp. 1254-78.
17. Kim KW, Choi BI, Han JK, Kim TK, Kim AY, Lee HJ, et al. Postoperative anatomic and pathologic findings at CT following gastrectomy. Radiographics. 2002;22:323-36.
18. Kumar RR, Kim JT, Haukoos JS, Macias LH, Dixon MR, Stamos MJ, et al. Factors affecting the successful management of intra-abdominal abscesses with antibiotics and the need for percutaneous drainage. Dis Colon Rectum. 2006;49:183-9.
19. Yuan X, Liu W, Ye L, Wu M, Hu B. Combination of endoscopic incision and balloon dilation for treatment of a completely obstructed anastomotic stenosis following colorectal resection: A case report. Medicine (Baltimore). 2019;98(26):e16292.

20. Frager D, Rovno HD, Baer JW, Bashist B, Friedman M. Prospective evaluation of colonic obstruction with computed tomography. Abdom Imaging. 1998;23(2):141-6.
21. Dijkstra FR, Nieuwenhuijzen M, Reijnen MM, van Goor H. Recent clinical developments in pathophysiology, epidemiology, diagnosis and treatment of intra-abdominal adhesions. Scand J Gastroenterol. 2000;232:52-9.
22. Berl S, Dawkins A, Di Santis D. The small bowel feces sign. Abdom Radiol. 2016;41(4):794-5.
23. Della Seta M, Kloeckner R, Pinto Dos Santos D, Walter-Rittel TC, Hahn F, Henze J, et al. Pneumatosis intestinalis and porto-mesenteric venous gas: a multicenter study. BMC Med Imaging. 2021;21(1):129.
24. Ghahremani GG, Jimenez MA, Rosenfeld M, Rochester D. CT diagnosis of occult incisional hernias. AJR Am J Roentgenol.1987;148(1):139-42.
25. Weinstein S, Osei-Bonsu S, Aslam R, Yee J. Multidetector CT of the postoperative colon: Review of normal appearances and common complications. Radiographics. 2013;33:515-32.
26. Ogilvie JW, Ricciardi R. Complications of perineal surgery. Clin Colon Rectal Surg. 2009;22(1):51-9.
27. Smith-Behn J, Arnold M, Might J. Use of computerized tomography of the abdominal wall in the diagnosis of partial post-operative wound dehiscence. Postgrad Med J. 1986;62(732):947-8.
28. Zhang L. Incidence of abdominal incisional hernia in developing country: a retrospective cohort study. Int J Clin Exp Med. 2015;8(8):13649-52.
29. Itatsu K, Yokoyama Y, Sugawara G, Kubota H, Tojima Y, Kurumiya Y, et al. Incidence and risk factors for incisional hernia after abdominal surgery. Br J Surg. 2014;101(11): 1439-47.
30. Brown SR, Goodfellow PB. Transverse versus midline incisions for abdominal surgery. Cochrane Database Syst Rev. 2005:CD005199.
31. Gayer G, Lubner MG, Bhalla S, Pickhardt PJ. Imaging of abdominal and pelvic surgical and postprocedural foreign bodies. Radiol Clin North Am. 2014;52:991-1027.
32. Manzella A, Filho PB, Albuquerque E, Farias F, Kaercher J. Imaging of gossypibomas: pictorial review. AJR Am J Roentgenol. 2009;193:S94-101.
33. Hwang S, Jung DH, Jwa EK, Kim Y. Preemptive pyloroplasty for iatrogenic vagus nerve injury in intrahepatic cholangiocarcinoma patients undergoing extensive left-sided lymph node dissection: a retrospective observational study. J Yeungnam Med Sci. 2022;39(3):235-43.
34. Tolan DJM, Harris KM, Prasad D, Mehta SP. The esophagus. In: Brittenden J, Tolan DJM (Eds). Radiology of the postsurgical abdomen. London: Springer-Verlag; 2012. pp. 41-71.
35. Swanson JO, Levine MS, Redfern RO, Rubesin SE. Usefulness of high density barium for detection of leaks after esophagogastrectomy, total gastrectomy and total laryngectomy. AJR Am J Roentgenol. 2003;181:415-20.
36. Upponi S, Ganeshan A, D'Costa H, Betts M, Maynard N, Bungay H, et al. Radiological detection of post-oesophagectomy anastomotic leak: a comparison between multidetector CT and fluoroscopy. Br J Radiol. 2008;81:545-8.
37. Rubesin SE. Postoperative esophagus. In: Gore RM, Levine MS (Eds). Textbook of Gastrointestinal Radiology, 4th edition. Philadelphia: Elsevier-Saunders; 2015. pp. 449-61.
38. Lamb PJ, Griffin SM, Chandrashekar MV, Richardson DL, Karat D, Hayes N. Prospective study of routine contrast radiology after total gastrectomy. Br J Surg. 2004;91:1015-9.
39. Gayer G, Barsuk D, Hertz M, Apter S, Zissin R. CT diagnosis of afferent loop syndrome. Clin Radiol. 2002;57:835-9.
40. Tolan DJM, Harris KM, Prasad D, Mehta SP. The stomach and duodenum. In: Brittenden J, Tolan DJM (Eds). Radiology of the postsurgical abdomen. London: Springer-Verlag; 2012. pp. 72-126.
41. Carucci LR. Postoperative stomach and duodenum. In: Gore RM, Levine MS (Eds). Textbook of Gastrointestinal Radiology, 4th edition. Philadelphia: Elsevier-Saunders; 2015. pp. 630-56.
42. Quigley S, Colledge J, Mukherjee S, Patel K. Bariatric surgery: a review of normal post-operative anatomy and complications. Clin Radiol. 2011;66(10):903-14.
43. Baba A, Yamazoe S, Dogru M, Okuyama Y, Mogami T, Kobashi Y, et al. Petersen hernia after open gastrectomy with Roux-en-Y reconstruction: a report of two cases and literature review. Springerplus. 2015;4:753.
44. Pieroni S, Sommer EA, Hito R, Burch M, Tkacz JN. The "O" sign: a simple and helpful tool in the diagnosis of laparoscopic adjustable gastric band slippage. AJR Am J Roentgenol. 2010;195:137-41.
45. Sandrasegaran K, Maglinte DD, Rajesh A, Tann M, Kopecky KK. CT findings for postsurgical blind pouch of small bowel. AJR Am J Roentgenol. 2006;186:110-3.
46. Broder JC, Tkacz JN, Anderson SW, Soto JA, Gupta A. Ileal pouch-anal anastomosis surgery: imaging and intervention for post-operative complications. Radiographics. 2010;30(1): 221-33.
47. Macklin CS, Brittenden J, Jayne D, Tolan DJM. The colon. In: Brittenden J, Tolan DJM (Eds). Radiology of the post surgical abdomen. London: Springer-Verlag; 2012. pp. 255-93.
48. Mulé S, Colosio A, Cazejust J, Kianmanesh R, Soyer P, Hoeffel C. Imaging of the postoperative liver: review of normal appearances and common complications. Abdom Imaging. 2015;40(7):2761-76.
49. Guthrie JA, Salahudeen HM, Lodge JPA. The liver. In: Brittenden J, Tolan DJM (Eds). Radiology of the post surgical abdomen. London: Springer-Verlag; 2012. pp. 187-226.
50. Terminology Committee of the International Hepato-Pancreato-Biliary Association. Terminology of liver anatomy and resections. Oxford University: HPB (Oxford). 2000;2:333-9.
51. Kele PG, de Boer M, van der Jagt EJ, Lisman T, Porte RJ. Early hepatic regeneration index and completeness of regeneration at 6 months after partial hepatectomy. Br J Surg. 2012;99(8):1113-9.
52. Zappa M, Dondero F, Sibert A, et al. Liver regeneration at day 7 after right hepatectomy: global and segmental volumetric analysis by using CT. Radiology. 2009;252(2):426-32.
53. Petrovai G, Truant S, Langlois C, Vullierme MP, Belghiti J, Vilgrain V. Mechanisms of splenic hypertrophy following hepatic resection. Oxford University: HPB (Oxford). 2013;15(12):919-27.
54. Hoeffel C, Azizi L, Lewin M, Laurent V, Aubé C, Arrivé L, et al. Normal and pathologic features of the postoperative biliary tract at 3D MR cholangiopancreatography and MR imaging. Radiographics. 2006;26(6):1603-20.
55. Boraschi P, Donati F. Biliary-enteric anastomoses: spectrum of findings on Gd-EOB-DTPA-enhanced MR cholangiography. Abdom Imaging. 2013;38(6):1351-9.

56. Kaman L, Sanyal S, Behera A, Singh R, Katariya RN. Comparison of major bile duct injuries following laparoscopic cholecystectomy and open cholecystectomy. ANZ J Surg. 2006;76(9):788-91.
57. Radunovic M, Lazovic R, Popovic N, Magdelinic M, Bulajic M, Radunovic L, et al. Complications of Laparoscopic Cholecystectomy: Our Experience from a Retrospective Analysis. Open Access Maced J Med Sci. 2016;4(4):641-6.
58. Hjelmqvist B. Complications of laparoscopic cholecystectomy as recorded in the Swedish laparoscopy registry. Eur J Surg Suppl. 2000;585:18-21.
59. Gorsi U, Gupta P, Kalra N, Kang M, Singh R, Gupta R, et al. Multidetector computed tomography evaluation of postcholecystectomy complications: A tertiary care centre experience. Trop Gastroenterol. 2015;36(4):236-43.
60. Tonolini M, Ierardi AM, Patella F, Carrafiello G. Early cross-sectional imaging following open and laparoscopic cholecystectomy: a primer for radiologists. Insights Imaging. 2018;9:925-41.
61. Moran J, Del Grosso E, Wills JS, Hagy JA, Baker R. Laparoscopic cholecystectomy: imaging of complications and normal post-operative CT appearance. Abdom Imaging. 1994;19:143-6.
62. Sood R, Sharma D, Sharma G, Kaushik S. Post cholecystectomy common bile duct dilatation and associated symptomatology. J Family Med Prim Care. 2020;9(7):3464-9.
63. Lohan D, Walsh S, McLoughlin R, Murphy J. Imaging of the complications of laparoscopic cholecystectomy. Eur Radiol. 2005;15(5):904-12.
64. Desai NS, Khandelwal A, Virmani V, Kwatra NS, Ricci JA, Saboo SS. Imaging in laparoscopic cholecystectomy: what a radiologist needs to know. Eur J Radiol. 2014;83(6):867-79.
65. Tripathi M, Chandrashekar N, Kumar R, Thomas EJ, Agarwal S, Bal CS, et al. Hepatobiliary scintigraphy: an effective tool in the management of bile leak following laparoscopic cholecystectomy. Clin Imaging. 2004;28:40-3.
66. McGahan JP, Stein M. Complications of laparoscopic cholecystectomy: imaging and intervention. AJR Am J Roentgenol. 1995;165:1089-97.
67. Park MS, Kim KW, Yu JS, Kim MJ, Kim KW, Lim JS, et al. Early biliary complications of laparoscopic cholecystectomy: evaluation on T2-weighted MR cholangiography in conjunction with mangafodipirtrisodium–enhanced 3D T1-weighted MR cholangiography. AJR Am J Roentgenol. 2004;183:1559-66.
68. Patel N, Jensen K, Shaaban A, Korngold E, Foster B. Multimodality Imaging of Cholecystectomy Complications. Radiographics. 2022;42(5):1303-19.
69. Jagadesham VP, Sheridan M, Lodge JPA, Brittenden J. The biliary tree. In: Brittenden J, Tolan DJM (Eds). Radiology of the post surgical abdomen. London: Springer-Verlag; 2012. pp. 153-85.
70. Thurley PD, Dhingsa R. Laparoscopic cholecystectomy: postoperative imaging. AJR Am J Roentgenol. 2008;191: 794-801.
71. Shamiyeh A, Wayand W. Laparoscopic cholecystectomy: early and late complications and the treatment. Langenbecks Arch Surg. 2004;389:164-71.
72. Sandrasegaran K, Maglinte DD, Howard TJ, Lappas JC. Surgery for Chronic Pancreatitis: cross-sectional imaging of postoperative anatomy and complications. AJR Am J Roentgenol. 2005;184:1118-27.
73. Levine M and Carucci L. Imaging of Bariatric Surgery: Normal Anatomy and Postoperative Complications. Radiology. 2014; 270(2):327-41.
74. Yamauchi FI, Ortega CD, Blasbalg R, Rocha MS, Jukemura J, Cerri GG. Multidetector CT evaluation of the postoperative pancreas. Radiographics. 2012;32:743-64.
75. Gaballah A, Kazi I, Zaheer A, Liu PS, Badawy M, Moshiri M, et al. Imaging after Pancreatic Surgery: Expected Findings and Postoperative Complications. Radiographics. 2024; 44(1):e230061.
76. Hashimoto M, Koga M, Ishiyama K, Watarai J, Shibata S, Sato T, et al. CT features of pancreatic fistula after pancreaticoduodenectomy. AJR Am J Roentgenol. 2007;188:W323-7.
77. Hashimoto N, Yasuda C, Ohyanagi H. Pancreatic fistula after pancreatic head resection: incidence, significance and management. Hepatogastroenterology. 2003;50:1658-60.
78. Liu Y. Postoperative reactive lymphadenitis: A potential cause of false-positive FDG PET/CT. World J Radiol. 2014;6(12):890-4.
79. Mortelé KJ, Lemmerling M, de Hemptinne B, deVos M, deBock G, Kunnen M. Postoperative findings following the Whipple procedure: determination of prevalence and morphologic abdominal CT features. Eur Radiol. 2000;10:123-8.
80. Riediger H, Makowiec F, Schareck WD, Hopt UT, Adam U. Delayed gastric emptying after pylorus preserving pancreatoduodenectomy is strongly related to other postoperative complications. J Gastrointest Surg. 2003;7:758-65.

CHAPTER 27

Shivanand Gamanagatti, Dipin Sudhakaran, Smita Manchanda

Portal Hypertension: Imaging and Intervention

IMAGING OF PORTAL HYPERTENSION

INTRODUCTION

Portal hypertension (PHT) is defined as an increase in portal pressure above the normal range of 6–10 mm Hg or as pressure gradient > 5 mm Hg between portal and hepatic veins, as evaluated by hepatic vein cannulation. PHT is considered clinically significant when the pressure gradient is > 10–12 mm Hg.[1]

Portal hypertension is of hemodynamic importance, since it leads to range of complications such as gastrointestinal hemorrhage, ascites, portal-systemic encephalopathy, hepatorenal syndrome, hepatopulmonary syndrome, and spontaneous bacterial peritonitis.[2,3]

CAUSES OF PORTAL HYPERTENSION[4]

Causes of PHT are divided into prehepatic, intrahepatic, and posthepatic causes **(Table 1)**.

ANATOMY OF PORTAL SYSTEM[5]

The liver has dual blood supply, 70% of blood flow is via the portal vein and remaining 30% is via the hepatic artery. Approximately, 50% of oxygen demand is met by the portal vein and 50% by the hepatic artery. Portal blood carries nutrient-rich, oxygen-poor blood to the liver whereas hepatic artery carries oxygen rich, nutrient-poor blood to the liver.

Portal and hepatic blood merge within the portal sinusoids, which drain into hepatic veins and then to the systemic venous system, i.e., inferior vena cava (IVC).

The portal vein is formed by the confluence of the superior mesenteric vein (SMV) and splenic vein (SV) posterior to the neck of pancreas. It courses superiorly and laterally to enter the liver at the porta. Other tributaries include inferior mesenteric vein (IMV) and right and left gastric veins, which drain into portal circulation **(Fig. 1)**.

Work-up[6,7]

Laboratory Studies

Aimed at identifying the causes of cirrhosis (the most common cause of PHT), laboratory studies include **(Box 1)**.

Imaging Studies

Duplex-Doppler ultrasonography:[8-11] Ultrasound (US) is used as screening modality for evaluating portal hypertension, since it is a safe and cost-effective method.

TABLE 1: Causes of portal hypertension.

Prehepatic causes	Intrahepatic causes	Posthepatic causes
Caused by obstruction of the portal, splenic, or superior mesenteric veins	Caused by intrinsic diseases of the parenchyma	Caused by diseases obstructing the blood outflow from the liver
• Portal vein thrombosis/extrahepatic portal vein obstruction • Congenital origin, such as aplasia or hypoplasia • Infection, such as pylephlebitis • Splanchnic arteriovenous fistula	• Cirrhosis due to various causes • Congenital hepatic fibrosis • Noncirrhotic portal fibrosis/ idiopathic portal hypertension	• Budd–Chiari syndrome • Veno-occlusive disorder

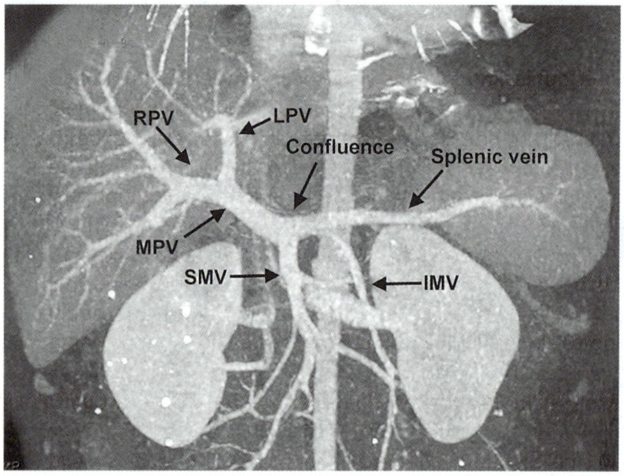

FIG. 1: Coronal three-dimensional (3D) maximum intensity projection (MIP) image of CT portography showing anatomy of spleno-portal axis.

(IMV: inferior mesenteric vein; LPV: left branch of portal vein; MPV: main portal vein; RPV: right branch of portal vein; SMV: superior mesenteric vein)

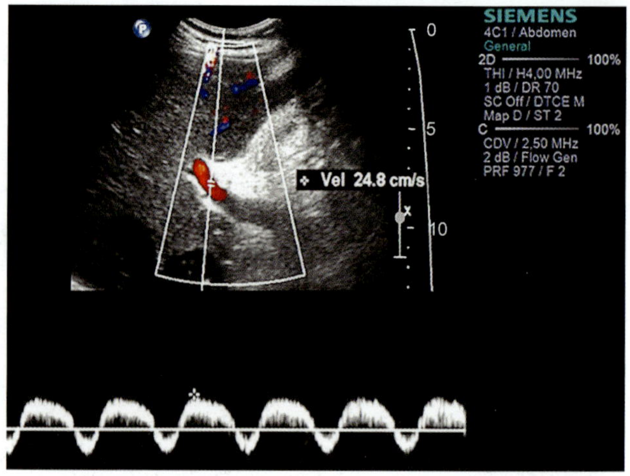

FIG. 2: Ultrasound Doppler image showing typical waveform of main portal vein exhibiting continuous hepatopetal (antegrade) flow with undulation due to respiratory and cardiac variation.

BOX 1 Laboratory studies for the work-up of cirrhosis.

- Liver function tests including albumin and prothrombin time
- Viral hepatitis serologies
- Platelet count
- Iron indices
- Antinuclear antibody, antimitochondrial antibody, anti-smooth muscle antibody
- α-1-antitrypsin deficiency
- Ceruloplasmin alone or along with 24-hour urinary copper in selective cases

It helps in identifying the patency of portal vein, direction of portal flow (hepatopetal or hepatofugal), also helps in diagnosing cavernoma formation of main portal vein (MPV), splanchnic vein thrombosis.

Limitations of US include:

- Reproducibility of findings is challenging.
- Portal hemodynamics is affected by several variables such as circadian rhythm, meals, and medications.
- Substantial interobserver and intraobserver discrepancy.

Normal Doppler Findings of Portal Vein

The portal vein has a typical Doppler waveform and exhibits continuous hepatopetal (antegrade) flow. The normal flow velocity range is 15–18 cm/sec. Mild undulation due to respiratory and cardiac variation in the waveform is a common finding **(Fig. 2)**.

Technique of Doppler of Portal System

Doppler evaluation of the splenoportal axis can be extremely challenging, due to the altered anatomy, blood flow conditions, bowel gas, and the type of changes that happen in a diseased liver. Doppler examination should be performed following overnight fasting because bowel gas may interfere with evaluation of SMV and retroperitoneal collaterals **(Table 2)**.

TABLE 2: Checklist of typical Doppler evaluation of splenoportal axis (Figs. 3A to F).

Structures	Parameters
Hepatic veins	Patent/Not patent
IVC	Patent/Not patent
Liver	Size and echotexture, any space occupying lesion
Splenoportal axis (MPV/splenic vein/SMV)	• Patent/Not patent • Diameter—dilated/normal • Direction of flow (hepatopetal/ hepatofugal) • Respiratory variation of MPV (present or absent)
Collaterals	• Present/Absent • Location—intrahepatic/extrahepatic
Spleen	Size—enlarged/normal
Ascites	Present/Absent
Left renal vein	Patent/Not patent

(IVC: inferior vena cava; MPV: main portal vein; SMV: superior mesenteric vein)

Challenges of Doppler evaluation include:

- Acquiring a suitable angle of insonation
- Altered depth of the vessels
- Slow flow velocities due to disease process
- Amount of tissue movement due to respiration

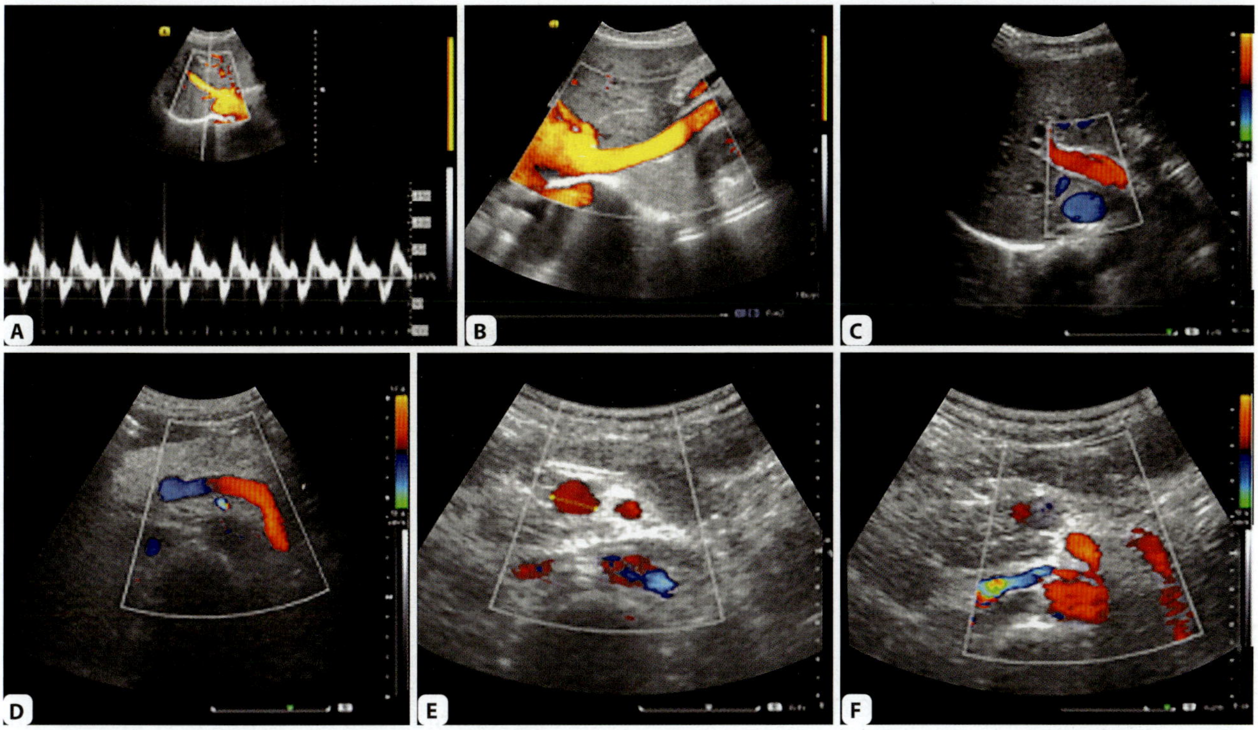

FIGS. 3A TO F: Power Doppler images showing normal Doppler findings to look at during scanning in setting of portal hypertension: (A) Patency of hepatic vein; (B) Patency of inferior vena cava (IVC); (C) Patency of main portal vein (MPV); (D) Patency of splenic vein; (E) Patency of superior mesenteric vein (SMV); (F) Patency of left renal vein (LRV).

In PHT, Doppler signal demonstrates a low frequency shift and low amplitude and there is an increase in noise from tissue movement. Hence, it is very important to optimize the imaging parameters and sonographic technique to increase the frequency shift and to increase the signal amplitude.

Optimization of Sonographic Technique

Angle of Insonation

Single most useful adjustment that improves the Doppler signal quality is to decrease the angle of insonation. Ideally, the angle of insonation should be <60°. In routine clinical practice, it is difficult to achieve this angle due to restrictions related to vessel position, body habitus, ribs, and gas.

Useful modifications for improving the angle include:

- Roll the patient into left lateral decubitus position to move the liver away from the ribs and displace bowel gas.
- Use a small footprint phased array transducer to visualize vessels through intercostal space.

Color Frequency

Current ultrasound machines come with transducers having multiple Doppler frequencies. This offers the sonographer a chance to increase the frequency shift or increase the amplitude of the returning echoes depending on conditions within the body.

A higher incident frequency will produce a greater frequency shift but subject to higher rates of attenuation thereby decreasing penetration and reducing signal amplitude. Hence, when scanning deep abdominal vessels, a lower frequency should be used to overcome problems of poor penetration.

Optimization of the Received Signal

The scale or pulse repetition frequency (PRF) needs to be set appropriately to optimize the display of Doppler signal received. In cirrhosis, blood flow rates are very low, hence the scale (PRF) should be set low enough to display these small frequency shifts.

One can use the zoom facility that significantly improves resolution and frame rate by reconfiguring the beam forming for a smaller field of view.

Respiration

Smart use of respiration can be very helpful. Performing Doppler in arrested inspiration may hamper the detection of flow as the increase in intra-abdominal pressure can halt or even reverse the flow in diseased portal venous system. Hence, scanning should be done with arrested expiration or gentle respiration even if flow is not seen.

Presets

It is recommended to use vendor presets as a starting point and also it is advocated that each department generate a dedicated preset for abdominal vascular studies.

Pathophysiology of Doppler Findings in Portal Hypertension

Cirrhosis is a mixture of fibrosis and regeneration that alters the normal liver architecture. Cirrhosis leads to obstruction to blood flow in distal sinusoids due to perisinusoidal collagen deposition and fibrosis. This obstruction reduces flow from the portal veins and hepatic artery into the hepatic veins. This increases arterial resistance and leads to an increase in arterial flow into the portal vein via existing and new anastomoses that result from the fibrotic scarring. The net result of this obstruction to venous outflow and increase in arterial to portal vein flow manifests as increase in portal vein pressure, drainage of blood away from the liver (hepatofugal flow) via collateral pathways.

Ultrasound Criteria for Detecting Portal Hypertension

Portal Vein Diameter

Portal vein diameter is a luminal measurement made at the level where the portal vein enters the porta. A portal vein diameter of 13 mm or more is abnormal and an indicator of PHT. While it has good specificity, it has a sensitivity of only about 40% **(Fig. 4)**.

This lack of sensitivity is due to collateral pathways, which partially decompress the system. Portal vein size normally varies with respiration and loss of this variation can also be used to identify PHT. Less than 20% variation in diameter with respiration is reported as having 80% sensitivity and 100% specificity.

Although this is a sensitive test for PHT, in practice obtaining reliable and reproducible measurements can be difficult as many of these patients have poor ultrasound access and limited ability to comply with instructions.

Flow Reversal or Hepatofugal Flow

This is relatively uncommon in the portal vein and is a poor marker for PHT being seen in only 1–8% of cases of PHT **(Fig. 5)**. When present, it is usually associated with a reduction in the vein diameter. It is highly dependent on the severity of the disease and the location of collaterals (if a paraumbilical collateral exists, forward flow is usually maintained because the shunt is beyond the level of the portal vein).

Splenomegaly and Ascites

Splenomegaly develops in most, but not all cases, of PHT but it is of little use due to the large number of alternative causes **(Figs. 6A and B)**.

Ascites is not usually caused by uncomplicated PHT. It is often secondary to underlying liver disease with liver cell failure and is insensitive, as it tends to be a late complication.

Portosystemic Venous Collaterals

Collaterals have up to 90% sensitivity and excellent specificity for PHT. Paraumbilical collaterals have a specificity of 100% for PHT. Collaterals have predictable locations making them a very practical sign for the diagnosis of PHT. Clues to their presence and location can also be found from changes in the flow patterns in the portal venous system.

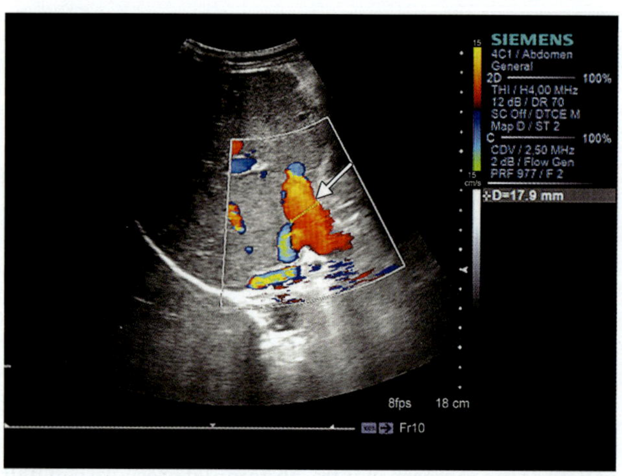

FIG. 4: Doppler ultrasound image showing dilated main portal vein (arrow) in a cirrhotic patient, which measures 17.9 mm at porta.

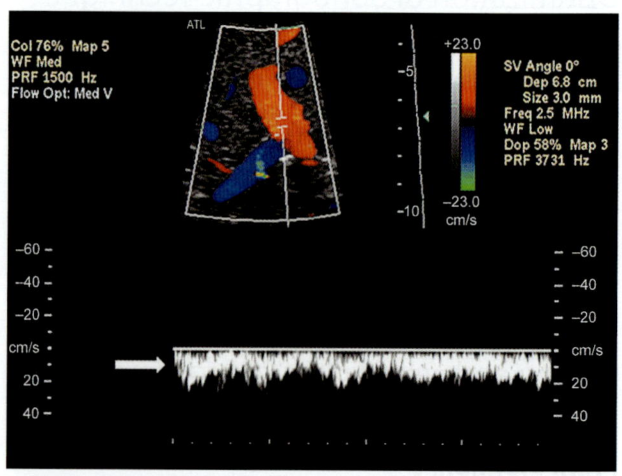

FIG. 5: Doppler ultrasound image showing dilated main portal vein with reversal of flow (arrow) on spectral waveform suggestive of hepatofugal flow.

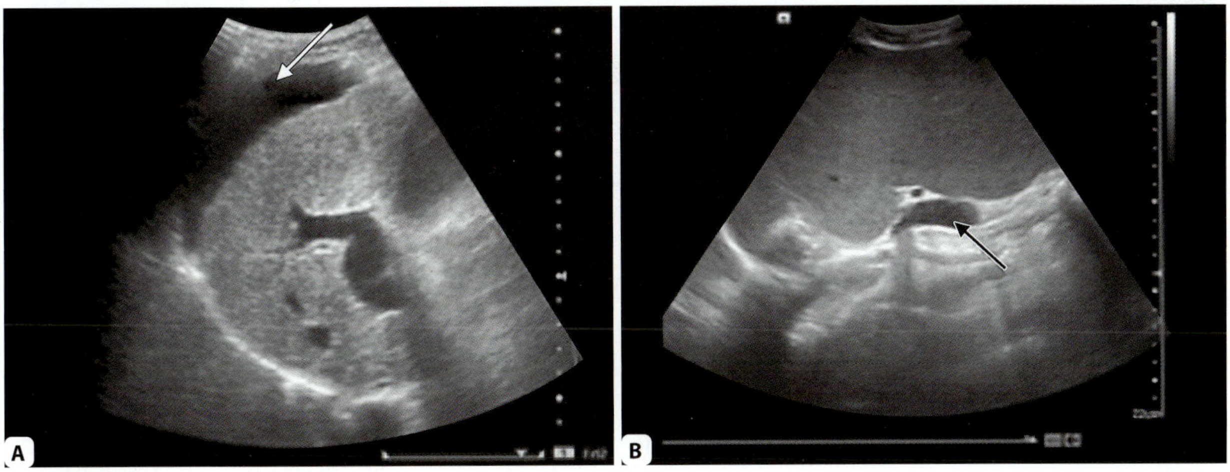

FIGS. 6A AND B: Ultrasound images of a cirrhotic patient showing shrunken liver with nodular surface, dilated splenoportal axis, splenomegaly (black arrow) and ascites (white arrow).

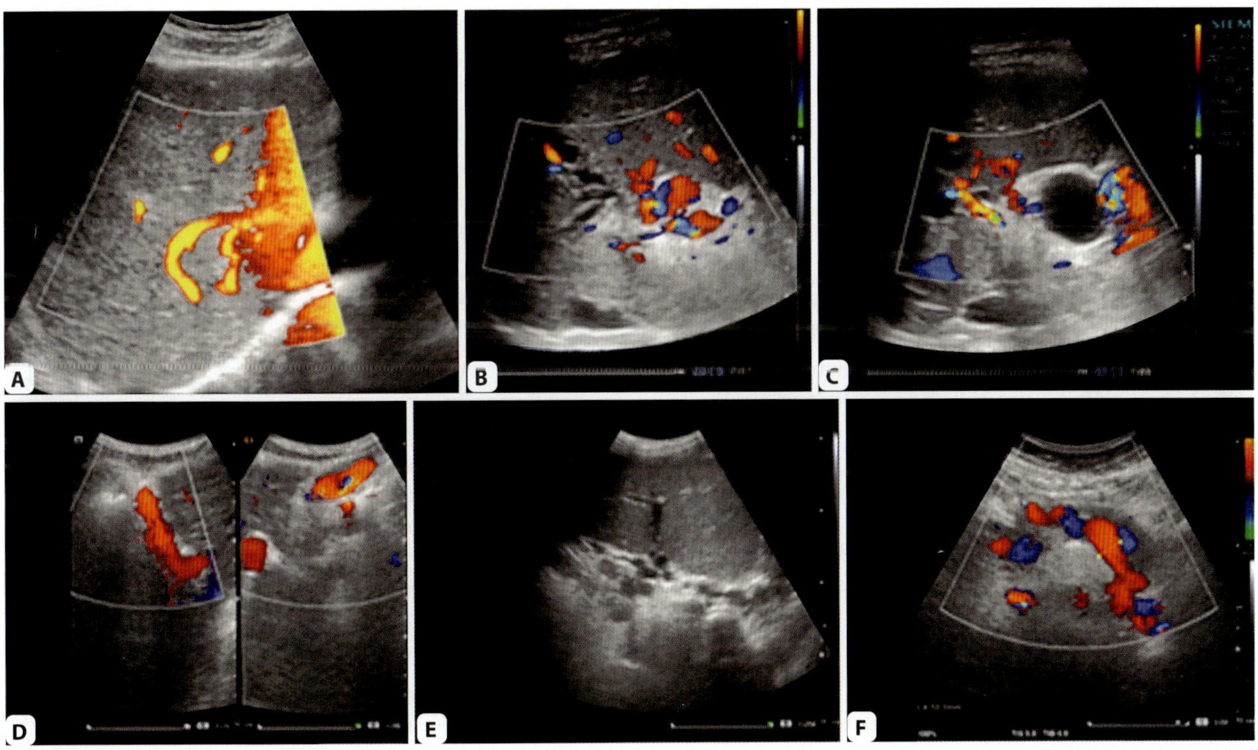

FIGS. 7A TO F: Doppler ultrasound images showing collaterals in various location: Intrahepatic veno-venous collaterals (A), at porta (B), pericholecystic (C), paraumbilical (D), lienorenal location (E), and mesenteric location (F).

The collaterals most frequently detected with ultrasound are the **(Figs. 7A to F)**:

- Paraumbilical
- Splenorenal
- Gastroesophageal

Other less common collaterals, such as mesenteric and pericholecystic **(Figs. 7A to F)**, may also be found **(Box 2)**.

Computed Tomography[12,13]

Computed tomography (CT) is not the prime diagnostic tool in patients with PHT, and is usually done as a second-line technique to ultrasound with color Doppler imaging. Main limitations of CT include inability to provide information about flow direction, portal flow rates or pressure gradients, and radiation issue. CT findings practically depend

BOX 2 Teaching points: Ultrasonography (USG) features of portal hypertension.

- *Portal vein diameter >13 mm*: High specificity; low sensitivity
- Variation in portal vein diameter with respiration <20%
- *Hepatofugal flow*: Poor marker because if a paraumbilical collateral exists forward flow is usually maintained
- *Splenomegaly*: Less useful because of a large number of alternative causes
- *Ascites*: Not usually seen in uncomplicated cases
- *Collaterals*: High sensitivity and specificity. Good practical sign due to predictable locations

upon morphologic changes rather than flow dynamic changes.

Indications for CT, in patients with known PHT:
- To demonstrate the main collateral pathways
- To identify possible causes of PHT
- To identify and characterize focal lesions like hepatocellular carcinoma (HCC).

Examination Technique

Multidetector computed tomography (MDCT) permits improved timing of contrast injection, excellent outlining of collateral pathways, and better detection of accompanying liver lesions in patients with PHT.

Scan parameters and protocols with respect to different MDCT scanners are mentioned in **Table 3**.

The volume of contrast to be used differs depending upon the iodine strength in the contrast medium. If the iodine strength is 300 mg/mL, the recommended volume is 120–150 cc, whereas if iodine strength is 370 mg/mL, then 80–100 cc is required. Also, as a standard for liver imaging using MDCT, nonionic contrast medium is used with an injection rate of 4–5 cc/sec, using a pressure injector. Therefore, it is important to customize the injection rate protocols and volume of contrast based on the iodine concentration of contrast media.

Oral Contrast

The positive oral contrast interferes with evaluation of varices. Hence, it is suggested to use water as a neutral contrast agent that helps in better depiction of varices. Patients are advised to take about 1–1.5 L water, 30 minutes before the start of CT examination; to distend the stomach and the proximal bowel loops. Precontrast scans are generally not required; however, in patients with suspected HCC or hypervascularized liver lesions, may be useful if hemorrhage or calcifications are suspected. In the case of dual-energy scanners, virtual noncontrast images can be obtained from the arterial phase data without subjecting the patient to additional radiation for obtaining the unenhanced scan.

TABLE 3: Scan parameters and protocols with respect to different multidetector computed tomography (MDCT) scanners.

Parameter	4 slices	16 slices	64 slices
Detector collimation (mm)	4 × 1.25	16 × 0.625	64 × 0.6
Slice thickness (mm)			
• Arterial phase	1.25	1	1
• Venous phase	1.25	1	1
Arterial delay	• Bolus tracking/ automated trigger • Empirical delay: 25–30 seconds		
Venous delay	65–70 seconds	60 seconds	50–60 seconds

For optimal visualization of the splenoportal axis, scanning should start 45–50 seconds following contrast injection. In patients with PHT, this time delay must be increased up to 65–70 seconds, because of slower opacification of the portal branches.

For suspected HCC, a multiphasic technique should be used with injection of 100 mL of contrast at a flow rate of 4–5 mL/s using a power injector.

Display Technique[13]

Computed tomography images are usually assessed based upon axial sections. In patients with PHT because of development of complex collateral pathways further assessment using interactive cine display is very helpful and will resolve most of the fundamental diagnostic issues.

In certain cases, multiplanar reformats (MPRs)/ volume rendering techniques (VRTs) and thin slab maximum intensity projection (MIP) are valuable for better understanding of the collateral pathways **(Figs. 8A and B)**.

Magnetic Resonance Imaging[14-16]

- Provides morphologic information comparable to CT scan when ultrasound findings are inadequate.
- MRI angiography also helps in localizing and defining the extent of the presence of portosystemic collaterals **(Figs. 9A to D)**.
- Special MR techniques (like phase contrast) also offer quantitative information about portal venous flow.

Magnetic resonance portography has few benefits over other imaging techniques used for evaluation of PHT. Doppler ultrasonography is inexpensive and noninvasive, provides quantitative information on portal blood flow, but it is operator dependent and may be unsatisfactory when a proper acoustic window is not available. CT portography can demonstrate the portal venous system in a short time,

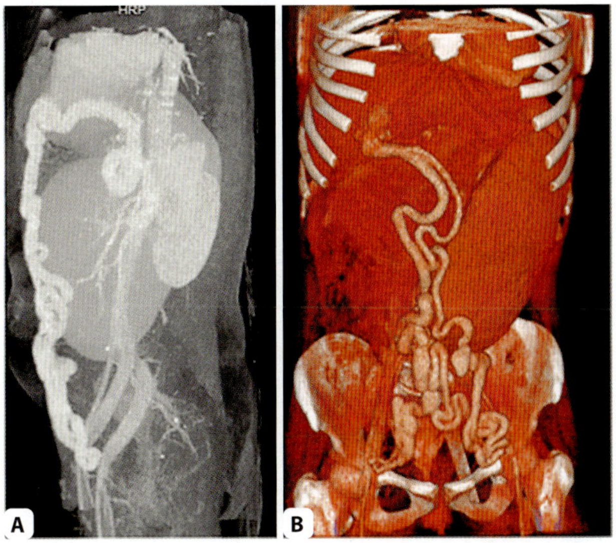

FIGS. 8A AND B: Thin Slab maximum intensity projection (MIP) (A) and volume rendered technique (VRT) (B) images showing dilated tortuous paraumbilical vein, showing advantages of these techniques in understanding of the collateral pathways.

but this technique is associated with ionizing radiation and requires administration of a large amount of contrast agent.

Magnetic Resonance Technique

Nonenhanced MR angiography using time-of-flight (TOF) and phase-contrast (PC) techniques can demonstrate the portal venous system, but is limited by its long data acquisition time, motion and flow artifact, and in-plane saturation.

However, contrast-enhanced MR portography overcomes flow artifacts and saturation effects. MR portograms reconstructed by MIP post-processing technique and source images, provide detailed information about the portal venous system **(Figs. 9A to D)**.

Magnetic Resonance Protocol

Magnetic resonance imaging is performed with a 1.5- or 3-T superconducting scanner using a torso-phased array coil. A three-dimensional (3D) fast spoiled gradient recalled pulse sequence with minimum repetition time and echo

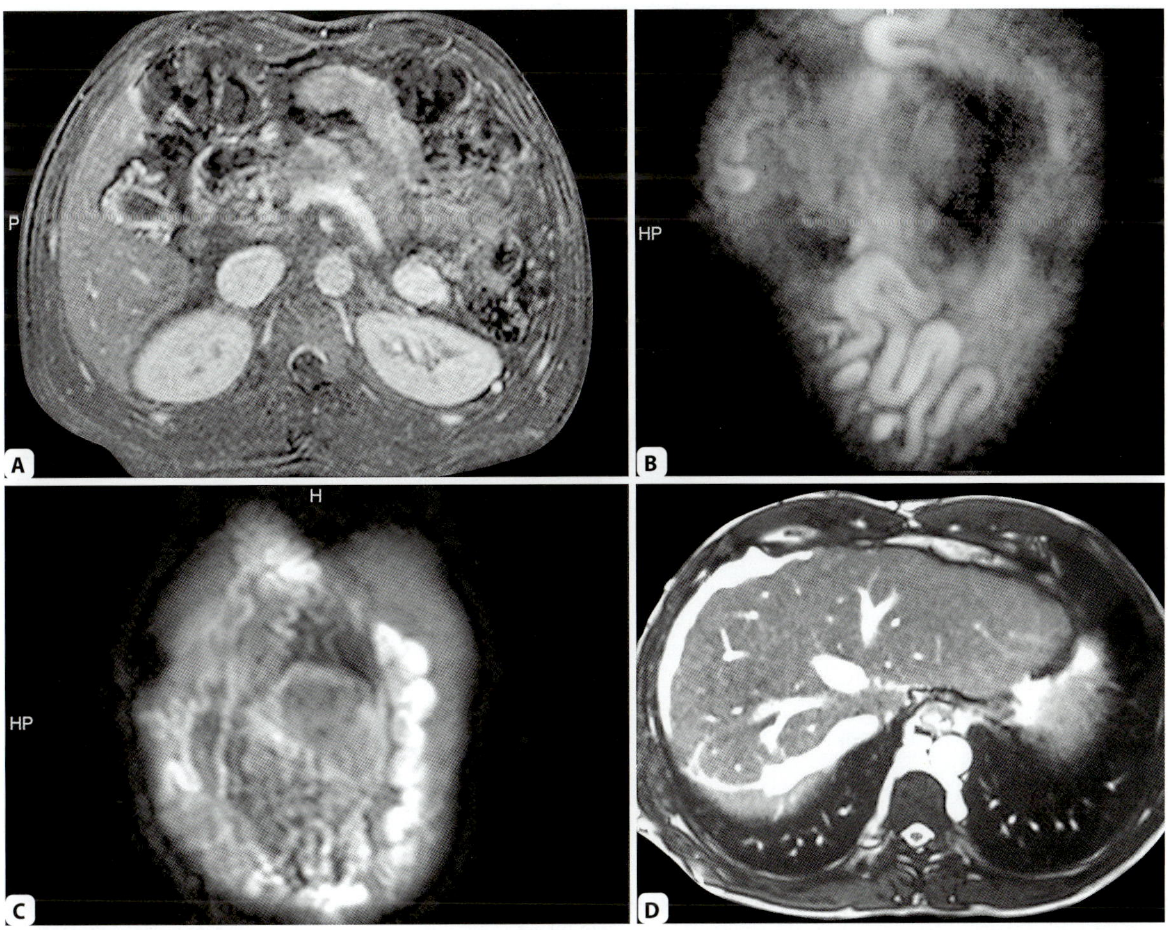

FIGS. 9A TO D: MR images showing various collateral pathways; pericholecystic (A), paraumbilical (B), abdominal wall (C) and intrahepatic veno-venous collaterals (D).

time should be used. An optimized slab volume is placed in the axial plane on a coronal localizer extending from the dome of diaphragm to inferior part of the kidneys and the acquisition is performed during a single breathhold period of 13–15 seconds. An intravenous bolus of 0.2 mmol/kg of gadolinium is injected either using a pressure injector or manually. Gadolinium injection is immediately followed by a 15-mL saline flush. Three repetitive acquisitions (performed within separate breathhold of 13–15 seconds) for portal venous phase imaging are obtained after a delay of 45–50 seconds after the start of contrast injection.

HEMODYNAMIC MEASUREMENT OF PORTAL PRESSURE[17]

Procedures (Fig. 10)

- Portal pressure measurement by direct puncture of portal vein is not generally done due to invasive nature and there is high risk of associated anesthetic and bleeding complications.
- However, most commonly indirect pressure measurement that closely matches the direct portal pressure is used, which is popularly known as "hepatic venous pressure gradient (HVPG) measurement".
- In this procedure, through transfemoral route or more commonly through transjugular route, a Swan-Ganz balloon catheter is placed into the right hepatic vein and free hepatic venous pressure (FHVP) is measured without inflating the balloon.
- In the next step, the balloon is inflated using either diluted contrast or room air, occluding the hepatic vein outflow completely and occluded hepatic venous pressure or wedged hepatic venous pressure (WHVP) is measured **(Figs. 10A and B)**.
- The wedged pressure value minus free venous pressure value gives HVPG.

Interpretation (Table 4)

- Normal HVPG is <5 mm Hg.
- Complications of PHT such as variceal bleeding, ascites, or hepatorenal syndrome are seen when HVPG exceeds 10 mm Hg.
- If there is HVPG < 10 mm Hg and complications of PHT are present, then one should suspect noncirrhotic portal hypertension (NCPH).

MORPHOLOGIC SIGNS OF PORTAL HYPERTENSION

Direct signs include dilatation of splenoportal axis, i.e., MPV diameter > 13 mm, SV diameter > 10 mm **(Figs. 11A and B)**. If there are adequate venous collaterals, splenoportal axis may not show significant dilatation.

TABLE 4: Interpretation of HVPG findings.

Causes	FHVP	WHVP	HVPG
Prehepatic	Normal	Normal	Normal
Hepatic presinusoidal	Normal	Normal to ↑	Normal to ↑
Sinusoidal	Normal	↑↑	↑↑
Postsinusoidal	Normal	↑↑	↑↑
Posthepatic	↑↑	↑↑	Normal to ↑

(FHVP: free hepatic vein pressure; HVPG: hepatic vein pressure gradient; WHVP: wedged hepatic vein pressure)

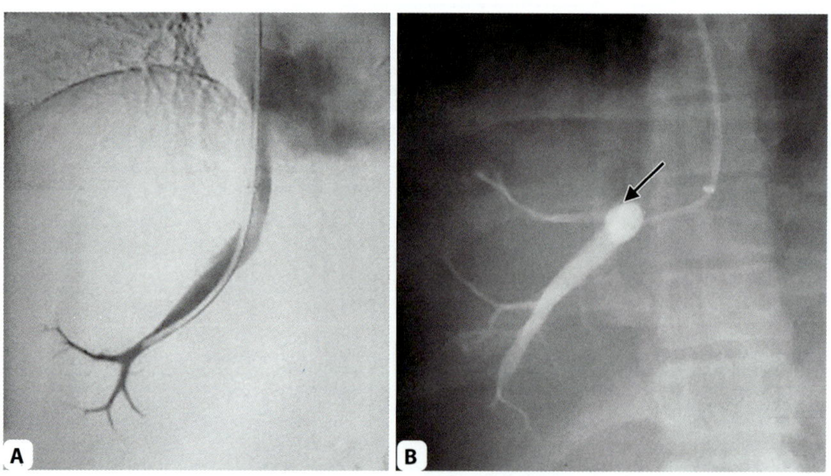

FIGS. 10A AND B: Digital subtraction angiography (DSA) spot images showing steps of hepatic venous pressure gradient (HVPG) measurement; cannulation of the right hepatic vein (A) for measuring the free hepatic venous pressure (FHVP) followed by inflation of balloon catheter (B) (arrow) and measuring the wedged hepatic venous pressure (WHVP).

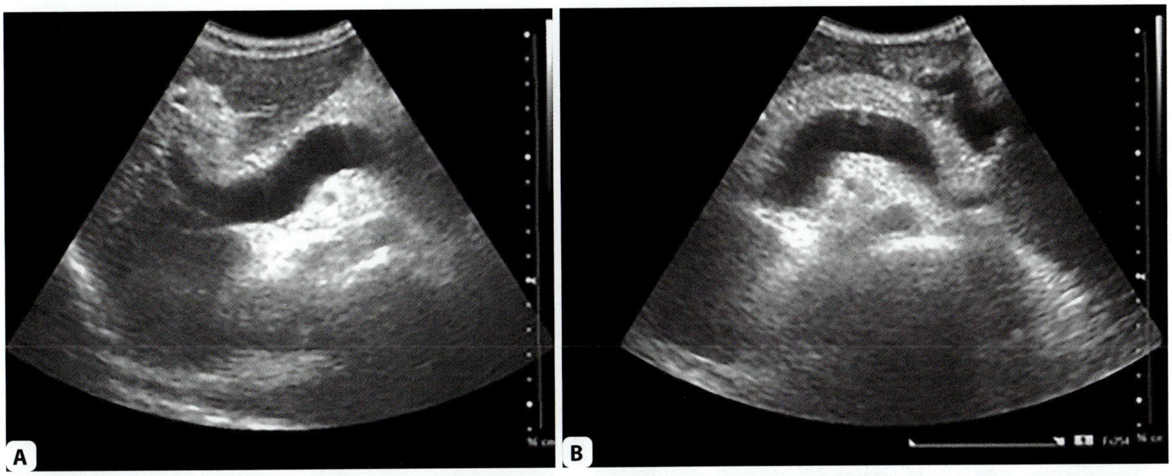

FIGS. 11A AND B: Ultrasound images showing dilated entire splenoportal axis; (A) Dilated main portal vein (MPV) and (B) Dilated splenic vein.

TABLE 5: Normal portosystemic communications (Figs. 12A to D).

Location	Portal veins	Systemic veins
Lower esophagus	Left gastric vein	Azygos
Stomach	Short gastric or gastroepiploic	Left renal
Spleen	Splenic	Left renal or adrenal
Rectum and anal canal	Superior rectal vein	Middle and inferior rectal vein
Umbilicus	Paraumbilical veins	Superior and inferior epigastric veins
Bare area of liver	Portal vein branches	Inferior phrenic vein
Retroperitoneum	Tributaries of splenic, pancreatic, and colic veins	Renal, suprarenal, gonadal, and paravertebral veins

Collateral Pathways[18,19]

In healthy humans, congenitally originated connections exist between portal and systemic circulation **(Table 5)**. In the setting of PHT, these connections get dilated leading to formation of varices at various sites within the body.

These varices are divided into two groups **(Table 6)**:
1. Gastroesophageal varices
2. Ectopic varices

In long-term, these varices develop large spontaneous shunts **(Table 7)**, which are categorized into intrahepatic, transhepatic, and extrahepatic shunts.

VARICES

Esophageal and Paraesophageal Varices

The most common varices encountered in PHT are esophageal varices (50%). Esophageal varices are located within the wall of the lower esophagus, whereas paraesophageal varices are located outside the esophageal wall. These are the most common varices to bleed in PHT due to high pressure and high volume of blood that they carry and account for high mortality due to spontaneous hemorrhage.

Gastric and Perigastric Varices

Gastric varices are less common than esophageal varices (5–33%), drain either into the left renal vein through spontaneous gastrorenal shunt or directly into the IVC through a spontaneous gastrocaval shunt. Risk of bleeding is low as compared to esophageal varices, but the severity of bleeding is much higher due to their large size.

Ectopic Varices

They account for 2–5% of variceal bleeding, have a fourfold increased risk of bleeding as compared to esophageal varices and are associated with a high mortality rate. These varices are difficult to treat and there is no established standard treatment. When hemorrhage arises from these ectopic varices, it is challenging to control by any method, and the bleeding may be potentially lethal.

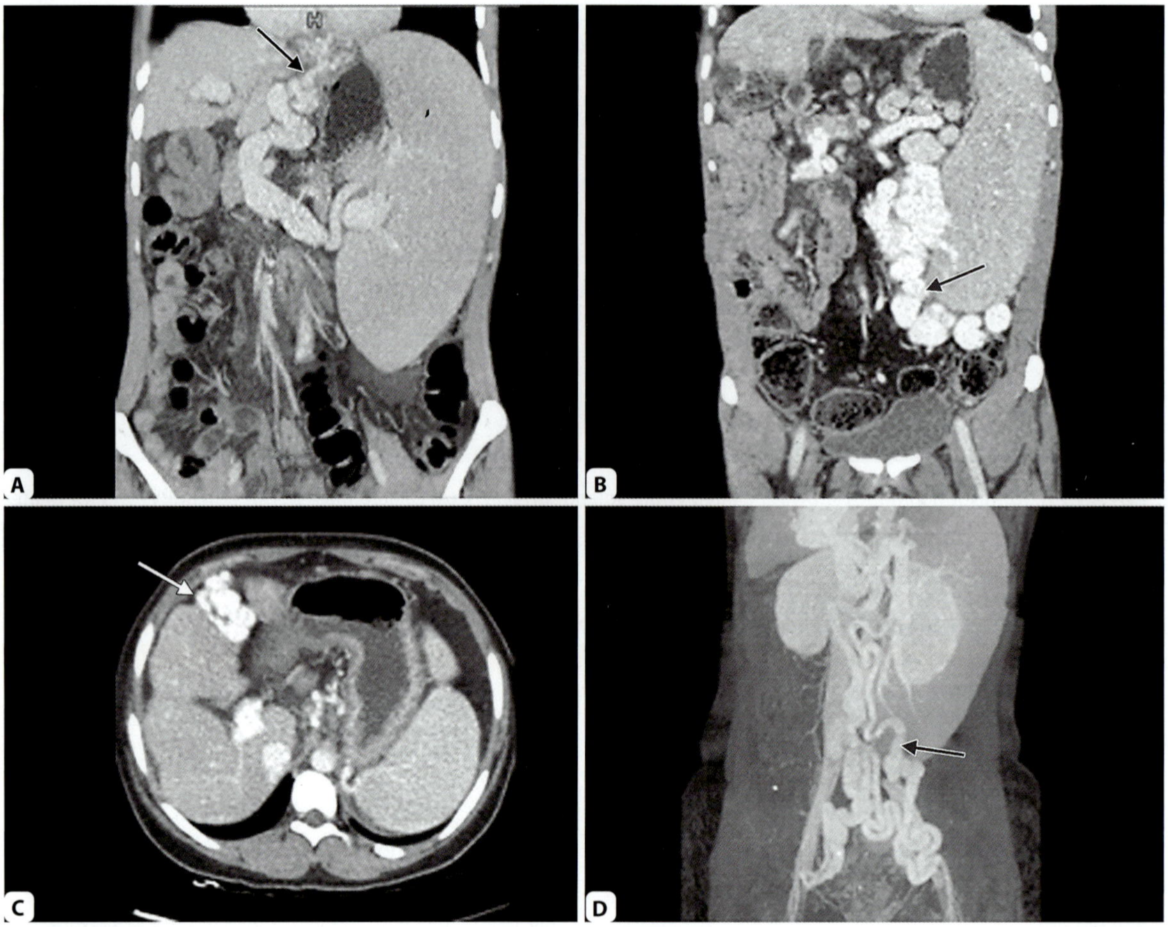

FIGS. 12A TO D: CT images showing various normal portosystemic communications; at lower end of esophagus (A), in retroperitoneum (B) and at umbilicus (paraumbilical veins) (C and D).

TABLE 6: Gastroesophageal and ectopic varices (Figs. 13 and 14).

Gastroesophageal varices	Ectopic varices
Esophageal	Duodenal
Paraesophageal	Jejunoileal
Gastric and perigastric	• Colonic • Pancreatic • Mesenteric • Vesical • Pericholecystic • Retroperitoneal • Rectal/Perirectal

TABLE 7: Spontaneous shunts (Figs. 15A to C).

Intrahepatic	Transhepatic	Extrahepatic
Rare	Recanalized paraumbilical vein	Gastrorenal; splenorenal; gastrocaval

Associated Findings

The most important associated findings in PHT are splenomegaly and ascites. Other associated findings are small bowel edema, thickening of the gallbladder wall, increased density within mesenteric fat (misty mesentery) and omentum. In addition, patients with PHT, especially those with hypersplenism, have an increased incidence of splenic artery true aneurysms due to hyperkinetic circulation, which may be seen as incidental finding on imaging.

Splenomegaly

Splenomegaly develops in most, but not all cases, of PHT; however, it is of little use due to the large number of alternative causes. The size of the spleen does not correlate with degree of PHT. Also, if splenomegaly is absent, PHT cannot be ruled out. Siderotic Gamna-Gandy nodules that represent small foci of perifollicular and trabecular hemorrhage may be seen as multiple faint hyperechoic foci on ultrasound or multiple faint

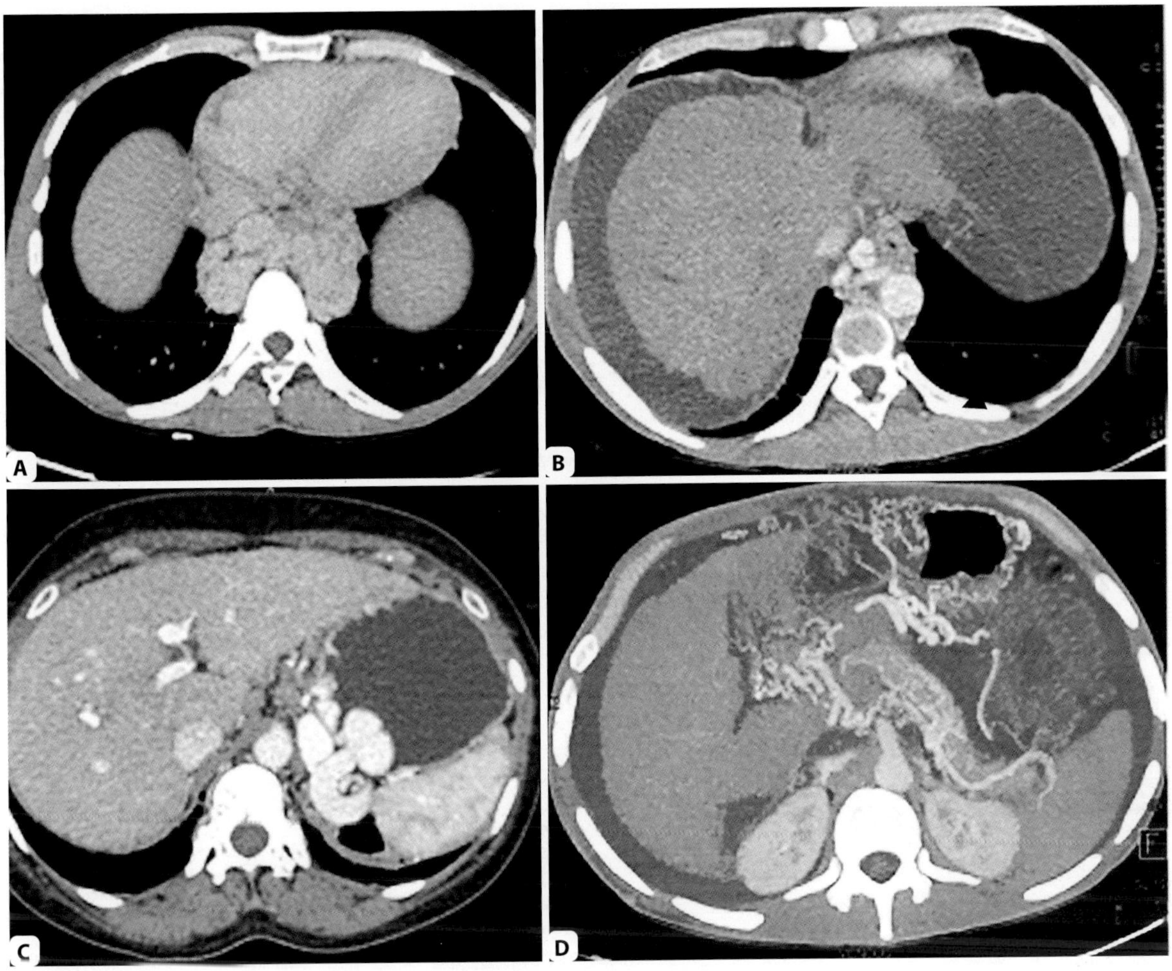

FIGS. 13A TO D: Axial CT images showing various gastroesophageal varices; Paraesophageal (A), esophageal (B), fundal (C), and perigastric (D) locations.

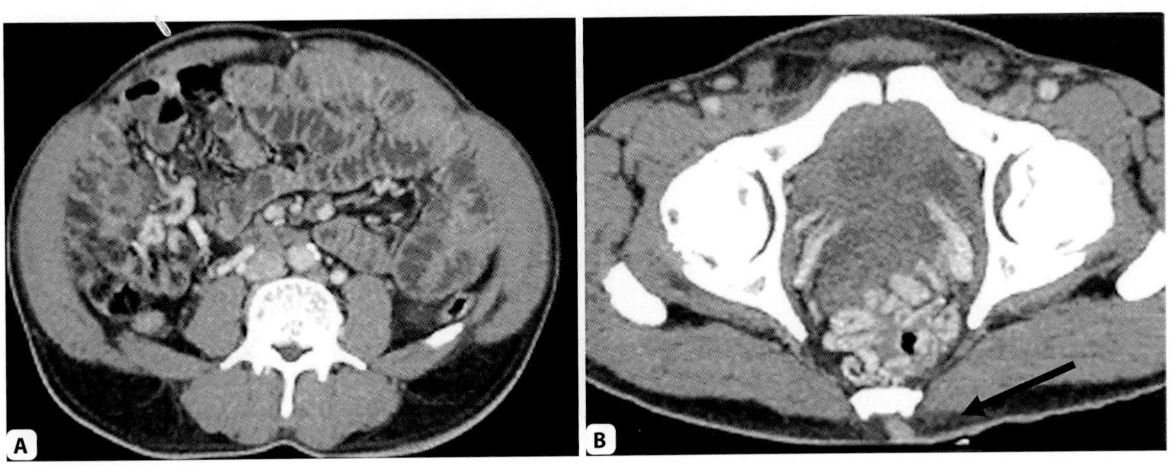

FIGS. 14A TO D: *Continued*

Continued

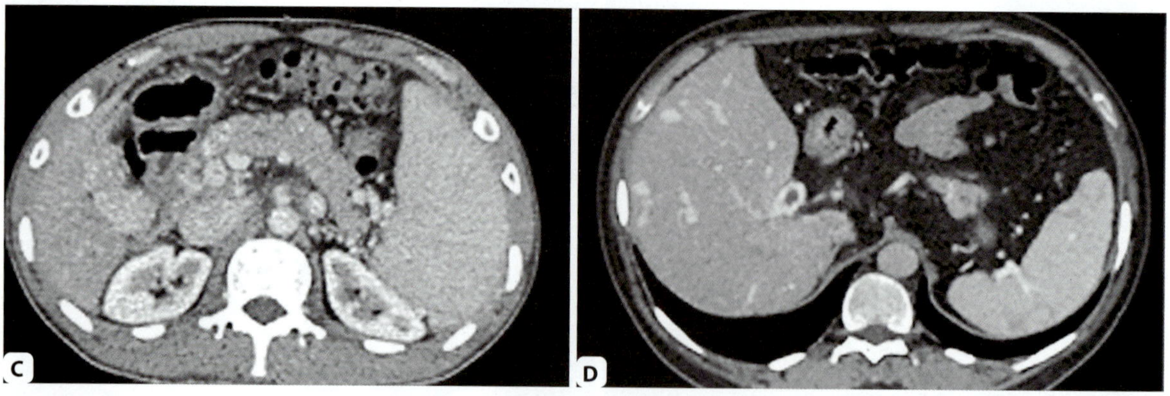

FIGS. 14A TO D: Axial CT images showing ectopic varices; colonic (A), rectal (B), pericholecystic (C), and pericholedochal locations (D).

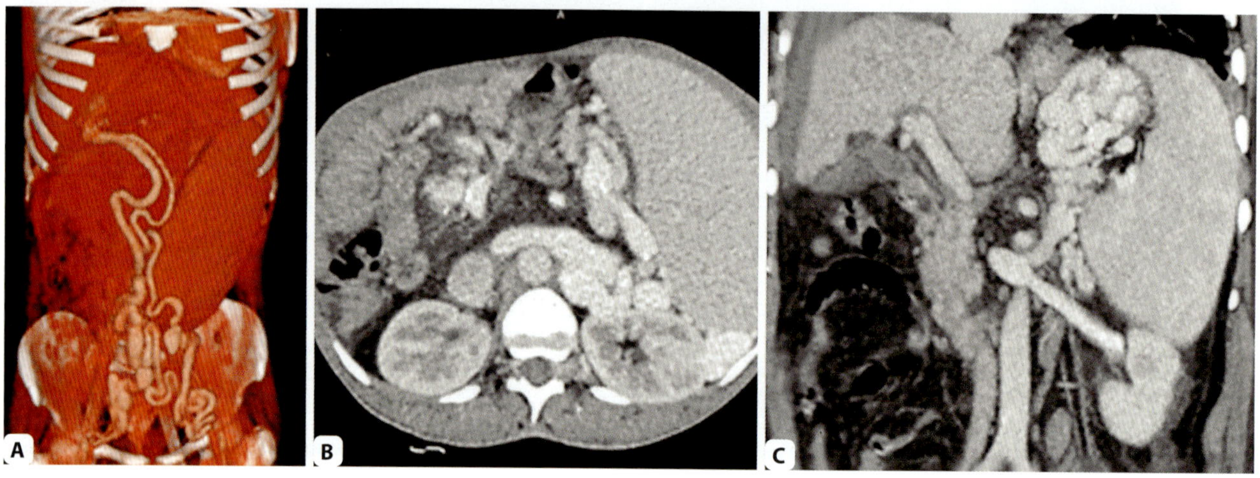

FIGS. 15A TO C: CT images showing spontaneous shunts; recanalized paraumbilical (transhepatic shunt) (A), splenorenal (B), and gastrorenal (C) shunts.

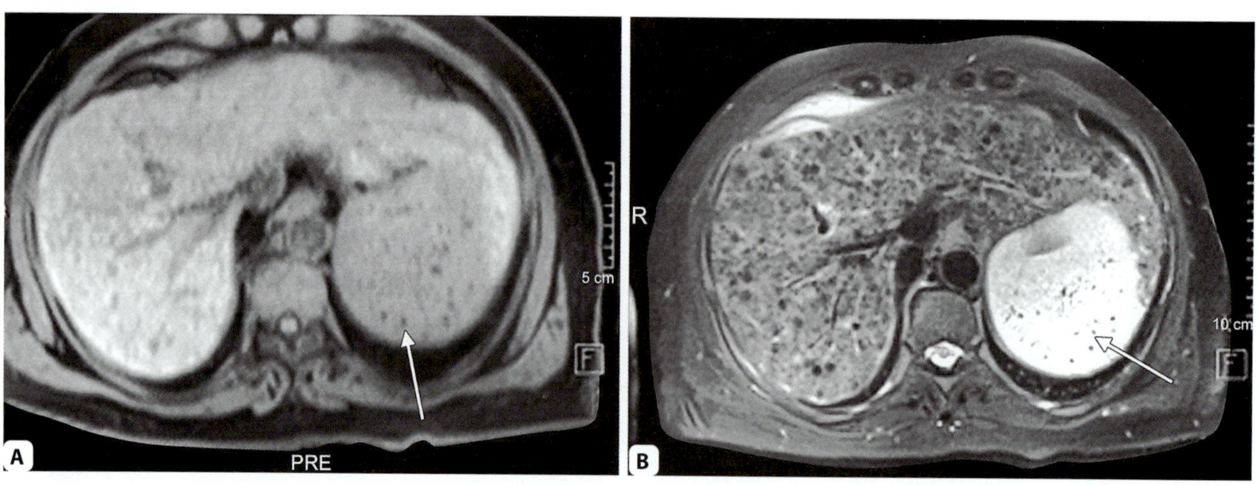

FIGS. 16A AND B: Axial T1-weighted (T1W) and T2-weighted (T2W) MR images (A and B) showing multiple low signal intensity foci (arrow) scattered in enlarged spleen in a cirrhotic patient.

calcifications on CT. They are seen as multiple low signal foci 3–8 mm in size on gradient echo sequences of MR images **(Figs. 16A and B)**.

Ascites is not usually caused by uncomplicated PHT. It is often secondary to underlying liver diseases with liver cell failure and increase in sinusoidal pressure leading to an increase in fluid in the space of Disse with resultant ascites. In prehepatic PHT, liver function remains normal, and ascites is minimal.

SPECIFIC SITUATIONS

Intrahepatic Portal Hypertension

Cirrhosis of liver: Imaging features are described under the chapter on Diffuse Liver Diseases. Sonography can differentiate intrahepatic from extrahepatic PHT in majority of cases and can also detect the presence of splenomegaly and ascites. Evaluation of the liver by ultrasound may reveal changes of cirrhosis such as coarsened echotexture with or without altered echogenicity, nodularity of liver surface, presence of regenerating nodules, and reduction in the number of visible portal or hepatic veins. Reduction of liver size with a combination of segmental hypertrophy and atrophy in the form of caudate to right lobe ratio >0.65 and reduction of the transverse diameter of segment IV.

Noncirrhotic portal hypertension: Includes a spectrum of diseases of diverse causes **(Box 3)**.

The most common causes of NCPH are noncirrhotic portal fibrosis (NCPF) and extrahepatic portal vein obstruction (EHPVO). These constitute one-third of all cases of PHT in India.[20,21] The fundamental cause in both NCPF and EHPVO is thought to be vascular origin. However, the exact etiopathogenesis of the two conditions is not known, but a common pathway with different outcomes has been advocated and is depicted in **Flowchart 1**.

Basically, in a genetically susceptible patient, a trigger point such as infection or prothrombotic episode can incite thrombosis in the portal system. In EHPVO, a major thrombotic event in early life leads to occlusion of the MPV with resultant cavernoma formation. Whereas in NCPF, repeated events of microthrombi in later life leads to occlusion of small- and medium-sized venous channels with resultant presinusoidal fibrosis.

Noncirrhotic portal fibrosis: This condition was first described by Banti in the late 19th century and was originally identified in India as an etiological factor of portal hypertension in the mid-20th century. NCPF is seen in patients during their third to fourth decade of life and especially more common in individuals of low socioeconomic background.[20,21]

There are well-established guidelines for making the diagnosis of NCPF **(Box 4)**.

Imaging findings include normal size liver with normal echogenicity, splenomegaly, patent hepatic veins, dilated splenoportal axis, and presence of varices **(Figs. 17A to D)**. Few specific ultrasound findings are also described (which are difficult to document), such as echogenic thick-walled portal branches, narrowing or cuff of the peripheral portal vein branches classically described as "withered tree" appearance.[21,22]

Management: Prognosis is generally excellent in NCPF, since liver functions are well-preserved. Main concern is usually prevention/control of variceal bleeding which is the major cause of death in these patients.

BOX 3 Causes of noncirrhotic portal hypertension.

- Extrahepatic portal venous obstruction (EHPVO)
- Noncirrhotic portal fibrosis (NCPF) or idiopathic portal hypertension (IPH)
- Nodular regenerative hyperplasia
- Partial nodular transformation
- Congenital hepatic fibrosis
- Schistosomiasis
- Peliosis hepatis

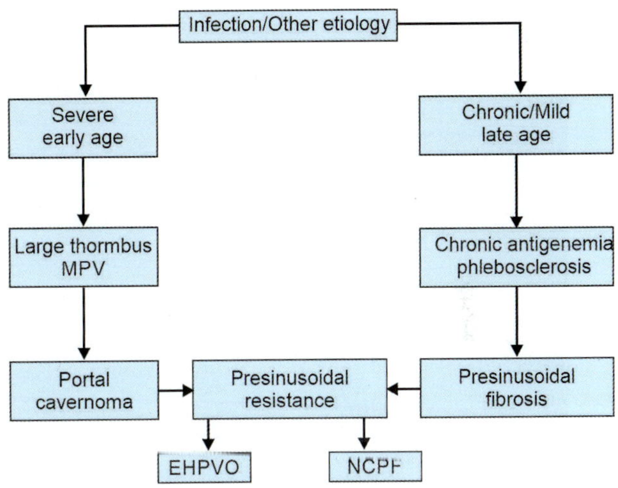

FLOWCHART 1: Etiopathogenesis of extrahepatic portal venous obstruction and noncirrhotic portal fibrosis.

(EHPVO: extrahepatic portal venous obstruction; MPV: main portal vein; NCPF: noncirrhotic portal fibrosis)

BOX 4 Guidelines for the diagnosis of NCPF.

- Presence of splenomegaly
- Normal liver function tests
- Varices on upper GI endoscopy
- Patent portal and hepatic veins on Doppler
- Normal or mildly elevated WHVP; and markedly elevated intrasplenic and portal vein pressure
- No evidence of cirrhosis on liver biopsy

(GI: gastrointestinal; NCPF: noncirrhotic portal fibrosis; WHVP: wedged hepatic venous pressure)

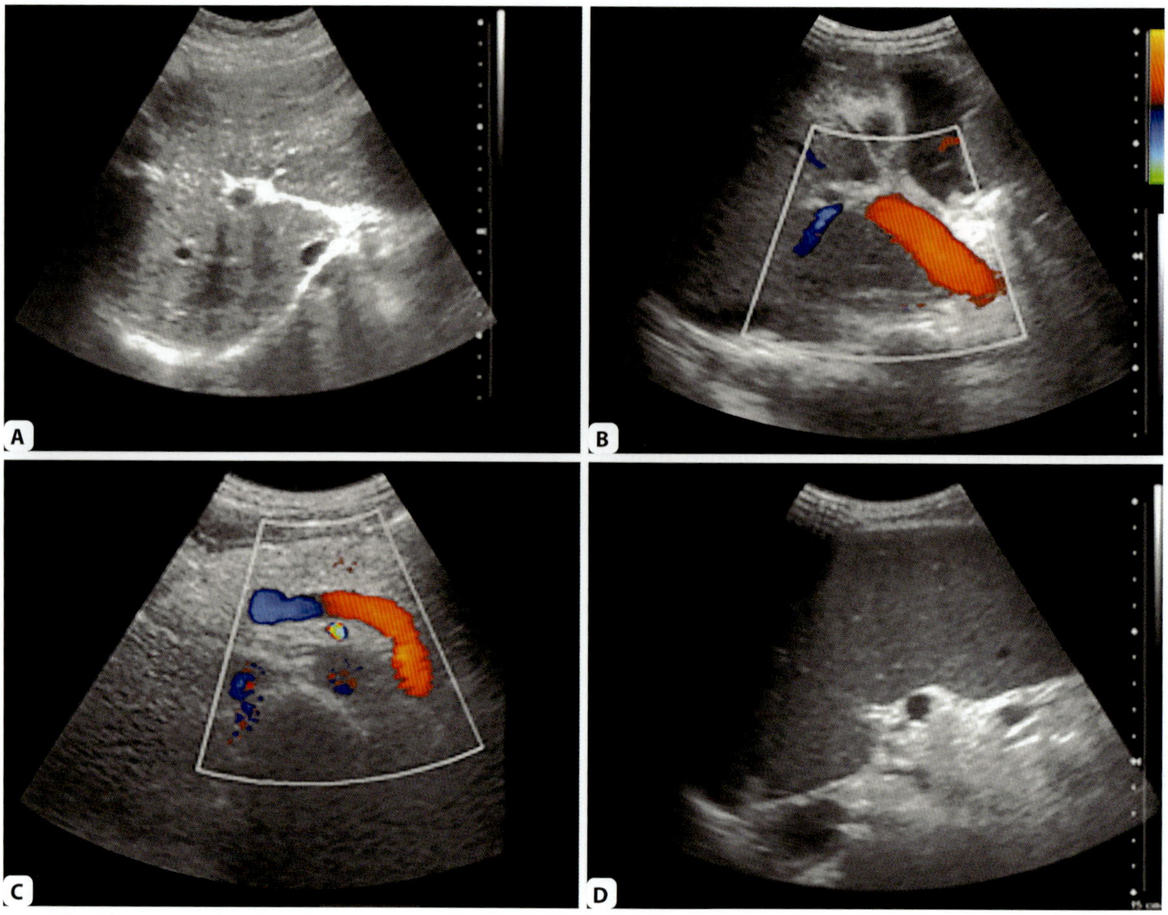

FIGS. 17A TO D: Ultrasound and Doppler images of noncirrhotic portal fibrosis (NCPF) patient showing normal size liver with normal echotexture (A), dilated main portal vein (MPV) (B), splenic vein (C), and splenomegaly (D).

PREHEPATIC CAUSES

Extrahepatic Portal Vein Obstruction[23,24]

Definition

Extrahepatic portal vein obstruction is an important cause of upper gastrointestinal bleeding in the pediatric age group, caused by thrombotic event in early life resulting in cavernoma formation.

The disease process may involve only the MPV and its branches at porta or may extend to involve the SV and upper portion of the SMV. Splenoportal confluence is the most common site to get involved in this disease process, whereas the entire SPA is involved in only 10% of cases.

The etiopathogenesis of EHPVO is not known in nearly 50% of patients. Possible causes include neonatal sepsis, omphalitis, umbilical vein catheterization, dehydration, multiple exchange transfusions, and hypercoagulable states.

These patients may present anywhere between 6 weeks and adulthood with well-controlled variceal bleeding and massive splenomegaly. Generally, liver function tests (LFTs) are normal in young patients with EHPVO. Infrequently, these patients may present with jaundice due to portal biliopathy. Hemodynamically, wedged HVPG is normal since the block is (presinusoidal hepatic); however, direct intrasplenic pressure is significantly increased in these patients.

Portal cavernoma cholangiopathy (earlier portal biliopathy) refers to biliary abnormalities (intrahepatic/extrahepatic) either due to compression of bile ducts by prominent paracholedochal and epicholedochal varices or due to ischemic injury (stricture formation) **(Fig. 18)**. Although imaging biliary abnormalities have been described in 80–100% of cases, but only a few patients present with jaundice or pain.[25]

Imaging modalities: Currently, ultrasonography with Doppler is the best imaging modality to evaluate EHPVO patients **(Fig. 18)**. Invasive and direct splenoportography provides information about the portal venous system to identify the site of obstruction, extent of disease, and extent of collateral circulation, however, this procedure is now obsolete **(Fig. 19)**. The more advanced techniques such as computed tomographic portography and MR portography of the upper abdomen are performed only if Doppler is of suboptimal quality **(Figs. 20A to D)**.

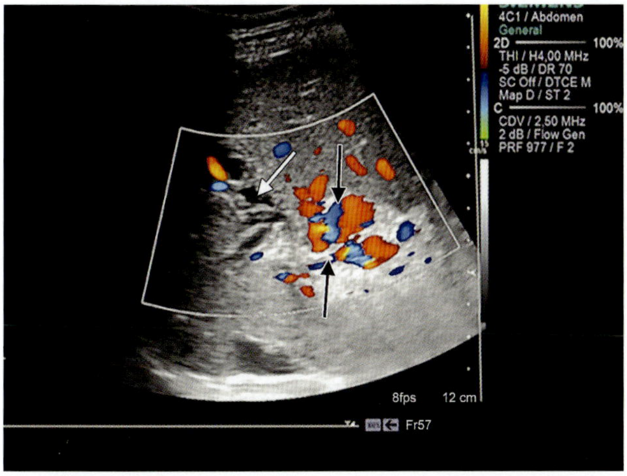

FIG. 18: Doppler ultrasound image showing multiple collaterals at porta (black arrow) replacing the main portal vein (MPV) with dilatation of intrahepatic biliary radicles suggestive of portal biliopathy (white arrow).

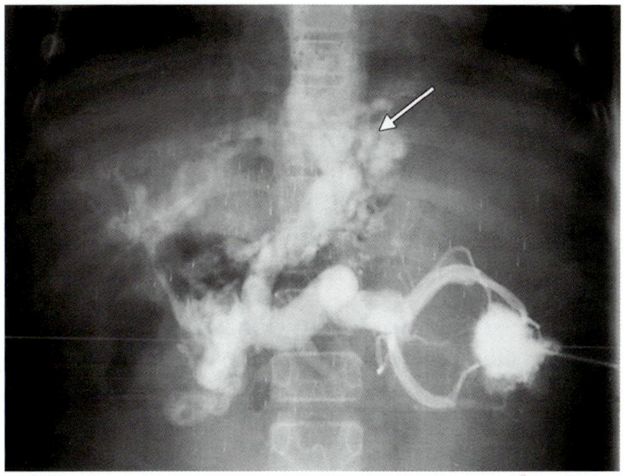

FIG. 19: Spot image of direct splenoportography showing patent and dilated splenoportal axis with varices supplied by the left gastric vein (arrow).

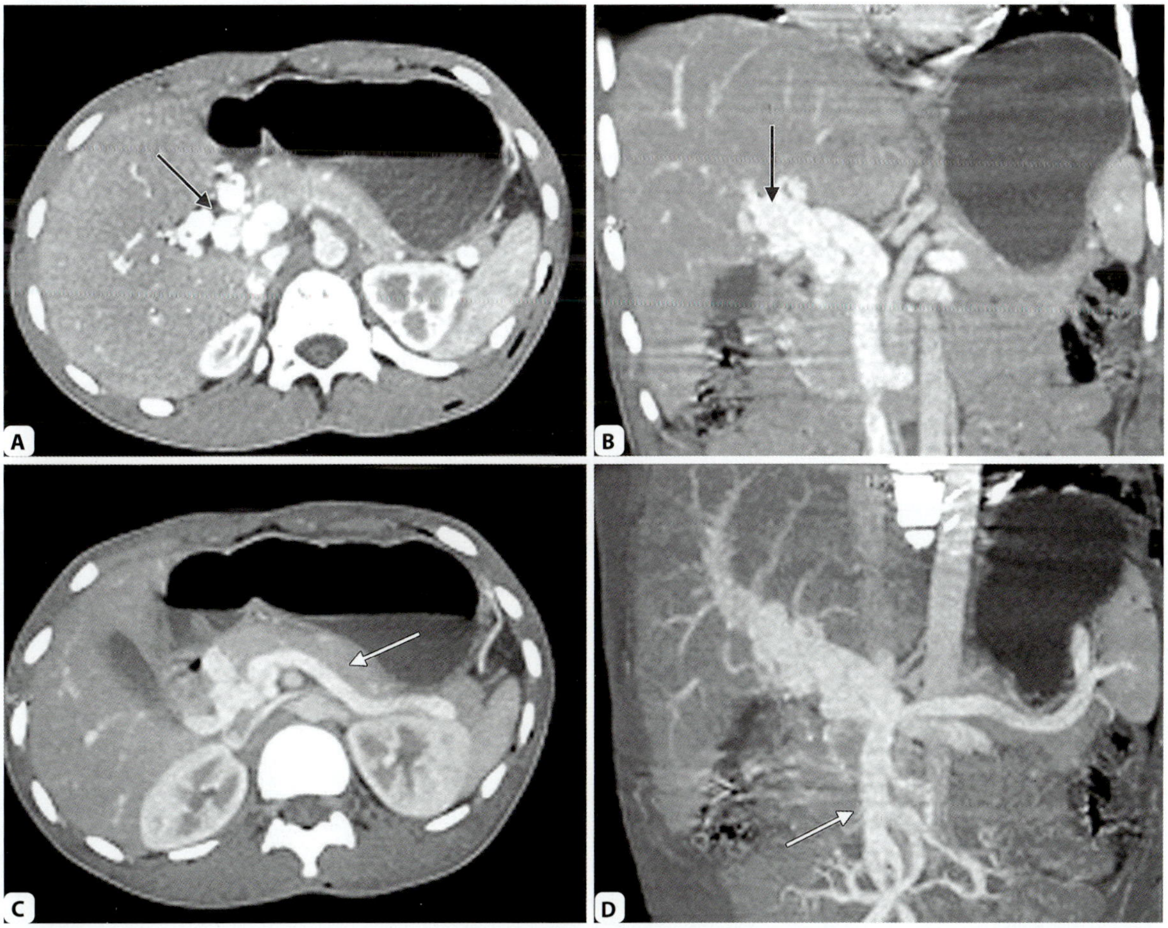

FIGS. 20A TO D: CT portography images showing multiple collaterals at porta (arrow) (A and B) replacing the main portal vein (MPV) with patent splenic (C) (arrow) and superior mesenteric vein (D) (arrow).

Imaging findings: MPV is replaced by echogenic fibrosis and multiple collaterals around the porta classically described as cavernoma formation **(Figs. 21A and B)**. Sometimes, one may see recanalized portal vein or dominant collateral at porta. CT and MR portography are used as problem-solving modalities when Doppler findings are inconclusive.

Other risk factors for development of acute portal vein include infectious disease (e.g., sepsis, cholangitis, and pancreatitis), neoplasms, hypercoagulable states, and surgery.

Contrast-enhanced CT/CT portal venography can exhibit a filling defect, i.e., thrombosis that occludes the portal vein lumen either partially or completely **(Figs. 22A and B)**. Indirect signs include the presence of cavernous transformation of the portal vein and the presence of portosystemic collateral vessels.

It is important to differentiate bland thrombus from malignant thrombus in cirrhotic patients. Bland thrombus will not enhance on postcontrast studies and will not distend the lumen **(Figs. 22A and B)**. Whereas malignant thrombus distends the lumen and shows enhancement like the primary index lesion, classically described as "Threads-streaks" **(Figs. 23A and B)**. Malignant lesion shows diffusion restriction on diffusion-weighted MRI.

Treatment and Prognosis

Prognosis is generally good in EHPVO, since liver functions are well-preserved. Main concern is usually prevention/control of variceal bleeding which is the major cause of death in these patients. Endoscopic therapy is the first line of treatment for variceal bleeding. However, surgery is reserved for patients with variceal bleeding who fail to respond to endoscopic management. Other indications for surgery include patients with ectopic variceal bleeding, portal biliopathy and growth retardation **(Table 8)**.

Portal Vein Thrombosis[26-28]

Cirrhosis is an important risk factor for development of splanchnic vein thrombosis in cirrhotic patients, either due to development of portal venous hypertension or stasis of blood flow in portal circulation.

Left-sided Portal Hypertension

Left-sided portal hypertension (LSPH) is a special form of PHT that occurs due to obstruction of the SV in isolation and presents with bleeding from isolated gastric varices. The main cause of LSPH is SV thrombosis and pancreatic disease is the most common etiology. This entity is usually thought of in situations of gastrointestinal bleeding with normal

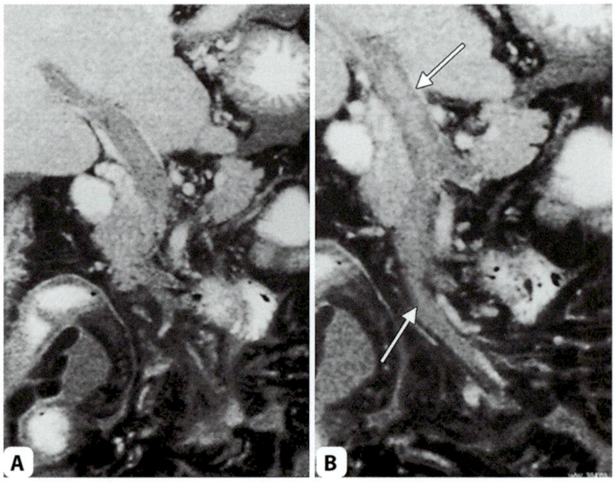

FIGS. 22A AND B: Coronal thin slab maximum intensity projection (MIP) image showing long segment nonenhancing filling defect (A) within the main portal vein extending into superior mesenteric vein (B) (arrows).

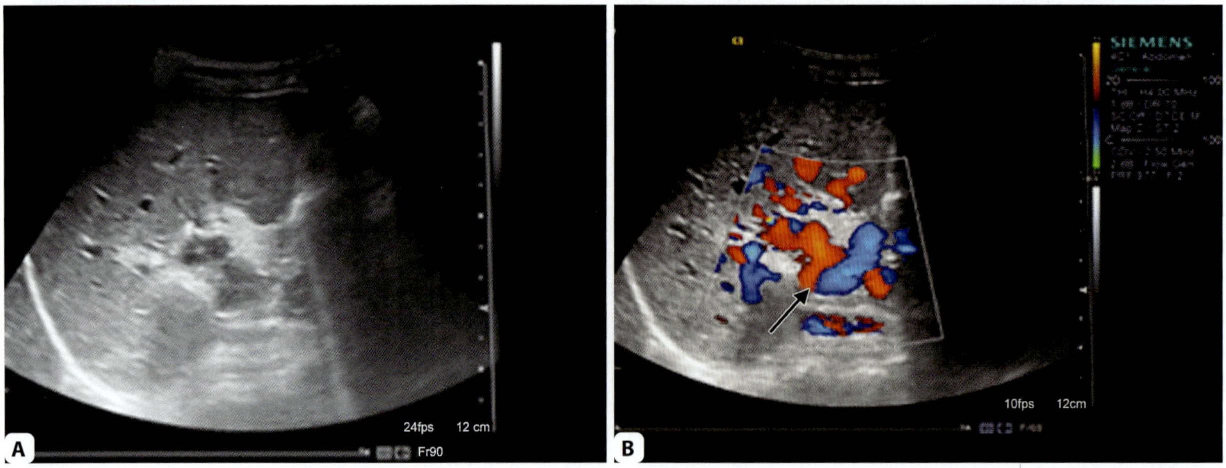

FIGS. 21A AND B: Doppler ultrasound images showing multiple collaterals at porta replacing the main portal vein (B) (arrow) with small size liver having normal echotexture (A).

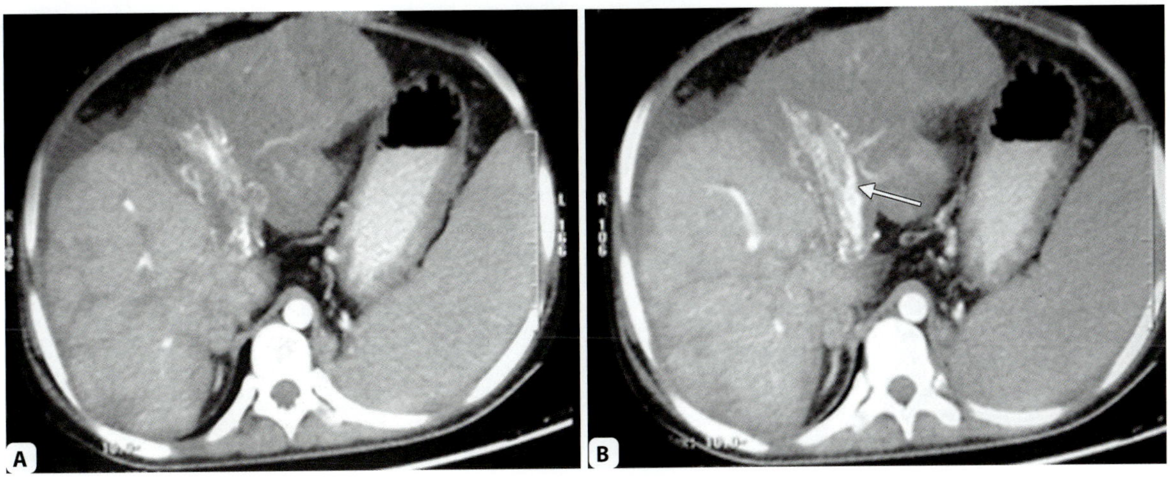

FIGS. 23A AND B: Axial CT images in arterial phase showing large infiltrative mass in left lobe of liver (A) with enhancing tumor thrombus in left portal vein (B) giving streaks and thread appearance (arrow).

TABLE 8: Comparison of NCPF and EHPVO.[24]

	NCPF	EHPVO
Epidemiology	Low > high socioeconomic status	Low >> high socioeconomic status
Age of onset	Third to fourth decade	First to second decade
Sex predilection	M = F	
Etiology	Infections/prothrombotic states/drugs and toxins/ immunogenic/genetics	Infection/prothrombotic states/congenital
Liver parenchymal architecture	• Maintained • Differential atrophy may be seen	Maintained
Characteristic hallmark	*Obliterative portovenopathy*: Segmental and patchy periportal/perisinusoidal fibrosis. Medium and small portal veins involved	Cavernous transformation of portal vein
Clinical complaints	• Hematemesis/Malena • Transient ascites	• Variceal bleeding • Transient ascites
Liver function test	Normal or near normal	Normal
Splenomegaly	May be seen	Common
Ultrasound	Prominent SPA. Dilated PV with thick walls and cutoff of intrahepatic 2nd and 3rd degree PV branches (withered tree appearance)	Portal veins replaced by bunch of collaterals (cavernoma)
Endoscopy	• Esophageal varices present • Gastric varices may be present • Portal hypertensive gastropathy is rare	• Esophageal varices present • Gastric varices and portal hypertensive gastropathy may be present
Hemodynamics	WHVP/FHVP/HVPG—normal	WHVP/FHVP/HVPG—normal
Prognosis	• Good—as liver function preserved • Portal biliopathy—less common • Hepatic encephalopathy—absent	• Good—as liver function preserved • Portal biliopathy—common • Hepatic encephalopathy—may be seen

(EHPVO: extrahepatic portal venous obstruction; FHVP: free hepatic venous pressure; HVPG: hepatic venous pressure gradient; NCPF: noncirrhotic portal fibrosis; PV: portal vein; SPA: splenoportal axis; WHVP: wedged hepatic venous pressure)

liver function and unexplained splenomegaly. At times, LSPH may be difficult to diagnose both endoscopically and radiologically. On imaging, there is thrombosis or severe attenuation of SV with extensive collaterals all around the stomach **(Figs. 24A and B)**. If repeated gastric variceal bleeding complicates this condition, splenectomy is considered.[29]

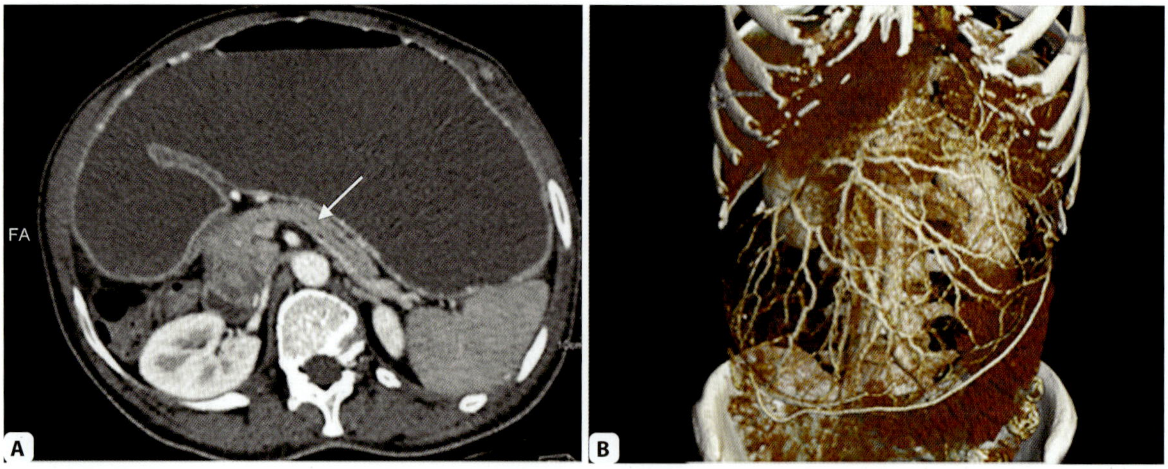

FIGS. 24A AND B: Axial CT (A) and coronal volume rendering technique (VRT) (B) image showing severely attenuated and splenic vein (arrow) and is replaced by extensive collaterals around the stomach (B).

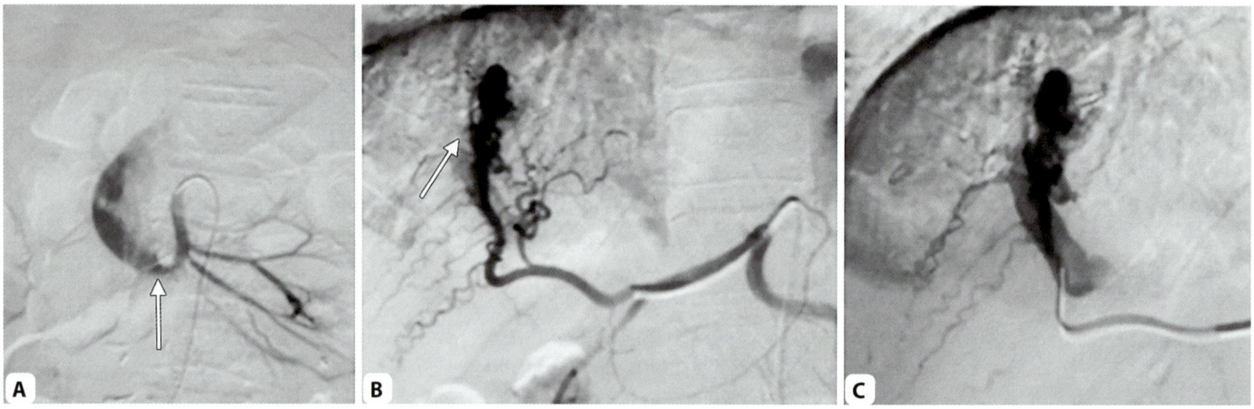

FIGS. 25A TO C: Digital subtraction angiography (DSA) spot images (A to C) showing fistulous communication between superior mesenteric artery and superior mesenteric vein (A) (arrow). Fistulous communication between right hepatic artery and right portal vein suggestive of arterioportal fistula (B and C) (arrow) as a prehepatic causes of portal hypertension.

Splanchnic Arterioportal Fistula

Arterioportal fistula (APF) is rare, occurring mainly from a ruptured pseudoaneurysm communicating with the portal system either due to iatrogenic cause or due to penetrating trauma. This entity is encountered increasingly due to rising numbers of percutaneous transhepatic procedures. The predominant symptoms are due to complications of PHT, most commonly variceal bleeding. Angiography remains the gold standard **(Figs. 25A to C)**. However, duplex ultrasonography is a useful screening tool. CT angiography helps in pretreatment planning such as delineating the artery involved, level and diameter of communication, and to see the extent of varices.

Broadly, surgery is the treatment of choice for large extrahepatic fistula, whereas embolization is ideal for intrahepatic fistulas and small extrahepatic fistula. Embolization is also beneficial for patients with comorbidities who carry high risk of surgical mortality. Main goal of treatment is to occlude the fistula and maintain the arterial flow.[30]

Posthepatic Causes of Portal Hypertension

Budd-Chiari syndrome: Imaging findings and interventions are described in detail in a separate chapter.

RADIOLOGICAL INTERVENTIONS IN PORTAL HYPERTENSION

INTRODUCTION

The role of radiologists in the management of PHT was earlier confined to diagnosis and treatment planning. However, with the advancements in the field of interventional radiology various minimally invasive techniques have evolved in the management of portal hypertension and its complications such as recanalization techniques, shunt creation, and variceal bleeding control. Thus, with these technical advances, there is a paradigm shift in the role of radiologist from only diagnosis to the management of PHT.

The management of PHT and its complications requires a multimodality approach including medical and endoscopic management and surgical and nonsurgical (minimally invasive radiological techniques) methods to reduce portal pressure. Surgical methods carry significant morbidity and mortality in these groups of patients.

Interventions in Portal Hypertension

Primary aim is to reduce the portal pressure and thereby reduce the complications related to PHT such as variceal bleed, ascites, hydrothorax, and hepatorenal syndrome.

Secondary aim (in cases where it is difficult to bring down the portal pressure) is to deal with the complications of PHT such as esophageal and gastric varices, refractory ascites, and encephalopathy.

The radiologic interventions in PHT are broadly categorized in **Box 5**.

Transjugular Intrahepatic Portosystemic Shunts

Transjugular intrahepatic portosystemic shunts (TIPSs) involve the creation of a low resistance conduit between the portal vein and hepatic vein by deploying an intrahepatic stent. The procedure is done under fluoroscopic and ultrasound guidance, under conscious sedation or general anesthesia depending upon patients' condition. Prophylactic antibiotics may be given, and coagulation defects must be corrected prior to the procedure.

Technique: The procedure starts with a puncture of the right internal jugular vein for venous access under sonographic guidance. A 10-F long vascular sheath is placed across the right heart into the IVC. Initial cavogram is obtained to look for the status of IVC and the ostium of hepatic vein. Diagnostic angiographic catheter is then introduced into one of the hepatic veins (preferably right hepatic vein). At this stage, baseline hepatic vein wedge pressure is obtained using balloon catheter occluding the hepatic vein outflow. After getting access into the right hepatic vein, this catheter is exchanged with a long metallic cannula with 7-F vascular sheath over the metallic guidewire. This metallic cannula is then wedged against the hepatic vein wall close to the ostium and gentle contrast study is done to look for retrograde visualization of intrahepatic portal vein branches. USG or direct transhepatic portography may also be used to visualize the portal vein and branches in difficult cases with distorted anatomy. Then using a combination of coaxial system of 16-G metallic cannula with 7-F sheath and 21-G Chiba needle with 4-F catheter, hepatic parenchyma is entered through hepatic vein wall. Using either fluoroscopic landmark of the portal vein or USG guidance, access into the portal vein is made using 21-G Chiba needle with 4-F catheter loaded over it. This is the most critical step of TIPS that utmost care should be taken not to breach the liver capsule to prevent life-threatening intraperitoneal bleed. The preferable site of portal vein puncture is at the portal vein bifurcation or within 2 cm of portal vein bifurcation. Once portal vein access is obtained, a portogram is obtained to look for splenoportal axis anatomy and variceal status. The parenchymal tract is dilated using angiographic balloon catheters (diameter 8–10 mm) and specially designed TIPS stent (uncovered segment in portal vein and covered segment in hepatic parenchyma and hepatic vein) is deployed to maintain the patency of the tract. Polytetrafluoroethylene (PTFE)-covered stents are preferred over bare stents as they show improved long-term patency of the shunt and prevent portobiliary fistula.[31-33] Customized TIPS stent graft has a small, uncovered part (2 cm), which is to be kept in the portal vein to promote good inflow and avoid portal vein thrombosis **(Figs. 26A to E)**.

The established indication for TIPS is in the management of patients with cirrhosis and PHT complicated by recurrent/refractory variceal bleeding and refractory ascites. Refractory acutely bleeding varices and complicated chronic/acute Budd–Chiari syndrome is among the optional indications **(Box 6)**.[34]

Absolute contraindications for TIPS placement include congestive cardiac failure, severe pulmonary hypertension, unrelieved biliary obstruction, pre-existing hepatic encephalopathy, etc. **(Box 7)**.[35]

Variceal bleeding is a major cause of death in cirrhotic patients and correlates with PHT. Many studies have demonstrated the efficacy of TIPS in controlling and preventing massive life-threatening variceal hemorrhage. It is recommended to reduce the HVPG below 12 mm Hg in controlling variceal bleeding. TIPS is also beneficial in preventing bleeding from hypertensive gastropathy.[35]

BOX 5 Radiologic intervention in portal hypertension.

Interventions that reduce portal blood pressure:
- Transjugular intrahepatic portosystemic shunts (TIPSs)
- Recanalization of hepatic venous outflow
- Partial splenic embolization
- Recanalization of occluded/thrombosed portal veins or tributaries
- Occlusion of arterioportal shunts (congenital/acquired)
- Revision of occluded surgical or radiological shunts

Interventions to control the symptoms of portal hypertension:
- Percutaneous transhepatic variceal embolization [balloon-occluded antegrade transvenous obliteration (BATO)]
- Balloon occluded retrograde transvenous obliteration (BRTO) of gastric varices

Occlusion of surgical or radiologic shunts in refractory encephalopathy

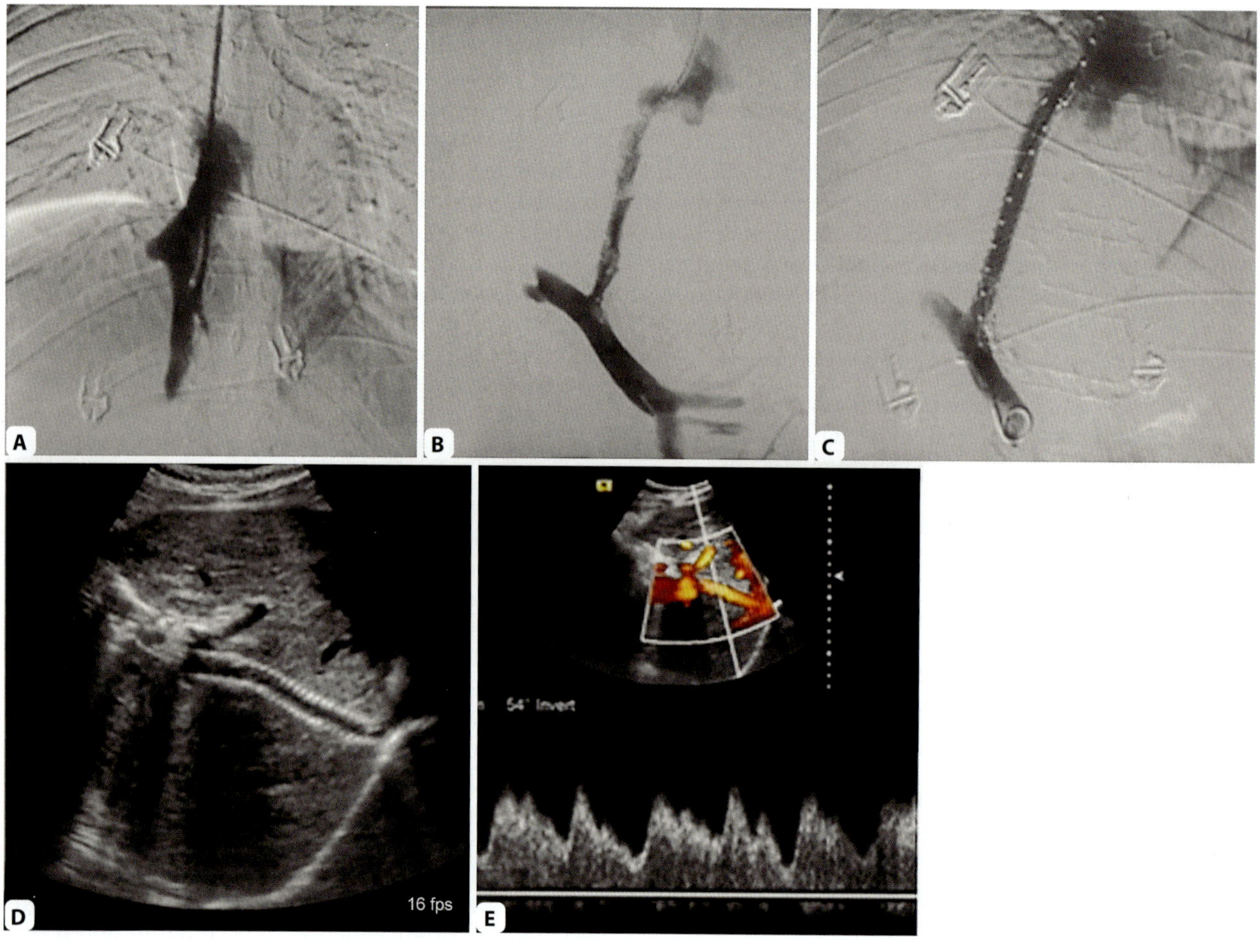

FIGS. 26A TO E: Transjugular intrahepatic portosystemic shunts (TIPS) performed in a cirrhotic patient with uncontrollable variceal bleeding: (A) Initial cavogram showing normal caliber inferior vena cava (IVC) and hepatic vein; (B) A parenchymal tract is made from the hepatic vein to the portal vein; (C) Post-TIPS venogram showing free flow of contrast through the stent graft; (D and E) USG and color Doppler showing TIPS stent with optimal flow.

BOX 6 Indications for transjugular intrahepatic portosystemic shunts (TIPS).

- Refractory cirrhotic ascites
- Refractory acutely bleeding varices
- Portal hypertensive gastropathy
- Bleeding gastric varices
- Refractory hepatic hydrothorax
- Hepatorenal syndrome
- Budd–Chiari syndrome
- Veno-occlusive disease
- Hepatopulmonary syndrome

BOX 7 Contraindications of transjugular intrahepatic portosystemic shunts (TIPS).

Absolute:
- Right-sided heart failure
- Biliary tract obstruction
- Uncontrolled infection
- Pulmonary hypertension
- Chronic recurrent disabling hepatic encephalopathy
- Hepatocellular carcinoma involving hepatic veins

Relative:
- Severe liver failure (Pugh score > 12)
- Portal vein thrombosis
- Multiple hepatic cysts

Refractory ascites reflects severe PHT and advanced liver dysfunction and is associated with very poor outcome and survival. TIPS will decrease the need for repeated large volume paracentesis in patients with refractory ascites. However, in view of poor functional status of such patients and the higher risk of hepatic encephalopathy, TIPS is recommended for those who are intolerant to repeated paracentesis. Similarly in cases of refractory hepatic hydrothorax, TIPS is only recommended for those whose effusion is not controlled by diuretics and sodium restriction. In cases of Budd-Chiari syndrome TIPS or direct intrahepatic portosystemic shunt (DIPS) is recommended in cases with moderate severity and those who failed to respond to anticoagulation.[34]

Complications of Transjugular Intrahepatic Portosystemic Shunts

Immediate complications are procedure related, such as hematoma, arrhythmia, stent displacement and shunt thrombosis. Uncommon life-threatening complications include hemoperitoneum, cardiac failure, liver ischemia, and sepsis. Chronic complications include congestive cardiac failure, portal vein thrombosis, chronic recurrent encephalopathy, TIPSitis and TIPS dysfunction. TIPS dysfunction is defined as loss of decompression of the portal system due to occlusion or stenosis of the shunt. The best indicator of it is reappearance of symptoms such as variceal bleeding and ascites and can be demonstrated by imaging.

Follow-up Evaluation after Transjugular Intrahepatic Portosystemic Shunts

All TIPS patients should receive close follow-up under both interventional radiologist and hepatologist. Regular noninvasive imaging by ultrasound is imperative. Follow-up protocol include US Doppler at 1 month, 3 months, 6 months after TIPS; and 6 months thereafter or when clinical symptoms worsen. This should be continued for at least 5 years. Thereafter, the patency rates remain stable.[36]

Doppler results are considered abnormal if either of one is seen:

- An absolute stent velocity is <50 or > 200 cm/s.
- The stent velocity gradient is > 50 cm/s.
- The portal vein velocity < 30 cm/s.
- There is presence of flow reversal in the portal vein distal to the shunt.

Interventions in Hepatic Venous Outflow obstruction (Budd–Chiari Syndrome)

Budd-Chiari syndrome is a heterogeneous group of disorders characterized by hepatic venous obstruction at the level of hepatic veins, IVC or right atrium. Hepatic venous outflow increases sinusoidal pressure, PHT, and decreased liver perfusion which in turn leads to progressive liver failure. The manifestations can range from fulminant acute liver failure to chronic liver disease depending on factors such as extent and acuteness of obstruction and adequacy of remaining collateral circulation. The etiology of obstruction in western population is primarily thrombosis (bland or tumor). Membranous web-like obstruction of hepatic veins and IVC is seen commonly in the Asian population.

Medical therapy including anticoagulation for preventing recurrence and extension of thrombosis and measures to control ascites, and gastrointestinal bleeding has poor long-term outcomes. Surgical options in Budd-Chiari syndrome include creation of a portosystemic shunt and liver transplant. Portosystemic surgical shunts can only partially decompress the portal system and feasibility of liver transplant depends largely on availability of a donor.

Percutaneous techniques in Budd-Chiari syndrome include transluminal balloon angioplasty of hepatic veins and/or IVC and stent placement. Percutaneous interventions can restore physiologic hepatic venous outflow and help in resolution of venous congestion, improvement in hepatic function, and arresting hepatic destruction. Hepatic venous recanalization techniques are feasible if the occlusion is short segment with a large patent segment.

Transjugular approach is preferred for approaching the hepatic veins. Once the hepatic venous ostium is accessed, an attempt is made to negotiate a guidewire across the stenosis followed by balloon angioplasty of the narrowed segment. Transjugular approach may fail in cases with tight stenosis at the ostium. Percutaneous transhepatic approach is preferred in such cases which involves USG-guided puncture of the patent segment of hepatic veins and negotiating the guidewire across stenosis into the IVC. The guidewire is then snared through the transjugular route and procedure is completed by transjugular route to avoid making larger tracts in the liver. Successful angioplasty is seen as free flow of contrast across the stenosis, reduction in pressure gradients and collapse of intrahepatic veno-venous collaterals **(Figs. 27A to C)**. Metallic stents are deployed in cases of insufficient response and rapid restenosis following balloon angioplasty **(Figs. 28A to F)**. Good medium-term outcome is noted following angioplasty provided adequate anticoagulation is maintained.[36-38]

Inferior vena cava stenosis secondary to liver congestion in Budd-Chiari syndrome gets resolved after successful venous decompression procedures. However, primary caval stenosis that occludes hepatic venous outflow must be addressed by IVC angioplasty. IVC angioplasty is performed by femoral or jugular approach **(Figs. 29A to D)**. Caval stenting is needed, if angioplasty fails.

Long-segment occlusion of hepatic veins is difficult to reopen and has higher chances of reocclusion and this subgroup of patients requires creation of a portosystemic shunt. TIPS and DIPS are being increasingly performed in such scenario with gratifying results.[39,40]

Partial Splenic Embolization

Partial splenic embolization (PSE) is performed to decrease portal venous inflow, thereby decreasing the portal pressure. It is performed by super-selective catheterization of splenic arterial branches and embolization using polyvinyl alcohol particles or glue **(Figs. 30A to D)**. PSE is efficacious in reducing the episodes of variceal bleeding. It also helps in decreasing splenic size and in improving hematologic

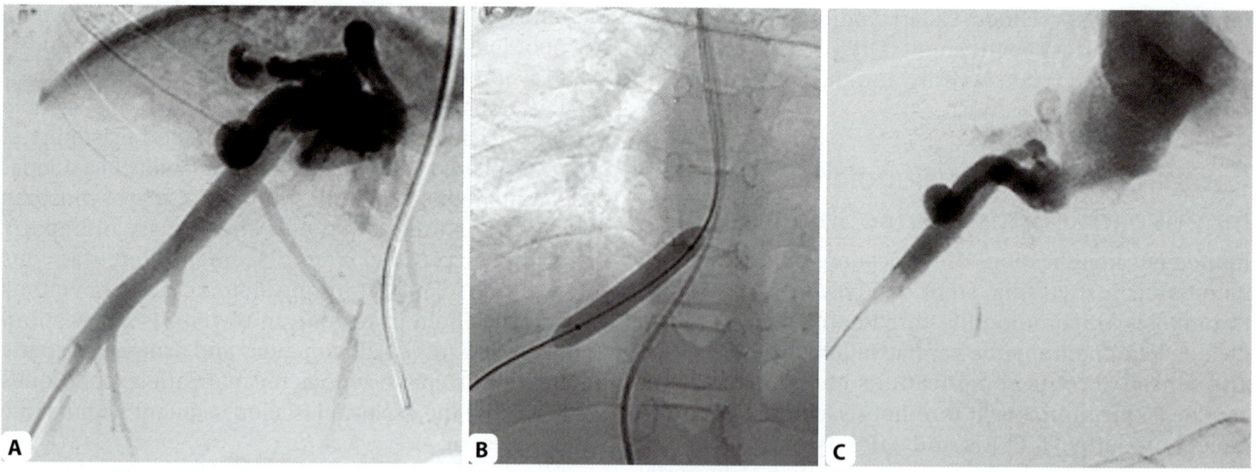

FIGS. 27A TO C: Hepatic vein angioplasty in a patient with Budd–Chiari syndrome: (A) Hepatic venogram (percutaneous approach) shows complete occlusion at the ostium with multiple venous collaterals; (B) Balloon angioplasty of the stenosed ostium; (C) Postangioplasty hepatic venogram showing free flow of contrast into inferior vena cava (IVC).

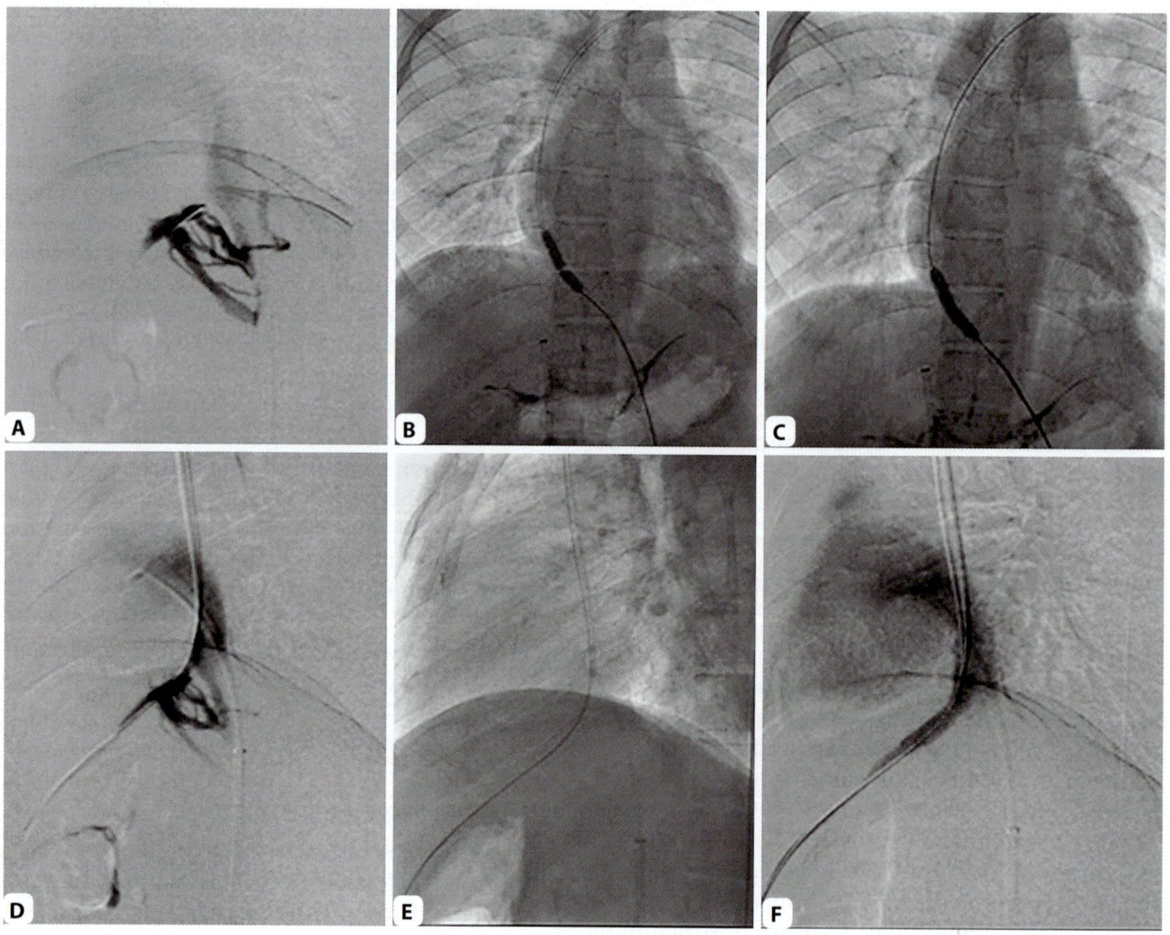

FIGS. 28A TO F: Hepatic vein stenting: (A) Hepatic venogram showing stenosis at ostium with multiple collaterals; (B and C) Balloon angioplasty; (D) Postangioplasty showing residual stenosis with persistent collaterals; (E and F) Stent deployment and subsequent study showing free flow of contrast with disappearance of collaterals.

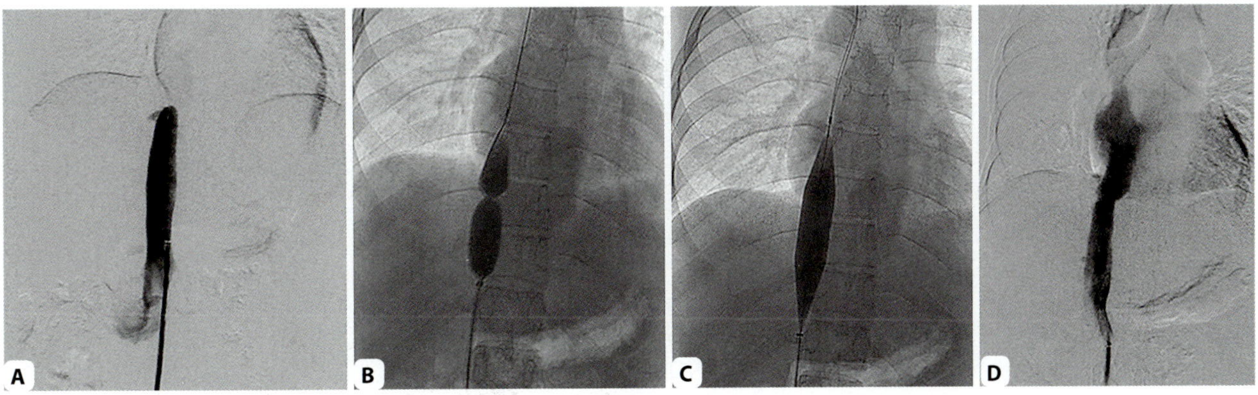

FIGS. 29A TO D: Inferior vena cava (IVC) angioplasty: (A) Cavogram showing total occlusion below cavoatrial junction; (B and C) Angioplasty using balloon catheter; and (D) Postangioplasty cavogram showing free flow of contrast into right atrium.

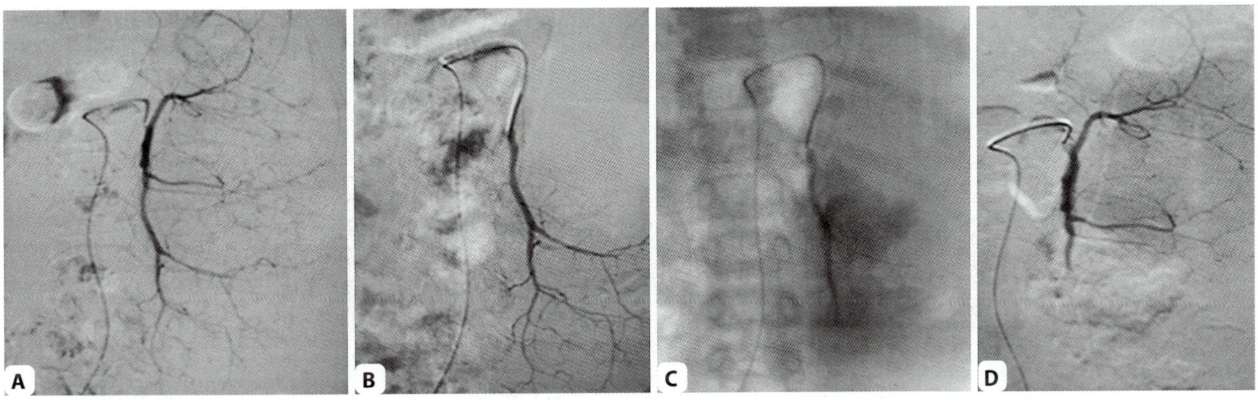

FIGS. 30A TO D: Partial splenic embolization in a patient with hypersplenism: (A) Splenic arteriogram showing parenchymal branches; (B) Selective run of lower branch of splenic artery; (C) Embolization of lower part of spleen using polyvinyl alcohol (PVA) particles; and (D) Postembolization study showing decreased perfusion in lower part.

parameters and hepatic protein synthesis.[41] PSE is a safe, simple, and effective alternative for splenectomy in hypersplenism.[42] It causes partial necrosis of splenic parenchyma with minimal risk of complications such as liver abscess and sepsis. Splenic artery embolization can also be used in management of bleeding gastric varices secondary to SV thrombosis.[43]

Recanalization of Occluded/Thrombosed Portal Veins or Tributaries

Portal hypertension can be caused by obstruction of the portal vein or its tributaries. It can be due to inflammatory stenosis, bland thrombus or due to tumor infiltration. In both benign and malignant conditions, patients present with variceal bleeding, ascites, or abdominal pain. These symptoms can be relieved by recanalization of occluded vessels, which can be achieved by angioplasty and stenting through transjugular, transhepatic, or transsplenic route.[44,45] Anastomotic strictures of portal vein can also be treated by angioplasty **(Figs. 31A to D).**

Occlusion of Arterioportal Shunts (Congenital/Acquired)

Arterioportal shunts can cause PHT by increased portal flow. Etiology of arterioportal shunts may be congenital malformation, trauma, tumors, aneurysms, and surgery or hepatic interventions. Such patients may rarely present with gastrointestinal bleeding, ascites, heart failure, and splenomegaly. Transarterial embolization of feeding arteries by coils, glue, or other closure devices depending on the size of the fistula is the preferred treatment in such cases **(Figs. 32A to D)**.[46]

Revision of Occluded Surgical or Radiological Shunts

Surgically created portosystemic shunts for PHT may be complicated by thrombosis and occlusion. Surgical treatment of such cases is difficult and carries a high morbidity. Occluded leno-renal shunts and mesocaval shunts can be successfully recanalized by endovascular route **(Figs. 33A to E)**.[47,48]

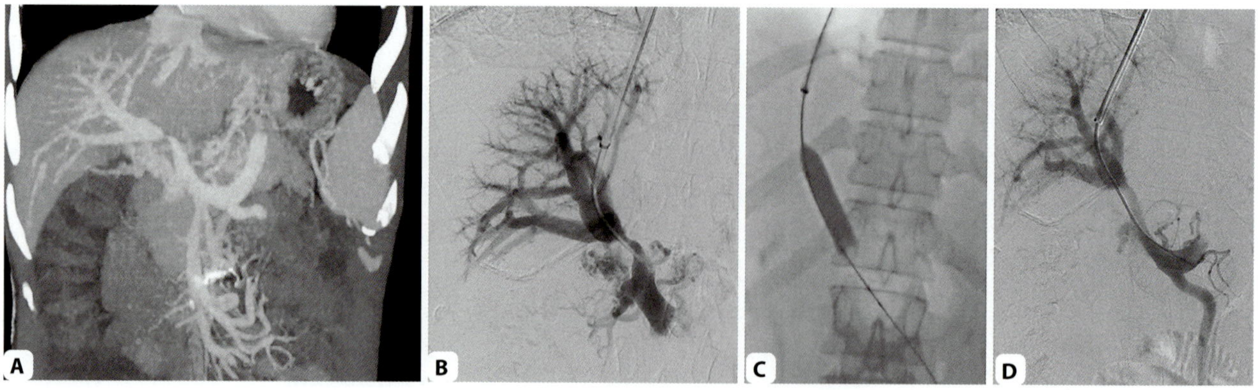

FIGS. 31A TO D: Recanalization of tubercular stenosis of portal vein: (A and B) CT portogram (A) and transjugular portogram (B) showing short segment stenosis of main portal vein; (C) Balloon dilatation of the stenosis; (D) Postangioplasty run showing improvement in diameter of stenotic segment.

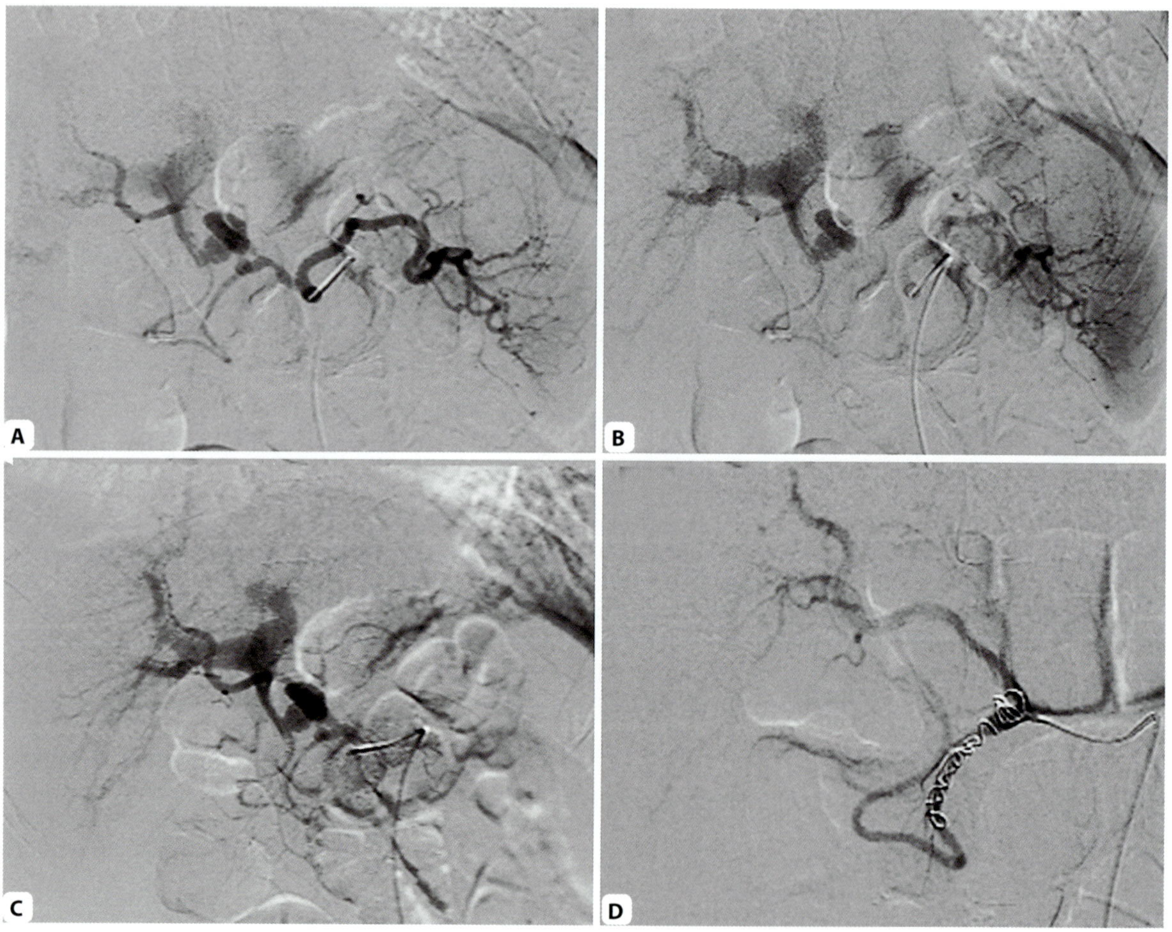

FIGS. 32A TO D: Occlusion of arterioportal shunts: (A and B) Celiac angiogram showing pseudoaneurysm of gastroduodenal artery communicating with portal vein; (C) Selective hepatic angiogram prior to embolization showing pseudoaneurysm; (D) Postembolization study showing complete isolation of pseudoaneurysm and disappearance of abnormal shunt.

Balloon-occluded antegrade transvenous obliteration (BATO) uses an antegrade approach (i.e., from the portal veins). It is generally used to access the gastric varices in the absence of a gastrorenal shunt and can be performed either through transhepatic [percutaneous transhepatic obliteration (PTO)] and trans-TIPS (if a TIPS already exists).

Percutaneous Transhepatic Variceal Embolization

Percutaneous transhepatic variceal embolization was introduced as a technique to manage bleeding esophagogastric varices by Lunderquist and Vang in 1974.[49]

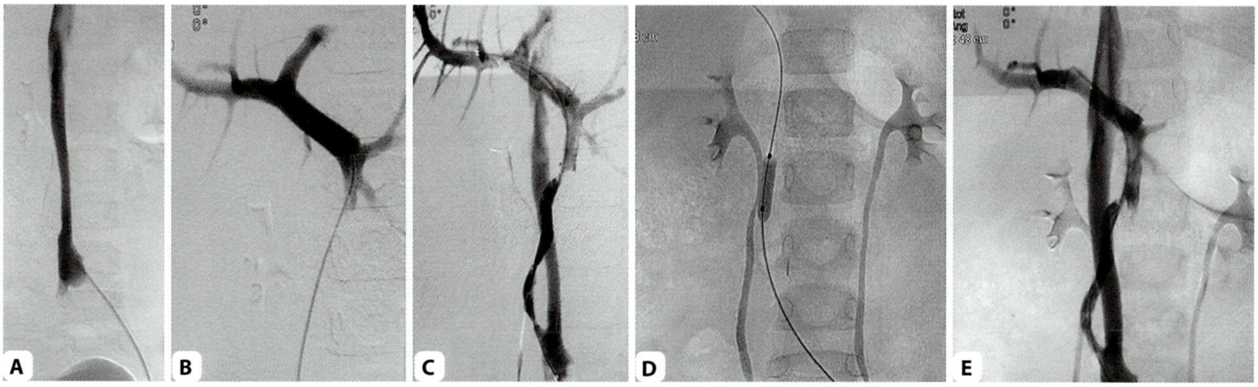

FIGS. 33A TO E: Mesocaval shunt revision: (A) Cavogram showing normal inferior vena cava (IVC); (B and C) Portogram done after advancing the catheter into portal vein through mesocaval shunt showing stenosis in the shunt; (D) Balloon dilatation of stenosis; (E) Subsequent portogram showing improved flow of contrast through the shunt.

Subsequent studies had shown excellent immediate success rate of 70–90%. Recurrent bleeding rate of 30–65% was noted in those studies since the procedure alone does not address the basic issues of PHT and hepatic insufficiency.[50-54] Subsequently, the procedure was recommended in acute settings when the variceal bleeding was not controlled by endoscopic sclerotherapy, vasopressin infusion, and balloon tamponade.[55] It can also be used in the management of bleeding gastric varices, which are difficult to localize by endoscopy.[56,57]

The technique starts with percutaneous transhepatic puncture of the intrahepatic branch of portal vein with ultrasound or fluoro-guidance and advancement of catheter into the SV. Diagnostic splenoportography is then performed to delineate the feeding veins, varices, and draining veins. The common veins feeding the gastric varices are the left gastric, short gastric, and posterior gastric veins. Subsequently, the feeding vein is selectively catheterized, and venography is performed to assess the size of the varices, velocity of flow and the size of gastrorenal shunt. Based on this data variceal sclerotherapy is performed with cyanoacrylate mixed with lipiodol. In cases with large gastrorenal shunts with rapid venous drainage, the gastrorenal shunts must be occluded with angiographic balloon catheter prior to sclerotherapy. The track in the hepatic parenchyma is embolized using gelfoam and steel coils at the end of the procedure **(Figs. 34A to D)**. BATO can also be performed through pre-existing TIPS **(Figs. 35A to D)**.

Variceal embolization can also be done with a trans-splenic route in which the access into the portal system is through the SV with the rest of the procedure being the same. The trans-splenic route is especially helpful in cases with preexisting portal vein thrombosis **(Fig. 36)**.[58]

Balloon-occluded Retrograde Transvenous Obliteration of Gastric Varices

Patients of PHT are often complicated by bleeding from esophagogastric varices. Although less common, gastric variceal rupture often leads to profuse bleeding and is difficult to manage with endoscopic and surgical technique.[59] BRTO is a novel technique in the management of gastric varices with major gastrosystemic shunts. It involves obliteration of gastric varices using sclerosants after occluding the communicating shunts with angiographic balloon catheter. Contrast-enhanced computed tomography (CECT) of the abdomen is commonly performed for planning the procedure. The diameter of major shunts is assessed using CECT to calculate the size of balloon catheter which can occlude it. Gastrorenal shunt is commonly encountered. Other shunts such as gastrocaval and gastropericardiophrenic are also rarely seen **(Table 9)**.

The procedure is commonly performed with an access through the right femoral vein. After cannulating the left renal vein, guidewire is advanced into the left adrenal vein which is a common channel to gastrorenal shunt. Along the guidewire the balloon catheter is advanced into the shunt and inflated to block the shunt. Contrast study through the catheter is done to see the opacification of gastric varices. Some of the varices may show leaking collaterals which can be dealt by deploying microcoils or gelfoam pledgets after selective catheterization. Subsequently, the sclerosant mixed with contrast [e.g., 5% ethanolamine oleate with lipiodol or sodium tetradecyl sulfate (STS) with contrast medium like Iomeron] is injected into the varices through the balloon catheter. The STS foam used in our institute is created by mixing the room air; STS and lipiodol at a ratio of 3:2:1, respectively. The angiographic balloon is kept inflated for a variable time ranging from 1 to 24 hours for adequate thrombosis to occur in the varices. After a period to allow thrombi formation, the hemolyzed blood with the remaining sclerosant is aspirated and the balloon is deflated, and catheter removed. If free flow of blood is seen in aspirate, a supplemental dose of sclerosant can be injected. Amount of sclerosant and duration of application is up to the discretion of the radiologist, and it varies with the size and extent of varices. Rarely, varices may show multiple shunts and balloon occlusion of all the shunts would be

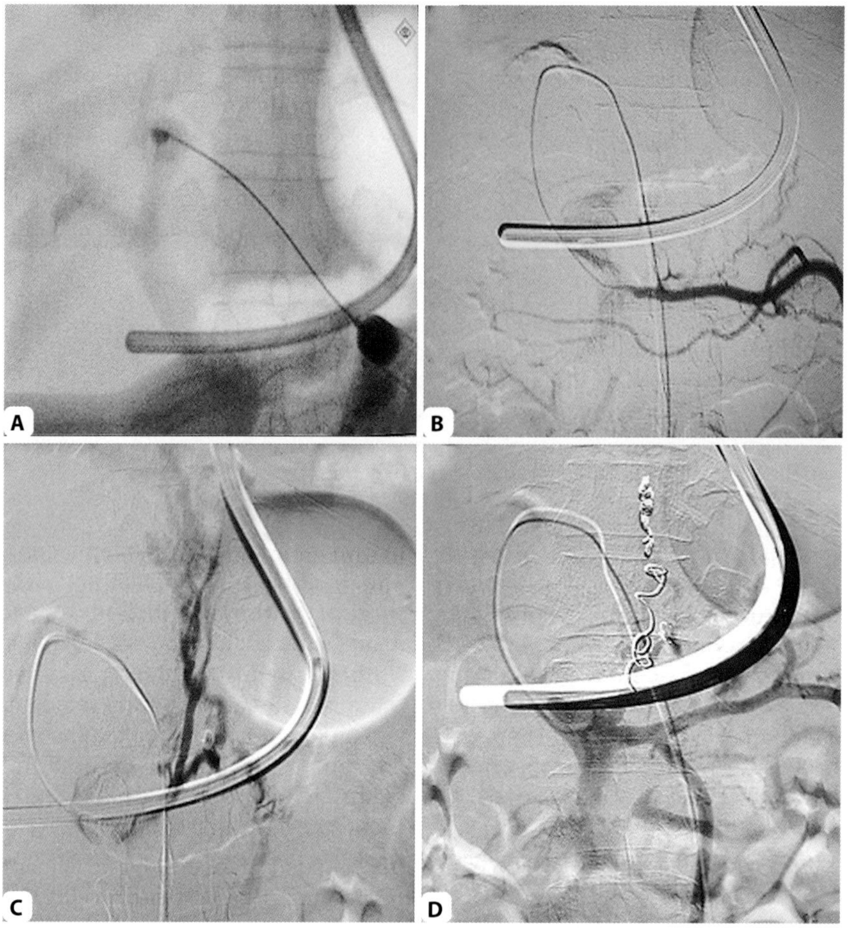

FIGS. 34A TO D: Balloon-occluded antegrade transvenous obliteration (BATO) using percutaneous transhepatic approach: (A and B) Percutaneous transhepatic portogram showing portal vein and branches; (C) Selective angiogram of coronary vein is showing gastric varices; (D) Feeding vein is occluded by deploying stainless steel coils.

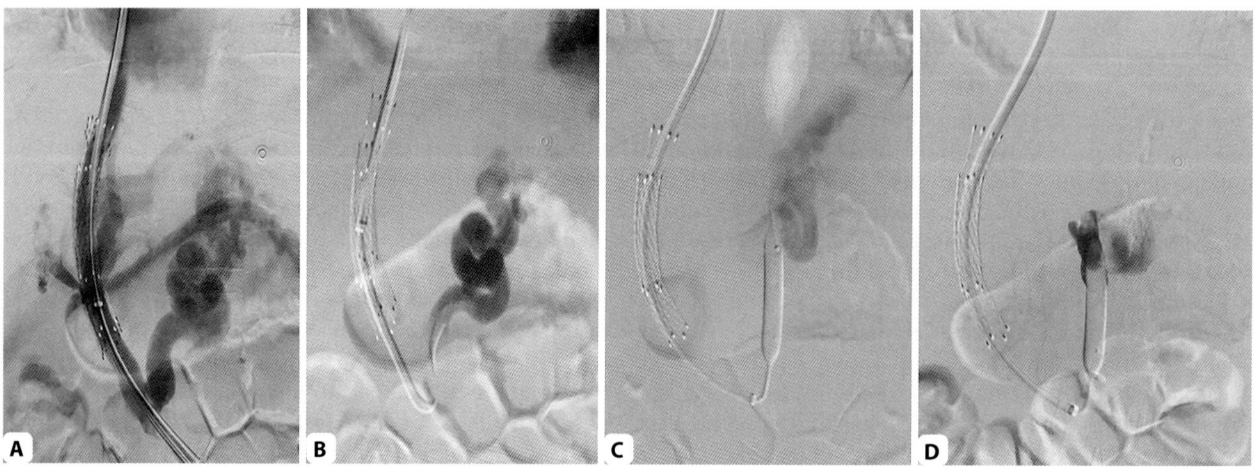

FIGS. 35A TO D: Balloon-occluded antegrade transvenous obliteration (BATO) through pre-existing transjugular intrahepatic portosystemic shunts (TIPS): TIPS portogram showing dilated left gastric vein (A) and esophageal varices (B); Embolization of the varices was performed, after balloon occlusion of left gastric vein (C) to reduce the forward flow in varices, using glue (D) resulting in near complete obliteration of esophageal varices.

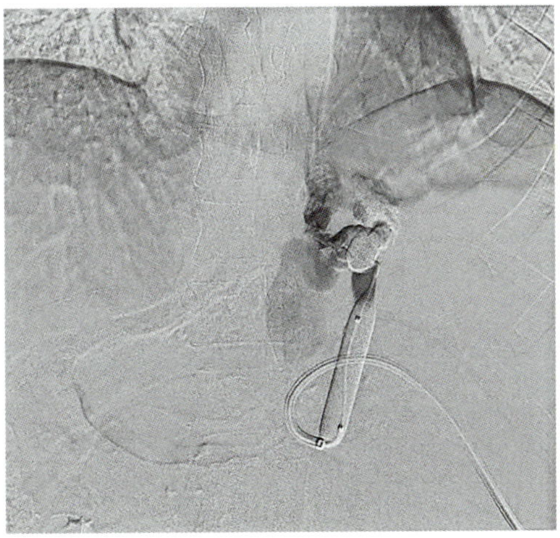

FIG. 36: Digital subtraction angiography (DSA) spot image showing technique of transsplenic fundal variceal obliteration; Glue was injected into the fundal varices after accessing the splenic vein under combined ultrasound fluoroscopic guidance followed by placing vascular sheath into the short gastric vein. Note: Forward flow through the short gastric vein was reduced using a balloon catheter.

required in such cases. CT scan is performed after 2–4 days for immediate response. Follow-up with CT or endoscopy every 3–6 months is done depending on different patient factors **(Figs. 37A to D)**.

TABLE 9: Teaching points—Kiyosue classification of varices.[60,61]

Based on venous outflow	Based on venous inflow
Type A: It has a shunt with a single draining vein	*Type 1*: Gastric varices are supplied by a single afferent gastric vein
Type B: It has a shunt with multiple collateral draining veins	*Type 2*: Gastric varices are supplied by multiple afferent gastric veins
Type C: It has both a gastrocaval and gastrorenal shunt	*Type 3*: By single or multiple gastric veins with coexistent gastric veins that are directly contiguous with the shunt, but do not contribute to the varices
Type D: It has multiple small draining veins and no shunt	

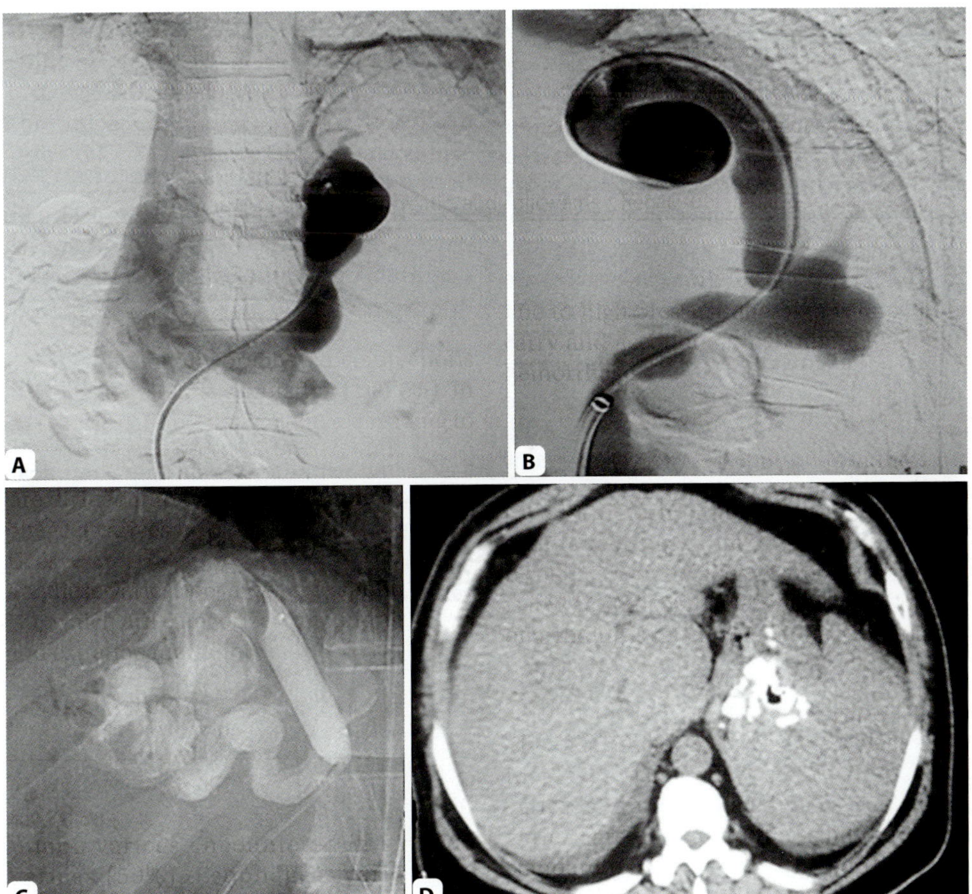

FIGS. 37A TO D: Balloon-occluded retrograded transvenous obliteration (BRTO) of gastric varices: (A and B) Fundic gastric varices are approached through large gastrorenal collaterals of left renal vein; (C) Sclerosing agent (STS) mixed with lipiodol is injected into the varices with the balloon inflated and kept for about 3 hours; (D) Follow-up noncontrast computed tomography (NCCT) scan is showing lipiodol cast formation within the varices in fundal region of stomach.

TABLE 10: Comparison of classical BRTO and modified BRTO techniques.[69]

BRTO	PARTO	CARTO
Indwelling occlusive balloon inflated for hours with injection of sclerosing agents	Indwelling balloon catheter is replaced with a vascular plug with injection of sclerosing agents	Coils are used instead of indwelling balloons or vascular plugs with injection of gelfoam
	Advantage: • Short time • No need to embolize collateral veins	*Advantage*: If the shunt size (larger shunt up to 30 mm), shunt angle, or vessel tortuosity where BRTO/PARTO is not conducive
Limitations: • Lengthy procedure times • Risk of balloon rupture • Risk of pulmonary embolism	*Limitations*: • Size limit of the plug • Additional cost of the plug • Additional gelfoam and contrast media is administered into the IGVs because plug cannot block the liquid or foam sclerosants completely	*Limitations*: Need multiple detachable coils instead of one plug—hence costlier

(BRTO: balloon occluded retrograde transvenous obliteration; CARTO: coil-assisted retrograde transvenous obliteration; IGVs: isolated gastric varices; PARTO: plug-assisted retrograde transvenous obliteration)

Since the introduction of the technique by Kanagawa et al., BRTO has been widely performed as a minimally invasive technique to manage gastric fundal varices.[62-67] The technique has an excellent efficacy of 81–100% and relapse rate of 0–10% reported in literature.[63-68] Complications reported include technique-related errors such as coil migration, balloon malposition, and extension of thrombus outside the varices. Renal failure secondary to hemolysis is a known complication with the use of ethanolamine oleate and can be prevented by administration of haptoglobin. Development of ascites, pleural effusion, hepatic encephalopathy, and worsening of esophageal varices are also observed in occasional patients depending on their preprocedure functional status.[68]

Recently, several modified BRTO techniques have been described to overcome some of the problems associated with conventional BRTO. These include plug-assisted retrograde transvenous obliteration (PARTO) and coil-assisted retrograde transvenous obliteration (CARTO). The comparison of BRTO with these techniques is given in **Table 10**.

Occlusion of Surgical or Radiologic Shunts in Refractory Encephalopathy

In few patients of advanced cirrhosis, the surgical portosystemic shunts (or TIPS) can cause or aggravate hepatic encephalopathy. In such scenarios, therapeutic occlusion of the shunts can be achieved by surgical or endovascular route. Endovascular route is preferred because its minimally invasive nature is favored in a sick patient. Using an endovascular approach different occlusion devices are used depending on the size of shunt vessels. Large lumen shunts are closed with larger devices such as Amplatzer vascular plugs **(Figs. 38A to D)**.

CONCLUSION

Portal hypertension is of hemodynamic importance and associated with life-threatening complications. Imaging plays a vital role in identifying the etiology, level, and extent of PHT. Various interventional procedures help to reduce the portal pressure, and also the morbidity and mortality associated with PHT.

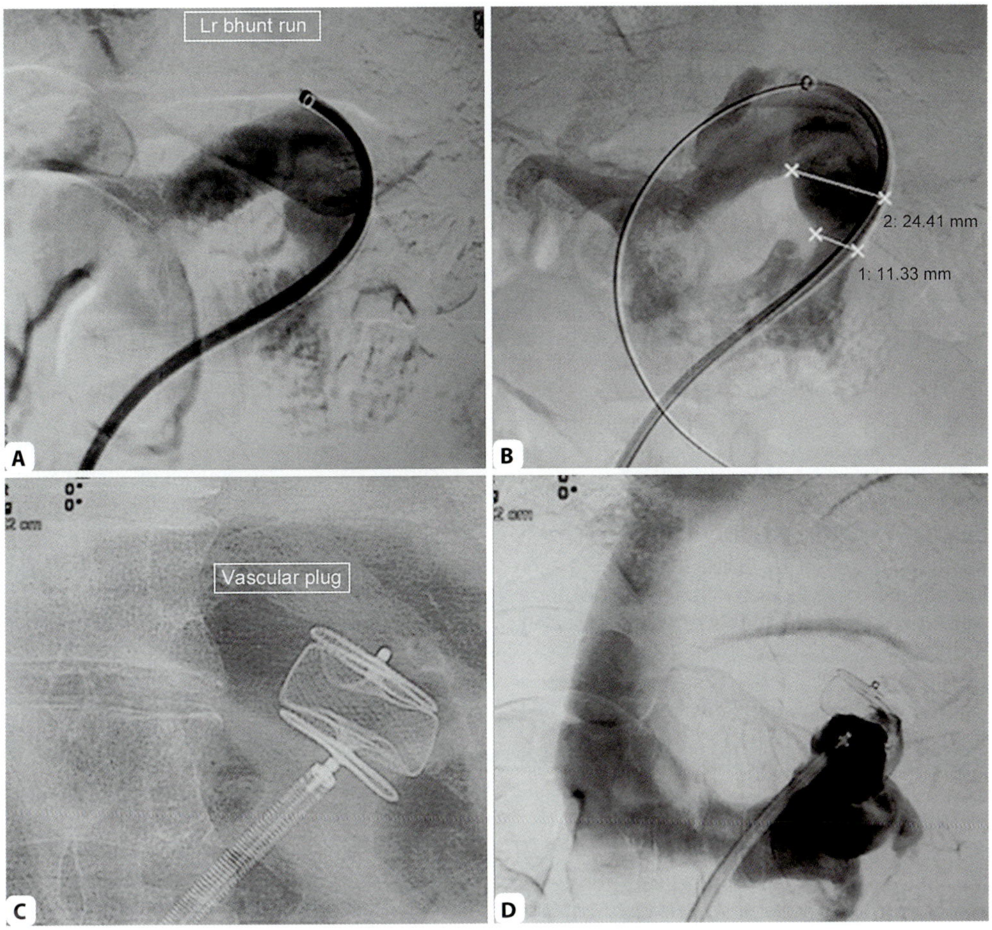

FIGS. 38A TO D: Occlusion of surgical shunts in refractory encephalopathy: (A and B) The surgically created lienorenal shunt for the extrahepatic portal vein obstruction (EHPVO) was accessed through the left renal vein. Contrast study showing the large patent shunt, diameter is approximately 11 mm; (C) Deployed vascular plug (16 mm diameter) at the level of shunt close to the renal vein; (D) Post-shunt closure contrast showing complete closure of the shunt and patent left renal vein.

REFERENCES

1. Kumar A, Sharma P, Sarin SK. Hepatic venous pressure gradient measurement: time to learn! Indian J Gastroenterol. 2008;27(2):74-80.
2. Peck-Radosavljevic M, Trauner M, Schreiber F. Austrian Society of Gastroenterology and Hepatology. Austrian consensus on the definition and treatment of portal hypertension and its complications. Endoscopy. 2005;37(7):667-73.
3. Sanyal AJ, Bosch J, Blei A, Arroyo V. Portal hypertension and its complications. Gastroenterology. 2008;134(6):1715-28.
4. DeLeve LD, Valla DC, Garcia-Tsao G. American Association for the Study Liver Diseases. Vascular disorders of the liver. Hepatology. 2009;49(5):1729-64.
5. Schmidt S, Demartines N, Soler L, Schnyder P, Denys A. Portal vein normal anatomy and variants: implication for liver surgery and portal vein embolization. Semin Intervent Radiol. 2008;25(2):86-91.
6. Brůha R, Petrtýl J. Evaluation and treatment of portal hypertension. Cas Lek Cesk. 2016;155(2):22-6.
7. Procopet B, Cristea VM, Robic MA, Grigorescu M, Agachi PS, Metivier S, et al. Serum tests, liver stiffness and artificial neural networks for diagnosing cirrhosis and portal hypertension. Dig Liver Dis. 2015;47(5):411-6.
8. Zwiebel WJ. Sonographic diagnosis of hepatic vascular disorders. Semin Ultrasound CT MR. 1995;16(1):34-47.
9. Görg C, Riera-Knorrenschild J, Dietrich J. Colour Doppler ultrasound flow patterns in the portal venous system. Br J Radiol. 2002;75;919-29.
10. Kuskal JB, Newman PA, Sammons LG, Kane RA. Optimizing Doppler and colour flow US: application to hepatic sonography. RadioGraphics. 2004;24:657-75.
11. Wachsberg RH, Bahramipour P, Sofocleus CT, Barone A. Hepatofugal flow in the portal system: pathophysiology, imaging findings and diagnostic pitfalls. Radiographics. 2002;22:123-40.
12. Kang HK, Jeong YY, Choi JH, Choi S, Chung TW, Seo JJ, et al. Three-dimensional multi-detector row CT portal venography

in the evaluation of portosystemic collateral vessels in liver cirrhosis. Radiographics. 2002;22(5):1053-61.
13. Calhoun PS, Kuszyk BS, Heath DG, Carley JC, Fishman EK. Three-dimensional volume rendering of spiral CT data: theory and method. Radiographics. 1999;19:745-64.
14. Prince MR, Grist TM, Debatin JF. Portal Venous System. 3D Contrast MR Angiography, 3rd edition. New York: Springer-Verlag; 2003. pp. 171-84.
15. Leyendecker JR, Rivera E, Washburn WK, Johnson SP, Diffin DC, Eason JD. MR angiography of the portal venous system: techniques, interpretation, and clinical applications. Radiographics. 1997;17:1425-43.
16. Kim HC, Bae SH, Choi CS, Kim EA, Kim IJ, Cho SY, et al. MR portography. J Korean Radiol Soc. 1994;31(6):1121-5.
17. Bosch J, Abraldes JG, Berzigotti A, García-Pagan JC. The clinical use of HVPG measurements in chronic liver disease. Nat Rev Gastroenterol Hepatol. 2009;6(10):573-82.
18. Sharma M, Rameshbabu CS. Collateral pathways in portal hypertension. J Clin Experimen Hepatol. 2012;2(4):338-52.
19. Arora A, Rajesh S, Meenakshi YS, Sureka B, Bansal K, Sarin SK. Spectrum of hepatofugal collateral pathways in portal hypertension: an illustrated radiological review. Insights into Imaging. 2015;6(5):559-72.
20. Bissonnette J, Rautou PE, Valla DC. Idiopathic non-cirrhotic portal hypertension: An update. Presse Med. 2015;44(10):1009-15.
21. Arora A, Sarin SK. Multimodality imaging of obliterative portal venopathy: what every radiologist should know. Br J Radiol. 2015;88(1046):20140653.
22. Sarin SK, Kumar A, Chawla YK, Baijal SS, Dhiman RK, Jafri W, et al. Members of the APASL Working Party on Portal Hypertension. Noncirrhotic portal fibrosis/idiopathic portal hypertension: APASL recommendations for diagnosis and treatment. Hepatol Int. 2007;1(3):398-413.
23. Arora A, Sarin SK. Multimodality imaging of primary extrahepatic portal vein obstruction (EHPVO): what every radiologist should know. Br J Radiol. 2015;88:1052.
24. Sarin SK, Khanna R. Non-cirrhotic portal hypertension. Clin liver dis 2014;18(2):451-76.
25. Baskan O, Erol C, Sahingoz Y. Portal biliopathy, magnetic resonance imaging and magnetic resonance cholangiopancreatography findings: a case series. Gastroenterol Rep (Oxf). 2016;4(1):68-72.
26. Rajesh S, Mukund A, Arora A. Imaging diagnosis of splanchnic venous thrombosis. Gastroenterol Res Pract. 2015;2015:101029.
27. Chawla YK, Bodh V. Portal vein thrombosis. J Clin Exp Hepatol. 2015;5(1):22-40.
28. Yerdel MA, Gunson B, Mirza D, Karayalçin K, Olliff S, Buckels J, et al. Portal vein thrombosis in adults undergoing liver transplantation: risk factors, screening, management, and outcome. Transplantation. 2000;69(9):1873-81.
29. Köklü S, Coban S, Yüksel O, Arhan M. Left-sided portal hypertension. Dig Dis Sci. 2007;52(5):1141-9.
30. Lumsden AB, Allen RC, Sreeram S, Atta H, Salam A. Hepatic arterioportal fistula. Am Surg. 1993;59(11):722-6.
31. Angermayr B, Cejna M, Koenig F, Karnel F, Hackl F, Gangl A, et al. Survival in patients undergoing transjugular intrahepatic portosystemic shunt: ePTFE-covered stentgrafts versus bare stents. Hepatol Baltim Md. 2003;38(4):1043-50.
32. Bureau C, Pagan JCG, Layrargues GP, Metivier S, Bellot P, Perreault P, et al. Patency of stents covered with polytetrafluoroethylene in patients treated by transjugular intrahepatic portosystemic shunts: long-term results of a randomized multicentre study. Liver Int Off J Int Assoc Study Liver. 2007;27(6):742-7.
33. Cejna M, Peck-Radosavljevic M, Thurnher SA, Hittmair K, Schoder M, Lammer J. Creation of transjugular intrahepatic portosystemic shunts with stent-grafts: initial experiences with a polytetrafluoroethylene-covered nitinol endoprosthesis. Radiology. 2001;221(2):437-46.
34. Boyer TD, Haskal ZJ, American Association for the Study of Liver Diseases. The role of transjugular intrahepatic portosystemic shunt in the management of portal hypertension. Hepatol Baltim Md. 2005;41(2):386-400.
35. Boyer TD. Transjugular intrahepatic portosystemic shunt: current status. Gastroenterology. 2003;124(6):1700-10.
36. Cura M, Cura A, Suri R, El-Merhi F, Lopera J, Kroma G. Causes of TIPS dysfunction. AJR Am J Roentgenol. 2008;191(6):1751-7.
37. Fisher N, McCafferty I, Dolapci M, Wali M, Buckels J, Olliff S, et al. Managing Budd-Chiari syndrome: a retrospective review of percutaneous hepatic vein angioplasty and surgical shunting. Gut. 1999;44(4):568-74.
38. Cura M, Haskal Z, Lopera J. Diagnostic and interventional radiology for Budd-Chiari syndrome. Radiogr Rev Publ Radiol Soc North Am Inc. 2009;29(3):669-81.
39. Michl P, Bilzer M, Waggershauser T, Gülberg V, Rau HG, Reiser M, et al. Successful treatment of chronic Budd-Chiari syndrome with a transjugular intrahepatic portosystemic shunt. J Hepatol. 2000;32(3):516-20.
40. Ochs A, Sellinger M, Haag K, Nöldge G, Herbst EW, Walter E, et al. Transjugular intrahepatic portosystemic stent-shunt (TIPS) in the treatment of Budd-Chiari syndrome. J Hepatol. 1993;18(2):217-25.
41. Koconis KG, Singh H, Soares G. Partial splenic embolization in the treatment of patients with portal hypertension: a review of the english language literature. J Vasc Interv Radiol JVIR. 2007;18(4):463-81.
42. Alwmark A, Bengmark S, Gullstrand P, Joelsson B, Lunderquist A, Owman T. Evaluation of splenic embolization in patients with portal hypertension and hypersplenism. Ann Surg. 1982;196(5):518-24.
43. Saugel B, Gaa J, Phillip V, Schmid RM, Huber W. Splenic artery embolization in a woman with bleeding gastric varices and splenic vein thrombosis: a case report. J Med Case Reports. 2010;4(1):247.
44. Yamakado K, Nakatsuka A, Tanaka N, Fujii A, Isaji S, Kawarada Y, et al. Portal venous stent placement in patients with pancreatic and biliary neoplasms invading portal veins and causing portal hypertension: initial experience. Radiology. 2001;220(1):150-6.
45. Shan H, Xiao X-S, Huang M-S, Ouyang Q, Jiang Z-B. Portal venous stent placement for treatment of portal hypertension caused by benign main portal vein stenosis. World J Gastroenterol WJG. 2005;11(21):3315-8.
46. Vauthey JN, Tomczak RJ, Helmberger T, Gertsch P, Forsmark C, Caridi J, et al. The arterioportal fistula syndrome: clinicopathologic features, diagnosis, and therapy. Gastroenterology. 1997;113(4):1390-401.

47. López-Medina A, Peiró J, Gonzalez de Garay M, Antoñana MA, Sustacha J, Grande D. Treatment of occluded distal splenorenal shunts with endovascular stents: a report of two cases. Cardiovasc Intervent Radiol. 2001;24(3):194-7.
48. Lorenz JM, Funaki B, Denison G. Balloon dilatation of a distal splenorenal shunt in a child. AJR. 2005;184(6):1915-6.
49. Lunderquist A, Vang J. Transhepatic catheterization and obliteration of the coronary vein in patients with portal hypertension and esophageal varices. N Engl J Med. 1974;291(13):646-9.
50. Bengmark S, Börjesson B, Hoevels J, Joelsson B, Lunderquist A, Owman T. Obliteration of esophageal varices by PTP: a follow-up of 43 patients. Ann Surg. 1979;190(4):549-54.
51. Benner KG, Keeffe EB, Keller FS, Rösch J. Clinical outcome after percutaneous transhepatic obliteration of esophageal varices. Gastroenterology. 1983;85(1):146-53.
52. Lunderquist A, Börjesson B, Owman T, Bengmark S. Isobutyl 2-cyanoacrylate (bucrylate) in obliteration of gastric coronary vein and esophageal varices. AJR Am J Roentgenol. 1978;130(1):1-6.
53. Smith-Laing G, Scott J, Long RG, Dick R, Sherlock S. Role of percutaneous transhepatic obliteration of varices in the management of hemorrhage from gastroesophageal varices. Gastroenterology. 1981;80(5 pt 1):1031-6.
54. L'Herminé C, Chastanet P, Delemazure O, Bonnière PL, Durieu JP, Paris JC. Percutaneous transhepatic embolization of gastroesophageal varices: results in 400 patients. AJR Am J Roentgenol. 1989;152(4):755-60.
55. Sos TA. Transhepatic portal venous embolization of varices: pros and cons. Radiology. 1983;148(2):569-70.
56. Kwak HS, Han YM. Percutaneous transportal sclerotherapy with N-butyl-2-cyanoacrylate for gastric varices: technique and clinical efficacy. Korean J Radiol Off J Korean Radiol Soc. 2008;9(6):526-33.
57. Tian X, Wang Q, Zhang C, Liu F, Cui Y, Liu F, et al. Modified percutaneous transhepatic variceal embolization with 2-octylcyanoacrylate for bleeding gastric varices: long-term follow-up outcomes. AJR Am J Roentgenol. 2011;197(2):502-9.
58. Gong GQ, Wang XL, Wang JH, Yan ZP, Cheng JM, Qian S, et al. Percutaneous transsplenic embolization of esophageal and gastrio-fundal varices in 18 patients. World J Gastroenterol. 2001;7(6):880-3.
59. Sarin SK, Lahoti D, Saxena SP, Murthy NS, Makwana UK. Prevalence, classification and natural history of gastric varices: a long-term follow-up study in 568 portal hypertension patients. Hepatology. 1992;16(6):1343-9.
60. Sabri SS, Saad WE. Balloon-occluded Retrograde Transvenous Obliteration (BRTO): Technique and Intraprocedural Imaging. Semin Intervent Radiol. 2011;28(3):303-13.
61. Philips CA, Ahamed R, Rajesh S, George T, Mohanan M, Augustine P. Beyond the scope and the glue: update on evaluation and management of gastric varices. BMC Gastroenterol. 2020;20(1):361.
62. Kanagawa H, Mima S, Kouyama H, Gotoh K, Uchida T, Okuda K. Treatment of gastric fundal varices by balloon-occluded retrograde transvenous obliteration. J Gastroenterol Hepatol. 1996;11(1):51-8.
63. Hirota S, Matsumoto S, Tomita M, Sako M, Kono M. Retrograde transvenous obliteration of gastric varices. Radiology. 1999;211(2):349-56.
64. Matsumoto A, Hamamoto N, Nomura T, Hongou Y, Arisaka Y, Morikawa H, et al. Balloon-occluded retrograde transvenous obliteration of high-risk gastric fundal varices. Am J Gastroenterol. 1999;94(3):643-9.
65. Koito K, Namieno T, Nagakawa T, Morita K. Balloon-occluded retrograde transvenous obliteration for gastric varices with gastrorenal or gastrocaval collaterals. AJR Am J Roentgenol. 1996;167(5):1317-20.
66. Kiyosue H, Mori H, Matsumoto S, Yamada Y, Hori Y, Okino Y. Transcatheter obliteration of gastric varices: Part 2. Strategy and techniques based on hemodynamic features. Radiogr Rev Publ Radiol Soc North Am Inc. 2003;23(4):921-37.
67. Ninoi T, Nishida N, Kaminou T, Sakai Y, Kitayama T, Hamuro M, et al. Balloon-occluded retrograde transvenous obliteration of gastric varices with gastrorenal shunt: long-term follow-up in 78 patients. AJR Am J Roentgenol. 2005;184(4):1340-6.
68. Arai H, Abe T, Takagi H, Mori M. Efficacy of balloon-occluded retrograde transvenous obliteration, percutaneous transhepatic obliteration and combined techniques for the management of gastric fundal varices. World J Gastroenterol. 2006;12(24):3866-73.
69. Kim DJ, Darcy MD, Mani NB, Park AW, Akinwande O, Ramaswamy RS, et al. Modified Balloon-Occluded Retrograde Transvenous Obliteration (BRTO) Techniques for the Treatment of Gastric Varices: Vascular Plug-Assisted Retrograde Transvenous Obliteration (PARTO)/Coil-Assisted Retrograde Transvenous Obliteration (CARTO)/Balloon-Occluded Antegrade Transvenous Obliteration (BATO). Cardiovasc Intervent Radiol. 2018;41(6):835-47.

Index

Page numbers followed by *b* refer to box, *f* refer to figure, *fc* refer to flowchart, and *t* refer to table.

A

B

C

D

E

H

I

J

K

L

M

N

O

P

R

S

T

U